CONTACT LENS PRACTICE

Third Edition

CONTACT LENS PRACTICE

By

ROBERT B. MANDELL, O.D., Ph.D.

Professor of Physiological Optics and Optometry
School of Optometry
University of California
Berkeley, California

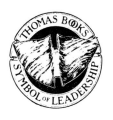

CHARLES C THOMAS • PUBLISHER
Springfield • Illinois • U.S.A.

Published and Distributed Throughout the World by
CHARLES C THOMAS • PUBLISHER
2600 South First Street
Springfield, Illinois, 62717, U.S.A.

© *1965, 1974, and 1981, by* CHARLES C THOMAS • PUBLISHER
ISBN 0-398-04494-5
Library of Congress Catalog Card Number: 81-1541

First Edition, First Printing, 1965
First Edition, Second Printing, 1966
First Edition, Third Printing, 1968
First Edition, Fourth Printing, 1969
First Edition, Fifth Printing, 1971
Second Edition, First Printing, 1974
Second Edition, Second Printing, 1976
Second Edition, Third Printing, 1977
Second Edition, Fourth Printing, 1979
Third Edition, First Printing, 1981

*With THOMAS BOOKS careful attention is given to all details
of manufacturing and design. It is the Publisher's desire to
present books that are satisfactory as to their physical qualities
and artistic possibilities and appropriate for their particular use.
THOMAS BOOKS will be true to those laws of quality that
assure a good name and good will.*

Library of Congress Cataloging in Publication Data

Mandell, Robert B.
    Contact lens practice.

    Bibliography: p.
    Includes index.
        1. Contact lenses. I. Title.   [DNLM: 1. Contact
lenses. WW 355 M271c]
RE977.C6M25   1981   617.7'523   81-1541
ISBN 0-398-04494-5   AACR2

Printed in the United States of America
OK-1

CONTRIBUTORS

SOLON M. BRAFF, O.D. *El Monte, California*

ROBERT FLETCHER, M.Sc., TECH., F.B.O.A., F.S.M.C. *Professor and Head, Department of Ophthalmic Optics and Visual Science, The City University, London.*

ANTONIO R. GASSET, M.D. *Chairman of Ophthalmology, Miami Eye Institute, Miami, Florida.*

ROBERT GRAHAM, O.D. *Professor Emeritus.*

MICHAEL G. HARRIS, O.D., M.S. *Senior Lecturer, School of Optometry, University of California, Berkeley, California.*

PHILLIP R. HAYNES, O.D. *Editor,* Encyclopedia of Contact Lens Practice.

KENNETH A. POLSE, O.D., M.S. *Professor of Optometry, School of Optometry, University of California, Berkeley, California.*

MORTON D. SARVER, O.D., M.S. *Professor of Optometry, School of Optometry, Unisity of California, Berkeley, California.*

PREFACE TO THE THIRD EDITION

The field of contact lens practice has reached a new level of maturity. The hope that a single lens would reign supreme over all the others has been abandoned and replaced by a more realistic outlook towards fitting principles. The hydrogel lens has become an accepted part of the contact lens armamentarium and is now being used in numbers equal to hard contact lenses. However, the prediction by some that soft contact lenses would soon replace hard lenses has not come true, nor does it appear likely to do so in the near future. Various modifications have been made to soft contact lenses, and significant improvements have been accomplished. Nevertheless, the limitations of this lens modality have now been recognized. A few years of experience has unveiled new problems that were never seen before with hard contact lenses. Several corneal changes pathognomonic of a badly fitting soft lens are now recognized, and in many cases, corrective procedures can now be recommended. Other corneal changes are less well understood and present many puzzles for our contact lens research in the upcoming years.

Another prediction of former times was that the contact lens field would soon be overrun by new materials. Many new materials, which sounded ideal for contact lenses, invariably showed some drawbacks. In most cases, this reflects our lack of understanding of corneal physiology and, in particular, the physiology of tears. Very often materials that are optimal in all other respects as a contact lens do not wet properly, and this deficiency prevents the success of the lens. Nevertheless, many new hard lens materials have been discovered or synthesized that demonstrate permeability to oxygen and carbon dioxide. These hard gas-permeable lenses show the greatest promise for advancement within the next few years.

A critical question that remains to be answered is what factors are necessary to design an extended wear lens successfully. Many patients seem to tolerate extended wear with ease, whereas others show adverse responses of severe magnitude. It would appear that contact lenses, in many cases, can abuse the eye severely, but as long as the lens is removed at night, the eye is capable of recovery. However, when the lens is worn twenty-four hours per day, the eye does not have this opportunity to restore itself, and the lens can no longer be tolerated.

The major goal of this text remains the same: to provide a detailed contact lens fitting guide for practicing optometrists and ophthalmologists and to provide a comprehensive text for students. I have eliminated some of the older materials and rearranged the chapters to give the book a more logical flow. By consolidating some of the material, it has been necessary only to expand the number of chapters from 32 to 34. I have once again tried to restrict the more theoretical concepts of contact lenses to Chapter 6 on the theory of fitting and to Chapter 34 on optics.

I have always considered it a unique opportunity to be part of a field that is growing and developing at such a rapid pace. There are many puzzles remaining to be solved, and we have much to look forward to in the future of this dynamic field.

R.B.M.

ACKNOWLEDGMENTS

It would not have been possible to complete this edition in a relatively short production time without the efforts of Doctor Emily Holden. Her assistance in working on all phases of this revision made possible the extensive review that was undertaken. Her dedication to the enormous task of coordinating the completion of this edition is gratefully acknowledged.

Since the introduction of this text, seventeen years ago, I have received an abundance of materials and help from friends and colleagues. I wish particularly to thank the following: Doctors Gary Andrasko, Robert S. Arner, Charles A. Bayshore, Irving M. Borish, Solon M. Braff, Roy Brandreth, Donald Brucker, Thomas Brungardt, L. Dean Clements, William Feinbloom, E. J. Fisher, Ed Gary, Martin Gellman, Joe B. Goldberg, Stanley Gordon, Lorance W. Harwood, Richard M. Hill, H.D.E. Ins, Lester E. Janoff, George Jessen, Barry Kissack, Henry A. Knoll, Joseph Krezanoski, John Levene, George Mertz, Carl Moore, Robert Morrison, Harold Moss, Rosalie Nash, Richard Neumaier, Maurice Poster, Roy Rengstorff, Preston Richmond, Dale A. Rorabaugh, Alfred A. Rosenbloom, Charles R. Shick, Charles Stewart, Peter Urrea, Don C. West, and Milton York.

I especially wish to thank Doctors Don and Joan Korb for contributing sections of material to this edition.

In addition, the following companies have provided considerable assistance: Allergan Pharmaceuticals, American Optical, Barnes-Hind Laboratories, Bausch and Lomb, Calcon Laboratories, ConCise Contact Lens Co., Cooper Vision, Inc., Morrison Laboratories, Soft Lens, Inc., Syntex Ophthalmics, and Wesley-Jessen.

A special thanks to my colleagues also involved in contact lenses at the University of California: Morton Sarver, Michael Harris, and Robert Lester. Merton Flom made several suggestions about the section on binocular vision, and Henry Peters provided considerable help in the form of materials on aniseikonia. Larry Stark gave invaluable advice on biomaterials. I have reserved a special thanks to Irving Fatt for his help and guidance in corneal physiology and to Kenneth Polse for our many years of collaboration and mutual support.

Another special thanks goes to Bob Tarr and Pat Charley at the Multimedia Services at the University of California School of Optometry and to my secretary, Pat McGlinchy, for calmly holding everything together.

CONTENTS

CONTACT LENS PRACTICE

SECTION I

INTRODUCTION

Chapter 1

HISTORICAL DEVELOPMENT

ROBERT GRAHAM

CONTACT LENSES ARE the smallest, the least visible, and in certain optical respects the finest of all devices for correcting refractive errors of the eye. Consequently, they have come to occupy an increasingly significant place in the work of improving human vision. Their growing importance makes it appropriate to inquire into the origins and development of these very valuable ophthalmic resources.

Modern contact lenses are the result of a long tradition of optical innovations and are not the work of one person alone. Before considering this history, it would be well to define the modern contact lens and to keep this definition in mind during the historical discussion that follows.*

CONTACT LENS

A contact lens is a small, shell-like, bowl-shaped glass or plastic lens that rests on the eye, in contact with the cornea or the sclera, or both, serving as a new anterior surface of the eye and/or as a retainer for fluid between the cornea and the contact lens; it is ordinarily used to correct refractive errors of the eye.

Contact lenses are usually divided into two types (Figure 1.1):

1. *Corneal contact lens.* A contact lens that rests primarily on the cornea rather than on the sclera.

2. *Scleral contact lens.* A contact lens that fits over both the cornea and the surrounding sclera, used with or without an auxiliary fluid to fill the space between the lens and cornea.

In addition, they can be classified according to material:

1. *Hard gas-permeable,* e.g. cellulose acetate butyrate.

2. *Hard nonpermeable,* e.g. polymethylmethacrylate.

3. *Soft gas-permeable,* e.g. hydrogel and silicon elastomer.

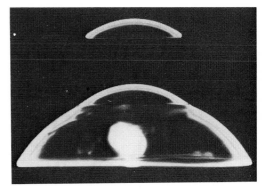

Figure 1.1. Major types of hard contact lenses: (*top*) corneal contact lens; (*bottom*) scleral or haptic contact lens.

*Definitions for contact lenses were taken from the *Dictionary of Visual Science*, by Schapero, Cline, and Hofstetter with permission of the authors.

5

DA VINCI

As far as known records reveal, Leonardo da Vinci was the first person to conceive of neutralizing the cornea by substituting for it a new refracting surface. About AD 1508, he sketched and described several forms of contact lenses which would accomplish this end.[1] Some of his devices were enormous and complex (Figure 1.2); some were simple and made by cutting "little round ampules" of glass in two. One of the halves was to be filled with water "if you want to look with only one eye." He clearly suggested the concept of corneal neutralization and replacement upon which all contact lenses function.

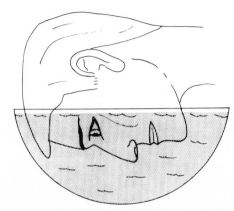

Figure 1.2. A hollow glass semispheroid filled with water. One type of contact lens described by da Vinci.

DESCARTES

The first individual to suggest placing a lens directly upon the cornea without scleral contact was Rene Descartes. In 1636, he described and illustrated a contact lens as one of his *Ways of Perfecting Vision.*[2] Concerning his illustration (Figure 1.3) he wrote the following:

If one applies directly against the eye a tube full of water, like E F, at the end of which there is a glass G H I, whose shape is exactly like that of the skin B C D, . . . there will no longer be any refraction at the entry of this eye.

The tube full of water must have required external support, instead of being self-supporting as are present corneal lenses. Descartes actually had a grossly elongated corneal lens resting within the limbus of the eye. His proportions were poor, but his principle was quite correct.

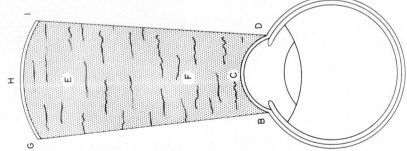

Figure 1.3. Contact lens described by Descartes.

THOMAS YOUNG

In 1801, Thomas Young wrote the following:

I take out of a small botanical microscope, a double convex lens, of eight-tenths radius and focal distance, fixed in a socket one-fifth of an inch in depth; securing its edges with wax, I drop into it a little water, nearly cold, till it is three-fourths full, and then apply it to my eye, so that the cornea enters half way into the socket, and is everywhere in contact with the water. My eye immediately becomes presbyopic, and the refractive power of the lens, which is reduced by the water to a focal length of about 16 tenths, is not sufficient to supply the place of the cornea, rendered inefficacious by the intervention of the water; but the addition of another lens, of five inches and a half focus, restores my eye to its natural state, and somewhat more. I then apply the optometer, and I find the same inequality in the horizontal and vertical refractions as without the water; and I have, in both directions, a power of accommodation equivalent to a focal length of four inches, as before.[3]

It is evident that Young, too, grasped and utilized the principle of fluid neutralization of most of the corneal refracting power. His device and his description of it may be said to be the antecedent of hydrodiascopes as well as of contact lenses.

HERSCHEL

Sir John F. W. Herschel wrote the following in 1823:

The strict method, applicable in all such cases (of irregular cornea), would be to adapt a lens to the eye, of nearly the same refractive power and having its surface next to the eye an exact intaglio facsimile of the irregular cornea, while the external should be exactly spherical of the same general convexity of the cornea itself: for it is clear that all the distortions of the rays at the posterior surface of such a lens would be exactly counteracted by the equal and opposite distortions at the cornea itself.

Should any very bad cases of irregular cornea be found, it is worthy of consideration whether at least a temporary distinct vision could not be procured, by applying in contact with the surface of the eye some transparent animal jelly contained in a spherical capsule of glass; or whether an actual mold of the cornea might not be taken and impressed on some transparent medium.[4]

Herschel has a place in the evolution of corneal lenses, not because he made or described corneal lenses as such, but because his widely circulated proposals pointed out that corneal lenses were optically feasible.

The preceeding concepts notwithstanding, the first contact lenses known to have been worn on the cornea were not devised until 1888. At that time two men, working independently, invented adhering lenses that could be worn in contact with the eyes.

FICK

In a treatise entitled *A Contact Spectacle*,[5] A. Eugen Fick described the first contact lenses with refractive power known to have actually been worn.* He wrote the following:

... it is certainly not superfluous to look for another means (than spectacles) to correct the dif-

---

*In 1887, F. A. Muller, a maker of artificial eyes, blew a thin glass shell with transparent corneal portion to protect a cornea from desiccation due to lagophthalmos. This device, closely resembling a contact lens, was worn successfully for many years and must have been transparent.[6] The purpose of this device was to protect the eye, not to serve as a lens; thus it should not be considered as the first contact lens which was worn.

ferent types of irregular astigmatism. The most radical means would obviously be to substitute for the cornea another regularly curved surface. This can really happen now, and I shall show in these papers that I have succeeded to exclude the faulty cornea from its total dioptrical powers with a very small glass bowl and to increase the minimum visual acuity of an eye from 1/30 to 1/6 without contraction of the visual field. ...

The contact spectacle consists of a thin, very small glass bowl bounded by concentric and parallel sphere segments. ...

The same is placed on the eye, and the space between the little glass and the eyeball is filled with a liquid which has the same refractive index as the cornea.

The "bowl bounded by concentric and parallel sphere segments" can only have the simple form characteristic of corneal lenses; it could not have the scleral flange or compound construction found in scleral contact lenses. Figure 1.4 represents what Fick has here specified. Later Fick discusses scleral contacts, which he describes quite differently from the other lens.

I began my investigation to determine through animal experiments whether or not and for how long one may place a contact lens onto the eyeball without the same receiving damage. As experimental animals, large rabbits proved themselves preferentially suitable. From one of those animals, I lifted away the lids and nictitating membranes of the eyeball and filled the pocket so obtained with a paste of gypsum [plaster of Paris]. After congelation has taken place, such a mold of the eyeball shows that the radius of curvature of the cornea does not differ essentially from that of the sclera and that the eyeball of the rabbit is a practically perfect sphere. Thereafter I had very small glass basins blown after these gypsum casts, whose shape became ever simpler, until finally after numerous trials, I abandoned the casts completely and was satisfied with preparing glass bubbles of 21, 20 and 19 mm. diameter and to break off a segment, the base of which had only a few mm. distance from the middle point of the sphere. From a great number of such very small bowls, I selected then for each individual rabbit the one most suitable.

Here it is unmistakably clear that many of the devices that Fick used in his early investigations were simple segments of hollow glass spheres. Certain subsequent devices, for trial on

himself and others, were made by modified techniques, using casts of human cadaver eyes.

Friedrich Muller of Wiesbaden, writing at the University of Marburg in 1920,[7] recorded the dimensions of some of Fick's corneal lenses:

Completely new ways for the correction of refractive anomalies of the cornea were undertaken by A. E. Fick in the year 1888. He eliminated the optically useless cornea from the dioptric system and substituted for it a spheric-anastigmatic glass cornea-contact spectacle—which is directly placed upon the cornea and is held fast on the same by adhesion and capillary attraction of the tear fluid in all motions of the eyeball. This idea of A. E. Fick's, to replace the conical cornea by a new one made out of glass, has with time become fundamental for the correction of keratoconus. The contact spectacle consists of a thin sphere of glass of about 8 mm. radius of curvature with parallel surfaces and a basal diameter equal to that of a natural cornea.

The preceding leaves no doubt that Fick's sphere segments were not larger than a cornea, were placed directly upon the cornea, and were true corneal lenses.*

In his 1888 article, Fick also described his later and preferred contact lenses.[5] These were the first scleral lenses intended to correct refractive errors (Figure 1.5).

I decided to prepare the contact spectacle in an optically usable form; that means to have it ground. Unfortunately, all prerequisites were lacking here in Zurich, and I contacted via letter Professor

---

*For further information on this point *see* Graham, R.: The evolution of corneal contact lenses, *Am. J. Optom.*, *36*(2):55–72, 1959.

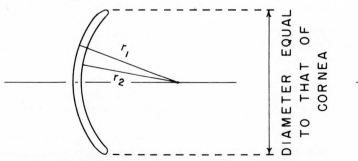

Figure 1.4. Corneal contact lens described by Fick.

Abbe in Jena, asking him to have some contact spectacles made for me. He was good enough to satisfy my request. The specification which so far was found most satisfactory for the preparation of contact lenses reads as follows:

"A glass cornea of 8 mm. radius of curvature sits with a base of 7 mm. radius (14 mm. across) on the glass sclera; the latter is 4 mm. wide and corresponds to a sphere with a radius of curvature of 15 mm.; the glass cornea has parallel walls, ground and polished on the in- and out-sides; similarly, the free edge of the glass sclera is also ground and polished; weight of the contact lens, approximately 0.5 g."

It is not difficult to see why Fick began with corneal lenses, for these are the simpler type. Neither is it difficult to see why he preferred lenses with scleral flanges after he had access to them. The addition of these flanges provides better support and distribution of the lens weight than can be achieved with simple corneal lenses. Weight was always a serious problem with glass corneal lenses, which are approximately twice the weight of plastic lenses.

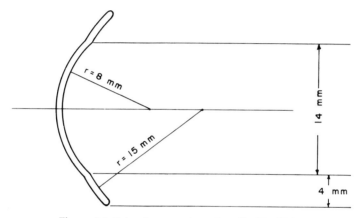

Figure 1.5. Scleral contact lens described by Fick.

KALT

On March 20, 1888, P. Panas presented to the Académie de Médecine in Paris a report on a lens devised by E. Kalt. The report was published in the *Bulletin of the Academie*.[8] The most pertinent passages state the following:

The method which Mr. Kalt presents [for correcting conical cornea] has the advantage of correcting the cornea immediately, through suppression of the cone and correction of the anomaly of refraction. It consists of the use of glass shells, similar to those which are sometimes employed in the treatment of symblepharon. These glasses, the size of enamel shells which serve for ocular prostheses, have a radius of curvature similar to that of the cornea. They are well borne for several hours by this membrane, and the feeble irritation which these provoke subsides quickly after their removal. They follow the motions of the eye and adhere nicely to the bulb thanks to the atmospheric pressure. The cornea, being very thinned, conforms exactly to the concavity and finds itself, from so doing, straightened out. If the curvature of the glass is correctly chosen, one can bring about a state of emmetropia and, what is the important thing, the vision is improved over the whole extent of the visual field.

A patient who could hardly count fingers shown to him at 50 cm. distance, saw his vision improved immediately in this way, so that he could read at 5 M. distance letters of 26 mm. height. He could also read then a newspaper.

Thus the optical correction is brought about in a manner quite satisfactory. The future only will show to what degree the effect is curative. These results obtained in the Poor People's Clinic on two patients, said M. Panas, were ready to be published when a paper by Dr. Fick was brought to our attention, which appeared in the *Archiv fur Augenheilkunde*, the copy of March, 1888. The author, who has employed a similar method, has arrived at absolutely the same results as far as keratoconus is concerned.

Ocular prostheses of a size sometimes employed in the treatment of symblepharon are smaller than regular prostheses, else there would have been no occasion to mention this special condition. Kalt, like Fick, used corneal lenses; however, unlike some of Fick's corneal lenses, Kalt's lenses pressed against the conus, instead of arching over the center of the cornea.

In 1893, M. A. Chevallereau reported a discussion at the Society of Ophthalmology of France:

Mr. Abadie: . . . to better his condition (keratoconus) I recommended the patient to wear . . . the contact lenses recommended by Mr. Sulzer. He is very satisfied with them.

Mr. Kalt: I will allow myself to remind Mr. Abadie that the optical treatment of keratoconus has been simultaneously recommended by Mr. Fick, in Switzerland, and by myself in France about 1887, through a communication to the Academy of Medicine, and not by Mr. Sulzer.

Mr. Sulzer: The idea of applying lenses to the cornea is much older than Mr. Kalt thinks. It dates from the past century. But the practical realization of the idea has encountered great difficulties. The lenses used by Mr. Fick gave insufficient optical results because of the irregularity of their surface, and Mr. Kalt's lenses, because they lacked a scleral flange, adhered too little to the eye to be useful.

Mr. Kalt: Mr. Sulzer says that my shells adhered insufficiently to the cornea and did not lie close. Mr. Sulzer does not seem to take into account that adherence is obtained by atmospheric pressure,

just as it happens for two wet glass plates. . . . [9]

In 1937, Emile Haas wrote the following in the *Bulletin of the Société d'Ophtalmologie de Paris:*

After his first experiments* and to have, as he says, a "better transparency," Mr. Kalt asked an optical glass manufacturer to construct for him "thin cut crystal glasses, built according to the curvature of the normal cornea as measured with Javal's ophthalmometer and checked on a casting of corpse's eye." Thanks to Mr. Kalt, I had the possibility to examine the plaster cast and also three of the glasses that were delivered to him. These glasses consisted of corneal parts only, segments of spheres, whose diameters at the base were 11, 11.5 and 13 mm., respectively. Examined with the two faces in air, they have convergent effects of approximately 1.5, 1.5 and 2 diopters respectively. Their polish is satisfactory, their refraction very regular. Examined in Javal's ophthalmometer all three show an anterior face free of astigmatism and a radius of curvature of 7.9 mm. Evidently they were ground, probably all three by means of the same ball and the same basin. The difference in their power must be due to the slightly different thicknesses. Mr. Kalt did not tell me which optician had made them.

It is evident that they must have held—if they held—only by atmospheric pressure, since their diameter is precisely of the order of magnitude of the palpebral opening. The difficulties of their removal, which were indicated by Mr. Kalt, are thus explained, as are also the difficulties of their insertion. It is probable that one and the other might have been greatly facilitated by pneumatic suction.[10]

In the preceding excerpt Haas recorded explicitly the principal specifications of some of the first powered corneal lenses (Figure 1.6). It is worth noting that these same specifications were used when corneal lenses were later reintroduced in plastic.

ORIGIN OF THE TERM CORNEAL LENSES

The first use of the term *corneal lenses* appears in the year 1889. In that year August Müller employed the word "Hornhautlinsen" (corneal lenses) in his inaugural thesis.[11] However, the lenses he described

would be termed scleral lenses today.

---

*A communication to me from R. A. Dudragne of Paris, who knew Kalt, states that Kalt's first experiments were made with segments cut from the bottoms of test tubes.

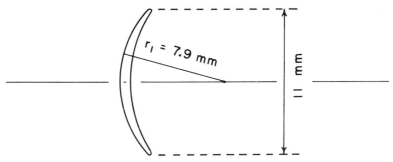

Figure 1.6. Lens described by Kalt (thickness unknown).

IMPROVED SCLERAL LENSES

For sixty years (1888 to 1948) after their introduction, scleral lenses were the type of contact lenses most used. The majority of these lenses were blown from semi-molten glass by the Muller organization of Wiesbaden and by others or were ground and polished by the Carl Zeiss Company of Jena. During this period, Josef Dallos, improving on Cza-pody's work (1929) with molding, introduced techniques for taking impressions of the anterior portion of living eyes without gross insult:

Models prepared by making a cast of the living eye show absolutely that on the surface of the eyeball, only the center of the cornea approaches the surface of a sphere and that it flattens out toward the limbus.... It is noted besides this that the curvature of the scleral conjunctiva usually changes in every meridian.[12]

Thereafter, lenses could be made to conform more accurately to individual sclerae and were consequently more tolerable. They remained, however, a rarity as a means of correcting vision, being substantially limited to keratoconus and other cases of extreme refractive error. Even in these cases the wearing time was rarely more than a few hours. This situation continued until optical plastics came into use.

GLASS CORNEAL LENSES

Glass corneal lenses, made by the Carl Zeiss Optical Works of Jena, were described in 1912 and 1923.[13,14] They were also used and described by Weve of Utrecht in 1932.[15-17] However, they were not widely used. Since corneal lenses must cling to the front of the cornea with only the support of fluid adhesive force alone, the weight and irregular surfaces of the glass lenses were serious impediments to any wide use. Consequently, they were soon, and for many years almost totally, supplanted by sclerals.

NEW SUBSTANCES

William Feinbloom was the first American to utilize the newer synthetic plastics for contact lenses. Their lightness, workability, and compatibility with ocular tissues were advantageous factors. In 1936, he had developed and described lenses in which the scleral portions were made of opaque, molded resin. The corneal portions were of glass and were inserted into the plastic scleral band.[18]

In 1936, Rohm and Haas Company introduced transparent methyl methacrylate in the United States.*

In 1938, John Mullen and Theodore Obrig developed techniques for making scleral lenses of the new substance.[19] Contact lenses made of this new material were free from limitations of heavy refractory glass lenses. Their manufacture did not employ blowing of semi-molten material or slow grinding and polishing processes; plastics may be turned on a lathe. They may also be shaped and reshaped at low temperatures, scraped, routed, drilled or buffed, quickly finished to a high polish, and made thinner than is possible with fragile glass. The reduced thickness causes less weight and diminished ocular sensation.

MINIMUM CLEARANCE SCLERAL LENSES

All the previously mentioned scleral lenses held a pool of artificial fluid between lens and cornea.† Stagnation of this fluid usually led to temporary corneal edema and to clouding just a few hours after lens insertion.

In 1937, Dallos mentioned glass scleral lenses with "only a capillary touch between the glass and the cornea." With scleral lenses subsequently made of highly workable plastic, it became possible for others to achieve the infinitesimal and very precise separation between cornea and lens necessary to hold liquid in the interspace. In 1943, Norman Bier perforated such lenses to allow ingress and egress of natural tears, thus greatly ameliorating the corneal clouding that had been so characteristic of prior sclerals.[21,22]

PLASTIC CORNEAL LENSES

The weight of glass had been a far more serious detriment to corneal lenses than it had been to sclerals. With the advent of optical plastics, the weight could be halved.‡ In 1947, Kevin Tuohy redeveloped and began the manufacture of corneal lenses, making them out of clear plastic instead of glass.[23-25]

Plastic corneal lenses, at the time of their introduction, were made with total diameters of 10.8 mm. to 12.5 mm. They provided better appearance and greater average success in performance than the plastic scleral lenses, which preceded them.

MICRO-CORNEALS

In Germany, in 1952, Wilhelm Sohnges began to use a diminutive lens with less than half the bulk of the Tuohy corneal lenses.[26,27] After refinement by himself and two collaborators, John Neill and Frank Dickinson (who, each in his own country, had made similar lenses), the diminutive lenses were made about twice as flat, with respect to the corneas on which they rested, as the earlier plastic corneal lenses.§ The edges were rounded, not tapered. These micro-corneal

---

*I. G. Farbenindustrie A. G. applied for a patent in Germany in 1935 to cover the making of "adhering lenses and contact lenses of polymerization products" such as celluloid.

†For a time Muller-Welt made a glass scleral lens that did not require artificial fluid.[20]

‡The specific gravity of the plastic used is 1.12; of the glass, 2.52.

---

§Early corneals were made 0.1 to 0.2 mm longer in radius than the cornea. Micros were usually 0.2 to 0.3 mm flatter and as much as 0.6 mm flatter.

contact lenses (frequently referred to as micro-lenses) were usually made without a bevel and were essentially a small Kalt type of lens made of plastic. The diminished size and thickness and the wider departure from the corneal curve permitted greater tear circula-tion to the cornea than was achieved with earlier plastic corneals. As a consequence, the earlier and larger type was largely super-seded by micro-lenses with gratifying im-provement in performance in most instances.

CORNEAL CONFORMITY

The early plastic corneal lenses were fit-ted longer in radius than the corneas on which they rested. However, in 1955 a new principle was introduced, which is now used in fitting the majority of corneal lenses. According to this principle of fitting, the lens should con-tact the cornea quite uniformly except at the very periphery of the lens. This is commonly spoken of as "contouring the cornea," "paral-leling the cornea," or "corneal alignment."

This method was originally advocated by Sohnges, Moss, and Bier.[28] It is interesting to note that this approach would appear to have been anticipated by an invention patented by George Butterfield (No. 2,544,246, application filed 1950). In this he states: "... the concave side of the lens approximates the surface of a paraboloid ... providing a lens whose contact surface is very close to the shape of the eye-ball" (Figure 1.7). Whether the Butterfield

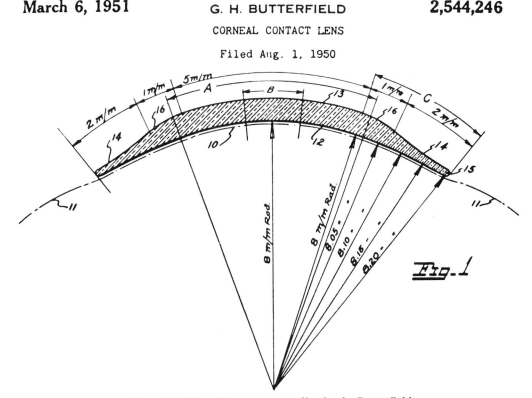

March 6, 1951　　　G. H. BUTTERFIELD　　　**2,544,246**

CORNEAL CONTACT LENS

Filed Aug. 1, 1950

Figure 1.7. Figure from patent application by Butterfield.

lens suffered from lack of "ski" effect and resultant tightness around the edge from too great size and thickness (he shows a lens covering the whole cornea), from the latent period, which often occurs between the time of an invention and its wide utilization, or from other causes, it was not until later that there was widespread adoption of approximately conforming lenses.

These examples illustrate how develop-ments occur as different minds converge toward similar solutions to current problems. Developments seldom occur solely as a result of the salient points mentioned in histories. More often they arise as the result of many increments contributed by numerous imaginative minds. The actuality is often like a slow journey on foot. History does not recount each step of the journey, only the landmarks passed.

REFERENCES

1. da Vinci, L.: *Codex of the Eye, Manuscript D* (circa 1508). For translation and illustrations, *see* Hofstetter, H. W., and Graham, R.: Leonardo and contact lenses, *Am. J. Optom.*, *30*(1):41–44, 1953.

2. Descartes, R.: Methods of correcting vision (in French), in his *Discours de la Méthode*, 1636, Discours 7, La Dioptrique, p. 147. For translation and illustrations, *see* Enoch, J. M.: Descartes' contact lens, *Am. J. Optom.*, *33*(2): 7–85, 1956.

3. Young, T.: On the mechanism of the eye, *Philos. Trans. R. Soc. Lond.*, [Biol. Sci.] 91:23–88, 1801. Reprinted in *Survey Ophthalmol.*, *6*(4): 383–391, 1961.

4. Herschel, J. F. W.: Light, *Encyclopaedia Brittanica*, 6th ed., 1823.

5. Fick, A. E.: Eine Contactbrille, *Arch. f. Augenheilk.*, *18*:279–289, 1888. For one translation into English *see Arch. Ophthalmol.*, *17*(2):215–226, 1888.

6. Mann, I.: History of contact lenses, *Trans. Ophthalmol. Soc. U.K.*, *58*, *Pt. 1*:109–136, 1938.

7. Muller, F. E.: *Über die Korrektion des Keratokonus und anderer Brechungsanomalien des Auges mit Müllerschen Kontaktschalen.* Inaugural dissertation. Marburg, Germany, University of Marburg, 1920, p. 6.

8. Panas, P.: Presentation of instruments and apparatus, Pt. 4, *Bull. Acad. Med., Ser. 3*, *19*:400–401, March 20, 1888. (A discussion of Kalt's use of shells of glass against keratoconus.)

9. Chevallereau, M. A.: Traitement du kératocone, *Bull. 35, Mem. Soc. Franc. Ophthal.*, *11*:385–392, 1893.

10. Haas, E.: Les verres de contact: rapport présenté à la Séance plénière du 14 Novembre, 1937, *Bull. Soc. Ophthalmol. Fr.*, pp. 74–76, 1937.

11. Müller, A.: *Spectacle lenses and corneal lenses* (in German), Inaugural dissertation, Kiel, Germany, University of Kiel, 1889.

12. Dallos, J.: Über Haftglaser u. Kontaktschalen, *Klin. Monatsbl. Augenheilkd.*, 91:640, 1933. For first English translation *see Arch. Ophthalmol.*, *15*(4):617–623, 1936.

13. von Rohr, M., and Boegehold, H.: *Das Brillenglas als Optisches Instrument.* Berlin, Springer, 1934, p. 17.

14. von Rohr, M.: On the available means for correcting cases of considerable anisometropia, *Trans. Opt. Soc. Lon.*, *24*(2):92–96, 1922–1923.

15. Weve, H. J. M.: Diathermieverfahren zur Behandlung der Netzhautablösung, *Ber. Versamml. Deutsch. Ophth. Gesellsch.*,49: 110, 1932.

16. Weve, H. J. M.: *Ber. Versamml. Deutsch. Ophth. Gesellsch.*, Leipzig, May 19, 1932.

17. Weve, H. J. M.: Die genezing der netviesloslating met behulp van diathermie, *Ned. Tijdschr. Geneeskd.*, 76:3591–3599, 1932.

18. Feinbloom, W.: A plastic contact lens, in *Trans. Amer. Acad. Optom.*, *10*:37–44, Chicago, Aug., 1936.

19. Obrig, T., and Salvatori, P.: *Contact Lenses*, 3rd ed. New York, Obrig Laboratories, 1957, p. 188. Also Mullen, J. E.: *Contact Lens*, U. S. Patent 2,237,744.

20. Obrig, T., and Salvatori, P.: *Contact Lenses*, 3rd ed. New York, Obrig Laboratories,

1957, pp. 158, 753.

21. Bier, N.: *Contact Lens Routine and Practice*, 2nd ed., London, Butterworths, 1957, pp. 6, 191–192.

22. Bier, N.: U.K. patent 592,055.

23. Nugent, M. W.: The corneal lens, a preliminary report, *Ann. West. Med. Surg.*, 2(6):241, 1948.

24. Graham, R.: The corneal lens, a progress report, *Am. J. Optom*, 26(2):75–77, 1949.

25. Tuohy, K. M.: The birth of an idea, *Optom. World*, 50(22):14–20, 1963. Woehlk was apparently working with corneal lenses

at the same time as Tuohy, but appears not to have had his work described in the literature.

26. Dickinson, F.: A report on a new corneal lens, *The Optician*, 128(3303):3–6, 1954.

27. Dickinson, F.: Notes on a new German corneal contact lens, *Am. J. Optom.*, 31(7):378–381, 1954.

28. Bier, N.: *Contact Lens Routine and Practice*, 2nd ed., London, Butterworths, 1957, pp. 143, 200. This was apparently not presented in the literature until 1956. The contour lens, *The Optician*, 132:397, 1956.

ADDITIONAL READINGS

Davis, H. E.: Contact lens trends—past and future, *Contacto*, 20(3):39–40, 1976.

Deeson, A. F. L.: A brief history of the development of contact lenses, *The Disp. Opt.*, 30(5): 140–143, 1978.

Dickinson, F.: The microlens attains its majority, *Contact Lens*, 4(4):22, 1973.

Endore, M. A.: Origin and early history of contact lenses, *Optom. World*, pp. 26, 30, 32, 52, Jan. 1948.

Genco, L.: The history of contact lenses, *Optom. Monthly*, 70(8):49–53, 1979.

Goodlaw, E. I.: How corneal contacts were born,

Cont. Lens Forum, 3(9):31, 1978.

Knoll, H. A.: Kevin Tuohy: thirty years of corneal contacts, *Cont. Lens Forum*, 1(7):11, 13, 1976.

Knoll, H. A.: William Feinbloom: pioneer in plastic contact, *Cont. Lens Forum*, 21(8):29, 31, 32, 1977.

Knoll, H. A., Harrington, B., and Williams, J. R.: Two years' experience with hydrophilic contact lenses, *Am. J. Optom. Arch. Am. Acad. Optom.*, 47(12):1000–1006, 1970.

Larke, J. R.: Hydrophilic gel lenses in Czechoslovakia, *Contact Lens*, 1(6):10–15, 1968.

Chapter 2

ANATOMY AND PHYSIOLOGY OF THE CORNEA

CORNEA PROPER

THE CORNEA IS THE transparent structure that constitutes the first and principal optical component of the eye. The cornea has been classically considered as composed of five layers: *epithelium, Bowman's membrane, stroma, Descemet's membrane,* and *endothelium* (Figure 2.1).

EPITHELIUM

The epithelium is about 50 μm thick and forms the outermost 10 percent of the total corneal thickness. It consists of five or six layers of cells that are divided into three types: *basal, wing,* and *surface cells.* The basal cells are arranged in a single layer on the basal membrane[1] and are columnar with flat bases. The next three layers are composed of wing cells of a polyhedral shape, which become flatter in the layers towards the surface. The most superficial layer consists of large, flattened surface cells (Figure 2.2). The different cell layers represent stages of cell development. The columnar-shaped cells are formed in the basal layer, pushed towards the surface, and replaced by new cells. As the cells move outward, they gradually flatten and become desquamated but are not keratinized.

On gross examination the surface of the epithelium appears to be smooth, but with the aid of scanning electron microscopy, it can be shown that the surface actually has a rather uneven texture (Figure 2.3).[2-4] The cells have many microvilli and minute folds, or microplicae, which are ½ to ¾ μm high (Figure 2.4).[5,6] It has been said that their function is to aid in holding the tear film on the corneal surface, but this is questionable. The plicae have

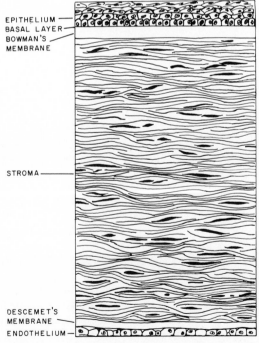

Figure 2.1. Schematic sectional view of the cornea.

16

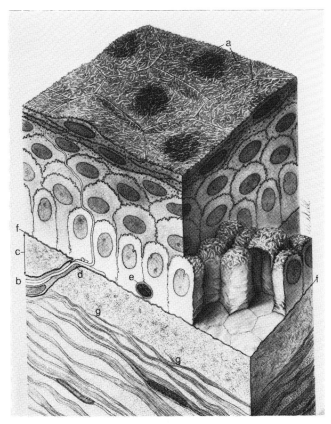

Figure 2.2. Three-dimensional drawing of the corneal epithelium. The five layers of cells forming this epithelium are shown. The drawing brings out the polygonal shape of the basal and surface cells and their relative size. The wing cell processes fill the spaces formed by the dome-shaped apical surface of the basal cells. The turnover time for these cells is seven days, and during this time the columnar basal cell is gradually transformed into a wing cell, then into a thin, flat surface cell. During this transition the cytoplasm changes and the Golgi apparatus becomes more prominent. Numerous vesicles develop in the superficial wing and surface layers, and glycogen appears in the surface cells. The intercellular space separating the outermost surface cells is closed by a zonula occludens, forming a barrier that prevents ingress of the precorneal tear film into the corneal stroma. The cell surface shows an extensive net of microplicae (a) and microvilli, which may be involved in the retention of the precorneal film. A corneal nerve (b) passes through Bowman's layer (c); it loses its Schwann sheath near the basement membrane (d) of the basal epithelium. The nerve then passes between the epithelial cells toward the superficial layers as a naked nerve. A lymphocyte (e) is seen between two basal epithelial cells. The basement membrane is seen at f. Some of the most superficial corneal stromal lamellae (g) are seen curving forward to merge with Bowman's layer. The regular arrangement of the corneal stromal collagen differs from the random disposition of that in Bowman's layer. From M. J. Hogan, J. A. Alvarado, and J. Esperson, *Histology of the Human Eye*, 1971. Courtesy of W. B. Saunders, Co., Philadelphia, Pennsylvania.

been shown to be covered by acid mucopoly-saccharides, which are the major component of the basal layer of the tear film.

The epithelial cells are bound together

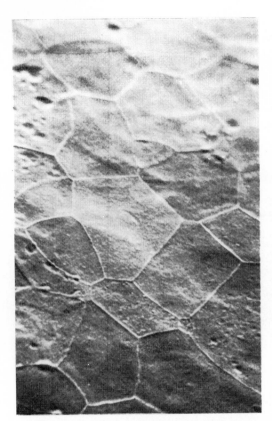 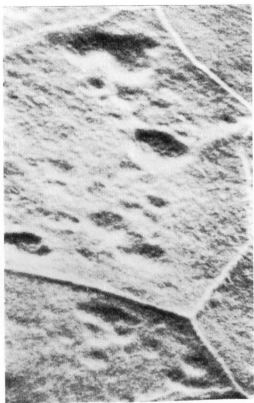

Figure 2.3. Surface of the epithelium by scanning electron microscopy: (*left*) human cornea air dried, magnified about 1,600 times (reduced 18%); (*right*) human cornea air dried, magnified 3,700 times (reduced 18%). Courtesy of Spencer, Matas, and Hayes.

by their interdigitations, by attachment devices, or desmosomes, and by the zonula occludens. The *desmosomes* are points of attachment between cells where the cell membrane becomes thickened and many fibrils are attached.[7] The fibrils are known as tonofibrils. The zonulae have been identified by Liegl[8,9] between the surface cells of the corneal epithelium. The zonulae are composed of a fusion of the outer protein layers of the membranes of two adjacent cells. This fusion occludes the intercellular space, which is normally 10 to 20 nm, and may run continuously around the circumference of a cell. The zonula occludens determines the degree of permeability of the corneal epithelium to water-soluble substances and drugs.

A corneal contact lens will tend to rest directly on portions of the epithelial surface. Theoretically, the lens is separated from the epithelium by the tear layer, but actually this condition rarely, if ever, exists for the entire lens surface. If the bearing is not excessive, the lens can be supported by the epithelium without injury. The cells in the epithelium are linked to one another by protoplasmic connections and fine intercellular processes, all of which lend support to the epithelium and aid in its resistance to mechanical abrasion by a contact lens.[10] The cells are not normally keratinized, however, and can be damaged by a poorly handled lens.

It is not surprising that a properly fitted contact lens should have little abrasive effect on the epithelium. The epithelium must normally withstand the rubbing action of the

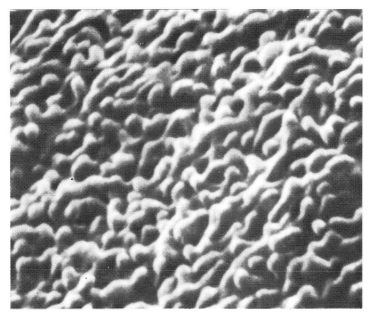

Figure 2.4. Microplicae of the corneal epithelium: rabbit cornea, freeze dried. (x20,000) Courtesy of Spencer, Matas, and Hayes.

lids, which occurs during blinking, and it is not greatly affected by vigorous massage through the lids. The superficial layers are normally shed with such actions, and the cells are rapidly replaced by the inner layers.

Observations of the mitotic rate and of the movement of radioactively labeled cells indicate that the time from division to desquamation for normal epithelial cells is less than one week.[11,12] It is likely, however, that wearing a corneal lens will cause more than normal desquamation, and the cornea must adapt to this condition. The cornea has the capacity to replace epithelial cells at a very rapid rate if necessary, as is seen following superficial corneal injuries. Small abrasions of the epithelial layer are covered rapidly by a gliding and flattening motion of the adjacent cells.[13] Usually within twenty-four hours the denuded areas have been replaced.

It has been proposed that variations in the fragility of the epithelium play a large part in determining whether contact lenses will produce corneal abrasions under normal conditions of wear. Cochet has designed an epithelial fragility test, which may be used to screen potential contact lens wearers,[14] but its validity is doubtful.

BASEMENT MEMBRANE OF THE EPITHELIUM

The basement membrane of the epithelium assists the epithelium in adhering to Bowman's membrane. The elasticity of the basement membrane seems to play an important role in the cohesion and regularity of the corneal epithelium and in preserving the smooth curvature of the cornea.[15] Like the epithelium, the basal layer regenerates after injury, but its rate is much slower.

The basement membrane is about 30 to 60 nm in thickness. Fibrils from the adjacent membrane anchor the layer firmly to the stroma.

The epithelial cells are attached to the basement membrane by structures very similar to half of a desmosome, which are called *hemidesmosomes*. If the epithelium is torn loose, the basement membrane usually remains. If the basement membrane is also destroyed, it is found that the epithelium regenerates and covers the injured area without the reformation of the basement membrane. It may require months before the new basement membrane is formed, and during that period the epithelium can be easily dislodged. This is the most probable explanation for the occurrence of recurrent erosion.[16-19]

BOWMAN'S MEMBRANE

Bowman's membrane is a thin sheet, 8 to 14 μm thick, consisting of a condensed outer layer of the stroma from which it cannot be isolated. It is composed of irregularly arranged collagen fibers and is highly resistant to injury, pressure, and infection. It is completely acellular. Unlike the epithelium (and Descemet's membrane), Bowman's membrane will not regenerate when damaged but is replaced by a permanent scar or opacity, hence the importance of arresting any complication arising from an epithelial abrasion caused by a contact lens.

STROMA (SUBSTANTIA PROPRIA)

The stroma comprises 90 percent of the total corneal thickness. It consists of tapelike bands of parallel collagen fibrils, known as *lamellae*, and cells (Figure 2.5a). There are between 100 and 200 lamellae, which vary in thickness from 1.3 to 2.5 μm. They run parallel to the surface and to each other across the cornea from limbus to limbus.[13,20]

The lamellae in the center of the central and deep stroma cross at nearly right angles to each other. Near the corneal surface they may interlace somewhat. At the corneal periphery, they sometimes divide and intermingle with some circular lamella found at the limbal region.

Collagen fibrils lie parallel to each other and for any given lamella are of nearly uniform diameter, which varies from about 19 nm in the anterior layer to 35 nm near the posterior stroma.

Apparently, the fibers of the lamella have high tensile strength and are embedded in a springy ground substance, which keeps them apart and prevents their compression.[20] This arrangement allows the transfer of substances through the tissues for adequate nutrition.

Nearly all the nutritional substances to the stroma arrive by diffusion through the endothelium from the aqueous humor. Only a very slight amount to the corneal periphery comes from the limbal capillaries. There is some evidence that glucose enters the stroma at a rate that is greater than can be explained by diffusion alone.[21]

Two types of cells are found within the stroma, the *wandering cells* and the *keratocytes*, or corneal corpuscles. The keratocytes lie between or possibly within the lamellae and parallel to the surface.[10] They are modified fibroblasts with many processes. The wandering cells are few in number and are a type of leukocyte or reticuloendothelial cell.

DESCEMET'S MEMBRANE

Descemet's membrane (posterior elastic lamina) is a strong, structureless layer, 10 to 15 μm in thickness, which is secreted by the endothelium (Figure 2.5b). It is resistant to

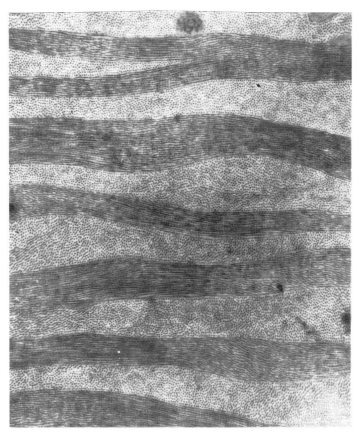

Figure 2.5a. The stroma of the human cornea as viewed with the electron microscope. From M. A. Jakus, Further Observations on the Fine Structure of the Cornea, *Investigative Ophthalmology*, 1(2):202–225, 1962.

trauma and pathology. Among its properties is the ability to take elastic tissue stains; the tendency for its cut edges to roll outward (showing its elasticity); its imperviousness to invasion by blood vessels, cells, and other formed elements; and its apparent resistance to pathological processes in the body.[22] Descemet's membrane is elastic; however, it is not composed of elastin but rather of collagen.

ENDOTHELIUM

The most posterior layer of the cornea, the endothelium, consists of a single layer of flattened cells, 5 μm high by 20 μm wide (Figure 2.5b).

The cells are attached weakly to Descemet's membrane by hemidesmosomes and to each other by interdigitation, desmosomes, and a zonula occludens near the anterior chamber. The zonulae close the intracellular space from the anterior chamber. The cytoplasm facing the anterior chamber is modified to form a terminal web, which is rich in fibrils. In marked contrast to the epithelium, endothelial cells are infrequently, if ever, replaced as a normal process during adult life. When disrupted, they may be replaced by the spread-

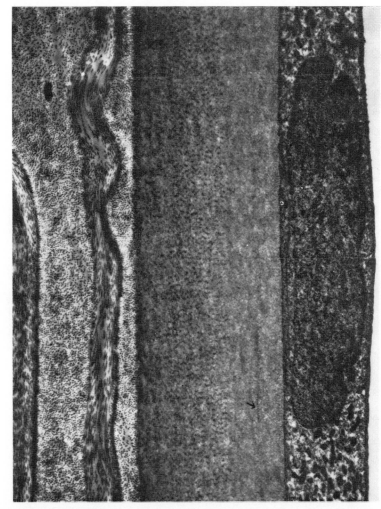

Figure 2.5b. Descemet's membrane and endothelium (*to right*) with deeper layer of the stroma. From M. A. Jakus, Further Observations on the Fine Structure of the Cornea, *Investigative Ophthalmology*, 1(2):202–225, 1962.

ing of healthy cells. The cells may reach double their normal size, as can be seen by slit-lamp biomicroscopy. The endothelial cell density decreases with age and as the result of trauma from cataract surgery, corneal transplantation, and intraocular lens implantation.

LIMBUS

The limbus is the transition zone, approximately 1 mm. wide, in which the cornea is joined with the conjunctiva and the sclera. It differs structurally from the cornea proper and contains blood vessels and lymphatics, which are not normally found in the cornea. The physiological functioning of the cornea is dependent upon the limbus, from which the cornea receives part of its nutrients. The limbal region is especially significant in fitting contact lenses because it is so closely connected to the cornea proper and because some contact lenses bear directly on the limbus.

The limbus differs in its histological structure from the cornea in that it has only two layers, the stroma and the epithelium. Bowman's membrane stops short in a rounded edge at the limbus, and Descemet's membrane is continuous with a similar structure secreted by the endothelium of the trabecular meshwork. The stroma is broken by fingerlike processes from the sclera, the papillae, which run radially (1.5 to 2 mm. apart) from the sclera and merge into the cornea. The papillae contain blood vessels and lympahatics.[24] The epithelium of the limbus is thicker than in the cornea. It contains about ten layers of cells that project down radially and fill the spaces between the papillae.

VASCULAR SUPPLY

Normally, other than at the limbus, the cornea is avascular. The limbus is supplied with arterioles derived from the anterior ciliary arteries. Just before reaching Bowman's membrane the arterioles terminate as capillary loops (in the papillae) and form venules, which in turn lead into a venous plexus. Anterior ciliary veins lead from the venous plexus.

Aqueous veins run from the paralimbal region towards the equator of the eye and, by way of the trabecular meshwork, are connected with the anterior chamber. They contain intraocular fluid mixed with small quantities of blood. This fluid is emptied into the conjunctival or episcleral veins. Pressure on the sclera, produced, for example, by a cotton-tipped applicator or chemical or physical irritation, causes an increase of red blood cells in the aqueous veins due to reversed blood flow. The pressure caused by lid closure or blinking is also sufficient to reverse flow in the aqueous vein or in its recipient vessel. Neill suggested that the pressure of a scleral contact lens on the sclera or limbus could produce the same result and be a possible cause of the corneal edema sometimes found when contact lenses are worn.[25] Ascher[26] found experimentally that scleral lenses at times provoked a reversal in aqueous flow, an increased red-cell content, cyanosis, and stagnation in the part of the vessel covered by the scleral portion of the lens. Corneal lenses produced no changes in the aqueous veins.

THICKNESS

From measurements of central corneal thickness for 224 eyes, von Bahr found that the mean thickness was 0.56 mm.,[27] with no significant difference with age or sex. From the standard deviation of the sample, he predicted statistically that the range for normal corneal thickness of the population would be 0.46 to 0.67 mm. The average corneal thickness for eight cases of hyperopia was also 0.56 mm., while in twelve cases of myopia over 4.00 D. the thickness was significantly less, with an average of 0.52 mm. Maurice concludes from the results of various investigators that the average central corneal thickness is about 0.53 mm.[20]

Mandell and Polse[28] used a modified pachymeter with an automatic recording system to measure the corneal thickness at 5° intervals along the horizontal meridian of sixteen eyes of normal patients (Figure 2.6). The mean value for the central (minimum) thickness for normals was 0.506 mm. (range 0.43 to 0.56 and S. D. ±0.04). The mean value for normal corneas is slightly lower than other figures that have been presented in the literature and probably occurs because they were using the *minimum* thickness measurement from each series on a cornea, whereas other inves-

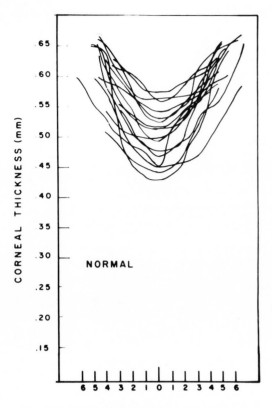

CORNEAL THICKNESS (mm)

.65
.60
.55
.50
.45
.40
.35
.30
.25
.20
.15

NORMAL

6 5 4 3 2 1 0 1 2 3 4 5 6

DISTANCE FROM THINNEST POINT (mm)

Figure 2.6. Mean corneal thickness for the horizontal meridian of sixteen eyes. From R. B. Mandell and K. A. Polse, Keratoconus: Spatial Variation of Corneal Thickness as a Diagnostic Test, *Archives of Ophthalmology*, 82(2):182–188, 1969.

tigators have measured at a constant corneal position.

Measurements of corneal thickness have, for the most part, been confined to experimental studies where they may be used as an index of various physiological changes. Corneal thickness is to a great extent determined by corneal hydration, and anything that tends to increase the water content of the cornea will cause an increase in corneal thickness.[29]

It is known that the cornea thickens soon after a contact lens is first worn. This is due to edema caused by interference with the normal physiological processes. The amount of corneal thickening can be correlated with other corneal reactions to contact lens wear, such as clouding and subjective symptoms of haze.[20]

Some attempts have been made by contact lens practitioners to measure corneal thickness by attaching a dial gauge to a biomicroscope and measuring the distance traveled to focus first on the epithelium and then on the endothelium. This method does not give results to an acceptable degree of accuracy, which explains some of the unusual variation in the measurements reported. It should also be noted that the apparent thickness measured is not equal to the true thickness, because the image of the endothelium through the cornea is optically displaced in relation to the index of refraction of the cornea.

MECHANICAL PROPERTIES

The eye of the contact lens wearer is subjected to several forces that are not often exerted on the normal eye. This is especially so during removal of a contact lens. In this act the lids are drawn tightly against the cornea in a squeezing action. Such action does no harm to the cornea because the stroma is a flexible membrane of high tensile strength. The construction of the eye is analogous to an inflated football.[20] It provides a spherical shape together with high resistance to shock. Experiments in which the globe is inflated from a compressed air cylinder show that the eye can withstand very high pressures before bursting. There is a safety factor of about one hundred times above normal intraocular pressure before the eye bursts.

The eye returns to normal very quickly following deformation as can be illustrated by movies of a pattern of circles reflected from the eye. It is possible to demonstrate this by a simple experiment. Stretch the lids across the cornea (which duplicates the action of contact lens removal) by placing the index finger at the outer canthus and pulling temporally and at the same time view a visual acuity chart. It will be noted that blurring and distortion of the chart occur due to the induced and irregular corneal toricity that has been induced. When the finger is released, the reappearance of normal acuity takes place in only a fraction of a second.

TRANSPARENCY

To maintain its vital function as an optical medium of the eye, the cornea must have a high degree of transparency. This it achieves by its unique structure and physiology. A contact lens may interfere with many of the normal processes that maintain corneal transparency, and it is necessary that the contact lens practitioner be thoroughly informed as to the nature of the mechanisms that control these processes.

THEORIES OF CORNEAL TRANSPARENCY

A classical explanation for the transparency of the cornea is based upon the regularity of the collagen fibrils in its lamellar structure. It has been pointed out, however, that other tissues, such as tendons, have fibers that are uniformly arranged and yet are opaque.[22] Also, Cogan suggests that perhaps the uniform arrangement of the collagen fibrils primarily serves the function of tensile strength and has little to do with the corneal transparency.[22]

If the refractive index of the cornea were uniform, it would make no difference whether the fibrils were regularly arranged or not. This, however, is not the case. Maurice has found there is a definite difference in refractive index between the collagen fibrils and the ground substance.[20] He determined the refractive index of the collagen fibrils (from measurements of their birefringence) to be 1.47. By calculating the difference between the refractive index of the whole stroma and that for dried collagen, he obtained a refractive index of 1.354 for the ground substance.

A theory of corneal transparency has been proposed by Maurice,[30] which he calls the *lattice theory*. This postulates that the corneal stroma consists of a two-dimensional lattice of collagen fibrils, regularly and uniformly oriented and having a higher refractive index than the surrounding interstitial substance. The spacing of the fibrils of the lattice is less than that of the wavelength of light. From the phenomenon of interference, waves of light striking the cornea are scattered from the individual fibrils and cancel one another in all directions, except that of the beam which falls on the tissue. The lattice is thus transparent in the direction of the incident beam, and destructive interference eliminates any light scattered in other directions. Lack of regular lamellar structure and alteration of the crucial distance between the fibrils would alter the interference relationship and cause a decrease of transparency.

The principal advantage of Maurice's theory is that it accounts satisfactorily for the loss of transparency due to hydration and swelling of the cornea. Francois and Rabaey have shown that as the cornea swells the diameter of the collagen fibril does not increase but that the swelling appears to take place between the fibrils and tends to separate them further.[31] If the collagen fibers that form the lattice are displaced during corneal hydration, the normal light interference relationship is destroyed, and corneal transparency is lost. Maurice's theory also explains the rapid change in transparency caused by pressure on the cornea and the equally rapid restoration of the transparency on release of that pressure.

Potts has pointed out that assuming the lattice theory of corneal transparency is correct, this phenomenon is unique and not duplicated anywhere else in the body.[32] Electron microscopy fails to show any such structural organization in the lens and corneal epithelium, and hence, these organs must depend for their transparency on some other mechanism, possibly that of optical homogeneity.

Schwartz and Keyserlingk have shown that the distance between the collagen fibers ranges from 10 to 40 nm.[33] They feel that the regularity of the collagen fibers is not sufficient to account for Maurice's theory of transparency and suggest that it is due to the small and regular diameter fibers. This viewpoint is also taken by Goldman[34] and co-workers, which is based on the concepts of Benedek.[35]

Casperson and Engstrom[36] have suggested that the corneal transparency could be due to a smooth gradient of refractive index from one corneal fibril to the next. Potts,[32] however, has raised the questions of whether the smooth gradient would actually result in transparency and how the gradient would be maintained.

RELATION TO WATER CONTENT

Corneal transparency is closely related to corneal water content. The stroma normally stays in a state of *deturgescence* or partial dehydration at about 78 percent water. It has been shown experimentally that when the excised cornea is stripped of its epithelium and endothelium, it imbibes water profusely, thus increasing greatly in weight.[37] The cornea then becomes translucent.

OSMOTIC THEORY

This early theory presumed that the osmotic pressures of the precorneal film on the anterior corneal surface and of the aqueous on the posterior corneal surface were higher than the osmotic pressure of the cornea.[38] The epithelium and endothelium would act as semipermeable membranes (Figure 2.7a). Water that entered the cornea via the perilimbal vessels would tend to be drawn out in the direction of the hypertonic fluids, i.e. towards the tear layer and aqueous. It was shown later that the osmotic pressure of the tears and aqueous were not appreciably greater than the stroma.[39] Although the control of water content in the stroma cannot be explained by osmotic forces alone, the corneal epithelium does act as though it were an excellent semipermeable membrane. In addition, the epithelium and endothelium serve as barriers to the excessive flow of water into the stroma.

The tear osmolarity* is an important factor in maintaining the normal hydration state of the cornea. The normal tears are equivalent to about 0.91 NaCl solution.[40] If the cornea is bathed with solutions of lower salt concentration, it will produce corneal swelling (Figure 2.7b).[41] This would be the condition, for example, when someone is swimming in a freshwater pool and opens his eyes under water for a period of time. Higher salt

---

*Osmolarity and tonicity are synonyms that are used to describe the force created by an imbalance of salts or other substances on two sides of a membrane.

concentrations will cause some corneal thinning and may be used to reduce corneal edema (Figure 2.7b). It has been shown that corneal swelling can be produced by tearing, which is caused either by chemical or mechanical stimulation (Figure 2.7c).[42,43] It is assumed that during lacrimation, the tear osmolarity is lower than normal, which causes the water to enter the cornea and produce edema. This phenomenon is thought to play an important role in contact lens adaptation (*see* Chapter 6).

Changes in the osmolarity of the tears are also thought to occur under several other conditions. When the eye is open, the tear osmolarity is higher due to evaporation into the atmosphere. This evaporation is much less than would take place were the external layer of the tear film not composed of an oily substance. When the eyes are closed, the tear osmolarity is lowered and hence a slight corneal thickening is produced. When the eyes are opened following sleep, the cornea thins over a period of about one hour,[44,45]

and the recovery to baseline corneal thickness after awakening is logarithmic (Figure 2.7d). Mertz also found that there was considerable variability among subjects in amount of overnight swelling that occurred.[46] He hypothesized three possible mechanisms for this variability: (1) variation in the level of oxygen or hypotonicity in the closed-eye environment, (2) variation in the cornea's ability to adapt to the relatively hypoxic or hypotonic closed eye environment, or (3) variation in completeness of eyelid closure during sleep. The maximum corneal swelling that is produced by tearing alone is equal to about 4 percent.

The tears in the meniscus of the lid margin (representing the open-eye condition) have an osmolarity about 5 percent greater than the tears in the fornix (representing the closed-eye condition).[47] This is adequate to explain the corneal hydration changes that occur, although the change has not been measured directly.[48-50]

THE PUMP THEORY (ACTIVE CONTROL)

The osmotic theory of Cogan and Kinsey has now been virtually replaced by a theory that postulates the action of a *metabolic pump* in the endothelial cells and perhaps, to a lesser extent, the epithelium. Water and electrolytes are actively secreted out of the stroma. The actual mechanism is debatable, however, and there is disagreement as to which particular corneal layers are most involved. Evidence favors the endothelium as the chief

site of activity.[51,52] The endothelium is less of a barrier to water than is the epithelium and allows a certain leakage of aqueous fluid into the stroma. This fluid must be compensated for by an active process of water removal, or else the stroma would swell. The oxygen supply normally available for the aqueous is sufficient to maintain an effective pump mechanism in the endothelium (Figure 2.8).

RELATION TO POLYSACCHARIDES

It would appear that there is a definite relationship between corneal hydration and polysaccharides and that the polysaccharides and collagens determine, to a certain extent, corneal transparency.[52,53] There would also

appear to be an association between polysaccharides and avascularity because structures that are rich in polysaccharides (cornea, cartilage, vitreous) are devoid of blood vessels. In addition, the elimination of certain poly-

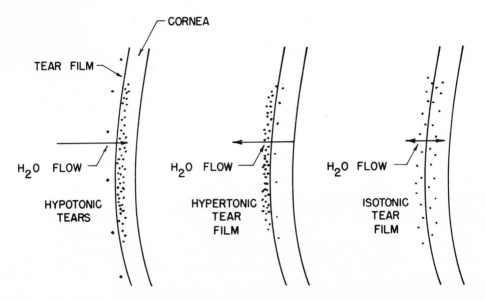

Figure 2.7a. Cornea as a semipermeable membrane. Direction of fluid flow depends upon tear tonicity.

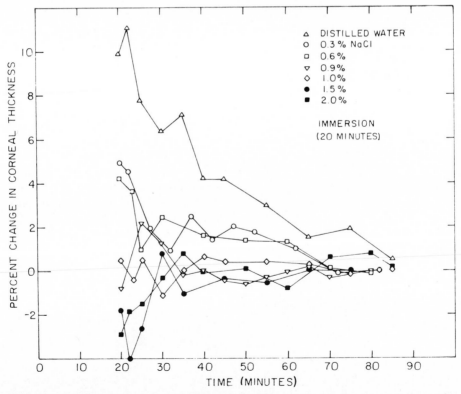

Figure 2.7b. Corneal recovery from swelling produced by immersing the cornea in lower than normal salt concentration for twenty minutes. From R. S. Chan and R. B. Mandell, Corneal Thickness Changes from Bathing Solution, *American Journal of Optometry and Physiological Optics*, 52:465–469, 1975.

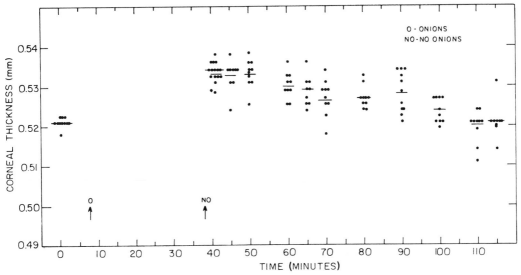

Figure 2.7c. Corneal swelling produced by tearing from exposure to onions (O) and return to normal after their removal (NO).

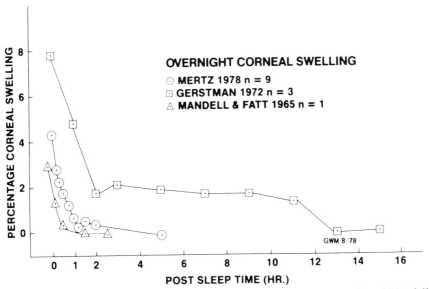

Figure 2.7d. Data for overnight corneal swelling (from Mertz,[46] Gerstman,[121] and Mandell and Fatt[45]).

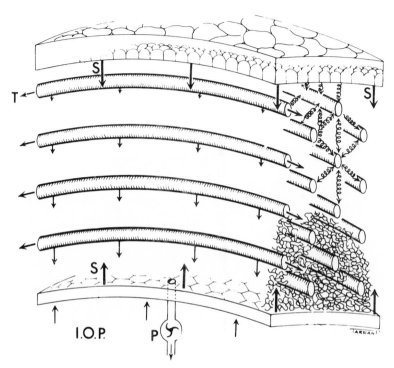

Figure 2.8. Schema of forces within the cornea. The ground substance is shown enmeshing the collagen fibrils at the bottom right, but its expansile component is represented functionally, upper right, by the compressed springs. The tension (*T*) of the individual fibrils creates a centrally directed pressure, rising cumulatively from the outside to the inside of the stroma, where it is balanced by the intraocular pressure. This would compress the ground substance unevenly across the thickness and cause a displacement of the majority of the fibrils towards the endothelial surface. However, the endothelial pump mechanism (*P*) maintains a suction (*S*) in the stromal tissue fluid. The suction acting on the epithelial and endothelial surfaces tends to establish a uniform compression of equal distribution and leading to the formation of a regular lattice on which the transparency of the tissue depends. The compression of the ground substance is manifested as the swelling pressure, 60 mm. Hg, when fluid is allowed free access to the stroma. From D. M. Maurice, Clinical Physiology of the Cornea, *International Ophthalmology Clinics*, 2(*3*):561–572, 1962.

saccharides by hyaluronidase results in corneal vascularization.[22] Cogan has suggested that, because of the polysaccharide content, the cornea has the property of acting as a reversible sponge, imbibing and discharging water in response to varying hydrostatic and osmotic pressure.[22] Ruptures and distortions are prevented from occurring because the cornea is allowed to adapt itself to changes in tension.

METABOLISM

Metabolism of glucose provides the biological energy required by the cornea for growth and cellular activity. In addition, it provides for the maintenance of the normally dehydrated state of the cornea, which is necessary for transparency. Two processes are involved, *aerobic glycolysis* and *anaerobic glycolysis*. Metabolism of glucose in the presence of oxygen produces lactic acid, which, in the presence of certain enzymes, is oxidized to carbon dioxide and water. Under anaerobic conditions, the cornea does not further oxidize the lactic acid; therefore, the amount of lactic acid accumulated is a measure of anaerobic glycolysis.

SOURCES OF METABOLITES

Since the cornea is devoid of blood vessels, some mechanism must be provided in order to supply the metabolites needed for cell life and to remove the waste products. This is accomplished by the movement of water and dissolved materials into, through, and out of the cornea by one of three possible routes: the limbal blood supply, the aqueous, and the tears. Two processes serve this function: the transfer of dissolved species by convective flow, and the diffusion of dissolved species in the absence of convective flow. Convective flow takes place as the result of a pressure from the aqueous humor, whereas diffusion takes place without a pressure gradient and results in a movement of solutes without a flow of water. In this way substances in high concentration are moved to an area of low concentration. From various experiments it has been found that the flow of water either through the cornea or along its length is very slow.

LIMBUS

The capillary bed at the limbus has the potential to supply the cornea with all the soluble constituents of the blood. However, very little of these can be brought to the central area of the cornea by means of a fluid flow, due to the high resistance by the cornea. Some substances, namely, plasma, proteins, and small ions such as sodium, are passed into the cornea by diffusion, but the limbus does not supply any appreciable amount of oxygen to the cornea. Near the center of the cornea, the major supply of all substances comes from the anterior and posterior faces.

ANTERIOR AND POSTERIOR FACES

The cornea receives most of its needed materials from the aqueous and tears. Because of the high resistance to the flow of water in the cornea, the principal mode of supply is diffusion. Each substance is supplied in relation to its concentration in the aqueous, cornea, and tears with the movement in the direction of lower concentration.

The oxygen is obtained primarily from the tears (via the atmosphere) with smaller amounts contributed by the other sources.

The cornea exhibits a high rate of aerobic glycolysis, without which it cannot function normally.[54-57] About nine-tenths of the reactions requiring oxygen are confined to the epithelial layers, there being very little aerobic glycolysis in the stroma.[54,55,58-60]

The rate of oxygen uptake by the living cornea is about 4.8 μl per hour per cm.[2][61,62] Fatt and Bieber[63] have performed a series of calculations to show the concentration of oxygen at different layers of the cornea, which occur as a

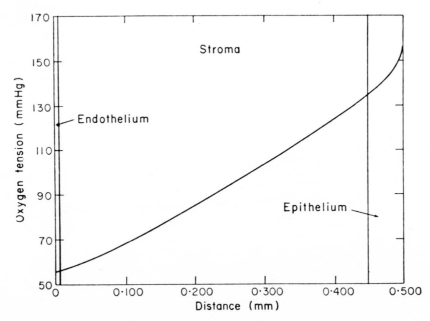

Figure 2.9. Concentration of oxygen at different layers of the cornea that occurs as a result of diffusion from the atmosphere. From I. Fatt and M. T. Bieber, The Steady State Distribution of Oxygen and Carbon Dioxide in the *In Vivo* Cornea, 1. The Open Eye in Air and the Closed Eye, *Experimental Eye Research*, 7(1):103–112, 1968.

result of diffusion from the atmosphere (Figure 2.9).

It should be noted that the quantity of carbon dioxide leaving the cornea is approximately four times the amout entering (Figure 2.10).[64] Only part of this excess can be accounted for by corneal metabolism. The balance is apparently due to a gradient of carbon dioxide across the cornea from the aqueous (about 55 mm. Hg partial pressure) to the atmosphere (only a trace), so that the cornea acts as a release route.

During sleep, the oxygen supply to the cornea comes from the vascular bed of the palpebral conjunctiva.[65] Fatt and Bieber have calculated the concentration of oxygen when the eyes are closed (Figure 2.11).[63] In addition, they have shown the carbon dioxide level in this condition. It may be noted that the carbon dioxide level rises only slightly and does not reach a level that will cause interference with normal metabolism.[66]

The oxygen uptake of the endothelium is much less than that of the epithelium, but it is of great importance in maintaining the corneal thickness and transparency. The lower uptake of the endothelium is a consequence of the thinness of the layer, since, on the basis of the cell volume, the metabolic activity is similar to that of the epithelium. Langham has demonstrated that the aqueous humor is a source of oxygen for the endothelium.[55]

CONTACT LENSES AND METABOLISM

Many of the symptoms that accompany the wearing of contact lenses can be traced to an interference with the normal metabolic processes of the cornea. These disturbances can be brought about in several ways, and the exact mechanism is not always understood.

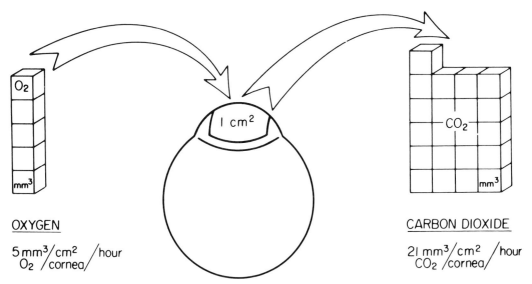

Figure 2.10. The volume of oxygen entering and carbon dioxide leaving a square centimeter of corneal surface area per hour. From R. M. Hill, The Physiology of Soft Contact Lens Systems, in M. Ruben (Ed.), *Soft Contact Lenses*, 1978. Courtesy of John Wiley & Sons, Inc., New York, New York.

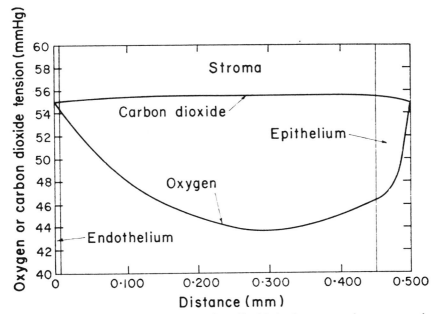

Figure 2.11. Concentration of oxygen and carbon dioxide in the cornea when eyes are closed. From I. Fatt and M. T. Bieber, The Steady State Distribution of Oxygen and Carbon Dioxide in the *In Vivo* Cornea, 1. The Open Eye in Air and the Closed Eye, *Experimental Eye Research*, *7(1):103–112, 1968.*

Abnormal effects caused by deprivation of atmospheric oxygen in the cornea have been reported for human subjects, rabbits, and guinea pigs when wearing contact lenses.[67-70]

These effects are attributed to the diminished aerobic metabolism of the active epithelial cells, upon which both epithelium and stroma appear dependent for energy.

Smelser and Chen,[70] in experiments with scleral lenses on guinea pigs, found that the concentration of lactic acid in the cornea rose rapidly after the contact lens was in place, indicating a decrease in the aerobic metabolism. There was a coincident decrease in corneal transparency and an increase in corneal thickness with the increase of lactic acid concentration. Smelser and Ozanics had observed in earlier experiments that after a scleral contact lens was worn for a short time the normal glycogen store of the cornea disappeared, which suggested that the cornea suffered from relative anaerobic conditions.[69] Hirano observed in rabbits that a decrease in epithelial glycogen occurred within three hours after wearing corneal contact lenses.[71] Other effects on corneal metabolism also have been evaluated.[72,73]

Polse and Mandell first quantified the amount of corneal swelling due to anoxia at the corneal surface.[59] This experiment was accomplished by fitting tight goggles to human subjects and filling the space behind with nitrogen (Figure 2.12).[61] By mixing various quantities of nitrogen and oxygen together, the rate of corneal swelling can be found for various oxygen pressures. At some minimal level of oxygen, the cornea no longer shows swelling.

The typical corneal swelling response to low oxygen levels is an increase in thickness for two to three hours, followed by stabilization or a thickness decrease, indicating adaptation (Figure 2.13).* The mechanism of adaptation is subject to conjecture, since control of hydration in the cornea is not completely

---

*The partial pressure of oxygen simply indicates the pressure of the proportion of air that is composed of oxygen. Since air normally has an atmospheric pressure of 760 mm. Hg, oxygen, which occupies approximately 20 percent of the air, will have a partial pressure of 155 mm. Hg.

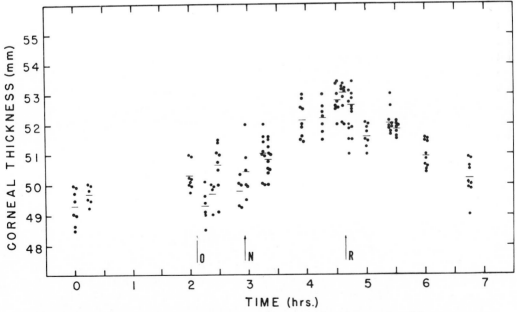

Figure 2.12. Corneal swelling due to anoxia at the corneal surface produced by exposure to nitrogen gas. Goggles placed on eye (*O*) and nitrogen gas started (*N*). Goggles removed and eye exposed to air (*R*). From R. B. Mandell, K. A. Polse, and I. Fatt, Corneal Swelling Caused by Contact Lens Wear, *Archives of Ophthalmology*, 83(*1*):3–9, 1970.

understood. There are significant differences in the minimum oxygen requirement for individuals. The threshold to swelling is between 23 mm. Hg and 37 mm. Hg, depending upon the allowance made for contaminating factors, which are difficult to control (Figure 2.14). The individual thresholds for 95 percent of the subjects vary ±8.7 mm. Hg from the mean value. These results are in close agreement with those found previously in animal studies using various histochemical measures of oxygen deprivation.[74,75]

The amount of corneal swelling at low oxygen levels is less than might be expected. Corneal swelling at the 0.95 percent O_2 level (6.9 mm. Hg) varies among individuals between 2.4 percent and 7.3 percent. These limits are within the range commonly found clinically for both hard and soft contact lens patients,[6,77] and it suggests that many contact lens wearers may be exposed to very low oxygen levels.

Mandell et al. described the corneal swelling response to hard contact lenses as having essentially the same characteristics as were found at low oxygen levels.[61] They postulated that the stabilization or reversal of the swelling response was due to the cessation of tearing as adaptation occurred. This response could also be explained as due to corneal adaptation to low oxygen levels.

The question remains as to what level of oxygen tension is needed at the precorneal surface of a contact lens wearer to avoid interference with the normal corneal physiology. An oxygen tension as low as 7 mm. Hg may be tolerable for short time periods, even

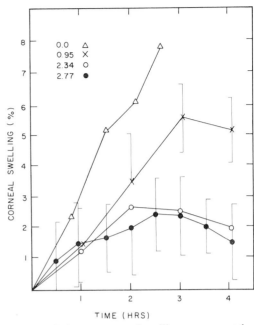

Figure 2.13. Average corneal swelling response at the three oxygen concentrations (0.95%, 2.34%, and 2.77% oxygen) and at the zero oxygen level (100% nitrogen).

though a level of about 35 mm. Hg might be necessary for longer periods. Consequently, significant differences may exist in the oxygen needs of an extended-wear contact lens patient as contrasted to a daily-wear patient. It must also be considered that the corneal oxygen requirement of the sleeping patient may be less than during the daytime.

Because of differences in their oxygen requirement some contact lens patients are basically more prone than others to corneal edema from contact lens wear.

NEUROLOGY

The corneal nerves are derived from the ciliary nerves (ophthalmic division of the trigeminal nerve), whose branches enter the sclera from the perichoroidal space behind the limbus. There are about seventy to eighty nerve bundles that penetrate at the posterior two-thirds of the cornea. Each bundle contains about twenty fibers, which vary in diameter from less than 1 to 4 μm. They proceed forward radially and divide dichotomously, gradually diminishing in size as they approach the anterior surface of the cornea. They penetrate Bowman's membrane and enter the epithelium. Rodger, in experiments on rab-

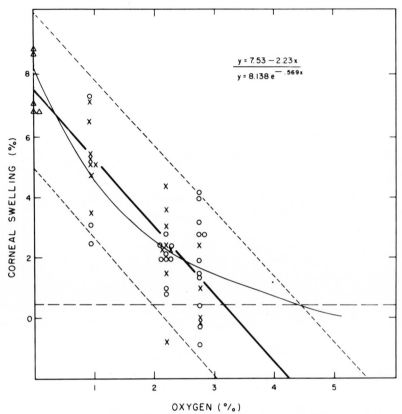

$$\frac{y = 7.53 - 2.23x}{y = 8.138\,e^{-.569x}}$$

Figure 2.14. Corneal swelling after four hours exposure to low oxygen levels. The linear regression line and confidence limits at two standard deviations are shown, together with the exponential regression line. The base line at 0.44 percent denotes average swelling in the control eyes. An X indicates one of two measurements at that same concentration for the same subject.

bits, found that the nerve fibers form networks at three levels, one within the stroma, occupying its whole width, one under Bowman's membrane, and one within the epithelium.[78] The nerve endings are most numerous in the epithelium. The nerve fibers have only free endings, and no specialized end organs are found (Figure 2.15).

The cornea is densely supplied with nerve fibers, having ten to fifty times as many fibers proportionately as the skin. Each nerve fiber may distribute its branches over as much as one-fourth of the corneal area so that there is considerable overlapping of the nerve supply. Because of this overlapping nerve distribution, the localization of corneal stimuli is relatively poor. It is only possible to tell whether a stimulus is up or down or temporal or nasal.

TESTING SENSIBILITY

Basic measurements of corneal sensibility date back to the researches of von Frey (1894), who used hairs of different calibers and lengths to stimulate the cornea. When a strand of hair is pressed against the cornea its elasticity produces a fairly constant force. The

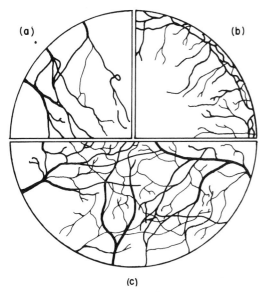

(a)

(b)

(c)

Figure 2.15. Innervation of the cornea. (*a*) Nerve bundles entering from the sclera; (*b*) episcleral pericorneal plexus; (c) plexiform arrangement in the stroma. Adapted from R. C. Rodger, The Pattern of the Corneal Innervation in Rabbits, *British Journal of Ophthalmology, 34(2)*:107–113, 1950.

force may be measured by pressing the hair against a scale. From his studies, von Frey concluded that the cornea possessed only the sense of pain, to which it was more sensitive than any other part of the body. Later investigators have differed in their opinion as to whether there exists tactile sensitivity in addition to pain sensitivity.

It has been difficult in the past to evaluate the different variables encountered in classifying the von Frey hairs. For clinical purposes it is frequently impractical to have a test battery of hairs of different values, for they can change with the moisture of the surrounding atmosphere. Boberg-Ans has designed an instrument (*corneal sensibilitometer*) to measure corneal sensitivity which has higher reliability.[79,80] It consists of a sleeve containing a single nylon thread 0.11 mm. in diameter, which may be extended to various lengths. When the length of the nylon thread is extended, it is more easily bent and exerts

less force. Thus, with a single nylon thread it is possible to provide the range of forces that are required for testing normal or pathological corneal sensitivity.

Corneal sensitivity is measured with the sensibilitometer by first touching the cornea with the thread fully extended. The thread is directed perpendicularly to the cornea and pressed with sufficient force to just cause a visible bend. If no sensation is reported, the thread is progressively shortened until a response is elicited. In this way it is possible to vary the force of the stimulus in a controlled manner from 10 mg. to 200 mg.

A modification of the Boberg-Ans apparatus has been introduced by Schirmer and Mellor.[81] They employ a double nylon thread, fused at each end, which feeds into a thin polyethylene tube. The length of the double thread may be altered; and in so doing, the force can be increased or decreased by the same principle used by Boberg-Ans. This method differs, however, in that the force exerted on the cornea can be controlled by watching the separation of the two threads rather than watching for the bend of a single thread.

An airstream has also been employed for evoking corneal response, although difficulties have arisen in attempting to measure small areas of the cornea.[80] With lowered corneal sensitivity it is necessary to employ high air pressure, which makes the airstream turbulent and interferes with the test.

A frequent method of testing corneal sensitivity is by means of a piece of finely twisted cotton in the form of a pointed brush. The cornea is lightly touched or stroked, and different painful sensations are evoked. This method only provides a *gross* measure of the presence or absence of sensation.

The most satisfactory clinical means at present of estimating corneal sensitivity is either the method of Schirmer and Mellor or the Boberg-Ans single nylon thread. It cannot be said, however, that these instruments are entirely satisfactory.

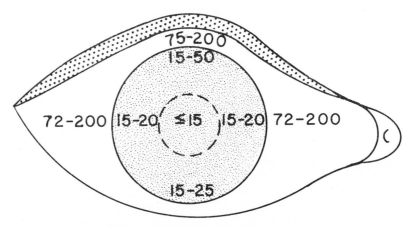

Figure 2.16. Normal sensitivity for different areas of the surface of the eye (mg.) Adapted from J. Boberg-Ans, Experience in Clinical Examination of Corneal Sensitivity, *British Journal of Ophthalmology*, *39(12)*:705–726, 1955.

SENSITIVITY

Touch and pain are both mediated by the bare nerve endings. Boberg-Ans found that the sensitivity of the central cornea for the eyes of normal young persons is 15 mg. or less (mg. referring to the force of the nylon thread). The sensitivity at the limbus is approximately 20 mg., and the conjunctiva varies between 72 and 200 mg. (Figure 2.16).

It was found that the horizontal meridian of the cornea is the most sensitive and that the temporal half appears to be more sensitive than the nasal half. The sensitivity corresponds with the density of the corneal nerve endings. It increases from the limbus to the central zone, at first very quickly obtaining a high value, and then increasing more slowly as the peak is reached.[82]

It has been shown that corneal sensitivity

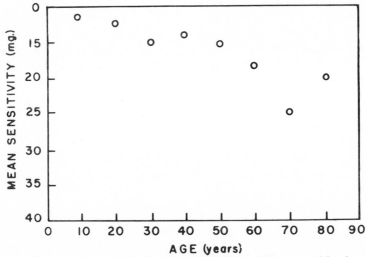

Figure 2.17. Mean corneal sensitivity by age groups, showing decrease with advancing years. Adapted from J. Boberg-Ans, Experience in Clinical Examination of Corneal Sensitivity, *British Journal of Ophthalmology*, *39(12)*:705–726, 1955.

decreases with age.[83] Boberg-Ans[79] found a high sensitivity during childhood (10 to 15 mg.) and a decrease with advancing years (25 to 39 mg.) (Figure 2.17).

CONTACT LENSES AND CORNEAL SENSITIVITY

Byron and Weseley,[84] using Frey hairs, reported a decrease in corneal sensitivity of their patients after four hours of contact lens wear. In a study by Boberg-Ans, corneal contact lenses worn by a group of patients were shown to produce a slight decrease in corneal sensitivity after one or two hours of wear, the average sensitivity falling from 25 to 72 mg.

Hamano tested corneal sensitivity on a small sample of prospective contact lens wearers and indicated that about 30 percent had high corneal sensitivity, 65 percent moderate sensitivity, and 5 percent low sensitivity.[85] His system of classification appears rather arbitrary, however. After the patients had worn contact lenses for a month, it was reported that they showed a general overall reduction in corneal sensitivity, but after twelve months of wear, sensitivity again approached normal.

Schirmer has developed a variation of the usual corneal sensitivity test for use with contact lens patients.[86] His "aesthesiometer" consists of a small plastic disc on the end of a wire, which is connected to a spring mechanism. The instrument is equipped with a scale from which readings may be obtained that can be converted into milligrams of force. Schirmer attempted to correlate the corneal sensitivity of fifty-six new contact lens patients with their success in wearing the lens with comfort. He concluded that prediction of contact lens tolerance appears possible from the measurements of corneal sensitivity.

Although the research that has been completed shows some relation between corneal sensitivity and ability to wear contact lenses, the results are far from conclusive. The ability to wear contact lenses depends upon a multitude of factors that have not been adequately controlled during most studies of corneal sensitivity. It is obvious that much additional information about corneal sensitivity is needed, and this may prove of considerable value in the prognosis of successful wearing of contact lenses.

From our present knowledge, corneal hypersensitivity cannot be considered a definite contraindication for the fitting of contact lenses. It is not even known, for example, that the person who is hypersensitive before he wears contact lenses continues to be hypersensitive after contact lenses are worn for a period of time. A contact lens patient with reduced corneal sensitivity, however, definitely needs closer observation than the normal patient to make certain that undetected abrasions do not occur.

Polse found that measurements of corneal touch threshold are not a useful indicator of disturbed corneal physiology.[87] However, sensitivity measurements may provide a useful guide to the process of adapting to contact lenses. During the adaptive process, there was a slow but steady decrease in corneal sensitivity over a two to three week period. Once the corneal touch threshold had increased approximately 100 percent, no further changes were noted.

Polse found that corneal swelling resulting from exposing the cornea to either an oxygen-free environment or a hypotonic solution does not change corneal sensitivity.[87] It was possible, however, to decrease corneal sensitivity by having these same subjects wear contact lenses. During daytime contact lens wear, the corneal touch threshold increased whether or not significant amounts of corneal swelling occurred. It was possible to alter corneal sensitivity during contact lens wearing without causing significant corneal swelling. Since sensitivity decreases are related to the time the lens is on, it seems that the change in corneal touch threshold accompanying contact lens wearing is not caused by metabolic disturbance to the cornea but rather by sensory adaptation as a consequence of continuous mechanical stimulation.

TEMPERATURE SENSATION

It is generally believed that heat receptors are absent from the cornea.[88] Lele and Wedell, however, do not agree and have shown that action potentials are evoked in the corneal nerves by the application of thermal stimuli.[89,90] In fact, it was found that the four primary modalities of common sensibility (touch, warmth, cold, and pain) were always evoked if the cornea was suitably stimulated. Kenshalo more recently has found that changes of the temperature of a solid body applied to the cornea were described by subjects as irritations rather than as warmth.[91] In comparison with the skin of the lip, forehead, and conjunctiva, the temperature had to be increased greatly before any sensation was experienced. He concluded that true heat sensations were not evoked, although the free endings in the cornea were sensitive to thermal sensation.

Krause's end-bulbs, thought to be specialized cold receptors, are found abundantly in the conjunctiva and limbus but not in the central cornea; however, there is some evidence that cold sensation is actually partly or wholly due to free nerve ending stimulation.[92] As with the pain sensation, sensations of cold are more acute in the horizontal meridian.

CORNEAL TEMPERATURE

The temperature of the cornea is relatively low compared to the rest of the eye or body. It is lowest at the corneal apex (92°F) and highest beneath the upper eyelid. The limbus is normally warmer than the cornea, due to its greater vascularity.

Occasionally, after a patient wears his contact lenses for a period of time he reports that they feel hot. This symptom appears to be associated with a lens that does not allow a proper tear circulation between the lens and cornea. Whether the heat sensation is actually correlated with a rise in the corneal temperature is doubtful.[93] It has often been *presumed* that, since a plastic contact lens could act as an insulator, it tends to raise the temperature of the cornea. Yet, Hill and Leighton have found an insignificant difference in the central corneal temperature before and after a corneal contact lens was worn on rabbits, providing that the lids remained open.[94] With lid closure, however, the temperature could be made to rise more than 6°F. This is illustrated in Figure 2.18, where the corneal temperature has been monitored during various closures of the lids. First shown is the initial temperature response of the cornea after insertion of the lens. There occurred a blepharospasm, which was followed by a slow period of relaxation of the lids and an opening of the fissure. A temperature rise accompanied the period of blepharospasm. Other temperature rises accompanied periods in which there were natural blinks and forced blinks. Figure 2.18 also gives the sizes of the palpebral aperture at all times so that they may be compared directly with the corneal temperatures that were present at the same times. These data may be used to illustrate the relationship between palpebral aperture size and corneal temperature for all lid positions (Figure 2.19). In general, the corneal temperature becomes lower for an increase in the lid aperture until a critical point of 7 mm. is reached; beyond this there is little further decrease in temperature.

Comparable data on corneal temperature for human subjects were obtained by Hill and Leighton (Figure 2.20).[94] The consequence of the increased temperature is an increase in corneal metabolism and consequent increased demand for oxygen (Figure 2.21).[95] This may

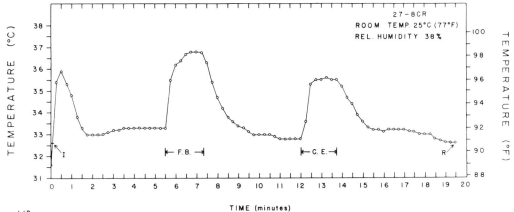

Figure 2.18. Complete time course of a corneal lens temperature experiment. (*I*) the insertion, (*FB*) the period during which the lids were kept forcibly closed by the animal, (*CE*) the period of natural lid closure, and (*R*) removal of the lens. Associated vertical lid apertures are shown below. From R. M. Hill and A. J. Leighton, Physiological Time Courses Associated with Contact Lenses—Temperature: 2. Animal Time Courses with Corneal Lenses, *American Journal of Optometry*, 41(1):3–9, 1964.

be clinically relevant when the lens-tear pump mechanism is performing marginally already and a poorly adapted contact lens wearer adopts an abnormal squinting lid posture. It may also present a challenge in the fitting of extended-wear contact lenses.

Hill and Leighton had the added advantage of receiving subjective reports in connection with the temperature changes.[94] They found that no subjective sensation of heat was reported when corneal temperature was elevated. This result is as expected and concurs with the results Kenshalo obtained when he compared the corneal sensitivity to heat with the sensitivity of the conjunctiva, forehead, and upper lip.[91] It may be noted from Figure 2.20 that normally the cornea that

bears a contact lens never reaches the temperature (108°F) which is required to evoke any thermal sensation on the basis of the results by Kenshalo.

What, then, causes the sensation of heat that sometimes accompanies contact lens wear? It is probable that the fit of the contact lens interferes with tear exchange behind the contact lens and affects corneal metabolism. This disturbance produces conjunctival hyperemia, thus raising the temperature in the adjacent sclera, which unquestionably is supplied with heat receptors. Patients are in many instances unable to specifically locate a sensation, and it would be natural for them to refer to the heat sensation as coming from the cornea, whether it actually does or not.

TEARS

SUPPLY

Tears are the mixture of the products from two sets of glands: (1) primary glands, which consist of the main lacrimal gland and about fifty small accessory lacrimal glands of

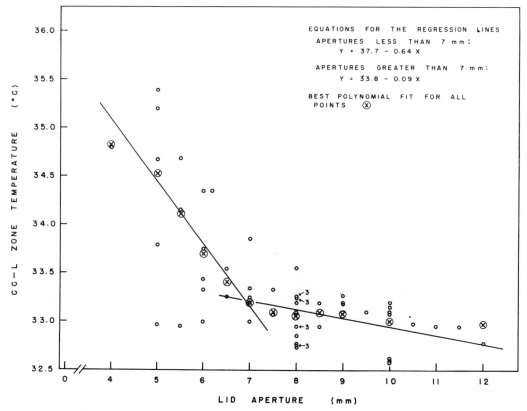

Figure 2.19. The lid aperture-temperature relationship for data of Figure 2.18. From R. M. Hill and A. J. Leighton, Physiological Time Courses Associated with Contact Lenses—Temperature: 2. Animal Time Courses with Corneal Lenses, *American Journal of Optometry*, 41(*1*):3–9, 1964.

Krause and Wolfring in the lids, and (2) secondary glands, which consist of the mucin-secreting goblet cells of the conjunctiva, the oil-secreting tarsal glands, and the glands of Zeis at the margin of the lids. The accessory and secondary lacrimal glands furnish the basic supply of the tear fluid. The main lacrimal gland is primarily an emergency organ, which reacts to emotion and sudden changes in the physical environment of the organism. The complete tear fluid is considered as the product of the lacrimal gland, the accessory lacrimal glands, the meibomian glands, and the mucous glands of the conjunctiva. Strictly speaking, the lacrimal fluid is the fluid secretion of the lacrimal gland without the admixture of the secretions of the other glands of the conjunctiva.

CONTENT

The normal tears contain about 1.8 percent dissolved solids with an osmotic pressure equivalent to a salt solution of 0.91 percent (actual sodium chloride content 0.65%). The chemical composition of the tears is very similar to that of blood plasma; the main exception is that it is slightly more dilute (98.2% water) and that the protein content is much smaller (albumin 0.4%, globulin 0.27%). The pH of the normal tears fluctuates significantly throughout the day (Figure 2.22).

Samples of tears taken from the eyes of

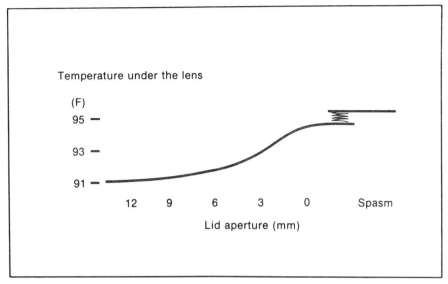

Figure 2.20. The increase in tear-cornea temperature under a contact lens as the lid is gradually closed and during blepharospasm. From R. M. Hill, How the Cornea "Takes the Heat," *International Contact Lens Clinic*, 5(6):65–67, 1978.

contact lens wearers both before and after fitting (Figure 2.23) reveal much about the impact of the lens upon the eye. The changes in tear sodium content during adaptation to a hard lens (Figure 2.24) reflect the increased reflex tearing caused by lid sensation and the return to normal as adaptation occurs. This effect has, of course, also been demonstrated for chloride ions and has been demonstrated to correlate well with the presence or absence

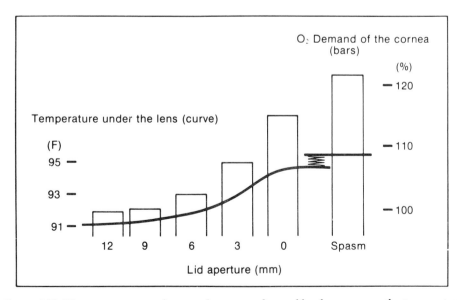

Figure 2.21. The commensurate increase in oxygen demand by the cornea as the temperature under a contact lens increases. From R. M. Hill, How the Cornea "Takes the Heat," *International Contact Lens Clinic*, 5(6):65–67, 1978.

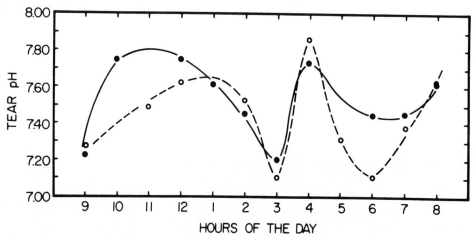

Figure 2.22. The tear pH values of a patient (a non–contact lens wearer) who was monitored throughout his waking hours on two different days. From R. M. Hill, The Physiology of Soft Lens Systems, in M. Ruben (Ed.), Soft Contact Lenses, 1978. Courtesy of John Wiley & Sons, Inc., New York, New York.

of edema.[96] For example, a hard lens wearer, during the initial adaptation period, manifested a fall in chloride concentration paralleling corneal swelling. After the first week, the tears became slightly chloride rich, and edema was absent (Figure 2.25). In contrast, a soft lens wearer showed no appreciable change in tear chloride content (Figure 2.26). Finally, tear protein concentrations (Figure 2.27), as well as glucose and cholesterol concentrations, have been shown to undergo the same drop and slow recovery to normal during adaptation to a hard contact lens. Callender and Morrison hypothesize that the change in all of the preceding solute concentrations contributes to the edema of initial hard contact lens adaptation by lowering the osmotic pressure of the tear fluid.[97]

An excess of albumin and globulin in the tears, in comparison with the corneal tissue fluid, produces a considerably lower surface tension, thus enabling the tears to spread easily and wet the epithelial surface. In addition, the tears cover microscopic irregularities of the epithelial surface and produce a smooth surface on the cornea.[98] The protein components of tears are conjugated with highly hydrated polysaccharides and have

good wetting properties on methyl methacrylate resin. Consequently, a contact lens will remain wet while in the eye, unless the surface of the lens has become hydrophobic by oily secretions deposited on the lens.[99]

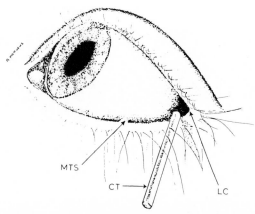

Figure 2.23. Lateral view of a patient's eye showing the collection of tear samples with a capillary tube (*CT*), from the inferior marginal tear strip (*MTS*) at the lateral canthus (*LC*). From M. Callender and P. E. Morrison, A Quantitative Study of Human Tear Proteins Before and After Adaptation to Non-flexible Contact Lenses, *American Journal of Optometry and Physiological Optics*, 51(12): 939–945, 1974.

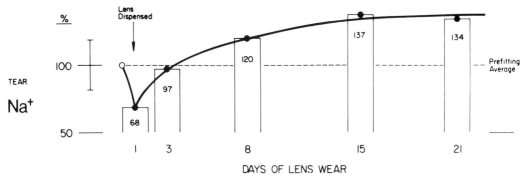

Figure 2.24. The tear sodium concentrations (smoothed function) of a new hard contact lens wearer. The value of 100 percent represents his prefitted mean. From R. M. Hill, The Physiology of Soft Lens Systems, in M. Ruben (Ed.), *Soft Contact Lenses*, 1978. Courtesy of John Wiley & Sons, Inc., New York, New York.

The constituency of the tear fluid varies in different locations, and it is given various names. The precorneal film is the layer of tear fluid about 5 to 12 μm thick that covers the cornea and which, at the corneal limbus, is continuous with the conjunctival fluid. The pre-

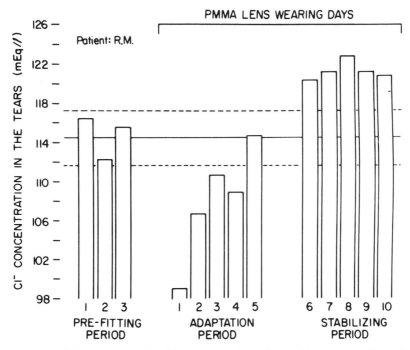

Figure 2.25. The daily mean tear chloride concentrations of a hard lens patient throughout his prefitting, initial adaptation, and stabilizing periods. The mean and standard deviation found for the total prefitting period are extended across the entire graph for comparison with the other two periods. From R. M. Hill, The Physiology of Soft Lens Systems, in M. Ruben (Ed.), *Soft Contact Lenses*, 1978. Courtesy of John Wiley & Sons, Inc., New York, New York.

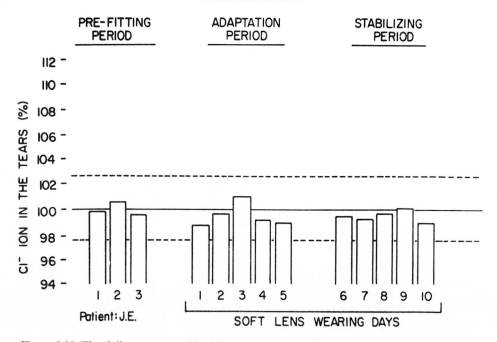

Figure 2.26. The daily mean tear chloride concentrations of a soft lens wearer throughout her prefitting, initial adaptation and stabilizing periods. The mean and standard deviation found for the total prefitting period are extended across the entire graph for comparison with the other two periods (100% = 121 mEq/liter). From R. M. Hill, The Physiology of Soft Lens Systems, in M. Ruben (Ed.), *Soft Contact Lenses*, 1978. Courtesy of John Wiley & Sons, Inc., New York, New York.

corneal film is composed of a mucoid layer, an intermediate watery (lacrimal fluid) layer, and an oily (sebaceous) layer on the surface (Figure 2.28).[100] These three layers are derived from the bulbar conjunctiva, where goblet cells produce the mucous secretion; the accessory lacrimal glands, which contribute the lacrimal layer; and the meibomian glands, situated at the tarsus, which produce the sebaceous layer.

There is evidence that the corneal epithelium has no goblet cells, and mucus cannot be found histochemically in any of the surface epithelium. The normal conjunctiva has many goblet cells, and most likely the mucous material comes from this source and is rubbed onto the corneal surface by the tarsal conjunctiva during the blink.[101] The importance of the mucous component of the tears has been made evident in several studies and has been found to play an essential

role in wetting the corneal surface.[101-103] If the mucus is experimentally removed from the epithelium, it is found that the cornea becomes hydrophobic (Figure 2.29). This principle may play an important role in the formation of dry spots (Figure 2.30).

The sebum is present on the lid margins and contributes towards producing the foam sometimes seen when a contact lens is worn. The sebaceous layer forms a protective film over the cornea and reduces tear evaporation to about 10 percent of what it would be without this layer.[92,104] Were the sebaceous layer not present, the cornea might dry between blinks. Even if the film were to almost completely evaporate, there would remain a thin mucoid layer adhering to the epithelium.[105]

The precorneal film is frequently replaced. It is essential that this medium be kept clear and uncontaminated to maintain its function

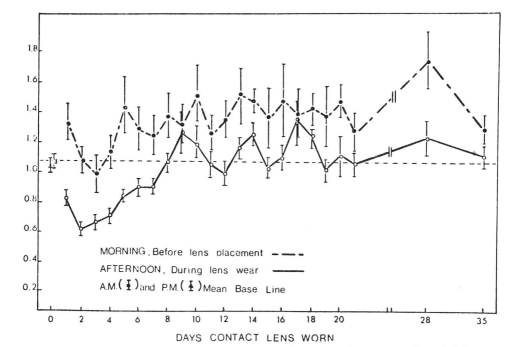

Figure 2.27. Graphical representation of the mean total tear protein concentration of eight subjects measured during the first 35 days of lens wear. From M. Callender and P. E. Morrison, A Quantitative Study of Human Tear Proteins before and after Adaptation to Non-flexible Contact Lenses, *American Journal of Optometry and Physiological Optics,* 5(12):939–945, 1974.

of providing a stable, transparent, viscous film with high wetting properties and a smooth surface to the epithelium. The normal tear volume is estimated at about 6 μl, and the average rate of turnover at about 1.2 μl per minute.[106,107]

The precorneal film usually contains very few cells, including desquamated cells from the cornea and conjunctiva, lymphocytes, and polymorphonuclear leukocytes.[92,108]

The normal bacterial flora of the tear fluid secretions is controlled by lysozyme in the tears, which, in normal physiological concentrations, can kill the common bacteria (staph., strep., etc.). Lysozyme is mycolytic and dissolves the bacterial membrane. The tear film also contains many immunoglobulins, which are thought to play an important role in the corneal defense mechanism.

TEAR TESTING

Tear Film Breakup

The precorneal film has all the characteristics of what is known in physics as a thin film. This means that the cohesive nature of the fluid and the adhesive forces to the body on which it stands (cornea) are greater than the gravitational force pulling the film down so the film remains in a static position until evaporation causes it to be disrupted.

Under certain conditions, the tear film is abnormal and becomes susceptible to drying.[109] When the lids are open, water evaporates

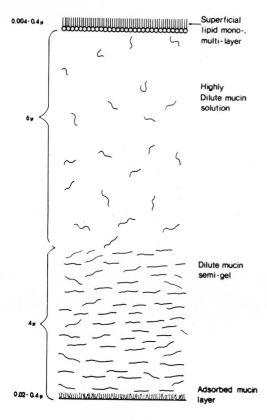

Figure 2.28. Layers of the precorneal film. From M. A. Lemp et al., The Precorneal Tear Film: 1. Factors in Spreading and Maintaining a Continuous Tear Film over the Corneal Surface, *Archives of Ophthalmology*, *83*(1):89–94, 1970.

from the tear film, and dry spots occur at various points on the cornea. This tear film *breakup time* (B.U.T.) may be used as an index of an abnormal tear formation. It is accentuated under pathological conditions, but occurs in nearly all patients under the following conditions:

If the eye is held open voluntarily so that no blinking occurs, it is usually found that in ten to thirty seconds, the tear film shows dry spots (Figure 2.31). The time at which the spots appear can be reduced by holding the lids apart (Figure 2.32).[110-112] The exact significance of the breakup time is not known.

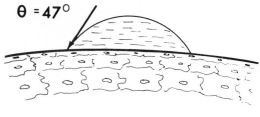

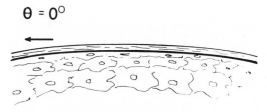

Figure 2.29. If the mucus is removed from the epithelium, it becomes hydrophobic. From M. A. Lemp et al., The Precorneal Tear Film: 1. Factors in Spreading and Maintaining a Continuous Tear Film over the Corneal Surface, *Archives of Ophthalmology*, *83*(1):89–94, 1970.

It is known, however, that when the cornea is suffering from localized pathology, a dry spot will occur in that area (Figure 2.33). For example, following an abrasion, it is found that the cornea soon heals and appears normal by means of the fluorescein stain. Careful observation of the tear layer will show, however, that a dry hole appears over the area of the abrasion in an abnormally short time. Any dry spot that occurs in less than ten seconds is probably pathological.[113] Hence, this technique can be used to detect improperly or incompletely healed abrasions and is the only diagnostic objective test of recurrent corneal erosion.

The test is performed simply by placing a drop of fluorescein in the eye and having the patient voluntarily keep the lids open. Some practice may be necessary to accomplish this. The patient is seated at the slit lamp, and the slit beam is widened to 2 to 3 mm. The black light is used, and the slit is scanned back and forth across the cornea.

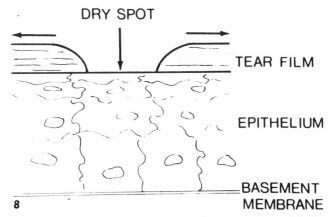

Figure 2.30. Formation of a dry spot due to absence of mucus on the epithelium. From M. A. Lemp et al., The Precorneal Tear Film: 1. Factors in Spreading and Maintaining a Continuous Tear Film over the Corneal Surface, *Archives of Ophthalmology, 83(1)*:89–94, 1970.

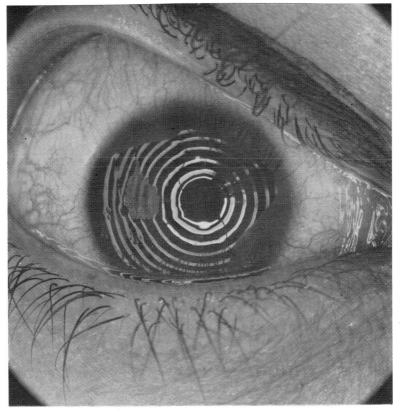

Figure 2.31. Dry spots on the cornea.

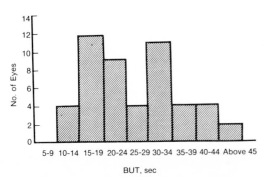

Figure 2.32a. Tear film breakup time (B.U.T.) in normal subjects varies between ten and forty-five seconds. From M. A. Lemp and J. R. Hamill, Jr., Factors Affecting Tear Film Break Up in Normal Eyes, *Archives of Ophthalmology*, 89(2):103–105, 1973.

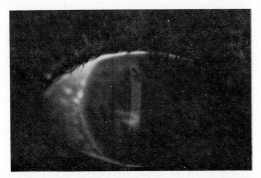

Figure 2.32b. Appearance of dry spots on the cornea with fluorescein and biomicroscope.

Schirmer Test

The most commonly used clinical test for evaluating the rate of tear flow is the Schirmer test. It gives an indication of either hypersecretion or hyposecretion of tears.

A filter paper 5 by 35 mm. long with the upper 5 mm. folded over is placed in the lower conjunctival fornix at a position one-third the horizontal length of the lid from the outer canthus. The normal tear secretion moistens 15 mm. of the strip (from the lid margin) in five minutes. The moistened paper is measured with a millimeter rule.

Since the Schirmer test was first introduced in the early part of the century, various types of blotter paper and modifications have been adopted.[85,114] The basic test procedure, however, remains the same.

Care must be taken that the lid is not disturbed before Schirmer's test is given. The biomicroscope examination, for example, should be performed after the Schirmer test. Care should also be taken when inserting the filter paper that it does not touch the cornea, otherwise the test has no value. The patient will experience pain, and reflex lacrimation will result.

Some normal variation in the results of the Schirmer test is expected. Henderson and Prough used a modified version of Schirmer's test in a study of 231 patients and found that the majority showed a difference of 3 mm. or less in the flow of tears from their two eyes.[114] Between the ages of fifteen and twenty-nine years, females exhibited a greater tear flow than males. Henderson and Prough also found that decrease in tear flow was in general parallel to increase in age. De Roeth, in studies on tears in 827 persons, concluded that tear production decreases with age, the fall being greatest between twenty and fifty, and that in all age groups, except for the thirty to thirty-nine year old group, females produced more tears.

FUNCTION OF THE EYELID

The eyelids apparently play a multiple role in meeting many needs of the eye. Some of the functions that have been suggested are the following: (1) protecting the eye from the entrance of foreign particles, (2) removing foreign matter, (3) pumping the lacrimal sac, (4) blocking the light during sleep, (5) supplying protection against trauma, (6) distributing the tear layer over the cornea.

The latter reason has not been particu-

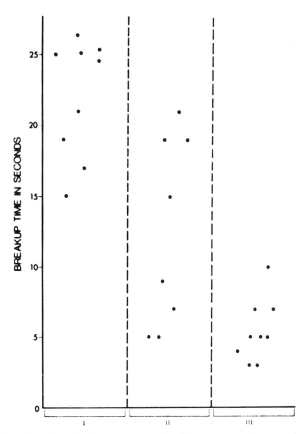

Figure 2.33. Breakup time for three groups of subjects: group 1, normal; group 2, low mucin; group 3, pathological dry eyes. From M. A. Lemp et al., The Precorneal Tear Film: 1. Factors in Spreading and Maintaining a Continuous Tear Film over the Corneal Surface, *Archives of Ophthalmology, 83(1)*:89–94, 1970.

larly emphasized and is probably the most important function of the eyelid. As the tears are produced, they collect in a meniscus that forms along the lid margins. This meniscus is prevented from spilling over the lid margin by the secretions of the meibomian glands. As the eyes are closed, the lid acts as a wiper and distributes a perfectly uniform layer of precorneal tear fluid. Once the fluid is deposited on the corneal surface, the cohesive forces hold it in place, and virtually no movement occurs. Due to evaporation and external contaminants, however, the film will be disrupted in fifteen or twenty seconds on the eye. Hence, a periodic system of renewal is necessary to insure continuous stability of the tear film.

Obviously, this system would not function efficiently if the blink rate were of the order of twenty to twenty-five seconds. In this case, the subject would experience some intermittent blurring, which would disrupt the efficiency of the system. Therefore, it is expected teleologically that the blink rate would be significantly shorter than this blur period. A rate of one blink every three to six seconds would adequately serve this purpose. If the blink rate were faster than this—say, every second—it would serve no functional purpose in the formation of the tear layer. It would exert an unnecessary effort on the muscles of the lid, and it could be noticeable to vision.

It should be noted that in many animals, particularly the rabbit, the blink is very infrequent, perhaps occurring only every few minutes. It is found in these animals that the tear layer is very irregular and undoubtedly interferes somewhat with vision.

BLINKING

Blinking plays an essential role in the ability of the eye to accept a contact lens. With the blink, the contact lens acts as a pump, interchanging the tears behind the lens and bringing fresh supplies of oxygen and nutrients to the cornea. Because of the importance of blinking, it is valuable to spend some time reviewing the anatomy of the eyelids.

The eyelids are controlled by two main sets of muscles. In the superior lid, the levator palpebrae superioris is the primary muscle that elevates the lid. This muscle starts at the back of the orbit near the small wing of the sphenoid. It has a tendinous origin and passes over the superior rectus, where the sheaths are fused. The belly of the muscle lies over the superior rectus. The tendon of the muscle fans out to form a large aponeurosis for the attachment to the lid. The fibers insert in front of the tarsus and into the skin of the lid. A few of the fibers go to the fornix of the conjunctiva.

Opposing this muscle is the main muscle that is used for eye closure, the *orbicularis oculus*. This muscle has its origin in the medical palpebral ligament and makes a complete sweep around the eye. It is divided into two portions—an orbital, or non-lid, portion, which is not used unless the eyes are forcibly closed, and a palpebral portion. The palpebral portion is in the third layer of the lid. It originates from the medial palpebral ligament and inserts in the lateral raphe. This muscle is used for the ordinary closure of the lid during blinking. It has two other parts: (1) Horner's muscle, or the lacrimal portion of the muscle, has its origin at the upper portion of the posterior lacrimal crest and may affect the drainage of the lacrimal sac by exerting pressure on the canaliculus and the lacrimal sac. (2) Riolan's muscle is the portion right behind the cilia follicles. This part of the muscle has the finest fibers, which are located on either side of the meibomian ducts in the lid margin. It insures good closure of the lid and keeps the margins close to the eye.

Blinking may be defined simply as a rapid closure of the eyelid. It occurs in a voluntary and involuntary form. The involuntary form is normally divided into two types, the spontaneous blink that occurs at regular periodic intervals of unknown origin and the reflex blink that is a response to various external stimuli.

The voluntary blink has the following characteristics: Both the upper and lower lids move together to close the palpebral fissure. The upper lid movement is predominantly downward but is somewhat nasal. The lower lid movement has a primary nasal direction due to the attachment of the muscle at the medial palpebral ligament. This lateral movement of the lower lid is difficult to see, except in high speed moving pictures.

The involuntary blink is similar to the voluntary blink except that quite often the closure is incomplete. These incomplete blinks occur in nearly all subjects, but their frequency is much greater for some people. The average rate of blinking is about twelve times per minute, or once every four to five seconds. Many contact lens wearers modify their blinking characteristics and begin to have incomplete blinks as a regular phenomenon. This usually leads to interference with the normal corneal physiology.

The total blink period takes from about 0.2 to 0.3 seconds, but the actual time that the lid is covering the pupil and blocking light from the retina is about 0.13 seconds. Normally this time is so short that the person is unaware that a blink has had any effect on his vision.

Sleep abolishes the involuntary blink, but resting with the eyes closed does not. Careful observation of the subject will show that there is a periodic twitching of the lid corresponding to the blink rate.

Each blink is normally accompanied by some movement of the eyes (Bell's phenomenon) (Figure 2.34).[115] The normal movement is considered up and temporal, but it has been shown that the movement occurs in many different directions for different individuals.

BELL'S PHENOMENON

The association of Bell's phenomenon with the functional success of contact lens wearing has been reported by Stewart,[116117] Mackie,[118] and Korb et al.[119]

Korb et al. evaluated 200 subjects under the age of fifty, using the following technique: With the patient's head in the primary position, fixation is directed to optical infinity. The observer, resting one hand on the patient's forehead, holds the upper lid with the thumb. The index finger of the other hand is used to depress the lower lid. With the lids thus immobilized the patient is then asked to close both eyes. The observer, positioned with his eye level slightly below that of the patient's, then observes the movement of the exposed eye. It is of particular importance in this technique to minimize the pressure required to control the upper lid during observation of the eye movements.

The most difficult problem is conveying to the patient the type of closure desired. If the concept of a slow, smooth closure such as occurs while falling asleep is not understood by the patient, the patient may look down while closing the lids. The eyes will then move down and the results will not be reliable.

Bell's phenomenon has a temporal oblique component associated with the upward move-

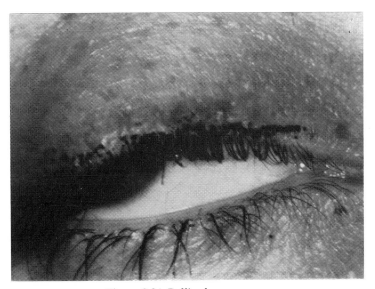

Figure 2.34. Bell's phenomenon.

ment in approximately two-thirds of all the eyes studied and a nasal component with approximately 20 percent.[112] A straight vertical movement was exhibited by 8 percent of the eyes with no oblique component present. A lateral or downward movement was only present in 3 percent of 185 subjects, while 7 percent demonstrated unreliable or inconsistent movements that did not lend themselves to classification. Approximately 90 percent of all eyes demonstrate a significant oblique component of 15 degrees or more associated with the upward movement.

When considering the eyes of each subject as a pair, the excursions are in the expected upward and temporal direction with relative symmetry for approximately 40 percent of all subjects.[112] Approximately 30 percent of all subjects demonstrate conjugate excursions where one eye moves temporally and vertically, while the other eye moves nasally and vertically.

REFERENCES

1. Teng, C. C., and Katzin, H. M.: The basement membrane of corneal epithelium, *Am. J. Ophthalmol.*, *36*(*7*):895–900, 1953.
2. Akus, M. A.: Ocular fine structure. Selected electron micrographs, London, Churchill, 1964.
3. Blümcke, S., and Morgenroth, K., Jr.: The stereo ultrastructure of the external and internal surface of the cornea, *Arch. Ophthalmol.*, *57*:11, 1967.
4. Jakus, M. A.: The fine structure of the human cornea, in Smelser, G. K. (Ed.): *The Structure of the Eye*, New York and London, Academic, 1961.
5. Blümcke, S., and Morgenroth, K., Jr.: The stereo ultrastructure of the external and internal surface of the cornea, *J. Ultrastruct. Res.*, *18*:502, 1967.
6. Beitch, I.: The induction of keratinization in the corneal epithelium, *Invest. Ophthalmol.*, *9*(*11*):827–843, 1970.
7. Pedler, C.: The fine structure of the corneal epithelium, *Exp. Eye Res.*, *1*(*3*):286–289, 1962.
8. Liegl, O.: Die funktionelle bedeutung der zellkontakte im hornhautepithel, *Ophthalmologica*, *157*(*5*):362–373, 1969.
9. Liegl, O.: Elektronenmikroskopische untersuchungen über die fluoresceinbarriere am intakten hornhautepithel, `Dtsch. Ophthalmol. Ges. Ber.*, *68*:220, 1968.
10. Jakus, M. A.: Further observations on the fine structure of the cornea, *Invest. Ophthalmol.*, *1*(*2*):202–225, 1962.
11. Hanna, C., and O'Brien, J. E.: Cell production and migration in the epithelial layer of the cornea, *Arch. Ophthalmol.*, *64*(*4*):536–539, 1960.
12. Teng, C. C.: Electron microscope study of the pathology of keratoconus, *Am. J. Ophthalmol.*, *55*(*1*):18–47, 1963.
13. Thomas, C. I.: *The Cornea*, Springfield, Thomas, 1955.
14. Cochet, P. et al., Fragilité mécanique et adaptation des verres de contact, *Soc. Ophthalmol. Ouest de la France Nantes*, Oct. 8, 1961, *C. R. Bull. Soc. Ophthalmol. Fr.*, *9*(*10*):810–814, 1961.
15. Offret, G., and Haye, C.: La membrane basale de l'épithélium cornéen. Étude histopathologique, *Arch. Ophthalmol. (Paris)*, *19*(*2*):126–159, 1959.
16. Khodadoust, A. A. et al.: Adhesion of regenerating corneal epithelium, *Am. J. Ophthalmol.*, *65*(*3*):339–348, 1968.
17. Blümcke, J. R., and Niedorf, H. R.: Formation of the basement membrane during regeneration of the corneal epithelium, *Z. Zellforsch. Mikrosk. Anat.*, *93*:84, 1969.
18. Varga, M.: The significance of the basal membrane in the regeneration of the corneal epithelium, *abstract Curr. Ophthalmol.*, *17*(*4*):229–300, 1973.
19. Goldman, F. N., Dohlman, C. H., and Kravitt, B.: The basement membrane in recurrent epithelial erosion, *Trans. Am. Acad. Ophthalmol. Otolaryngol.*, *73*(*3*):471–481, 1969.

20. Maurice, D. M.: The cornea and sclera, in Dauson, H. (Ed.): *The Eye*, New York, Academic, 1962, vol. 1, pp. 289–236.

21. Hale, P. N., and Maurice, D. M.: Sugar transport across the corneal endothelium, *Exp. Eye Res.*, 8(2):205–215, 1969.

22. Cogan, D. G.: Applied anatomy and physiology of the cornea, *Trans. Am. Acad. Ophthalmol. Otolaryngol.*, March–April, 329–359, 1951.

23. Maurice, D. M.: Clinical physiology of the cornea, *Int. Ophthalmol. Clin.*, 2(3):561–572, 1962.

24. Duke-Elder, S., and Wybar, K. C.: *System of Ophthalmololgy*, St. Louis, Mosby, vol. 2, *The Anatomy of the Visual System*, 1961, p. 114.

25. Neill, J. C.: Contact lens haze, *Am. J. Optom.*, 25(10):461–479, 1948.

26. Ascher, K. W.: Aqueous veins and contact lenses, *Am. J. Ophthalmol.*, 35(5) Part 2: 10–20, 1952.

27. von Bahr, G.: Corneal thickness: Its measurement and changes, *Am. J. Ophthalmol.*,42(2):251–266, 1956.

28. Mandell, R. B., and Polse, K. A.: Keratoconus: spatial variation of corneal thickness as a diagnostic test, *Arch. Ophthalmol.*, 82(2): 182–188, 1969.

29. Maurice, D. M., and Giardini, A. A.: Swelling of the cornea *in vivo* after the destruction of its limiting layers, *Br. J. Ophthalmol.*, 35(12):791–797, 1951.

30. Maurice, D. M.: The structure and transparency of the cornea, *J. Physiol. (Lond.)*, 136(2):263–286, 1957.

31. Francois, J., and Rabaey, M.: The anatomy of the cornea, in Duke-Elder, S., and Perkins, E. S. (Eds.): *The Transparency of the Cornea: A Symposium*, Springfield, Thomas, 1960, pp. 7–15.

32. Potts, A. M.: Some aspects of the interrelation between corneal hydration and corneal transparency, *Invest. Ophthalmol.*, 1(2):163–169, 1962.

33. Schwarz, W., and Keyserlingk, D. G.: Über die feinstruktur der menschlichen cornea, mit besonderer berucksichtigung des problems der transparenz, *Z. Zellforsch. Mikrosk. Anat.*, 7:540, 1966.

34. Goldman, J. N. et al.: Structural alterations affecting transparency in swollen human corneas, *Invest. Ophthalmol.*, 7(5):501–519, 1968.

35. Goldman, J. N., and Benedek, G. B.: The relationship between morphology and transparency in the nonswelling corneal stroma of the shark, *Invest. Ophthalmol.*, 6(6):574–600, 1967.

36. Casperson, T., and Engstrom, A.: Corneal transparency, *Nord. Med.*, 30:1279, 1946 (cited by Potts, *see* reference 32).

37. Davson, H.: *The Physiology of the Eye*, Philadelphia, Blakiston, 1949, pp. 46–48.

38. Cogan, D. G., and Kinsey, V. E.: The cornea v. physiologic aspects, *Arch. Ophthalmol.*, 28(4):661–669, 1942.

39. Mishima, S., and Maurice, B. M.: The effect of normal evaporation on the eye, *Exp. Eye Res.*, 1(1):46–52, 1961.

40. Farris, R. L., Kubota, Z., and Mishima, S.: Epithelial decompensation with corneal contact lens wear, *Arch. Ophthalmol.*, 85(6): 651–660, 1971.

41. Chan, R. S., and Mandell, R. B.: Corneal hydration changes caused by bathing the eye with solutions of different tonicities, in press.

42. Chan, R., and Mandell, R. B.: Corneal swelling caused by *allium cepa*, *Am. J. Optom.*, 49(9):713–715, 1972.

43. Mandell, R. B., and Harris, M.: Theory of the contact lens adaptation process, *J. Am. Optom. Assoc.*, 39(3):260–261, 1968.

44. Mishima, S.: Some physiological aspects of the precorneal tear film, *Arch. Ophthalmol.*,73(2):233–241, 1965.

45. Mandell, R. B., and Fatt, I.: Thinning of the human cornea on awakening, *Nature (Lond.)*,208(5007):292–293, 1965.

46. Mertz, G. W.: Overnight swelling of the living human cornea. *J. Am. Optom. Assoc.*, 51 (3):211–212, 1980.

47. Mishima, S., Kubota, Z., and Farris, R. L.: Tear flow dynamics in normal and keratoconjunctivitis sicca cases, *XXI Concilium Ophthal. Acta*, part 2, 1801, 1970.

48. Hill, R. M., and Uniacke, N. P.: Tear chemistry of a new contact lens wearer, *J. Am. Optom. Assoc.*, 40(3):294–296, 1969.

49. Lowther, G. E., Miller, R. B., and Hill, R. M.: Tear concentrations of sodium and potassium during adaptation to contact lenses, 1. Sodium Concentrations, *Am. J. Optom.*, 47(4):266–275, 1970.

50. Uniacke, N. P., and Hill, R. M.: Osmotic pressure of the tears during adaptation to contact lenses, *J. Am. Optom. Assoc.*, 41(11):932–936, 1970.

51. Harris, J. E.: The physiologic control of corneal hydration, *Am. J. Ophthalmol.*, 44(5):262–280, 1957.

52. Harris, J. E.: Factors influencing corneal hydration, *Invest. Ophthalmol.*, 1(2):151–157, 1962.

53. Anseth, A., and Laurent, T. C.: Polysaccharides in normal and pathologic corneas, *Invest. Ophthalmol.*, 1(2):195–201, 1962.

54. Kinoshita, J. H.: Some aspects of the carbohydrate metabolism of the cornea, *Invest. Ophthalmol.*, 1(2):178–186, 1962.

55. Langham, M.: Interrelationship of metabolism and deturgescence of the living cornea, *Invest. Ophthalmol.*, 1(2):187–194, 1962.

56. Hill, R. M., and Fatt, I.: Oxygen uptake from a limited volume reservoir by *in vivo* human cornea, *Science*, 142(3597):1295–1297, 1963.

57. Hill, R. M., and Fatt, I.: Oxygen depletion of a limited reservoir by human conjunctiva, *Nature (Lond.)*, 200:1011, 1963.

58. de Roeth, A., Jr.: Respiration of the cornea, *Arch. Ophthalmol.*, 44(5):666–676, 1950.

59. Polse, K. A., and Mandell, R. B.: Critical oxygen tension at the corneal surface, *Arch. Ophthalmol.*, 84(4):505–508, 1970.

60. Hill, R. M., and Fatt, I.: How dependent is the cornea on the atmosphere?, *J. Am. Optom. Assoc.*, 35(10):873–875, 1964.

61. Mandell, R. B., Polse, K. A., and Fatt, I.: Corneal swelling caused by contact lens wear, *Arch. Ophthalmol.*, 83(1):3–9, 1970.

62. Kohra, T.: On the metabolism of the cornea, *Acta Soc. Ophthal. Jap.*, 39:1429, 1935.

63. Fatt, I., and Bieber, M. T.: The steady state distribution of oxygen and carbon dioxide in the *in vivo* cornea, 1. The open eye in air and the closed eye, *Exp. Eye Res.*, 7(1):103–112, 1968.

64. Hill, R. M.: The Physiology of Soft Lens Systems, in Ruben, M. (Ed.): *Soft Contact Lenses*, New York, John Wiley, 1978, pp. 41–50.

65. Langham, M. E.: Utilization of O_2 by the component layers of the living cornea, *J. Physiol. (Lond.)*, 117(4):461–470, 1952.

66. Fatt, I., Hill, R. M., and Takahashi, G. H.: Carbon dioxide efflux from the human cornea, *in vivo*, *Nature (Lond.)*, 203(4946):738–740, 1964.

67. Langham, M. E., and Taylor, I. S.: Factors affecting the hydration of the cornea in the excised eye and the living animal, *Br. J. Ophthalmol.*, 40(6):321–340, 1956.

68. Smelser, G. K.: Relation of factors involved in maintenance of optical properties of cornea to contact lens wear, *Arch. Ophthalmol.*, 47(3):328–343, 1952.

69. Smelser, G. K., and Ozanics, V.: Structural changes in corneas of guinea pigs after wearing contact lenses, *Arch. Ophthalmol.*, 49(3):335–340, 1953.

70. Smelser, G. K., and Chen, D. K.: Physiological changes in cornea induced by contact lenses, *Arch. Ophthalmol.*, 53(5):565–679, 1955.

71. Hirano, J.: Histochemical studies on the corneal changes induced by corneal contact lenses, *Jap. J. Ophthalmol.*, 3(1):1–8, 1959.

72. King, J. E., Augsburger, A., and Hill, R. M.: Quantifying the distribution of lactic acid dehydrogenase in the corneal epithelium with oxygen deprivation, *Am. J. Optom.*, 48(12):1016–1020, 1971.

73. Uniacke, C. A. et al.: Physiological tests for new contact lens materials, 1.: Quantitative effects of selected oxygen atmospheres on glycogen storage, LDH concentration and thickness of the corneal epithelium, *Am. J. Optom.*, 49(4):329–332, 1972.

74. Uniacke, C. A., and Hill, R. M.: The depletion course of epithelial glycogen with corneal anoxia, *Arch. Ophthalmol.*, 87(1):56–59, 1972.

75. Uniacke, C. A., Augsburger, A., and Hill, R. M.: Epithelial swelling with oxygen insufficiency, *Am. J. Optom.*, 48(7):565–568, 1971.

76. Bailey, I. L., and Carney, L. G.: Corneal changes from hydrophylic contact lenses, *Am. J. Optom.*, *50*:299, 1973.

77. Polse, K. A., Sarver, M. D., and Harris, M. H.: Corneal edema and vertical striae accompanying the wearing of hydrogel lenses. *Am. J. Optom.*, *52*:185, 1975.

78. Rodger, R. C.: The pattern of the corneal innervation in rabbits, *Br. J. Ophthalmol.*, *34*(2):107–113, 1950.

79. Boberg-Ans, J.: Experience in clinical examination of corneal sensitivity, *Br. J. Ophthalmol.*, *39*(12):705–726, 1955.

80. Boberg-Ans, J.: On the corneal sensitivity, *Acta Ophthalmol.*, *35*:149–162, 1956.

81. Schirmer, K. E., and Mellor, L. D.: Corneal sensitivity after cataract extraction, *Arch. Ophthalmol.*, *65*(3):433–436, 1961.

82. Strughold, H.: Sensitivity of cornea and conjunctiva of the human eye and the use of contact lenses, *Am. J. Optom.*, *30*(12):625–630, 1953.

83. Jalavisto, E., Orma, E., and Tawast, M.: Ageing and relation between stimulus intensity and duration in corneal sensitivity, *Acta Physiol. Scand.*, *23*:224–233, 1951.

84. Byron, H. M., and Weseley, A. C.: Clinical investigation of corneal contact lenses, *Am. J. Ophthalmol.*, *51*(4):675–694, 1961.

85. Hamano, H.: Topical and systemic influences of wearing contact lenses, *Contacto*, *4*(2):41–48, 1960.

86. Schirmer, K. E.: Assessment of corneal sensitivity, *Br. J. Ophthalmol.*, *47*(8):488–492, 1963.

87. Polse, K. A.: Etiology of corneal sensitivity changes accompanying contact lens wear, *Invest. Ophthalmol. Vis. Sci.*, *17*(12):1202–1206, 1978.

88. Nafe, J. P., and Wagoner, K. S.: The insensitivity of the cornea to heat and pain derived from high temperatures, *Am. J. Psychol.*, *49*(4):631–635, 1937.

89. Spooner, J. D.: *Ocular Anatomy*, London, Hatton, 1957, p. 19.

90. Lele, P. P., and Weddell, G.: Sensory nerves of the cornea and cutaneous sensibility, *Exp. Neurol.*, *1*:334–359, 1959.

91. Kenshalo, D. R.: Comparison of thermal sensitivity of the forehead, lip, conjunctiva and cornea, *J. Appl. Physiol.*, *15*(6):987–991, 1960.

92. Records, R. E.: *Physiology of the Human Eye and Visual System*, Hagerstown, Harper & Row, 1979, pp. 33–55.

93. Hill, R. M., and Leighton, A. J.: Temperature changes of human corneas and tears under contact lenses: 3. Ocular sensation, *Am. J. Optom.*, *42*(10):584–588, 1965.

94. Hill, R. M., and Leighton, A. J.: Physiological time courses associated with contact lenses — temperature: 2. Animal time courses with corneal lenses, *Am. J. Optom.*, *41*(1):3–9, 1964.

95. Hill, R. M.: How the Cornea "Takes the Heat," *Int. Cont. Lens Clin.*, *5*(6):65–67, 1978.

96. Schmidt, P. P., Schoessler, J. P., and Hill, R. M.: Effects of hard lenses on the chloride ion of the tears. *Am. J. Optom.*, *51*:84, 19.

97. Callender, M., and Morrison, P. E.: A quantitative study of human tear proteins before and after adaptation to non-flexible contact lenses. *Am. J. Optom. Physiol. Opt.*, *51*(12):939–945, 1974.

98. Ridley, F.: The tears, in Ridley, F., and Sorsby, A. (Eds.): *Modern Trends in Ophthalmology*, New York, Hoeber, 1940, vol. 1, Chap. 36, pp. 382–387.

99. Hind, H. W., and Szekely, I. J.: Wetting and hydration of contact lenses, *Contacto*, *3*(3):65–68, 1959.

100. Wolff, E.: The muco-cutaneous junction of the lid-margin and the distribution of the tear fluid, *Trans. Ophthalmol. Soc. U. K.*, *66*:291–308, 1946.

101. Lemp, M. A., Dohlman, C. H., and Holly, F. J.: Corneal desiccation despite normal tear volume, *Ann. Ophthalmol.*, *2*(3):258–261, 284, 1970.

102. Lemp, M. A. et al.: Dry eye secondary to mucus deficiency, *Trans. Am. Acad. Ophthalmol. Otolaryngol.*, *75*(6):1223–1227, 1971.

103. Iwata, S. et al.: Evaporation rate of water from the precorneal tear film and cornea in the rabbit, *Invest. Ophthalmol.*, *8*(6):613–619, 1969.

104. Mishima, S., and Maurice, D. M.: The oily layer of the tear film and evaporation

from the corneal surface, *Exp. Eye Res.*, *1(1)*:39–45, 1961.

105. Wolff, E.: *The Anatomy of the Eye and Orbit*, 4th ed., New York, Blakiston, 1954, p. 212.

106. Mishima, S. et al.: Determination of tear volume and tear flow, *Invest. Ophthalmol.*, *5(3)*:264–276, 1966.

107. Mishima, S.: Some physiological aspects of the precorneal tear film, *Arch. Ophthalmol.*,*73(2)*:233–241, 1965.

108. Norn, M. S.: The conjunctival fluid, its height, volume, density of cells, and flow. *Acta Ophthalmol.*, *44(2)*:212–222, 1966.

109. Lemp, M. A. et al.: The precorneal tear film: 1. Factors in spreading and maintaining a continuous tear film over the corneal surface, *Arch. Ophthalmol.*, *83(1)*: 89–94, 1970.

110. Nron, M. S.: Desiccation of the precorneal film: 1. Corneal wetting time, *Acta Ophthalmol.*, *47(4)*:865–880, 1969.

111. Norn, M. S.: Desiccation of the precorneal film: 2. Permanent discontinuity and dellen, *Acta Ophthalmol.*, *47(4)*:881–889, 1969.

112. Girard, L. J., and Moore, C. D.: Dry spots of the cornea, in Luntz, M. H. (Ed.): *Proceedings of the First South African International Ophthalmology Symposium*, London and Toronto, Butterworth, 1969, p. 25.

113. Lemp, M. A., and Hamill, J. R., Jr.: Factors affecting tear film break up in normal eyes, *Arch. Ophthalmol.*, *89(2)*:103–105, 1973.

114. Henderson, J. W., and Prough, W. A.: Influence of age and sex on flow of tears, *Arch. Ophthalmol.*, *43(2)*:224–231, 1950.

115. Bell, C.: On the motions of the eye, in illustration of the uses of the muscles and nerves of the orbit, *Philos. Trans. R. Soc. Lond. [Biol. Sci.]*, 168, 1923.

116. Stewart, C. R.: Bell's phenomenon and corneal lenses, *Br. J. Physiol. Opt.*, *25(1)*:50–60, 1970.

117. Stewart, C. R.: Functional blinking and corneal lenses, *Am. J. Optom.*, *45(10)*:687–691, 1968.

118. Mackie, I.: Blinking mechanisms in relation to the development of lesions at the corneal limbus at three o'clock and nine o'clock with contact lens wear, Contact Lens Symposium, 21st International Congress of Ophthalmology, Mexico City, 1970, published by Basel Karger.

119. Korb, D. R., Korb, J. E., and Herman, J. P.: in press.

120. Chan, R. S., and Mandell, R. B.: Corneal thickness changes from bathing solutions. *Am. J. Optom. Physiol. Opt.*, *52*:465–469, 1975.

121. Gerstman, D. R.: The biomicroscope and Vickers image splitting eyepiece applied to clinical variation in human central corneal thickness, *J. Microscopy*, *96*:385–388, 1972.

122. Hogan, M. J., Alvarado, J. A., and Esperson, J.: *Histology of the Human Eye*, Philadelphia, Saunders, 1971.

ADDITIONAL READINGS

Adler, I. N., Wlodyga, R. J., and Rope, S. J.: The effects of pH on contact lens wearing, *J. Am. Optom. Assoc.*, *39(11)*:1000–1001, 1968.

Andrews, J. S.: The meibomian secretion, *Int. Ophthalmol. Clin.*, *13(1)*:23, 1973.

Aquavella, J.: Corneal physiology and the contact lens, *Cont. Intraoc. Lens Med. J.*, *1(1–2)*:121–125, 1975.

Bron, A. J.: Anterior corneal mosaic, *Br. J. Ophthalmol.*, *52*:659–669, 1968.

Burns, R. P., and Roberts, H.: Effect of contact lenses on corneal metabolism, *Symp. Ocular Pharm. & Ther. Trans. New Orleans Acad. Ophthalmol.*, pp. 73, 1970.

Carney, L. G., and Hill, R. M.: Other hydrophilic lens environments: pH, *Am. J. Optom.*, *53(9)*: 456–458, 1976.

Cochet, P., and Liotet, S.: Tears and contact lenses, *Les Cahiers des Verres de Contact* (Translation by W. F. Coombs), *11*:7, 1966.

Collin, H. B.: Clinical conditions affecting the basement membrane of the corneal epithelium, *Austr. J. Optom.*, *60(7)*:234, 1977.

Collin, H. B., and Larson, H. D.: Rupture of Descemet's membrane of the cornea, *Int. Cont. Lens Clin.*, *5(4)*:27, 1978.

Cope, W. T., Wolbarsht, M. L., and Yamanishi, B. S.: The corneal polarization cross, *J. Opt. Soc. Am.*, *68(8)*:1139–1141, 1978.

Corazza, J. P.: Palpebral tension, *Contacto*, *21(1)*: 20–22, 1977.

Dutesco, N.: La fragilité de l'épithélium cornéen (translation), unpublished paper, 1971.

Ebbers, R. W., and Sears, D.: Ocular effects of a 325nm ultraviolet laser, *Am. J. Optom. Physiol. Opt.*, *52*:216–223, 1975.

Ehlers, N.: The precorneal films-biomicroscopical, histological, and chemical investigations, *Acta Ophthalmol.*, Supp., No. 81, Copenhagen, 1965.

Ehlers, N., and Hansen, F. K.: Further data on biometric correlations of central corneal thickness, *Acta Ophthalmol.*, *54(6)*:774–778, 1976.

Fatt, I., Bieber, M. T., and Pye, S. D.: Steady state distribution of oxygen and carbon dioxide in the *in vivo* cornea of an eye covered by a gas-permeable contact lens, *Am. J. Optom. Arch. Am. Acad. Optom.*, *46(1)*:13–14, 1969.

Fatt, I., and Harris, M. G.: Refractive index of the cornea as a function of its thickness, *Am. J. Optom. Arch. Am. Acad. Optom.*, *50(5)*:383–386, 1973.

Fatt, I., and Hill, R. M.: Oxygen uptake from a reservoir of limited volume by the human cornea *in vivo*, *Science*, *142(3597)*:1295–1297, 1963.

Feldman, G. L.: Physiology of hard and soft contact lens wear, *Cont. Lens Med. Bull.*, *3(1)*:14–18, 1970.

Finkelstein, I. S.: The biophysics of corneal scatter and diffraction of light induced by contact lenses, *Am. J. Optom. Arch. Am. Acad. Optom.*, Part I, *29(4)*:185–208, 1952; Part II, *29(75)*: 231–259, 1952.

Freeman, R. D.: Oxygen consumption by the component layers of the cornea, *J. Physiol.*, *225*:15–32, 1972.

Furukawa, R. E.: Slit lamp fluorophotometry, *Opt. Engin.*, *15(4)*:321, 1976.

Furukawa, R. E., and Polse, K. A.: Changes in tear flow accompanying aging, *Am. J. Optom. Physiol. Opt.*, *55(2)*:69–74,. 1978.

Gould, H. L., and Guibor, P.: Contact lens wearer and lacrimal secretion, *Cont. Lens Med. Bull.*, *6(2–3)*:6–10, 1973.

Green, K.: Anatomic study of water movement through rabbit corneal epithelium, *Am. J. Ophthalmol.*, *67(1)*:110–116, 1969.

Greiner, J., Covington, H. I., and Allansmith, M.

R.: The human limbus—A scanning electron microscopic study, *Arch. Ophthalmol.*, *97(6)*: 1159–1165, 1979.

Grosvenor, T.: Physiological factors in contact lens wearing, *Optom. Weekly*, 13–19, March 31, 1966.

Hamano, H.: Scanning electron microscopic findings of wearing contact lens on rabbit cornea epithelium (Eng. Abst.), *J. Jap. Contact Lens Soc.*, *13(6)*:35–42, 1971.

Hamano, H.: Bio differential interference microscopic observations on anterior segment of eye, *Folia Ophthalmol. Japonica*, *30(9)*:229, 1979.

Hanna, H. L., Jr.: Cytological contraindications in contact lens wear, *Contacto*, *23(1)*:15–23, 1979.

Hill, R.: The "modal" tear, *Cont. Lens Forum*, p. 63, Feb. 1980.

Hill, R. M.: Corneal physiology and the contact lens, *2nd AOA Cont. Lens Symp.*, April 10–12, 1965.

Hill, R. M.: Comments on contact lens adaptation: osmotic pressure of the tears, *J. Cont. Lens Soc. Am.*, *4(4)*:15–21, 1970.

Hill, R. M.: The quest for oxygen, *J. Cont. Lens Soc. Am.*, *7(4)*:29–31, 1974.

Hill, R. M.: Tear cholesterol and your contact lens patient, *Austr. J. Optom.*, *58(8)*:300–303, 1975.

Hill, R. M.: The physiology of contact lens systems, *J. Am. Optom. Assoc.*, *47(3)*:284, 1976.

Hill, R. M.: The closed eye environment:pH, *Am. J. Optom.*, *53(11)*:718–719, 1976.

Hill, R. M.: The pH mystique, *Int. Cont. Lens Clin.*, *5(2)*:27, 1978.

Hill, R. M.: Oxygen demand: The same for every cornea?, *Int. Cont. Lens Clin.*, *6(3)*:45–48, 1979.

Hill, R. M.: Conjunctival competition?, *Int. Cont. Lens Clin.*, *6(6)*:255, 1979.

Hill, R. M., and Fatt, I.: Oxygen deprivation of the cornea by contact lenses and lid closure, *Am. J. Optom. Arch. Am. Acad. Optom.*, *41(11)*:678, 1964.

Hill, R. M., and Young, W.: Cholesterol levels of human tears: case reports, *J. Am. Optom. Assoc.*, *44(3)*:424–428, 1973.

Holden, B. A., and Zantos, S. G.: The corneal endothelium and contact lenses, *Int. Cont. Lens Clin.*, *5(1)*:29, 1978.

Holly, F. J.: Formation and stability of the tear film, *Int. Cont. Lens Clin.*, *13(1)*:73. 1973.

Holly, F. J.: The preocular tear film—Chapter 5, *Cont. Intraoc. Lens Med. J.*, *4(4)*:134, 1978.

Holly, F. J., and Lemp, M. A.: Wettability and

wetting of corneal epithelium, *Exp. Eye Res.*, 11:239–250, 1971.

Holly, F. J., and Lemp, M. A.: Surface chemistry of the tearfilm; implications for dry eye syndromes, contact lenses, and ophthalmic polymers, *J. Cont. Lens Soc. Am.*, 5(1):12, 1971.

Holly, F. J., and Lemp, M. A.: Tear physiology and dry eyes, *Survey Ophthalmol.*, 22(2):69, 1977.

Hori, M., and Hamano, H.: Histochemical approach to corneal epithelial changes induced by intralamellar lens implant, *Contacto*, 19(1): 24–27, 1975.

Hung, G., Hsu, F., and Stark, L.: Dynamics of the human eyeblink, *Am. J. Optom. Physiol. Opt.*, 54(10):678, 1977.

Hurwitz, J. J., Maisley, M. N., and Welham, R. A. N.: Quantitative lacrimal scintillography I. Method and physiological application, *Br. J. Ophthalmol.*, 59:308–312, 1975.

Hurwitz, J. J., Maisley, M. N., and Welham, R. A. N.: Radiography in functional lacrimal testing, *Br. J. Ophthalmol.*, 59:323–331, 1975.

Huth, S., Hirano, P., and Leopold, I. H.: Calcium in tears and contact lens wear, *Arch. Ophthalmol.*, 98:122–125, 1980.

Hypher, T. J.: Uptake and loss of tears from filter paper discs employed in lysozyme tests, *Br. J. Ophthalmol.*, 63:251–255, 1979.

Iwata, S.: Biophysico-chemical aspects on contact lens, *J. Jap. Contact Lens Soc.*, 21(7):208, 1979.

Jauregui, M. J., and Fatt, I.: Estimation of the *in vivo* oxygen consumption rate of the human corneal epithelium, *Am. J. Optom.*, 49(6):507–511, 1972.

Jumblatt, M. M., Maurice, D. M., and McCulley, J. P.: Transplantation of tissue—cultured corneal endothelium, *Invest. Ophthalmol.*, 17(12): 1135, 1978.

Kame, R. T., Takemura, R. K., and Mukai, G. T.: Tear breakup time and the Schirmer tear test, *J. Am. Optom. Assoc.*, 47(12):1535–1538, 1976.

Katz, J., and Kaufman, H. E.: Corneal exposure during sleep (Nocturnal Lagophthalmos), *Arch. Ophthalmol.*, 95(3):449–453, 1977.

Kempster, A. J., Larke, J. R., and Marsters, J. P.: The effect of hypertonic saline on human corneal hydration, *Br. J. Physiol. Opt.*, 30(1):16–19, 1975.

Khorazo, C., and Thompson, R.: The bacterial flora of the normal conjunctiva, *Am. J. Ophthalmol.*, 18:1114–1116, 1935.

Kikkawa, Y.: Effects of the contact lens on the corneal metabolism, *Contacto*, 14(3):43–50, 1970.

Kikkawa, Y.: Biological rhythm in corneal thickness (Eng Abst), *Folia Ophthalmol. Japonica*, 26(7):723–728, 1975.

Knoll, H. A., and Williams, J.: Effects of hydrophilic contact lenses on corneal sensitivity, *Am. J. Optom. Arch. Am. Acad. Optom.*, 47(7):561–563, 1970.

Kuwabara, T.: Current concepts in anatomy and histology of the cornea, *Cont. Intraoc. Lens. Med. J.*, 4(2):101, 1978.

Laing, R. A., Sandstrom, M., and Leibowitz, H. L.: *In vivo* photomicrography of the corneal endothelium, *Arch. Ophthalmol.*, 93(2):143–145, 1975.

Landsman, L. A.: Clinical observation of micro dry spots on the cornea, *Opt. J. Rev. Optom.*, 114(4):86, 1977.

Laule, A. et al.: Endothelial cell population changes of human cornea during life, *Arch. Ophthalmol.*, 96(11):2031, 1978.

Leach, N. E.: Corneal hydration changes during the normal menstrual cycle—a preliminary study, *J. Repro. Med.*, 6(5):15–18, 1971.

Lemp, M. A.: Surfacing the precorneal tear film, *Ann. Ophthalmol.*, 5(7):819–826, 1973.

Lemp, M. A., Goldberg, M., and Roddy, M. R.: The effect of tear substitutes on tear film breakup time, *Invest. Ophthalmol.*, 14(3): 255–258, 1975.

Lemp, M. A., and Szymanski, E. S.: Polymer absorption at the ocular surface, *Arch. Ophthalmol.*, 93(2):134–136, 1975.

McDonald, J. E.: Surface phenomena of the tear film, *Am. J. Ophthalmol.*, 67(1):56–64, 1969.

McDonald, J. E., and Brubaker, S.: Meniscus-induced thinning of tear films, *Am. J. Ophthalmol.*, 72(1):139–146, 1971.

McEwen, W..K, et al.: Filter-paper electrophoresis of tears. III. Human tears and their high molecular weight components, *Am. J. Ophthalmol.*, 45(1):67–70, 1958.

Mackie, I. A., and Seal, D. V.: Quantitative tear lysozyme assay in units of activity per microlitre, *Br. J. Ophthalmol.*, 60(1):70–74, 1976.

Millodot, M.: Studies on the sensitivity of the cornea, *The Optician*, 157(4067):267–271, 1969.

Millodot, M.: Diurnal variation of corneal sensitivity, *Br. J. Ophthalmol.*, 56(11):844–847, 1972.

Millodot, M.: Objective measurement of corneal sensitivity, *Acta Ophthalmol.*, 51(3):325–334, 1973.

Millodot, M.: Do blue-eyed people have more sensitive corneas than brown-eyed people? *Nature*, *255(5504)*:151–152, 1975.

Millodot, M.: Effect of the length of wear of contact lenses on corneal sensitivity, *Acta Ophthalmol.*, *54(6)*:721–730, 1976.

Millodot, M.: The influence of age on the sensitivity of the cornea, *Invest. Ophthalmol.*, *16(3)*: 240–242, 1977.

Millodot, M.: Effect of long-term wear of hard contact lenses on corneal sensitivity, *Arch. Ophthalmol.*, *96(7)*:1225–1227, 1978.

Millodot, M., Henson, D. B., O'Leary, D. J.: Measurement of corneal sensitivity and thickness with PMMA and gas-permeable contact lenses, *Am. J. Optom. Physiol. Opt.*, *56(10)*:628–632, 1979.

Mishima, S.: Corneal thickness, *Survey Ophthalmol.*, *13(2)*:57–96, 1968.

Mishima, S.: Some applications of slit lamp microphotometry, *Cont. Intraoc. Lens Med. J.*, *(1–2)*: 46–57, 1975.

Norn, M. S.: Outflow of tears and its influence on tear secretion and break up time (B.U.T.), *Acta Ophthalmol.*, *55(4)*:674–682, 1977.

Norn, M. S., and Opauszki, A.: Effects of ophthalmic vehicles on the stability of the precorneal film, *Acta Ophthalmol.*, *55(1)*:23–34, 1977.

Pfister, R., and Burstein, N.: The normal and abnormal human corneal epithelium surface: a scanning electron microscope study, *Invest. Ophthalmol. Vis. Sci.*, *16(7)*:614–622, 1977.

Pfortner, T. et al.: Immunological action on the precorneal tear film with the use of contact lenses, *Int. Cont. Lens Clinic*, *4(6)*:65–74, 1977.

Pitts, D. G., and Gibbons, W. D.: Corneal light scatter measurements of ultraviolet radiant exposures, *Am. J. Optom. Arch. Am. Acad. Optom.*, *50(3)*:187–194, 1973.

Polse, K. A.: Measurement of corneal sensitivity— Part I, *Optom. Weekly*, *68(45)*:1380–1381, 1977.

Polse, K. A.: Measurement of corneal sensitivity— Part II, *Optom. Weekly*, *68(46)*:1404–1406, 1977.

Chapter 3

CORNEAL TOPOGRAPHY

CLASSICAL CONCEPT OF CORNEAL CONTOUR

TRADITIONALLY, the external corneal contour has been described as consisting of two zones.[1] In the center is a spherical or toric zone known as the corneal cap,* which is 4 to 5 mm. in diameter. Surrounding the corneal cap is an annular peripheral zone, which flattens progressively towards the sclera (Figure 3.1a).

The corneal cap may be defined as the central corneal area of maximum and constant meridional curvature. It is limited by the positions where the radii of curvature increase more than 0.05 mm. This definition is arbitrary and based on the fact that 0.05 mm. is about the limit of accuracy that can be obtained for corneal radius measurements. The radius of the corneal cap is normally between 7.2 and 8.7 mm. (average 7.9) with small amounts of toricity.[2]†

The peripheral corneal zone is the annular portion that surrounds the cap and that forms the remainder of the cornea. The radius of curvature at the inner border of the peripheral corneal zone is 0.05 mm. longer than the radius of the cap, and it gradually lengthens to about 14 mm. at the junction with the sclera.[3]

The size of the corneal cap or the size of the overall cornea is usually expressed in terms of the diameter. In referring to the cornea, the term diameter is reserved for the width of the chord that spans a given arc, whereas the term radius always refers to the curvature of the arc.

The size of the peripheral corneal zone is specified in terms of its width as projected directly (isometrically) onto the diameter chord (Figure 3.1). Hence, two widths of the peripheral zone must be added to the cap diameter to equal the overall diameter of the cornea. For example, a cornea having a 5 mm. cap diameter and a peripheral zone width of 2.5 mm. will have an overall diameter of 10 mm.

---

*The term central zone is often used synonymously with corneal cap, but since the central zone is also used to refer to the central portion of a contact lens, the author has adopted the corneal cap designation when referring to the cornea.

†Very often corneal curvature is expressed in terms of refractive power, rather than radius, as, for example, on the scales of most keratometers. With the radius known, corneal power is found by the formula for the power of a single refracting surface

$$F = \frac{n-1}{r}$$

where
F = corneal power (D.)
n = index of refraction of cornea
r = radius of curvature of cornea (M.)

An assumption must be made for the index of refraction of the cornea. The value 1.3375 has been adopted for the Bausch and Lomb Keratometer, and the value 1.336 has been adopted for the American Optical Ophthalmometer. Conversion tables for radius and power eliminate the need for calculations. Tables distributed by contact lens companies are nearly always based on an assumed index of 1.3375 and hence present a slight error when used with the American Optical Ophthalmometer. A conversion table for indices 1.3375 and 1.336 is presented in Appendix 1.

ORIGIN OF CLASSICAL CORNEAL CONCEPT

The question arises, is the two-zone concept of the corneal contour valid?

The origin of the classical corneal classification appears to have come from Aubert,[1]

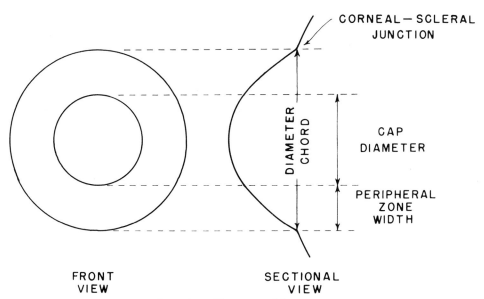

Figure 3.1a. The zones of the cornea.

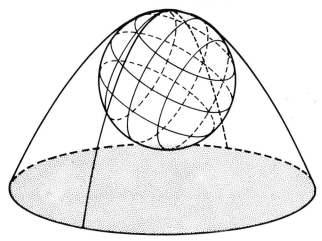

Figure 3.1b. The central cornea has only an instantaneously spherical curvature at the most central point.

who, on the basis of six measurements on each of four subjects, described the cornea as having an optic part and a basilar part. This classification was further supported by Ericksen[4] in a study in which he used the Javal-Schiøtz ophthalmometer to measure the corneal periphery of twenty-four eyes. Ericksen described the corneal cap as having a width of 4 mm. in the horizontal meridian. He defined the cap as that area in which the corneal power does not vary more than 1.00 D. from the central measurement. Further evidence for a two-zone cornea was found by Gullstrand[5] using the method of photokeratoscopy. Gullstrand described the corneal cap as essentially spherical.

These studies by early investigators showed definite central corneal areas of constant curvature. Later investigators found the corneal contour to be more like that of a conic,[6,7] flattening at an increased rate towards the periphery but with no sharp cutoff point for the cap. Thus, the limits of the corneal cap are determined only by arbitrary definition.

If the corneal cap is defined as the area within which the corneal power does not decrease more than 1.00 D., the average cap will be about 4 mm. in diameter. If the power is allowed to vary 2.00 D., the average cap will be about 6 mm. in diameter.

The concept of a two-zone cornea has been a convenient system of classification for anatomical purposes but has been misleading for contact lens practice. The corneal cap is often regarded as truly spherical, and contact lens fitting procedures are based on that premise. This misconception is due to the frequency in which it is stated, without qualification, that the cornea has two zones. The corneal cap is described as "approximately spherical"[8] or "of fairly uniform radius of curvature."[9] Its width is given as between 4 and 6 mm. It must be understood that significant variation in corneal curvature occurs in the central cornea, with only the central point having an instantaneous spherical curvature (Figure 3.1b). The two-zone concept is an arbitrary division for convenience.

CORNEAL CONTOUR MEASUREMENTS

Considerable controversy has arisen over the exact form of the corneal contour because the results of measurements by various investigators have been inconsistent.* Apparently, much of the disagreement is due to the inaccuracies in some of the methods used for corneal measurements. Recent research has determined many reasons for errors in corneal measurements and has greatly modified the classical concept of corneal contour.[15]†

An accurate measurement of the corneal contour is not easily accomplished. The cornea constantly moves, is sensitive to touch,

pliable, and susceptible to harm by many forms of radiation. In addition, the cornea has an aspherical surface that should ideally be measured at many separate positions. If a 2 to 3 mm. area is used for a single measurement, the curvature obtained will be a function of the many curvatures within this area, and considerable error will be introduced into the measurement.

Many methods of corneal contour measurement have been employed, including some that are only applicable to laboratory conditions, including modified keratometry,[18-20] Moiré keratometry,[21,22] interferometry,[23] electronic keratometry,[24] ultrasound,[25] stereo-

---

*In addition to the classical two-zone description of the corneal contour, the cornea has been described as elliptical,[6] parabolic,[10] and hyperbolic.[11,12] Bier[13] and others reported the existence of a so-called negative zone between the cap and peripheral zone. However, such a zone does not appear to be present.[3,14]

---

†No attempt has been made to cover all the early literature available on corneal contour measurement as adequate summaries are available.[16,17]

photogrammetry,[26] profile photography,[27] and photokeratoscopy.[28,29] Objections to most of these methods are based on their need for several approximations.

KERATOMETER

The corneal curvature is commonly and easily measured clinically with a keratometer.[30] This measurement is restricted to a small central corneal area and is not representative of the entire corneal contour. In fact, the only portions of the cornea actually used for a keratometer measurement are two small areas for a given meridian, or a total of four small areas for the two principal meridians (Figure 3.2).* The separation of the two areas in each meridian varies as a function of the corneal radius of curvature and the dimensions and position of the keratometer mire target. These distances are shown in Figure 3.3. With the American Optical Ophthalmometer the corneal areas measured are separated by a distance that, on the average, is about 0.5 mm. less than that with the Bausch

and Lomb Keratometer. For example, with a 7.94 mm. radius cornea, the average separations of the areas measured by Bausch and Lomb Keratometers and American Optical Ophthalmometers are 3.1 mm. and 2.6 mm. respectively. The smallest corneal area is measured by the Gambs keratometer.[31]

There have been several attempts to use a keratometer to measure peripheral corneal curvatures,[32-44] but it has generally been recognized that the keratometer was designed to measure only the radius of the corneal cap and that peripheral corneal measurements are approximations.[45,46] The accuracy can be improved with special techniques,[47,48] but a standard keratometer is nevertheless of little value in measuring the entire corneal contour.

Relationship of K Reading to Corneal Contour

A keratometer is designed for use in measuring a spherical surface. When it is used to measure the central corneal curvature, the

---

*Basic principles of the keratometer are discussed in Chapter 33.

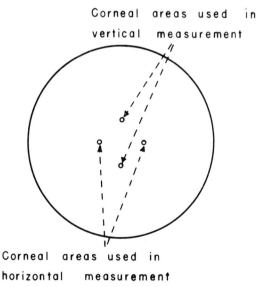

Corneal areas used in
vertical measurement

Corneal areas used in
horizontal measurement

Figure 3.2. Corneal areas used for keratometry measurements.

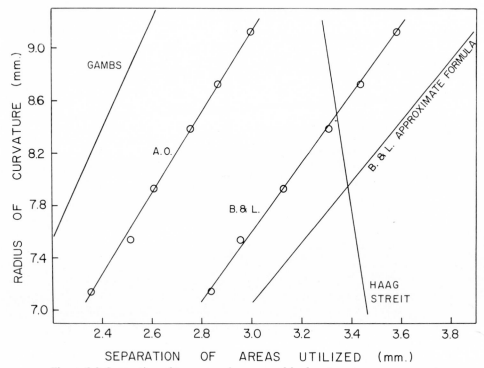

Figure 3.3. Separation of two corneal areas used for keratometry measurements.

assumption must be that the central portion of the cornea is spherical. If the cornea has a spherical cap with a width of at least 3.5 mm., the measurement will be valid.[49] However, if the central cornea is aspherical, as so often occurs, the measurement will be in error. The magnitude of the error is related to the rate of peripheral corneal flattening. This may be understood by considering some basic characteristics of corneal contour.[50]

For the sake of simplicity, a cornea that has only two curvatures will be considered. Care must be taken in the construction of the corneal curvatures, as an error at this point has given rise to many misconceptions in the study of contact lenses.

A common, but incorrect, method of illustrating the corneal curvatures is shown in Figure 3.4a. The corneal cap is drawn with a center of curvature at C_1 and limited by points a and b. The center of curvature, C_2, for the peripheral curve, is incorrectly placed directly behind C_1, and curves are drawn from points a and b to the periphery. This method of corneal construction implies that the cornea has a dip at points a and b, where the cap meets the segments of the peripheral curve.

Figure 3.4b shows the corneal centers of curvature in their proper relationship.[44] From the limit of the corneal cap (a), a line should be drawn through the center of curvature, C_1. The center of curvature C_2, must lie on this line; otherwise a smooth transition to a different curvature will not be possible. Both the cap and the peripheral curve will now be perpendicular to the line bC_1 at b. Since the radius of the peripheral curve is longer than the radius of the cornea cap, its center of curvature must lie behind C_1 and off the optic axis of the cornea. Only one side of the peripheral curve can be constructed in this way, and the procedure must be repeated for the other side. Figure 3.4c shows how the cornea is properly constructed, using two seg-

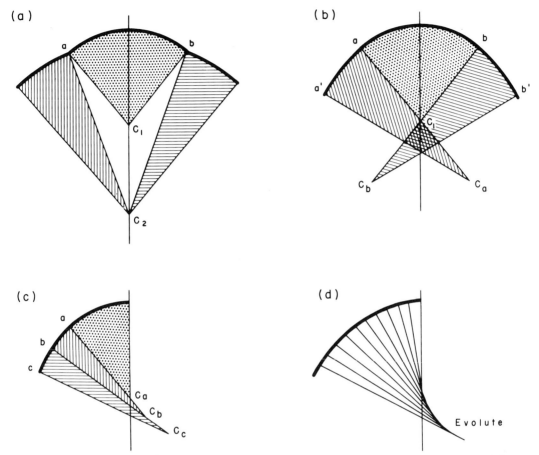

Figure 3.4. Construction of the peripheral corneal curvatures, (*a*) incorrect, (*b*) correct, (*c&d*) addition of more radii.

ments for the peripheral curve. Each segment is drawn in sequence by repeating the process shown in Figure 3.4b. Since the peripheral curve of the actual cornea has a consistently varying radius of curvature, the center of curvature is constantly changing to a new position. All the centers of curvature form a locus of points that extends from the center of curvature of the corneal cap to an off-axis position. This locus of centers of curvature for a constantly varying curve is known as an evolute. The general appearance of a corneal evolute is shown in Figure 3.4d.

If a keratometer is used to measure an

aspherical cornea, the central portion of the cornea will be interpreted to be spherical. The degree of error will be related to the rate of flattening of the cornea away from the apex. In Figure 3.5 an aspherical cornea is shown in relation to the keratometer mires. Light from the mires will be reflected from two corneal areas, a and b, to the keratometer. The actual radii of the cornea at positions a and b are represented by aC_a and bC_b. For simplicity, assume that the cornea is symmetrical so that aC_a and bC_b are equal.

The radius of curvature that is measured with the keratometer will not be the actual

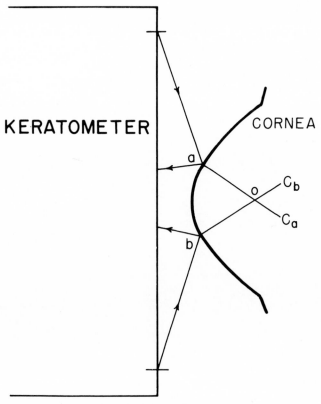

Figure 3.5. Effect of central corneal asphericity on keratometer measurement. Radius $\overline{aC_a}$ is measured as $\overline{ao}$

radius of the cornea at the positions a and b. Instead, the keratometer will indicate the curvature to be more nearly that of the corneal apex, which has a shorter radius. This occurs because the keratometer interprets the area between a and b to be circular. The radius of the circle is determined by the slope of the cornea at a and b. The perpendicular bisectors of the cornea at a and b represent the radii of this circle. Their intersection, o, represents the center of the circle, the radius of which is read from the keratometer. Thus, the radius of the cornea as measured by the keratometer will be equal to ao and bo, rather than aC_a or bC_b. The radius measured will be insignificantly longer than the radius of the corneal apex.

The predicted relationship between the keratometer measurement and the corneal contour has been substantiated experimentally. Fifteen corneas were measured by using both the small-mire keratometer (*see* the section on small-mire keratometry) and the standard keratometer. Thirteen of these corneas showed no significant difference between the apical curvatures and the curvatures as found by the standard keratometer. The two remaining corneas measured 0.75 D. and 0.87 D. flatter than their true apical curvatures. These corneas both had apexes that were greatly decentered from their lines of sight, which appears to be the reason for the keratometer errors. When the normal keratometer is used to measure the corneal periphery, it has the error of making the corneal cap appear abnormally large and the corneal periphery appear abnormally steep (Figure 3.6).[53-56]

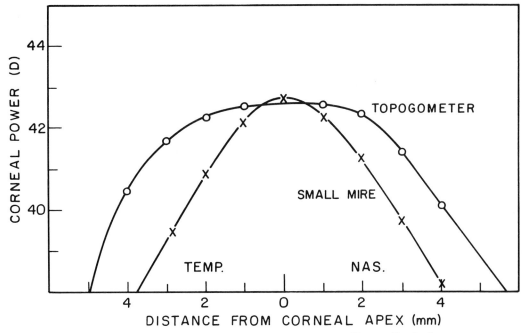

Figure 3.6. Corneal contour measured by the topogometer and by small-mire keratometry.

Peripheral Keratometry

The curves of a contact lens must have an optimum relationship with the cornea to allow the needed interchange of tear fluid behind the lens. This relationship is probably fulfilled by a number of possible curves for the lens. If sufficient information were available about the total contour of the cornea, it would seem possible to select the ideal curves for the contact lens to go with that particular cornea. To accomplish this, better methods have been developed to measure the total corneal contour rather than only the very central cornea.

Unfortunately, all methods that have been developed to measure the total corneal contour have various disadvantages. Even the most sophisticated devices have been shown to have limited accuracy by the standards we commonly apply to corneal measurements. The instrument most commonly utilized on a clinical basis to determine the corneal contour is the keratometer.

In order to determine corneal contour with a keratometer, it is necessary to take a series of peripheral corneal measurements. As shown previously the peripheral cornea is even more aspherical than has generally been realized. Since the keratometer was designed only to measure spherical surfaces, the interpretation of peripheral keratometer readings is a most difficult and complicated problem.

Advocates of peripheral keratometry have more or less ignored the complexities of this analysis in favor of arbitrary rules of thumb. Calculations are performed incorrectly as a rule, and yet all claim a large measure of success. Unfortunately, peripheral keratometry cannot be reduced to simple interpretation because the cornea is such a vastly complicated curve. Accurate peripheral corneal measurements are only possible if the keratometer is modified so that it measures a very small area of the cornea (*see* a later section on the size of measurements).

Many devices have been developed that

can be attached to the keratometer to provide a fixation target for the subject and allow peripheral readings to be made. The most elaborate device of this type cannot compensate for the errors inherent in peripheral keratometry.

The author originally developed a method to utilize the keratometer to measure the size of the corneal cap. The technique required that the cornea have a true cap, that is, an area of constant curvature. Later experiments have revealed that the assumption of a corneal cap is not valid. Therefore, for most corneas this technique cannot be used.

Let us assume for the moment that we have an instrument that can measure the corneal curvature to any accuracy desired. What then would be our method for determining the characteristics of the contact lens that would best fit this cornea? Unfortunately, we have no research whatsoever that can give us any clue to the solution of this problem. To illustrate this dilemma, consider the following hypothetical case. A cornea has a curvature of 43.00 D. for its cap, which measures 2 mm. in diameter. From the edge of the cap, the cornea begins to flatten at a rapid rate on the nasal side until approximately halfway to the periphery, after which the rate of flattening increases gradually. Temporally, the cornea flattens gradually in a regular fashion all the way to the periphery. In the superior meridian the cornea retains the same curvature until near the periphery, when it suddenly flattens very rapidly. Inferiorly the cornea retains the same curvature until it reaches the limbus. Which areas of the cornea should now be considered in making the selection of the contact lens? Obviously, the decision would have to be arbitrary, and none would be adequate to give any known relationship between the contact lens and the cornea.

To further complicate the problem, two additional factors must be considered—that of the relationship of the lens curve to the corneal curve and the inaccuracy of the peripheral curves of the contact lenses that are received from the laboratory.

The simple problem of relating the cornea to the peripheral curve of the contact lens will be used here to illustrate. It was shown previously that the centers of curvature for the peripheral areas of the cornea fell off the axis of symmetry (*see* Figure 3.4). However, contact lenses are made with the centers for all the curves on the axis of symmetry. Consequently, even if a contact lens is made with the same curvatures as the cornea, it will not have the same *contour* as the cornea. This is illustrated in Figure 3.4, where Figure 3.4a represents the contact lens and Figure 3.4b represents the cornea.* After testing both valid and invalid methods of peripheral keratometry on hundreds of contact lens patients, it is the author's conclusion that other methods of fitting are both more efficient and accurate.

Small-mire Keratometry

In a study of corneal contours, a standard Bausch and Lomb Keratometer was modified so that curvature measurements of approximately 1 mm. areas of the cornea could be taken.[57] New mires were made by drilling apertures into the mire target with a separation of 26 mm. instead of the standard 64 mm. separation of the original mires. The apertures that formed the new mires were transilluminated by the lighting system of the keratometer. A 2.25 *Δ* prism was placed behind the standard lateral doubling prism of the keratometer so as to bring the small-mire images seen by the operator into a position that would allow measurements.

To calibrate the small-mire keratometer, measurements were made on a series of precision steel balls, and a conversion table was constructed. The exact corneal area to be utilized during small-mire keratometry was found by measuring the mire reflection area

---

*The enigma has also been responsible for the lack of validity for various contact lens "computers" that have been marketed.

on steel balls with an apparatus constructed for this purpose.[58]

Corneal Measurements

Measurements were made of the central and peripheral corneal curvatures by having subjects fixate a series of spots that had been painted on the mire target. Fluorescent paint was used, and the spots were illuminated with fluorescent light during the measurements. Since the spots were luminous, they could easily be seen even though they were within the subject's near point of accommodation. The fixation points were placed at 2.5° intervals, subtended at an assumed point for the eye's center of rotation of 13 mm. behind the cornea. The position assumed to be the center of rotation is not critical, since the measured corneal area is only a function of the radius of the corneal cap and the rate of change in the curvature of the corneal periphery.*

Three series of measurements were made and averages taken for each subject at a single test period.

Results

The results of the corneal curvature measurements by small-mire keratometry are plotted in Figure 3.7 in terms of the corneal power for each corneal position measured in the horizontal meridian.[59,60] Each curve represents an individual cornea and is shaped

---

*The paradox that the measured corneal position does not depend upon the position of the eye's center of rotation is explained in reference 47. Some investigators who apparently fail to understand this paradox have needlessly mounted keratometers on apparatus that allows the keratometer to be moved to different positions in order to take peripheral corneal measurements.

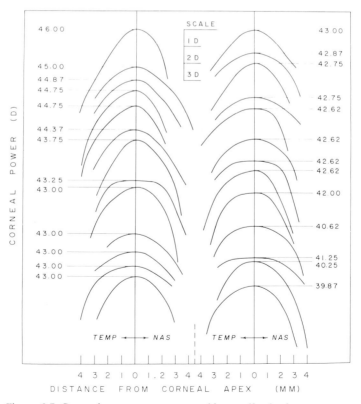

Figure 3.7. Corneal contours as measured by small-mire keratometry.

opposite to the actual corneal contour, i.e. if a cornea is spherical, its curve will be a straight horizontal line. The diameter of a corneal cap is represented by the width of the straight horizontal line segment at the center of each curve, and a cornea without a cap will not have a straight horizontal line segment. As the cornea flattens, its curve moves downwards at a rate that increases with greater corneal flattening.

The curves shown in Figure 3.7 indicate the high degree of variability for corneal contour from subject to subject. Twenty-one of the twenty-six subjects were found not to have corneal caps. Of the five remaining subjects, the corneal caps ranged from 2 to 3.75 mm. in width. Five corneas flattened symmetrically towards the periphery. Sixteen corneas flattened more on the nasal side than on the temporal side, whereas five others had the opposite relationship. The apex, or point of maximum corneal curvature, was decentered temporally up to 1.1 mm. from the line of sight for twelve subjects and decentered nasally up to 1 mm. for ten subjects. In four subjects the apex coincided with the line of sight.

These results indicate that the classical concept of a two-zone cornea occurs as the exception rather than the rule. Most corneas do not have a cap, and their central areas can be best approximated by an ellipse.* The rate of flattening begins slowly, and it gradually increases towards the periphery. Abrupt changes in the rate of flattening do not frequently occur.

The average corneal flattening is 0.93 D. nasally and 0.81 D. temporally at positions 2 mm. from the apex and 2.64 D. nasally and 1.87 D. temporally at positions 3 mm. from the apex. There is no significant correlation between the curvature at the apex and the rate of peripheral flattening (Figure 3.8). Corneas with large caps usually show a low rate of peripheral flattening. The rate of peripheral flattening is simply a continuation of a trend that begins at the central cornea.

Measurements of the vertical corneal mer-

*The semimeridians for the corneas' central areas could be closely approximated by ellipses. However, the peripheral portions of the corneas flattened too rapidly to also fit the ellipses. A meridional section of the total cornea cannot be closely approximated by any conical curve.

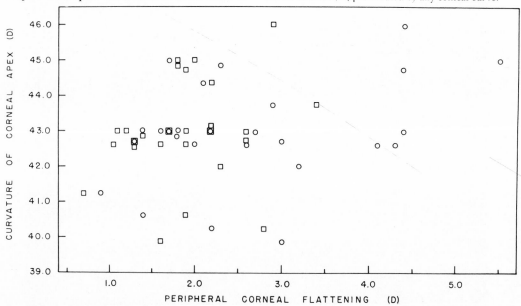

Figure 3.8. Relationship between curvature at corneal apex and rate of peripheral corneal flattening 3 mm. from apex.

idian were taken for the twenty-six subjects of the study. It was found that less regularity of curvature exists in the vertical meridian than in the horizontal meridian.

Exceptions to the average corneal contour are frequent, and each cornea must be considered as a separate entity. It is possible for the apex to be decentered in any direction and for the peripheral flattening to follow almost any course. The importance of considering individual corneal variability in the fitting of contact lenses cannot be overemphasized, since corneal variations affect the fit of a contact lens.

PHOTOKERATOSCOPY

Photokeratoscopy is a very old method of measuring corneal contour. It was introduced by Gullstrand[5] in 1896.[61,62] Many of the disadvantages recognized in the early years of its development tend to be ignored in its more recent use.[20,53-68]

Basically, the principle of photokeratoscopy is the same as the principle of keratometry, that is, to determine the relationship between the size of a target (object) and the size of its virtual image formed by the cornea, which acts as a convex mirror.[69] From this relationship the unknown radius of cor-

neal curvature can be determined by using optical formulas for mirrors. The advantage of the photokeratoscope compared with the keratometer is that its target may be composed of many parts, acting as separate objects, whose images may be used to measure curvatures over a large corneal area.

One type of photokeratoscope consists of a flat target (object) of black and white concentric rings, which is placed a few inches in front of the eye. Improved photokeratoscopes have aspherical targets (Figure 3.9).[70,71] A camera in an aperture at the center of the target

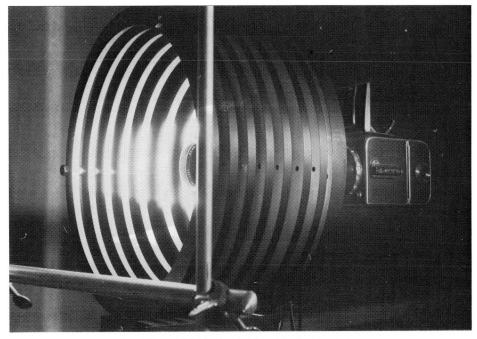

Figure 3.9. Author's photokeratoscope.

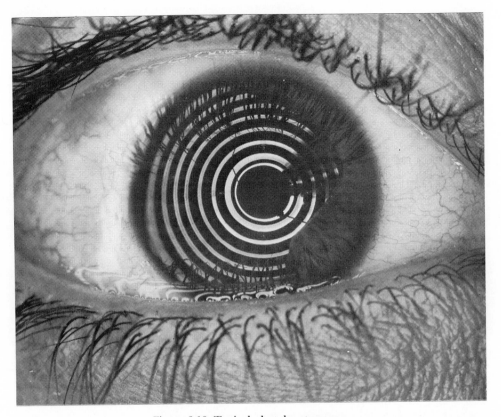

Figure 3.10. Typical photokeratogram.

is used to photograph the corneal image for a permanent record.

The radius of curvature for a given part of the cornea is a function of the separation of the target rings in the corneal image, which have been reflected from that corneal area (Figure 3.10). With the magnification of the camera known, the ring separations of the corneal image can be determined from the photograph.

The photokeratoscope does not measure the curvatures at all points on the cornea, but it does measure the curvatures at about ten small areas in each meridian where light from the target rings is reflected from the cornea. The total corneal area that is measured depends upon the size and shape of the object surface of the photokeratoscope. Hemispherical and cylindrical targets can be used to measure curvatures of nearly the whole

cornea, whereas the more easily constructed flat targets (the original type, which is still common today) can only be used to measure the central 7 mm. of the cornea.

A significant advance occurred in photokeratoscopy with the introduction of a method that allows a complete description of the corneal toricity from measurements of any three meridians.[71]

The photokeratoscope has occasionally been purported to have a greater accuracy than the ophthalmometer. However, this has not been substantiated experimentally.[28,72]

There is variation in values found by successive measurements on a steel ball with the photokeratoscope. Apparently, the most important factor is the difficulty of obtaining constant results with the film used for the keratograph.[73] Values of the corneal curvatures are determined by measuring the separations of the rings on the keratograph. Under magnification, these rings will have borders that are not sharply demarcated, but which are blurred due to the film grain. The exact position of the border of the ring is difficult to locate. If a second keratograph is made, the same position for the border must be used for measuring the ring separations. Variability in determining the position of the border can be reduced by the use of a photoelectronic scanning device (micro-densitometer). However, a slight rotation of the keratograph results in a reading that varies significantly from the original reading. Whether or not the microdensitometer is used,

additional variability may come from differences in the photosensitive material on the film or from differences in film shrinkage during development.

Thus, there are many sources of error that can cause a variation in repeated readings on a steel ball; consequently, these same errors must occur when the photokeratoscope is used to measure corneal curvatures.[17] In addition, new problems are added, such as alignment and fixation.[23] Perhaps this is the reason that Knoll found the accuracy of the photokeratoscope values to be uncertain above 0.20 mm.[3] Under ideal laboratory conditions this accuracy can be greatly improved.

TEMPLATE MEASUREMENTS

One of the oldest methods of determining the curvature of an optical surface is to match the surface with templates. Templates can be used to measure ophthalmic lens surfaces to an accuracy of better than

0.25 D. It has occasionally been suggested that the template principle also be used in measuring the corneal curvatures at various positions to determine the total contour.[74] Two general methods of testing this sugges-

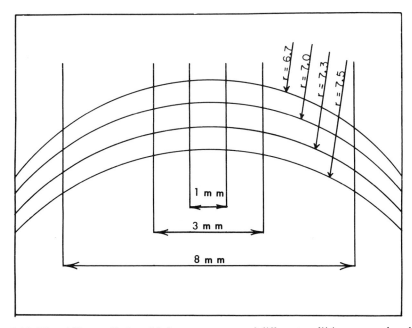

Figure 3.11. The ability to distinguish between curves of different radii increases when larger arcs are compared.

tion have been tried: the direct and the indirect. In the direct method a photograph or shadowgraph is taken of the eye from a lateral position, giving a profile replica of the cornea.[75,76] The photograph is enlarged and compared to templates.[17,77] In the indirect method an impression (mold) is taken of the eye, and a positive cast made from the impression. Templates are then applied to the positive cast,[78] or the cast is photographed, and the resulting picture is compared to templates.[79] If circular templates are compared to the aspherical corneal curve, a match is not possible for the entire cornea. Measurements of corneal arcs over 1 mm. in length would have considerable error due to the corneal asphericity. In order to determine the corneal contour, it is necessary to match templates to several small arcs of the corneal contour.

Unfortunately, the accuracy of the template method is very low when used to measure *small* arcs of a curve. This is illustrated in Figure 3.11, where it is shown that two curves with only slightly different radii may be distinguished easily if large portions of the curves are compared, but they appear nearly identical if only small arcs are compared.

Even when profile corneal photographs are enlarged as much as 100 times, it is difficult to match a template to a small area of the cornea. If the curvature is measured by matching a template over a 1 mm. corneal arc, the accuracy is found to be about ± 4.00 D.[73] If the measurement is taken over a 3 mm. arc, the accuracy can only be increased to about ± 2.00 D. In addition to these experimental results, it has been shown mathematically that higher accuracies in measuring the corneal contour are not to be expected from the template method.[73] Consequently, profile photography is of little value in the measurement of the corneal contour.

STEREOPHOTOGRAMMETRY

If a cornea is anaesthetized and covered with talcum powder, it is possible to take a stereoscopic photograph of its surface. The corneal contour can be reconstructed by the stereophotogrammetric methods used in aerial photography of ground contour.[26,80]

Bonnet and Cochet reported that in using this method, the mean error of the height found for the corneal topography is rarely more than 0.03 mm.[19] However, these measurements are of *relative corneal heights,* which gives much lower accuracy figures when interpreted in terms of radii of curvature.

OTHER METHODS

Other methods that have been used in attempts to measure corneal contour include mechanical tracing with a pantograph type of apparatus, ultrasonics, biological sectioning of the cornea, or measurements with an optical spherometer. None of these has yet proved sufficiently accurate.

CORNEAL STABILITY

There is a long history of research supporting the concept that the contour of the normal cornea is stable over short time periods.[81,82] However, a few investigators postulated that a force from the lids or ocular muscles might be capable of changing the corneal contour.[83-85] Corneal contour changes are known to occur as the result of pathological conditions such as keratoconus, meibomian cysts, and bilateral monocular diplopia.[86-88] There have been reports of corneal contour changes as a result of changes in convergence, pupil diameter, ambient temperature, and time of day and as an effect of miotics or mydriatics.[28,89] Suzuki has shown by an indirect method that very slight changes occur in the corneal curvature during systole and diastole.[90]

As a whole, the short-term stability of the cornea appears to be very high, unless external pressure is applied.[91,92]

Corneal stability studies are rare because of the difficulties in obtaining accurate measurements of the cornea.[93-97] When a difference occurs in the corneal measurements, which are taken at various times, it is difficult to determine if the difference is due to actual corneal curvature changes or to instrument error.[98-100]

A change in the curvature of the cornea can be easily demonstrated by measuring the cornea with a keratometer before and after manually pulling the lids taut.

Mandell and St. Helen investigated corneal stability with a new high accuracy photokeratoscope to determine the influence of accommodation, convergence, pupil size, eye position, lid position, lid closure, miotics, and rubbing.[43] Significant changes in corneal curvature occurred as a result of lid forces, digital pressure, and rubbing.

The results of these experiments are summarized in Table 3.1. Of a total of fifty-two experiments, thirteen showed corneal changes which were statistically significant (numbers in parentheses), representing the conditions of "Force Open," "Digital Pressure," "Rubbing," and "Lid Pull." For the other variables, no significant corneal change occurred. Forcing the lids open, "Lid Pull" or direct "Digital Pressure" produced a corneal curvature increase in the meridian for which the pressure was applied (vertical) and a decrease at 90 degrees from this meridian (Figures 3.12, 3.13, and 3.14).

Rubbing the eye caused a general distor-

TABLE 3.1

Subject	Hold Open	Force Open	Voluntary Open	Digital Pressure	Temporally Fixated	Nasally Fixated	Downwardly Fixated	Upwardly Fixated	Accommodation	Convergence	Miotic	Blink	Voluntary Lid Squeeze	Rubbing	Lid Pull
B.Q.	1		1												
A.A.	2	(2)	1		1	1	1			1					(1)
R.M.	1	(1)	1	(2)	1	1	1	1							(4)
M.K.	1	1	1									1			
G.L.		3	1					1	1	1		1	1	(1)	
R.W.		2	1					1		1			1	(1)	
J.W.		1	1					1	1	1				(1)	

tion that remained for several minutes and probably represents a disruption of the tear layer or epithelial surface (Figure 3.15).

CORNEAL DIMENSIONS

CORNEAL DIAMETER

Most investigators of corneal diameter have assumed that a measurement of the visible iris diameter is probably a close approximation of the true corneal diameter. Values that have been reported for the visible iris diameter usually fall between 10.5 and 13.5 mm.[101] and are smaller than the measurements made from eye molds or from contact lenses[102] which have been fitted to the eye. Some discrepancy is to be expected between these two methods of measuring the cornea, since the outer border of the iris does not necessarily have a definite relation to the outer border of the cornea.

Obrig and Salvatori[103] found average corneal diameter values of 12 mm. for the vertical and 13.6 mm. for the horizontal meridians. Their data for 1,000 eyes are presented in Table 3.2. In all cases except one, the cornea was found to be oval, with the vertical meridian measuring 0.5 to 3.0 mm. smaller than the horizontal meridian. The diameters were measured by taking a mold of the eye and making a positive cast which was measured with a pair of calipers. They found that with only a few exceptions the corneas showed definite "points" on the nasal and temporal margins which fell on a horizontal line bi-secting the cornea. These points have been observed by other investigators and are called *corneal notches*. They are generally considered to occur in only a small percentage of corneas. If the notches do indeed occur in most corneas, then their inclusion in the diameter of the cornea will make the findings of Obrig and Salvatori larger than would be expected from other methods.

The author measured total corneal diameters for twelve subjects from profile photographs.[27] The mean size for the total diameter was 12.08 mm., and the standard deviation was ±0.48 mm. These values are in accord with values obtained by anatomical measurements.

The author determined what relationship existed between the size of the corneal diameter as measured from the profile view and the size of the iris as measured from the front view. The correlation between the hand method and the profile photograph was +0.60, the profile view giving a value that, on the average, was 0.7 mm. larger than the value obtained from the visible iris diameter measurement.

The visible iris diameter is inversely related to the corneal power (Figure 3.16).

SAGITTA

The mean value for the corneal sagitta of twelve subjects was found to be 2.59 mm. and the standard deviation ±0.22 mm.[27] It is interesting to note that the sagittal depth obtained by profile photography is consider-ably smaller than values reported for the depth of the anterior chamber, which are obtained by measuring the distance from the corneal surface to the anterior surface of the crystalline lens.

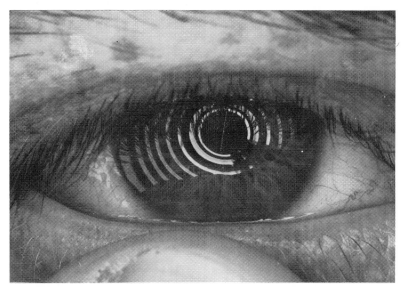

Figure 3.12. Corneal distortion caused by direct digital pressure.

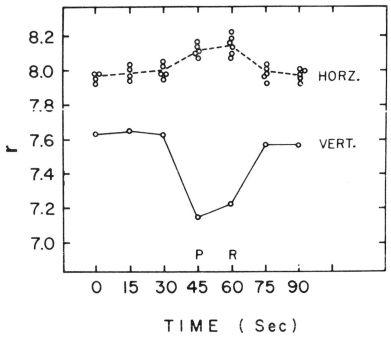

Figure 3.13. Graph of corneal distortion caused by direct digital pressure. *r* is corneal radius, *P* pressure applied, and *R* pressure released.

CORNEAL-SCLERAL JUNCTION

Figure 3.17 shows profile photographs of the horizontal meridians of corneas. Attention is directed to the corneal-scleral junction where it may be seen that instead of an abrupt change, there is a smooth transition between the two curves. It may also be noted that it is extremely difficult to detect a single point for the junction, although this task is somewhat easier on the original photographs.

The average angle for the corneal-scleral junction is only about 12 degrees.[27]

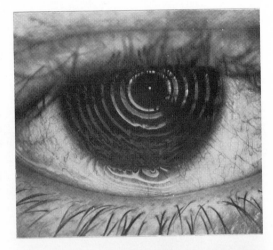

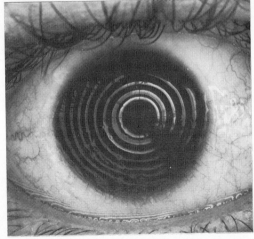

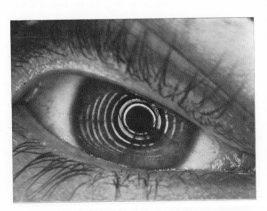

Figure 3.14. Corneal distortion caused by stretching the lid.

Figure 3.15. Temporary corneal distortion caused by ten seconds of eye massage through the lid: (a) fifteen seconds after massage, (b) one minute after massage.

CORNEAL APEX

It is well known that the apex of the cornea does not generally coincide with the line of sight or the geometric center of the cornea.[42,62,104,105] The locations of the corneal apexes for the right eyes of seven adults are giv-

en in Table 3.3. In each case the apex was decentered from the line of sight, but a directional trend does not exist. The curvature is slightly greater at the apex than at the line of sight. The mean difference was 0.13 D. for the ver-

TABLE 3.2

CORNEAL DIAMETERS (OBRIG AND SALVATORI)

Horizontal Diameter (mm.)	Vertical Diameter (mm.)							Total	Per Cent
	10.5	11.0	11.5	12.0	12.5	13.0	13.5		
15.0				3	8	14	12	37	3.7
14.5		1	5	19	30	22	1	78	7.8
14.0		5	22	139	75	21		262	26.2
13.5	3	15	41	143	49	6		257	25.7
13.0	5	51	81	88	16	1		242	24.2
12.5	12	35	26	4				77	7.7
12.0	4	27	10					41	4.1
11.5	6							6	0.6
Total	30	134	185	400	174	64	13		
Per Cent	3	13.4	18.5	40.0	17.4	6.4	1.3		

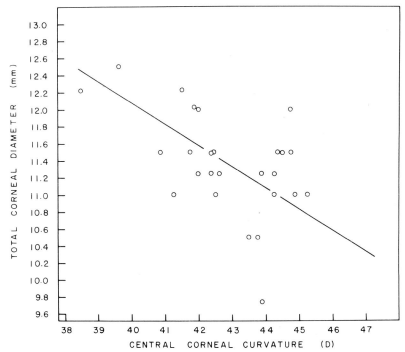

Figure 3.16. Relationship between total corneal diameter and central corneal (keratometer) power.

tical meridian and 0.36 D. for the horizontal meridian. There was not a significant reduc-tion in corneal toricity at the apex, as has been reported.[81]

Contact Lens Practice

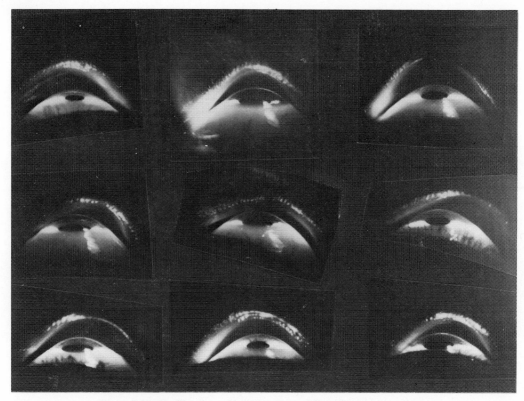

Figure 3.17. Profile view of horizontal meridians for nine corneas.

TABLE 3.3

Subject	L.O.S.	Apex	Difference	Apex Position
G.L ...	45.37/94	45.50/92	0.13	5° Temp.
	43.80	44.50	0.70	5° Inf.
D.A. ...	45.50/73	45.50/63	0.0	9° Nas.
	44.37	45.00	0.62	5° Sup.
R.H. ..	44.25/115	45.00/90	0.75	9° Temp.
	43.62	44.00	0.37	5° Inf.
R.W. ..	44.33/88	44.95/84	0.62	14° Temp.
	41.62	42.00	0.38	5° Sup.
R.P. ...	45.00/78	45.12/81	0.12	5° Nas.
	44.50	44.40	−0.10	5° Sup.
M.C. ..	41.87/112	42.37/95	0.50	0°
.	42.50	42.75	0.25	9° Inf.
J.A. ...	42.37/86	42.40/80	0.03	5° Temp.
	40.75	40.87	0.12	5° Inf.

REFERENCES

1. Aubert, H.: Nähert Sich die Hornhautkrummung am meisten der Ellipse, *Pfluegers Arch.*, *35*:597–621, 1885.

2. Stenstrom, S.: Investigation of the variation and the correlation of the optical elements of human eyes (translated by D. Woolf), *Am. J. Optom.*, *25*(5):218–232, 1948.

3. Knoll, H.: Corneal contours in the general population as revealed by the photokeratoscope, *Am. J. Optom.*, *38*(7):389–397, 1961.

4. Tscherning, M.: *Physiologic Optics*, Philadelphia, 1904, *The Keystone* (translated by Carl Weiland).

5. Helmholtz, H.: *Physiological Optics, Menasha, Banta, 1924, vol. I, p. 211 (translated by James Southall).*

6. Noto, F.: Studies on the form of anterior corneal surface, *Acta Soc. Ophthalmol. Jap.*, *65*(3):447–468, 1961.

7. Berg, F.: Vergleichende Messungen der Form der vorderen Hornhautfläche mit Ophthalmometer und mit photographischer Methode, *Acta Ophthalmol.*, *7*:386–423, 1929.

8. Duke-Elder, S., and Wybar, K. C.: *System of Ophthalmology: The Anatomy of the Visual System*, St. Louis, Mosby, 1961, vol. 2, pp. 92–94.

9. Tour, R. L.: Symposium: Contact lenses, definition: Anatomy and physiology of the cornea, *Trans. Am. Acad. Ophthalmol. Otolaryngol.*, *66*(3):278–285, 1962.

10. Reynolds, A. E., and Kratt, H. J.: The photoelectronic keratoscope, *Contacto*, *3*(3):53–59, 1959.

11. *The Ophthalmometer*, Optical Developments, Bausch and Lomb, Inc., Dec., 1939.

12. Hamilton, C. B.: An investigation of corneal profiles, *Contacto*, *7*(3):9–16, 1963.

13. Bier, N.: A study of the cornea in relation to contact lens practice, *Am. J. Optom.*, *33*(6):291–304, 1956.

14. Evershed-Martin, L.: The sanctity of corneal clarity and some contact lens fallacies, *Br. J. Physiol. Opt.*, *16*(1):24–25, 1959.

15. McMonnies, C. W.: New thinking on old thinking—corneal curvature, *Austr. J. Optom.*, *50*(1):8–17, 1967.

16. Levene, J. R.: An evaluation of the hand keratoscope as a diagnostic instrument for corneal astigmatism, Part II, *Br. J. Physiol. Opt.*, *19*(4):237–251, 1962.

17. Stone, J.: The validity of some existing methods of measuring corneal contour compared with suggested new methods, *Br. J. Physiol. Opt.*, *19*(4):205–230, 1962.

18. Mandell, R. B.: Keratometry and contact lens practice, *Optom. Weekly*, *456*(18):69–75, 1965.

19. Bonnet, R., and Cochet, P.: New method of topographic ophthalmometry—its theoretical and clinical applications, *Am. J. Optom.*, *39*(5):227–251, 1962.

20. Bennett, A. G.: A new keratometer and its application to corneal topography, *Br. J. Physiol. Opt.*, *21*(4):234–238, 1964.

21. Mandell, R. B.: Corneal curvature measurements by the aid of Moiré fringes, *J. Am. Optom. Assoc.*, *373*(3):219–242, 1966.

22. Mandell, R. B., and York, M. A.: A new calibration system for photokeratoscopy, *Am. J. Optom.*, *46*(6):410–417, 1969.

23. Clark, B. A.: *The Determination of Corneal Topography*, Master's thesis, University of Melbourne, 1966.

24. Westheimer, G. A.: A method of photoelectric keratoscopy, *Am. J. Optom.*, *42*(5):315–320, 1965.

25. Mandell, R. B.: Unpublished study.

26. Bertotto, E. V.: The stereophotogrammetric study of the anterior segment of the eye, *Am. J. Ophthalmol.*, *3*(5):573–579, 1948.

27. Mandell, R. B.: *Morphometry of the Human Cornea*, Doctoral thesis, Indiana University, 1962.

28. Reynolds, A. E.: Corneal topography as found by photo-electronic-keratoscopy, *Contacto*, *3*(8):229–233, 1959.

29. Levene, J. R.: The true inventors of the keratoscope and photokeratoscope, *Br. J. Hist. Sci.*, *2*:324, 1965.

30. Brungardt, T. F.: Contact lens clinic (keratometer readings), *Optom. Weekly*, *59*(7):47–48, 1968.

31. Lehmann, S. P.: Corneal areas utilized in keratometry, *The Optician*, *154*(3989):261–264, 1967.

32. May, M. C.: Investigation of corneal curvature, *Contacto*, *1(1)*:7–9, 1957.

33. Bayshore, C. A.: Exploration of the corneal curvature, *Contacto*, *3(7)*:188–190, 1959.

34. Jessop, D. G.: Plotting corneal topography, *Contacto*, *5(2)*:69–74, 1961.

35. Grosvenor, T.: Clinical use of the keratometer in evaluating the corneal contour, *Am. J. Optom.*, *38(5)*:237–246, 1961.

36. Jessop, D. G.: Peripheral corneal readings— corneal isopters, *Contacto*, *7(2)*:7–16, 1963.

37. Jessop, D. G.: Corneal topography, *Contacto*, *5(10)*:325–332, 1961.

38. Luneburg, R. J.: Method of analysis of peripheral keratometry findings, *Optom. Weekly*, *60(33)*:25–30, 1969.

39. Watkins, J.: Scllentecorel by the four "C" method, *Contacto*, *8(1)*:27–28, 1964.

40. Jessop, D. G.: Para-central readings and apical clearance fitting, *Contacto*, *9(1)*: 10–13, 1965.

41. Handal, J. P.: Some considerations concerning corneal topography and determination of contact lens base curves, *Contacto*, *7(6)*:8–15, 31–32, 1963.

42. Wallace, H.: Systems of analyzing peripheral corneal topography—a comparison, *Opt. J. Rev. Optom.*, *105(22)*:33–35, 1968.

43. Mandell, R. B., and St. Helen, R.: Stability of the corneal contour, *Am. J. Optom.*, *45(12)*:797–806, 1968.

44. Mandell, R. B., and St. Helen, R.: Position and curvature of the corneal apex, *Am. J. Optom.*, *46(1)*:25–29, 1969.

45. Weymounth, F.: *Laboratory Experiments in Physiological Optics*, Los Angeles College of Optometry, 1953.

46. Bier, N.: The fallacy of ophthalmometry, *Br. J. Physiol. Opt.*, *21(4)*:224–233, 1964.

47. Mandell, R. B.: Reflection point ophthalmometry, *Am. J. Optom.*, *39(10)*:513–537, 1962.

48. Cochet, P., and Barbara, G.: Topographic ophthalmometry and contact lenses, *Survey Ophthalmol.*, *9(3)*:358–359, 1964.

49. Prijot, E. et al.: Topographic variations of the curvature radius of the cornea—its importance for the prescription of corneal lenses (in Fr.), *Bull. Soc. Belge. Ophthalmol.*, *138*:429–437, 1964.

50. LeGrand, Y.: Studies on the human cornea: Application to the aphakic eye, in Giles, G. H. (Ed.): *Transactions of the International Ophthalmology and Optometry Congress*, London, Lockwood, 1961.

51. Mandell, R. B.: Methods to measure the peripheral corneal curvature, Part 3: ophthalmometry, *J. Am. Optom. Assoc.*, *33(12)*:889–892, 1962.

52. Mandell, R. B.: Methods to measure the peripheral corneal curvature, Part 2: Geometric construction and computers, *J. Am. Optom. Assoc.*, *33(8)*:585–589, 1962.

53. Sampson, W. G. et al.: Topographical keratometry and contact lenses, *Trans. Am. Acad. Ophthalmol. Otolaryngol.*, *69(5)*:959–969, 1965.

54. Girard, L. J. et al.: Corneal topography, in King, J. H., and McTigue, J. W. (Eds.): *The Cornea World Congress*, Washington, Butterworths, 1965, pp. 617–626.

55. Sampson, W. G. et al.: Topographical keratometry and contact lenses, *Trans. Am. Acad. Ophthalmol. Otolaryngol.*, *69(5)*:959–970, 1965.

56. Soper, J. W. et al.: Corneal topography, keratometry, and contact lenses, *Arch. Ophthalmol.*, *67(6)*:753–760, 1962.

57. Mandell, R. B.: Small mire ophthalmometry, paper read before the annual meeting of American Academy of Optometry, Miami, Florida, 1962.

58. Mandell, R. B.: Corneal areas utilized in keratometry, *Am. J. Optom.*, *41(3)*:150–153, 1964.

59. Mandell, R. B.: Corneal contour and contact lenses, paper read before the annual meeting of the American Academy of Optometry, Chicago, Illinois, 1963.

60. Mandell, R. B.: Keratometry and contact lens practice, *Optom. Weekly*, *56(18)*:69–75, 1965.

61. Wittenberg, S.: Appendix to Part I, in Gullstrand, Allvar: *Photographic-Ophthalmometric and Clinical Investigations of Corneal Refraction*, translated by William M. Ludlam, *Am. J. Optom.*, *43(3)*:198–214, 1966.

62. Chiquiar-Arias, M.: Apex of the cornea and directed keratometry, *Contacto*, *5(6)*:201–204, 1961.

63. Ritz, N. W.: Keratoscopic photographs of the cornea, *The Optician*, *144(3744)*:657–

659, 1963.

64. Ludlam, W. M., and Henberg, J. W.: Photo-keratoscopy, *Can. J. Optom.*, *28*(2):47–50, 1966.

65. Cochet, P. et al.: Photokeratoscopy, an element in corneal biometry (in Fr.), *Bull. Soc. Ophtalmol. Fr.*, *66*:1094–1104, 1966.

66. Wittenberg, S., and Ludlam, W. M.: Derivation of a system for analyzing the corneal surface from photokeratoscopic data, *J. Opt. Soc. Am.*, *56*(11):1612–1615, 1966.

67. Cochet, P.: Presenting a recent photo-kerametric method, *Contacto*, *12*(2):12–19, 1968.

68. Ludlam, W. M. et al.: Photographic analysis of the ocular dioptric components, *Am. J. Optom.*, *44*(5):279–296, 1967.

69. Brown, N.: A simplified photokeratoscope, *Am. J. Ophthalmol.*, *68*(3):517–519, 1969.

70. Townsley, G.: New equipment and methods for determining the contour of the human cornea, *Contacto*, *11*(4):72–81, 1967.

71. York, M.A.: *A System of Photokeratoscope Calibration and Its Application in the Study of Corneal Development*, Master's thesis, University of California, 1968.

72. Blair, W. A.: Photo-electronic keratoscopy testing, *Contacto*, *4*(7):217–227, 1960.

73. Mandell, R. B.: Methods to measure the peripheral corneal curvature—Part I, Photokeratoscopy, *J. Am. Optom. Assoc.*, *33*(2):137–139, 1961.

74. Daily, L., Jr., and Kaily, R. K.: Modification of corneal contact lenses, *Int. Ophthalmol. Clin.*, *1*(2):441–494, 1961.

75. Martin, W. F.: Fitting of contact lenses utilizing a new photographic method, *Contacto*, *11*(1):44–46, 1967.

76. Bitonte, J. L., and Bitonte, J. A.: The corneopter-corneograph—a new topographic instrument, *Contacto*, *11*(4):6–10, 1967.

77. Mandell, R. B.: Profile methods of measuring corneal curvature, *J. Am. Optom. Assoc.*, *32*(8):627–631, 1961.

78. Salvatori, P.: The elusive corneal cap; paper read before the American Academy of Optometry, Miami, Florida, 1962.

79. Elliott, D. O.: Drafting the requirements for a minimum clearance corneal contact lens, *Am. J. Optom.*, *33*(11):602–603, 1956.

80. Rzymkowsky, J.: Stereophotographic and stereophotogrammetric reproduction of the cornea and sclera of the living eye (translated by W. P. Schumann), *Am. J. Optom.*, *31*(8):416–422, 1954.

81. Ludlam, W. M.: Human experimentation and research on refractive state, in Hirsch, M. J. (Ed.): *Synopsis of the Refractive State of the Eye; A Symposium*, Minneapolis, Burgess, 1967, pp. 13–25.

82. Young, T.: On the mechanism of the eye; the Bakerian lecture, *Philos. Trans. R. Soc. Lond.* [*Biol. Sci.*], *91*:23–88, 1801.

83. Leroy, C. J. A.: Recherches sur l'influence exercée par les muscles de l'oeil sur la forme normale de la cornée humaine, in Masson, G. (Ed.): *Mémoires d'Ophtalmometrie*, Paris, 1890.

84. Marin-Amat, M.: Les variations physiologiques de la courbure de la cornée pendant la vie; leur importance et transcendance dan la réfraction oculaire, *Bull. Soc. Belge Ophtalmol.*, *113*:251–293, 1956.

85. López-Lacarrère, J.: La córnea inestable, *Arch. Soc. Oftal. Hispano-Americana*, *15*:552–556, 1955.

86. Javal, E.: Variation rythmiques de la courbure de la cornée, *Séances et Mem. Soc. Biol.*, *36*:581, 1884.

87. Mandell, R. B.: Bilateral monocular diplopia following near work, *Am. J. Optom.*, *43*(8):500–504, 1966.

88. Ormond, A. W.: Notes on three cases of acquired astigmatism associated with meibomian cysts, *Br. J. Ophthalmol.*, *5*:117–118, 1921.

89. Weale, R. A.: On corneal curvature, *The Optician*, *148*(3844):552–557, 1964.

90. Suzuki, I.: Corneal pulsation and corneal pulse waves, *Jap. J. Ophthalmol.*, *6*(4):6–10, 1962.

91. Fairmaid, J. A.: The constancy of corneal curvature, *Br. J. Physiol. Opt.*, *16*(1):2–23, 1959.

92. Daily, L., and Coe, R. E.: Lack of effect of anesthetic and mydriatic solutions on the curvature of the cornea, *Am. J. Ophthalmol.*, *53*(1):49–51, 1962.

93. Bronstein, L.: Experiments in keratometry, *Contacto*, *6*(10):298–301, 1962.

94. Clark, B. A. J.: Autocollimating photo-keratoscope, *J. Opt. Soc. Am.*, 62(2):169–176, 1972.
95. El Hage, S. G.: Suggested new methods for photokeratoscopy, a comparison for their validities—Part 1, *Am. J. Optom.*, 48(11):897–911, 1971.
96. El Hage, S. G., and Berny, F.: Contribution of the crystalline lens to the spherical aberration of the eye, *J. Opt. Soc. Am.*, 63(2):205–211, 1973.
97. Mandell, R. B., and St. Helen, R.: Mathematical model of the corneal contour, *Br. J. Physiol. Opt.*, 26(3):183–197, 1971.
98. Kikkawa, Y.: Diurnal variation in corneal thickness, *Exp. Eye Res.*, 15(1):1–9, 1973.
99. Alezzandrini, A. A. et al.: Radius of the unstable corneal curvature (in Sp.), *Arch. Oftal. B. Air.*, 37:148–151, 1962.
100. Löpping, B., and Weale, R. A.: Changes in corneal curvature following ocular convergence, *Vision Res.*, 5(4):207–215, 1965.
101. Duke-Elder, S.: *Textbook of Ophthalmology*, reprint, St. Louis, Mosby, 1946, vol. 1, p. 40.
102. Bier, N.: *Contact Lens Routine and Practice*, 2nd ed., London, Butterworths, 1957, p. 130.
103. Obrig, T.: *Contact Lenses*, 2nd ed., Philadelphia, Chilton, 1947, pp. 22–23.
104. Chiquiar-Arias, M.: Central vs. directed keratometry for base curve determination of contact lenses, *Contacto*, 11(2):15–17, 1967.
105. Chiquiar-Arias, M.: Measuring the true apex of the cornea with the keratometer, *Contacto*, 4(6):195–198, 1960.

ADDITIONAL READINGS

Alsbirk, P. H.: Corneal thickness I. Age variation, sex difference and oculometric correlations, *Acta Ophthalmol.*, 56(1):95, 1978.

Alsbirk, P. H.: Corneal thickness II. Environmental and genetic factors, *Acta Ophthalmol.*, 56(1):105, 1978.

Azen, S. P. et al.: A comparison of three methods for the measurement of corneal thickness, *Invest. Ophthalmol.*, 18(5):535–538, 1979.

Ball, R., Smolen, D., and Zacks, J. L.: Postnatal changes in corneal curvature, *Am. J. Optom. Physiol. Opt.*, 53(4):165–167, 1976.

Bibby, M. M.: The Wesley-Jessen System 2000 Photokeratoscope, *Cont. Lens Forum*, 1(7):37–45, 1976.

Bibby, M. M., and Townsley, M. G.: Analysis and description of corneal shape, *Cont. Lens Forum*, 1(8):27–35, 1976.

Bibby, M. W., and Townsley, M. G.: Corneal contour: the things to know, *Cont. Lens Forum*, 2(1):45–53, 1977.

Binder, P. S., Kohler, J. A., and Rorabaugh, D. A.: Evaluation of an electronic corneal pachometer, *Invest. Ophthalmol. Vis. Sci.*, 16(9):855, 1977.

Blueston, R. et al.: Lacrimal immunoglobulins and complement quantified by Couter-immunoelectrophoresis, *Br. J. Ophthalmol.*, 59(5):279–281, 1975.

Bonavida, B., and Saspe, A. T.: Human tear lysozyme: I. Purification, physicochemical and immunochemical characterization, *J. Lab. Clin. Med.*, 70(6):951–962, 1967.

Bonavida, B., and Saspe, A. T.: Human tear lysozyme. II. Quantitative determination with standard Schirmer strips, *Am. J. Ophthalmol.*, 66(1):70–75, 1968.

Bowman, K. J., and Carney, L. G.: The effect of non-contact tonometry on corneal topography, *J. Am. Optom. Assoc.*, 49(12):1389, 1978.

Brown, S. I. and Dervichian, D. G.: Hydrodynamics of blinking—*in vitro* study of the interaction of superficial oily layer and the tears, *Arch. Ophthalmol.*, 82(4):541–547, 1969.

Brubaker, R., Puffer, M. J., and Neault, R. W.: Basal precorneal tear turnover in the human eye, *Am. J. Ophthalmol.*, 89(3):369–376, 1980.

Brubaker, S. and McDonald, J. E.: Meniscus-induced thinning of tear films, *Am. J. Ophthalmol.*, 72(1):139, 1971.

Brungardt, T.: The relationship of corneal curvature to corneal diameter, *Optom. Weekly*, 67(29):803–805, 1976.

Brungardt, T. F.: Sagittal height of the cornea, *Am. J. Optom.*, 42(9):525, 1965.

Brungardt, T. F.: K readings versus valid corneal curvature values, *J. Am. Optom. Assoc.*, 46(3):

230–233, 1975.

Brungardt, T. F.: The split ball experiment, *Cont. Lens Forum*, p. 54, Feb. 1980.

Carney, L. G., and Hill, R. M.: Human tear pH, *Arch. Ophthalmol.*, *94(5)*:821–824, 1976.

Carney, L. G., and Hill, R. M.: Tear pH: hydrophilic lenses and the closed eye, *Int. Cont. Lens Clin.*, *3(4)*:30–31, 1976.

Carney, L. G., and Hill, R. M.: Human tear pH—how individualized?, *Austr. J. Optom.*, *60(7)*:258, 1977.

Carney, L. G., and Fullard, R. J.: Ocular irritation and environmental pH, *Austr. J. Optom.*, *62(8)*: 335, 1979.

Clark, B. A. J.: Mean topography of normal corneas, *Austr. J. Optom.*, *57(4)*:107–114, 1974.

El Hage, S. G. et al.: Evaluation of corneal thickness induced by hard and flexible contact lens wear, *Am. J. Optom. Physiol. Opt.*, *51(1)*:24–33, 1974.

El Hage, S. I., and Leach, N. E.: Central and peripheral corneal thickness changes induced by "on K", steep, and flat contact lens wear, *J. Am. Optom. Assoc.*, *46(3)*:296–302, 1975.

Enoch, J. M.: Techniques for evaluating scleral curvature and corneal vault, *Cont. Lens J.*, *8(5)*:19, 1979.

Filderman, I. P.: Precision measurement of the corneal topography, *J. Am. Optom. Assoc.*, *47(9)*: 1169–1170, 1976.

Forst, G.: Experiments with the tear film break-up time, *Optom. Suppl.*, p. 51, Jan. 1976.

Francois, J. et al.: Disposition of the collagen structures in the corneal stroma, *Cont. Intraoc. Lens Med. J.*, *1(1–2)*:13–28, 1975.

Frankel, S. H., and Ellis, P. P.: Effect of oral contraceptives on tear production, *Ann. Opthalmol.*, *10(11)*:1585–1588, 1978.

Freedman, A. J.: Using aerial reconnaisance for the design of PMMA contact lens base curve and optic diameter and for monitoring cornea changes, *Contacto*, *22(2)*:32, 1978.

Freeman, J. M.: The punctum plug: evaluation of a new treatment for the dry eye, *Trans. Am. Acad. Ophthalmol. Otolaryngol.*, *79(6)*:874–879, 1975.

Freeman, R. D.: Corneal radius of curvature of the kitten and the cat, *Invest. Ophthalmol.*, *19(3)*:306–308, 1980.

Fry, G. A.: Analysis of photometric data, *Am. J. Optom. Physiol. Opt.*, *52(5)*:305–312, 1975.

Hansen, F. K.: A clinical study of the normal human central corneal thickness, *Acta Ophthalmol.*, *49(1)*:82–89, 1971.

Hasegawa, S.: A comparison of slitlamp photographs of corneal thickening before and five hours after wearing of hard contact lenses, *J. Jap. Cont. Lens Soc.*, *16(10)*:133–134, 1974.

Hirano, A.: Stereoscopic observations and analytical study over the Placido images, *Folia Ophthalmol. Jap.*, *28(1)*:5–10, 1977.

Itoi, M.: A new photokeratometry system, *J. Jap. Cont. Lens Soc.*, *21(5)*:171, 1979.

Kawara, T.: Corneal topography using Moiré contour fringes, *Applied Optics*, *18(21)*:3675, 1979.

Kiely, P. M., and Carney, L. G.: Influence of lid pressure on corneal topography, *Austr. J. Optom.*, *61(11)*:390, 1978.

Kiely, P. M., and Carney, L. G.: Influence of ophthalmic solutions on corneal contour, *Austr. J. Optom.*, *61(1)*:6, 1978.

Knoll, H. A.: The stability of the shape of the human cornea, *Am. J. Optom. Physiol. Opt.*, *53(7)*:359–361, 1976.

Kuyama, J.: A new photokeratometer for contact lens in clinic, *J. Jap. Cont. Lens Soc.*, *21(3)*:80, 1979.

Lo Cascio, G.: Contribution to the knowledge of the curvature of the sclera in the forward section of the eye, *Ann. di Otta. e Clin. Ocul.*, April 1934.

Mandell, R. B., and St. Helen, R.: Position and curvature of the corneal apex, *Am. J. Optom. Arch. Am. Acad. Optom.*, *46(1)*:25–29, 1969.

Chapter 4

CONSULTATION, EXAMINATION, AND PROGNOSIS

MICHAEL G. HARRIS

CONSULTATION

IT IS ADVISABLE to conduct a preexamination consultation with each potential contact lens wearer. The consultation serves two purposes. It gives the patient an opportunity to receive valid information about contact lenses, and it gives the fitter the opportunity to determine whether the patient appears to be a suitable candidate for wearing contact lenses.[1] Indiscriminate fitting of contact lenses to all patients will only leave the practitioner with a large number of problem cases.

A properly conducted consultation may save the fitter and the patient considerable time and expense and will help avoid the unhappy aftermath of a fitting failure. If, from the consultation, the patient appears to be a good candidate for contact lenses, the information exchanged will better prepare the patient for the actual fitting and will reduce the amount of time that would otherwise be required later in the examination.

During the consultation it is important that the patient's confidence be gained and that good rapport be established immediately,[2-4] but the fitter must, from the beginning, avoid overstating the advantages and minimizing the disadvantages of contact lenses.

Much of the consultation must invariably be devoted to answering many of the patient's questions. These questions normally concern his chances of successfully wearing contact lenses.

ABILITY TO WEAR CONTACT LENSES

Not all patients fitted with contact lenses can wear them successfully. Estimates of the unsuccessful portion of patients fitted vary from 3 to 30 percent.[5-15] These estimates differ because various practitioners use different and often vague criteria for judging the success of their patients. Reports of 90 percent success are certainly far too high.

Some fitters included among their "successful" patients those who had not returned with a complaint or a request for a fee reduction.[6]

Sarver and Harris evaluated patient success by the five criteria of adequate wearing time, good comfort, proper vision, normal patient appearance, and lack of significant ocular tissue changes (Table 4.1).[11] After one year of lens wear, 72.9 percent of the corneal contact lens patients were successful by these criteria even though a higher percentage passed each individual criterion (Table 4.2). It would appear that many of the figures that show a high percentage of success probably include many patients who failed one or more of these criteria or who no longer wore their lenses. The patient should be advised that many factors affect the chances for success, perhaps the most important being need and motivation.

COMFORT OF CONTACT LENSES

It is not often that a real sensation of pain occurs in either the fitting or wearing of contact lenses. There is, however, a definite touch sensation that may be irritating during the adjustment period. Many patients report that after a brief adjustment period they are not aware that their contact lenses are being worn. On the other hand, a large number of patients report that they continue to experience a slight touch sensation but that it is not particularly annoying. The patient should not be misinformed that he will be totally unaware of his lenses once he adapts to them.[16] In cases where comfort is a problem, gel lenses may be of benefit.

VISION

Some myopic contact lens wearers report that their vision seems improved when they wear contact lenses rather than spectacles.[17-19] This might be expected because, compared to spectacle lenses, contact lenses produce a slight increase in magnification of the retinal image, are free from the obstruction of the spectacle frame, produce a slight increase in light from increased transmission, and cause fewer optical aberrations that affect vision. An examination often shows, however, that these effects do not necessarily improve the measurable visual acuity. Any increase in magnification of the retinal image by contact lenses in comparison to spectacles is not significant, except for higher lens powers. The spectacle frame is psychologically annoying but actually causes little obstruction of the visual field.[20,21] The increased light transmission through the lenses is not sufficient to make a detectable change in visual acuity. The one factor that does make considerable difference, however, is the quality of the retinal image. With contact lenses the patient views through the optical center of the lens at nearly all times, thus avoiding the aberrations that are encountered when viewing through the periphery of spectacle lenses. This becomes particularly important in prescriptions of higher power.

When contact lenses are worn, the patient usually experiences increased sensitivity to light.[22,23] Hence, the visual field appears brighter. The same sensation occurs when there is an irritation to the eye such as that which occurs in conjunctivitis. It is possible that the contact lenses give the patient a feeling that objects appear brighter, and he reports this as improved vision. This report is sometimes made even when the measurable acuity is actually lower for the patient when he wears contact lenses than when he wears spectacles.[24]

In a significant proportion of cases, visual acuity will be noticeably lower in the patient wearing contact lenses.[25] This can usually be traced to an astigmatic refractive error, which remains after correction with contact

TABLE 4.1

CRITERIA OF A SUCCESSFUL PATIENT RESPONSE

1. Wearing time. The patient must be able to wear his lenses regularly and continuously for a minimum period of eight hours.
2. Comfort. The patient may experience no more than a slight lens awareness, slight photophobia in sunlight, and/or an occasional foreign body sensation.
3. Vision. The patient must report no significant blur, flare, or edge reflections, and his visual acuity must be within one Snellen line of the visual acuity achieved with his best spectacle lens correction. He must report no significant spectacle blur following lens removal.
4. Ocular tissue changes. The cornea (and other ocular tissues) must be free of any significant disturbances. Only slight peripheral corneal staining, faint central corneal clouding immediately upon removing the lenses, and corneal curvature changes not exceeding ± 0.75 D.K. are acceptable.
5. Normal appearance of the patient. There must be no squinting or significant alteration in either head posture, blinking pattern, or eye injection.

From Sarver, M. D., and Harris, M. G.: A standard for success in wearing contact lenses, *Am. J. Optom., 48(5)*:382-385, 1971.

lenses. Hyperopes rarely report that their vision seems better with contact lenses, unless

TABLE 4.2

SUCCESSFUL RESPONSE TO CORNEAL CONTACT LENSES

Criteria	*(N = 122)* Number Meeting the Criteria	Percentage Meeting the Criteria
Wearing time	106	86.8
Comfort	111	91.0
Vision	117	95.9
Ocular tissue changes	106	86.8
Appearance	114	93.4
Total criteria	89	72.9

From Sarver, M. D., and Harris, M. G.: A standard for success in wearing contact lenses, *Am. J. Optom., 48(5)*:382-385, 1971.

their refractive error is high, in which case they receive considerable increase in the useful field of view.[20]

Vision with gel (soft) lenses may not be as good as vision with corneal lenses.[26-29] Since gel lenses conform to the cornea, they tend not to correct corneal astigmatism. Also, vision may fluctuate with gel lenses due to changes in their state of hydration or lens positioning.

LENGTH OF ADJUSTMENT PERIOD

It usually takes about two weeks before the patient can wear hard contact lenses for extended periods with confidence; about two to four weeks are required before the physiological adaptation is complete, and about two months usually pass before the patient is fully adapted.[30-33] The adaptation time may vary for different individuals and different fitting techniques.[34-42] A few patients adapt so readily that they are comfortable in only a few days and are completely adapted in two weeks, but others, who have difficult adjustment problems, may not adapt fully for several months.[43] Adaptation seems to be faster for gel lens wearers than corneal lens wearers and sometimes full-time wear is achieved in only a few days.

APPEARANCE

Corneal and gel contact lenses can rarely be detected when worn, and scleral lenses are only visible under certain conditions. It is possible to make some changes in the apparent eye color of patients with light irises by using tinted contact lenses. For patients with dark irises, tinted contact lenses do not affect the eye color. Opaque lenses with artificial iris coloring may be used.

SAFETY

Although a contact lens can be broken while on the eye, occasions when this occurs are rare, and no eye damage has been reported from this cause. It is very likely that corneal lenses can be an important factor in protecting the cornea from injury by various flying objects (Figure 4.1).[6,44-50] This, of course, should not be considered as a suggestion that contact lenses be substituted for safety spectacle eyewear. The potential disadvantages and dangers of contact lenses have also been the subject of many reports.[51-61]

Rengstorff gave a report concerning documentation of eyes that have been protected by contact lenses.[62,63] Prior to his survey, he was able to find twenty-one references in the literature (sixty-two instances) concerning protection of eyes by contact lenses. Rengstorff and Black designed a questionnaire, which was sent to a number of optometrists and ophthalmologists. As a result of this questionnaire, an additional 63 cases were reported, for a total of 125 cases. These cases were classified into the following categories: sports, twenty-five cases; automobile, fourteen cases; workshop, thirty cases; miscellaneous, thirty-two cases; and chemical, twenty-four cases. There were *no* cases reported in which an eye was seriously injured while wearing a contact lens. In almost all cases reported, the contact lens was broken, but in *no* case was the eye damaged (Table 4.3).

It should be pointed out that the overwhelming majority of serious problems associated with contact lens wear result from patients not following proper lens care and hygiene and/or not having regular follow-up examinations.

It should be explained to the patient that it is impossible for a contact lens to become

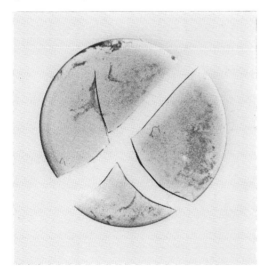

Figure 4.1. Contact lens which, while worn, was broken by the tip of a fishing pole. No corneal damage resulted.

TABLE 4.3

DOCUMENTED CASES OF EYES WEARING CONTACT LENSES PROTECTED FROM SERIOUS INJURIES

Circumstances	Previously Reported Cases (Before 1972)*	(From Rengstorff) New Cases†	Total
Sports	15	10	25
Automobile	8	6	14
Workshop	19	11	30
Miscellaneous	15	17	32
Chemical	5	19	24
TOTAL	62	63	125

* From literature.

† A survey of a few hundred optometrists and ophthalmologists was conducted. They were asked to report any cases where a contact lens *damaged* or *protected* the eyes from injury.

All replies indicated that contact lenses minimized or completely protected the eyes from a more serious injury. The abrasions referred to in this report were minor and healed completely.

lost behind the eye, as this is prevented by the cul-de-sac. It is surprising how many patients express this fear. A lens has even become embedded in the upper lid with no serious effects.[64,65]

OCCUPATION

The need to wear contact lenses for occupational purposes may stem from either their cosmetic or functional advantages over spectacles. The most enthusiastic reception to the wearing of contact lenses has probably been in the theater, television, and movie industries, where the use of spectacle lenses might well limit an actor's career. Contact lenses often have been used to make an apparent change in eye color so that the actor's eye coloring might better fit the needs of a specific part.[66] It is common for newscasters and others who appear before camera lights to prefer contact lenses; they thus avoid the undesirable highlights of light reflection from spectacle lenses.

The use of contact lenses by professional and amateur sports contestants has been well publicized.[67-69] Some caution, however, must be exercised in recommending contact lenses to athletes. If the sport is one in which the contestant is exposed to a great deal of dust, he may find corneal contact lenses intolerable, although he may be an excellent candidate for scleral lenses or gel lenses. This category would include such sports as baseball and track.

Corneal or gel contact lenses are valuable in sports such as gymnastics, boating, archery, tennis, badminton, bowling, fencing, golf, handball, and squash. Occasionally, they can be worn successfully for swimming, but there is a considerable chance that they will be lost. Scleral lenses are usually necessary for swimming, diving, and waterpolo. Scleral or gel lenses are often better in contact sports. Many coaches of basketball and football teams will not allow their players to wear corneal lenses unless they have replacement lenses on hand in case of loss during the game.

A particular danger in sports presents itself when darkly colored corneal lenses are worn for snow skiing. The cold atmosphere makes the lenses seem unusually comfortable and may mask the effect of damaging exposure of the bulbar conjunctiva to the strong ultraviolet light. Corneal lenses are acceptable only if they are worn in conjunction with goggles, which give protection to the entire eye.

Contact lenses are advantageous in an occupation that exposes the wearer to radical shifts in temperature, as would occur when going in and out of a walk-in refrigerator. In moving from cold to warm areas, moisture condenses on spectacle lenses, necessitating removal and cleaning. There is no noticeable effect when contact lenses are subjected to the same temperature change. Contact lenses are also of value to those who are bothered by rain, ocean spray, or mist.

When driving a motor vehicle, properly fitted contact lenses pose no difficulties, but loose or annoying contact lenses can distract the driver's attention from the road, which might predispose him to accidents.[70-72] License examination in all states provides that vision correction with contact lenses is acceptable.

Observing through any type of monocular or binocular microscope is easier with contact lenses, but the same advantages of increased field of view can usually be obtained by equipping the microscope with a long relief eyepiece designed for spectacle wearers.

Some occupations pose problems for the contact lens wearer and definitely contraindicate their use. These include mining, pneumatic drilling, sandblasting, or any other type of work where dust or fine particles are present. In addition, many sprays and fumes cause considerable irritation to the eyes when contact lenses are worn and may even increase the cornea's susceptibility to abrasion.[48]

Most commercial airlines do not allow members of the flight crew to wear contact lenses while on duty. This restriction is imposed on the airlines by the Federal Aviation Agency for Class 1 and 2 (airline transport and commercial) pilots, but certain exceptions are made upon review and approval by the FAA.[73] For instance, in monocular aphakia an experienced pilot could be allowed to wear a contact lens. The restrictions on contact lenses for flying personnel are designed primarily for safety reasons. Loss of a lens during flight from windblast or vibration could prove particularly dangerous.[74] Even if a second pair of lenses were available, the pilot would be disabled for an interval of time, which could be critical.

There is some evidence that eyes are more sensitive to abnormal pressure with contact lenses, and they could become more uncomfortable at high altitudes.[75] Diamond has summarized the hazards of wearing contact lenses during flight as follows:

(1) The threat of wearing loss of one or both lenses producing visual confusion; (2) Lens intolerance forcing removal; (3) Spectacle blur on transition to spectacles; (4) Bubble formation under the lens on reduced barometric pressure or rapid decompression; (5) Problems of presbyopia, and aggravation of decreased accommodation; (6) Residual astigmatism affecting visual acuity; and (7) The threat of acute incapacitation by corneal complications.[76]

The United Kingdom and most overseas airways similarly restrict the wearing of contact lenses by the flight crew.

Flight attendants for most airlines are allowed to wear contact lenses but are usually required to meet the following provisions:

1. The unaided vision, without contact lenses or other correction, must be quite sufficient (better than 20/100) to carry out all their normal duties on an aircraft, enabling them to cope in any emergency without glasses of any kind, including contact lenses.

2. They must be fully accustomed to wearing the lenses for the requisite number of hours without irritation or upset.

In a survey by the author, it was found that approximately 10 to 15 percent of the flight attendants on the major United States airlines were wearing contact lenses.

MYOPIA CONTROL

Occasionally myopia control has been credited to the wearing of contact lenses .[77-80] Although support of this was apparently presented as early as 1946,[81] its greatest impetus was felt after a report and subsequent publication on the subject by Morrison in 1957.[82] Morrison reported that his contact lens patients did not need subsequent changes in their prescriptions. Unfortunately this preliminary report received unusually extensive publicity and was largely responsible for a nearly nationwide feeling at that time that contact lenses did indeed stop myopia progression. There is no reason to question the validity of Morrison's observations, but his implication that contact lenses had stopped his patients' myopia was not warranted by the study.

More recently, orthokeratology has been advocated as a means of reducing or eliminating the existing myopia.[78,83-96] Orthokeratology has been defined as a system that "reduces, modifies or eliminates a visual defect by the programmed application of contact lenses or other related procedures."[85]

At present there is no conclusive evidence to indicate that contact lenses stop or retard the rate of myopia progression or that they can permanently reduce existing myopia (*see* Chapter 31).[97]

FEES

It is often stated that the patient's motivation in wearing contacts is closely related to whether or not he is required to pay a total fee before the fitting process has begun. There is little doubt·that there is some truth in this belief. A patient will likely give more thought to choosing contact lenses when he must also consider his pecuniary interests. Many practitioners, however, do allow the patient to make payments on an extended time basis and do not feel that it makes any difference in the patient's motivation. They feel that a patient who is motivated only by the large fee that he paid will very likely stop wearing the lenses at a later date.

It is sometimes advisable not to quote a total fee if there is some doubt as to the successful outcome of the fitting. It may be necessary to try several different types of lenses before the optimum fit is obtained, and the fee must be altered proportionately.

A few people have the opinion that after the initial payment the overall cost of upkeep for contact lenses will be less than the cost of their spectacles. This is thought to be due to fewer necessary changes in contact lenses over a period of time. It is found, however, that the expense for the upkeep of contact lenses usually make their long-term cost greater than for spectacle lenses. Contact lens wearers must have their eyes and lenses examined at more frequent intervals than spectacle wearers.

LENS LOSSES

Losses are relatively few if a reasonable amount of care is exercised. One survey indicated that there are 635.8 lost or damaged corneal lenses per each 1000 corneal lens wearers during the first year of wear, while there are 572.2 gel lenses lost or damaged for each 1000 gel lens wearers during the first year.[98] Over 60 percent of the gel lens losses were due to careless handling. One-third of these were lost while inserting or removing the lenses. Contact lenses may be insured by various insurance programs, which usually operate on a deductible basis.

EXAMINATION

A thorough eye and vision examination is a necessity in fitting contact lenses. This examination should include all tests normally done in an eye examination with special emphasis on certain parts of the examination.

HISTORY

A complete patient history is probably the most important part of the examination. Among the areas covered in the history are the following:

1. The patient's reasons for seeking contact lenses
2. History of eye injury, disease, or surgery
3. Systemic health history
4. Medications presently being taken and reasons for them
5. Any ocular or vision problems

The patient's reason for seeking contact lenses may be ascertained during the consultation but should be recorded as part of the history. The major reasons for seeking contact lenses are (1) cosmetic, (2) sports, (3) occupation, (4) high refractive error or other visual needs, (5) corneal irregularity, or (6) myopia control.

Careful documentation of any former history of ocular injury is important for both legal and professional reasons. If the injury has only recently occurred, consultation should be made with the patient's previous practitioner to determine if any unknown factors exist that should delay or contraindicate the fitting. Any injury to the cornea or anterior segment of the eye should be completely healed before the contact lens is worn.

Any history of past or present eye diseases, infections, or inflammations should be noted. Active conditions should be under control before contact lenses are prescribed. Medical consultation may be advisable.

A history of eye surgery should be explored to determine the residual effects that may be present. If the corneal nerves have been severed in the course of surgery, there will be reduced sensitivity of the cornea, and the natural protective device of alarm against irritation by a contact lens is lost.[99] If the cornea is completely devoid of sensation, it may be that contact lenses should not be prescribed or at least special precautions should be taken.

Surgery of the extraocular muscles may produce scar tissue on the bulbar conjunctiva or near the limbal area, but seldom does this interfere with the wearing of corneal lenses. If scar tissue remains on the cornea itself, it does not usually interfere with a corneal contact lens unless the scar is excessive and raised considerably above the normal contour of the cornea. Contact lenses usually prove very successful after cataract surgery or corneal transplants.

Many systemic diseases and medications affect the eyes and corneas. Consultation with the patient's physician may be advisable before fitting contact lenses if systemic problems exist.

EXTERNAL EXAMINATION

A careful examination should be conducted to confirm any ocular conditions described in the history and to detect those unknown to the patient. The routine methods of external ocular examination employ the penlight, biomicroscope, and ophthalmoscope. If any condition exists that does not prevent the wearing of contact lenses but which is unknown to the patient, it should be pointed out to him so that he will not feel later that the condition resulted from wearing contact lenses. A photographic record of the eye is of considerable value for later comparison. Careful notation of all findings should be made.

Biomicroscopy

The external examination cannot be considered complete without a thorough biomicroscopic examination.[100-103] The biomicroscope allows minute scrutiny of the cornea, lids, conjunctiva, and precorneal fluid and will often allow the examiner to detect ocular anomalies that otherwise would escape notice. (The reader is referred to Chapter 33 for the methods used.) The cornea should be examined for scars, signs of former disease, evidence of abnormal growths, and dryness.[104] The tears should be examined for excessive debris or secretions that could collect on a contact lens. The lids and conjunctiva should be examined for any abnormalities or signs of inflammation, with particular attention to the lid margins for signs of blepharitis marginalis.

If any evidence of corneal inflammation is reported in the history, the cornea should be searched for remnants of former corneal vascularization. When the cornea has once become vascularized during an inflammation, the vessel walls never regress, even though the condition is cured and the cornea appears normal. The vessel walls rarely cause any visual disturbances and may be undetected unless a careful biomicroscopic examination is conducted. Recognition of the remnants of the blood vessels is important because it indicates a predisposition to corneal vascularization following any corneal injury when the contact lenses are worn. Although no new vessels may be formed, the old vessels may become easily engorged with blood, and the patient may feel that a new increase in vessel formation has occurred. The patient should be told of the possibility for recurrence of vessel formation, but this is not necessarily a contraindication for wearing contact lenses.

EXAMINATION OF VISUAL FUNCTION

A routine examination should include the following tests:

Visual Acuity

The patient's visual acuity with the old and new spectacle prescriptions should be measured so that a later comparison can be made with the visual acuity achieved with contact lenses. The patient's impression of the difference in acuity with spectacles and contact lenses may not be in accordance with the acuity difference that actually exists.

Refraction

The method of refraction may be that customarily used by the fitter. It is convenient to record the final prescription in minus cylinder form for ordering the contact lenses.

Binocularity and Accommodation Tests

Particular attention should be given to tests for phorias and accommodative amplitude.

ADDITIONAL TESTS

Keratometry

As mentioned in Chapter 3, the keratometer measurement, while reasonably accurate for refraction purposes, has lower validity for contact lens work. Therefore, great care should be taken to avoid further error in the corneal curvature measurement. Even the experienced practitioner is likely to commit errors while taking a keratometer measurement. This has not presented any difficulty when the measurement was used for ordinary refractive work because the measurement was taken to determine the degree of toricity that existed on the cornea, and toricity is somewhat easier to measure than the absolute value of the corneal curvature. For example, assume that a keratometer is out of adjustment and always reads 0.50 D. too high. This will have little effect on the measurement of the corneal toricity, since values for the two principal meridians will both be 0.50 D. too high, and the difference will be essentially the true amount. On the other hand, when the corneal curvature is measured for contact lens fitting, the absolute values are of prime importance. The measurements can only be accurate if close attention is given to all the factors that may influence the keratometer reading. The keratometer must be periodically calibrated and adjusted for maximum accuracy. Techniques for this procedure as well as proper methods to be used in keratometer measurements are given in Chapter 33.

There is some question about the number of keratometer measurements needed to obtain maximum accuracy. Tests have shown that little is to be gained by taking more than three measurements of each principal meridian. The quickest and most accurate method is to take the median value of the three readings. The median value is simply the middle value of the three readings. If two of the three readings have the same value, then the median value is that of the two equal readings.

Peripheral Keratometry

The curvature of the peripheral cornea affects the design of corneal contact lenses. Several methods have been suggested to determine the entire corneal contour from keratometer measurements of the corneal periphery. While peripheral keratometry could be reasonably accurate, it is not accurate as performed with present instrumentation. Instruments other than the keratometer are available for the measurement of corneal contour, including the photokeratoscope,[105] the topogometer,[106] and the corneopter.[107] Devices of this type have not yet been shown to be superior to the keratometer and/or diagnostic contact lenses in determining the contact lens specifications (*see* Chapter 3).

Corneal Diameter

The corneal diameter has an effect on the specifications of the contact lens prescribed, especially lens diameter. When being measured, the corneal diameter is assumed to equal the diameter of the iris, and for simplicity the actual measurement is made of the visible iris diameter.

Whenever corneal diameter is mentioned in reference to contact lens fitting, it may be assumed that the term refers to the diameter in the horizontal meridian.

The actual measurement of the corneal diameter is made with a P.D. ruler in a way

similiar to that used in measuring the interpupillary distance. The ruler should be held as close to the cornea as possible in order to reduce the small parallax error (Figure 4.2). Although special instruments are available for more exact measurements of the corneal diameter,[108] they are unnecessary. For practical purposes, only the relative size of the cornea needs to be known.

Pupil Diameter

Contact lenses must be designed to cover the pupil adequately. The pupillary diameter can be measured with a P.D. ruler. Of interest for contact lens fitting is the maximum diameter that the pupil attains under low illumination. This measurement is extremely difficult to take accurately, since the pupil size will fluctuate with varying emotions and external stimuli. It is usually sufficient to classify pupil size as small, medium or large on the basis of its maximum diameter.

Pupil	Size
Small	Less than 3 mm.
Medium	3 to 6 mm.
Large	Larger than 6 mm.

Devices are available for the accurate measurement of pupillary diameter,[109] but considering the pupil's continuous fluctuation, these devices are hardly necessary.

Palpebral Aperture Height

The palpebral aperture height is another important factor in determining corneal contact lens dimensions.[110] With the patient relaxed and fixating straight ahead, a measurement should be made of the maximum vertical distance when the lids are separated (Figure 4.3a). This measurement may be difficult to take accurately, since the lid aperture is under voluntary control, and patients have a tendency to squint when the ruler is placed near their eyes. This dimension can sometimes be determined more accurately by estimation when the patient is in a more natural situation. This may be done by noting the

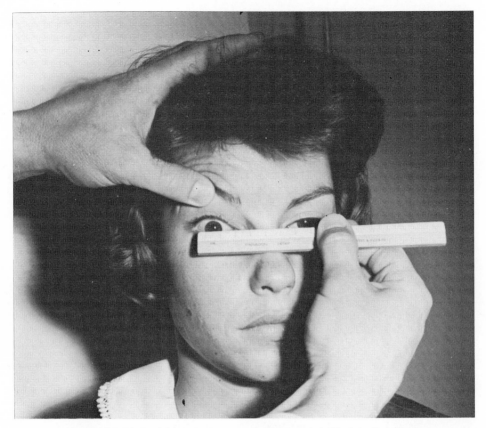

Figure 4.2. Method to measure corneal diameter (visible iris diameter).

difference in the height of the aperture and the corneal diameter in the vertical meridian. From the value measured for the visible iris diameter, an estimate can be made with reasonable accuracy of the palpebral fissure height (Figure 4.3b).

Lids

The eyelids play an important role in designing and fitting contact lenses.[111-113] An estimate of the lid tension can be made by grasping the lid between the thumb and forefinger, giving a very slight pull, and observing the resiliency as the lid springs back into place. Although this measurement is rather gross, with experience it may be used to detect lids that are unusually loose or tight.

A determination of the blink rate should be made when the patient is unaware that it is being done. It should be noted whether the rate is unusually slow or fast; the normal rate ranges between ten to fifteen blinks per minute. The blink amplitude, length, and completeness should also be noted. Many patients who blink improperly have difficulty with contact lenses.[114,115]

Corneal Sensitivity

Corneal sensitivity tests should be performed in cases where it is suspected that sensation may be absent or greatly diminished. If the cornea is found to be of less than normal sensitivity, precautions must be taken to check the patient's cornea frequently for possible abrasions that are undetected by the patient. Various methods are available for a gross detection of corneal sensitivity, including the use of the Cochet-Bonnet anesthe-

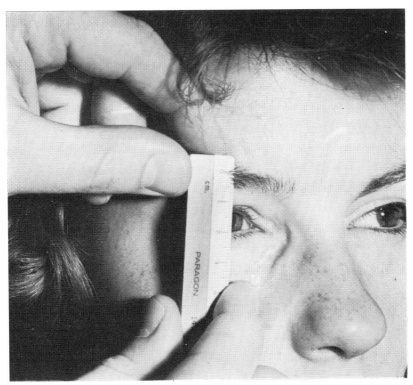

Figure 4.3a. Method of measuring palpebral aperture height.

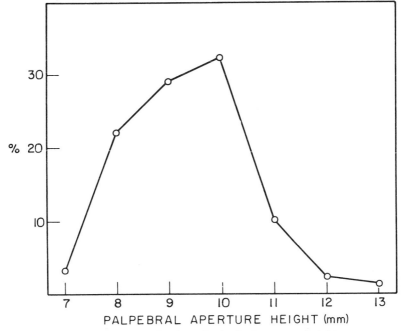

Figure 4.3b. Distribution of palpebral aperture heights.

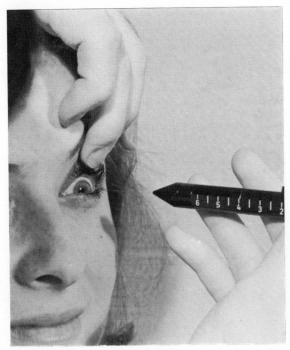

Figure 4.4. Method of measuring corneal sensitivity with the Cochet-Bonnet anesthesiometer.

siometer (Figure 4.4).[116-120] None has been shown to be definitive in predicting success in wearing of contact lenses, although Koetting has shown that patients with extremely fragile corneas are more likely to be contact lens failures than patients with less fragile corneas (*see* Chapter 2).[116]

Tearing

An insufficiency of tearing may limit a patient's ability to wear contact lenses. This can be measured with the Schirmer tear test (Figure 4.5).[121,122]

DIAGNOSTIC LENS FITTING

The fitting of diagnostic contact lenses as part of the examination is an extremely valuable technique in determining whether a patient should be fitted with contact lenses, and if so, what type of lens is best for the patient.[123-126] It may not be advisable to fit patients who react adversely to the diagnostic lenses.[126] In addition, a proper diagnostic lens fitting can save time and effort in determining the proper lens type and dimensions needed for the patient.

Record Form

The fitting of contact lenses is an extensive procedure, and more than passing consideration must be given to an adequate record system. A disorganized record will cause the practitioner considerable loss of time when a search must be made for the specifications of former lenses or for a review of past history. Regular types of refraction records are normally inadequate, and a large double page 8.5 × 11 inch record is usually needed to contain all the information necessary.

A special record form designed specifically for use with contact lens patients will help to insure that all information is recorded and will give adequate medicolegal protection. Several good record forms[127-131] are available, an example of which is illustrated in

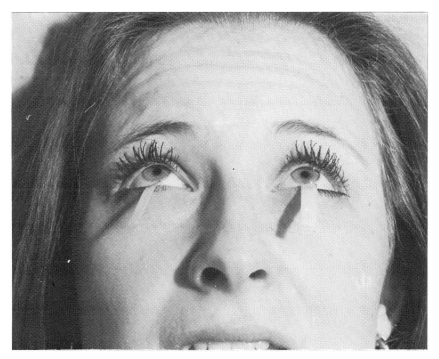

Figure 4.5. Method of measuring tear sufficiency with the Schirmer test.

Figures 4.6 to 4.8.* This first page of the record provides space for all data pertaining to the history and the eye examination, the second page is for recording routine progress examinations, the third page provides space for recording the results of later visits, and the fourth page provides space for the sys-tematic recording of all lens specifications on a continuing basis, including how the lens was ordered, when it was received, and what adjustments were subsequently made. The use of this record form will be discussed in greater detail in later chapters.

PROGNOSIS

During the consultation and the examination, the patient must be evaluated for his chances of successful contact lens wear. Many factors are related to a person's ability to wear contact lenses successfully.

MOTIVATION

The desire on the part of the patient to wear contact lenses is one of the most important factors in predicting a successful fitting .[2,3,132-139] A highly motivated patient can often tolerate discomfort and other problems that would be insurmountable to the patient with only a superficial motivation. Motivation can be tested by explaining the disadvantages of contact lenses and the extensive fitting procedure. Of course the disadvantages should not be stressed to such a point that the patient

*This form was designed by Drs. Morton Sarver and Robert Lester.

NAME   AGE   PHONE   DATE

ADDRESS   CITY   POSTAL ZONE

| Previous Rx. | Distance or Reading | R. | | | Add. | R. | | Lens Type | |
| | | L. | | | | L. | | | |

| Rx.1 CONTACT LENS Rx | | | DATE | | Rx.2 PURPOSE | | | | | DATE | |

Distance or Reading	R.		20/	add	R.		Sphere	Cylinder	Axis	Prism	Decenter	Base Curve	V.A.
	L.		20/		L.	R.							20/
						L.							20/

Above is / is not Max. V.A. finding

Reasons for Contact Lenses:	Cosmetic		Sports			Add.	Seg. Ilgt.	Seg. Width	Seg. Dec.	Total Dec.	Vert. Center
Irregular Cornea	High refractive error		Aphakia		R.						
					L.						

Other

| Lens Type | | | Tint | | Size | | Shape | |

REMARKS:

| Mounting Type | | | | Bridge | Temple | | P.D. |

| Fitted by | Disp. by | Instructor | | Charge | Dep. | | Bal. |

CONTACT LENS HEALTH HISTORY   0 - No Comment   X - Explanation in Remarks above

BLEPHARITIS	ALLERGIES	SINUS	PINGUECULA	PTERYGIUM	EYE SURGERY
EYE INJURIES	EYE DISEASE	EYE DRUGS	DIABETES	THYROID	
CONDITION OF TEETH	KIDNEYS	PRESENT MEDICATION		OTHER	

ANATOMICAL FEATURES: IRIS COLOR   EYES: DEEPSET   AVERAGE   PROMINENT

SLIT–LAMP EXAMINATION: R   L

EXAMINED BY   CLINICAL INSTRUCTOR

VISUAL AND GENERAL HEALTH HISTORY

Faculty   Student   Employee   Other

| Visual Acuity | Old Rx. | R. | L. | O.U. | No Rx. | R. | L. | O.U. |

FUNDUS, MEDIA, LIDS, ETC.

Contraindications for Contact Lenses:

Pupillary Reflexes		Direct	Consensual	Near	Cover Test	Versions	Conv. N.P.	P.D. /
Ophtalmometry		R.				L.		
Static Skiametry		R.				L.		
Subj. Test.	Max V.A. 20/ O.U.	R.			20/	L.		20/
	20/20 Binoc. V.A.	R.			20/	L.		20/
Heterophoria		Eso.	Exo.	Hyper.		Vertical Vergences	Supra.	
Vergences at 6 M.		Pos.	Neg.				Infra.	
Accommodative Amplitude		R.				L.		
Dynamic Skiametry		R.				L.		
Cross Cylinder	Monocular	R.				L.		
	Binocular	R.				L.		
Tentative Near Rx.		R.			V.A.	L.		V.A.
Fusional Supp. Conv.						Accom.-Conv. Gradient		
Vergences at 40 cm.		Pos.				Neg.		
Relative Accommodation		Neg.				Pos.		

Figure 4.6. Contact lens record form, page 1.

is frightened. An honest and factual discussion will prove worthwhile.

Motivation is closely related to the reasons for wanting contact lenses.[140] Many people dislike the appearance of spectacles and therefore do not want to wear them. Their motivation for wearing contact lenses is a twofold desire to see well and to improve their appear-

CONTACT LENS PROGRESS EXAMINATIONS

Clinician	1		2		3		4		5	
Date										
Maximum wearing time	hrs.		hrs.		hrs.		hrs.		hrs.	
Wearing time this examination	hrs.		hrs.		hrs.		hrs.		hrs.	

Fluorescein pattern
Corneal staining
Lens position   R
Lid position

(Sketch pattern of fit in
green and blue, lens position
in red, lid positions in black,   L
accent trouble area in green.)

Symptoms (record time of occurrence)
1. Burning	8. Irritation
2. Hotness	9. Itching
3. Injection	10. Lacrimation
4. Veiling	11. Blurring
5. Halos	12. Lid edema
6. Poor V.A.	13. Edge reflec.
7. Flare	14. Other

Visual acuity through contacts	R	20/		20/		20/		20/		20/	
	L.	20/		20/		20/		20/		20/	
Best Sph. Refraction	R	add	20/	add	20/	add	20/	add	20/	add	20/
through Contact Lenses	L.	add	20/	add	20/	add	20/	add	20/	add	20/
Best Sph-Cyl Refraction	R	add	20/	add	20/	add	20/	add	20/	add	20/
Through Contact Lenses	L.	add	20/	add	20/	add	20/	add	20/	add	20/

Slit-Lamp Exam

Ophthalmometer readings after removing contacts:
Mires   Clear   -   Distorted

DISCHARGE EVALUATION

Average daily wearing time:	Maximum wearing time:		
Full wearing reached in weeks.	Discharge visual acuity: R 20/	L 20/	OU 20/
Patient reaction:	Very satisfied	Satisfied	Dissatisfied
Comments:			
Date of patient discharge:			
Insurance discussed: Date:		Initials:	

STATEMENT BY PATIENT: I have been instructed in the proper methods of insertion, removal, use and care of my contact lenses and have read and do hereby agree to abide by the rules stated in "The Care and Wearing of Your Contact Lenses." I also have the names, addresses and telephone numbers of my clinicians should I need to call upon them.

Lenses delivered to me: Date: Signed:

Figure 4.7. Contact lens record form, page 2.

ance. The greater a patient's need for contact lenses, either visual or psychological, the more likely it is that his motivation will be high.

Unfortunately, people vary considerably in their overt enthusiasm during an inter-view, and it is not always possible to evaluate the patient's true motivation adequately during the short time of this initial contact. Fitters are often surprised at the changing attitudes of their patients once the fitting is under

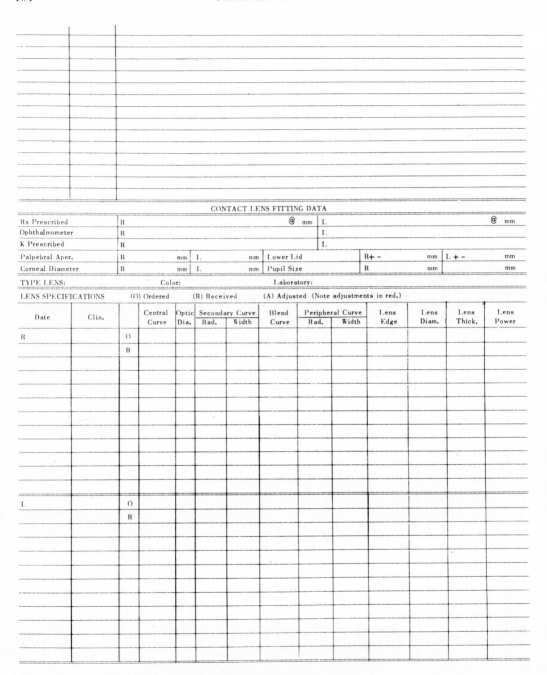

Figure 4.8. Contact lens record form, page 4.

way. Many patients have only a temporary need for contact lenses, and their enthusiasm wanes with the fading of the need. Evidence of this is that of the 10 million people fitted with contact lenses in the past fifteen years, only 3.8 million are wearing lenses today.[98]

An example is seen in those who abandon their contact lenses after establishing marital ties. In other cases motivation increases after the initial stages of the fitting. This may occur when the patient is especially apprehensive about the wearing of contact lenses and later finds that they are much easier to wear than he anticipated. Other patients gain motivation after they have been fitted when they find that better optical performance is gained by the use of contact lenses.

A larger proportion of females desire contact lenses for cosmetic reasons, and a greater percentage of females are successful contact lens wearers than males.[141] This is not to say, however, that women are always more motivated than men to wear contact lenses for cosmetic reasons.

PERSONALITY

Personality is one of the most complex factors related to predicting a patient's chances of successful contact lens wear. Many investigators have written about the relationship of personality and contact lens wear with little conclusion.[3,142-149] It was shown, however, that the personalities of patients seeking contact lenses do not differ significantly from those of patients seeking spectacles.[147] Also, many contact lens wearers undergo a change in personality after being fitted.[146,148]

Confident and dominating patients are sometimes very fearful of the fitting process and react quite differently than would be suspected. Meek individuals often show considerable confidence once they learn just what is involved in the wearing of contact lenses. Fear on the part of the patient is generally a normal reaction and can be disposed of by proper handling. However, patients who are timid and unsure of themselves are more likely to be unsuccessful contact lens wearers than patients who are independent and confident.[147]

Patients who show undue regard for their health and who are apparently plagued with minor ailments that they enjoy describing at length are often unwilling to tolerate the minor discomforts which accompany the normal adjustment process in contact lens wear.

FORMER CONTACT LENS WEARERS

A patient who was dissatisfied with a previous contact lens fitting but wishes to try again presents a special problem. Care must be taken to establish, as far as possible, the reason for the previous failure. Some patients have been fitted with older types of lenses that proved unsuccessful, and these patients offer reasonable risks for a new fitting attempt. Other patients may be unsuited to wear contact lenses but attempt to place the blame for failure on their former practitioner. An attempt should be made to secure all information about the patient from the former fitter, as it will often reveal the source of the difficulty. The fact that the patient has been fitted with contact lenses previously does not in itself tend to make the patient unsuccessful at the present fitting.[150]

MONOCULAR WEAR

It is possible in cases of monocular aphakia, anisometropia, and various corneal anomalies that a contact lens correction will be needed in only one eye. A single contact lens can be used for this purpose, although the patient is often not sufficiently motivated to wear the lens if the other eye has good vision.

MANUAL DEXTERITY

It should be noted whether the patient has sufficient manual dexterity to handle small corneal lenses.

HYGIENE

Patients who exhibit poor hygiene and grooming may be poor candidates for contact lenses, especially gel lenses. Since wearing contact lenses requires proper hygiene and proper lens care, careless patients may not be suited for contact lenses.

REFRACTIVE ERROR

Usually patients with higher refractive errors are highly motivated to wear contact lenses, but it is a common mistake to assume that high refractive error will insure that the patient has strong motivation. Patients with high myopia seem more likely to be unsuccessful than patients with moderate myopia, probably because of the greater difficulty in designing and fitting their contact lenses.[141] Myopes of less than 1.00 D. and patients with uncorrected visual acuity of 20/60 or better are less likely to be good patients since their vision is adequate without correction.[141] Hyperopes are well motivated if they are dependent upon their glasses for much of their daily activities. High astigmats can usually be fitted adequately but may need special lenses that require greater skill and longer fitting periods. They should understand the special nature of their correction so that they will know why their fitting takes longer than others.

The best patients for contact lenses are those whose visual condition is such that contact lenses will provide a higher level of visual acuity or visual efficiency than spectacles.

BINOCULARITY

A phoria of sufficient magnitude to cause subjective symptoms with spectacle lenses may cause the same difficulty with contact lenses, although there is evidence that some patients who must have prism in their spectacle corrections to see comfortably do have comfortable vision without prism in contact lenses.[151] Vertical phorias of up to 2Δ can be corrected with prism corneal contact lenses, but lateral phorias can only be corrected by prism scleral lenses. However, an exotrope or high exophoria may be aided by wearing an overminus correction in contact lenses, just as he would by wearing the same in spectacle lenses.[152]

It is usually advantageous to have the patient take any necessary visual training before the contact lenses are fitted so that symptoms will not be attributed to the wearing of contact lenses. Consideration should also be given to the optical effects of contact lenses on heterophoria. A myopic patient is

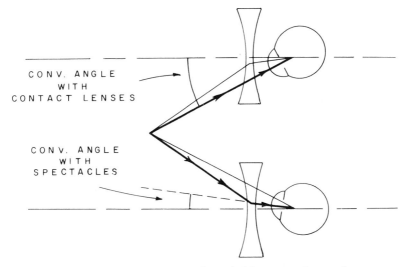

CONV. ANGLE
WITH
CONTACT LENSES

CONV. ANGLE
WITH
SPECTACLES

Figure 4.9. A myope must converge more through his contact lenses than was necessary through his spectacles.

required to converge more through his contact lenses than was necessary through his spectacle lenses, whereas the converse is true for a hyperope (Figure 4.9).[153]

Contact lenses may also be valuable in obtaining binocularity when patients have significant aniseikonia with spectacle lenses.[154]

ACCOMMODATION

A myopic patient must accommodate more with contact lenses than with spectacle lenses to observe an object clearly at a finite distance, while the hyperopic patient accommodates less with contact lenses.[153,155-157] Consequently, this problem should be considered when fitting a myope with insufficient accom-

modation. This applies particularly to beginning presbyopes who are still able to get along without a plus addition for near vision in their spectacle lenses. It may be found that a plus addition is necessary when wearing contact lenses.

ANATOMICAL CONSIDERATIONS

Anatomical features and eye dimensions seem to have little effect on success with contact lenses, although patients with very large or small palpebral apertures have been found more likely to be failures.[141]

The following conditions seem favorable to contact lens wear.

1. Lids of average tension, shape, and posi-

tion. A normal blink rate. Blinking should result in the complete closure of the eyelids.

2. Cornea of average curvature with low toricity. Corneas that are spherical or highly toric are more difficult to fit.

3. Pupil of small or average diameter.

It is sometimes claimed that the patient's skin pigmentation has some bearing on the prognosis for wearing contact lenses. Darker pigmented individuals are said to adapt to the lenses more readily than those of lighter pigmentation,[158] but there is little evidence for this hypothesis.

HEALTH CONSIDERATIONS

The advisability of fitting a patient with contact lenses may be dependent upon the patient's ocular and general health. Many health problems lower the probability of success for contact lens wearers.[150]

Ocular Conditions

Some eye pathology may eliminate the possible use of contact lenses; some may dictate that only limited use will be possible, and some will indicate that only certain types of contact lenses will be feasible. Each pathological condition should be considered separately.

Surgery

Surgery performed on the extraocular muscles may produce scar tissue on the bulbar conjunctiva or near the area of the limbus, but seldom does this interfere with the wearing of corneal lenses. If scar tissue remains on the cornea itself, it does not usually interfere with a corneal contact lens unless it is excessive and raised considerably above the normal contour of the cornea. Contact lenses usually prove very successful after cataract surgery, corneal transplant, or other corneal surgery.

Keratitis and Conjunctivitis

Patients with old, inactive cases of keratitis may achieve better vision when fitted with contact lenses.[159] However, extreme caution must be exercised; the lenses may irritate the cornea and expose it again to the disease. If this occurs, the lenses should be removed and not used again. Conjunctivitis, while a much less serious disease, causes considerable irritation and discomfort to the wearer of contact lenses. When the disease is persistent, contact lenses should probably not be prescribed, although patients with periodic conjunctivitis attacks can often wear their lenses successfully when their eyes are normal;[160] the lenses do not appear to aggravate the condition. Prior to the fitting, the patient should be made to understand that he will not be able to wear the lenses comfortably while his conjunctivitis is active.

Keratitis Sicca

Patients who have inadequate tear circulation react variably to the wearing of contact lenses. In some patients the condition is aggravated, apparently because the lack of sufficient tears fails to provide a lubricating action between the lens and cornea. In others the condition is improved, apparently because protection is provided against a rapid evaporation of the small quantity of tears that is present on the cornea. If corneal lenses cannot be worn, a fluid scleral lens or a gel lens may prove effective.[161-167]

Trachoma

Old, inactive cases of trachoma will usually be helped by the wearing of contact lenses, as they provide some protection for the cornea against the scarring that is often present on the lids. Also, contact lenses will usually provide better vision than spectacles for these patients.

Corneal Ulcers

Scleral contact lenses have aided in the healing of the corneal ulcers.[168,169] Gel lenses can be used as bandage lenses to relieve the

Herpes Zoster

Iliff and Naquin successfully fitted a six-year-old girl who had a corneal graft after an attack of herpes zoster ophthalmicus. [168]

Keratoconus and Keratoglobus

Cases involving keratoconus and keratoglobus have been most successful in wearing contact lenses (*see* Chapter 30).

Pinguecula and Pterygium

A small pinguecula should normally cause no difficulty in the wearing of corneal lenses, but a large pinguecula that is near the limbus may be irritated by the lenses and cause considerable discomfort. If a pterygium is present, it is not advisable to have the patient wear contact lenses, and even after its surgical removal, it is sometimes doubtful if the lenses are advisable. If the pterygium should recur, as occasionally happens, contact lenses will undoubtedly be blamed, whether or not they actually contributed to the condition.

Iritis, Iridocyclitis, or Uveitis

Patients with iritis, iridocyclitis, or uveitis should normally not be fitted with contact lenses because the added irritation may activate the condition. Even if the lenses are not the precipitating factor in the recurrence of the disease, they will usually be blamed if they are being worn when the exacerbation occurs.[158,173]

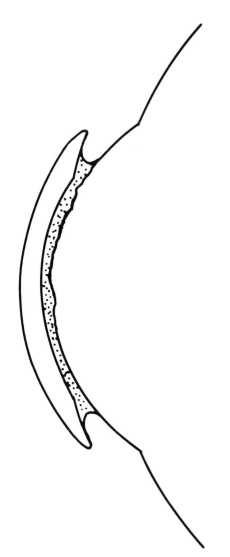

Figure 4.10. Contact lens on irregular cornea. Tear fluid fills the irregularity.

Glaucoma

Scleral lenses are definitely not to be worn when the patient has glaucoma because they often press on the aqueous veins (*see* Chapter 2), which may further interfere with the aqueous outflow and precipitate an acute attack.[174] The status of corneal and gel lenses is less definite. Some advocate that corneal lenses are not harmful and may actually produce a massaging effect on the cornea, which increases the flow of aqueous from the ante-

pain of corneal ulcers and aid in their healing .[162,164,170-172] Contact lenses may be of exceptional benefit to a patient who develops corneal irregularity or scarring from ulcers. Here the contact lens effectively replaces the irregular cornea with a new surface (Figure 4.10). Care must be taken, however, that the lenses be well fitted so that no corneal irritation occurs.

rior chamber .[175-178] Others feel that the risk of contact lenses for these cases is too great and that they should never be worn.[138] Further information is needed before a definite conclusion can be made.

Ocular Albinism

Several investigators have reported fitting contact lenses to ocular albinos in an attempt to improve vision and reduce the other ocular complications of albinism.[179-189] Iliff and Naquin fitted two albinos and found no improvement in the visual acuity of albinos fitted with pinhole contact lenses.[185-189,190] Grayson and Boling propose that a pinhole (cosmetic) contact lens will reduce glare and increase visual acuity, especially if a high myopic error is present.[190] It may also reduce the nystagmus. It has often been reported that a pinhole scleral contact lens provides the best correction for an albinotic patient. This is based on the assumption that light passing through the iris and sclera is scattered in the eye and produces a veiling effect. This light would be absorbed by the opaque portion of the pinhole lens. The value of pinhole lenses seems somewhat dependent on the age at which they are fitted. The results seem best when they are fitted to infant albinos. However, pinhole contact lenses do not always improve an albino's visual acuity, since his lowered visual acuity is also due to faulty retinal pigmentation and not just to the scattering of light within the eye.[17,188]

Nystagmus

Iliff and Naquin reported three cases of nystagmus in which contact lenses made no improvement in visual acuity.[168] Others feel that patients with nystagmus and a significant refractive error will benefit from contact lenses because the lenses tend to remain centered with respect to the line of sight.[190]

The effect of contact lenses on nystagmus cannot be generalized; it will depend upon the cause of the nystagmus. If the nystagmus occurs as a result of a lesion in the nervous system, the type of visual correction will have no effect on its magnitude. If the nystagmus results from a visual defect and that defect can be corrected as effectively with contact lenses as with spectacles, there is a fair chance that the contact lenses will also decrease the nystagmus. Pinhole contact lenses fitted in infancy may be of value in reducing or eliminating nystagmus.[186,187,191]

Other Conditions

In addition to the more common pathological conditions already described, contact lenses have been successfully fitted to correct the distorted cornea of arrested mustard gas keratitis,[192,193] to prevent symblepharon in inflammatory conditions of the conjunctiva,[161,194] to maintain clarity of the cornea during prolonged surgery,[195] to improve vision in scarred corneas,[196,197] and to treat amblyopia.[198] Gel and scleral lenses have been used to aid in the treatment of bullous keratopathy,[162,164] ocular pemphigus,[166,199] and corneal burns.[199]

Cosmetic contact lenses have been fitted to patients with iris coloboma and aniridia.[200,201]

The fitting of specially tinted contact lenses has been advocated as aiding color-blind patients,[168,202] although regular contact lenses have no effect on color discrimination.[203] The proposed effect of the lenses was not given.

Lid Conditions

Chalazion or Hordeolum

Any active lid inflammation will usually be greatly irritated by contact lenses. A chalazion should be corrected before fitting contact lenses. Patients with a history of recurrent hordeola will probably not be able to wear contact lenses with comfort and should be discouraged from the fitting.

Meibomianitis

Excessive sebaceous secretions may be produced by the meibomianitis, and they will collect in the precorneal fluid and eventually coat the contact lens. This will produce discomfort as well as interference with vision. The condition should be cured before contact lenses are fitted.

Entropion, Ectropion, and Trichiasis

Patients with these conditions will usually benefit from wearing contact lenses because they protect the cornea from the mechanical abrasion of the lids. A scleral or a gel lens is often preferable.

Blepharitis Marginalis

If the blepharitis is chronic, it will be aggravated by contact lenses. The condition should be treated and allowed to heal before contact lenses are fitted.

Other Lid Conditions

Other lid conditions can also be aggravated by contact lenses and cause a patient to be uncomfortable while wearing contact lenses.

Systemic Disorders

Respiratory Disorders

A number of conditions including rhinitis, sinusitis, hay fever, and asthma tend to produce conjunctival injection and cause discomfort when contact lenses are worn. Such conditions should be cured before contact lenses are prescribed. If these conditions are chronic and recurrent, the patient should be advised not to wear his contact lenses during an active attack.

ALLERGY. Patients with allergies, especially respiratory allergies, are more likely to be unsuccessful contact lens wearers than patients without allergies.[138,150] This may even be true after the allergy has become inactive or following desensitization therapy.[204] These allergies usually cause ocular symptoms such as photophobia, itching, lacrimation, and burning. These are the same subjective symptoms that make contact lens wearers unsuccessful.[205]

An allergy to the plastic material of the lens itself has not been demonstrated, although it is often blamed for the inability of some patients to wear contact lenses. Patients may, however, develop allergies to contact lens solutions.

Allergies to soaps and cosmetics may also affect the ability to wear contact lenses successfully.[206]

COMMON COLD. A patient who has chronic colds should be advised that his contact lenses cannot be worn comfortably while he has a cold.

Diabetes

Since most diabetics experience a general retardation of the healing process and are prone to corneal staining when contact lenses are worn, contact lenses are not to be recommended, except under very controlled conditions.[12,207]

Endocrine Changes

Women undergo changes in their endocrine system during pregnancy that can affect the ability to wear contact lenses.[12,208,209] These endocrine changes alter the fluid balance of the body and can cause significant corneal changes, since the cornea is about 75 percent fluid. It may be best to postpone fitting contact lenses until the pregnancy is terminated and the fluid balance returns to normal.

Similar endocrine changes occur during menses and may cause otherwise properly fitting contact lenses to become uncomfortable.[138] Also, changes in the endocrine balance during the menopause can cause tear flow to vary and affect the comfort of contact lenses.[138]

Other Systemic Disorders

Other systemic disorders may adversely affect the eyes and the ability to wear contact lenses successfully. Among these are disorders of the thyroid gland, the kidneys, the teeth, and the skin.

Medication

The practitioner must ascertain detailed information about any medications or drugs being taken by a prospective contact lens wearer, especially why the medication is being taken and any possible ocular side effects.

Ocular Medication

The use of ocular medication may indicate an ocular condition wherein contact lenses should not be worn. Cosmetic gel lenses cannot be worn while any ocular medication, prescription, or over-the-counter drug is being used.[210]

Systemic Medication

Many systemic medications and drugs affect the eyes and can affect a patient's success with contact lenses.[211] Orally taken antihistamines and decongestants can have a drying effect on the tears and the cornea[138] and cause a keratitis with related symptoms. Oral contraceptives alter the fluid balance of the body and can have a similar effect on the corneas and contact lens wear as does pregnancy.[208,209,212-219]

REFERENCES

1. Remba, M. J.: "Doctor, can I wear contact lenses?" *Optom. Weekly*, *55*(*37*):31–34, 1964.
2. Sarver, M. D.: Psychological management of the contact lens patient, *Second A.O.A. Contact Lens Symposium*, pp. 55–72, 1965.
3. Racusen, F. R., Corral, E., and McGee, T. F.: An exploratory investigation of factors associated with success or failure in contact lens wearing, *Am. J. Optom.*, *41*(*4*): 232–240, 1964.
4. Dowaliby, M.: An optometrist learns to wear contact lenses, *Optom. Weekly*, *54*(*14*):611–613, 1963.
5. Rosen, D. M.: Cause of contact lens wearing failure, *Optom. Weekly*, *54*(*40*):1877–1878, 1963.
6. Wesley, N. K.: Apprehension of opportunity, *Am. J. Optom.*, *41*(*1*):37–44, 1964.
7. Westsmith, R. A.: Patients' acceptance of corneal microlenses, *Am. J. Ophthalmol.*, *46*(*6*):869–872, 1958.
8. Girard, L. J.: *Corneal Contact Lenses*. St. Louis, Mosby, 1964, pp. 271–272.
9. Deas, R. H.: A method of designing corneal contact lenses, in Girard, L. J. (Ed.): *Corneal and Scleral Contact Lenses, Proceedings*

of the International Congress, St. Louis, Mosby, 1967, pp. 273–275.
10. Sanning, F. B.: Statistical survey of factors that determine success or failure in the wearing of contact lenses, in Girard, L. J. (Ed.): *Corneal and Scleral Contact Lenses, Proceedings of the International Congress*, St. Louis, Mosby, 1967, pp. 170–173.
11. Sarver, M. D., and Harris, M. G.: A standard for success in wearing contact lenses, *Am. J. Optom.*, *48*(*5*):382–385, 1971.
12. Debrousse, and Barbier: Concerning over 300 attempts to fit contact lenses, *Survey Ophthalmol.*, *12*(*3*):344–345, 1967. Translated from *Bull. Soc. Ophthalmol.*, *46*:1058–1068, 1966.
13. Morrison, R. J.: Measured corneal curvature and corneal contact lens prescribing, *The Optician*, *162*(*4185*):12–13, 1971.
14. Morrison, R. J.: A survey of 1,000 consecutive contact lens patients, *J. Am. Optom. Assoc.*, *43*(*2*):79–183, 1972.
15. Liuzzi, S.: Statistical analysis of contact lens wearers in the Bahia Blanca area, *Contact Lens*, *3*(*2*):30–31, 1971.
16. Cohen, D. P.: Psychology and contact lenses,

Optom. Weekly, 50(44):2165–2166, 1959.

17. Dickinson, F.: On the preservation of the most precious benefit of contact lens correction, *Contacto, 11(2)*:12–14, 1967.

18. May, C. H.: A comparative study of visual performance before and after wearing contact lens, *Contacto, 4(2)*:51, 1960.

19. Gumpelmayer, T. F.: Special considerations in the fitting of corneal lenses in high myopia, *Am. J. Optom.,, 47(11)*:879–886, 1970.

20. Peterson, J. E., and McDonell, D. H.: A study of the effect of contact lenses, spectacle prescriptions, and unaided vision on the horizontal motion and form fields, *The Oregon Optometrist, July-Oct.*:9–12, 1962.

21. Brombach, T. A.: Visual fields and contact lenses, *Contacto, 5(8)*:265, 1961.

22. Miller, D. et al.: Glare sensitivity related to use of contact lenses, *Arch. Ophthalmol., 78 (4)*:448–450, 1967.

23. Millodot, M.: Variation of visual acuity with contact lenses (a function of luminance), *Arch. Ophthalmol., 82(4)*:461–465, 1969.

24. Bailey, N. J.: Personal communication.

25. Loring, J. H.: Visual acuity in five selected contact lens cases not correctible to standard acuity, *Optom. Weekly, 49(43)*:2031–2032, 1958.

26. Grosvenor, T.: Visual acuity, astigmatism and soft contact lenses, *Am. J. Optom., 49(5)*: 407–412, 1972.

27. Larke, J. R., and Sabell, A. G.: A comparative study of the ocular response to two forms of contact lens—Part 2, *The Optician, 162(4188)*: 10–17, 1971.

28. Sarver, M. D.: Vision with hydrophilic contact lenses, *J. Am. Optom. Assoc., 43(3)*: 316–320, 1972.

29. Grosvenor, T.: Soft lens patient selection and criteria for success, *J. Am. Optom. Assoc., 43(3)*:330–333, 1972.

30. Harris, M. G., and Mandell, R. B.: Contact lens adaptation: osmotic theory, *Am. J. Optom., 46(3)*:196–202, 1969.

31. Mandell, R. B., and Harris, M. G.: Theory of the contact lens adaptation process, *J. Am. Optom. Assoc., 39(3)*:260–261, 1968.

32. Miller, R. B.: Tear concentrations of sodium and potassium during adaptation to contact lenses—II. Potassium observations. *Am. J. Optom., 47(10)*:773–779, 1970.

33. Uniacke, N. P., and Hill, R. M.: Osmotic pressure of the tears during adaptation to contact lenses, *J. Am. Optom. Assoc., 41(11)*: 932–936, 1970.

34. Berman, M. R.: Central corneal curvature and wearing time during contact lens adaptation, *Optom. Weekly, 63(6)*:132–135, 1972.

35. Arroyo, J. C.: Fourteen hours' wear in three days, *Contact Lens, 3(3)*:26–27, 1971.

36. Mandell, R. B.: Contact lens adaptation, *J. Am. Optom. Assoc., 42(3)*:231, 1971.

37. Polse, K. A., and Mandell, R. B.: Contact lens adaptation, *J. Am. Optom. Assoc., 42(1)*: 45–50, 1971.

38. Jackson, W. R.: Some physio-chemical and biochemical factors influencing contact lens adaptability, *S. Afr. Refr., 18(4)*:14–16, 21, 1971.

39. Jackson, W. R.: Physiochemical and biochemical factors affecting contact lens adaptability, *Br. J. Physiol. Opt., 26(2)*:109–110, 1971.

40. Hill, R. M.: Comments on contact lens adaptation: Osmotic pressure of the tears, *J. Cont. Lens Soc. Am., 4(4)*:15–21, 1970.

41. Masnick, K.: A preliminary investigation into the effects of corneal lenses on central corneal thickness and curvature, *Austr. J. Optom., 54(2)*:38–60, 1971.

42. Masnick, K.: A preliminary investigation into the effects of corneal lenses on central corneal thickness and curvatures—Part 2, *Austr. J. Optom., 54(3)*:87–98, 1971.

43. Brungardt, T. F., and Potter, C. E.: Adaptation to corneal contact lenses: profile of clinical tests, *Am. J. Optom., 49(1)*:41–49, 1972.

44. Blackstone, D.: Comments on the latest U.S. contact lens survey, *The Optician, 151(3914)*: 344–345, 1966.

45. Blackstone, M. R.: Contact lenses as eye protector, *The Optician, 154(3997)*:469, 1967.

46. Brown, D. V.: Traumatic fracture of plastic contact lenses, *Arch. Ophthalmol., 72*:319–322, 1964.

47. Robinson, L.: Contact lenses are eye savers, *Contacto, 10(3)*:7–14, 1966.

48. Simpson, W.: Environmental factors involved

in wearing contact lenses, *Optom. Week-ly*, 46(50):2067, 1955.

49. Schwartz, A., and Glatt, L. D.: Contact lenses for children and adolescents—a survey, *J. Am. Optom. Assoc.*, 32(2):143–146, 1960.

50. Cohen, J. M.: Corneal protection through contact lenses (letter to the editor), *Optom. Weekly*, 55(4):30–31, 1964.

51. O'Rourke, P. J.: Traumatic fracture of contact lens with corneal injury, *Br. J. Ophthalmol.*, 55(2):125–127, 1971.

52. Dixon, J. M., and Lawaczeck, E.: Some disadvantages of contact lenses, *Eye, Ear, Nose and Throat Mon.*, 43(9):62–63, 1964.

53. Donn, A.: Pros and cons of contact lenses, *Sight Sav. Rev.*, 37(2):83–86, 1967.

54. Evershed-Martin, L.: Contact lenses—their use in correction and therapy, *Contacto*, 11 (2):18–21, 1967.

55. Gyorffy, I.: Contact lenses, are they dangerous to the eyes? *Can. J. Optom.*, 28(1):22–24, 1966.

56. Ashline, J. W., and Ellis, P. P.: Endophtalmitis and contact lenses, *Am. J. Ophthalmol.*, 66(5): 960–961, 1968.

57. Allen, J. H.: Who's afraid of the little green bug? The Fourth Conrad Berens Memorial Lecture, Oct. 19, 1971, *Contact Lens Med. Bull.*, 5(1):2–14, 1972.

58. Diamond, S.: Medical complications of contact lenses and their aeromedical implications, *Aerosp. Med.*, 38(7):739–741, 1967.

59. Golden, B. H., Fingerman, L. H., and Allen, H. F.: Pseudomonas corneal ulcers in contact lens wearers. Epidemiology and treatment, *Arch. Ophthalmol.*, 85(5):543–547, 1971.

60. Taub, R. G.: Pathology induced by contact lenses and their treatment, *Opt. J. Rev. Optom.*, 109(7):23–24, 1972.

61. Bigger, J. F., Meltzer, G., Mandell, A., and Burde, R. M.: Serratia marcescens endophthalmitis, *Am. J. Ophthalmol.*, 72(6): 1102–1105, 1971.

62. Rengstorff, R. H., and Black, C. J.: Eye protection from contact lenses, *J. Am. Optom. Assoc.*, 45(3):270–275, March 1974.

63. Rengstorff, R. H.: Eye protection from contact lenses, *S. Afr. Opt.*, 30(1):31–38, March 1975.

64. Bloodworth, C. E.: Case history of a contact

lens embedded in the upper eyelid, *Contact Lens*, 2(8):7–8, 1970.

65. Smalling, O. H.: Embedment of inverted corneal contact lens, *J. Am. Optom. Assoc.*, 42(8):755, 1971.

66. Greenspoon, M. K.: History of the cinematic uses of cosmetic contact lenses, *Am. J. Optom.*, 46(1):63–67, 1969.

67. Gyorffy, I.: Sports and contact lenses— observation of 400 cases, *Contacto*, 4(11):495, 1960.

68. Runninger, J.: You can't hit 'em if you don't see 'em, *Optom. Weekly*, 62(14):309–313, 1971.

69. Berkow, J. W.: Preservation of sight in sports, *Md. State Med. J.*, 20(11):57–59, 1971.

70. Stone, J.: Contact lenses and driving, *The Ophthalmic Optician*, 10(6):268–270, 273, 1970.

71. Stone, J.: Contact lenses and driving—Part 2, *The Ophthalmic Optician*, 10(7):322–324, 337–339, 1970.

72. Stone, J.: Subjective comparison of the use of contact lenses and spectacles for driving, *Am. J. Optom.*, 47(12):952–965, 1970.

73. Davis, H. E.: Keep them flying! A dramatic presentation of interprofessionalism in action, *Contacto*, 15(2):12–15, 1971.

74. Wick, R. L., Jr.: Civil aviation and contact lenses, *Contacto*, 9(4):24–29, 1965.

75. Duquet, J.: Practicability of contact lenses for pilots, *J. Aviation Med.*, 23:477, 1952.

76. Diamond, S.: Contact lenses in aviation. *Aerosp. Med.*, 33:1361–1366, 1962.

77. Grant, S. C., and May, C. H.: Orthokeratology— a therapeutic approach to contact lens procedures, *Contacto*, 14(3):3–16, 1970.

78. Paige, N.: The plus lens increment—a system of myopia control and reduction, *Contacto*, 15(1):28–29, 1971.

79. Kelly, T. S. B.: Contact lens and myopia, *Contact Lens*, 3(7):10–18, 1972.

80. Kelly, T. S. B., and Butler, D.: The present position of contact lenses in relation to myopia, *Br. J. Physiol. Opt.*, 26(1):33–48, 1971.

81. Neill, J. C.: Contact lenses and myopia, in (Ed.): *Transactions of the International Ophthalmology and Optometry Congress*, London, Lockwood, 1962, pp. 191–197.

82. Morrison, R. J.: Contact lenses and the pro-

gression of myopia, *J. Am. Optom. Assoc.*, 28(12):711–713, 1957.

83. Ziff, S. L.: Orthokeratology, *J. Am. Optom. Assoc.*, 42(3):275, 1971.

84. Nolan, J. A.: Orthokeratology, *J. Am. Optom. Assoc.*, 42(4):355–360, 1971.

85. Ziff, S. L., and Wesson, M. D.: Orthokeratology-visual care, *Contacto*, 15(2):55–57, 1971.

86. Grant, S. C., and May, C. H.: Orthokeratology control of refractive errors through contact lenses, *J. Am. Optom. Assoc.*, 42(13): 1277–1283, 1971.

87. Grant, S. C., and May, C. H.: Orthokeratology the control of refractive errors through contact lenses, *The Optician*, 163 (4214):8–11, 1972.

88. Fontana, A. A.: Orthokeratology using the one piece bifocal, *Contacto*, 16(2):45–47, 1972.

89. Harris, D. H.: Developmental myopia and orthokeratology, *Contacto*, 16(2):49–57, 1972.

90. Grant, S. C., and May, C. H.: Effects of corneal curvature change on the visual system, *Contacto*, 16(2):65–69, 1972.

91. Grant, S. C., and May, C. H.: Refinements and advances in orthokeratology techniques, *Contacto*, 15(3):6–8, 1971.

92. Kemmetmueller, H.: The influence of contact lenses on myopia, *Contact Lens*, 3 (7):9–10, 1972.

93. Ziff, S. L.: Orthokeratology in relation to existing corneal curvatures, *South. J. Optom.*, 7(3):9–19, 30, 33–35, 37, 1965.

94. Kolles, B. A.: Ortho who? *Minn. Optom.*, Dec.:8–11, 1970.

95. Gates, R. C.: Orthokeratology and the Air Force, *Contacto*, 15(4):8–16, 1971.

96. Paige, N. A.: The rapid reduction of myopia by the plus lens increment method, *Opt. J. Rev. Optom.*, 107(23):17–18, 1970.

97. Bailey, N. J.: Possible factors in the control of myopia with contact lenses, *Contacto*, 2(5):114–117, 1958.

98. News Cues: Interesting contact lens data, *Optom. Weekly*, 63(45):25, 1972.

99. Welsh, R. C.: Contact lenses in aphakia, *Int. Ophthalmol. Clin.*, 1(2):401–440, 1961.

100. Girard, L. J., Soper, J. W., and Sampson, W. G.: Ophthalmological evaluation of a contact lens, *Trans. Ophthalmol. Soc. U.K.*, 87: 671–691, 1967.

101. Goodlaw, E. I.: Use of the bio-microscope in contact lens work, *Contacto*, 3(4):81, 1959.

102. Voss, E. H., and Caretti, J.: Contact lenses: fitting under slit lamp. Indications and contraindications, *Contacto*, 15(4):56–63, 1971.

103. Mayer, M. L., and Fridman, A. J.: Biomicroscopy in contact lens fitting, *Contact Lens*, 3(4):22–27, 1971.

104. Korb, D. R., and Korb, J. M. E.: Corneal staining prior to contact lens wearing, *J. Am. Optom. Assoc.*, 41(3):228–232, 1970.

105. Prechtel, L. A., and Wesley, N. K.: Corneal topography and its application to contact lenses, *Br. J. Physiol. Opt.*, 25(2):117–126, 1970.

106. Soper, J. W., Sampson, W. G., and Girard, L. J.: Corneal topography, keratometry, and contact lenses, *Arch. Ophthalmol.*, 67(6): 753–760, 1962.

107. Nolan, J. A.: Fitting with a corneal photograph, *Br. J. Physiol. Opt.*, 25(2):108–116, 1970.

108. Anderson, T. W.: Modified caliper for measuring corneal diameter, *Am. J. Ophthalmol.*, 59(6):1137, 1965.

109. Simons, S. J., Jr., and Ogle, K. N.: Pupillary responses to momentary light stimulation to eyes unequally adapted to light, *Am. J. Ophthalmol.*, 63(1):35–45, 1967.

110. Fox, S. A.: The palpebral fissure, *Am. J. Ophthalmol.*, 62(1):73–78, 1966.

111. Shanks, K. R.: The shape of the margin of the upper eyelid, related to corneal lenses, *Br. J. Physiol. Opt.*, 22(2):72–83, 1965.

112. Goldberg, J. B.: Current commentary about contact lenses, *Optom. Weekly*, 62(47):1096–1097, 1971.

113. Stewart, C. R.: Bell's phenomenon and corneal lenses, *Br. J. Physiol. Opt.*, 25(1): 50–60, 1970.

114. Korb, D. R., and Korb, J. E.: A new concept in contact lens design—Parts I and II, *J. Am. Optom. Assoc.*, 41(12):1023–1032, 1970.

115. Stewart, C. R.: Blinking and corneal lens wear, *J. Am. Optom. Assoc.*, 42(3):263, 1971.

116. Koetting, R. A.: A corneal abrasive resistance test, *Am. J. Optom.*, 42(8):475–485,

1965.

117. Koetting, R. A.: Useful auxiliary tests in contact lens examination, *J. Am. Optom. Assoc.*, 36(5):439–442, 1965.

118. Schirmer, K. E.: Assessment of corneal sensitivity, *Br. J. Ophthalmol.*, 47(8):488–492, 1963.

119. Schirmer, K. E.: Corneal sensitivity and contact lenses, *Br. J. Ophthalmol.*, 47(8):493–495, 1963.

120. Romero, H. A.: Fitting of a contact lens taking ocular sensitivity into consideration, *Contact Lens*, 3(3):24–25, 1971.

121. *Schirmer Tear Test*, Wayne, N.J., Tilden-Yates Co.

122. Tabak, S.: A short Schirmer tear test, *Contacto*, 16(2):38–42, 1972.

123. Arias, M. C.: A predetermined wearability contact lens fitting technique, *Contacto*, 4(9): 403–414, 1960.

124. Chang, T. C.: Psychological aspect of contact lens fitting, *Contacto*, 5(7):251–256, 1961.

125. Giraldi, O.: Dresser drawer wearing, *Contacto*, 4(3):93, 1960.

126. Koetting, R. A.: Conjunctival injection a factor in contact wearability, *Optom. Weekly*, 56:34–37, 1965.

127. Schapero, M.: A new contact lens record form, *Contacto*, 3(6):167–168, 1959.

128. Lester, R. W.: A new contact lens form, *Contacto*, 3(5):117–124, 1959.

129. Vodnoy, B. E.: Emphasis on the progress examination routine, in *Encyclopedia of Contact Lens Practice*, South Bend, Indiana, International Optics, 1959–1963, Chap. 12, pp. 30–39.

130. Moss, H. L.: Contact lens records, forms and routine, *J. Am. Optom. Assoc.*, 30:563–566, 1959.

131. Sarver, M. D.: Record keeping and patient control procedures for the contact lens case, in *Encyclopedia of Contact Lens Practice*, South Bend, Indiana, International Optics, 1959–1963, vol. 2, Chap. 5, pp. 7–23.

132. Katz, B.: The psychological approach to the contact lens patient, *Second A.O.A. Cont. Lens Symposium*, pp. 7–24, 1965.

133. Beacher, L. L.: The psychologic aspects in contact lens therapy, *J. Am. Optom. Assoc.*, 38(3):185–189, 1967.

134. Gyorffy, I.: The importance of motivation for the prescription and tolerance of contact lenses, *Contacto*, 12(2):20–23, 1968.

135. Iacono, G. D.: Psychological considerations in contact lens practice, *Contacto*, 4(6):205, 1960.

136. Newman, B.: Enthusiasm—the key to success with contact lens patients, *Optom. Weekly*, 55(48):15–17, 1964.

137. Paige, N. A.: The power of positive suggestion in fitting contact lenses, *Optom. Weekly*, 55(27):15–16, 1964.

138. Cole, O. W.: "If the contacts fit, why can't I wear them?" *Contacto*, 15(2):5–9, 1971.

139. Paige, N.: Positive psychological aspects of contact lens fitting, *Optom. Weekly*, 62(17): 378–380, 1971.

140. Berk, R. L.: The psychological impact of contact lenses on children and youth, *J. Am. Optom. Assoc.*, 34(15):1217–1222, 1963.

141. Harris, M. G., and Sarver, M. D.: The prefitting eye examination and failure in wearing contact lenses, *Am. J. Optom.*, 49 (7):565–568, 1972.

142. Beiman, J. A., and Blumenthal, D.: Personality study of contact lens patients, a preliminary report, *Optom. Weekly*, 51(9): 963–965, 1960.

143. Woolf, D.: Social and psychological impact of contact lenses on children and youth, *J. Am. Optom. Assoc.*, 34(14):1138–1143, 1963.

144. Gording, E. J., and Match, E.: Psychology and contact lenses, *J. Am. Optom. Assoc.*, 42(3):230, 1971.

145. Weiner, M.: A comparison of personality patterns of individuals requesting contact lenses and those rejecting them, *Optom. Weekly*, 55(15):21–28, 1964.

146. Gording, E. J., and Match, E.: Personality changes of certain contact lens patients, *J. Am. Optom. Assoc.*, 39(3):266–269, 1968.

147. Harris, M. G., and Messinger, J. H.: Personality traits and failure in wearing contact lenses, *Am. J. Optom.*, 50(8):641–646, 1973.

148. Gording, E. J.: Personality changes in contact lens patients, *Contacto*, 13(3):12–16, 1969.

149. Terry, R. L., and Zimmerman, D. J.: Anxiety induced by contact lenses and framed

spectacles, *J. Am. Optom. Assoc., 41*(3): 257–259, 1970.

150. Harris, M. G., and Sarver, M. D.: Health history and failure in wearing contact lenses, *J. Am. Optom. Assoc., 42*(6):550–553, 1971.

151. Thurmond, R. H.: The heterophoric patient, *Contacto, 3*(6):164–165, 1959.

152. Kennedy, J. R.: The lens correction of divergent strabismus, *Contacto, 15*(2):67–69, 1971.

153. Sampson, W. G.: Contact lenses and the AC/A ratio—applications in accommodative esotropia, *Contact Lens Med. Bull., 2*(3):9–15, 1969.

154. Taranto, E.: Aniseikonia. Relationship of the size of ocular images and visual acuity to achieve binocular vision, *Contacto, 15*(1): 50–51, 1971.

155. Robertson, D. M. et al.: Influence of contact lenses on accommodation—theoretic considerations and clinical study, *Am. J. Ophthalmol., 64*(5):860–871, 1967.

156. Hermann, J. S.: Oculographic determination of the accommodative requirement in hyperopia. Contact lenses versus spectacles, *Contact Lens Med. Bull., 4*(3):14–16, 1971.

157. Sampson, W. G.: Correction of refractive errors: Effect on accommodation and convergence, *Trans. Am. Acad. Ophthalmol. Otolaryngol., 75*(1):124–132, 1971.

158. Schapero, M.: Physical considerations in contact lens fitting, Part one: Determinations from the case history, *J. Am. Optom. Assoc., 33*(3):215–218, 1961.

159. Fontana, F. D.: Corneal scarring and contact lenses—a case in point, *Contacto, 4*(8):377, 1960.

160. Goldbert, J. B.: Current commentary about contact lenses (contraindication for contact lenses; contact lenses and allergic conjunctivitis; tear layer and precorneal film; keratoprosthesis aids aphakic patient; edge thickness controls for corneal lenses), *Optom. Weekly, 61*(13): 287–288, 1970.

161. Gasset, A. R., and Kaufman, H. E.: Hydrophilic lens therapy of severe keratoconjunctivitis sicca and conjunctival scarring, *Am. J. Ophthalmol., 71*(6):1185–1189, 1971.

162. Kaufman, H. E., Uotila, M. H., Gasset, A. R., Wood, T. O., and Ellison, E. D.: The medical uses of soft contact lenses, *Trans. Am. Acad. Ophthalmol. Otolaryngol., 75*(2):361–373, 1971.

163. Gould, H. L.: Therapeutic contact lenses, *Int. Ophthalmol. Clin., 10*(1):131–141, 1970.

164. Espy, J. W.: Management of corneal problems with hydrophilic contact lenses. A report of thirty cases, *Am. J. Ophthalmol., 72*(3):521–526, 1971.

165. Krejci, L.: Scleral gel contact lenses in treatment of dry eyes, *Br. J. Ophthalmol., 56*(5): 425–428, 1972.

166. Gould, H. L.: The dry eye and scleral contact lenses, *Am. J. Ophthalmol., 70*(1):37–41, 1970.

167. Schultz, R. O.: Management of disorders affecting the corneal stroma, *Survey Ophthalmol., 15*(5):317–324, 1971.

168. Iliff, C. E., and Maquin, H. A.: Contact lenses: Indications, *Trans. Am. Acad. Ophthalmol. Otolaryngol., 66*(3):303–305, 1962.

169. Heyman, L. S.: A flush fitting shell for an eight week old infant, *J. Contact Lens Soc. Am., 5*(1):26–27, 1971.

170. Watts, G. K.: Therapeutic uses of soft contact lenses, *The Optician, 16*(4178):17–18, 1971.

171. Leibowitz, H. M., and Rosenthal, P.: Hydrophilic contact lenses in corneal disease. I. Superficial, sterile, indolent ulcers, *Arch. Ophthalmol., 85*(2):163–166, 1971.

172. Buxton, J. N., and Locke, C. R.: A therapeutic evaluation of hydrophilic contact lenses, *Am. J. Ophthalmol., 62*(3):532–535, 1971.

173. Rosenthal, J. W.: Clinical pathology in contact lenses, *Int. Ophthalmol., Clin., 1*(2): 517–534, 1961.

174. Huggert, A.: Increase of the intraocular pressure when using contact glasses, *Acta Ophthalmol, 29*(4):475–481, 1951.

175. Raiford, M. B.: Examination for contact lenses, *Int. Ophthalmol. Clin., 1*(2):337–350, 1961.

176. Dyer, J. A.: Corneal contact lenses and ocular disease, *Minn. Med., 45*(1):27–33, 1962.

177. Kennedy, J. R.: Contact lenses in compli-

cated glaucoma, *Am. J. Optom.*, *39*(7):369–373, 1962.

178. Tortolero, J.: Glaucoma and contact lenses, *Contacto*, *8*(2):6–10, 1964.

179. Fonda, G.: Characteristics and low-vision corrections in albinism, *Arch. Ophthalmol.*, *68*(2): 754–761.

180. Edmunds, R. T.: Vision of albinos, *Arch. Ophthalmol.*, *42*:755–767, 1949.

181. Courtney, G. R.: *Ocular characteristics of the human albino*, Masters thesis in physiological optics at Indiana University, pp. 1–68, 1966.

182. Fonda, G., Thomas, H., and Gore, G. V., III: Educational and vocational placement, and low-vision corrections in albinism, *Sight Sav. Rev.*, *41*(1):29–36, 1971.

183. Ruben, M.: Albinism and contact lenses, *Contact Lens*, *1*(2):5–8, 1967.

184. Borish, I. M.: *Clinical Refraction*, 3rd ed., Chicago, Professional Pr., 1970, p. 127.

185. Meloan, J. B.: Albinism—a case report, *Am. J. Optom.*, *28*(8):435–437, 1951.

186. Hermann, J. S., and Koverman, J. J.: Prophylaxis of amblyopia in aniridia—the role of pinhole contact lenses, *J. Pediatr. Ophthalmol.*, *5*(1):48–52, 1968.

187. Sato, T., and Saito, N.: Contact lenses for babies and children, *Contacto*, *3*:419–424, 1959.

188. Gregersen, E.: Contact lenses in a series of weaksighted patients, *Acta Ophthalmol. (Kbh)*, *45*:119–126, 1967.

189. Hugill, G. E.: Contact lens practice in a provincial English hospital, *S. Afr. Refr.*, *19* (1):42–46, 1972.

190. Grayson, M., and Boling, R.: Clinical application of contact lenses, *Int. Ophthalmol. Clin.*, *1*(2):327–336, 1961.

191. Enoch, J. M., and Windsor, C. E.: Remission of nystagmus following fitting contact lenses to an infant with aniridia, *Am. J. Ophthalmol.*, *66*(2):333–335, 1968.

192. Williams, D.: Results with contact lenses, *Arch. Ophthalmol.*, *44*:481, 1950.

193. Gyorffy, I.: Therapeutic contact lenses from plastic, *Br. J. Ophthalmol.*, *34*(2):115–118, 1950.

194. Klein, M., and Millwood, E. G.: Control of experimental corneal infection with medicated semi-solid contact cap and disc,

195. Lewis, E. L.: Protective corneal lens for prolonged procedures, *Am. J. Ophthalmol.*, *45*(6):922, 1958.

196. Flynn, M. A., and Esterly, D. B.: Contact lenses in Groenouw's dystrophy, *Am. J. Ophthalmol.*, *63*(5):991, 1967.

197. Siese, A.: Interesting contact lens case: Improving visual acuity with a contact lens, *The Optician*, *151*(3910):241–242, 1966.

198. Sellers, E.: The restoration of visual function in cases of amblyopia utilising contact lenses, *Br. J. Physiol. Opt.*, *26*(2):130–142, 1971.

199. Ruedemann, A. D., and Jardon, F.: Ten years' experience with scleral lenses, *Trans. Am. Ophthalmol. Soc.*, *68*:245–276, 1970.

200. Tomlinson, K.: The therapeutic value of contact lenses in cases of ocular abnormalities, *The Optician*, *163*(4212):8–11, 1972.

201. Alleger, C.: The case of the artificial iris, *Optom. Weekly*, *62*(3):55–57, 1971.

202. Zeltzer, H.: The x-chrom lens, *J. Am. Optom. Assoc.*, *42*(9):933–939, 1971.

203. Schwartz, I., and Wienke, R. E.: Effect of contact lenses upon the red/green ratio, *Contacto*, *3*(11):379, 1959.

204. Fein, B. T.: Allergy and contact lenses, *Tex. Med.*, *56*(8):665–666, 1960.

205. Taub, S. J.: Allergic manifestation of the eye and adjacent structures, *Eye, Ear, Nose and Throat Mon.*, *44*(1):71, 1965.

206. McConnell, J.: Cosmetics and contact lenses, *Contacto*, *11*(1):40–43, 1967.

207. Shnider, H. A.: Diabetes mellitus and contact lenses, *J. Am. Optom. Assoc.*, *36*(8):706–709, 1965.

208. Chappell, G. H.: General after-care procedures and the contact lens patient—Part 3, *The Optician*, *163*(4231):10–14, 1972.

209. Rosenwasser, H. M.: Aetiology of systemic oedema and its effect on contact lens wearing, *The Optician*, *163*(4127):8–10, 1972.

210. Mulrooney, G.: Soft contact lenses, cosmetics and medication, *Can. J. Optom.*, *33* (3):74, 1971.

211. Rosenwasser, H. M.: Effects of diuretics and

infection with Ps. Pycocyanea treated with Streptomycin, *Br. J. Ophthalmol.*, *37*(1): 30–36, 1953.

tranquillisers on the wearing of contact lenses, *Opt. J. Rev. Optom.*, *100*(*22*):41–45, 1963.

212. Kennedy, J. R.: After-care of contact lenses, *Contacto*, *15*(*2*):42–46, 1971.

213. Koetting, R. A.: The influence of oral contraceptives on contact lens wear, *Am. J. Optom.*, *43*(*4*):268–274, 1966.

214. Koetting, R. A.: The influence of oral contraceptives on contact lens wear, *Aust. J. Optom.*, *49*(*7*):200–205, 1966. Reprinted from Am. J. Optom., *43*(*4*):268–274, 1966.

215. Goldberg, J. B.: A commentary on oral con-

traceptive therapy and contact lens wear, *J. Am. Optom. Assoc.*, *41*(*3*):237–241, 1970.

216. Ridley, H. D.: Oral contraceptives: their manifestations, *J. Optom.*, *3*(*1*):9–10, 1971.

217. Sabell, A. G.: Oral contraceptives and the contact lens wearer, *Br. J. Physiol. Opt.*, *25*(*2*):127–137, 1970.

218. Sartoris, R.: The pill: ocular manifestations, *S. Afr. Refr.*, *18*(*4*):67–68, 1971.

219. Moss, H. L., and Polishuk, A.: Oral contraceptives and contact lenses, *J. Am. Optom. Assoc.*, *43*(*6*):654–656, 1972.

ADDITIONAL READINGS

Applegate, R. A.: Changes in the contrast sensitivity function induced by contact lens wear, *Am. J. Optom. Physiol. Opt.*, *52*(*12*):840–846, 1975.

Applegate, W. W.: Who benefits from contact lens insurance?, *Cont. Lens Forum*, *2*(*6*):29–31, 1977.

Arons, I. J.: Soft lenses today, *Int. Cont. Lens Clin.*, *4*(*3*):42, 1977.

Arons, I. J.: Soft lens update, *Int. Cont. Lens Clin.*, *5*(*3*):54, 1978.

Arons, I. J., and Little, A. D.: The soft lens market today: view from outside, *Optical Index*, *50*(*2*): 20–30, 1975.

Backman, H.: Vision in aviation, *Optom. Weekly*, *63*(*33*):805, 1972.

Backman, H., and Bolte, C.: Chronic allergic conjunctivitis and its effect on contact lenses, *Optom. weekly*, *65*(*31*):831, 1974.

Backman, H. A.: Identification of patient intolerance to contact lenses, *Opt. J. Rev. Optom.*, *114*(*4*):59, 1977.

Bailey, N. J.: All is vanity?, *Cont. Lens Forum*, *2*(*2*):45–47, 1977.

Barasch, K. R., and Morrison, R.: The overwearing syndrome and its care, *Cont. Lens Clin.*, *1*(*2*): 83–87, 1974.

Barber, J., and Malin, A. H.: Hypnosis and suggestion for fitting contact lenses, *J. Am. Optom. Assoc.*, *48*(*3*):379, 1977.

Barber, J. C.: Management of the patient with dry eyes, *Cont. Intraoc. Lens Med. J.*, *3*(*4*):10, 1977.

Bayshore, C. A.: Rigid lenses: an overview, *J. Am. Optom. Assoc.*, *50*(*3*):317, 1979.

Beacher, L. L.: A guidance program for contact lens patients, *Opt. J. Rev. Optom.*, *106*(*1*):27–28,

1969.

Berry, R.: Contact lenses for contact sports, *Optom. Mgmt.*, *11*(*3*):16–19, 1975.

Bowers, L. T.: The contact lens Rx: release it or not?, *Optom. Mgmt.*, *15*(*1*):125, 1979.

Boyce, J. W.: Contact lenses now not later, *J. Opt. (New Zealand)*, pp. 6–9, March/April 1977.

Breschkin, J.: The philosophy of contact lens fitting—updated, *J. Am. Optom. Assoc.*, *47*(*3*):283, 1976.

Broe, D. J.: Fitting modalities, design vs. material, *Cont. Lens J.*, *11*(*4*):9, 1978.

Carney, L. G., and Woo, G. C.: Comparison of accommodation with rigid and flexible contact lenses, *Am. J. Optom. Physiol. Opt.*, *54*(*9*):595, 1977.

Consumer Reports: Soft contact lenses—they have their limitations, *Consumer Reports*, *37*(*5*):272–278, 1972.

Cordrey, P.: Arc flash and the contact lens wearer—a modern myth, *The Disp. Opt.*, *29*(*18*):74–77, 1977.

Crossen, R. J.: Safety of contact lenses in industry, *Cont. Intraoc. Lens Med. J.*, *3*(*3*):28, 1977.

Danker, F. J.: The contact lens industry of the future, *Cont. Lens Forum*, *3*(*1*):69, 1978.

De Jonge, J. K.: Case report: a lens is a lens is a lens, *Cont. Intraoc. Lens Med. J.*, *4*(*2*):94, 1978.

De Manzanos, A. M.: Variation in the cornea during the menstrual cycle and the effect on contact lenses, *The Optician*, *169*(*4377*):4–6, 1975.

Des Groseilliers, R. (translators): Contact lenses . . . are they dangerous to the eye?, *S. Afr. Opt.*, p. 42, Dec. 1966 *(original paper by Istvan Gyorffy, Budapest)*.

Dickinson, F.: The public and soft contact lenses, *Contacto*, 20(4):33–34, 1976.

Dixon, W. S.: Contact lenses: do they belong in the workplace?, *Occup. Health Saf.*, 47(3):37, 1978.

Dowaliby, M.: Eyewear for the contact lens wearer, *Opt. J. Rev. Optom.*, 113(6):33–37, 1976.

Eng, W. G.: Survey on eye comfort in aircraft: 1. Flight attendants, *Aviation, Space, Environ. Med.*, pp. 401–404, April 1979.

Farkas, P.: Hypnosis in contact lens practice, *Opt. Mgmt.*, 14(3):51, 1978.

Farkas, P.: What's in a brand name?, *Cont. Lens Forum*, 4(7):35–39, 1979.

Gauvreau, D. K.: Skydiving with Soflenses, *Cont. Lens Forum*, 2(11):59, 1977.

Goldberg, J. B.: Soft contact lens marketing trends, *Opt. Weekly*, 68(14):46–48, 1977.

Goldberg, J. V.: Contact lenses: pterygium and contact lenses, *Opt. J. Rev. Optom.*, 110(14):31–32, 1973.

Gording, E. J.: Psychology and contact lenses, *J. Am. Optom. Assoc.*, 47(3):286, 1976.

Gould, H.: How to remove contact lenses from comatose patients, *Am. J. Nurs.*, 76(9):1483–1485, 1976.

Hand, S. I.: Contact lens removal in the nonresponsive or incapacitated patient, *Med. Serv. Digest*, 28(4):17, 1977.

Harris, J. G., Wayda, R. A., and Kletzelman, J.: Changes in binocularity associated with wearing contact lenses in place of spectacles, *J. Am. Optom. Assoc.*, 46(3):271–272, 1975.

Hewett, L.: Clinical responsibility in fitting contact lenses, *Austr. J. Optom.*, 57(12):381–386, 1974.

Hicks, M.: Industrial hazards of contact lenses, *The Ophthalmic Optician*, 16(24):1061–1062, 1976.

Hill, J. F.: Tear analysis for successful contact lens wear, *Optom. Weekly*, 64(39):21–24, 1973.

Hill, R. M.: The cornea's need to "breathe", *Int. Cont. Lens Clin.*, 3(4):60–61, 1976.

Hodd, F. A. B.: Public protection and contact lenses, *The Ophthalmic Optician*, 14(13):615, 1974.

Jagerman, L. S.: Effects of air travel on contact-lens wearers, *Am. J. Ophthalmol.*, 75(3):533, 1973.

Janoff, L. E.: A pilot study of the effect of soft contact lenses on intraocular pressure, *J. Am. Optom. Assoc.*, 48(3):303, 1977.

Josephson, J. E.: Hydrogel lens statistics drawn from private practice, *Int. Cont. Lens Clin.*, 5(3):26, 1978.

Kaplan, J.: The effect of contact lenses on visual function, *J. Am. Optom. Assoc.*, 47(3):288, 1976.

Kassalow, T. W.: Hypnosis and the optometrist, *Contacto*, 19(2):37–40, 1975.

Keiko, Y., and Keiichiro, K.: Changes in near points of accommodation when wearing soft contact lenses, *Cont. Intraoc. Lens. Med. J.*, 1(1–2):60–68, 1975.

Litvin, M. W.: The incidence of eye infections with contact lenses, *The Optician*, 174(4496):11–14, 1977.

McEachern, C. L.: Patient indoctrination, *J. Am. Optom. Assoc.*, 47(3):366, 1976.

McEachern, C. L.: Role/relationship of government in the contact lens field, *J. Am. Optom. Assoc.*, 50(3):276–277, 1979.

Malin, A. H.: A survey of patient handling of contact lenses, *J. Am. Optom. Assoc.*, 42(2):158–159, 1971.

Malin, A. H.: Suggestion and hypnosis for fitting contact lenses, *Int. Cont. Lens Clin.*, 2(3):39–42, 1975.

Mandell, R. B.: Why does the lens color look different on my eye?, *Int. Cont. Lens Clin.*, 1(4):36–37, 1974.

Mor, E.: Motivation and coping behavior in adaptation to contact lenses, *J. Pers. Assess.*, 37(2):136, 1973.

Morgan, E. H.: The professional liability problem and optometry, *J. Am. Optom. Assoc.*, 42(2):160–164, 1971.

Mulrooney, G.: Soft contact lenses, cosmetics, and medication, *Can. J. Optom.*, 33(3):74, 1971.

Nicolitz, E., and Flanagan, J. C.: Orbital mass as a complication of contact lens wear, *Arch. Ophthalmol.*, 96(12):2238–2239, 1978.

O'Neil, J.: Use of contact lenses in the industrial environment, *Cont. Intraoc. Lens Med. J.*, 3(3):30–32, 1977.

Older, J. J.: Encysted corneal contact lens presenting as an eyelid mass, *Ann. Ophthalmol.*, 11(9):1393–94, 1979.

Ong, J., and Mauney, M. C.: Classificational distribution and characteristics of contact lens clinic patients, *Am. J. Optom. Physiol. Opt.*, 51(11):857–861, 1974.

Ong, J, and Bowling, R.: Effect of contact lens on cornea and lid of a 10-year wearer, *Am. J. Optom. Arch. Am. Acad. Optom.*, 49(11):932–935, 1972.

Paris, A.: The use of hypnosis in contact lens

adaptation—a case report, *Optom. Weekly*, 66(3): 59–61, 1975.

van Bijsterveld, O. P. et al.: Contact lens tolerance and oral contraceptives, *Ann. Ophthalmol.*, 10(7): 947, 1978.

SECTION II

HARD LENSES

Chapter 5

BASIC PRINCIPLES OF CORNEAL LENSES

C ORNEAL CONTACT LENSES usually have been named and classified either by (1) *lens type*—the physical construction of the lens or (2) *fitting philosophy*—the fitting relationship between the lens and the eye.* If the first classification is used and only the physical design of contact lenses is considered, lenses may be conveniently divided on the basis of the number of curves on the concave surface into four basic types: *monocurve, bicurve, tricurve, and multicurve* lenses. In addition, a large variety of special contact lens designs are available. Lenses are produced in bifocal form, as pinhole apertures, in nonrotational designs, with toric surfaces, and with many other optional features for various purposes. These lenses will be discussed in later chapters and are mentioned here only to bring attention to the diversity of lenses produced.

It is possible to make any of the basic lens types with a variety of dimensions. These dimensions should be varied according to the characteristics of the patient's eye and the fitting philosophy that is followed. In the description of basic lens types that follows, some average figures are given for the dimensions of the lens variables. These figures are intended only to familiarize the reader with the general construction of the lenses and should not be interpreted as norms to be used in fitting. A more detailed description of methods to select the dimensions of the lens variables will follow in later chapters.

BASIC LENS TYPES

MONOCURVE LENS

Construction

From the standpoint of construction, the monocurve lens is the simplest type of con-

*The author, in hopes of alleviating undue confusion in fitting terminology, has employed three distinguishing categories: lens types, fitting philosophies, and fitting methods. Lens type refers to actual lens construction, fitting philosophy pertains to the relationship of the lens to the eye, and fitting method refers to the technique used to arrive at the specifications for the lens.

tact lens. It is essentially a miniature meniscus lens, which has a single curve on both the convex and concave surfaces. A typical monocurve lens is illustrated in Figure 5.1. The convex surface is termed either the front or anterior surface, and the concave surface the back or posterior surface. (Occasionally, the latter is called the ocular surface.) At the periphery the two surfaces are contoured to form a smooth and rounded edge.

125

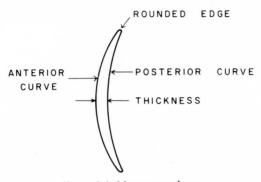

Figure 5.1. Monocurve lens.

BICURVE LENS

Construction

The bicurve lens is similar to the monocurve lens but has an additional curve at the periphery of the posterior surface that is concentric to the central curve (Figure 5.2). The central curve area is referred to as the optical zone. The peripheral curve always has a longer radius of curvature (said to be flatter) than the optical zone radius.

The width of the peripheral curve of a bicurve lens is specified by the band width of the curve as it appears from a straight ahead (isometric) projection. This method of specification has a practical advantage in describing the dimensions of the contact lens. It is then possible to add the band widths of the curves to the optical zone diameter to obtain the total diameter. This simple system would

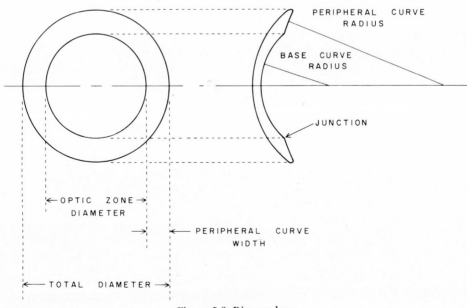

Figure 5.2. Bicurve lens.

not be possible were the peripheral curve width expressed in terms of its chord width (Figure 5.3). It must be noted, however, that since the peripheral curve is given in terms of a single band width it must be added twice to the optical zone diameter to find the total diameter. Hence, for a bicurve lens the following results:

T.D.   = Total diameter
O.Z.D.   = Optical zone diameter
P.C.W.   = Peripheral curve width
   T.D.$_{bicurve}$ = O.Z.D. + 2(P.C.W.)

Dimensions

1. *Total diameter.* The average is about 8.8 mm. but may range from 7.5 to 10 mm.

2. *Center thickness.* For a lens of average dimensions and plano power, the thickness is about 0.18 mm. It varies with the total diameter, power, and widths and with radii of the optical zone and peripheral curve.

3. *Optical zone.* Usually varies between 7.0 and 8.0 mm. in width and has a radius that is between 7.3 and 8.8 mm.

4. *Peripheral curve.* Usually between 0.2 and 1.2 mm. in width, with a radius that is 1.0 to 5.0 mm. longer than the optical zone radius.

TRICURVE LENS

Construction

If an additional curve is added to the periphery of a bicurve lens, it will form a tricurve lens (Figure 5.4). The third curve surrounds the other two curves and is known as the *peripheral curve.* The middle curve is known as the *secondary curve* or as the *intermediate curve.* Some authors prefer, however, to call all the curves peripheral curves except the optical zone, and to number them the first peripheral curve and second peripheral curve. Unfortunately, for those who use this system there has not always been agreement as to which direction the order of numbering should follow. Although there is generally no confusion regarding the meaning of the commonly used terms for contact lens parameters, some more precise terms have been recommended by the American National Standards Institute as given in Table 5.1.

The total diameter of a tricurve lens (T.D.$_{tricurve}$) is equal to the diameter of the optical zone (O.Z.D.) plus twice the widths of the intermediate curve (I.C.W.) and peripheral curve (P.C.W.). That is—

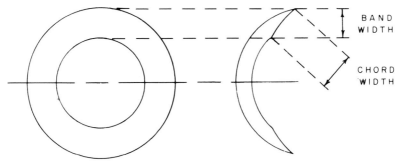

Figure 5.3. Peripheral curve width is expressed in terms of the band width rather than the chord width.

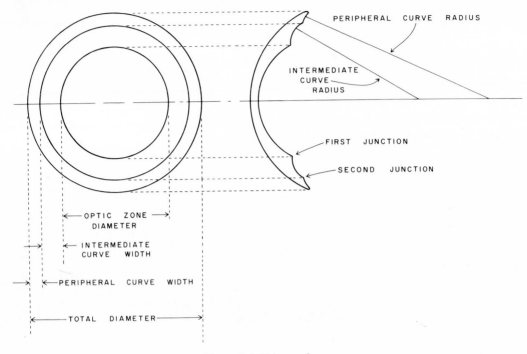

Figure 5.4. Tricurve lens.

$$T.D._{tricurve} =$$
$$O.Z.D. + 2(I.C.W.) + 2(P.C.W.)$$

Dimensions

1. *Total diameter.* The average is about 9.2 mm., but it may range from about 8.8 to 10.0 mm.

2. *Center thickness.* For a lens of average thickness and plano power, the thickness is about 0.18 mm. It varies with the total diameter, power, and widths and radii of the optical zone and peripheral curves.

3. *Optical zone.* Usually varies between 7 and 8 mm. in width with a radius between 7.3

TABLE 5.1
AMERICAN NATIONAL STANDARDS INSTITUTE
Z80–1972 TERMINOLOGY

Commonly Used Term	*ANSI Term*
Optic Zone Diameter	Posterior Optic Zone Diameter (P.O.Z.D.)
Front Optic Zone	Anterior Optic Zone Diameter (A.O.Z.D.)
Intermediate Curve Width	Posterior Secondary (Intermediate) Curve Width (P.S.C.R.)
Peripheral Curve Width	Posterior Peripheral (Bevel) Curve Curve Width (P.P.C.R.)
Total Diameter	Diameter (D)
Base Curve Radius	Posterior Central Curve Radius (P.C.C.R.)
Intermediate Curve Radius	Posterior Secondary Curve Radius (P.S.C.R.)
Peripheral Curve Radius	Posterior Peripheral Curve Radius (P.P.C.R.)
Junction	Transition Zone
Front Peripheral Curve Radius	Anterior Peripheral Curve Radius (A.P.C.R.)

and 8.8 mm.

4. *Intermediate curve.* Usually between 0.2 and 1.2 mm. in width with a radius that is 1.0 to 2.0 mm. longer than the optical zone radius.

5. *Peripheral curve.* Usually between 0.2 and 0.6 mm. in width with a radius that is 1 to 4 mm. longer than the radius of the intermediate curve.

MULTICURVE LENS

If a contact lens has more than two peripheral curves it is classified as a *multicurve* lens (Figure 5.5). Such a lens is rarely used except for special fitting requirements, the best example of which is keratoconus. All curves of a multicurve lens except the central curve are called peripheral curves and are numbered beginning with the curve adjacent to the optical zone and progressing towards the periphery. The dimensions of the multicurve lens will be given under the various topics in which it is applicable.

GENERAL LENS FEATURES

Blend

It is sometimes desirable to smooth the transition point, which is the *junction* of adjacent curves on the posterior surface of a lens. This process is known as *blending.* A blend differs from an actual lens curve in that it does not have a distinct curvature but merely tends to smooth one curve into another as illustrated in Figure 5.6.

Front Bevel

Very often negative power lenses have excessively thick edges. A thick edge is undesirable from the standpoint of comfort and fitting characteristics. There is a tendency for the superior lid to catch the edge during blinking and move the lens about. Edge thickness can be reduced by tapering the front surface at the edge so that it approaches the back surface as illustrated in Figure 5.7. This tapering is known as a front or anterior bevel. Sometimes a true curve is used at the position of the front bevel, which is then called a front or anterior peripheral curve.

Posterior Bevel

A few laboratories use the term bevel to refer to a tapering of the back surface of the lens towards the front surface in the area near the edge. In most instances what is called the posterior bevel is actually another spherical curve at the periphery of the posterior surface. The term bevel has been generally replaced by peripheral curve when used in reference to a true curve. Since there is no general agreement as to what denotes the difference between a bevel and a peripheral curve, the term bevel in this text will be used to refer only to the front taper.

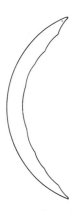

Figure 5.5. Multicurve lens (peripheral curves exaggerated).

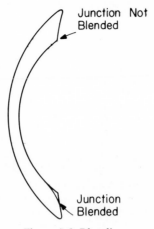

Junction Not
Blended

Junction
Blended

Figure 5.6. Blending.

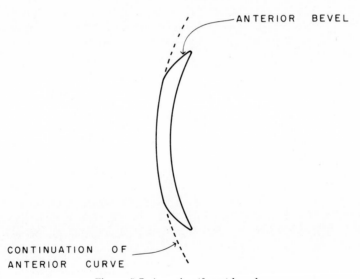

ANTERIOR   BEVEL

CONTINUATION   OF
ANTERIOR   CURVE

Figure 5.7. Anterior (front) bevel.

TRADE NAMES FOR CONTACT LENSES

Some caution is necessary in interpreting the description of lenses made by various laboratories. One manufacturer may call a given lens a bicurve, and another may call a nearly identical lens a tricurve. What one company calls a curve another may call a blend. To add to this confusion, many optical companies use trade names for their own versions of the basic lens types. A lack of consistency for these names has caused more than one neophyte fitter to conclude that there are many more types of lenses than actually exist.

STANDARDIZED LENS DIMENSIONS

A source of confusion for categorizing contact lenses results from various attempts by manufacturers to standardize contact lens dimensions. Early in the development of corneal lenses many laboratories advocated a single set of dimensions for each lens type. For instance, one laboratory listed the bicurve as having a diameter of 9.5 mm., whereas a second laboratory said that the bicurve was 9.2 in diameter. Actually, the bicurve lens, or any other lens type, can and should be made in any diameter necessary to meet the requirements of the individual eye to which it is to be fitted. The reason some laboratories preferred one set of dimensions for each lens type was that it simplified the manufacturing process. It also simplified the teaching of contact lens fitting procedures. The latter reason was particularly important in the early development of corneal lenses because the laboratories provided the first contact lens education to many practitioners.

GENERAL FITTING REQUISITES

Generally, in order for a contact lens to be worn successfully, (1) it must correct the wearer's visual anomaly, and (2) it must be made comfortable and physiologically compatible with the eye. These requisites are fulfilled by choosing the proper dimensions for the contact lens.

OPTICAL REQUISITES

To provide adequate visual acuity, a contact lens must accurately correct for the patient's refractive error. In addition, the optical portion of the lens must cover the major portion of the pupillary area.

Vision is best when the contact lens is centered in front of the pupil and the optical zone diameter is larger than the pupil. Vision is not materially affected, however, as long as approximately three-fourths of the pupillary area is covered by the optical zone of the lens. Consequently, the lens can move back and forth across the cornea within limits and not interfere with vision.

PHYSIOLOGICAL REQUISITES

Contact lenses that are improperly fitted bring about a variety of symptoms which are due to the irritation of the cornea and surrounding structures. While these symptoms are usually looked upon with contempt by the patient, they do serve as a warning that the normal physiological processes of the eye have been disturbed. Unfortunately, the warning system is not always reliable, and a lens that feels comfortable momentarily is not necessarily a correct lens from the standpoint of physiology. It may require days or weeks before ocular changes occur that would prove the lens unsuitable. Consequently, the patient's subjective symptoms cannot be considered the only guide to lens selection. The contact lens must be designed in such a way that it will interfere minimally with the normal function of the eye and its adnexa. If this fitting criterion is fulfilled, the lens selected will be comfortable and allow unrestricted wear.

GENERAL FITTING RULES

The physiological requisites for successful contact lens wear are usually satisfied by three general fitting rules: tears must be exchanged between the lens and the cornea, excessive lens weight must not be borne on small corneal areas, and the lens must not move excessively.

Tear Exchange

Exchange of tears from outside to between the contact lens and the cornea is necessary to maintain the normal metabolism of the cornea and thus allow the contact lens to be tolerated for a normal wearing time. The cornea depends in part upon the tears to bring it nutrient materials and to carry away its metabolic wastes. Stagnation of the tears under a contact lens will cause subjective symptoms of discomfort and objective signs of physiological corneal trauma.

It has been known for some time that a lens that contours the cornea too closely does not allow adequate tear flow and can only be tolerated for a short period. An extreme example of this can be demonstrated by casting a mold of the cornea and then constructing a corneal lens from the mold. This lens quickly produces signs of interference with the corneal metabolism. Consequently, at least some part of the contact lens should not parallel the cornea in order to provide a channel for tear flow.

Excessive Lens Weight on the Cornea

There is a tendency for a contact lens to more or less float on the layer of tears that covers the cornea, but at least part of the lens is touching the cornea proper at all times. The lens touch should not be limited to one or two small corneal areas. The lens should be made to follow the corneal contour closely enough so that its weight is distributed over a large area. On the other hand, some space must exist between the lens and cornea to allow for tear circulation. Consequently, the lens should deviate from the corneal contour to the minimum degree that will still provide space for tear circulation behind the lens.

The distribution of the contact between the lens and cornea is known as the bearing relationship. A lens is tolerated best which has a fairly large bearing area that gradually shifts from point to point across the cornea as the lens is moved during the course of normal lid and eye movements.

Lens Movement

Some movement of a contact lens on the cornea is necessary in order to allow the circulation of tear fluid behind the contact lens, but a lens that moves excessively may cause mechanical trauma to the cornea. The amount of trauma will depend upon the weight of the lens per unit area of bearing surface and the amount of lens movement. Mechanical corneal trauma may thus be reduced by increasing the bearing area or reducing the total lens weight. Lenses that are lighter, that is, either smaller or thinner, can usually be supported more successfully on smaller corneal areas.

It may also be found that a lens that moves excessively bumps against the lid and limbus and causes irritation. Contact lens wearers vary considerably in their ability to tolerate a lens that constantly bumps against the lids. For some wearers the bumping causes no particular disturbance, whereas for others the lens becomes intolerable.

FORCES AFFECTING THE LENS FIT

Several forces act together to hold a contact lens against the cornea. Other forces constantly act to move the lens or eject it from the eye. A correct balance of these forces is necessary in order to have a properly fitting lens.

Of the various factors that control the adherence of the lens to the cornea, three are most important: fluid attraction forces, gravity, and the lids. In addition, frictional forces tend to hold the lens in position on the eye.

FLUID ATTRACTION

The force of attraction between the lens and the cornea is inversely related to the thickness of the tear layer.[1] If the contact lens exactly parallels the cornea, the tear layer thickness is minimal, and the attraction is greatest. If any curve on the lens is made flatter than the cornea, the distance between the periphery of that curve and the cornea is increased. The attractive force between the lens and cornea is reduced, and the lens will move more easily.

If any curve on the lens is steeper than the cornea, it tends to make the lens adhere more to the cornea. This is not adequately explained on the basis of fluid attraction forces. Since the cornea is compressible, a suction effect may occur after the lens has been pressed against the cornea during blinking. Much further study is needed to understand the exact effect of these forces.

GRAVITY

The effect of gravity on a contact lens is most easily analyzed by use of the concept of the center of gravity. The center of gravity is the property that tends to make the object act as though all of its weight were concentrated at that one point. For a contact lens the position of the center of gravity is near the posterior surface or actually behind the lens. The exact position depends upon the diameter, power, base curve, and thickness of the lens.[2]

When the center of gravity is towards the front surface of a lens, there is a great tendency for the lens to drop below the center of the cornea (Figure 5.8). This occurs because the lens has little corneal support above the center of gravity. When the center of gravity is behind the contact lens there is less tend-

ency for the lens to drop. The center of gravity is now below a large lens area, which is supported by the cornea.

The center of gravity shifts towards the front surface when there is an increase in positive power, a decrease in lens diameter, an increase in thickness, or a flattening of the base curve. Consequently, these are all factors which will decrease the adherence of the lens to the cornea.

The center of gravity moves towards the back surface or behind the lens when there is an increase in negative power, an increase in lens diameter, a decrease in thickness, or a steepening of the base curve. Changes in these factors are commonly used to make a lens adhere better to the cornea.

LID FORCE

Some contact lenses ride in a position such that the superior lid covers a small portion of the lens. The lens is thus held against the cornea by direct pressure. This force contributes to, but is not necessary to, holding the lens upon the eye. Lenses of small diameter that ride between the lids will adhere to the cornea unless they are caught at the edge by the lids and ejected.

FRICTION

A contact lens will tend to remain stationary on the eye because of frictional forces. This is largely due to the viscosity of the precorneal film. If the precorneal layer is thin, friction may also occur directly between the surface of the lens and the cornea.

It is possible that variations in the viscosity of the precorneal film occur, which greatly affect the frictional forces. It may be sufficient to influence lens riding position. When the eye is irritated, the tear flow from the lacrimal gland is increased. These tears have a much different composition from the normal precorneal film, which is more viscous. The lens will be loose for two reasons: because of the greater tear volume and because of the reduced viscosity of the precorneal film.

The stability of the lens is also increased with an increase in the total surface area of the lens. This is due in part to greater frictional resistance to lens movement and to the greater area of adhesion between the precorneal film and the lens.

From the analysis of the forces affecting the fit of a contact lens, it is possible to evaluate the effect of changes in each of the lens variables.

The adherence of a contact lens to the cornea is increased by the following:

1. Increasing optical zone diameter or total diameter

2. Decreasing the radius of the optical zone

3. Decreasing the radius of the intermediate or peripheral curve

4. Decreasing the lens thickness

The adherence of a contact lens is de-

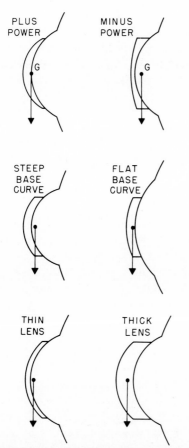

Figure 5.8. The center of gravity (*G*) of a contact lens is farther towards the front surface for a lens (*top*) that has more plus power, and (*center*) that has a flatter base curve, and (*bottom*) that is thicker.

creased by the following:

1. Decreasing the optical zone diameter or total diameter
2. Increasing the radius of the optical zone

3. Increasing the radius of the intermediate or peripheral curve
4. Increasing the lens thickness

FITTING PHILOSOPHIES

Each of the basic lens types may be fitted to the eye on the basis of various bearing and dimensional relationships. The proposed relationship is called the fitting philosophy.

Some practitioners tend to use one fitting philosophy to the near exclusion of the others. The greatest success, however, is achieved by the practitioner who uses all fitting philosophies to his greatest advantage. For some patients, a particular philosophy will be most suitable for fitting a lens. For other patients, a number of fitting philosophies will be equally effective.

Modern fitting philosophies are the outgrowth of trial and error. Little scientific investigation preceded the introduction of most philosophies, and those which proved clinically effective remain popular. This empirical approach has established no particular principle by which to fit a contact lens so that it will be worn successfully. It is now generally agreed, however, that, regardless of the philosophy followed, the lens dimensions should be varied according to the size and morphology of the wearer's eye.

FITTING PHILOSOPHY FOR MONOCURVE LENS

The monocurve lens is rarely used in present-day contact lens practice but much can be learned from a study of the wearing problems associated with this lens type.

The monocurve lens does not conform well to the cornea. As was stated in Chapter 3, the cornea is usually aspherical in shape, even in the center. If a monocurve lens has a spherical posterior surface with a curvature equal to the curvature of the central cornea, the lens will come to rest on the flattened corneal periphery. A closed area filled with tears will remain between the center of the lens and the cornea (Figure 5.9 *top*). Fluid attraction forces hold the lens firmly against the cornea, and it is difficult for tears to pass under the lens periphery. Consequently, to provide tear circulation, the monocurve lens is usually made with a posterior curve of longer radius of curvature (flatter) than that

of the central cornea.* It is then found that the lens tends to rest principally on the central cornea and has clearance at the corneal periphery (Figure 5.9 *bottom*). During the act of blinking, the lens is rocked back and forth on the cornea by the lids. This rocking helps to circulate the tears through the space between the lens and the cornea. There is considerable clearance between the edge of the lens and the cornea. Consequently, a tendency exists for the edge to irritate the superior lid during the act of blinking. It is even possible that the lids will eject the lens if the

---

*If the back surface radius of the monocurve lens is longer than the radius of the cornea, the lens is often said to have a flat fit or to be fitted flatter than the cornea. If the back surface has a shorter radius than the cornea, the lens is said to have a steep fit or to be fitted steeper than the cornea.

patient moves his eyes excessively or blinks rapidly.

The monocurve lens is poorly tolerated due to the heavy bearing (touch) of the lens on the central corneal area. The lens moves a great deal and often abrades the central cornea. Apparently, the long-term effect of central bearing and abrasion produces an irritation that becomes intolerable, and the patient can no longer wear the lenses. This intoler-ance to contact lenses, which develops after a period of comfortable wear, has been called corneal exhaustion, a poorly qualified term, since the processes that cause the phenomenon are not understood. The variety of problems associated with wearing monocurve lenses is responsible for the near extinction of this lens type in present day fitting techniques.

FITTING PHILOSOPHIES FOR BICURVE LENS

The criteria for a contact lens that is physiologically compatible with the eye are much better fulfilled by a lens of the bicurve type than by a monocurve lens. The bearing area of the bicurve lens is distributed fairly evenly over the central cornea by making the central zone of the lens *approximately* the same curvature as the central cornea. The peripheral curve of the lens is designed so as to provide clearance between the peripheral part of the lens and the cornea. A pool of tears collects beneath the peripheral curve. As the lens is rocked back and forth by the action of the lids, the tears are passed under the central portion of the lens. In this manner the lids and lens work together as a pump and exchange some tear fluid behind the lens with each blink.

The use of a peripheral curve does not insure adequate tear exchange. If the optical zone radius of the lens is much steeper than the cornea, tears may be blocked from the optical zone of the lens. If the peripheral curve of the lens does not flatten as much as the cornea, there will not be sufficient clearance to provide tear exchange. If either of these curves is given a radius that is longer than certain limits, the lens will be too loose and will move excessively on the cornea. The lens must be designed to strike a balance between that shape which parallels the cornea contour closely enough to distribute its weight over a large corneal area and a shape which will differ from the corneal curvature sufficiently to allow tear exchange.

There are many specific fitting philosophies that may be followed in determining the specifications of a bicurve lens. Two philosophies are very popular and will be introduced here, but they are discussed at length in later chapters: the *modified contour philosophy* and the *palpebral aperture philosophy.*

Modified Contour Philosophy

The modified contour philosophy is a principle of fitting contact lenses so that they closely parallel the corneal contour. To accomplish this, the lens is made with a relatively small optical zone diameter and a wide peripheral curve. The optical zone radius is very nearly equal to the radius of the central cornea. The peripheral curve radius is only slightly flatter (about 1.0 to 3.0 mm.) than the optical zone radius. It is given the minimum flattening that will allow a sufficient space between the lens and cornea to provide a reservoir of tears (Figure 5.10a).

A bicurve lens fitted according to the modified contour philosophy is supported on the cornea principally at the optical zone area. However, by making the peripheral curve closely parallel the corneal contour, some additional lens support is contributed by the

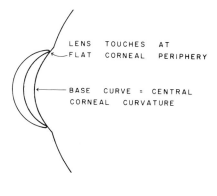

LENS   TOUCHES   AT
FLAT   CORNEAL   PERIPHERY

BASE   CURVE = CENTRAL
CORNEAL   CURVATURE

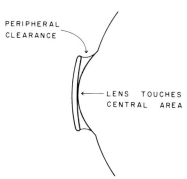

PERIPHERAL
CLEARANCE

LENS   TOUCHES
CENTRAL   AREA

Figure 5.9. Monocurve lens fitted with back sur-face radius (*top*) equal to the radius of the central cornea and (*bottom*) flatter than the cornea.

peripheral curve.

Generally, the fitting philosophy for a tricurve follows the general principles of the contour philosophy for bicurve lenses.

Since the cornea flattens more and more towards the periphery, it follows that a con-tact lens must also have a greater flattening towards the periphery to provide corneal clearance. Theoretically, a tricurve lens is an attempt to contour the cornea better while still fulfilling the basic criteria of an accept-able lens. In general, there is a tendency to use the tricurve lens when a larger total diam-eter is desired. Some fitters advocate that every contact lens should be designed as a tricurve lens, but there has been no controlled research to support this claim. A bicurve lens has, by

experience, been found to provide adequate clearance for a large proportion of corneas. It is possible to fit bicurve lenses and then convert them into tricurve lenses by a simple modification.

Palpebral Aperture Philosophy

A bicurve lens fitted according to the palpebral aperture philosophy has a relatively large optical zone diameter with a narrow, flat peripheral curve (Figure 5.10b). The opti-cal zone is usually designed to parallel the central cornea. The peripheral curve serves only to provide a space for tears and does not aid in supporting the lens on the cornea. It is usually 2 to 5 mm. flatter than the optical zone radius. The lens is designed so as to ride within the lid aperture. It is usually of the bicurve type, although other lens types are sometimes used. The palpebral aperture phi-losophy differs from the modified contour philosophy in that sometimes the base curve radius is made shorter than the radius of the central cornea. This steep fit helps to keep the lens centered within the palpebral aperture. The palpebral aperture philosophy is suitable for most eyes, but may be particu-larly useful when the following conditions exist:

1. The cornea is small
2. The palpebral aperture is small

Comparison of Modified Contour and Palpebral Aperture Philosophies

The modified contour and palpebral phi-losophies of fitting bicurve lenses are proba-bly the most commonly used general fitting philosophies. Many practitioners adopt one of these philosophies and use it for all their patients. Other fitters adopt one or the other philosophy for most of their patients but use the alternate philosophy when it better meets the requirements of a given patient. Many patients can be fitted equally well on the

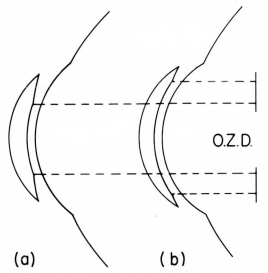

O.Z.D.

(a)   (b)

Figure 5.10. Bicurve lens fitted according to the (*a*) modified contour philosophy, and (*b*) palpebral aperture philosophy.

curve must be used to avoid excessive clearance from the cornea.

Thus, the primary determinant of lens design is the total diameter, and the P.C.W. generally increases with a larger total diameter. It is emphasized, however, that this is only a general relationship; there is not a fixed peripheral curve for a given lens diameter. The specific peripheral curve width and radius are determined by other factors.

Contact lens fitters commonly refer to lens diameter in qualitative terms as small or large without agreement as to their exact meaning. In this text there will be an arbitrary division of lens diameter into three groups as follows:

Large	> 9 mm.
Medium	8–9 mm.
Small	< 8 mm.

basis of either philosophy, but a few will be fitted better by one philosophy than the other. Other patients are not suitable subjects for fitting by either philosophy, and one of the other philosophies to be discussed later should be used.

Actually, the modified contour and palpebral aperture philosophies represent artificial constructs, which are convenient for teaching purposes. In practice the two philosophies represent extremes in a continuum for which there is no sharp boundary. The primary determinant of lens design is the total diameter. If a lens is relatively small, most of the lens area will be occupied by the optical zone in order to cover the pupillary area and fulfill the optical requirements. Hence the peripheral curve must be narrow in width, which dictates that it must be relatively flat. A larger lens, conversely, can have a larger optical zone diameter for optical purposes, but has a practical limit to the optical zone diameter due to physiological considerations. Hence, it must have a wider peripheral curve. In this case, a steeper peripheral

In general, a bicurve lens fitted according to the modified contour philosophy will more nearly parallel the cornea than a lens fitted according to the palpebral aperture philosophy. The lens bearing will be distributed over a larger corneal area. At the same time, because the lens contours a larger corneal area, it is slightly more difficult to fit. It is important to select both the optical zone and peripheral curve radii with care. If the palpebral aperture philosophy is followed, it is only necessary to fit the optical zone radius and use a flat peripheral curve.

In general, a contact lens fitted according to the modified contour philosophy is slightly larger in total diameter than the lens fitted by the palpebral aperture philosophy. This gives the lens greater stability. However, for eyes with small corneas and/or small palpebral aperture heights, a smaller lens, fitted according to the palpebral aperture philosophy, is usually preferred. This is especially true if the eye also has a very large pupil. In this case the optical zone of the lens is necessarily large, whereas the total diameter of the lens must remain small (Table 5.2).

FITTING METHODS

For each of the fitting philosophies, two methods can be used to determine the dimensions of the contact lens to be prescribed: the *keratometer method* (a method of direct measurement) and the *trial lens method.* In the keratometer method, measurements are taken of each eye to determine those characteristics which influence the fit of the lens, and the final lenses are ordered from these data. In the trial lens method, a series of lenses with various dimensions are tested on the patient's eye in an attempt to arrive at the best fit by a systematic trial and error system.

In the succeeding chapters, the keratometer method (Chapter 7), the trial lens method (Chapter 8), and various philosophies with both methods (Chapter 7) will be discussed.

TABLE 5.2
SUMMARY OF AVERAGE SPECIFICATIONS
(All in mm.)

| Lens Type | | Bicurve | | Tricurve |
Size	Small	Medium	Large	Mod. Contour
Total D	8	8–9	9	8.6–10
O.Z.	6–7.4	6.5–8	7–8	7–8
I.C.W.	—	—	—	0.4–1.1
I.C.R.	—	—	—	9–10.5
P.C.W.	0.3–0.5	0.3–0.5	0.5–1.0	0.3–0.5
P.C.R.	9–17	9–17	10–12	10.5–15
Function of P.C.	Tear Reservoir Only	Tear Reservoir Only	Tear Reservoir Only	Tear Reservoir and Lens Support
Lid Relation	Lens Rides Free of Lid	Lens Rides Free of Lid	20% of Lens Beneath Lid	20% of Lens Beneath Lid
Application	General Use Preferred for Smaller Eyes with Large Pupils	General Use	Large Eyes	Large Eyes

REFERENCES

1. Wray, L.: An elementary analysis of the forces retaining a corneal contact lens on the eye, *The Optician, 146(3780)*:239–241; *(3785)*:374–376, 1963.

2. Gordon, S.: Factors determining the physical and physiological fit of corneal type contact lenses, in *Encyclopedia of Contact Lens Practice*, South Bend, Indiana, International Optics, 1959–1963, vol. 2, Chap. 6, pp. 1–34.

ADDITIONAL READINGS

Arner, R. S.: The invariants of corneal contact lens fitting, *Optom. Weekly*, 56(30):13–19, 1965.

Bailey, N. J.: Contact lens design—a survey, *Am. J. Optom.*, 45(2):96–102, 1968.

Chiquiar-Arias, M.: Contact lens base curve determination—by central or peripheral keratometry, *Optom. Weekly*, 56(48):35–39, 1965.

Cinefro, J.: Importance of thickness in contact lens fitting, *Contacto*, 5(3):101–105, 1961.

Cummings, D. G.: A new photographic method of fitting contact lenses, *Contacto*, 11(1):6–8, 1967.

Dallos, J.: Individually-fitted corneal lenses made to corneal moulds, *Br. J. Ophthalmol.*, 48(9):510–512, 1964.

Davis, H. E.: Small contact lenses, *Contacto*, 8(4): 12–15, 1964.

Davis, H. E.: Why the small contact lens? *Br. J. Physiol. Opt.*, 21(4):215–218, 1964.

Dickinson, F.: Some aspects of contact lens technique in optometric education, *Contacto*, 13(4):37–41, 1969.

Evershed, M. L.: The search for a common factor in successful contact lens prescribing, *Br. J. Physiol. Opt.*, 21(4):200–202, 1964.

Goldberg, J. B.: Current commentary about contact lenses (an assessment of lens size), *Optom. Weekly*, 61(3):47, 1970.

Goldberg, J. B.: Transition zone between optic diameter and bevel, *Contacto*, 6(3):79–80, 1962.

Gordon, S.: An evaluation of small, thin contact lenses, *Optom. Weekly*, 55(5):21–25, 1964.

Gordon, S. P.: The peripheral fit of corneal lenses, *The Optician*, 159(4125):451–453, 1970.

Hamilton, C. B.: A new method of determining size, *Contacto*, 11(1):27–28, 1967.

Hartstein, J.: Practical points in contact lens fitting, *Eye, Ear, Nose and Throat Mon.*, 46(8): 1004–1005, 1967.

Hersh, D.: A system of contact lens nomenclature, *Opt. J. Rev. Optom.*, 98(9):29–31, 45, 1961.

Hodd, F. A.: A design study of the back surface of corneal contact lenses—Part 3, *The Ophthalmic Optician*, 7(1):14–16, 19–21, 39, 1967.

Isen, A. A.: Two complementary techniques for fitting small corneal lenses, *Optom. Weekly*, 54(51): 2355–2358, 1963.

Jessen, G. N.: Medium and large lens fitting techniques, *Contacto*, 11(1):37–39, 1967.

Jessop, D. G.: Tear layer reduction factor, *Contacto*, 5(5):189–191, 1961.

Koetting, R. A.: The steep/flat lens, *Contacto*, 13(2):44–45, 1969.

Koltun, L. J.: Small, thin lenses—a critical appraisal, *Can. J. Optom.*, 31(1):51–57, 1969.

Lichtman, W. M.: An approach to contact lenses in a "sophisticated era," *Opt. J. Rev. Optom.*, 107(11): 25–26, 1970.

McCormack, H. G.: Desirability of a positive vertical clearance, *Contacto*, 8(4):29–40, 1964.

Martin, W. F., and Jensen, R. D.: Size and peripheral curve factors in contact lens fitting, *Contacto*, 4(5):155–158, 1960.

Mills, P. V.: The "apex" contact lens, *Trans. Ophthalmol. Soc. U.K.*, 87:729–732, 1967.

Morrison, R.: Small, thin contact lens use, *Optom. Weekly*, 54(18):853–855, 1963.

Moss, H. I.: A review of the small corneal lenses and the lens-cornea relationship, *Austr. J. Optom.*, 48(2):47–51, 1965.

Pennington, N.: A comparison of three corneal lens forms, *Austr. J. Optom.*, 52(8):229–237, 1969.

Rocher, P., and Francois, J.: Choice of the total diameter of a contact lens, *Contacto*, 12(2):30–35, 1968.

Rosenthal, P.: Corneal contact lenses: Large or small? *Arch. Ophthalmol.*, 76:631–632, 1966.

Sarver, M. D.: Comparison of small and large corneal contact lenses, *Am. J. Optom.*, 43(10): 633–652, 1966.

Schlossman, A.: The ophthalmological advanced fitting contact lens symposium—Part 2, *Eye, Ear, Nose and Throat Mon.*, 45(1):94, 118, 1966.

Sellers, E.: Towards calculated accuracy—a contact lens philosophy, *Austr. J. Optom.*, 49(12):355–360, 1966.

Shnider, H. A.: The role of the contact lens diameter, *Contacto*, 11(1):65–70, 1967.

Sloan, D. P., Jr.: Small lens fitting, *Contacto*, 11(1): 61–64, 1967.

Steele, E.: Problems associated with the fitting of corneal contact lenses, *Br. J. Physiol. Opt.*, 19(3): 171–177, 1962.

Thomas, P. F.: Apical clearance in contact lens design, *The Ophthalmic Optician*, 10(5):216–218, 1970.

Ullen, R. L.: A contact lens fitting procedure, *Optom. Weekly*, *53*(*45*):2225–2229, 1962.

Vodnoy, B. E.: Some principles for corneal contact lens practice, *Am. J. Optom.*, *42*(*10*):619–625, 1965.

Wakita, S.: Some factors for the determination of the size of contact lens, *Contacto*, *6*(*2*):37–40, 1962.

Warren, G. T.: The single contact lens—an often-overlooked solution, *Opt. J. Rev. Optom.*, *107*(*12*): 31–34, 1970.

Wesley, N. K.: A study of comparative fitting methods, *Contacto*, *13*(*4*):58–62, 1969.

Williams, C. E.: The minimum compression concept, *Contacto*, *11*(*2*):61–65, 1967.

Chapter 6

THEORY OF CONTACT LENSES

As stated in Chapter 5, a contact lens must fulfill certain optical and physiological requisites. Factors affecting the optical performance of a contact lens are fairly well established. Contact lenses follow the laws of optics, and these are generally known. It is the physiological and physical aspects of a contact lens that are not well understood.

OXYGEN SUPPLY

Of principal interest in contact lens fitting is whether or not a given contact lens will provide at least the minimum oxygen need of a cornea. The oxygen can be supplied by the exchange of tears behind a contact lens with freshly oxygenated tears outside the lens or, in some cases, by direct transmission through the lens material. There has been considerable confusion associated with this topic, which may be attributed to the difficulty of the measurements and the variations in techniques that have been used.

LENS PERMEABILITY AND OXYGEN REQUIREMENT

Basically, it is possible to determine whether or not a given contact lens has sufficient permeability to supply the oxygen need of the cornea by one of two methods:

1. *In vivo.* The lens to be tested may be placed on the eye for a standard period of time. The lens is then removed, and the oxygen requirement of the cornea is measured with a polarographic oxygen electrode.

2. *In vitro.* The oxygen need of corneas for the population was first established by exposing subjects to low oxygen levels until a threshold for corneal swelling was determined. Lens permeabilities can now be measured *in vitro* and calculations made to determine whether the lens can supply the required corneal oxygen need.

In Vivo Measurement Technique

This method was introduced and developed by Hill,[1] using a method originally developed by Hill and Fatt.[2] It is usually conducted on rabbits, but may also be done on humans.[3] Since the results are generally comparable, the rabbit model has been adopted as a standard laboratory procedure.[4] The test is based upon changes in the rate at which oxygen is taken up from the atmosphere by the cornea before and after a contact lens is worn. Oxygen is normally consumed by the cornea at a rate of approximately 4 to 5 μl per square cm. of corneal area per hour.[5] After a lens that reduces the oxygen supply to the cornea is worn, it produces what Hill has termed an oxygen debt, so when the lens

142

is removed, the rate of oxygen uptake is much higher.

In order to make this a practical test that is easily understood, Hill expresses the oxygen consumption after the lens is worn in terms of an "equivalent oxygen percentage" (E.O.P.).[6] This value is based upon an experiment by Hill in which he first measured the rate of oxygen uptake on a number of rabbits who did not wear contact lenses (Figure 6.1).[7] He then placed goggles on the rabbits, through which he passed oxygen mixed with nitrogen in known concentration. When the goggle was removed, he measured the oxygen uptake rate. This was repeated for several concentrations of oxygen. It was then possible to ignore the calculation for oxygen uptake rate altogether and simply express the oxygen uptake rate in terms of oxygen concentration that was present under the goggles just before polarography was taken.

Pressing the polarographic electrode against the cornea produces a typical graph, which is illustrated in Figure 6.2a. After a contact lens is inserted, it is found that the polarographic record will drop faster, indicating that a lower oxygen concentration was present under the lens. It is now simply a matter of matching up the curves produced under various oxygen concentrations to those produced by contact lenses in order to establish the oxygen level beneath the contact lens (Figure 6.2b). Of course, there is a risk in the assumption that the oxygen level under the goggle is the same as that beneath the contact lens, but the differences are probably insignificant.

The equivalent oxygen level is expressed in terms of percent atmospheric oxygen at sea level and is easily compared to a normal of about 21 percent. This attempt to simplify the interpretation of the results may, indeed,

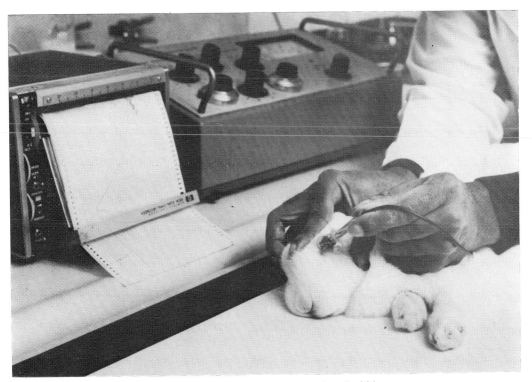

Figure 6.1. Measurement of oxygen uptake of rabbit cornea.

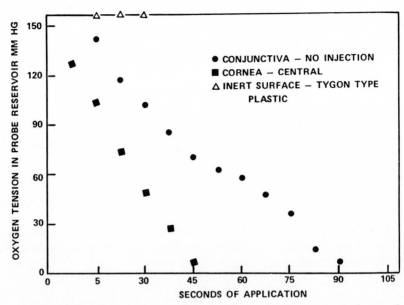

Figure 6.2a. Graphical representation of fall in oxygen tension in sensor membrane when the probe is pressed against three different surfaces. From R. M. Hill and I. Fatt, Oxygen Measurements under a Contact Lens, *American Journal of Optometry*, 41(6):382–387, 1964.

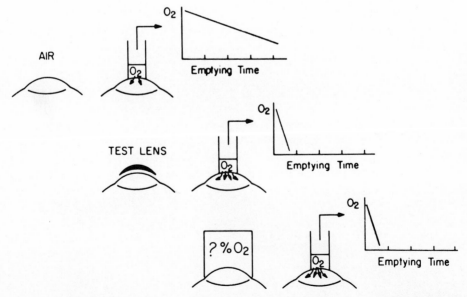

Figure 6.2b. Method of measuring the equivalent oxygen percentage of a lens on the cornea. From R. M. Hill and W. H. Jeppe, Hydrogels: Is a Pump Still Necessary?, *International Contact Lens Clinic*, 2(4):28, 1975.

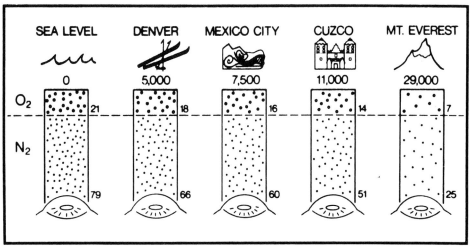

Figure 6.3. A schematic model of the progressive scarcity of oxygen available to the lens pump as a patient travels to higher and higher altitudes. From R. M. Hill, Perils of the Pump, *International Contact Lens Clinic*, 3(3):49, 1976.

lead to possible errors. The normal atmosphere contains about 21 percent oxygen at sea level and also contains 21 percent oxygen at higher altitudes. However, the available oxygen to the cornea at higher altitudes is less. This occurs because the total pressure of all gases at the higher altitude is reduced. Hence, an expression of oxygen in percentage does not describe the true oxygen pressure adequately, except at sea level (Figure 6.3).

If the oxygen concentration is expressed as an oxygen pressure in millimeters of mercury, no such error occurs. It should be recalled that the total pressure exerted on the earth by the atmosphere at sea level is 760 mm. Hg. There is approximately 21 percent oxygen in air. The pressure that is exerted by the oxygen component may be determined by simply taking 21 percent of 760 mm., or 159 mm. Hg. (Actually, the value usually adopted is slightly less than 21%, or 155 mm. Hg.) At higher altitudes, such as in the mountains, the atmospheric pressure might be only 600 mm. Hg. At that altitude, again the oxygen pressure is found by taking 21 percent of 600 mm. Hg, or 126 mm. Hg.

In Vitro Method

The second method for determining whether a contact lens provides sufficient oxygen at the corneal surface requires two parts. First, the corneal oxygen need must be determined for the population. Second, the oxygen that passes through a contact lens is measured directly and compared to the corneal need.

The minimum corneal oxygen need is determined by having the subject wear a pair of goggles, through which is passed a mixture of oxygen and nitrogen. The oxygen percentage is lowered in each experiment until corneal thickening is produced. The threshold for corneal thickening represents the minimum level of oxygen, below which an interference occurs in the normal corneal physiology. A description of the measurement instrumentation is given in Chapter 24.

The typical corneal swelling responses to various low oxygen levels is shown in Figure 6.4. In general, the cornea swells for two to three hours and then stabilizes or reduces slightly, indicating adaptation. The mechanism of adaptation is subject to conjecture, since control of hydration is not completely

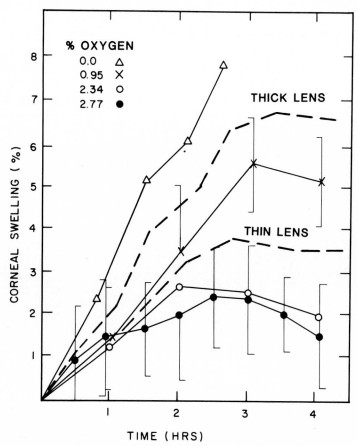

Figure 6.4. Average corneal swelling response at 3 oxygen concentrations and for a thick and thin hydrogel lens.

understood. These curves are very similar to those produced when subjects wear contact lenses and suggest that oxygen is the primary factor responsible for corneal swelling when contact lenses are worn. Further evidence to support this hypothesis was presented by Polse and Mandell in another experiment,[8] in which the swelling was eliminated in contact lens wearers by exposing the eye to hyperbaric oxygen. It was assumed that this raised the oxygen concentration behind the lens to a level above the minimum corneal need.

The minimum level of oxygen that is needed at the cornea varies with the individual between 2 and 5 percent. It is possible to differentiate between subjects with low and

high oxygen need by the simple test of wearing a low permeability soft contact lens and closing the eyes for a period of three hours. Subjects with high oxygen need show evidence of corneal edema by biomicroscopy. A more exact measurement, if needed, can be taken by pachymetry.

The permeability of contact lens materials to oxygen may be measured directly by using one of various oxygen-sensitive electrodes. In simplest terms, the technique requires that a known oxygen supply be placed on one side of the lens with the electrode on the opposite side of the lens. The arrangement is such that oxygen can only pass to the electrode by going through the lens and is blocked from any other route. The apparatus differ in several ways. Some electrodes are very sensitive and fast, whereas others are less sensitive and slow, requiring up to twenty-four hours for a measurement. In some apparatus, the lens surface away from the electrode is exposed to gaseous oxygen, whereas in others the oxygen is dissolved in solution. Because of the differences in technique, there have been many inconsistencies and gross errors in the literature. Measurements that have been obtained by one technique and have been compared to another technique are generally valueless because of the sensitive nature of the measurement. The most valid measurements are those taken on the same apparatus so that one material may be compared directly to another. A common apparatus used for this measurement is produced by Schema Versatae and used by various contact lens researchers and laboratories. The apparatus consists of an electrode upon which the contact lens is placed and which has a curvature that approximates the lens curvature (Figure 6.5). The apparatus directly measures the amount of oxygen that passes through a lens at a given thickness. Hence, the measurement is one of *transmission*, or *transmissivity*, as it is known in engineering. Note that the transmissivity depends upon not only the characteristics of the material itself but also the thickness of the lens. Multiplying this value by the thickness of the lens gives a more useful value, which is independent of lens thickness and which is called *permeability*. Permeability is a more useful measure because it allows a direct comparison between various materials that are used for contact lenses without regard to their thickness. Hence, a permeability value requires no statement about lens dimensions,

whereas the transmissivity value should be accompanied by a thickness specification.

Some further errors occur in the measurement of contact lens transmissivity because often only the center thickness of the lens is considered in calculating permeability. Obviously, if a lens has significant plus or minus power, there will be differences in thickness. Since oxygen passes through all parts of the lens, the effective thickness is the average of the integrated thicknesses across the lens. Fatt has calculated the correction factors that should be applied for lenses having significant power, in order to convert center thickness to an average thickness (Figure 6.6a).[9]

The characteristics of gas transmission through a contact lens are analogous to light transmission through a spectacle lens. If a spectacle lens of absorptive material is made in high-minus power, it is noted that the center portion, which is very thin, shows a very light coloration in contrast to the periphery, where the coloration is very dark. This indicates that greater absorption of light occurs through the thicker part of the lens. If the flow of oxygen is compared to light transmission, the transmissivity for oxygen is less where the lens is thicker. This is true even though the absorptive property (permeability) of the lens is the same everywhere.

Figure 6.6b shows a comparison of the equivalent oxygen level for lenses of various permeabilities and different thicknesses. Table 6.1 shows the permeabilities for many commonly used contact lens materials. Once the permeability value is known, it may be referred to Figure 6.6b to determine how much oxygen is transmitted for a lens of a given thickness. Remember, if the lens has significant power, the average thickness must be used, rather than center thickness.

LENS TEAR PUMP

The original theory of tear circulation beneath a contact lens was that tears were collected in the space between the peripheral curve and cornea, then gradually passed

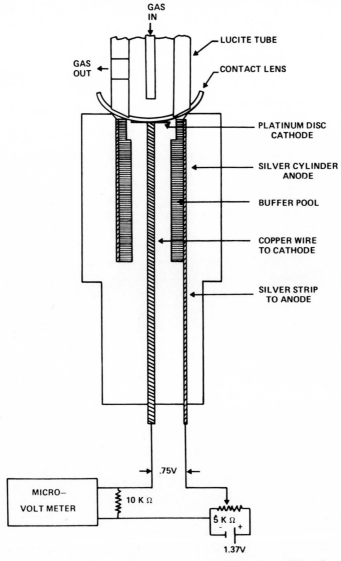

Figure 6.5. Schema Versatae device for measurement of the permeability of a contact lens.

beneath the lens to the the bottom portion from where the tears were expelled. It is very likely that there is no actual tear flow beneath the contact lens, but only a tear interchange from outside to beneath the contact lens during blinking.

In an experimental study by Hill and Lowther,[10] it was shown that various contact lenses, which were placed on the corneas of rabbits and not allowed to move, all influ-ence the oxygen uptake of the rabbit corneas differently over a short time period. However-er, it was found that if a lens remained sta-tionary on the cornea for more than a short period of time, it made no difference thereaf-ter whether the lens was on K, steeper than K, or flatter than K. Once the oxygen that was originally between the lens and the cor-nea was used by the cornea, no significant additional oxygen diffused under the lens

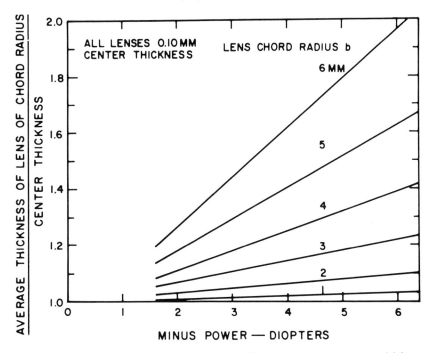

Figure 6.6a. Average thicknesses for lenses of significant power when center thickness and chord diameter are known.

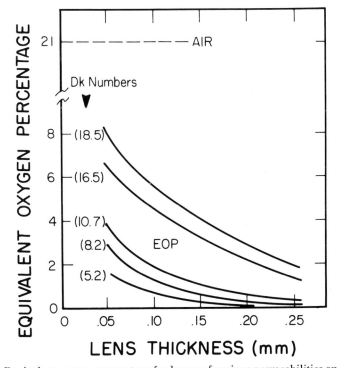

Figure 6.6b. Equivalent oxygen percentage for lenses of various permeabilities and thicknesses.

TABLE 6.1
PERMEABILITY OF HARD MATERIALS

Lens	DK
C.A.B.	
Hydrocurve	4.5
Rynco	
Danker	
Wöhlk	
Polycon (Syntex)	4.3
"A" Lens	10.5
Boston Lens	10.5
Menicon	4.8

from the edge. The important conclusion is that no significant oxygen can diffuse into the central portion of the lens from the edge while the lens remains stationary.

Tears are exchanged only at the time of the blink when the lens is driven downward by the upper lid until either the lower lid or limbus is contacted.

This can be easily demonstrated on any contact lens wearer. Hold the patient's upper lid so that it is not allowed to make contact with the lens. Next, place a small drop of fluorescein on the lower sclera and let the drop move slowly until it strikes the lens. The fluorescein will penetrate behind the peripheral curve (Figure 6.7) but will not enter behind the optic zone, even if the lid is held for several minutes (Figure 6.8). Now let the patient make one blink, and it will be found that the fluorescein has penetrated behind the optic zone (Figure 6.9).

The oxygen supply in the small reservoir behind the contact lens is not constant but is increased with each blink as new tears are exchanged under the lens (Figure 6.10). After the blink the oxygen pressure falls in the lens reservoir as oxygen is consumed by the cornea. According to Fatt,[11] the amount of oxygen that is pumped to the lens reservoir becomes fixed shortly after a lens is inserted (as soon as ten seconds or after about five blinks). The amount of oxygen passed under the lens with each blink then becomes dependent on only three factors:

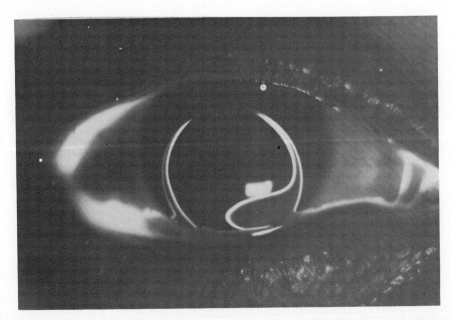

Figure 6.7. Preparation for pump demonstration. Fluorescein placed at lower rivus climbs edge meniscus.

1. Frequency of the blink

2. Percent of new tears exchanged with the blink

3. Volume of the tear reservoir behind the lens

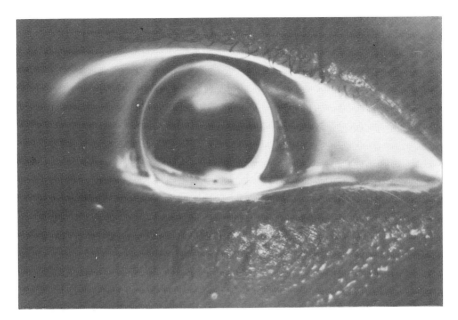

Figure 6.8. Fluorescein enters the peripheral curve but not the optic zone.

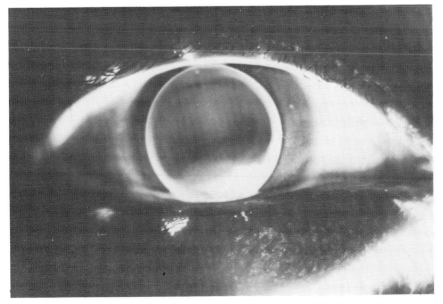

Figure 6.9. After one blink, the fluorescein penetrates behind the optic zone.

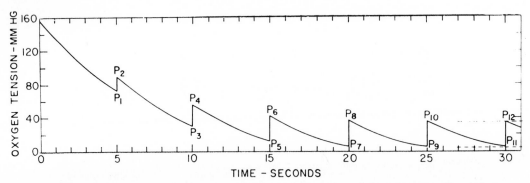

Figure 6.10. Oxygen tension under a contact lens as a function of time. Lens was inserted at t=0; blink period is five seconds. The fractional tear volume replaced by a blink is 0.2, and the equivalent reservoir thickness is 0.35 x 10 cm. From I. Fatt, Oxygen Tension under a Contact Lens during Blinking, *American Journal of Optometry*, 46(9):654–661, 1969.

The Frequency of Blinking

Fatt and Hill have measured the oxygen tension behind a lens as a function of blink frequency.[12] They show that the oxygen tension drops about 40 percent when the blink is changed from once per second to once each four seconds (Figure 6.11).

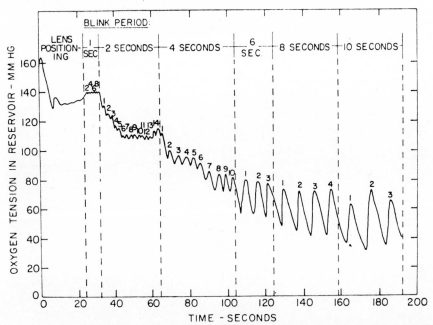

Figure 6.11. Oxygen tension in the tear reservoir between a human cornea and a corneal lens as influenced by the period between blinks. Individual blinks, at a given blink period, are numbered on the curve. From I. Fatt and R. M. Hill, Oxygen Tension under a Contact Lens during Blinking: A Comparison of Theory and Experimental Observation, *American Journal of Optometry*, 47(1):50–55, 1970.

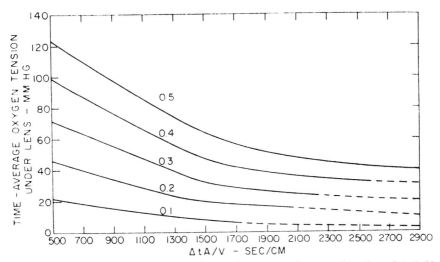

Figure 6.12. The time-average oxygen tension under a contact lens as a function of Δt A/V and the fractional tear volume replenishment (Δt is the time between blinks, A is the lens area, and V is the tear reservoir volume). The dashed portion of the curves indicates that the oxygen tension under the lens will be zero for a significant time between blinks. From I. Fatt and R. M. Hill, Oxygen Tension under a Contact Lens during Blinking: A Comparison of Theory and Experimental Observation, *American Journal of Optometry*, 47(1):50–55, 1970.

Percent Tears Exchanged

Cuklanz and Hill found for one set of lens conditions that approximately 20 percent of the tears were exchanged with each blink.[13,14] As the percentage exchanged is increased, the oxygen tension behind the lens goes up, as illustrated for another set of lens conditions by Fatt and Hill (Figure 6.12).[11]

Tear Volume Behind Lens

The tear volume behind the optical zone of the contact lens is an important variable in determining the oxygen tension behind the lens. The greater the tear volume, the more oxygen that will be available. Thus, a lens that exactly parallels the cornea will have a smaller oxygen supply than either a lens flatter or steeper than the cornea. Hill has shown this to be true in both theory and experiments.[14] This outstanding study has been often misinterpreted by some who feel it proves that a lens should be fitted steeper than the cornea. It proves no such thing.

Hill and others show only that in the static condition, the lens that parallels the cornea will have the minimum oxygen reservoir.[10,14-16] This research does not consider the percentage of tears exchanged and the blink rate, which are probably more important factors in the practical situation.

Theory of Tear Exchange

On the downward excursion, tears are forced upward between the lens and cornea through the channel formed by the peripheral curve (Figure 6.13). At the same time, stagnant tears are forced out from the sides of the lens. As the eye is opened following the blink, the lid pulls the lens with its supply of fresh tears to a high position, from which the lens drops to its riding position (Figure 6.14).

While the major pumping action probably occurs as described during the downward movement of the lens, it is recognized that other pump actions may be active. For exam-

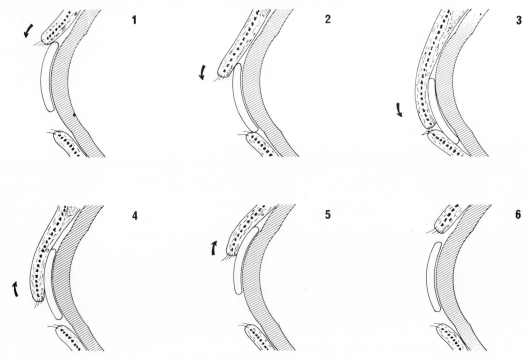

Figure 6.13. Excursion of a contact lens during a blink. (1) The superior lid makes contact with the lens. (2) The lens is forced down to the lower corneal position. (3) The lens is forced past the lower limbus and the lid covers the lens. (4) The superior lid starts an upward movement. (5) Lens begins to drop from lid. (6) Lens falls free of lid.

ple, as the lens is pulled to a high position on the cornea, the volume in the post-lens reservoir is increased due to greater lens standoff on the corneal periphery. As the lens drops to the central cornea where the corneal curvature more nearly matches the base curve, the post-lens reservoir will be reduced. This change in volume by itself will cause a pumping action to take place.

Role of Peripheral Curve

The exact method of function for the peripheral curve is not known but may be attributed to either or both of the following:

1. Provides a means to produce lens pumping

2. Carries a reservoir of oxygenated tears, which is moved across the cornea with the lens

LENS PUMPING. As the upper lid passes over the top portion of the lens, the upper junction acts as a fulcrum to lift the lower lens edge slightly from the cornea (Figure 6.15). This provides an opening for the easy access of tears. The force of the lens being driven downward would pass tears under the lower edge, with the tears behind the lens being forced out the sides, which is the only opening that remains.

RESERVOIR OF OXYGENATED TEARS. The pool of tears that is formed between the peripheral curve and the cornea is large enough to allow diffusion and some mixing of oxygenated tears. As the lens is moved across the cornea during a blink, the peripheral curve area is moved back and forth to cover nearly all of the cornea.

For the normal cornea, there is not enough lens movement to allow the peripheral curve

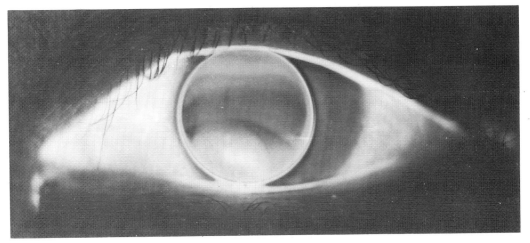

Figure 6.14a

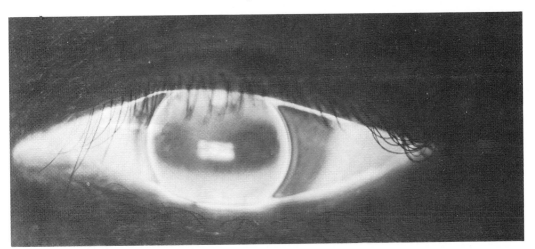

Figure 6.14b

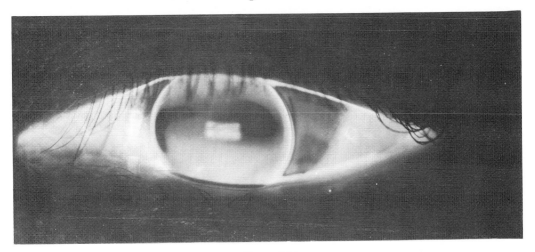

Figure 6.14c

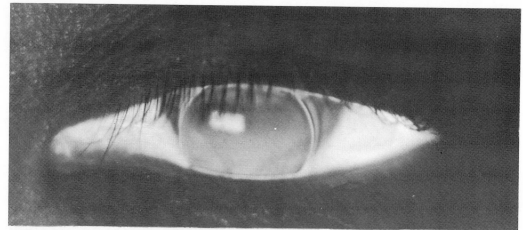

Figure 6.14d

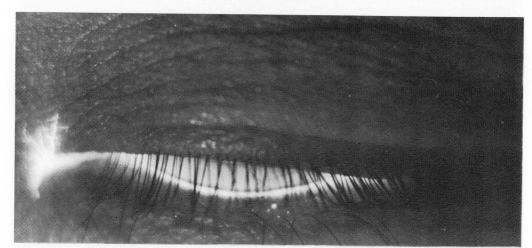

Figure 6.14e

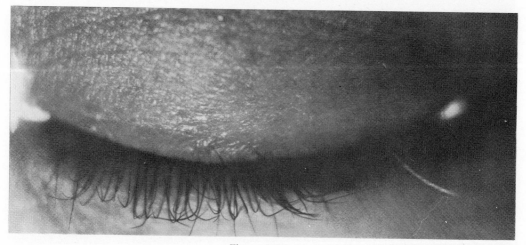

Figure 6.14f

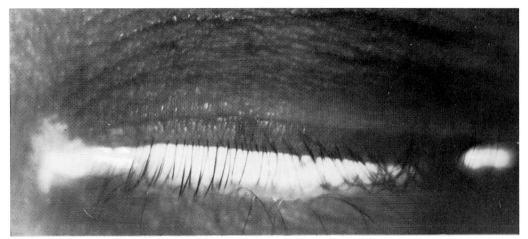

Figure 6.14g

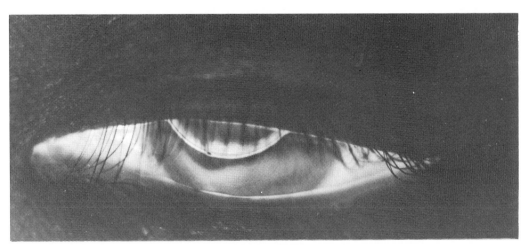

Figure 6.14h

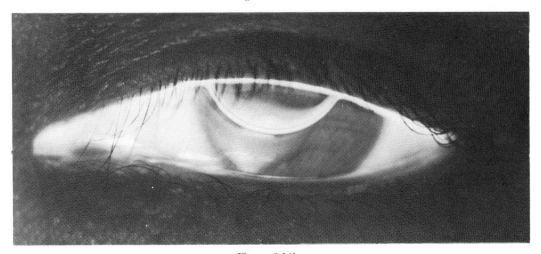

Figure 6.14i

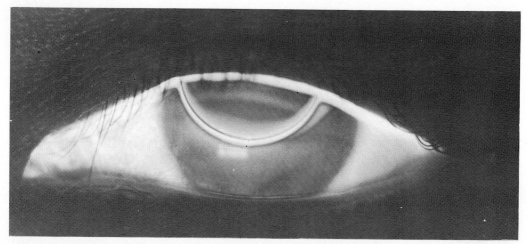

Figure 6.14j

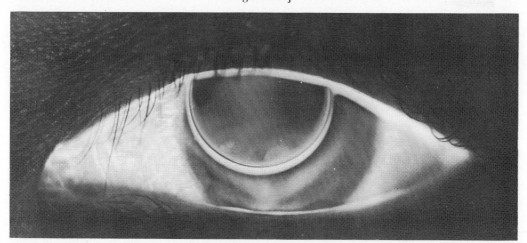

Figure 6.14k

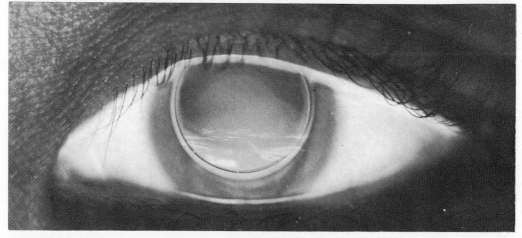

Figure 6.14l

Figure 6.14. Lens position during blinking. Note how lens moves below lower limbus just before eye closure.

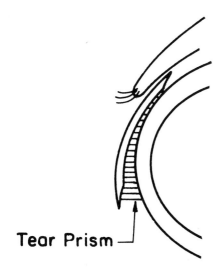

Tear Prism ⌐

Figure 6.15. Formation of tear prism produced by lid pressure on upper lens edge.

to cover the central region of the cornea at any time. For example, given a cornea that is 12 mm. in chord diameter, a lens would have to be less than 7.0 mm. in diameter to expose all corneal areas during the lens excursions to the limbus (Figure 6.16).

However, assume a lens has an optic zone of 7 mm. diameter and a peripheral curve 0.5

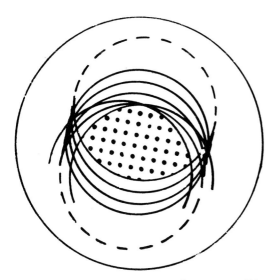

Figure 6.16. As lens moves on the cornea, all but the central cornea is covered by the peripheral curve.

mm. wide. Also, assume that as the lens moves it is pushed by the lid so that the peripheral curve moves beyond the limbus and that the junction of the optic zone stops at the limbus. In this case, the peripheral curve during its excursions would cover all but the central 0.66 mm. of the cornea. Hence, it is possible for the peripheral curve to pass over nearly all of the corneal area during the lens movement.

WHICH THEORY IS CORRECT? It is well established that some lens pump action takes place during the blink. However, one clinical condition is difficult to explain by this theory. When adequate oxygen is not supplied to the cornea, edema is produced. In a hard lens wearer, the edema typically is confined to a round or oval spot in the area behind the center of the lens. If a complete exchange of tears occurs with each blink, why is the oxygen supply less at the corneal area behind the center of the lens? If it is assumed that the tears behind the optic zone are stagnant between blinks, one should expect the corneal area that has the least clearance by the contact lens to have the lowest oxygen supply. Yet, the corneal edema usually occurs behind the area of lens-corneal clearance. This might be explained by assuming a greater resistance to tear flow occurs behind the central region of the optic zone.

If the peripheral curve serves also to carry a reservoir of oxygenated tears to different regions of the cornea, one would predict an area of corneal edema exactly where it is— behind the center of the optic zone, regardless of the lens riding position. It would also explain why the area of corneal edema often assumes an oval shape, since this would indicate that fewer excursions of the lens would occur laterally than vertically.

Each of the functions of the peripheral curve is dependent on movement of the lens, which must occur during a blink. Edema in the central cornea usually can be eliminated by flattening or widening the peripheral curve. Each of these would tend to increase lens movement, increase the channel between the edge and the cornea, and increase lens rocking.

ADAPTATION

In the jargon of the contact lens field, "adaptation" is a vague term used to describe the amelioration of ocular reactions that occur during the first few weeks of contact lens wear. The term is often applied to an unknown physiological process which is thought to occur in the cornea during the same period that allows it to tolerate the contact lens better. To give the cornea time to adapt, the new contact lens wearer usually follows a graduated wearing schedule for several weeks until all-day wear is achieved. If this wearing schedule is exceeded greatly, edema and/or a central corneal abrasion may be produced. When a corneal contact lens is first worn by an unadapted subject, there is corneal swelling. The corneal swelling is manifested clinically as corneal edema, which in gross form may be seen with the biomicroscope. The swelling may be accurately determined in the laboratory by measuring the increase in corneal thickness that always accompanies swelling.

Mandell and Harris isolated lacrimation as one of the factors contributing to corneal thickening during contact lens adaptation.[17,18] They measured an increase in corneal thickness of up to 3 percent caused by tearing in one eye when a contact lens was worn on the contralateral eye or on the ipsilateral sclera. This corneal thickening was not found when the experiment was repeated on subjects who had worn contact lenses for a period of several weeks. Corneal thickening produced by tearing from exposure to a noxious stimulus such as onions is comparable to that found by mechanical irritation.[19] These results support the theory that tearing alone can be responsible for mild corneal edema. The unadapted wearer secretes excess lacrimal fluid, which has a lower tonicity than the normal tear film and which causes water movement into

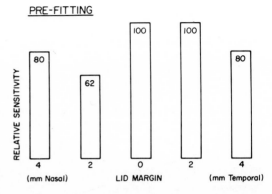

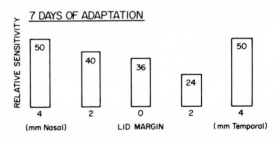

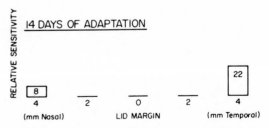

Figure 6.17. The change of sensitivity across the lower lid margin (0 being the lens impact site for central gaze) with the introduction and continuing wear of a hard contact lens.

the cornea. Direct measurements of the tonicity change have now been made, which verify this hypothesis.

Mandell and Harris proposed that the contact lens adaptation process may be accounted for by the decrease in tearing accompanying neural adaptation of the receptors in the lid margins to stimulation by a contact lens (Figure 6.17). The time course of this neural adaptation was shown by Lowther and Hill to coincide with that of the contact lens adaptation process.[20]

Another possible explanation for the increased corneal thickness could be the increased rate of circulation of the tears over the cornea. This might wash away some unknown substance in the precorneal film at a greater than normal rate. The unlikelihood of this is shown when the cornea was "washed" by drops of 1.0% sodium chloride solution; no significant change in corneal thickness was found.[21] The most plausible theory that has been suggested seems to be that excessive secretion of lacrimal fluid yields tears of lower than normal tonicity, which causes the corneal swelling.

Mandell, Polse, and Fatt performed several experiments on the changes of corneal thickness that accompanied contact lens wear.[22,23] They increased the accuracy and reliability of the apparatus for corneal thickness measurements by introducing several modifications and by the addition of an automatic recording system.[24]

A number of unadapted subjects were fitted with contact lenses. Some lenses were designed to fit well, while other lenses were purposely made to fit poorly, i.e. loose or tight. During the first weeks of contact lens wear, the subjects were seen daily for measurements of corneal thickness, keratometry, biomicroscopy, and other routine tests. Some subjects were tested continuously throughout the first few days of contact lens wear.

Summary of Results

Lenses that were optimally fitted by the usual clinical criteria produced minimum amounts of corneal swelling and no tight symptoms. Corneal swelling on the first day of contact lens wear usually peaked at about three hours after lens insertion and then reduced (Figure 6.18a). Corneal swelling for an unadapted subject was limited to 3 or 4 percent on the first day, and the subject would show no corneal swelling after the adaptation period. This suggests that excess tearing was responsible for the initial swelling, which disappeared following neural adaptation of the lids.

Subjects with 5 to 7 percent swelling on the initial day of contact lens wear all had reduced swelling by the end of the first day but did not return to normal (Figure 6.18b). The swelling that remained may have been due to prolonged tearing or a second mechanism.

Lenses fitted tightly by the usual clinical criteria produced maximum amounts of corneal swelling and tight symptoms. The swelling remained after the subject had passed through the adaptation period and may be attributed to a second mechanism (Figure 6.19). With very tight lenses, the swelling curve closely approximated that of a cornea in an oxygen-free environment. Under these conditions, the lens could not be tolerated for long periods of time and produced reversible pathology of the cornea. Lenses that produced between 4 and 9 percent swelling in three hours are hypothesized to allow some tear exchange, although in an inadequate amount to provide the oxygen needs of the cornea.

Evidence that the depletion of oxygen under a contact lens causes tight symptoms was first presented in the classical study by Smelser,[25] who showed that an absence of oxygen beneath a scleral contact lens gave rise to halos within four hours. Later, clinicians and investigators found corneal edema in some corneal contact lens wearers, which they assumed was due to the same cause.[26-29]

These studies indicated that the oxygen concentration under a contact lens influences the amount of corneal edema. However, there are a number of other factors that might lead to corneal edema such as changes in tear proteins, carbon dioxide accumulation beneath the lens, and mechanical pressure. Polse

CORNEAL SWELLING (EDEMA)

FIRST DAY

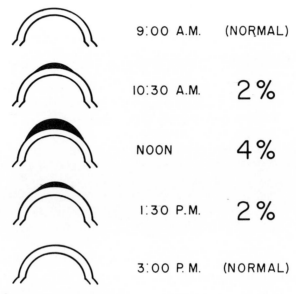

9:00 A.M.   (NORMAL)

10:30 A.M.   2%

NOON   4%

1:30 P.M.   2%

3:00 P.M.   (NORMAL)

Figure 6.18a. Corneal swelling on first day of contact lens wear peaks at about three hours and then subsides.

and Mandell proved that the oxygen concentration under a contact lens was the factor responsible for corneal edema by measuring corneal swelling under various oxygen tensions while all other contact lens variables were held constant.[30]

No change in corneal thickness was observed when a cornea fitted with a tight lens was subjected to a high oxygen atmosphere (Figure 6.20).

Therefore, there are at least two factors that may cause corneal swelling when contact lenses are worn. One is an initial increase in lacrimation, which probably causes a change in tear film osmolarity, and the other is caused by a lack of oxygen under the contact lens.

Blinking Effects

One factor not measurable in these exper-

iments is the effect of blinking. The rate of tear exchange depends upon the characteristics of the blink. Most new contact lens wearers pass through three stages of blinking. First there is an initial fast phase, which occurs immediately after the lenses are inserted. The lids are closed with maximum force, and the interblink period is very short. After a period of approximately an hour, the blinking rate decreases, and closure occurs with a minimum of force, representing the second or slow phase of blinking. After adaptation is complete, the blinking returns to normal, representing the third phase (Figure 6.21).

It is possible that, during the second phase, blinking is suppressed to the point that the tear exchange rate is reduced, and the oxygen supply to the cornea temporarily falls below that which will be provided later with

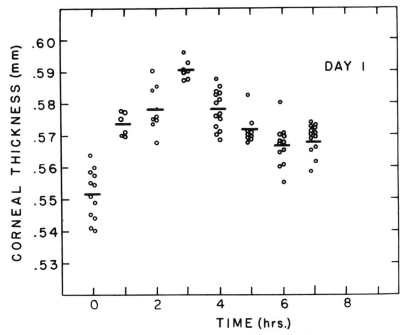

Figure 6.18b. Subjects with 5 to 7 percent swelling on first day of contact lens wear do not return to normal thickness at the end of the day. From R. B. Mandell and K. A. Polse, Corneal Thickness Changes as a Contact Lens Fitting Index—Experimental Results and a Proposed Model, *American Journal of Optometry*, 46(7):479–491, 1969.

the same lens. Some subjects experience this problem, which is manifested by swelling on the first day of contact lens wear that is greater than 4 percent (attributed to tear tonicity), but no swelling occurs after the lenses are worn for a period of weeks. It has been reported that some subjects have tight symptoms after the adaptation period, which are alleviated by teaching the subject to blink normally. These patients are fixed at stage two of blinking until training advances them to stage three.

A Physiological Model

On the basis of these experiments, Mandell and Polse propose a model to explain certain contact lens wearing results. They propose a theory that a change in tear osmolarity is the primary mechanism of the adaptation process, with blinking playing a possible secondary role. They find three distinct responses in the corneal swelling that occurs during the adaptation period.

In response 1 the unadapted patient shows an initial swelling of 2 to 4 percent on his first day of contact lens wear. The swelling reaches a peak value in about three hours and is then reduced so that in six hours the cornea has resumed its normal thickness (R1 in Figure 6.22a *top*).

If the contact lens is worn daily, the swelling is gradually decreased each day until at two weeks no swelling occurs (R1 in Figure 6.22a *bottom*).

Patients with response 1 have lenses that interfere minimally with the interchange of tears beneath the contact lens. The initial swelling of 2 to 4 percent can be attributed to tear osmolarity changes, which are temporary. Patients in response 1 show minimum or no symptoms and signs of adaptation.

In response 2 the unadapted patient shows

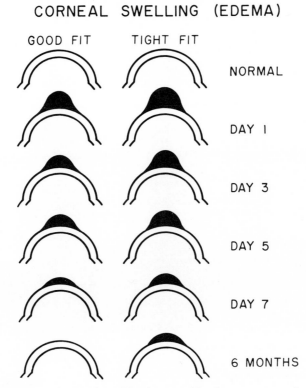

Figure 6.19. Comparison of corneal swelling in eye with adequate tear exchange (good fit) to eye with inadequate tear exchange (tight fit).

an initial swelling of 5 to 8 percent on his first day of contact lens wear. The swelling reaches a peak in about three hours and is then reversed by 2 to 4 percent, but the cornea may or may not return to its original thickness. Response 2 occurs as a result of adding the edema produced by tearing to that produced by an oxygen deficiency. The resultant curve is shown in Figure 6.22b.

Patients with response 2 typically exhibit spectacle blur, edema, and tight symptoms, and these effects are correlated with the degree of corneal swelling.

Patients with response 2 have lenses that interfere with the interchange of tears beneath the contact lens to a degree which does not allow an adequate oxygen supply in the tear layer for normal corneal physiology. On the first day of contact lens wear, the swelling is the result of both a tear tonicity decrease and oxygen deprivation. By the end of the first day, the tearing effect may be eliminated and only swelling from oxygen deprivation remains. After adaptation is completed, no hump occurs in the swelling curve because there is no tear effect. Swelling occurs that may be attributed to oxygen deprivation alone. This interference may be caused by a lens that has a tight-fitting relationship or may occur as the result of an inadequate pumping force or rate of blinking.

These causes may be differentiated after adaptation is complete. The subject with inadequate blinking will have no corneal swelling when blinking has returned to normal. However, the subject with a tight-fitting relationship will continue to have corneal swelling each day the contact lenses are worn,

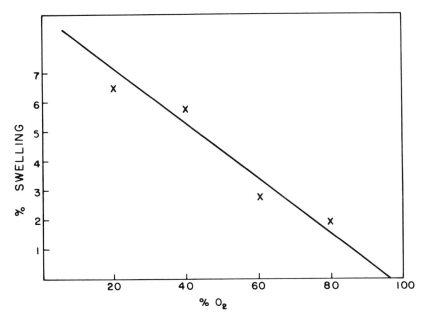

Figure 6.20. By raising the oxygen level in the surrounding atmosphere, it is possible to eliminate corneal thickening from a tight contact lens.

even after adaptation appears to be completed. This swelling will be less than about 8 percent. Patients with swelling of 5 to 8 percent may have constant wearing problems but are able to continue wearing their contact lenses. If a second problem is superimposed, the lenses will probably become intolerable.

In response 3 the unadapted patient shows an initial swelling of greater than 8 percent in three hours. This indicates that a very tight fit causes minimum or no tear exchange

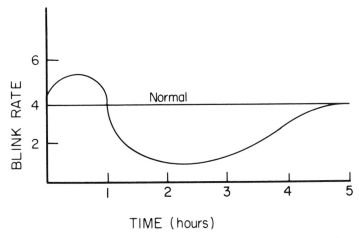

Figure 6.21. The three phases of blinking that occur on the first day of contact lens wear. Phase 1 is rapid and lasts about an hour. Phase 2 is slower than normal and lasts from three to five hours. Phase 3 is a return to normal blink rate.

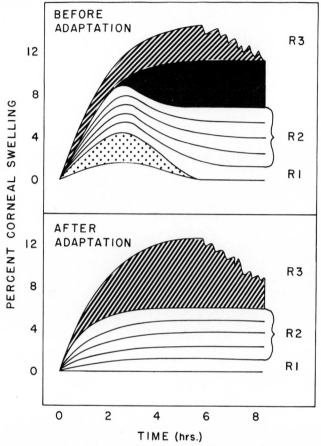

Figure 6.22a. Mandell-Polse model of corneal swelling responses to contact lenses. Response 1 (R1) indicates minimum interference with tear exchange, response 2 (R2) indicates interference with tear exchange and oxygen deprivation below basic corneal requirement, and response 3 (R3) indicates minimum or no tear exchange and oxygen deprivation at a level that will not allow cornea to tolerate the contact lens.

and that oxygen deprivation results in marked corneal swelling. The upper limit of swelling (about 10% in three hours) represents complete oxygen deprivation beneath the contact lens. Since for safety purposes subjects having response 3 cannot be allowed to wear their contact lenses for long periods of time, the later portions of their curves are unknown. An interesting feature of subjects having response 3, but at the lower level of swelling in that group, is that on the first day of contact lens wear the lenses are intolerable. However, after adaptation is complete and the

tearing effect is eliminated, the swelling may be reduced to an amount that allows the lenses to be tolerated. However, wearing time may be very short, and this patient will be predisposed to wearing problems.

Rapid Adaptation

It is possible to have a patient wear contact lenses all day on the first day of wear providing that he does not have a tight fit. At the present time a tight fit can only be evaluated by determining the corneal swelling.

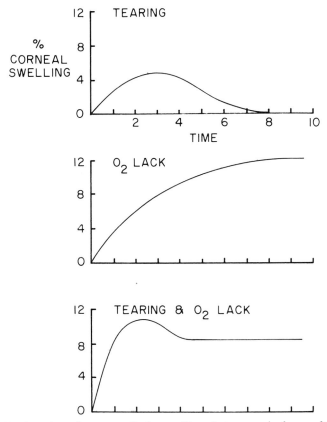

Figure 6.22b. Explanation of response 2: the swelling that occurs is the result of adding the edema produced by tearing to that produced by an oxygen deficiency.

The maximum swelling that results from a tight fit occurs three hours after the lenses are inserted. Hence, this is the time at which the patient should be evaluated for the acceptability of the lens. There are presently two clinical techniques to evaluate corneal swelling: keratometry and biomicroscopy.

KERATOMETRY

As corneal swelling occurs there is often an accompanying increase in the central corneal curvature as measured with a keratometer. Unfortunately, the reliability of the keratometer method is low, so swelling may also occur without any keratometric changes.[31] This occurs because the area of swelling is between the keratometer mire reflection positions or because the swelling produces aspheric corneal contour, which does not produce a change in the keratometer reading.

BIOMICROSCOPY

Biomicroscopy may be used to detect corneal edema, the most favorable method being sclerotic scatter. Unfortunately, the corneal edema cannot be seen until the swelling reaches 4 to 6 percent. However, a knowledge of this can be utilized to guide the clinical procedure. If, on the first day of contact lens wear, no corneal edema can be seen after three hours of wear, it may be concluded that less than 6 percent corneal swelling has occurred. Hence, no (or minimal) oxygen interference is present, and the patient may be allowed to continue wearing his lenses.

LENS DESIGN

LENS-CORNEA RELATIONSHIP

Opinion has varied over what is the optimum relationship between the curves of a contact lens and the cornea. This relationship has been determined for the most part by trial and error, and there is no exact theory that allows the fitter to predict exactly the effects of selecting specific lens dimensions. However, such a theory is developing as more data are collected.

The lens fit is usually considered first in the static condition with the lens centered on the cornea.

Optical Zone

In Chapter 3, it was shown that the cornea has an aspherical shape similar to an ellipse. Much can be determined about the fitting relationship by finding how the curves of a contact lens relate to this surface. If an average apical corneal curvature of 43.00 D. and an average rate of peripheral flattening is assumed, one can find first what the measurement of this cornea will be with a keratometer and how various lenses will fit to it.

A typical cornea with average peripheral flattening is shown in Figure 6.23. This cornea with an apex curvature of 43.00 D. theoretically would measure 42.87 D. with a keratometer. If a lens is now superimposed on the cornea, the interrelationship of the optical zone and the peripheral curve with the cornea can be found.

If the optical zone diameter is assumed to be 7 mm., the radius that most nearly parallels the cornea can be calculated by finding the curve which is the same distance from the cornea at both its center and its edges. To do this, one can assume that the cornea includes a normal tear layer of 10 μm thickness (which is what is actually measured with a keratometer) and that this tear layer remains after the lens is in place.

By calculation, the radius which most nearly parallels the cornea is found to be 7.87 mm., which is equivalent to a base curve of 42.87 D.

Thus, the base curve that most nearly parallels the cornea is, paradoxically, nearly equal in radius to the base curve measured by the keratometer (*see* Chapter 3).

Hence, for an average cornea, the best means for achieving an alignment fit when the optical zone diameter is 7 mm. is to order the contact lens base curve with the same radius as that measured on the cornea with the keratometer. However, if the base curve of the contact lens is made larger in diameter, it now rests on a flattened area of the cornea that is further from the apex (Figure 6.24), and the relationship just described no longer

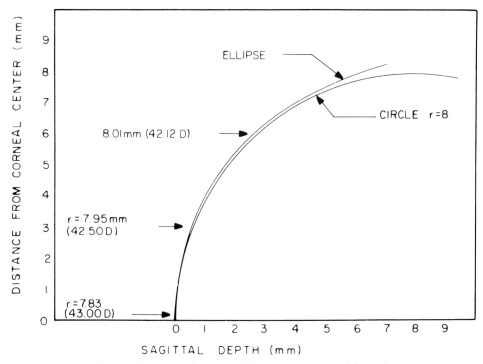

Figure 6.23. A typical cornea with an average rate of flattening.

holds. Again, a calculation for the lens can be made which most nearly parallels the larger corneal area. If the corneal area has a chord diameter of 7.4 mm., the radius for the base curve, which creates an alignment fit, should be 7.92 mm., which corresponds to a power of 42.66 D. If the chord diameter of the optic zone is increased to 7.8 mm., the base curve that would most nearly produce an alignment fit has a radius of 7.95 corresponding to 42.41D.

These values are very nearly those found by Harrison and Kubo in a practical study of this relationship using trial lenses (Figure 6.25).[32]

This theoretical relationship applies to a spherical cornea. If any corneal toricity exists, the relationship is somewhat altered. As the corneal toricity is increased, there is slightly greater bearing on the flatter corneal meridian near the margins of the optic zone. This reduces the apical clearance slightly between the lens and the cornea.

In a practical situation it is usually found that a lens fitted *on K* with an optic zone diameter of 7 mm. will closely parallel the corneal contour (alignment fit). If a larger optic zone is used, then the lens will produce a slight apical clearance between the lens and the central cornea, a relationship favored by most contact lens practitioners. It should be remembered that these relationships hold only for the average cornea and that considerable variation will be found clinically, which is justification for the use of trial lenses.

Peripheral Curve

It is difficult to quantify the space between the contact lens peripheral curve and the cornea. The implied meaning for the commonly used clinical term *corneal clearance* is the linear separation of the lens and cornea. However, the only common method of describing a contact lens peripheral curve is

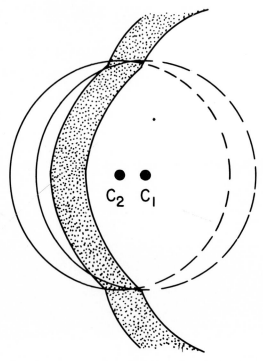

C_2 C_1

Figure 6.24. Base curve of contact lens is represented by a circle through the cornea. As the circle is moved to the left, representing a larger optic zone diameter, the fit becomes steep.

by its radius of curvature. From this expression, it is not possible to describe adequately the corneal clearance, even though the curvature of the peripheral cornea is known. In addition, for given lens dimensions, a change in peripheral curve width does not bring about a predictable change in the corneal clearance.

The latter problem may be illustrated by a hypothetical corneal model of ellipsoidal shape and two contact lenses, one with a relatively steep peripheral curve and the other with a relatively flat peripheral curve (Figure 6.26). Suppose the lenses were 9 mm. in diameter. Large separations would exist between their edges and the cornea. If the lenses were instead made 10 mm. in diameter (by increasing the peripheral curve widths while retaining the same peripheral curve radii), the space

between the edge of the steeper peripheral curve and the cornea would be reduced, whereas the space between the flatter peripheral curve and the cornea would be increased. Unfortunately, in clinical circumstances, the fitter cannot accurately determine what relationship exists between the peripheral curve of a contact lens and the cornea; hence, he cannot consistently predict the effect of differences in peripheral curve width on the corneal clearance (and the fitting characteristics of the lens).

Simple hypothetical corneal models may be used to illustrate mathematical transformations of corneal clearance from radial to linear terms. These transformations show relationships that explain certain clinical phenomena.

Linear clearance between the peripheral curve of a contact lens and the cornea varies as a function of the curvatures of the cornea and the curvatures and sizes of the zones of the contact lens. The position for the measurement of corneal clearance may be referred to either the cornea or the lens.

Linear clearance (d) is here defined as the distance from the posterior lens surface to the cornea, along the normal to the cornea at the point of reference (Figure 6.27). A similar concept that is now used is *edge lift*, defined as the distance from the edge of the posterior surface of the contact lens to the extension of the base curve, along the normal to the extended base curve.

To calculate linear clearance, place a hypothetical contact lens with an optical zone exactly duplicating the curvature of the corneal cap upon a corneal model (Figure 6.28). Neglecting tear thickness, or assuming that the calculations apply to the surface of the tear layer, the optical zone of the lens would be in exact alignment with the cornea. The peripheral curve of the contact lens has a radius of curvature, r_3, that is longer than r_1 but shorter than r_2. The center of curvature for the peripheral curve of the contact

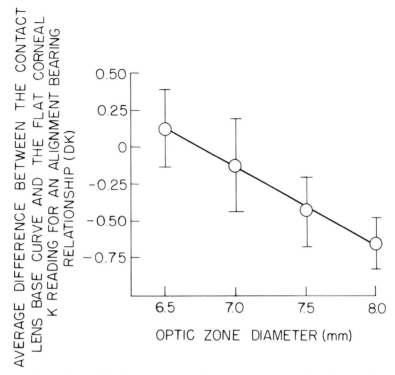

Figure 6.25. The relationship between contact lens base curve and optic zone diameter for alignment fitting. From M. G. Harris and R. S. Kubo, The Relationship between the Contact Lens Base Curve and Optic Zone Diameter for Alignment Fitting, *American Journal of Optometry*, in press.

lens is C_3, which lies on the axis of symmetry for both the lens and the cornea.

Figure 6.29 shows the linear clearances that were calculated for two lens positions relative to h, the chord diameter of the corneal cap: $h + 1$ mm. and $h + 2$ mm., and the radii $r_2 = r_1 + 2$ mm. and $r_3 = r_1 + 1$ mm.

From Figure 6.29, it may be seen that for the lens positions selected and the lenses used the linear clearance of the peripheral curve

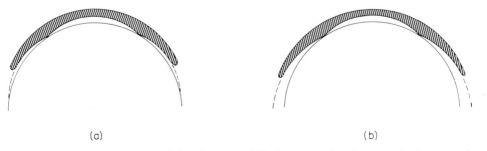

Figure 6.26. Increasing the peripheral curve width decreases the clearance for lens *a* and increases the clearance for lens *b*.

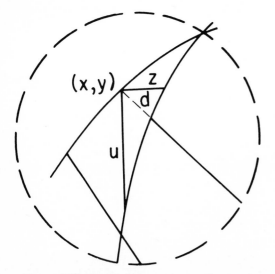

Figure 6.27. Linear clearance is the distance from the posterior lens surface along the normal to the cornea.

is less for lenses with optical zones of longer radii. This relationship holds for the practical dimensions anticipated for contact lenses and explains one enigma of contact lens practice. Most clinicians report from experience that the optimum difference between the base curve and the peripheral curve radii of a contact lens is one that varies as a direct function of the base curve radius. From this, it has been sometimes deduced that the rate of peripheral corneal flattening must be greater for corneas of longer central radius. Yet, direct measurements of corneal contour show no correlation between central corneal curvature and rate of flattening for the corneal periphery. The results of the calculations for Figure 6.29 explain the incongruity of the clinical results and make them compatible with experimental corneal measurements. They also show why contact lenses cannot be used to measure the corneal contour.

In order to predict which contact lens will produce a given lens-cornea relationship, the linear clearance must be known. Its calculation, even with simplified conditions, is too extensive to be practical. Calculations that allow for all the complexities of the human corneal contour (assuming it can be measured) compound the problem. However, it is possible to design contact lenses with constant amounts of edge lift.

To summarize, the results of calculations

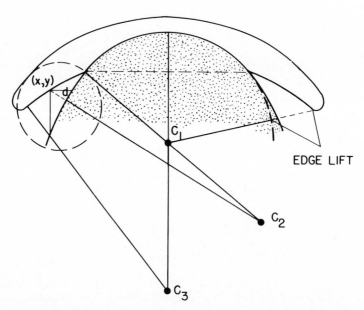

Figure 6.28. Hypothetical contact lens on a corneal model.

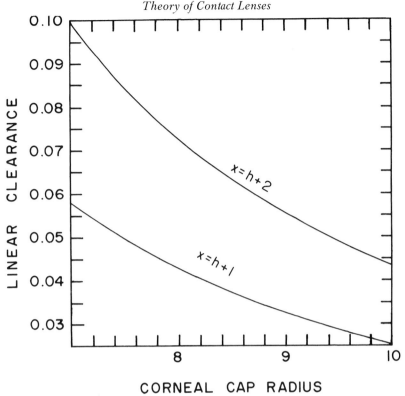

Figure 6.29. Linear clearance calculated for two lens positions using hypothetical corneas and contact lenses (all dimensions in millimeters).

for the linear clearances between contact lenses and a hypothetical cornea show the following: (1) the effect of differences in peripheral curve width on the corneal clearance cannot be consistently predicted clinically and (2) the clinical observation that the optimum peripheral curve radius of a contact lens is one which varies as a direct function of the base curve radius is found to be due to the geometry of the contact lens rather than to a correlation between the central corneal curvature and the rate of peripheral corneal flattening.

Diameter

Since the introduction of corneal contact lenses, there has been a trend towards the use of smaller diameters. There is some clinical evidence that smaller lenses produce fewer physiological disturbances of the cornea than do larger lenses.

It is interesting to examine the rationale that is usually given for the use of a smaller lens diameter. The statement is made that the diameter of the contact lens has been reduced in order to interfere less with normal cornea physiology. This occurs because the smaller contact lens covers less corneal area and hence interferes less with the atmospheric oxygen that is entering the cornea.

If a contact lens diameter is reduced, for example, from 10 mm. to 8 mm., the area is reduced by a factor of 36 percent. This would seem to be a large difference when compared to the total area of the cornea. The original lens covered about 60 percent of the corneal area (the original 10 mm. lens). A reduction in lens size, to 8 mm., would expose about 15 to 20 percent more of the cornea.

This explanation for the success of smaller lenses was made some time after the success of this lens had been realized. There is, however, no evidence that the lens area is actually the most important attribute of the smaller lens. Other factors may operate concurrently to produce the desirable effects achieved with smaller contact lenses, namely, lid pressure on the lens and the efficiency of the tear pump.

The most obvious result of reducing the lens diameter is to eliminate some of the force applied to the lens by the superior lid when the lens is in the centered position. This has been mentioned by several authors, although the difficult problem of evaluating the effect to the cornea has not been solved. During the blink, the lid force is transferred to the lens and onto the cornea, but following the blink, the smaller lens drops free of the lid and rides within the palpebral aperture. Hence, for the majority of time, the lens is free of the lid. This can be expected to have less long-term distortion effects on the cornea.

When using smaller diameter lenses, certain types of fitting relationships between the lens and the cornea seem to produce even more edema than is normally found with larger lenses. Even though these effects occur in only a small percentage of patients, it indicates that some factor other than lens diameter influences the amount of oxygen received by the cornea.

MINIMUM EDGE THICKNESS

A knowledge of edge thickness calculations is valuable for determining the minimum center thickness of a positive power lens which will allow sufficient edge thickness.

From a practical standpoint, the calculation of edge thickness for a contact lens is most often needed in determining whether it is possible to manufacture a lens of given specifications. It is not uncommon for contact lens companies to receive orders for lenses that are impossible to make because they will not have sufficient edge thickness.

In all positive power lenses, and in some negative power lenses with peripheral curves, the anterior and posterior surfaces approach each other in the periphery so that their intersection represents a theoretical limit to the total diameter. At this limit, the lens has an edge thickness of zero. If the size of the lens is to be larger than its theoretical limit and the surface curvatures cannot be changed, the center thickness must be increased; otherwise, the lens cannot be made (Figure 6.30). If the center thickness is reduced, the lens cannot be made unless it is also reduced in diameter. For practical purposes, the possibility that a lens cannot be manufactured is controlled by choosing a center thickness that is more than the anticipated minimum. Unfortunately, this means that superfluous weight will be added to the positive power lenses, which in most cases are already heavier than what is desired. Thus, it is important to choose

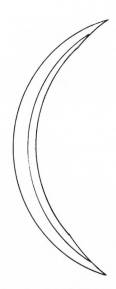

Figure 6.30. If lens diameter needs to be made larger, the center thickness must be increased, otherwise the lens cannot be made.

the minimum center thickness for a lens of positive power which will result in the minimum acceptable edge thickness.

Although an edge thickness of zero would be the theoretical minimum, practically speaking, a lens cannot be made with zero edge thickness, for the edge would be too sharp to be comfortable (knife edge). It has been found that an edge thickness before finishing of approximately 0.12 mm. is optimum.

In most cases, lenses of negative power will have sufficient edge thickness for any needed center thickness. An exception is found when a lens of low negative power has a very large diameter and a very flat peripheral curve. Here again, it is possible to choose lens variables that make an impossible lens design.

The thickness of a contact lens edge varies as a function of every geometric variable of the lens, and its computation by usual methods is too lengthy to be of direct value to the practitioner or manufacturer. With the aid of computers, however, the calculation may be reduced to a practical process.

PERIPHERAL CURVE

When designing a lens, certain aspects of the peripheral curve should be considered to produce a minimum lens thickness. As a peripheral curve of constant width is flattened, the edge thickness is reduced. For example, for a lens of average specifications, a change in peripheral curve radius from 10 to 12 mm. reduces edge thickness from 0.17 to 0.13 mm. (Figure 6.31).

As a peripheral curve of constant radius is increased in width from 0.2 to 0.5 mm., the edge thickness is reduced from 0.20 to 0.15 mm. (Figure 6.32). As lens diameter is increased, the same peripheral curve will produce less edge thickness (Figure 6.33).

These interrelationships are too laborious to be calculated by hand and are generally done with the aid of a computer.

FORCES RETAINING THE CONTACT LENS ON THE CORNEA

There have been only a few studies that attack the very difficult problem of analyzing the forces which hold a contact lens on the eye. This problem is made difficult because of a lack of knowledge of many factors.

The corneal contact lens is held in place by a balance of forces.[33,34] The main force that holds the lens against the cornea is the fluid force produced by the tear layer.[35] This force is determined by the physical characteristics of the tear layer and by the geometric relationship between the posterior lens curvature and the cornea.[36-38] Opposing this force are external forces produced by eye movements and by the action of the lids during closure. In addition, gravity plays a role that can assume major importance in some cases.

FLUID FORCES

The primary force that holds the contact lens against the cornea is surface tension.[39] This force is manifested on a contact lens by the tear meniscus, which is concave at the edge of the lens, indicating that the pressure of the post-lens tear fluid is negative compared with the atmospheric pressure (Figure 6.34). Mackie et al. have pointed out that if

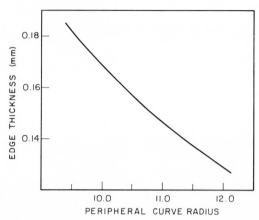

Figure 6.31. Relationship between peripheral curve radius and edge thickness for a lens of average specifications: back vertex power, −2.75; center thickness, 0.15; diameter, 8.5; P.C.W., 0.5; and base curve, 8.50.

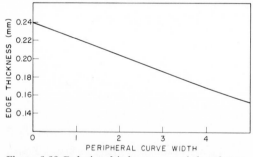

Figure 6.32. Relationship between peripheral curve width and edge thickness for lens of average specifications: back vertex power, −2.75; center thickness, 0.15; diameter, 9.5; P.C.R., 11; and base curve, 8.50.

the lids are drawn back from the cornea when a corneal lens is *in situ*, the lens may be seen to move down slowly to a slightly lower position, but it will not, in the majority of the cases, lie over the limbal regions (Figure 6.35).[40] If the lens is now pushed down slightly from this position and then released, it can frequently be seen to move upwards against gravity. However, when a contact lens is placed on the wetted surface of a smooth spherical ball, it moves downwards under the influence of

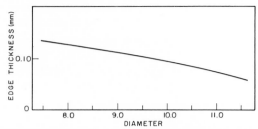

Figure 6.33. Relationship between lens diameter and edge thickness for lens of average specifications: back vertex power plano, P.C.R. 12.25, P.C.W. 0.5, center thickness, 0.20, and base curve 8.50.

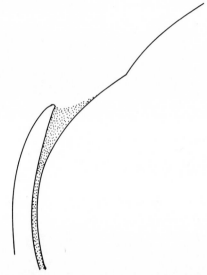

Figure 6.34. Tear meniscus at the lens edge is concave, indicating that pressure of post-lens tear fluid is negative.

gravity until it is at the lowest point on the ball. It does not become detached, but clearly there is no force attempting to keep the lens in the perpendicular position.

The additional fluid force when the lens is on the cornea is produced by the relationship between the lens and corneal curvatures. If the lens base curve is steeper than the cornea, there is a greater tendency for the lens to center on the eye. This occurs because the radius of the curvature of the peripheral cornea is longer than the central cornea. Therefore, as the lens is moved away from

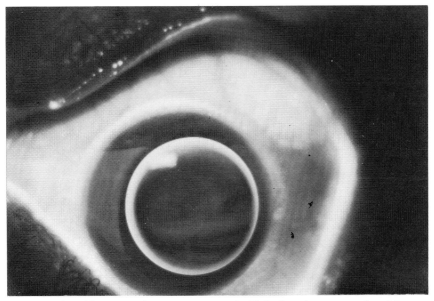

Figure 6.35. Lid pressure is not necessary to hold the lens in a centered position.

the corneal center, the lens must be lifted to move it onto the peripheral cornea. This lens lift is done against the negative pressure behind the lens. As long as the inertia of the moving lens is within the control of negative pressure, there is a tendency for the lens to be drawn back to the central zone by the negative pressure. In a similar way, during lateral eye movement, the lens must be lifted against negative pressure to move it from the center of the cornea. The lens is once again pulled back towards the center by the control of negative pressure. Kikkawa points out that although the tears cover the whole surface of the lens after a blink, it is not necessary to consider that the lens is immersed in a lake of tears.[41] The tear meniscus around the lens edge is concave, while the pre-lens tear film is slightly convex.

LID FORCE

The force of the lids during blinking is clearly larger than the fluid force holding the lens against the eye. The lens tends to move with the lid during the downward phase of the blink and the lens tends to move up as the upper lid is raised. From that point, the lens may fall completely free of the lid, whereupon lid influence is no longer active. At this point, gravity takes over.

GRAVITY

The influence of gravity on the lens begins as soon as the lens is free of the upper lid. The influence of gravity will be determined by the mass of the lens. In general, a lens with greater mass will be pulled downward with greater force. A contact lens that is free of lid forces is mainly controlled in position by the interaction between the opposite forces of gravity and the fluid force.

The balance of forces between the contact lens and the cornea can be easily disturbed. For example, when a corneal lens is made of glass, the increase in weight makes the lens drop to a low position because of gravity. This occurs regardless of the geometric relationship between the lens and the cornea because the force of gravity is now much greater than any fluid force attracting the lens to the eye.

REFERENCES

1. Hill, R. M., and Fatt, I.: How dependent is the cornea on the atmosphere?, *J. Am. Optom. Assoc.*, 35(10):873–875, 1964.
2. Hill, R. M., and Fatt, I.: Oxygen deprivation of the cornea by contact lenses and lid closure, *Am. J. Optom. Arch. Am. Acad. Optom.*, 41:678, 1964.
3. Jauregi, M. J., and Fatt, I.: Estimation of the *in vivo* oxygen consumption rate of the human corneal epithelium, *Am. J. Optom.*, 49:507–511, 1972.
4. Hill, R. M.: The cornea's need to "breathe," *Int. Cont. Lens Clin.*, 3(4):60–61, 1976.
5. Hill, R. M., and Fatt, I.: Oxygen uptake from a reservoir of limited volume by a human cornea *in vivo*, *Science*, 142(3597):1295–1297, 1963.
6. Hill, R. M.: The cohabitations of a cornea, *Int. Cont. Lens Clin.*, 17(1):22–25, 1980.
7. Hill, R. M.: Oxygen permeable contact lenses: how convinced is the cornea?, *Int. Cont. Lens Clin.*, 4(2):34–36, 1977.
8. Polse, K. A., and Mandell, R. B.: Hyperbaric oxygen effect on corneal edema caused by a contact lens, *Am. J. Optom. Arch. Am. Acad. Optom.*, 48(3):197–200, 1971.
9. Fatt, I.: The definition of thickness for a lens, *Am. J. Optom. Physiol. Opt.*, 56(5):324–337, 1979.
10. Hill, R. M., and Lowther, G. E.: Respiratory ophthalmometry, *Am. J. Optom.*, 45(3):152–159, 1968.
11. Fatt, I.: Oxygen tension under a contact lens during blinking, *Am. J. Optom.*, 46(9):654–661, 1969.
12. Fatt, I., and Hill, R. M.: Oxygen tension under a contact lens during blinking: a comparison of theory and experimental observation, *Am. J. Optom.*, 47(1):50–55, 1970.
13. Cuklanz, H. D., and Hill, R. M.: Oxygen requirements of contact lens systems, 1. Comparison of mathematical predictions with physiological measurements, *Am. J. Optom.*, 46(9):662–665, 1969.
14. Cuklanz, H. D., and Hill, R. M.: Oxygen requirements of corneal contact lens systems, *Am. J. Optom.*, 46(3):228–230, 1969.
15. Cuklanz, H. D., and Hill, R. M.: Tear space volumes of spherical and toric cornea—contact lens systems, 1. Mathematical models and physiological effects under static conditions, *Am. J. Optom.*, 45(11):719–733, 1968.
16. Cuklanz, H. D., and Hill, R. M.: Tear volumes between contact lens and cornea, *J. Am. Optom. Assoc.*, 40(3):284–286, 1969.
17. Mandell, R. B., and Harris, M. G.: Theory of the contact lens adaptation process, *J. Am. Optom. Assoc.*, 39(3):260–261, 1968.
18. Harris, M. G., and Mandell, R. B.: Contact lens adaptation: osmotic theory, *Am. J. Optom.*, 46(3):196–202, 1969.
19. Chan, R. S., and Mandell, R. B.: Corneal swelling caused by *Allium cepa*, *Am. J. Optom. Arch. Am. Acad. Optom.*, 49(9):713–715, 1972.
20. Lowther, G. E., and Hill, R. M.: Sensitivity threshold of the lower lid margin in the course of adaptation to contact lenses, *Am. J. Optom.*, 45(9):587–594, 1968.
21. Mishima, S., and Maurice, D. M.: The effect of normal evaporation on the eye, *Exp. Eye Res.*, 1(1):46–52, 1961.
22. Mandell, R. B., and Polse, K. A.: Corneal thickness changes as a contact lens fitting index—experimental results and a proposed model, *Am. J. Optom.*, 46(7):479–491,

1969.

23. Mandell, R. B., Polse, K. A., and Fatt, I.: Corneal swelling caused by contact lens wear, *Arch. Ophthalmol., 83*:3–9, 1970.

24. Mandell, R. B., and Polse, K. A.: Keratoconus: spatial variation of corneal thickness as a diagnostic test, *Arch. Ophthalmol., 82*(2): 182–188, 1969.

25. Smelser, G. K., and Chen, D. K.: Physiological changes in cornea induced by contact lenses, *Arch. Ophthalmol., 53*(5):676–679, 1955.

26. Sarwar, M.: Corneal veiling, *Br. J. Physiol. Opt., 11*(3):167–169, 1954.

27. Korb, D. R.: Corneal transparency with emphasis on the phenomenon of central circular clouding, in *Encyclopedia of Contact Lens Practice*, 1963, vol. 4, suppl. 20, Appendix B, pp. 106–115.

28. Mazow, B.: *Synopsis of Corneal Contact Lens Fitting for Optometrists*, Minneapolis, Burgess, 1962, Am. Acad. Optom. Ser., vol. 2.

29. Miller, D., and Exford, J.: Effect of corneal contact lenses on corneal thickness: a case study, *Contact Lens*, Middlesex, England, 1967, p. 5.

30. Polse, K. A., and Mandell, R. B.: Hyperbaric oxygen effect on corneal edema caused by a contact lens, *Am. J. Optom., 48*(3): 197–200, 1971.

31. Hazlett, R.: *Changes in corneal thickness, corneal curvature, and corneal transparency associated with contact lens wear*, Master's thesis, Indiana University, 1969.

32. Harris, M. G., and Kubo, R. S.: The relationship between the contact lens base curve and optic zone diameter for alignment fitting, *Am. J. Optom.*, in press.

33. Miller, D.: An analysis of the physical forces applied to a corneal contact lens, *Arch.*

Ophthalmol., 70(6):823–829, 1963.

34. Rocher, P.: New considerations on the adherence of contact lenses to the eye, *Contacto, 12*(1):51–56, 1968.

35. Lowther, G. E., and Hill, R. M.: Fluid forces associated with contact lens systems, *J. Am. Optom. Assoc., 38*(10):847–850, 1967.

36. Gordon, S.: Factors determining the physical and physiological fit of corneal type contact lenses, in *Encyclopedia of Contact Lens Practice*, South Bend, Indiana, International Optics, 1959–1963, vol. 2, Chap. 6, pp. 1–34.

37. Wray, L.: An elementary analysis of the forces retaining a corneal contact lens on the eye—Part 1, *The Optician, 146*(3780):239–242, 1963; Part 2, The Calculation of the force of attraction between Curved Plates Enclosing a Thin Liquid Film, *146*(3783): 318–322, 1963; Part 3, Practical Considerations, *146*(3785):374–376, 378, 1963.

38. Poster, M.: Hydro-dynamics of corneal contact lens, *Am. J. Optom., 41*(7):422–425, 1964.

39. Yorke, H. C.: Determination of the forces retaining a contact lens on the eye, *Br. J. Physiol. Opt., 26*(1):75–87, 1971.

40. Mackie, I. A.: Factors influencing corneal contact lens centration, *Br. J. Physiol. Opt., 25*(2):87–103, 1970.

41. Kikkawa, Y.: The mechanism of contact lens adherence and centralization, *Am. J. Optom., 47*(4):275–281, 1970.

42. Hill, R. M., and Fatt, I.: Oxygen measurements under a contact lens, *Am. J. Optom., 41*(6):382–387, 1964.

43. Hill, R. M., and Jeppe, W. H.: Hydrogels: is a pump still necessary?, *Int. Cont. Lens Clin., 2*(4):28, 1975.

44. Hill, R. M.: Perils of the pump, *Int. Cont. Lens Clin., 3*(3):49, 1976.

ADDITIONAL READINGS

Allaire, P. E., Allison, S. W., and Gooray, A. M.: Tear-film dynamics and oxygen tension under a circular contact lens, *Am. J. Optom. Physiol. Opt., 54*(9):617, 1977.

Atkinson, T. C. O.: The design of the contact lens periphery, *The Ophthalmic Optician, 15*(1):14,

1975.

Berger, R. E.: Effect of contact lens motion on the oxygen tension distribution under the lens, *Am. J. Optom. Physiol. Opt., 51*(7):441–456, 1974.

Berger, R. E.: A surface tension gradient mechanism for driving the pre-corneal tear film after a blink, *J. Biomechanics*, 7:225, 1974.

Berglund, J. H.: Tears: their need and movement with contact lenses, *Opt. Weekly*, 60(9):35–36, 1969.

Bibby, M.: Factors affecting peripheral curve design part II: specifying for reproducible performance, *Am. J. Optom. Physiol. Opt.*, 56(10):618–627, 1979.

Bibby, M.: Sagittal depth considerations in the selection of the base curve radius of a soft contact lens, *Am. J. Optom. Physiol. Opt.*, 56(7): 407–413, 1979.

Bibby, M.: An evaluation of edge lift as a specification in contact lens design, *Int. Cont. Lens Clin.*, 6(6):270, 1979.

Bibby, M. M.: Factors affecting peripheral curve design, *Am. J. Optom. Physiol. Opt.*, 56(1):2–9, 1979.

Bibby, M. M., and Gellman, M.: Tear layer thickness: a rationale for base curve selection, *Int. Cont. Lens Clin.*, 3(3):62–70, 1976.

Bibby, M. M., and Tomlinson, A.: Corneal clearance at the apex and edge of a hard corneal lens, *Int. Cont. Lens Clin.*, 4(6):50, 1977.

Bieber, M. T., and Fatt, I.: Steady state distribution of oxygen and carbon dioxide in the *in vivo* cornea of an eye covered by a gas-permeable contact lens, *Am. J. Optom. Am. Acad. Optom.*, 46(1):3–14, 1969.

Carney, L. G.: Effect of hypoxia on central and peripheral corneal thickness and corneal topography, *Austr. J. Optom.*, 58(2):61–65, 1975.

Clarke, C.: Contact lenses at high altitude: experience on Everest south-west face 1975, *Br. J. Ophthalmol.*, 60(6):479–480, 1976.

Decker, M., Polse, K. A., and Fatt, I.: Oxygen flux into the human cornea when covered by a soft contact lens, *Am. J. Optom. Physiol. Opt.*, 55(5):285, 1978.

Efron, N., and Carney, L. G.: Oxygen levels beneath the closed eyelid, *Invest. Ophthalmol. Vis. Sci.*, 18(1):93, 1979.

Efron, N., and Carney, L. G.: Oxygen tension measurements under soft contact lenses with blinking, *Int. Cont. Lens Clin.*, 6(6):250, 1979.

Ehlers, N., and Sperling, S.: A technical improvement of the Haag-Streit pachometer, *Acta Ophthalmol.*, 55(2):333–336, 1977.

Eng, W. G.: Low atmospheric pressure effects on wearing soft contact lenses, *Aviat. Space Environ. Med.*, Jan. 1978.

Fatt, I.: Steady-state distribution of oxygen and carbon dioxide in the *in vivo* cornea I. The open eye in air and the closed eye., *Exp. Eye Res.*, 7:103, 1968.

Fatt, I. Steady-state distribution of oxygen and carbon dioxide in the *in vivo* cornea II. The open eye in nitrogen and the covered eye, *Exp. Eye Res.*, 7:413, 1968.

Fatt, I., Ruben, M., and Morris, J.: Changes in oxygen permeability, *The Optician*, 173(4478):15, 1977.

Fitzgerald, J. K., and Jones, D. P.: Oxygen flux data can be misleading, *Int. Cont. Lens Clin.*, 5(3):61, 1978.

Goldman, J. N., and Kuwabara, T.: Histopathology of corneal edema, *Int. Ophthalmol. Clin.*, 8(3):561, 1968.

Hamano, H.: Variation of oxygen tension *in vivo* with various materials, *Contacto*, 16(4):4–9, 1972.

Hamano, H.: Variation of oxygen tension in the aqueous humor under the contact lens, *J. Jap. Cont. Lens Soc.*, 17(5):65–68, 1975.

Hamano, H.: Change of oxygen tension in corneal stroma with various kinds of contact lenses, *Contacto*, p. 9, Jan. 1980.

Harsant, R.: A method of estimating the edge thickness of minus lenses, *The Disp. Opt.*, 30(2):54, 1978.

Hess, R. G., and Carney, L. G.: Vision through an abnormal cornea: a pilot study of the relationship between visual loss from corneal distortion, corneal edema, keratoconus and some allied corneal pathology, *Invest. Ophthalmol.*, 18(5):476–483, 1979.

Hill, R.: The unblinking eye, *Int. Cont. Lens Clin.*, p. 57, July/Aug. 1979.

Hill, R.: Optimizing the oxygen, *Cont. Lens Forum*, p. 35, Jan. 1980.

Hill, R., and Carney, L. G.: Tear pH: how predictable?, *J. Am. Optom. Assoc.*, 49(3):269–270, 1978.

Hill, R., and Carney, L. G.: Human tear responses to alkali, *Invest. Ophthalmol.*, 19(2):207, 1980.

Hill, R., and Terry, J. E.: Predestined edema?, *Cont. Lens Forum*, 3(4):41, 1978.

Hill, R. M.: Osmotic vulnerability, *Int. Cont. Lens Clin.*, 4(4):31, 1977.

Hill, R. M.: Probing the edema zone, *Int. Cont. Lens Clin.*, 6(5):29, 1979.

Hill, R. M.: Hard lens pumps: trickle or tide?, *Cont. Lens Forum*, 4(3):77, 1979.

Hirano, T.: Epithelial edema of the cornea caused by maintaining the eye in oxygen-deficient gaseous atmosphere in rabbits, *J. Jap. Cont. Lens Soc.*, *21(1)*:36–41, 1979.

Hirji, N. K.: Is corneal pachometry worth the effort?, *The Optician*, *176(4550)*:14, 1978.

Hirji, N. K.: Some aspects of the design of studies to evaluate the ocular response to contact lens wear, *Cont. Lens J.*, *8(2)*:13, 1979.

Hirji, N. K., and Larke, J. R.: Thickness of human cornea measured by topographic pachometry, *Am. J. Optom. Physiol. Opt.*, *55(2)*:97, 1978.

Hom, F. S.: Soft gelatin capsules II: oxygen permeability study of capsule shells, *J. Pharm. Sci.*, *64(5)*:851–857, 1975.

Loshaek, S., and Hill, R. M.: Oxygen permeability measurements: correlation between living-eye and electrode-chamber measurements, *Int. Cont. Lens Clin.*, *4(6)*:26–29, 1977.

Lowther, G. E., and Hill, R. M.: Corneal epithelium—recovery from anoxia, *Arch. Ophthalmol.*, *92(3)*: 231–234, 1974.

Mandell, R. B.: The problem patient: why must we blink?, *Int. Cont. Lens Clin.*, *1(2)*:44–45, 1974.

Mandell, R. B.: Is the contact lens-cornea relationship predictable?, *Int. Cont. Lens Clin.*, *1(3)*:30–32, 1974.

Miller, D.: Contact lens-induced corneal curvature and thickness changes, *Arch. Ophthalmol.*, *80(4)*: 430–432, 1968.

Nakayama, C.: Studies on the tear flow under hard contact lenses by fluorescein cinematography (Eng. abstract), *J. Jap. Cont. Lens Soc.*, *18(2)*:25–30, 1976.

Peterson, J. F., and Fatt, I.: Oxygen flow through a soft contact lens on a living eye, *Am. J. Optom. Arch. Am. Acad. Optom.*, *50(2)*:91–93, 1973.

Polse, K. A.: Corneal edema and curvature changes, *Optom. Weekly*, *66(30)*:795–796, 1975.

Polse, K. A.: Importance of oxygen in contact lens wear, *J. Am. Optom. Assoc.*, *47(3)*:285, 1976.

Chapter 7

FITTING METHODS AND PHILOSOPHIES

The specifications for contact lenses may be determined by making a series of measurements of the patient's ocular dimensions or by systematically evaluating one or a series of test lenses (usually called trial lenses) on the eye. This chapter will emphasize the first method, known as the method of direct ordering, although it should be recognized that many principles of the trial lens procedure may be involved. Chapter 8 will explain the trial lens procedure in greater detail.

To order a contact lens directly, it is necessary to measure certain corneal and lid dimensions and to predict the probable influence of each on the fit of the contact lens. A large number of measurements must be considered, which makes it difficult to state simple rules for the fitting process. Generally, one of two approaches is followed: either the fitter attempts to customize the lens design so that it conforms precisely to the patient's needs or he chooses from a number of standard lens designs available from the various laboratories. In either case, it should be recognized that the first lens ordered is always a tentative selection. The fitting process is not completed until the lens has been evaluated following the adaptation period. A number of lens changes or modifications may be needed before the fitting process is accomplished.

SELECTION OF CUSTOM LENSES

TOTAL DIAMETER

The total diameter of a contact lens is determined by the corneal diameter and the vertical separation of the lids when the eye is open. Other factors are occasionally considered.

Corneal Diameter

Corneal diameter is determined by measuring the horizontal length of the visible iris diameter. Although the cornea itself extends somewhat beyond the bounds of the iris, the discrepancy is small and, for practical purposes, can be ignored (*see* Chapter 3). The diameter of the cornea will usually range from 10 to 12.5 mm. From this measurement a tentative size for the lens can be determined from Table 7.1. The fitter may wish to make the total diameter 0.2 mm. larger than the values given in Table 7.1 because lens diameter can be reduced, but a new lens has to be made if an increase in total diameter is required.

Lid Position

If the vertical separation of the lids is relatively small, the lens should be less than the average total diameter. Some fitters measure the palpebral aperture height with a P.D.

TABLE 7.1

For Corneal Diameter of:	Use Lens Diameter of:
10.0 mm.	8.2 mm.
10.5 mm	8.4 mm.
11.0 mm.	8.6 mm.
11.5 mm.	8.8 mm.
12.0 mm.	9.0 mm.
12.5 mm.	9.2 mm.
13.0 mm.	9.4 mm.

rule held vertically and close to the face. The average aperture size measured by this method is approximately 9.5 mm. When the aperture is less than 9.0 mm., the corneal lens diameter should be reduced 0.4 mm. from the value given in Table 7.1.

It is not difficult to estimate the vertical separation of the lids by inspection. In fact, the estimate may be more valid than the fairly inaccurate measurement with a P.D. rule, since people have a tendency to squint when the rule is placed near the eye. Figure 7.1 shows the normal relationship of the lids to the cornea. The margin of the superior lid usually crosses the limbus at about the ten and two o'clock positions. The inferior lid will normally just graze the edge of the lower limbus.* For every 0.5 mm. that the lids are estimated to be closer together than their normal positions, the total diameter of the contact lens should be reduced by 0.2 mm.

Lid Tension

Lid forces may affect the positioning of the contact lens, but the lack of any accurate method to evaluate the lid tension has made the measurement of this variable difficult. Some authorities feel that if the lids are tight, a large lens is necessary; others feel tight lids indicate the need for a small lens. There is better agreement when the lids are loose, for in this case most fitters feel that the lens should always be made 0.2 to 0.4 mm. larger than normal.

Refractive Power

Many fitters use larger diameters (0.2 to 0.4 mm.) for plus power contact lenses. Plus power lenses are somewhat heavier than average, and the larger diameter gives the lens better adherence providing thickness remains minimal.

POSTERIOR OPTICAL ZONE DIAMETER

The posterior optical zone should be as large as or larger than the pupil of the eye. To allow for lens movement, the optical zone diameter is usually made slightly larger than the maximum pupil diameter.

———————

*Care should be taken that the patient's head is not tipped forward or backward, as this will alter the lid position.

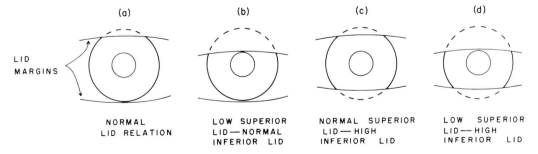

Figure 7.1. Relationship of the lids to the cornea.

For maximum pupil diameter of	*Use optic zone diameter of*
Less than 6 mm. (small)	7.0 mm. (small)
6 to 7 mm. (average)	7.4 mm. (average)
Larger than 7 mm. (large)	7.8 mm. (large)

In the selection of the optical zone diameter,

it should be noted that the optical zone can be made smaller by a modification of the lens but cannot be made larger unless a new lens is made. When there is any doubt of the correct diameter, a larger size should be used.

POSTERIOR OPTICAL ZONE RADIUS

The radius of the posterior optical zone (base curve) is usually made equal to the radius of the flatter principal meridian of the cornea as measured with a keratometer. In this way an attempt is made to achieve near parallelism between the optical zone of the lens and the flatter corneal meridian.

The power of the flatter principal corneal meridian measured with the keratometer is called the *K* value. A contact lens is said to be fitted *on K* if its optical zone has the radius of the *K* value. This is often erroneously interpreted to mean that the optical zone of the lens is fitted parallel to the corneal cap. This would only hold true if the corneal cap were as large as the optical zone diameter of the lens and if the keratometer measurement of the corneal cap radius were valid (Figure 7.2). It is unlikely that these two requirements will be fulfilled. It is found that a lens that is

fitted on *K* may actually be steeper or flatter than the central cornea.

The inability to predict the exact relationship that will exist between the optical zone radius of the lens and the cornea is one of the primary objections to fitting contact lenses by the method of direct ordering. Nevertheless, if the optical zone radius is always made equal to the *K* reading, the difference between the curvature of the flattest corneal meridian and the contact lens can never be very great. The *K* reading is the best estimate of the optical zone radius that will parallel the cornea.

The average cornea flattens rapidly towards the periphery, and the optical zone of the lens should be flattened accordingly. If an attempt is made to achieve near parallelism between the lens and the cornea and if it is desired to have approximately the same lens—cornea relationship for all eyes, it is neces-

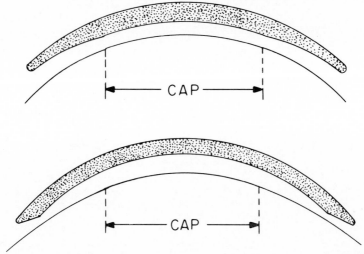

Figure 7.2. Even when the optical zone of a contact lens has the same radius as the central cornea, the two curves are parallel only if the optical zone is as small as the corneal cap (*top*).

TABLE 7.2

Optical Zone Diameter (mm.)	Optical Zone Radius
7.0 (Small)	0.5 mm. steeper that K
7.4 (Average)	on K
7.8 (Large)	0.05 mm. flatter than K

TABLE 7.3

CONVERSION TABLE
(Diopters to Radius in Millimeters)

Diopters	Radius	Diopters	Radius
37.25	9.060	45.25	7.459
37.50	9.000	45.50	7.418
37.75	8.940	45.75	7.377
38.00	8.882	46.00	7.337
38.25	8.824	46.25	7.297
38.50	8.766	46.50	7.258
38.75	8.710	46.75	7.219
39.00	8.654	47.00	7.181
39.25	8.599	47.25	7.143
39.50	8.544	47.50	7.105
39.75	8.491	47.75	7.068
40.00	8.438	48.00	7.031
40.25	8.385	48.25	6.995
40.50	8.333	48.50	6.959
40.75	8.282	48.75	6.923
41.00	8.232	49.00	6.888
41.25	8.182	49.25	6.853
41.50	8.133	49.50	6.818
41.75	8.084	49.75	6.784
42.00	8.036	50.00	6.750
42.25	7.988	50.25	6.716
42.50	7.941	50.50	6.683
42.75	7.895	50.75	6.650
43.00	7.849	51.00	6.618
43.25	7.803	51.25	6.585
43.50	7.759	51.50	6.553
43.75	7.714	51.75	6.522
44.00	7.670	52.00	6.490
44.25	7.627	52.25	6.459
44.50	7.584	52.50	6.429
44.75	7.542	52.75	6.398
45.00	7.500	53.00	6.368

sary to flatten the optical zone radii of lenses with larger optical zone diameters. Table 7.2 shows average amounts of flattening that should be made to optical zone radii for this purpose.

Power or Radius?

The curvature of the optical zone of a contact lens is often expressed in terms of diopters, just as the corneal power is expressed in diopters when read from the keratometer. It might be stated, for example, that a lens fitted on *K* to a 40.00 D. cornea has an optical zone with a power of 40.00 D. Correctly speaking, however, a lens that has the same radius of curvature on its posterior surface as the cornea has on its front surface will not have the same dioptric power because the index of refraction for the contact lens is not the same as for the cornea. To avoid this error, the curvatures for the contact lens surfaces should ideally be given in terms of radius rather than power. The keratometer measurement of the dioptic power of the cornea can be converted into the radius of curvature by using the optical formula for the power of a single refracting surface.[*]

$$r = \frac{n - 1}{F}$$

This radius value should be used for the optical zone of a lens that is to be fitted on *K*. Useful values for this conversion are given in Table 7.3. (Such tables are usually available

from contact lens companies in separate form and can be placed in convenient places for reference.)

It is common practice for practitioners to order the optical zone radius of a lens in terms of diopters to avoid the conversion. Optical companies will accept the order given in this way, but it should be realized by the practitioner that this is not the correct specification. Although power values may be used for ordering the optical zone curvature with no difficulty, using this power value incorrectly has led to many errors in other calculations. Use of the radius value in its correct form is preferred.

---

[*]It is well to remember that the keratometer "measures" the radius of curvature of the cornea and that this value has been converted to a power value on the instrument scale.

Deviations from Parallelism

Occasionally purposely making the optical zone of the contact lens either steeper or flatter than the cornea is desirable. This is most often done for highly toric and spherical corneas.

A lens that is fitted on K to a highly toric cornea will tend to rest mainly on the flattest corneal meridian. If the cornea is flattest in the horizontal meridian, the vertical corneal meridian will have considerable clearance from the lens because of its greater curvature. The overall effect of this lens-cornea relationship is to produce a very loose lens due to the small area of lens-cornea contact. In addition, since the edge of the lens stands away from the cornea in the vertical meridian, it presents considerable impedance to the lid. There is usually discomfort to the wearer because of lid irritation. As the lid moves, the lens tends to rock up and down across the horizontal meridian. This rocking effect can actually be seen during blinking by viewing the patient's eye from the side.

One approach to fitting the highly toric cornea is to decrease the optical zone radius. A lens fitted steeper than K can usually be tolerated on a highly toric cornea. The lens must be flatter than the steepest corneal meridian so that a channel is provided for the tear flow. Several rules have evolved for determining the amount of steepening that is necessary for various amounts of corneal toricity. It is very common to fit the optical zone of the lens so that its radius is steeper than flat K by one-third to one-half the difference in radius between the steepest and flattest corneal meridians. This rule works satisfactorily for moderate amounts of toricity, that is, in the range between 1.00 and 2.00 D.

When corneal toricity is above 2.00 D., it becomes increasingly difficult to achieve a satisfactory fit with a contact lens having a spherical optical zone. To avoid the problem of fitting a spherical optical zone on the toric cornea, the optical zone of the lens is sometimes made toric to give better overall parallelism. This is discussed further in Chapter 9.

In fitting a contact lens to a perfectly spherical cornea, there is no natural channel for tear flow as there is when corneal astigmatism is present. A lens that is fitted on K to a spherical cornea may block tear exchange in the central corneal area and eventually cause metabolic disturbances. It is therefore desirable to fit the contact lens with a slightly flatter optical zone than would ordinarily be used. As a general rule for a spherical cornea, the optical zone may be flattened 0.05 mm. from that which would be given according to Table 7.2.

PERIPHERAL CURVES

Number and Width

The selection of the number of peripheral curves for a lens, that is, whether a lens is to be a bicurve or tricurve, is to some extent arbitrary. One method of selection is based on the total lens diameter. A diameter of 9.0 mm. is set as an arbitrary limit for the bicurve lens, and larger lenses are automatically made in tricurve form.* In limiting the total diameter of a bicurve lens, a limit is automatically placed on the width of the peripheral curve. Since the smallest optical zone that is recommended is 7.0 mm., the peripheral curve of a bicurve lens is limited to a width of 1.0 mm.

$$\text{T.D.}_{\text{bicurve}} = \text{O.Z.D.} + 2(\text{P.C.W.})$$

$$\text{P.C.W.} = \frac{9.0 - 7.0}{2} = 1.0 \text{ mm.}$$

If a lens is 9.0 mm. or larger in total diameter, it is made in the form of a tricurve. The easiest method for the selection of the various

*There is nothing, of course, that would prevent the fitter from making bicurve lenses larger than 9.0 mm. or tricurve lenses smaller than 9.0 mm. in total diameter if he so desires.

curves for a tricurve is to make the peripheral curve standard. One common peripheral curve that is used has a width of 0.4 mm. and a radius of 12.25 mm. The intermediate curve width may be found by subtracting the width of the peripheral curve and the optical zone diameter from the total diameter.

$$2(\text{I.C.W.}) = \text{T.D.} - \text{O.Z.D.} - 2(\text{P.C.W.})$$

For example, when a tricurve lens has a total diameter of 9.0 mm., an optical zone diameter of 7.4 mm., and a peripheral curve width of 0.4 mm., the intermediate curve width would be 0.4 mm.

Radius of the Peripheral Curve

The radius of the peripheral curve can be within a range desired by the fitter, but it must be at least 0.8 mm. longer than the radius of the optical zone. A peripheral curve that is less than 0.8 mm. flatter than the optical zone radius is impractical and also difficult to manufacture.

If the lens is to be a bicurve, the peripheral curve may be given a standard radius that is 2 mm. flatter than the optical zone radius. For example, if the optical zone radius is 7.85 mm., the peripheral curve radius will be 9.85 mm. (usually rounded to 10.0 mm.).

For a tricurve, the intermediate radius might be 1.4 mm. flatter than the base curve and the peripheral curve made with a standard 12.25 mm. radius. Either of these curves can be varied to any dimensions desired by the fitter, within reasonable limits. Intermediate curves are sometimes made anywhere from 0.8 to 2.0 mm. flatter than the base curve, and peripheral curves are made with a radius from 10 to 15 mm. and occasionally longer. After a lens has been finished, the peripheral curves may be widened or flattened, but they cannot be narrowed or steepened without constructing a new lens. The recommended values given for these dimensions were selected with this point in mind. Some fitters wish to vary the peripheral curve radius according to various other lens dimensions. There has been considerable disagreement on the need to vary the peripheral curve.

BLEND

Specification of the blend is rather arbitrary, as illustrated by this classification by Haynes[1] in which blends are divided into three types (Figure 7.3).

1. *Unblended junction.* The junction between two adjacent zones is sharp and no distortion can be seen.

2. *Light blend.* The junction between the two adjacent zones is slightly rounded, but it can be clearly demonstrated that there are two distinct adjacent zones with specific radii. Its maximum width is 0.2 mm.

3. *Medium blend.* Maximum width is 0.4 mm.

4. *Complete blend.* There is a definite blurred area at the junction, and it is almost impossible to differentiate the two adjacent zones with their specified two radii (also termed a heavy blend).

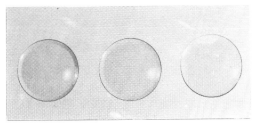

Figure 7.3. Blending of peripheral curve. *Left,* light blend; *center,* medium blend; and *right,* heavy blend.

As Haynes points out, the problem with the preceding qualitative description of blends is that there are many intermediate blend steps between the touch blend and the so-called complete blend. Therefore, it is desirable to have a more quantitative specification. One accepted technique is to specify the radius of the blending tool and the width of the blend.

In most cases only touch blends should be ordered from the laboratory. The blend can also be widened at a later time if it is found to be necessary. If a complete blend is ordered, it will make verification of the lens an almost impossible task.

CENTER THICKNESS

The center thickness is one of the most important dimensions of the lens. If the lens is too thin, it will be flexible and unstable. If the lens is too thick, it will be too heavy and will not fit properly.

The correct center thickness for a lens is based partly on the geometry of the lens shape and partly on the lens material. Some experience with the plastic used for contact lenses is necessary before one can determine a correct lens thickness. The calculations for the center thickness of a lens must consider all the variables of the lens (Chapter 34).

This can be done most easily by the laboratory.

Most laboratories publish thickness tables, which can serve as a guide to the practitioner when ordering (Appendix 3). These tables are only approximations, and they should serve only as a rough guide for the thickness selection.

If the lens thickness is not specified in the order, the manufacturer will follow his own recommended thickness table. After a few lenses have been ordered, the practitioner can judge whether or not the lenses are too thin or too thick.

POWER

Calculation of the exact contact lens power involves the use of numerous equations. Fortunately, for clinical purposes, a few simple rules normally suffice in replacing the equations. Only these rules will be presented here, leaving the more theoretical and exact calculations for Chapter 34.

Short Method of Power Calculation

Under certain limited conditions a short method can be used to find the refractive power that is needed for a contact lens:

1. When the patient's spectacle lens correction is less than 4.00 D.
2. When the contact lens is fitted on K

It should be realized, however, that the short method of calculating contact lens power is not exact and may produce large errors in a few cases.

In using the short calculation method, the spectacle lens correction (or refraction) must be specified in minus cylinder form. If the spectacle lens correction is in plus cylinder form, it must be converted to the minus cylinder form before proceeding.

The cylindrical component is dropped from the spectacle lens correction in minus cylinder form and the spherical element is retained as the refractive power to be ordered in the contact lens.

For example—

1. Spectacle lens power $-3.00 - 0.50 \times 90$
   Contact lens power -3.00 sphere
2. Spectacle lens power $-3.00 + 0.75 \times 90$
   Contact lens power -2.25 sphere
3. Spectacle lens power $+2.00 - 0.25 \times 180$
   Contact lens power $+2.00$ sphere

Correction for High Refractive Powers

If the spectacle lens power exceeds ± 4.00 D., a simple modification of the short calculation method is needed to obtain an accurate contact lens power. It involves making an allowance for the effective power of the spectacle lens. If the spectacle lens is to be replaced by a contact lens, the power of the contact lens must differ from the power of the spectacle lens to still have the same effective power relative to the eye. The difference in power may be found either from a table of calculated values or by direct calculation.

Table of Effective Powers

A list of spectacle lens powers and their corresponding contact lens powers corrected for effective power differences is presented in Appendix 2. It may be noted from Appendix 2 that if the spectacle lens power is less than ±4.00 D., the difference in power for the spectacle lens and contact lens will be less than 0.25 D.; this difference can usually be ignored. Thus, effective power allowances are only significant when the spectacle lens power exceeds ±4.00 D. It may also be noted that for myopia, less minus power is required for a correction in contact lens form than is required for a correction in spectacle form; for hyperopia, more plus power is required when correcting with contact lenses. For example, if the spectacle lens has a power of −9.00 D., the corresponding contact lens power should be −8.06 D. (13 mm. vertex distance). If the spectacle lens power is +9.00 D., the corresponding contact lens power should be +10.19 D.

Calculation of Effective Power

Corrective lenses for the eye have the same effective power when their focal points coincide at the same position relative to the eye. For example, a +5.00 D. hyperope wears his spectacle lenses 13 mm. in front of the cornea. The focal length of the positive power lens is 200 mm., as shown in Figure 7.4. If a contact lens is to be substituted to correct the ametropia, its focal point must be the same distance behind the eye as the spectacle lens, that is, 187 mm. behind the cornea. The power of the contact lens will need to be 1000/187 = +5.34 D. The focal points of both lenses must coincide with the far point of the eye to correct for the ametropia.

If the refractive correction for ametropia is expressed in terms of the lens power in the spectacle plane, it is specified as the *spectacle plane refraction*. The power for a contact lens that is to correct ametropia is referred to as the *corneal plane refraction*,* since the contact lens rests directly on the cornea.

The change in power that is necessary

―――――

*Some authors use the term ocular refraction to represent what is here termed corneal plane refraction. Ocular refraction should refer to the correction necessary at the position of the principal plane, and though the difference in distance is small, it is significant for topics such as magnification, which will be discussed later.

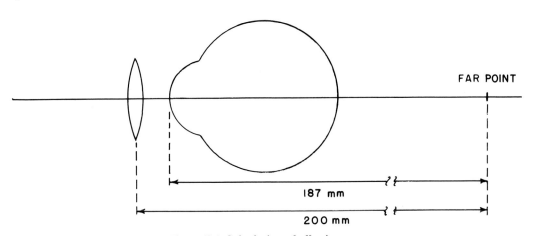

Figure 7.4. Calculation of effective power.

when substituting contact lenses at the corneal plane for ophthalmic lenses at the spectacle plane can be found by the standard effectivity formula.

$$F_c = \frac{F_s}{1 - dF_s} \qquad \text{(Formula 7.1)}$$

where

F_c = power of the contact lens
F_s = power of the spectacle lens
d = distance between spectacle lens and contact lens in meters.

For an astigmatic spectacle plane refraction, the effective power at the corneal plane must be calculated separately for each principal meridian.

Effect of the Fitting Relationship On Contact Lens Power

If the contact lens is not fitted on K, a further modification must be made to the short method of calculating contact lens power. If the contact lens is fitted steeper than K, it will be found that the tear fluid lens formed between the contact lens and the cornea contributes additional plus power to the power of the contact lens when it is worn on the eye. To correct the eye's refractive error properly, the power of the contact lens must be made with less plus or more minus by an amount equal to the plus power of the tear fluid lens.

When the contact lens is fitted flatter than K, the tear fluid lens formed between the lens and the cornea will contribute additional minus power to the contact lens. To correct the eye's refractive error properly, the power of the contact lens must therefore be made more plus or less minus by an amount equal to the minus power of the tear fluid lens. Two simple rules will serve to determine these corrections.

1. For every 0.25 D. that the optical zone curvature is greater than the corneal curvature, add -0.25 D. to the power of the correcting contact lens.

2. For every 0.25 D. that the optical zone curvature is less than the corneal curvature, add $+0.25$ D. to the power of the correcting contact lens.

In order to use these simple rules, the optical zone radius of the contact lens must be expressed in terms of diopters of power. As mentioned previously, this is not correct terminology, but it provides a convenient clinical rule. Its basis is explained in Chapter 34.

Examples

1. Corneal curvature   42.00 D.
   Spectacle lens power   − 1.50 D.
   Optical zone radius   42.50 D.
   Contact lens power   − 2.00 D.
2. Corneal curvature   43.50 D.
   Spectacle lens power   − 2.00 −1.00 × 180
   Optical zone radius   42.75 D.
   Contact lens power   − 1.25 D.
3. Corneal curvature   44.00 at 180 ⊃ 44.50 at 90
   Spectacle lens power   − 6.00 −1.00 × 180
   Optical zone radius   44.00 D.
   Contact lens power   − 6.00 D.
4. Corneal curvature   44.00 at 180 ⊃ 43.50 at 90
   Spectacle lens power   + 3.75 D.
   Optical zone radius   43.25 D.
   Contact lens power   − 4.00 D.

"Exact" Method of Power Calculation

The short method of calculating the contact lens power has the disadvantage of not properly accounting for the residual astigmatic refractive error that remains when a contact lens is worn.

Residual astigmatism is often present in contact lens wearers. In significant amounts it may interfere with visual acuity or cause asthenopia. When this occurs, one of the special types of contact lenses (Chapter 9) may be used to correct the residual astigmatism. Individual tolerance varies considerably, however, so there is no definite limit to the amount of residual astigmatism that can be allowed. Usually, astigmatism of less than 0.50 D. will be tolerated, but many sensitive individuals can stand none.

Whether a significant amount of residual astigmatism will be present when the contact lens is worn can be predicted with fair accuracy and used to modify the spherical power correction. The total astigmatism (A_t) of the eye is composed of corneal astigmatism (A_c)

plus residual astigmatism (A$_r$). When a contact lens is worn, corneal astigmatism is nearly eliminated. Residual astigmatism is determined by subtracting the corneal astigmatism from the total astigmatism.

$$A_t = A_c + A_r$$
$$A_r = A_t - A_c$$

Practically speaking, A$_t$ is the astigmatism from the refraction, corrected for the corneal plane. A$_c$ is the corneal astigmatism as found by the keratometer. If the corneal astigmatism is expressed as the corrective cylinder (in minus cylinder form), it may be subtracted from the refractive error to determine the power needed in the contact lens. For example, if the refractive error found at the corneal plane is $-2.25 -1.25 \times 180$ and the corneal astigmatism is -1.00×180, the correction that is necessary in the contact lens is -2.25 -0.25×180. Since the 0.25 D. of residual astigmatism is probably within the tolerance of the patient, the lens may be fitted with a power of -2.25 sphere. If, however, the corneal astigmatism were -0.25×180, the correction necessary in the contact lens would be -2.25 -1.00×180. With 1.00 D. of predicted astigmatism, it would not be advisable to fit the patient with a spherical contact lens; one of the special lens types should be used.

Some complication in the prediction of residual astigmatism occurs when the axes of the cornea and of the refractive correction do not coincide. If the axes are 90° apart, they may be made to coincide by converting the refractive correction to the opposite cylinder form.

The calculation of the contact lens power is most easily accomplished by the following system:

Steps

1. Record spectacle correction (corneal plane).
2. Record corneal cylinder, as found by keratometer, in minus cylinder form.
3. Check to see if cylinder axes of "1" and "2" coincide. If 90° apart, convert spectacle correction to plus cylinder form.
4. Subtract corneal cylinder from spectacle correction to find correction needed in contact lens.

Example

A. Ophth. 44.00 at 180
        43.00 at 90
    Corneal Plane Refraction $-2.25 -1.25 \times 180$

1. $-2.25 -1.25 \times 180$
3. $-3.50 + 1.25 \times 90$
2. $(-)-1.00 \times 90$

---

4. $-3.50 +2.25 \times 90$
    $-1.25 -2.25 \times 180$

Other examples of possible combinations of refractive error and corneal astigmatism follow.

B. Ophth. 39.00 at 180
        40.50 at 90
    Ref $-4.00 -1.50 \times 180$

1. $-4.00 -1.50 \times 180$
3.
2. $(-) -1.50 \times 180$
4. -4.00

C. Ophth. 42.25 at 180
        43.75 at 90
    Ref $-4.00 -1.50 \times 90$

1. $-4.00 -1.50 \times 90$
3. $-5.50 +1.50 \times 180$
2. $(-) -1.50 \times 180$
4. $-5.50 +3.00 \times 180$
    $-2.50 -3.00 \times 90$

D. Ophth. 44.00 at 180
        46.12 at 90
    Ref $-225 -1.25 \times 180$

1. $-2.25 -1.25 \times 180$
3.
2. $(-) -2.12 \times 180$
4. $-2.25 +0.87 \times 180$
    $-1.37 -0.87 \times 90$

E. Ophth. 43.00 at 180
        45.00 at 90
    Ref -400

1. -4.00
3.
2. $(-) -2.00 \times 180$
4. $-4.00 +2.00 \times 180$
    $-2.00 -2.00 \times 90$

F. Ophth. 41.00 at 180
        46.25 at 90
    Ref $+1.00 -4.25 \times 180$

1. $+1.00 -4.25 \times 180$
3.
2. $(-) -5.25 \times 180$
4. $+1.00 +1.00 \times 180$

G. Ophth. 42.50 at 180
        45.25 at 90
    Ref $-3.00 -275 \times 180$

1. $-3.00 -2.75 \times 180$
3.
2. $(-) -2.75 \times 180$
4. -3.00

If the correction that is necessary for the contact lens has a low astigmatic component, only a spherical correction is used in the contact lens. In such a case it is possible to make some allowance for the astigmatism that is uncorrected.

Whenever an astigmatic focus occurs in the eye, one position is found where the best image is formed. This is the circle of least confusion and occurs between the focal lines of two principal meridians. The circle of least confusion may be made to focus on the retina by correcting the eye with the equivalent sphere rather than using the astigmatic correction. The equivalent sphere is found by taking one-half the cylinder power and substituting this power sphere with the same sign.

Correction	Equivalent Sphere
-4.00 cyl.	-2.00 sphere
$-3.00 -2.50 \times 180$	-4.25 sphere
$-3.00 +1.75 \times 180$	-2.12 sphere

The contact lens power should always be the equivalent sphere to provide the best spherical correction.

EDGE

There is little point in giving specific directions to the laboratory for the *method* of finishing the contact lens edge. Most laboratories disregard all instructions and follow the manufacturing routine they feel works best. The practitioner has no control over the laboratories because he cannot determine whether or not his instructions were actually followed but can only tell if the finished lens is acceptable.

To insure that the laboratory will provide the best edge design, the practitioner should describe to the laboratory the characteristics of the edge desired for all lenses and should be critical in the edge inspection of each lens received (*see* Chapter 13).

FRONT BEVEL

Some practitioners feel that specifying whether a front bevel is needed or not should be a part of the lens order. They usually order a front bevel for all minus power lenses that exceed -4.00 D. It is the author's opinion that the practitioner should not be responsible for specifying whether a front bevel is needed, for this depends on many lens dimensions other than the lens power. Sometimes a -3.00 D. lens will require a bevel and a -5.00 D. will not. This can only be determined by a consideration of all the variables which contribute to edge thickness. This calculation can be made most easily by the laboratories.

The decision of whether or not a bevel is necessary can be made after lens inspection, without making any calculations. The final step in the manufacture of a contact lens is to shape and polish the edge. Prior to this step the lens should be inspected to see if a front bevel is necessary. Such inspection may be made by the laboratories, the lens can then be treated accordingly.

COLOR

Numerous tints are available for contact lenses (*see* Chapter 15).

SELECTION OF STANDARD LENSES

GENERAL CONSIDERATIONS

Many contact lens fitters believe that a custom-design lens for each patient is not necessary and that a standard contact lens construction can be used for a large number of contact lens patients. There is some experimental evidence to support this position.[2]

Diameter

It is questionable whether contact lenses need to be made in the minimum diameter steps of 0.1 mm. A lens must usually be varied by 0.4 mm. or 0.5 mm. in diameter in order to create a significant difference in the fitting characteristics. A large number of contact lens patients may be fitted adequately with an average size lens. Larger and smaller lenses may then be used for the more exceptional cases. Thus, a minimum of three diameters is probably necessary to meet the needs of a majority of patients. The author has somewhat arbitrarily chosen 8.3, 8.7, and 9.3 mm. diameter lenses, with the 8.7 mm. lens being used most often. This lens represents an average diameter in a conservative fitting approach. Larger lenses sometimes create corneal distortion when worn for long periods of time. Smaller lenses, however, are more difficult to handle for the patient, are less stable in terms of their physical dimensions, and seem to present no particular advantage over average diameter lenses with the exception of certain patients to be discussed later. There is a popular idea that a small contact lens will expose a greater area of the cornea to the atmosphere and therefore create less physiological interference. Even an extremely small lens of 5 mm. in diameter will create intolerable corneal edema if the lens does not produce a good pump (*see* Chapter 6). Small lenses have extremely narrow peripheral curves and often do not produce enough rocking action to create an adequate lens pump. They therefore become less advantageous in terms of corneal physiology than average size lenses. This is not to say that a small lens cannot be an adequate pump but only that the pump efficiency must be considered independently of the lens diameter.

An average diameter lens usually presents fewer optical problems and provides an adequate lens pump. However, the diameter should be made no larger than necessary for several reasons. First, a large diameter lens adds to the lens mass and creates a greater long-term distortion effect on the cornea. Second, a larger diameter lens has a more complex peripheral curve system and requires much greater accuracy in the selection of the peripheral curve. This idea may be explained as follows: When the peripheral curve is very narrow, its primary function is to provide space between the lens and the cornea for the action of the lens pump. It contributes little or nothing to the attraction between the lens and the cornea. However, a very wide peripheral curve must more closely contour the cornea. If it is fitted extremely flat, the lens will become very loose. Usually the radius of a wide peripheral curve must fall within a very narrow range.

Base Curve Relationship

For low corneal toricity, it is usually best to select a lens-cornea relationship of minimum apical clearance (Figure 7.5). This represents the best mechanical relationship between the lens and the cornea. However, it is not always possible to achieve. A lens that acts as an inadequate pump on the eye may have to be exchanged for one with apical touch. A lens that cannot be adequately centered on the eye may have to be exchanged for one with a steeper fit.

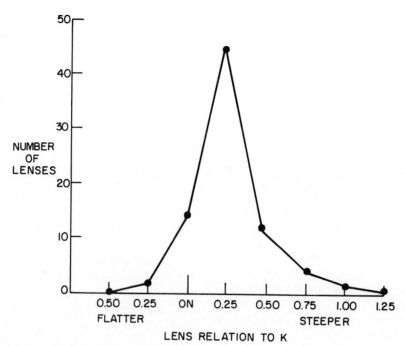

Figure 7.5. Distribution of base curve to cornea relationship in sample of lenses used by the author.

A slight apical clearance is probably desirable in fitting because it allows the lens to move about and not to place undue pressure on the corneal apex.

FITTING METHOD FOR REGULAR THICKNESS LENSES

Selection of Lens Dimensions

Lens Diameter

The lens diameter is determined by several eye dimensions, including the palpebral aperture height, the corneal diameter, and the corneal curvature. There is a high correlation between the corneal curvature and diameter, so in many fitting philosophies the lens diameter is based on corneal curvature alone. Most often very flat corneas are also relatively large corneas and may do better with a larger lens. However, a flat cornea with a small palpebral fissure will be better fitted with a small lens, so for atypical eye dimensions such as these, it is the palpebral aperture height that is most important in the

TABLE 7.4

DIAMETER

Palp Aperture	*Lens Diameter*
Large (> 11)	9.3
Medium (9-11)	8.8
Small (< 9)	8.3
If Cor. Diam. > 12	May use next
If Cor. Cur. Flatter 4200	larger diameter
If Cor. Diam. < 11	May use next
If Cor. Cur. Steeper 4400	smaller diameter

<table>
<tr><td colspan="2" align="center">TABLE 7.5</td></tr>
<tr><td colspan="2" align="center">BASE CURVE RELATIONSHIP</td></tr>
</table>

Cor. Toricity	Base Curve
Spherical	On K or 0.25 D. < K
0.25 to 1.00	On K or 0.25 D. > K
1.00 to 2.00	0.50 D. > K
> 2.00	ΔK/3

choice of lens diameter. A guide for the initial selection of the lens diameter is given in Table 7.4. Only three diameters are recommended as a starting point, which correspond to the lenses represented in the trial set in Table 7.6.

Base Curve

The base curve of the lens depends primarily on the corneal curvature according to Table 7.5. The base curve is modified somewhat according to the lens diameter. If the lens diameter selected first is 8.3 mm., start with a lens 0.25 D. steeper than would be used for larger diameter lenses.

Posterior Optic Zone Diameter

The posterior optic zone diameter is fixed by the lens diameter. Recommended O.Z.D.s are given in Table 7.6.

Peripheral Curve Radius

The peripheral curve radius varies with the base curve of the lens as shown in Table 7.7. These radii were selected on the basis of trial and error fitting as the steepest peripheral curves that do not give central corneal clouding in the majority of patients. Changes in the peripheral curves occur in steps of 0.3 mm. Greater accuracy is difficult to produce by the laboratory and is clinically insignificant. A change of at least 0.6 mm. is usually needed to produce a noticeable clinical effect.

TABLE 7.6a

MANDELL TRIAL SET

Power	8.3	Diameter 8.8	9.3
46.25	X		
46.00		X	
45.75	X		
45.50		X	
45.25	X		
45.00		X	
44.75	X		
44.50		X	
44.25	X·		
44.00		X	X
43.75	X		
43.50		X	X
43.25	X		
43.00		X	X
42.75	X		
42.50		X	X
42.25	X		
42.00		X	X
41.50		X	X
41.00		X	X
40.50		X	X
40.00			X
39.50			X

Center Thickness

Lens thickness selection depends on the inherent stability of the lens material and the lens dimensions. Normally the thickness is made as thin as possible consistent with the lens dimensions. For low minus lenses center thickness is usually kept at 0.13 mm. or greater to avoid lens flexing. Sample thicknesses for the trial set are given in Table 7.6. These center thicknesses are selected to give a uniform edge thickness of 0.11 mm. before finishing.

Trial Set

A recommended trial set is given in Table 7.6. It consists of thirty-one lenses in three diameters. Smaller lenses are available in steeper base curves, and larger lenses are available in the flatter base curves.

Contact Lens Practice

TABLE 7.6b
MEDIUM SET

Base Curve		Power	Diam.	O.Z.D.	Blend Width	I.C.W.		I.C.R.	P.C.W.		P.C.R.	tc
46.00	7.34	−3.00	8.8	7.5	0.1	0.15	/	8.7	0.4	/	9.9	.13
45.50	7.42	−3.00	8.8	7.5	0.1	0.15	/	9.0	0.4	/	10.2	.13
45.00	7.50	−3.00	8.8	7.5	0.1	0.15	/	9.0	0.4	/	10.2	.13
44.50	7.58	−3.00	8.8	7.5	0.1	0.15	/	9.0	0.4	/	10.2	.13
44.00	7.67	−3.00	8.8	7.5	0.1	0.15	/	9.3	0.4	/	10.5	.13
43.50	7.76	−3.00	8.8	7.5	0.1	0.15	/	9.3	0.4	/	10.5	.13
43.00	7.85	−3.00	8.8	7.5	0.1	0.15	/	9.3	0.4	/	10.5	.13
42.50	7.94	−3.00	8.8	7.5	0.1	0.15	/	9.6	0.4	/	10.8	.12
42.00	8.04	−3.00	8.8	7.5	0.1	0.15	/	9.6	0.4	/	10.8	.12
41.50	8.13	−3.00	8.8	7.5	0.1	0.15	/	9.6	0.4	/	10.8	.12
41.00	8.23	−3.00	8.8	7.5	0.1	0.15	/	9.9	0.4	/	11.1	.12
40.50	8.33	−3.00	8.8	7.5	0.1	0.15	/	9.9	0.4	/	11.1	.12

TABLE 7.6c
MEDIUM–SMALL SET

Base Curve		Power	Diam.	O.Z.D.	Blend Width	P.C.W.		P.C.R.	tc
46.25	7.30	−3.00	8.3	7.4	0.1	0.35	/	9.9	.13
45.75	7.38	−3.00	8.3	7.4	0.1	0.35	/	10.2	.13
45.25	7.46	−3.00	8.3	7.4	0.1	0.35	/	10.2	.13
44.75	7.54	−3.00	8.3	7.4	0.1	0.35	/	10.2	.13
44.25	7.63	−3.00	8.3	7.4	0.1	0.35	/	10.5	.13
43.75	7.72	−3.00	8.3	7.4	0.1	0.35	/	10.5	.13
43.25	7.80	−3.00	8.3	7.4	0.1	0.35	/	10.5	.13
42.75	7.89	−3.00	8.3	7.4	0.1	0.35	/	10.8	.12
42.25	7.99	−3.00	8.3	7.4	0.1	0.35	/	10.8	.12

TABLE 7.6d
LARGE SET

Base Curve		Power	Diam.	O.Z.D.	Blend Width	I.C.W.		I.C.R.	P.C.W.		P.C.R.	tc
44.00	7.67	−3.00	9.3	7.6	0.1	0.35	/	9.3	0.4	/	10.5	.14
43.50	7.76	−3.00	9.3	7.6	0.1	0.35	/	9.3	0.4	/	10.5	.14
43.00	7.85	−3.00	9.3	7.6	0.1	0.35	/	9.3	0.4	/	10.5	.14
42.50	7.94	−3.00	9.3	7.6	0.1	0.35	/	9.6	0.4	/	10.8	.14
42.00	8.04	−3.00	9.3	7.6	0.1	0.35	/	9.6	0.4	/	10.8	.14
41.50	8.13	−3.00	9.3	7.6	0.1	0.35	/	9.6	0.4	/	10.8	.14
41.00	8.23	−3.00	9.3	7.6	0.1	0.35	/	9.9	0.4	/	11.1	.13
40.50	8.33	−3.00	9.3	7.6	0.1	0.35	/	9.9	0.4	/	11.1	.13
40.00	8.44	−3.00	9.3	7.6	0.1	0.35	/	9.9	0.4	/	11.1	.13
39.50	8.54	−3.00	9.3	7.6	0.1	0.35	/	10.2	0.4	/	11.4	.13

FITTING METHOD FOR ULTRATHIN LENSES

If contact lenses of polymethyl methacrylate are made very thin, they will flex on the cornea and exhibit properties that are significantly different from those of thicker lenses.[3,4] Ultrathin lenses are useful for many patients, but they are especially effective as an alternative to lenses of regular thickness when there are any of the following problems:

1. Low riding position
2. Discomfort
3. Edema
4. Corneal distortion

The flexure of ultrathin lenses on the cornea presents an optical advantage for most patients because it tends to correct part of the residual astigmatism that is present with thicker lenses. However, lens flexure can be a disadvantage for patients who have the more uncommon types of astigmatism.

Lens Flexure

If a series of low minus lenses that vary only in center thickness is examined, the flexure property may be easily demonstrated. If the lenses are simply held by the edges between the fingers and gently squeezed, only those lenses having a center thickness of less than about 0.12 mm. can be easily flexed (Figure 7.6). If the lenses are high in minus power, flexure is less.

This same property of lens flexure occurs when a very thin lens is placed upon a toric cornea.[3,4] The lens tends to flex in a direction that would make it conform more closely to the corneal toricity. Harris demonstrated that for low minus lenses the critical center thickness below which a lens shows flexing on the eye is 0.12 mm.[5] As lenses are made progressively thinner, the flexing increases until, at about 0.06 mm., there is no longer sufficient plastic to retain good optics (Figure 7.7).[6]

As long as the lenses are of low minus powers, there is little or no difference in lens flexure for lenses of various diameters (Figure 7.8).[7] However, lens flexure decreases as the minus power increases (Figure 7.9). This is apparently a consequence of the increase in edge thickness, as high minus lenses of lenticular design will show greater amounts of flexing. The lack of relationship between lens diameter and amount of flexing would appear to suggest that flexing is not induced by lid

TABLE 7.7

PERIPHERAL CURVE RADII

	I.C.R.	Blend	P.C.R.
46.50			
46.25	8.7	9.3	9.9
46.00			
45.75			
45.50			
45.25	9.0	9.6	10.2
45.00			
44.75			
44.50			
44.25			
44.00			
43.75			
43.50	9.3	9.9	10.5
43.25			
43.00			
42.75			
42.50			
42.25	9.6	10.2	10.8
42.00			
41.75			
41.50			
41.25			
41.00			
40.75	9.9	10.5	11.1
40.50			
40.25			
40.00			
39.75			
39.50			
39.25	10.2	10.8	11.4
39.00			

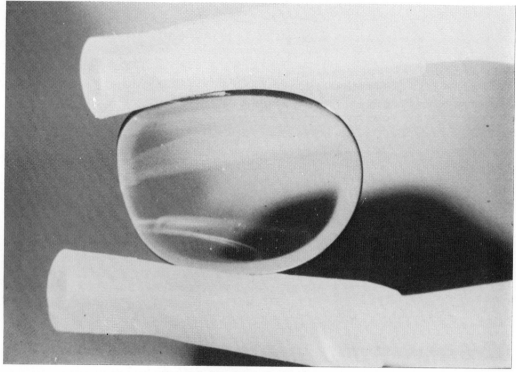

Figure 7.6. Flexure of an ultrathin lens.

pressure but is more likely related to the tear fluid attraction forces that hold the lens against the cornea.

The effect of lens flexure on reducing residual astigmatism is predictable and consistent with the optical effects expected from the amount of flexing.

Physical Design

An ultrathin contact lens is operationally defined as a lens that is sufficiently thin for flexure to occur when it is worn on a toric cornea. An ultrathin lens has both upper and lower limits to center thickness and certain restrictions on other lens parameters. The upper limit, by definition, is set when flexure no longer occurs on the cornea. The lower limit is set by the physical attributes of the plastic used. A polymethyl methacrylate (PMMA) lens of less than 0.06 mm. center

thickness is very difficult to manufacture. During polishing, the thin center heats excessively and tends to distort the plastic. This produces a detectable optical degradation for the wearer. For this reason, ultrathin lenses are generally made thicker than 0.06 mm.

Warping versus Flexing

It is important that an ultrathin lens be able to flex upon the eye without warping. The difference between warping and flexing must be clarified. When a regular hard contact lens of normal thickness warps, the lens becomes more or less permanently bent along one meridian. This has little effect on the power of the lens while the lens is off the eye because both surfaces are bent equally. If the lens is measured using a lensometer, there is no effect on the power. However, if

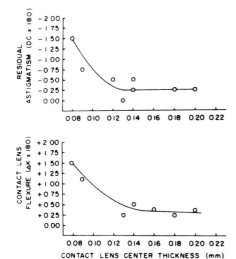

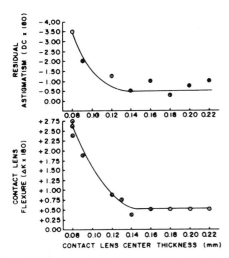

Figure 7.7. Contact lens flexure and residual astigmatism on a toric cornea for lenses of various center thicknesses, (*a*) on a 4.00 DK toric cornea, (*b*) on a 6.12 DK toric cornea. From J. G. Harris and C. S. Chu, The Effect of Contact Lens Thickness and Corneal Toricity on Flexure and Residual Astigmatism, *American Journal of Optometry,* *49(4)*:304–308, 1972.

the lens is measured with the radiuscope, it is found that the surfaces exhibit a toric shape. Because the toricity is equal for both surfaces, any cylindrical power effect on the front surface is canceled by the back surface so that there is no cylindrical power found when the lens is measured in the lensometer.

When a warped lens is placed on the eye, the lens holds its warped shape. The optical power of the back surface of the lens is nearly canceled out by the tear layer, but the toric curve on the front surface of the lens is not canceled and, hence, adds a cylindrical power effect to the lens system. If an overrefraction is performed with the lens on the eye, it is found that the patient now has residual astigmatism, which was not present before, and this may reduce visual acuity. In addition, as the lens rotates on the eye, the cylinder axis changes correspondingly. The distinguishing characteristic of a warped lens is that the change in shape is permanent and remains so while on the eye.

True warping is usually caused by faulty manufacturing techniques. It is most commonly produced by exerting excessive force on the lens button during manufacturing. This is caused either by a faulty holding mechanism for the lens button or by lathing techniques that are irregular or too fast. The warping is usually not manifested, however, until the lens is soaked or worn, when the induced strain is released as the lens is hydrated.

Flexing of a hard lens differs from warping in that a lens which flexes on the eye returns to its spherical shape when removed from the eye, just as a lens flexed between the fingers returns to its original shape when the pressure is released. The time required for the lens to change from the flexed to original shape depends upon the amount of flexure induced. Flexure on the eye is lost immediately when the lens is removed. Flexure between the fingers is greater and may require several minutes or longer before the lens returns to its spherical shape.

When the lens curvature is measured on a radiuscope, it may show a spherical surface, or it may appear to have a toric surface because it was squeezed prior to its place-

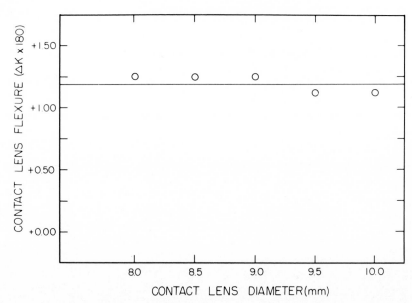

Figure 7.8. Contact lens diameter has little effect on contact lens flexure. From M. G. Harris and T. D. Appelquist, The Effect of Contact Lens Diameter and Power on Flexure and Residual Astigmatism, *American Journal of Optometry and Physiological Optics, 51(4):*266–270, 1974.

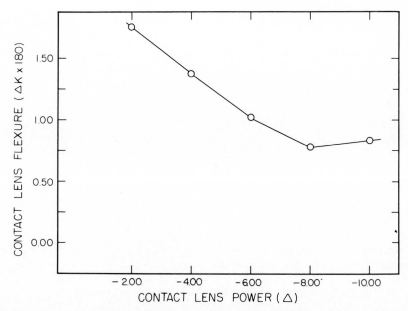

Figure 7.9. Contact lens flexure decreases for contact lenses of higher minus power. From M. G. Harris and T. D. Appelquist, The Effect of Contact Lens Diameter and Power on Flexure and Residual Astigmatism, *American Journal of Optometry and Physiological Optics, 51(4):*266–270, 1974.

ment on the instrument. However, in this case, the toric surface has no optical significance when the lens is placed on the eye because the lens flexure is then determined by the fluid forces exerted by the tears. In most cases, the lens flexure remains stable at the same axis as the corneal toricity. A warped lens, in contrast, will tend to rotate on the eye and produce variable vision.

It is usually found that the flexing of an ultrathin lens will produce a slight increase in visual acuity. This is due to the fact that the ultrathin lens produces with-the-rule astigmatism on corneas having with-the-rule toricities. Since the average contact lens patient has a small amount of against-the-rule residual astigmatism (about 0.50 D.), the ultrathin lens will counteract this and reduce or even eliminate the residual astigmatism.

Advantages

Ultrathin lenses have several advantages for most (but not all) contact lens patients. These advantages are better centering, better comfort, less edema, minimal corneal distortion, and improved vision.

Centering

A lens of regular thickness usually must be fitted steeper than K in order to achieve good centering. An ultrathin lens usually centers well on the cornea, even when fitted on K. This may be attributed to two factors. First, the ultrathin lens is extremely light in weight due to its thinness, so there is less gravitational effect pulling the lens downward. Second, there is much less lid force acting to move an ultrathin lens due to its overall thinness as well as its thin edge.

Comfort

The comfort of an ultrathin lens is generally better than that achieved by any other hard lens. This may be attributed to the thin edge and overall thinness of the lens, which presents a minimum obstacle to lid movement during blinking. This difference is most obvious when a patient who wears regular contact lenses switches to ultrathin lenses or an ultrathin lens is placed on only one eye and the patient is allowed to make a direct comparison to a regular thickness lens on the fellow eye.

New patients vary in their initial response to ultrathin lenses, with most doing very well. Others do no better than with regular lenses, but it is usually noted that after a few wearing periods the comfort for these patients is good. Patients who have the greatest initial response appear to be those who get a strong reflex to the first lens insertion and tear excessively. This washes the lens about and increases lid sensation. After the tearing subsides and the lens settles down, there is usually little or no sensation.

Minimal Edema

An ultrathin lens produces little edema primarily because it centers and moves well on the eye. In addition, some additional pumping has been claimed because the lens is flexed on the eye during blinking. This is doubtful, however.

Minimal Corneal Distortion

Because of its very light weight, the ultrathin lens causes minimal corneal distortion.

Vision

The patient will achieve the best visual acuity when he receives the proper optical correction and has the least amount of residual astigmatism, that is, astigmatism that remains when the contact lens is worn. The predicted residual astigmatism must be calculated by a different method for the three general types of lenses, the soft lens, the regular hard lens, and the ultrathin lens.

The best estimate of the residual astigmatism when a gel lens is worn is the amount of astigmatism that occurs in the spectacle correction (total astigmatism of the eye). Therefore, the most ideal condition for the use of a gel lens is when the spectacle astigmatism is zero, that is, when we have a spherical spectacle correction.

The residual astigmatism that occurs as a result of wearing rigid hard contact lenses may be determined simply by subtracting the keratometer astigmatism from the spectacle astigmatism as described in Formula 7.1.

The residual astigmatism of a hard flexible lens may be calculated from the values for a rigid hard lens and a soft lens. Before it is placed on the cornea, the flexible lens has characteristics that are essentially the same as those of a rigid hard contact lens. However, when it is placed on the cornea, it becomes flexible, more so than a rigid hard lens but less than a gel contact lens (Figure 7.10).[8] Since it will usually flex about one-third as much on the eye as a gel contact lens, the predicted residual astigmatism for an ultrathin lens would be about one-third of the way between the residual astigmatism of a rigid hard lens and a gel lens.

For example, if the residual astigmatism for a rigid hard lens is predicted to be −0.75 D. and the residual astigmatism for a gel lens is predicted to be zero, then the residual astigmatism for the hard flexible lens is predicted to be −0.50 D.

What happens for a typical eye? Assume that this eye has the following specifications:

Spectacle astigmatism:	−0.50 axis 180
Corneal astigmatism:	−1.00 axis 180
Predicted residual astigmatism:	
Rigid hard lens	
−0.50 axis 180 −	
(−1.00 axis 180)	+0.50 axis 180
Gel lens	−0.50 axis 180
Hard flexible lens	+0.12 axis 180

Theoretically, residual astigmatism will be zero whenever the lens flexing is such that the corneal astigmatism minus the flexing equals the spectacle astigmatism and they both have the same axis. Clinically, the residual astigmatism is usually reduced whenever the corneal astigmatism is in the same direction as the refractive astigmatism and the corneal astigmatism is at least 20 percent greater. This relationship usually occurs when there is with-the-rule astigmatism.

For against-the-rule astigmatism, it is often found that the refractive astigmatism is greater than the corneal astigmatism, a condition which results in increased residual astigmatism with lens flexing:

Spectacle astigmatism:	−1.00 axis 90
Corneal astigmatism:	−0.50 axis 90
Predicted residual astigmatism:	
Rigid hard lens	
−1.00 axis 90 −	
(−0.50 axis 90)	−0.50 axis 90
Gel lens	−1.00 axis 90
Hard flexible lens	−0.67 axis 90

Lens Design

Diameter

Ultrathin lenses may be made in any diameter within the usual limits for hard contact lenses. However, when lenses are less than 8.0 mm. in diameter, it is usually found that patients experience difficulty in handling them. They are difficult to insert and remove and difficult to pick up if dropped. In addition, the incidence of flare problems greatly increases. When lenses are made greater than 9.0 mm. in diameter, it is found that they generally perform well optically, but there is a higher incidence of edema. It is necessary to make other modifications in the lens design, such as a flatter base curve or flatter peripheral curve in order to achieve the same success in fitting.

The optimum lens diameter is found to

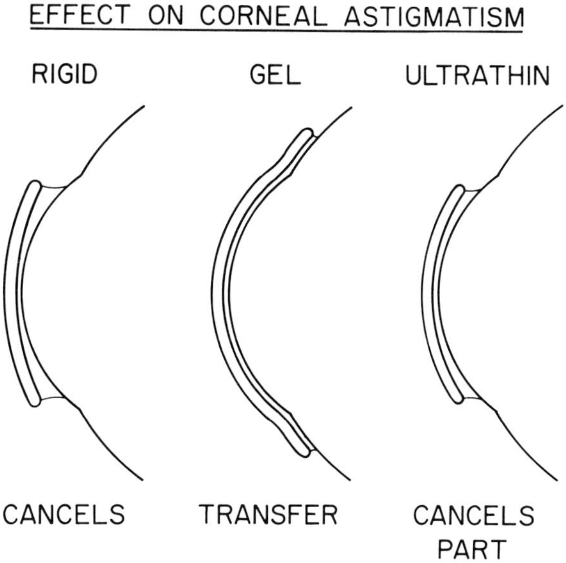

EFFECT ON CORNEAL ASTIGMATISM

RIGID   GEL   ULTRATHIN

CANCELS   TRANSFER   CANCELS PART

Figure 7.10. An ultrathin lens flexes more than a rigid lens but only about one-third as much as a gel lens on the eye.

be about 8.2 mm. for most patients. This lens diameter infrequently produces flare, is not particularly difficult to handle, and has riding characteristics that seem to be optimal. The total weight of the lens is dependent on both the diameter and thickness and somewhat secondarily on other lens dimensions. By keeping the lens relatively small in diameter it is possible to reduce its weight greatly. This is manifested clinically by the slow movement and good positioning of the lens, that is, if the lens is light enough, the tear fluid attraction forces tend to hold it in a centered position on the cornea. There is rarely a tendency for the lens to drop to a low position, a major problem with lenses of normal thickness. It is this riding characteristic which has been responsible for the excellent physiological results obtained with this lens.

The ultrathin lens needs to be made larger than an 8.2 diameter in patients who have a larger than normal pupil diameter or when there is a lens centering problem. Even here,

however, the practitioner should not be misled. Most patients who have a slightly larger than normal pupil diameter will still do well with lenses of 8.2 diameter. These may be successful even when the lens edge crosses the pupil margin, because the peripheral curve design of the ultrathin lens causes very little tear meniscus at the lens edge and, hence, little prism effect to direct light into the eye. For patients with very large pupils, however, flare may be exhibited, and then a larger lens is definitely indicated, usually about 8.7 mm. diameter. For higher minus power lenses it may be necessary to incorporate a lenticular design.

One of the other major problems that may require a larger than usual diameter is when the lens decenters laterally or superiorly on the cornea. In this case, a larger lens of ultrathin design may help to achieve centering.

Peripheral Curve Width

Since the ultrathin lens is designed for minimum thickness, there is usually very little variation possible in the selection of peripheral curve widths. It is necessary to have a peripheral curve width of 0.3 or 0.4 mm. in order to produce adequate tear exchange, but the peripheral curve cannot be made any wider with a standard diameter lens, or the optic zone will be so small that it will create visual problems.[9]

Peripheral Curve Radius

The radius of the peripheral curve is one of the most critical parameters to be selected because, for most lenses of low minus power, the peripheral curve cannot be made as flat as most fitters would choose for regular lenses. Because of mechanical limitations of the ultrathin lens, the fitter does not have the usual variety of peripheral curve radii open to him. This may be explained as follows: For a minus lens of normal center thickness, usually nearly any peripheral curve desired by the fitter can be ground onto the lens and still leave more edge thickness than is needed for finishing (Figure 7.11). In order to compensate for this, the peripheral portion of the front lens surface is beveled to produce either a thin or thick edge contour, according to the desires of the fitter (Figure 7.12). If this original lens is now visualized as reduced in center thickness to form a thin lens and the same peripheral curve is applied, there is just enough lens material remaining at the periphery to form a good edge contour (Figure 7.13). Next, if the center thickness is reduced even further and the peripheral curves are kept the same, the edge thickness will be reduced to zero, not leaving enough material

to form a proper edge contour. The only way this lens can be manufactured is by making the peripheral curve steeper to leave sufficient lens material at the periphery to form the edge (Figure 7.14). Hence, it is impossible to manufacture an ultrathin lens of low minus power unless a relatively steep peripheral curve or a very narrow peripheral curve width is used. Peripheral curve widths of less than 0.3 mm. in any radius are relatively ineffective. It is better to use steeper peripheral curves that are at least 0.3 to 0.4 mm. in width.

It is interesting that what appears to be a restriction on the peripheral curve of the ultrathin lens turns out to be a principal advantage; the steep peripheral curve gives the lens many of its excellent properties. Nearly all of the normal sensation produced by a contact lens comes from the edge, and the comfort of this lens is due to minimizing the obstacle to the lid produced by the lens edge. For example, a gel lens derives its excellent comfort from the fact that the edge lies in close apposition to the sclera and does not make contact with the lid. A hard lens begins to approach the comfort of a gel lens when the edge is kept close to the cornea and away from the lids. When the peripheral curve of the lens is relatively steep, the tip of the edge lies very close to the cornea. In addition, for maximum comfort it is necessary to have the edge as thin as possible without being sharp.

Fitting

An ultrathin lens may be fitted by either

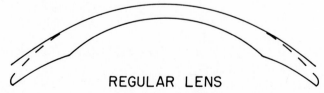

Figure 7.11. A regular center thickness lens can have nearly any peripheral curve radius and still leave more than enough edge thickness for finishing.

direct ordering or a trial lens method, depending on the preference of the fitter. The following procedure will serve as a guide to selection of either the first lens to be ordered or the first lens selected in the trial procedure:

1. Determine the base curve. The base curve is nearly always slightly steeper than K or on K and is selected on the basis of the keratometer reading. Remember that an important feature of the lens is that, because of its very light weight, it is not necessary to fit the lens very steep. Table 7.8 can be used as a guide to the initial lens selection.

2. Select diameter and optic zone. A larger ultrathin lens of about 8.7 mm. is usually needed for patients who have a problem of flare with the basic 8.2 lens diameter. Flare may occur either if the patient has a very large pupil or if the lens rides off the center of the cornea. Fortunately, flare is only an occasional problem with the 8.2 mm. diameter lens because the peripheral curve and edge are specifically designed to minimize flare problems. Trial sets in both the 8.2 and 8.7 diameters are given in Table 7.9. How large should the pupil be before an 8.7 mm. lens is used? This is always a difficult ques-

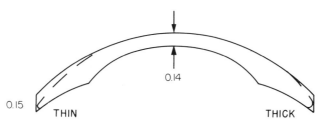

Figure 7.12. Regular center thickness lenses allow the fitter a wide choice of edge contours.

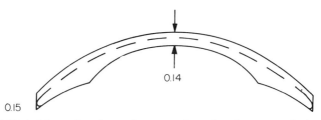

Figure 7.13. A thinner lens leaves just enough stock to form a good edge contour.

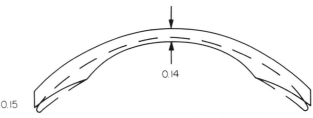

Figure 7.14. An ultrathin center thickness reduces the edge thickness to zero, requiring a steeper peripheral curve to leave enough stock for a good edge.

TABLE 7.8

FOR STEEP CORNEAS (> 44.00)		FOR FLAT CORNEAS (< 44.00)	
Keratometry/Astigmatism	*Base Curve*	*Keratometry/Astigmatism*	*Base Curve*
0 to 0.25 ΔK	0.25 Flatter than K	Sphere	0.25 Flatter than K
0.50 to 0.75 ΔK	On K	0.25 to 0.50 ΔK	On K
1.00 to 125 ΔK	0.25 Steeper than K	0.75 to 1.00 ΔK	0.25 Steeper than K
1.50 to 2.00 ΔK	0.50 Steeper than K	1.25 to 2.00 ΔK	0.50 Steeper than K
> 2.00 ΔK	$\frac{1}{3}$ ΔK	> 2,00 ΔK	$\frac{1}{3}$ ΔK

tion to answer for a number of reasons. Lighting conditions vary from office to office, and a patient measured in two different offices might well show two different diameters. Some patients have one pupil diameter under general lighting but quite different diameters under low light. Therefore, some fitters prefer to simply observe the pupil under different lighting levels and judge whether the pupil is of average or large diameter. Other fitters prefer to measure the pupil diameter exactly, and several very good gauges are available for this.

3. Calculate lens power. The usual methods for finding lens power in hard contact lenses also apply to ultrathin lenses.

Lens Appearance

Several differences will be noted immediately between the appearance of the ultrathin lens on the eye and the regular lens. The ultrathin lens should achieve good centering or be slightly high regardless of the base curve to cornea relationship. There is con-siderably less movement of the ultrathin lens than might be expected, and the lag is slower.

Principal Applications

The ultrathin lens has application in both problem cases and regular contact lens patients. It is particularly useful for those patients who suffer abnormal discomfort from a regular hard contact lens.

The ultrathin lens is also particularly useful for a patient who has a regular lens that rides low and causes edema and tight symptoms. In this case, the ultrathin lens will usually ride in a centered position on the cornea and provide normal tear circulation.

A principal application of the ultrathin lens is as a transition lens when a patient has induced corneal astigmatism as a result of wearing an improperly fitted regular hard contact lens. In this case, the reduced weight of the ultrathin lens allows the cornea to revert to its original shape with a minimum of visual inconvenience and discomfort to the patient during the transition period.

LID ATTACHMENT PHILOSOPHY

General Concepts

According to the lid attachment philosophy, the ideal contact lens should simulate the actions and movement of the tear layer. Since almost all tear layer movement is the result of upper lid actions, and since the tear layer may in effect be considered as attached to the upper lid, the ideal contact lens *should therefore be effectively attached to the upper lid* (Figure 7.15). This concept of lens perform-ance, in which the lens remains immobile without upper lid action but moves during blinking, as if the contact lens were attached to the upper lid, facilitates the act of blinking when contact lenses are worn and permits the successful training of blinking. The lid attachment philosophy has been used in PMMA lenses where large diameter lenses are needed and in some gas permeable lenses.

TABLE 7.9a
8.7 DIAMETER ULTRATHIN TRIAL SET

Base Curve		Power	Diam.	O.Z.D.	Blend Width	P.C.W.	P.C.R.	tc
46.50	7.26	−3.00	8.7	7.5	0.2	0.4	10.2	.09
46.00	7.34	−3.00	8.7	7.5	0.2	0.4	10.2	.09
45.50	7.42	−3.00	8.7	7.5	0.2	0.4	10.2	.09
45.00	7.50	−3.00	8.7	7.5	0.2	0.4	10.5	.09
44.50	7.58	−3.00	8.7	7.5	0.2	0.4	10.8	.09
44.00	7.67	−3.00	8.7	7.5	0.2	0.4	10.8	.09
43.50	7.76	−3.00	8.7	7.5	0.2	0.4	10.8	.09
43.00	7.85	−3.00	8.7	7.5	0.2	0.4	10.8	.08
42.50	7.94	−3.00	8.7	7.5	0.2	0.4	10.8	.08
42.00	8.04	−3.00	8.7	7.5	0.2	0.4	10.8	.08
41.50	8.13	−3.00	8.7	7.5	0.2	0.4	10.8	.08
41.00	8.23	−3.00	8.7	7.5	0.2	0.4	11.10	.08

TABLE 7.9b
8.2 DIAMETER ULTRATHIN TRIAL SET

Base Curve		Power	Diam.	O.Z.D.	Blend Width	P.C.W.	P.C.R.	tc
46.50	7.26	−3.00	8.2	7.0	0.2	0.4	9.9	.09
46.00	7.34	−3.00	8.2	7.0	0.2	0.4	10.2	.09
45.50	7.42	−3.00	8.2	7.0	0.2	0.4	10.2	.09
45.00	7.50	−3.00	8.2	7.0	0.2	0.4	10.2	.09
44.50	7.58	−3.00	8.2	7.0	0.2	0.4	10.2	.08
44.00	7.67	−3.00	8.2	7.0	0.2	0.4	10.2	.08
43.50	7.76	−3.00	8.2	7.0	0.2	0.4	10.5	.08
43.00	7.85	−3.00	8.2	7.0	0.2	0.4	10.5	.08
42.50	7.94	−3.00	8.2	7.0	0.2	0.4	10.5	.08
42.00	8.04	−3.00	8.2	7.0	0.2	0.4	10.8	.08
41.50	8.13	−3.00	8.2	7.0	0.2	0.4	10.8	.08
41.00	8.23	−3.00	8.2	7.0	0.2	0.4	10.8	.08

The Role of Blinking

Korb feels that an optimal blink for the closure of the lids is achieved without any spasm of the orbicularis or without any squeezing.[10] In addition, it is important that the eye exhibit Bell's phenomenon. Korb feels that good blinking habits must be trained to insure that the frequency and quality of the blink is adequate to achieve three specific functions of blinking as related to contact lens wear.

1. To maintain normal corneal wetting on those portions of the cornea not covered by the contact lens, particularly the nasal and temporal periphery

2. To effect an interchange of tears between the contact lens and the cornea

3. To maintain a clean and optically satisfactory anterior contact lens surface

The dropping movement, or lens lag, occurring after the opening phase of the blink, which is considered desirable in most fitting techniques, is purposely eliminated in the lid attachment philosophy for the following reasons:

1. Vision may blur during the lag of the

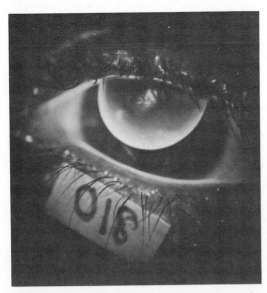

Figure 7.15. Lens fitted according to the lid attachment philosophy.

lens, which causes an inhibition of blinking or an alteration in the type of blink.

2. Blinking cannot be complete nor can blinking training be successful if the lens presents an ever-moving obstacle for the lid to hurdle. This is particularly true with palpebral aperture lenses, when blinking will often be inhibited to eliminate discomfort.

3. Although success may initially be achieved despite inhibition or alteration of blinking, the probability of edema and/or peripheral corneal staining occurring increases with time. All too often the long-term result involves corneal complications necessitating the discontinuance of contact lens wear.

Korb Lens Design

The five lens variables of most importance for correct contact lens performance in the lid attachment philosophy are as follows:

1. Peripheral lens contour
2. Edge contour
3. Edge thickness
4. Lens mass
5. Secondary radii and edge curvatures

The peripheral lens contour and the edge contour are closely related and are usually considered as a unit.

Peripheral Lens Contour

Korb considers the peripheral lens contour as that portion of the lens from the edge inward approximately 1.0 mm., as differentiated from the edge contour, which is only the outermost 0.2 mm. of the lens.

The peripheral lens contour is the most important factor in designing a lens that will adhere to the upper lid. Although the peripheral lens contour is usually considered to be predetermined by the optical power of the lens, it is possible to alter it by the use of special type of anterior lenticular constructions and by special edging techniques.

If the peripheral lens contour slopes away from the lid and towards the eye as with a high plus lens, the affinity of the lid for the lens is decreased. With a high minus lens, the peripheral lens contour and the edge contour are directed towards the lid, creating a broader area of contact between the lens and the lid and thereby increasing the affinity of the lens to the lid. In order to increase the adhesion of the lens to the lid, a broader area of lid-lens contact and an actual conforming of the peripheral lens contour to the lid contour are required. This may be achieved by the use of special lenticular constructions.

The Korb standard peripheral lens contour for a −3.00 D. lens is illustrated in Figure 7.16. Note that the lens profile resembles a plano lens and that the apex of the edge is located towards the anterior lens surface. Figure 7.17 illustrates a similar lens of −3.00 D. in which the anterior peripheral lens contour has been flattened by the use of a special lenticular flange. Note that despite the wedge effect (or minus peripheral lens contour) the edge contour is similar to the standard lens illustrated in Figure 7.16.

Edge Contour

The edge contour refers to the shape of

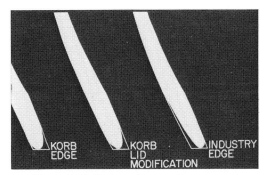

Figure 7.16. Korb optimum edge contour.

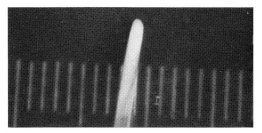

Figure 7.17. Korb lenticular edge contour.

the outermost 0.2 mm. of the lens. A sectional view of a standard edge contour for the Korb lens is shown in Figure 7.16 along with Mandell's optimum edge (industry), which has been symmetrically reduced to less than 0.10 mm., thus making it proportionate to Korb's edge. It is apparent that the Korb edge does not resemble those edge contours reported as desirable by others. The apex of the Korb edge is displaced as far towards the anterior surface as the usual apex is displaced towards the posterior surface.

Edge Thickness

Edge thickness is defined by Korb as that thickness measured at a point 0.2 mm. from the apex of the edge and measured prior to the beginning of the edging process. An edge thickness of 0.06 mm. ±0.01 mm. is used as the starting point for all lenses in the power range of plano to −6.00 D. However, variations in the nature of the peripheral lens contour may result in an increase in edge thickness of 0.01 to 0.04 mm.

The range of acceptable edge thicknesses for powers of plano to −6.00 D. varies from 0.05 to 0.12 mm. Edge thicknesses of less than 0.05 mm. will fray, while those greater than 0.12 mm. result in bridging of the lid from the cornea.

Lens Mass and Shape

The Korb philosophy strives for minimum mass in order to resist the pull of gravity and to maintain attachment to the upper lid. If the weight is increased, the peripheral lens contour must be redesigned to maintain lens adhesion to the upper lid. The standard center thickness required for the Korb technique for single cut lenses at diameters ranging from 8.2 to 9.4 mm. are given in Table 7.10. Lenses fitted by this technique, when used with appropriate secondary curvatures, will automatically result in the desired edge thickness of 0.05 ±0.005 mm. If a flatter peripheral lens contour (minus lenticular flange) is used to create additional lid adhesion, the center thickness is usually reduced to 0.11 mm. for plano, 0.10 mm. for −1.00, 0.09 mm. for −2.00, and 0.08 mm. for −3.00. It may, however, be maintained, as for single cut lenses, when necessary to eliminate lens flexing for visual reasons.

Plus lenses, and many plano and low minus power lenses, usually require a lenticular type of construction in order both to reduce weight and to create lid adhesion (Appendix 11). Carrier thicknesses of 0.09 to 0.12 mm. are usually indicated. Plano lenses may be as thin as 0.09 mm. However, plus lenses must be increased in center thickness in order to maintain a minimum 0.08 mm. and, preferably, a 0.11 mm. carrier thickness.

Secondary Radii

The critical specifications of this lens require lathe cut peripheral curves.

Diagnostic Lenses

The use of diagnostic lenses from stand-

TABLE 7.10

S-2 KORB TECHNIQUE (SINGLE CUT DESIGNS)
Plano to -6.00 Minus Thickness

Base	Plano 8.2	8.6	9.0	9.4	-1.00 8.2	8.6	9.0	9.4	-2.00 8.2	8.6	9.0	9.4	-3.00 8.2	8.6	9.0	9.4	4.00 8.2	8.6	9.0	9.4	-5.00 8.2	8.6	9.0	9.4	-6.00 8.2	8.6	9.0	9.4
7.40	-17	-18	-19	-21	-15	-14	-17	-18	-13	-13	-14	-15	-11	-12	-12	-13	-08	-08	-09	-09	-07	-07	-07	-07	06	06	06	06+
7.50	-17	-18	-19	-20	-15	-14	-17	-18	-13	-13	-14	-15	-11	-11	-12	-13	-08	-08	-08	-09	-07	07	07	-07	06	06	06+	06+
7.60	-17	-17	-18	-19	-14	-14	-16	-17	-12	-12	-13	-14	-11	-10	-11	-13	-08	08	-08	-09	-07	07	07	07	06	06+	06+	06+
7.70	-16	-17	-17	-18	-14	-14	-16	-17	-12	-12	-13	-14	-10	-09	-10	-12	08	08+	08	-08	07	07+	07	07	06+	06+	06++	06++
7.80	-16	-16	-17	-18	-14	-14	-16	-17	-12	12	-13	14	-10	-09	-10	12	08	08+	08	08	07+	07++	07+	06+	06+	06+	06++	06++
7.90	-15	-16	-16	-17	-13	-14	-15	-16	-12	12	-13	13	-10	09	10	14	08	08+	08+	08	07+	07++	07++	07++	06+	06++	06++	06++
8.00	-15	-16	-16	-16	-15	-13	-15	-16	-11	12	-12	13	10	09	10	11	08	08+	08+	08	07+	07++	07++	07++	06+	06++	06++	06++
8.10	-15	-16	-16	-16	-13	-13	-14	-15	11	12	12	13	10	09	10	10	08	08+	08+	08	07+	07++	07++	07++	06+	06++	06++	06++
8.20	-15	-16	-16	-16	-13	-13	-13	-15	11	11	12	12	10	09	09	10	08	08+	08+	08	07+	07++	07++	07++	06++	06++	L	L
8.30	-14	-16	-16	-16	-12	-12	-13	-14	11	11	12	12	09	09	09	09	07	07+	07+	07+	07+	07++	07++	07++	06++	06++	L	L
8.40	-14	-15	-15	-15	-12	-12	-12	-13	11	10	11	11	09	08	09	09	07	07+	07+	07+	07++	07++	06++	06++	L	06++	L	L
8.50	-13	-15	-15	-15	-11	-11	-12	-12	10	10	11	11	09	08	09	09	07	07+	07+	07+	07++	07++	06++	06++	L	L	L	L
8.60	-13	-14	-14	-15	-11	-11	-11	-11	10	10+	10	10	09+	08+	08	09	07	07+	07+	07+	07++	07++	06++	L++	L	L	L	L
8.70	-13	-14	-14	-15	-11	-11	-11	-11	10	10+	10	10	09+	08+	08	09	07	07+	07+	07+	07++	07++	06++	L++	L	L	L	L

I.e.: -11 = .05 edge plus or minus .005 mm.
I.e.: 11 = .06 edge plus or minus .005 mm.
I.e.: 11+ = .07 edge plus or minus .005 mm.
I.e.: 11++ = .08 edge plus or minus .005 mm.
I.e.: L = lenticular required.

TABLE 7.11

KORB TECHNIQUE DIAGNOSTIC LENSES

Diag. Set Code	Diam.	Opt. Zone	R2	Blend	R3	Lent.	Power	C.T.	Color
I	9.0	7.5	1.4	.7	.3/12.0	no	−3.00	.10	Blue
II	8.6	7.2	1.5	.7	.2/12.0	no	−3.00	.10	Green
III	8.2	6.8	2.3	1.0	.3/12.0	no	−3.00	.09	Clear
IV	8.2	7.2	1.5	.7	.2/12.0	7.6L/1.5f	−1.00	.11	Brown
V	8.6	7.2	1.5	.7	.2/12.0	7.4L/1.5f	+3.00	.17	Gray

All R2 (secondary radii), lenticular radii, and blend radii are expressed in mm. of curvature flatter than base curve.

ardized sets that use the specific lens variables conforming to this fitting philosophy is essential. The sets include single-cut and lenticular series and are constructed in diameters that vary in 0.4 mm. steps (Table 7.11). The diagnostic sets in the order of their frequency of use are the following:

1. 9.0 diameter, power −3.00, single cut
2. 9.0 diameter, power −1.00, lenticular series
3. 9.4 diameter, power −3.00, single cut
4. 8.6 diameter, power −3.00, single cut
5. 9.0 diameter, power +3.00, lenticular series

The frequency distribution of the final lens diameter for 1,000 patients was found to be the following:

Diameter	Percent
8.2	2
8.6	21
9.0	49
9.4	23
Above 9.4	5

Lens Selection Procedure

The first diagnostic lens selected in the initial fitting procedure should be a single-cut lens with a base curve that is from 0.15 to 0.20 mm. flatter than the flattest keratometric reading and with a diameter for an average eye of 9.0 mm. Korb's average base curve is 0.25 mm. flatter than the flattest keratometric reading, varying from a minimum of 0.15 mm. to as much as 0.70 mm.

flatter. For a larger eye, the diameter should be 9.4 mm., and for a smaller eye, 8.6 mm. Diameters of 9.8 and 8.2 mm. may occasionally be required.

Following insertion of the diagnostic lens, the continuation of blinking exercises will facilitate the settling of the lens. The first observation made in the analysis of the fit of the diagnostic lens should be the positioning of the lens. The lens *must* ride high and must remain attached to the upper lid. If lens lag occurs with the eye in the open position, the following procedures are followed in attempting to achieve upper lid attachment:

Analyze the blink and its effect on lens positioning. If partial blinking is flicking or pushing the lens down but a correct blink can maintain the superior position of the lens, then poor blinking is responsible for the lens lag, and the blinking training procedures must be repeated until correct blinking is firmly established.

A flatter base curve will frequently eliminate lens lag. Select and evaluate diagnostic lenses with flatter base curves, in steps of 0.10 mm. Often a lens 0.40 or 0.50 mm. flatter than the flattest keratometric reading is required to achieve the desired lens performance. When the fit of the base curve becomes too flat, the lens will lose its stability and will wobble on the cornea. If this occurs and lens lag has not been eliminated, other steps will have to be taken. The tendency is to resist using a flat enough base curve. This inhibition stems from conventional lens techniques and must be overcome in order to use the Korb philosophy to full advantage.

If the lens lag was not eliminated with correct blinking and/or flattening of the base curve, the lenticular series of diagnostic lenses must be used for lens attachment to the upper lid. The lenticular series is fitted according to the methods described previously, beginning with the base curve 0.15 to 0.20 mm. flatter than the flattest K.

Occasionally, a lens that remains marginally stable in the primary position of gaze will drop during lateral excursions of the eye. Blunting the apex of the lens edge will give the lens additional stability by altering the nature of the lens meniscus. If blunting the edge of a single-cut lens does not solve the problem, the use of a lenticular and, if

necessary, a blunt edge may be required.

If the lower lid is depressed by the examiner, a lens that usually remains attached to the upper lid may drop into the inferior fornix after the blink. If this occurs, it is likely that the lens will lag during normal vertical excursions. If the lens is a single cut, blunting of the lens edge and/or using a lenticular lens will be required.

LENS MOVEMENT. Because the movement of a properly designed lens occurs only during a blink, it can be observed only with the lower lid retracted. With the patient blinking slowly, the lens should move over the cornea and limbus and onto the sclera. The average lens moves approximately 6 mm., 3 mm. over the cornea and 3 mm. onto the sclera. If lens movement is insufficient and the lens does

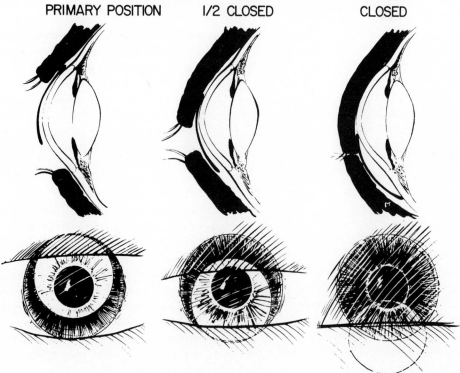

Figure 7.18. Fitting the Korb lens.

not move onto the sclera, try a diagnostic lens with a base curve 0.10 or 0.20 flatter. This lens should move more freely onto the sclera (Figure 7.18).

LATERAL CENTRATION. Failure of the lens to center is usually the result of one of the following: (1) Oblique eye movements during Bell's phenomenon, (2) Aspherical or "against-the-rule" cornea, (3) A small lens diameter. In each situation the first attempt at correction should be a lens of larger diameter. If this does not produce adequate centration, try a lenticular lens.

FLOURESCEIN PATTERN. The fluorescein pattern of the lens in its habitual position with the upper lid covering its superior portion should reveal relatively even bearing throughout the inferior 3 to 4 mm. portion. (If the lens is centered manually, it would appear very flat; however, evaluation in the centered position without the usual lid pressures is not meaningful.) The fluorescein standoff created by the secondary curvatures is usually significant only along the lateral aspects, since the inferior position of the lens shows marked standoff (Figure 7.19). The fluorescein pattern is of less value with this philosophy than with other techniques, since the lens is deliberately fitted flat to allow it to move onto the sclera during the blink.

INITIAL SENSATION. Once a diagnostic lens has been selected that satisfies the criteria of positioning, movement, and centration, consideration should be given to the patient's subjective sensation created by the lens. Corneal, scleral, and upper lid sensation should be *totally absent* with this philosophy of design upon initial lens insertion. Lens sensation is usually the result of lower lid feeling, which is present only during the adaptation period of approximately two weeks. After this adaptation period, a properly fitted lens should cause no sensation. To analyze lens sensation, depress the lower lid so that the lens cannot touch the lower lid as it moves during the blink. If there is no lens

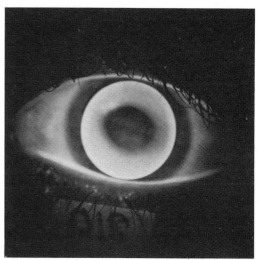

Figure 7.19. If Korb lens is centered, fluorescein pattern appears flat.

sensation created by both rapid and slow blinking with the lower lid depressed, the patient may be assured that adaptation for lower lid sensation will occur within two to three weeks after initial wearing begins. If sensation is present when the lower lid is retracted, it is usually caused by a base curve that is effectively too steep. The "binding" created when the lens passes over the peripheral cornea, limbus, or sclera during the blink causes the discomfort. To eliminate the sensation, use a flatter fit. Frequently a lens 0.40 to 0.60 mm. flatter than the flattest K is required to allow the lens to glide over the cornea and onto the sclera without binding. If it is impossible to eliminate the sensation during blinking, a successful fitting with Korb lenses will not be achieved. Whenever blinking creates discomfort, there will be an inhibition of the blink, which will subsequently result in three o'clock and nine o'clock staining, limited tear exchange, and eventual failure with contact lenses. When this occurs, contact lens fitting should be discontinued in all but one circumstance. If a lenticular lens evokes sensation but a nonlenticular of the same base curve and diameter is not felt, the source of the feeling is the *upper lid*, and adaptation will eliminate this sensation.

The limiting factor in determining final lens diameter is the creation of flare or other peripheral visual disturbances by the infringement on the pupillary area by the secondary curvatures or the lens edge.

FITTING SETS

By restricting the number of variables of a contact lens, it is possible to fit the patient directly from sets of 300 to 2,000 lenses rather than order individual lenses from the laboratory for each patient (Figure 7.20). The goal is to be able to fit the majority of patients, with only the more unusual case requiring a special order. Unfortunately, this philosophy often leads to compromises in lens design. Fitting sets usually contain medium or small diameter lenses, with only the larger sets containing a large diameter lens series.

Morrison has recommended a fitting set that has been standardized into five basic series.[11,12] All have the same peripheral curve width and same peripheral curve-base curve relationship:

Series I	9.3	8.3
Series II	8.8	7.8
Series III	8.3	7.3
Series IV	7.8	6.8
Series V	7.3	6.3

All lenses are engraved with base curve, power, and series number and stored in a cabinet that permits easy handling and organization. Four sets have been in use in clinical practice. They consist of either 300, 600, 900, or 1,800 lenses. Other laboratories offer various set sizes. Obviously, the larger the set, the greater the likelihood of having the proper base curve, power, and diameter.

THE FITTING PROCEDURE

Clinical Procedure

The author's clinical procedure is outlined as follows:

First Visit
1. Exam
2. Select trial lens (tables)
3. Insert trial lens
4. Wait ten to twenty minutes—no more
5. Check centering
    a. If lens low
       try 0.5 mm. larger diameter
       try B. C. steeper 0.25 D., 0.50 D., 0.75 D.
       try 0.5 mm. smaller diameter
    b. If lens high
       try smaller (0.5 mm.) and steeper (0.50 D.)
       try larger diameter
    c. If lens still cannot be made to center,

reduce thickness in Table 7.6
       0.4 mm. if greater than .14
       0.2 mm. if less than .14
6. Order lens

Follow-up Schedule

The lens should be evaluated after three hours of wear either on the same day the lens is fitted or on the following day. This may be accomplished by timing the patient's wearing schedule so as to precede the appointment time for the period desired.

There are numerous problems that may befall the new contact lens wearer. These are described in detail in Chapter 14. The primary test of the physiological corneal response at this time is the biomicroscopic examination for central corneal clouding (C.C.C.).

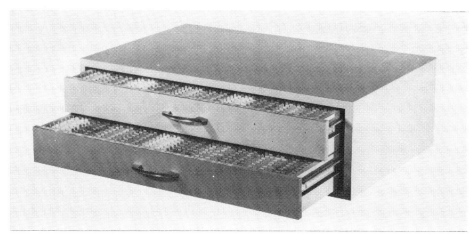

Figure 7.20. Fitting set. Courtesy of American Optical Co.

Possible results for this test are summarized in Table 7.12.

Additional Visits

Patient visits are normally scheduled for about one, five, eight, and fourteen days after lens delivery. This schedule is often modified according to progress of the individual patient (Table 7.13).

If the C.C.C. persists, an adjustment must be made to increase the tear exchange. The exact type of adjustment depends on the positioning of the lens.

A. If lens centers
  1. flatten P.C. to
    12 mm.
    15 mm.
    17 mm.
    (must use diamond tool)
  2. flatten I.C. to
    10 mm.
    10.5 mm.
    11 mm.
  3. reduce diameter
  4. fenestrate
B. If lens does not center, use a
  1. smaller diameter
    steeper base curve
    flatter P.C.
  2. larger diameter
    flatter P.C.

Additional discussion of follow-up care is given in Chapter 14.

ORDERING

Purchase plans vary with the companies. Information on this can be obtained directly from the manufacturer.

Special order forms, with spaces provided for all lens dimensions, are usually available from the contact lens manufacturers. Some forms do not provide adequate space, and on these the practitioner must add the necessary dimensions.

TABLE 7.12

Responses on First Day of Contact Lens Wear

(Mandell and Polse)

Corneal Swelling (Pachometer)	Response I 2% to 4%	Response II 5% to 8%	Response III Over 8%
Cause	a. Minimal tear exchange interference b. Temporary tear osmolarity changes c. Osmotically induced	a. Oxygen deprivation b. Tear tonicity decrease c. Tight fit and/or inadequate blink d. Metabolically and osmotically induced	a. Oxygen deprivation (Very tight fit) b. Primarily metabolically induced
Slit Lamp (Indirect)	none	Edema signs with Slit Lamp	Slit Lamp = edema (gross)
Keratometer	none	K changes less than 1.00 D.	K changes large
Central Corneal Clouding	Grade 0	Grade 1 or 2	Grade 3
Subjective Symptoms	Minimum or no symptoms of adaptation	Spectacle blur and tight symptoms	a. Severe discomfort b. Persistent spectacle blur c. Very severe tight symptoms
Symptom Peak	Swelling maximum after three hours wear and reduces to zero	Swelling reaches maximum in three hours and then reduces with continual wear	Very often patient unable to wear lenses over two hours
Prognosis	Generally no adjustments necessary. Cornea normal thickness after two weeks of controlled wear.	Patient may tolerate lenses if no other problem compounds the situation. Symptoms persist. Remedial changes in lens fit will generally resolve problem.	Very poor prognosis. Lens diameters must be changed. Corneal damage possible.

EXAMPLE ORDER

A complete order form is shown in Figure 7.21. The specifications given are for the following measurements of a hypothetical patient.

TABLE 7.13

Fit Evaluation

Day	Time Lenses Worn	Wearing Time	CCC Grade	Disposition
1 or 2	3	3	0	O.K.
			1	O.K.
			2	Alert
			3	Change lens
5	6	7	0	O.K.
			1	O.K.
			2	Alert
			3	Change lens
8	9	10	0	O.K.
			1	Alert
			2	Change lens
14	9	All day	0	O.K.
			1	Change lens

Refraction (Vertex distance 13 mm.)	O.D. −3.00 −1.00 × 180 O.S. + 15.00 −0.25 × 90 (Aphakia)
Keratometer	O.D. 42.25 43.00 at 90 O.S. 40.50 40.25 at 90
Corneal diameter	O.D. 12.0 O.S. 11
Pupil diameter	O.D. Average O.S. Small
Palpebral aperture	O.D. 9.5 O.S. 8.9
Lids	Normal position and normal tension

The patient has a congenital aphakia in the left eye with myopic astigmatism in the right eye. The left eye is slightly smaller and has a very slight ptosis. Lens specifications are given in Figure 7.21.

TABLE 7.14
LENS MODIFICATIONS

Lens Variable	Modification Possible	New Lens Necessary
Total diameter	Decrease	Increase
Optical zone diameter	Decrease	Increase
Peripheral curve radius	Increase (Flatten)	Decrease (Steepen)
Peripheral curve width	Increase (Must also decrease O.Z.D.)	Decrease (Must also increase O.Z.D.)
	Decrease (Must also decrease T.D.)	
Intermediate curve radius	Increase (Flatten)	Decrease (Steepen)
Intermediate curve width (if present)	Increase (Must also decrease O.Z.D. or P.C.W.)	Decrease (Must also increase O.Z.D.)
Blend width	Increase	Decrease
Front bevel width	Increase	Decrease
Power change	< ±1.00 D.	> ±1.00 D.
Surface polish	Yes (Minor)	Yes (Extensive)
Thickness increase or decrease	No	Yes
Change optical zone radius	No	Yes

Order Number_____

CONTACT LENS ORDER FORM

TO_____ Date_____Wanted_____

    NAME OF LABORATORY

PATIENT___*SMITH*_____ Do Not Fill After_____

		SPECIFICATIONS	(O) Ordered	(R) Received	(A) Adjusted	(G) Given	(M) Measured	(F) Final	(FO) Future Order

	Code	Type/Lab	PCCR or Series	POZD	PSCR	PSCW	Blend	PPCR	PPCW	AOZD	APCR or Edge	Diameter	Thickness	Power	Color	Lot No.	VA
O.D.	O	PMMA	7.99	7.4	8.85	0.7	10.5	12.25	0.4			9.6	0.18	-3.00	clear		20/
																	20/
O.S.	O	PMMA	8.39	7.0	X	X	None	8.5	0.85			9.2	✳	+15.50	clear		20/
																	20/

ADDITIONAL SPECIFICATIONS ☒,   MODIFICATIONS ☐,
REMARKS ☐

  O.D. Touch blend

✳ O.S. Minimum thickness

ORIGINAL ORDER......☒
ADDITIONAL LENSES...☐
MEMO LENSES.........☐
UNDER WARRANTY....☐
PLEASE REMAKE.......☐
PREVIOUS LENSES
    ENCLOSED...........☐
    TO COME ....☐
OTHER...............☐

Figure 7.21. Sample contact lens order form.

ALLOWANCE FOR MODIFICATIONS

It is frequently necessary to change the original contact lens dimensions after the lens has been worn by the patient. Some changes can be made by modifying the original lens, whereas other changes require that a new lens be made. Many fitters prefer to order lenses with total diameters and optical zone diameters that are slightly large, with peripheral curves which are slightly steep, and/or with little or no blends. Lenses ordered in this way will likely need only modifications

that can be made on the original lens. Dimensional changes that can be made on a lens and those which require a new lens are listed in Table 7.14.

REFERENCES

1. Haynes, P. R.: Quality control and inspection of contact lenses, in *Encyclopedia of Contact Lens Practice*, South Bend, Indiana, International Optics, 1959–1963, vol. 2, Chap. 23, pp. 8–64.
2. Sarver, M. D.: Comparison of small and large corneal contact lenses, *Am. J. Optom. Arch. Am. Acad. Optom.*, 37(10):633–652, Oct. 1966.
3. Gordon, S.: *Small Thin Contact Lenses*, Part I and II (monograph), Contact Lens Guild, Inc.
4. Bailey, N. J.: Residual astigmatism with contact lenses, Part 8, Possible sites, *Opt. J. Rev. Optom.*, 98(3):31–32, 1961.
5. Harris, M. G.: The effects of contact lens thickness and diameter on residual astigmatism: a preliminary study, *Am. J. Optom.*, 47(6):442–444, 1970.
6. Harris, J. G., and Chu, C. S.: The effect of contact lens thickness and corneal toricity on flexure and residual astigmatism, *Am. J. Optom.*, 49(4):304–308, 1972.
7. Harris, M. G., and Appelquist, T. D.: The effect of contact lens diameter and power on flexure and residual astigmatism, *Am. J. Optom. Physiol. Opt.*, 51(4):266–270, 1974.
8. Mandell, R. B.: Which lens will give the best vision, *Int. Cont. Lens Clin.*, 2(1):31–32, 1975.
9. Moore, C.: A new concept for fitting ultrathin lenses, *Int. Cont. Lens Clin.*, 1(3):47–55, 1974.
10. Korb, D. R., and Korb, J. E.: A new concept in contact lens design—Parts 1 and 2, *J. Am. Optom. Assoc.*, 41(12):1023–1034, 1970.
11. Morrison, R.: The series system of fitting contact lenses, *Optom. World*, 53(10):30–39, 1966.
12. Morrison, R.: A survey of 1,000 consecutive contact lens patients, *J. Am. Optom. Assoc.*, 43(2):179–183, 1972.

ADDITIONAL READINGS

Berglund, J.: The fitting set. Is it really a help in fitting?, *Int. Cont. Lens Clin.*, 1(4):38–47, 1974.
Brungardt, T.: Spectacle blur refraction: a routine test in patient contact lens care, *Int. Cont. Lens Clin.*, 1(4):72–81, 1974.
Brungardt, T.: Contact lens refraction—the time it takes, *Optom. Weekly*, 66(41):1121–1123, 1975.
Brungardt, T., and Sukoenig, M. R.: Evaluation of a fitting method for spherical PMMA contact lenses, *Optom. Weekly*, 68(26):804, 1977.
Brungardt, T.F.: Contact lens clinic—evaluating the fit, *Optom. Weekly*, 59(16):39–40, 1968.
Cole, O. W.: "If the contacts fit, why can't I wear them?", *Contacto*, 15(2):5–9, 1971.
Crook, T. G.: Fitting a flatter lens, *Optom. Weekly*, 66(3):29, 1975.
Defazio, A., and Lowther, G. E.: Inspection of back surface aspheric contact lenses, *Am. J. Optom. Physiol. Opt.*, 56(8):471–479, 1979.
Dexter, D. J.: Finding the K values, *Cont. Lens Forum*, 3(2):17, 1978.
Dickinson, F.: Notes on the wearing of microlenses, *Cont. Lens J.*, 9(1):31–35, 1975.
Goldberg, J. B.: Some characteristics of ellipsoidal corneal lenses, *Optom. Weekly*, 66(40):1098–1099, 1975.
Goldberg, J. B.: Questions and answers about ellipsoidal corneal lenses, *Optom. Weekly*, 66(30):800–802, 1975.
Goldberg, J. B.: Raising a low corneal lens fit, *Optical Index*, 51(2):42–44, 1976.
Goldberg, J. B.: Clinical management of VFL variable focus lens, *Cont. Lens Forum*, 2(7):27, 1977.
Gordon, S.: Designing a minimum-thickness hard

contact lens, *Cont. Lens Forum*, *1(2)*:41–53, 1976.

Hill, R. M.: Oxygen permeable contact lenses: how convinced is the cornea?, *Int. Cont. Lens Clin.*, *4(2)*:34–36, 1977.

Hodd, N. F. B.: The corneal lens today, *The Ophthalmic Optician*, *17(22)*:821, 1977.

Jenkin, L.: Further development of the ultra thin lens, *Contacto*, *20(1)*:36–38, 1976.

Jenkins, G.: The physiological fit, *S. Afr. Opt.*, *32(2)*:21–25, 1973.

Klauer, D. L.: Profile analysis of corneal contact lenses, *Cont. Lens J.*, *8(1)*:14–16, 1974.

Korb, D.: Fitting to achieve normal blinking and lid action, *Int. Cont. Lens Clin.*, *1(3)*:57–70, 1974.

Lichtman, W. M.: An approach to contact lenses in a "sophisticated era," *Opt. J. Rev. Optom.*, *107(11)*:25–26, 1970.

Mackie, I. A.: Management of keratoconus with hard corneal lenses with special reference to the lens lid attachment technique, *Cont. Lens J.*, *5(8)*:5, 1977.

Mandell, R. B.: The physiological response method of fitting, *Int. Cont. Lens Clin.*, *1(3)*:80–88, 1974.

Mandell, R. B.: What is fitting?, *Int. Cont. Lens Clin.*, *1(3)*:21–22, 1974.

Mandell, R. B.: Current thoughts on gel lenses: III which lens will give the best vision, *Int. Cont. Lens Clin.*, *2(1)*:31–32, 1975.

Martin, J. D.: A fitting challenge, *Cont. Lens Forum*, *4(3)*:49, 1979.

Moore, C.: Who should have a fitting set?, *Int. Cont. Lens Clin.*, *2(2)*:70–74, 1975.

Moore, C. F.: A new concept for fitting hard-flexible lenses, *Contacto*, *20(5)*:4–8, 1976.

Chapter 8

TRIAL LENS METHOD

IN THE TRIAL LENS fitting method the practitioner tries a series of contact lenses with known dimensions on the patient's eyes before the final lenses are ordered. The process continues until a lens is found that gives an optimum fit or that makes possible an interpolation of what the optimum lens dimensions should be. The procedure is not simply one of trial and error. By noting the fitting characteristics of each lens, it is possible to judge the changes that are necessary in the lens dimensions and to choose systematically other trial lenses. Many practitioners prefer other names for trial lenses, such as control lenses,[1] fitting lenses, or diagnostic lenses, to avoid the implication of a chance selection of the correct lens.

Advocates of the trial lens fitting method usually point out the disadvantages of the method of direct ordering. They stress the difficulty of evaluating all the characteristics of the eye that may influence the lens fit and point out that many structures, such as the lid, cannot be evaluated until a lens is placed on the eye. It has been demonstrated that a keratometer measurement of the central cornea has limited validity, and advocates of the trial lens are quick to mention this limitation.

Opponents of the trial lens fitting method claim that it is impossible to have enough lenses to fit every patient adequately. There is, in addition, a great deal of expense involved in keeping a large trial set, especially if the lens type currently used becomes obsolete and a new trial set with a different lens type must be purchased.

TRIAL LENS SETS

Trial lens sets may contain any number of lenses, but they are usually limited to about twenty. The minimum number that is generally considered to comprise a complete set would be about ten lenses, whereas the maximum number in a set which is commonly sold contains fifty. The sets are usually sold as a unit (Figure 8.1). Some practitioners carry very large trial sets of their own design, with many variations in each of the lens dimensions. These sets may contain up to several hundred lenses.

Many practitioners prefer to store the trial lenses in individual cases, which fit into a standard two by two (inch) slide case (Figure 8.2). This allows easy access to only one lens at a time, thus eliminating the chance of spilling the lenses. As surplus lenses are accumulated, they may be added to the fitting set.

MAINTENANCE OF TRIAL SET

Trial lenses should occasionally have the optical zone radius, surface polish, and edge finish checked. Lenses are often mishandled by new patients and become defective. The

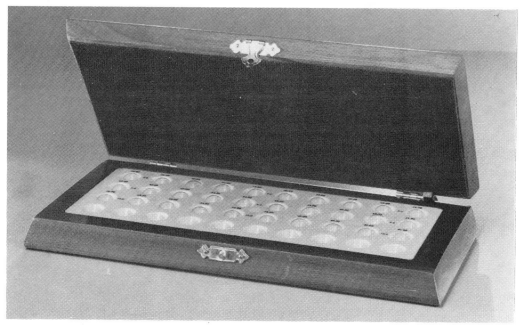

Figure 8.1. Trial lens set. Courtesy of Bausch and Lomb, Inc.

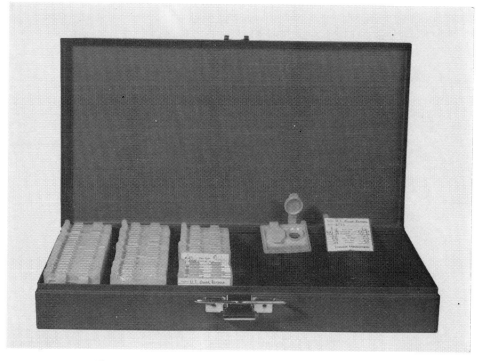

Figure 8.2. Trial lens set stored in a 2–by 2-inch slide case.

possibility also exists that they may be switched and several prescription lenses could thereby be incorrectly ordered.

REQUIREMENTS OF TRIAL SET

Every trial lens set is somewhat of a compromise, and none is ever completely adequate. The lenses should be designed to enable the practitioner to fit the greatest number of patients with the fewest lenses.[2] No two practitioners, however, will be likely to agree on the necessary lenses. The most sensible approach is to keep a medium-size trial lens set, which is adequate for most patients, and to borrow trial lenses from the laboratory for patients with unusual visual problems.

SAMPLE TRIAL LENS SET

In Table 8.1, the lens dimensions in a sample trial lens set are presented for use with the modified contour philosophy. Other trial sets are necessary for use with other fitting philosophies and will be presented later.

COLORS

Only light tints should be used. Darker colors may interfere with tests for the fitting characteristics of the lens. In addition to coloring the trial lenses, it is possible to scratch an identification mark on each lens.

DIAMETER

The lenses are made with a diameter of 9.1. This size is in the middle of the range for the total diameters commonly used in the modified contour philosophy.

POWERS

The power of the trial lenses is −3.00 D. This power is chosen to approximate the most frequently prescribed power for contact lenses.

Some difficulty is presented when the lenses of Table 8.1 are to be used for a patient whose refractive error is of positive power because the power of a contact lens may influence its fitting characteristics. If the trial lens is not very nearly the same power as the lens ordered for the patient, the patient's lens may not fit as the trial lens did. This problem is inevitable, however, regardless of the lens power put in the trial lenses. The trial lenses will never be the correct power for the majority of patients. For this reason, some fitters recommend that the trial lenses be of plano power. This produces the least difference from any positive or negative prescription which might be needed. On the other hand, these lenses will never be very close to any prescription, either, because few are of

TABLE 8.1

Base Curve		Power	Diam.	O.Z.D.	I.C.R.	I.C.W.	Blend	P.C.R.	P.C.W.	tc
46.50	7.26	−3.00	9.1	7.7	8.1	0.3	9.0	10.0	0.4	.12
46.00	7.34	−3.00	9.1	7.7	8.1	0.3	9.0	10.0	0.4	.12
45.50	7.42	−3.00	9.1	7.7	8.2	0.3	9.0	10.0	0.4	.12
45.00	7.50	−3.00	9.1	7.7	8.4	0.3	9.0	10.0	0.4	.12
44.50	7.58	−3.00	9.1	7.7	8.5	0.3	9.5	10.5	0.4	.12
44.00	7.67	−3.00	9.1	7.7	8.6	0.3	9.5	10.5	0.4	.12
43.50	7.76	−3.00	9.1	7.7	8.7	0.3	9.5	10.5	0.4	.12
43.00	7.85	−3.00	9.1	7.7	8.8	0.3	9.5	10.5	0.4	.12
42.50	7.94	−3.00	9.1	7.7	8.8	0.3	9.5	10.5	0.4	.12
42.00	8.04	−3.00	9.1	7.7	8.9	0.3	10.0	11.0	0.4	.12
41.50	8.13	−3.00	9.1	7.7	9.1	0.3	10.0	11.0	0.4	.12
41.00	8.23	−3.00	9.1	7.7	9.2	0.3	10.0	11.0	0.4	.12
40.50	8.23	−3.00	9.1	7.7	9.3	0.3	10.0	11.0	0.4	.12
40.00	8.44	−3.00	9.1	7.7	9.4	0.3	10.0	11.0	0.4	.12
39.50	8.55	−3.00	9.1	7.7	9.5	0.3	10.5	11.5	0.4	.12
39.00	8.65	−3.00	9.1	7.7	9.6	0.3	10.5	11.5	0.4	.12

plano power. Since most contact lens prescriptions are for low minus power, the greatest percentage of patients may be closely fitted with trial lenses having low minus power.

STORAGE OF TRIAL LENSES

It is usually most convenient to store contact lenses in a dry state. When the testing is completed the lenses should be cleaned and blotted dry with soft tissue. Drying a lens must be done carefully, or tiny scratches will be made on the lens with the tissue.

Some practitioners prefer to store their trial lenses in a container with soaking solution. Storage in soaking solution will help to sterilize the lenses; it will keep the lenses clean and eliminate the need to dry them.

Lenses should not be wet when placed in the case and then be allowed to dry before being used again. This will allow water impurities to dry and leave a hard deposit on the lens surface. It may also cause a lens to warp.

TRIAL SET FITTING METHOD

One may begin with a contact lens having average dimensions. This is placed on the eye, and, from its fitting characteristics, the differences needed in the next trial lens can be determined. Usually, however, the practitioner begins by taking a keratometer reading, which serves as a guide for choosing the optical zone radius of the first trial lens. Commonly, a lens is selected that has an optical zone on *K* or slightly steeper than *K*.

The lens is inserted by the practitioner (*see* insertion procedures), though a few practitioners let the patient insert the lens for the first time. They feel this gives the patient confidence, since he is naturally reluctant to let someone else "put a finger in his eye." It has been the author's experience that a skill-ful fitter can insert the lens much quicker and with much less manipulation of the eye than the patient can and that the sooner the lens is in place, the sooner the patient's appre-hension will be relieved.

It is quite natural for the patient to tear profusely when the contact lens is inserted for the first time. The lens will be washed around and will give the appearance of being very loose. Before any evaluation can be made of the lens fit, it is necessary to wait at least fifteen minutes; some practitioners prefer to wait longer. This depends upon how long the patient continues to tear.

LENS POSITION AND STABILITY

The lens position must be observed while the eye is in a relaxed and unirritated state. If the eye is tearing excessively, a false impres-sion of the fit will be made.

Tight and Loose Lenses

A tight lens is one that is stationary on the cornea and resists movement by exter-nal force. A loose lens moves freely on the cornea. Usually, there is a close relationship between the fit of the lens and its stability on the cornea. When the optical zone or peripheral zone of a lens is steeper than the cornea, the lens will tend to fit tightly. A lens that is flatter than the cornea will tend to fit loosely.

A tight lens, however, should not always be considered as synonymous with a steep lens nor a loose lens synonymous with a flat lens. Factors other than the lens-cornea rela-tionship may influence the stability of the lens. If a lens is relatively thin, it will have a tendency to fit tightly, whereas a thick lens may appear to fit loosely. If excessive tearing is present any lens may appear to fit loosely.*

The lens should first be observed when the eyes are in the straight ahead position. A well-fitted contact lens will tend to remain near one position. The lens will move dur-ing blinking, first downward, with the lid closure, then upward, with the lid with-drawal. With the lids fully opened, the lens drops slightly to its riding position; this movement is known as the *blink lag*. It then remains nearly stationary or drops very slowly.

The preferred riding position is for the geometric center of the lens to coincide with the line of sight. Such a lens is said to be centered. Most negative power lenses, how-ever, ride 1 to 2 mm. above the centered position, which is also satisfactory. Positive power lenses will often ride a millimeter or more below the centered position. It is usu-ally preferred that the lens not ride so low that it touches the lower lid. Some patients are not bothered, however, if the lens does touch the lower lid, and if the lens is worn comfortably in this position, it may be ac-ceptable.

A lens that lags below the inferior lid margin is definitely too loose.

Static Lag

If the eye is fixating straight ahead and the lids are drawn apart by the fitter, the lens will drop. A well-fitted lens falls 1 to 2 mm. in a smooth motion; a loose lens falls rapidly to the lower limbus (Figure 8.3), and a tight lens remains in a centered position.

Excursion Lag

As the eye makes lateral movements, the

---

*The reader should review the fitting principles pre-sented in Chapter 5.

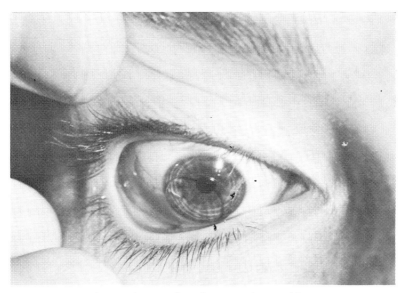

Figure 8.3. Loose lens drops to a low position.

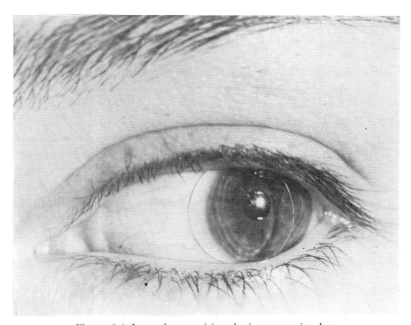

Figure 8.4. Loose lens position during excursion lag.

lens will tend to lag 1 to 2 mm. from a centered position. If the lens encroaches upon the sclera, it is too loose (Figure 8.4).

LENS MODIFICATION

It may be recalled from Chapter 5 that several possible changes can be made in a contact lens to alter the fitting relationship.

In general, when all the forces affecting a lens are considered, it may be tightened by the following procedures:

1. Increasing optical zone diameter or total diameter
2. Decreasing the optical zone radius
3. Decreasing the intermediate or peripheral curve radius
4. Decreasing the lens thickness

A contact lens may be loosened by the following methods:

1. Decreasing the optical zone diameter or total diameter
2. Increasing the optical zone radius
3. Increasing the intermediate or peripheral curve radius.
4. Increasing the lens thickness

The simple observation of lens movement will indicate whether a contact lens is excessively tight or loose but does not indicate what change should be made in the lens to correct an improper fitting relationship. This is determined by examining the bearing relationship between the lens and the cornea. The bearing relationship can be seen by means of the fluorescein test.

APPLICATION OF FLUORSCEIN IN FITTING CONTACT LENSES

In 1938, Obrig introduced the technique of adding a small quantity of sodium fluorescein solution to the tears, thus causing them to fluoresce a bright yellow-green color when viewed under ultraviolet light.[3] This makes it possible to view the tears that are present between the lens and cornea and to evaluate the fit of a contact lens *in situ*. The brightness of the fluorescent tears increases with the thickness of the tear layer and may be used to estimate the amount of clearance between the lens and cornea. If only ultraviolet light is allowed to shine on the cornea, any area under the lens that lacks fluorescein-stained tears appears black, thus indicating that at that position the lens is touching the cornea. Bubbles trapped beneath the lens also appear black and may be easily located.

Originally, fluorescein was used as a diagnostic aid in fitting scleral lenses, but it was later found to be equally helpful in evaluating the fit of corneal lenses. It may also be used to stain corneal abrasions to increase their visibility. Various other substances have been tried as substitutes for fluorescein, including milk, cresyl blue, and food coloring, but none has proved to be effective as a fitting guide.[4]

FLUORESCEIN SUBSTANCE

Fluorescein is an organic compound (resorcinolphthalein), which is inert and harmless to tissue. It has various applications in medicine. It may be injected directly into the anterior chamber to study ocular fluid movement. It is also used to study blood and lymph flow in the general circulation of the body.

FLUORESCEIN STORAGE

Fluorescein is available in several forms for storage, including liquid, powder, tablets, ointment,[5] or fluorescein-impregnated filter paper.[6] Selection of the form in which to keep fluorescein is governed principally by the necessity to maintain sterility.

Dangers of Fluorescein

The principal danger in the use of fluorescein is that it is easily contaminated by *Pseudomonas aeruginosa*, a highly virulent ocular pathogen. *Pseudomonas aeruginosa* (*Bacillus pyocyaneus*) cannot invade an intact cornea, but if the organism can gain entrance through a break in the epithelium, it may cause a corneal ucler of a most serious type, and it may totally destroy the eye.

Pseudomonas aeruginosa is commonly found on human skin and stools, in some eyes as a part of the normal conjunctival flora, and occasionally in the air and in well water.[7] It is frequently found in tap water, and it is not affected by ordinary soap.[8] Therefore, it is simple for *Pseudomonas* to contaminate ophthalmic solutions from various sources. Fluorescein stored in bottles that have been opened and retained for repeated use is very often contaminated with *Pseudomonas*.[8] Fortunately, no incident has been reported in which *Pseudomonas* was shown to have been transferred to the eye by fluorescein used specifically in fitting contact lenses. However, various reports have been made of corneal infection caused by the organism, infection which probably came from the contaminated fluorescein used to inspect corneal abrasions.[7]

Government Restrictions

Prior to 1953 there were no specific governmental regulations for the sterility of fluorescein and other eye medications. Even the major pharmaceutical companies were dispensing large quantities of eye solutions in a nonsterile state.[9] In 1953, however, the Pure Food and Drug Administration enacted regulations that required that all ophthalmic solutions be manufactured and packaged in a sterile condition.

Unfortunately, no chemical preservative commonly used in ophthalmic solutions, such as Zephiran®, chlorobutanol, or phenylmercuric nitrate, is effective in keeping fluorescein free from *Pseudomonas*,[7] but effective sterilization is possible by autoclaving. For this reason, keeping fluorescein in solution has been virtually discontinued in favor of the other methods of storage, in which sterility of the fluorescein is insured.

Fluorescein Strips

In 1951, Kimura demonstrated that fluorescein could be stored in dry form on thin strips of filter paper, which could be moistened to form the solution needed.[6] Each strip could be packaged separately and autoclaved so that it would remain sterile until opened. This method has proven by far to be the best for storing fluorescein in a sterile state, and the strips are now commercially available. Their low cost and ease of handling make the strips the most common method used today for the application of fluorescein.

Method of Using Fluorescein Strips

The fluorescein strip should first be moistened with ophthalmic irrigating solution. Care should be taken that the end of the irrigating bottle does not contact the fluorescein strip and introduce some fluorescein into the bottle of irrigating solution (Figure 8.5). Tap water is sometimes used, but irrigating solution is advantageous because it is sterile and its pH is adjusted to the alkaline side, which helps the fluorescein dissolve.[10] The patient's gaze should be directed downward, and the examiner then raises the patient's superior lid with the thumb, exposing the sclera. The wet fluorescein strip should be touched lightly to the superior sclera (Figure 8.6) and the solution allowed to mix with the tears. The patient is asked to blink a few times to circulate the fluorescein. He is then ready for observation under the ultraviolet lamp.

Occasionally, with an apprehensive patient, it is difficult to place fluorescein on the superior sclera, and it may be easier to have the patient look up and place the fluorescein strip in the lower fornix.

Care should be taken not to flood the eye with fluorescein. A single large drop is usually adequate. The brightness of the fluorescein beneath the tears is a function of the tear layer thickness and the fluorescein concentration. Too much fluorescein may give the appearance of a greater amount of clearance between the lens and cornea than actually exists. Also, the instillation of excessive fluorescein will sometimes precipitate extra tearing.

Care should be taken to avoid dripping the fluorescein on the patient's face or clothing, as it is extremely difficult to remove. A technique should be used for instilling the fluorescein, in which the hand is cupped in such a way as to catch any dripping from the strip.

Use of Wetting Solution with Fluorescein

It has been suggested that the fluorescein can be observed for longer periods in the eye if it is dissolved in wetting solution rather than irrigating solution. A mixture of wetting solution and fluorescein can be prepared

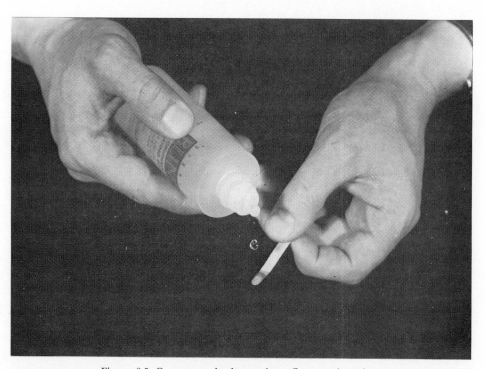

Figure 8.5. Correct method to moisten fluorescein strip.

PLATE I

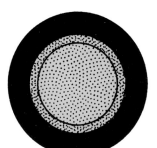

Fluorescein pattern: spherical cornea. Monocurve lens fitted steep.

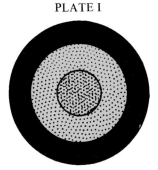

Fluorescein pattern: spherical cornea. Monocurve lens fitted flat.

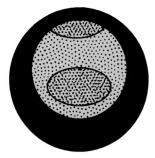

Fluorescein pattern: spherical cornea. Monocurve lens fitted flat. High riding position.

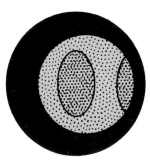

Fluorescein pattern: spherical cornea. Monocurve lens fitted flat. Nasal riding position.

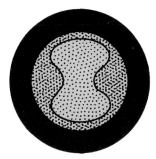

Fluorescein pattern: with-the-rule corneal toricity. Monocurve lens fitted slightly steeper than horizontal corneal meridian.

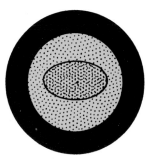

Fluorescein pattern: with-the-rule corneal toricity. Monocurve lens fitted slightly flatter than horizontal corneal meridian.

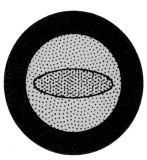

Fluorescein pattern: with-the-rule corneal toricity. Monocurve lens fitted much flatter than horizontal corneal meridian.

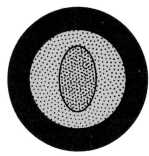

Fluorescein pattern: against-the-rule corneal toricity. Monocurve lens fitted slightly flatter than vertical corneal meridian.

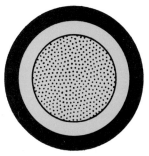

Fluorescein pattern: spherical cornea. Bicurve lens with O.Z. parallel to cornea and P.C. clearance.

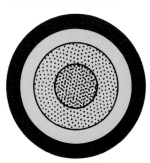

Fluorescein pattern: spherical cornea. Bicurve lens with O.Z. fitted flatter than central cornea.

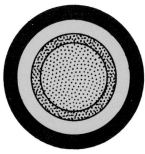

Fluorescein pattern: spherical cornea. Bicurve lens with O.Z. fitted steeper than central cornea.

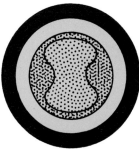

Fluorescein pattern: with-the-rule corneal toricity. Bicurve lens with O.Z. fitted slightly steeper than flattest corneal meridian.

PLATE II

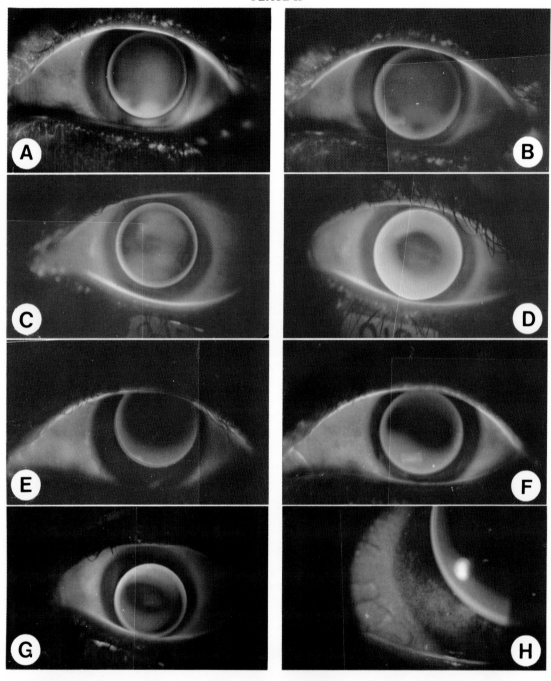

A) Small diameter bicurve lens with flat, narrow peripheral curve on a spherical cornea with minimum apical clearance.

B) Medium diameter bicurve lens with wide peripheral curve fitted on a spherical cornea with minimum apical clearance.

C) Bicurve lens fitted *on K* to with-the-rule toric (1.50 D) cornea.

D) Bicurve lens fitted 2.00 D flatter than K to a toric (1.00 D) cornea.

E) Bicurve lens fitted 1.50 D flatter than K to a spherical cornea.

F) Bicurve lens fitted *on K* to an oblique toric (2.50 D) cornea.

G) Low riding bicurve lens showing touch at lower periphery.

H) Peripheral (3 to 9 o'clock) corneal fluorescein stain.

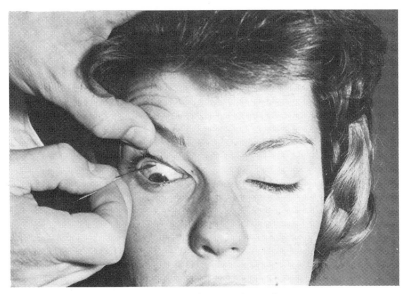

Figure 8.6. Placing fluorescein on the eye.

by soaking a few fluorescein strips in a small quantity of wetting solution. The solution is then instilled with an eyedropper. As an alternate method, it is possible to let a drop of wetting solution fall onto a dry strip from the bottle. It should be realized that the use of wetting solution, which is considerably more viscous than natural tear fluid, may create an abnormally thick tear layer.

FLUORESCENT EXAMINATION LAMPS

Various ultraviolet lamps are available that have been designed specifically for illuminating the fluorescein used in ophthalmic solutions, but many other types of ultraviolet lamps can be used for the same purpose. There are definite differences, however, in the amount of fluorescence that will be apparent when using the various lamps.

The most inexpensive "fluorescent" lamp consists of an incandescent source and a blue filter, which limits the transmitted light to the shorter wavelengths. It is available in flashlight form and has the advantage of portability, but it is disadvantageous in that it produces a minimum of fluorescence. A filter of Corning blue, No. 502, 503, or 554, has been recommended for screening the unwanted visible light.[4] Greater fluorescence can be obtained with ordinary fluorescent lamps (except those with pink or orange phosphers, which give them daylight spectral emission characteristics) when used with blue filters. The best results, however, are obtained by using ultraviolet fluorescent lamps, which have special phosphers that have a high emission, in the region of 300 mμ to 400 mμ, and which peak at about 350 mμ. Of course, ultraviolet germicidal lamps should never be used, as they have a high emission in the spectral region of 290 mμ and may cause injury to the eye.[11] With the long ultraviolet wavelengths emitted by lamps used in contact lens work, there is no possible damage to the eye, and the fitter need not be concerned about the length of exposure.

Commercial lamps that are commonly used for the observation of fluorescein under a contact lens are as follows:

1. Burton lamp—equipped with a +5.00 D. magnifying lens, which aids in viewing the contact lens (Figure 8.7).

2. American Optical fluorescent lamp.

3. American Optical Hague lamp—emits more light than is actually needed for contact lens purposes. This lamp is designed for use in cataract surgery.

4. Slit-lamp biomicroscopes usually have a short wavelength filter, which may be used to view the fluorescein pattern.

THE FLUORESCEIN PATTERN

The general appearance of the illuminated fluorescent tear layer under a contact lens is commonly referred to as the *fluorescein pattern.* It is best observed when only the light from the ultraviolet lamp is present (Figure 8.8).

Learning to evaluate fluorescein patterns requires a certain amount of practice and experience. Photographic reproductions and

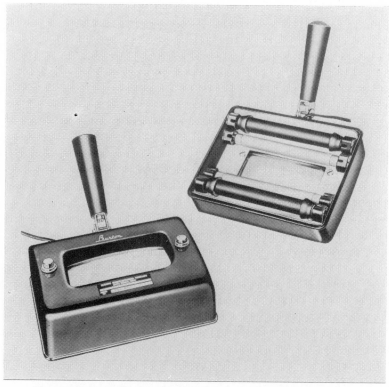

Figure 8.7. Burton lamp. Courtesy of Burton Manufacturing Co.

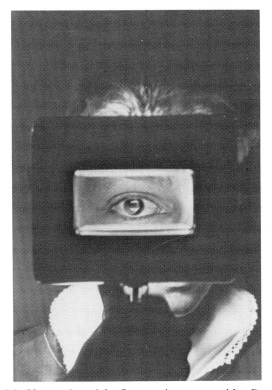

Figure 8.8. Observation of the fluorescein pattern with a Burton lamp.

drawings of fluorescein patterns often give rise to the misconception that their observation is not difficult. It must be appreciated, however, that the actual fluorescein pattern constantly changes as the lens moves on the eye with blinking, ocular movements, and gravity. Haynes et al. have listed various factors that contribute to the varying thickness of the tear layer behind the contact lens and, hence, to the appearance of the fluorescein pattern.[12]

1. Shape of the ocular surface of the contact lens

2. Topography of the cornea

3. Viscosity of the precorneal fluid

4. Wetting characteristics of the cornea and contact lens

5. Amount of tears

6. Gravity

7. Eye movements

8. Lid movements

Fluorescein patterns are usually illustrated with the contact lens in a centered position. Most fitters observe the pattern in the same way. If the lens does not center itself, the lower lid can be manipulated to bring the lens into a centered position.[13]

When the lens is in a centered position, the fluorescein pattern may appear to be very different from when the lens is moving freely.[14] These variations have prompted various authors to differentiate between a fluorescein pattern when the lens is centered (the *static pattern*) and when the lens is allowed to move freely (the *dynamic pattern*).

In evaluating any fluorescein pattern it should be remembered that the brighter the appearance of the fluorescein, the greater the thickness of the tear layer beneath the contact lens. Of course, some of the fluorescence seen comes from the tear layer formed on the anterior surface of the contact lens, but this tear layer is very thin and uniform and causes little interference with the pattern formed by the tears behind the lens.

Monocurve Lens Fluorescein Pattern

The appearance of fluorescein patterns are most easily observed with monocurve lenses that are fitted to a cornea having a spherical cap and a periphery that is flattened symmetrically in all meridians. The patterns are identical to those of the optical zone patterns in all other types of contact lenses.

As was illustrated previously, a monocurve contact lens cannot usually be made to parallel the cornea. If the lens has the same curvature as the central cornea, it will come to rest on the corneal periphery and will have the appearance of a steep lens. The fluorescein pattern will appear bright green in the center of the lens, indicating corneal clearance, and fade into a dark band at the lens periphery, indicating a lens touch in that area (Plate I). Since the cornea is somewhat compressible, the areas of touch will be greater than that predicted by a geometric illustration.

If the lens is flattened appreciably, it will tend to rest mainly on the central portion of the cornea and leave the lens periphery free of corneal contact. The fluorescein pattern will have a dark area in the center of the lens, where it touches the cornea, and a bright green pool will surround it (Plate I). This, of course, assumes that the lens has a centered position. In practice, the lens will probably rock in one direction until its periphery touches the cornea. Usually the lens will ride in a somewhat superior position and the fluorescein pattern will have two touch areas, one at the superior periphery (Plate I) and the other at the corneal apex, between which there will be an area of fluorescein pooling where the lens bridges the cornea. A similar pattern will be found if the lens lags downward or to either side (Plate I). This illustrates that a monocurve lens, which is much flatter than the central cornea, can effectively

be a steep lens when it rides onto the flattened corneal periphery.

The preceding examples illustrate only the possible variation in the appearance of the fluorescein pattern for a simple cornea and simple lens construction. As the contact lens moves over the cornea, the areas of touch are shifted and change rapidly in size, and the fluorescent areas vary in brightness as different amounts of tears are pumped under the lens. With more complicated corneal curvatures, the fluorescein pattern becomes much more difficult to interpret. Even if the central cornea is nearly spherical, some irregularity usually occurs in the corneal periphery. When a monocurve lens is fitted slightly steeper than the flattest meridian on a cornea that has with-the-rule toricity, there is a tendency for the periphery of the lens to bear more heavily on the horizontal or flattest corneal meridian. The fluorescein pattern for this condition shows dark areas in the periphery of the horizontal meridian corresponding to these touch areas (Plate I). If a flat lens is fitted to the same cornea, the touch area occurs at the central region and is elliptical, with the long axis horizontal (Plate I); the greater the degree of corneal toricity or the flatter the lens in relation to the cornea, the longer the ellipse (Plate I).

The fluorescein pattern of a lens that is fitted flat on a cornea with against-the-rule toricity will show just a 90° reversal of with-the-rule toricity.

False Fluorescein Patterns

Occasionally a fluorescein pattern may occur that appears to be just the opposite of what is expected and which is due to the absence of the fluorescein from its expected position. For example, if the lens fits steeply, as in Plate I, it is sometimes possible for the fluorescein to move over and around the contact lens without being able to flow beneath the lens. The whole lens remains dark, or a little fluorescein may collect at the bottom, giving the appearance of a flat fit. Suspicion of this type of fluorescein pattern is verified by instilling more fluorescein and in manipulating the lens by having the patient blink several times.

A lens may also appear dark, as in the preceding example, when it is fitted very flat. If only a little fluorescein has been placed on the eye, it may drain out from beneath the lens before it is observed, and the lens may appear dark. Again, this suspicion is tested by instilling more fluorescein.

Bicurve Lens

The fluorescein pattern formed by a bicurve lens will have two distinct zones, which correspond to the areas of the optical zone and peripheral curve. Its appearance can be most easily illustrated in the example of a bicurve lens that is placed upon a perfectly spherical cornea. If the optical zone of the lens has the same radius as the cornea, there will be perfect alignment (neglecting tear thickness) for the optical zone of the lens. This is seen in the fluorescein pattern as a dim and uniform glow of the fluorescein in the area of the optical zone, which indicates that only a thin layer of tears is present. In the position corresponding to the peripheral curve there will be a bright green band caused by the fluorescein of the thicker layer of tears in the space between the peripheral curve and the cornea (Plate I).

Unfortunately, most fluorescein patterns for bicurve lenses are not so easily analyzed. There are numerous variations for the pattern of an incorrectly fitted bicurve lens, and these can only be understood by having a detailed knowledge of the corneal contour and of possible lens-cornea relationships.

Interpretation of Pattern

The fluorescein pattern for a bicurve lens must be interpreted in terms of the simultaneous effects on all parts of the pattern, which are caused by the individual fitting relationships of the optical zone and peripheral curves of the lens. The bearing relationship of the peripheral curve of the contact lens can influence the fit of the optical zone, and conversely, the bearing relationship of the optical zone can influence the fit of the peripheral curve. For example, if the peripheral curve of the lens is considerably steeper than the cornea upon which it is worn, there will be bearing at the edge of the lens, and the entire optical zone will be held free of corneal contact. The fluorescein pattern will show clearance for the optical zone regardless of the relationship between the base curve of the lens and the cornea. Consequently, the fluorescein pattern for the optical zone can be misleading unless the peripheral curve is either parallel to or flatter than the cornea. Once the peripheral curve is made flatter than the cornea, however, further flattening has very little effect on the fit of the base curve, except that the lens may become loose and more difficult to judge.

It is also found that if the optical zone of the contact lens has a flatter curvature than the central cornea, the peripheral curve of the lens is held away from the cornea and gives the appearance in a fluorescein pattern of excessive flatness. Therefore, the fluorescein pattern for the peripheral curve can be misleading unless the optical zone is parallel to or steeper than the cornea.

To eliminate the confusion in interpreting fluorescein patterns caused by the interdependence of the various curves of a lens, Dunn and others have recommended the use of special bicurve trial lenses, which allow separate fluorescein evaluations of the fit for either the optical zone or peripheral curve of the lens.[15]

However, the technique of Dunn is seldom used in practice because of the time consumed in the lengthy trial lens procedure.

Practically, it has been found that the effect of the fit of one zone upon the fit of another zone is not as great as might be expected. For example, even if the peripheral curve of a lens is slightly steeper than the cornea, the lens will tend to compress the cornea so that the optical zone will be closer to the cornea than anticipated. Hence, small deviations from parallelism do not greatly affect the appearance of the fluorescein pattern, but any considerable bearing must be considered in the interpretation of fluorescein patterns.

It should be remembered that the effect of one zone upon the other in a fluorescein pattern will be a minimum when each curve is parallel to the cornea.

When an understanding has been gained about the influence of the various zones of the contact lens upon the total fluorescein pattern, it then becomes possible to estimate what the effect will be of a faulty fit of one zone upon the other. This procedure will then make it possible to derive more information from the observation of a single lens.

In order to obtain maximum information from the use of fluorescein in the trial lens testing procedure, most trial lenses are designed with peripheral curves that are somewhat flatter than would be needed to fit the average cornea. Consequently, when used for testing the majority of corneas, the trial lenses will have clearance of the peripheral curve or will have such a slight touch that little interference occurs with the fit of the optical zone. The peripheral curves are not made so flat that it is impossible to learn anything about their fit.

When the trial lens is placed on the cornea, the first observation that should be made is whether the peripheral curve has clearance. If there is considerable peripheral touch, a lens with flatter peripheral curve should be used. If such a lens is not available, a smaller lens can be used to reduce contact in the periphery.

Peripheral curve clearance can be verified if a bright fluorescein band is present for the entire area corresponding to the peripheral curve (Plate I). When the clearance of the periphery has been verified, an evaluation can be made of the fit for the optical zone.

As mentioned previously, the appearance of the optical zone for various corneas is analogous to the appearance of a small monocurve lens. However, because the optical zone is smaller than a monocurve lens, it is often possible to match the optical zone of the bicurve lens to the corneal curve so that the fluorescein pattern appears uniform over the entire optical zone. This is usually considered an ideal fit (Plate I). It is frequently found that the trial lens with an optical zone radius that is equal to the corneal curvature as found by keratometry gives the most uniform fluorescein pattern for the optical zone. This lens should be tried first.

If the original lens has apical touch (Plate I), a second trial lens should be used that has a radius of 0.05 mm. shorter. If the original lens has excessive apical clearance (Plate I), a second trial lens should be used with a radius that is 0.05 mm. longer. The trial lens should be changed in a systematic procedure until the optical zone radius that gives the most uniform fluorescein pattern is found.

Sometimes the contact lens that gives the most uniform fluorescein pattern has an optical zone radius which is 0.05 to 0.10 mm. longer than the curvature of the cornea as determined by the keratometer. This indicates either that the cornea has a very small cap and flattens rapidly towards the periphery or that the keratometer measurement is not valid for this cornea. This situation illustrates the need for verification of the fit of a lens by using fluorescein if the optical zone is to be fitted as nearly parallel to the cornea as possible.

Because of the flattening in the corneal periphery it will be found that, as a rule, lenses with larger optical zones will have to be flattened proportionately more in order to show near parallelism by the fluorescein test.

Basis for the Fluorescein Pattern of the Optical Zone

The appearance of the fluorescein pattern of the optical zone will depend upon the size of the corneal cap (if present), the size of the optical zone, and the curvatures of the optical zone and cornea. Since it is rare to find a corneal cap that is larger than 4 mm. and the optical zones of the trial lenses are 7.0 and 7.5 mm. in diameter, it is not theoretically possible to have exact parallelism between the optical zone of the lens and the cornea. It is found, however, that if the corneal cap is no more than 2 mm. smaller than the optical zone of the lens, it is possible to obtain a fluorescein pattern that appears to be uniform, indicating parallelism. Hence, the differences between the corneal curve and the optical zone of the contact lens are below the threshold of detectability by fluorescein.

If the cornea does not have a cap, it is not possible to obtain a fluorescein pattern of even bearing. The situation is analogous to trying to fit a large monocurve lens to the cornea. Touch must occur at either the center of the optical zone or at its periphery. Usually it is preferable to have a slight peripheral bearing.

Occasionally a lens will be fitted in such a way that the optical zone touches at both the center and the periphery. A fluorescein pattern will be seen in which there is central and peripheral touch in the optical zone with an annular zone of pooling between. While this pattern is occasionally interpreted as indicating the existence of a negative corneal zone (*see* Chapter 3), it may be explained simply as a consequence of the preceding fitting relationship. If a flatter base curve is used, it may be found that apical touch occurs so that the previous lens was the closest to parallelism and should be used.

Trial Lens Selection of the Peripheral Curve

Once a trial lens has been fitted to the cornea with the bearing relationship desired, attention should be directed again to the peripheral curve. If the trial lens procedure has been conducted properly, the peripheral curve will be either parallel to the peripheral cornea or too flat. If the curve is too flat, another lens may be tried, or an estimate can be made of how much steeper the curve should be and the lens ordered. When in doubt, it should be made too steep because it can be made flatter by a simple modification.

Often the peripheral curves on trial lenses are not correctly specified, and caution must be exercised not to place too much reliance on their values.

Optimum Fit of the Optical Zone

As stated previously, the ideal fluorescein pattern for a bicurve lens is usually considered to be one in which the optical zone has a thin, even layer of fluorescein and the peripheral zone has a brighter fluorescein layer indicating corneal clearance. Under certain conditions, however, the lens is purposely altered from this ideal fitting arrangement of *corneal alignment or parallelism*. The lens may be slightly steeper than the cornea to produce *apical clearance*, which is recognized by a slight pooling in the center of the optical zone, or the lens may be fitted slightly flatter than the cornea to produce *apical touch*, which is recognized by a slight darkening of the central 2 to 3 mm. of the optical zone.

When an attempt is made to fit a lens with its optical zone parallel to a cornea with low toricity, it is found that greater bearing will occur along the flattest meridian. Hence, in with-the-rule toric corneas, a slight pooling will occur in the superior and inferior portions of the optical zone, which increases with the amount of toricity.

Fluorescein Pattern for Toric Corneas

The appearance of the fluorescein pattern for a toric cornea will depend upon the amount of corneal toricity, the axes of the principal meridians, the curves on the posterior surface of the contact lens, and the position of the lens.

Assume a cornea with 2.00 D. of with-the-rule toricity. A contact lens that is centered on the cornea has an optical zone which is slightly steeper than the flatter (horizontal) corneal meridian. Since the vertical corneal meridian is steeper, a space exists between the lens and cornea at the superior and inferior periphery of the vertical meridian. This space will fill with tear fluid. The fluorescein pattern will show apical clearance in the horizontal meridian. A bright green area will be present at the top and bottom of the pattern, corresponding to the space between the lens and cornea at these positions (Plate I). This lens may not remain in a centered position. It may be moved to a high riding position. The fluorescein pattern will then show a touch area at the lower portion of the lens, which corresponds to the flattest (horizontal) corneal meridian. Another touch area will occur at the top of the lens, where it is touching the flattened corneal periphery. Between the two touch areas will occur a small zone of corneal clearance, which appears bright green. Fluid is often stagnated in this area and causes physiological trauma to the cornea.

If the lens is substituted by another having an optical zone equal in radius to the vertical corneal meridian, the lens will be steeper than the horizontal corneal meridian, and heavy bearing will occur at the horizontal periphery of the optical zone. The fluorescein pattern will show two dark bands of touch at these positions. The remainder of the lens will have a near parallelism to the cornea and will show an even fluorescein layer.*

If the lens is substituted by another having an optical zone radius that is in between the radii of the principal corneal meridians, the fluorescein pattern is again changed. Some bearing will still occur in the horizontal meridian at the periphery of the optical zone; however, it will be distributed over a larger corneal area. The bearing will occur over a large area of the horizontal meridian, and minimally in the periphery of the optical

---

*If the lens were fitted this way, the bearing in the horizontal meridian would cause corneal trauma.

zone. The fluorescein pattern will be a broad dumbbell or H figure.

By varying the optical zone radius of trial lenses, a lens may be found that best distributes the lens bearing over a large corneal area. The lens usually has a radius that is slightly steeper than the flattest corneal meridian. It can often be predicted by calculating one-third of the total corneal toricity and adding this to the flattest corneal meridian. For example, if the principal corneal meridians are 40.00 and 43.00 D., the optical zone radius of the lens tried first would be 8.23 mm. (41.00 D.). On the basis of the fluorescein pattern, further modifications of the optical zone radius are made.

When the corneal toricity is either against the rule or oblique, the same fitting rules apply as for with-the-rule toricity. The bearing areas of the fluorescein pattern will now be shifted to correspond to the principal corneal meridians.

False Fluorescein Patterns for Bicurve Lenses

As occurred for the monocurve lens, the fluorescein pattern of a bicurve lens may give invalid results. If either the optical zone or peripheral curve is too flat in relation to the cornea, the fluorescein may drain before the pattern is viewed. If either the optical zone or the peripheral curve is too steep, the fluorescein may be blocked from flowing behind the lens. In either case, the lens will look dark. Suspicion that this has happened should be verified by instilling more fluorescein.

Tricurve lenses

Tricurve lenses present fluorescein patterns that are similar to those of bicurve lenses. They differ in that the peripheral curve usually shows adequate clearance so that a bright band of fluorescein is present in the lens periphery. A touch area is usually present under the intermediate curve, which shows little or no fluorescence. The optical zone pattern may be interpreted in the same way as for bicurve lenses. The intermediate curve should show some area of clearance as the lens moves about on the cornea in order that pumping action may be executed.

Fluorescein Pattern for Ultrathin Lenses

The fluorescein pattern for an ultrathin lens appears more uniform than for a regular lens, apparently because the ultrathin lens conforms more closely to the cornea due to its flexibility. Even when the lens is slightly steeper than the cornea, there is almost always less central pooling than might be expected. A definite band of fluorescein should be noted at the position of the peripheral curve. This band is usually greater than expected based on the steep peripheral curves that are being used. An annulus of intermediate bearing will be noticed on most lenses. An attempt should be made to strive for a fluorescein pattern that has the most uniform bearing relationship. It is not necessary to use definite apical clearance, as is often found to be necessary with a regular contact lens. In fact, it is usually found that a slight central touch is tolerated with no difficulty.

Fluorescein Photography

It is possible to photograph the fluorescein pattern and obtain a permanent record of the lens bearing relationship (Plate II). Simple camera arrangements may be used for color or black and white photographs.

Accuracy of the Fluorescein Pattern

There is considerable disagreement between the advocates of the keratometer fitting method and the trial lens fitting method as to the accuracy by which the fluorescein pattern can be judged.

Bronstein tested the ability of a practitioner to use fluorescein to evaluate the fitting characteristics of contact lenses.[16] The examiner was experienced at interpreting fluorescein patterns and was confident of his proficiency with this technique. He was given a trial set of bicurve lenses, 9.2 mm. in total diameter with peripheral curves 0.4 mm. wide and 12.25 mm. in radius. The optical zone radii of the lenses varied from 7.5 mm. to 8.2 mm. The examiner was asked to place the lenses on a subject and determine which lenses most perfectly paralleled the cornea and also to determine the ranking of the trial lenses in terms of the optical zone radii.

The subject did not normally wear contact lenses but had worked with contact lenses and could wear them with little difficulty. His corneal curvature as measured by keratometry was 43.62 D. axis 90° and 43.87 D. axis 180°. Only the right eye was used for the experiment. The examiner placed each lens on the right eye of the subject and evaluated the fluorescein pattern. He categorized the optical zone radii according to one of five relationships to the cornea: very steep, steep, close to parallel, flat, and very flat. He then repeated the examination for all of the lenses and ranked them in order from the steepest to the flattest optical zone. Table 8.2 gives the optical zone radii of the trial lenses as measured with a microspherometer and the order in which they were ranked by the examiner.

TABLE 8.2

Correct Order as Measured on Microspherometer	Order Determined by Fluorescein Examination
7.50	7.50
7.55	7.70
7.61	7.78
7.65	7.65
7.70	7.61
7.73	7.55
7.78	7.73
7.86	7.92
7.92	7.95
8.00	8.00
8.08	8.20
8.10	8.16
8.16	8.10
8.20	8.08

The radius of curvature of the cornea as measured with the keratometer repeatedly was 7.73 mm. The optical zone radius of the contact lens that most nearly fitted the cornea, as determined by fluorescein and trial lenses, was 7.86 mm. From an examination of Table 8.2, it may be seen that the ability to rank the lenses by optical zone radii was not very good.

Bronstein states that the experiment was repeated several times with similar results obtained and concludes that it is extremely difficult to determine the curvature of the cornea accurately by examining the fluorescein patterns of trial lenses.

Bronstein's experiment points out several important facts about the fluorescein test, but his conclusions are not necessarily valid. The examiner's ability to select the trial lens with the correct optical zone radius is compared to the keratometer measurement, but there is no reason for assuming that the keratometer measurement is valid for this particular cornea. The optical zone radius of a contact lens that appears to parallel the cornea on the basis of the fluorescein test will almost always be longer than the corneal radius as measured with the keratometer.[17] The optical zone would have to be flatter than the central corneal curvature in order to parallel the larger corneal area.

In a study by Brungardt in which seventy-five beginning contact lens practitioners were asked to evaluate fluorescein patterns, the results indicated a good ability to evaluate fluorescein patterns.[18] The practitioners were given some training in the recognition of fluorescein patterns and were then divided into pairs and asked to find the lens from a trial set that most closely paralleled a subject's cornea. The criterion for the correct lens was that lens judged by Brungardt as having a parallel fit by the fluorescein test.

It was found that sixty-eight of the participants were able to find the correct contact lens that paralleled the cornea within an error of 0.25 D.

BIOMICROSCOPY

Even before fluorescein was used in evaluating the fitting characteristics of a contact lens, many practitioners learned to judge whether or not there was clearance between the contact lens and the cornea by observing if tears could be seen behind the lens with the biomicroscope.[19] Although it is possible to make a judgment of the lens-cornea relationship in this way, the transparency of tears, contact lens, and cornea makes their differentiation extremely difficult. The problem may be overcome, however, if the tears are stained with fluorescein. Modern types of biomicroscopes are usually equipped with a filter to transmit blue light, which will activate fluorescein,* and the general fluorescein pattern may then be viewed with the added advantage of the magnification provided by the biomicroscope.

METHODS OF OBSERVATION

Direct

With fluorescein in the tears and with the lids in a natural position, the fluorescein pattern of the lens is observed with the microscope at low power using diffuse blue illumination. The patient is allowed to blink normally so that there is a shifting of the

---

*In testing various biomicroscopes, it was noted that considerable variation exists in the capacity of their blue lights to activate the fluorescein.

lens, first upward as it is drawn with the lid and then downward from gravitational force until the lens stabilizes. It is difficult to evaluate the fit of the lens when it is in motion. After the lens stops moving, the tear fluid will continue in motion for a short time, as can be seen by watching the debris and bubbles moving between the lens and the cornea. By noting the size of the particles, their speed of movement, and the path that they follow, it is possible to determine the areas of clearance between the lens and cornea. Larger particles will be seen close to the edge and in positions of excessive clearance, whereas smaller particles will be found nearer the center of the contact lens and in positions of minimum clearance.[19] After each blink small bubbles will usually form at the bottom of the contact lens and move upward in the interspace between the contact lens and the cornea, mainly in the peripheral zone. They vary in size and the speed at which they move, and their paths also provide clues to the variation in depth of the pool of lacrimal fluid between the contact lens and the cornea. It should be understood, however, that the movements of the particles and bubbles do not necessarily indicate the actual flow of the tears under the contact lens.

Cross Section

Another method that is sometimes used for observing the tear layer with the biomicroscope is to view a cross section of the lens-cornea relationship. This is accomplished by using a narrow slit beam, which is directed at the cornea at an angle of at least 60° to the axis of the microscope in the same way as is used for normal sectional viewing of the cornea. It is then possible to see the various layers of the tears and contact lens. If the tears are stained with fluorescein, the appearance is that of a green layer representing the outer layer of tears on the lens, then a wider black layer, which is the contact lens, next another green layer representing the

tears between the lens and cornea, and then a bright greyish layer, which is the cornea. The fitting relationship between the lens and cornea can be judged by noting the thickness of the tear layer at various points. Several authors question the usefulness of this type of observation.[20,21] One of the greatest difficulties is in trying to view the lens under magnification when it is in constant motion. Korb found that three trained observers had difficulty in distinguishing trial lenses that were less than 0.15 mm. different in radius than the cornea when only a small corneal area was viewed at one time.[21] When the entire corneal area was viewed, however, it was possible to recognize differences in base curves of the lenses used of 0.05 mm. He points out that there was considerable difference between the usefulness of the various biomicroscopes for observation of contact lenses.

Korb makes the following conclusions about the use of the biomicroscope as an aid to fitting contact lenses.[21]

1. In some biomicroscopes the source of illumination is not of sufficient intensity to activate the fluorescein when a cobalt (blue) filter is used over the light source. While the standard white source does supply some illumination in the range required to activate fluorescein, a critical appreciation cannot be obtained unless the source is filtered with a cobalt or similar filter.

2. The corneal area that can be illuminated in a diffuse manner is frequently of small dimension. Thus, with the fluorescein filter it is impossible to illuminate the area required to view the entire cornea-lens relationship simultaneously.

3. The field of view diminishes quite rapidly as the magnification is increased. Thus, with many instruments it is not possible to utilize more than ten times magnification and still retain an adequate field of view. The microscope must therefore provide a wide field of view if the higher magnifications are to be used.

4. The number and choice of available

magnifications assume a more critical role than in normal biomicroscopy. As stated, it is important to observe the total area of the lens with black light. Many instruments are designed with only two magnifications, a high and a low. Usually the low is not adequate for the mentioned observations, offering little more than the standard black light magnifiers, while the high magnification severely limits the field of view.

It should also be noted that the observations of the section of the contact lens can be made in only one meridian at a time, and some instruments cannot be used for observation of any but the vertical meridian. The appearance of the structures viewed will vary with the angle and position of the illuminating slit and the microscope and with the amount of fluorescein that is present in the eye.

EVALUATION OF THE LENS EDGE

In addition to its use in evaluating the bearing relationships of the contact lens, the biomicroscope allows the observer to judge whether the lens edge is shaped in such a way that it does not injure the limbus. When the lens rides over the limbal area onto the sclera, it may press upon the bulbar conjunctiva, and this will show as a blanched streak in that area. If blanching occurs and it is apparent that the lens, under normal wearing conditions, rides so as to touch the limbus for extended periods, then the edge must be modified until the blanching no longer exists. This usually occurs in the case of a high riding lens. It may be verified by directing the patient to look downward and retracting the upper lid so that the pressure of the lower lid will push the lens up onto the upper limbal area. If the edge curve is not correctly shaped, there will be pressure of the edge of

the contact lens against the conjunctiva, which will be recognized by blanching of the limbal conjunctiva.[22]

It is also possible to detect a lens edge that is too thick by observation with the biomicroscope. Have the patient look up, then focus the slit and the microscope on the lower lid. Instruct the patient to move his eyes slowly downward and observe as the lens approaches the lower lid. If the lens is too thick, it will bump against the lower lid and will be supported as the eye moves down. The same thing can be seen by having the patient look straight ahead and gently retracting the upper lid so that it slides along toward the eyebrow without everting, until it passes the edge of the contact lens. Then slowly lift the lid up and let it down, and watch the lid pass over the edge of the contact lens.

LENS POWER

The trial lens fitting method greatly simplifies the procedure for finding the lens power for the final prescription. The contact lens should be worn for a sufficient period of time so that near normal tearing is resumed. With the lenses in place, a normal refraction is performed including both retinoscopy and subjective tests.

If the results of the refraction through the

contact lens show a spherical refractive error is present, the final lens prescription will be in spherical form. The true refractive error (R.E.) found by the refraction through the contact lenses is the sum of the then remaining refractive error and the lens power that was present in the trial lens.

$$\text{R.E.} = F_{measured} + F_{trial\ lens}$$

For example, if, through a trial lens of −3.00 D., a refractive error of −1.00 D. is found, the true refractive error of the patient would be −4.00 D. The final lens ordered for the patient should have a power of −4.00 D. If the refraction through the same trial lens had been +2.00 D., the final prescription would be −1.00 D.

If the refraction should be of higher power than 4.00 D., it is necessary to correct for the vertex distance. For example, the refraction through a trial lens of −3.00 D. sphere power is −8.00 D. The effective power of a −8.00 D. lens at the corneal plane is −8.75 D., assuming a vertex distance of 12 mm. The final prescription would be −8.75 (+) −3.00 or −11.75 D.

If the trial lenses are approximately −3.00 D., they will be near to the refractive error for the majority of contact lens patients. Small differences from the −3.00 D. power will not require any correction for vertex distance.

RESIDUAL ASTIGMATISM

One of the greatest advantages of the trial lens fitting method is that residual astigmatism can be determined before the final lenses are ordered. The refraction through the contact lens will show directly how much residual astigmatism will be present.

For example, if the refraction through a −3.00 D. lens is −1.00 −1.00 × 180 the final prescription should be −4.00 −1.00 × 180. The astigmatism will be the same for the final lens as it was for the refraction through the trial lens. A decision must be made if the residual astigmatism is of sufficient power to cause visual difficulty. If so, one of the special lenses must be used into which a cylindrical power can be incorporated.

If the residual astigmatism is less than 0.50 D. and can be ignored, the final prescription can be determined by two methods. It can be based on the equivalent sphere of the final refractive error. A subjective examination can be performed using only spherical lenses. The final prescription is the most positive power lens or least negative power lens that gives the patient the best acuity. The spherical lens subjective can be taken immediately following the spherocylindrical subjective when residual astigmatism is present. It is the usual method for arriving at the final spherical correction.

EXCESS ACCOMMODATION

Various authors have reported a tendency of a few patients to accommodate when a contact lens is worn for the first time.[23] This accommodation may cause the refractionist to overcorrect the myopic trial lens wearer or undercorrect the hyperopic wearer. After the wearer becomes adapted to his contact lenses, the accommodation is relaxed, and the patient then must have positive power added to his lenses. Accommodation should be suspected when the measured and predicted refractive error are not reasonably close.

SUMMARY OF TRIAL LENS PROCEDURE

1. Take keratometry measurement.
2. Select trial lens whose base curve is nearest to *K* value. Place lens on eye.
3. Allow patient to adapt to lens.
4. Observe lens dynamics.
5. Instill fluorescein and observe pattern.

6. Substitute new trial lens as determined by tests 4 and 5.

7. Perform refraction through trial len-ses.

8. Order special trial lenses from laboratory or final lenses.

REFERENCES

1. Moss, H. I.: The contour principle in contact lens fitting, *J. Am. Optom. Assoc.*, *29*(9):579–581, 1958.

2. Schapero, M.: The question of contact trial lenses. How many and what kind? *J. Am. Optom. Assoc.*, *34*(8):634–636, 1963.

3. Obrig, T. E.: *Contact Lenses*, 2nd ed. Philadelphia, Chilton, 1947, p. 153.

4. Lester, R. W.: Fluorescein and contact lenses, *Contacto*, *2*(4):91–95, 1958.

5. Morris, M. M.: A new method of fluorescein installation, *The Optician*, *142*:419, 1961.

6. Kimura, S. J.: Fluorescein paper, *Am. J. Ophthalmol.*, *34*(3):446–447, 1951.

7. Vaughn, D. G., Jr.: The contamination of fluorescein solutions, *Am. J. Ophthalmol.*, *39*(1):55–61, 1955.

8. Theodore, F. H.: Contamination of eye solutions, *Am. J. Ophthalmol.*, *34*(12):1764, 1951.

9. Theodore, F. H., and Minsky, H. J.: Lack of sterility of eye medicaments, *J.A.M.A.*, *147*:1381, 1951.

10. Krezanoski, J. Z., Hind, H. W., and Szekely, I. J.: Pharmaceutical aspects of contact lenses and their solutions, *J. Am. Pharm. Assoc.*, *NS2*(7):417–422, 438, 1962.

11. Cogan, D. G., and Kinsey, V. E.: Action spectrum of keratitis produced by ultraviolet radiation, *Arch. Ophthalmol.*, *35*(6):670–677, 1946.

12. Brungardt, T. F., Pollock, E. D., and Haynes, P. R.: Use of fluorescein in the fitting of contact lenses, in *Encyclopedia of Contact Lens Practice*, South Bend, Indiana, International Optics, 1959–1963, vol. 1, Chap.

10, pp. 3–44.

13. Feinbloom, W.: Personal demonstration, 1958.

14. Chiquiar-Arias, V.: Reshaping the cornea in keratoconus, *Contacto*, *8*(1):6–10, 1964.

15. Dunn, G. M.: Independent curve corneal fitting, *The Optician*, *138*:501–503, 1959.

16. Bronstein, L.: The accuracy of fluorescein for determining corneal curvature, *Contacto*, *3*(6):170–171, 1959.

17. Dickinson, F.: The role of the keratometer: a survey of fifty cases, *Contacto*, *6*(6):160–161, 168–169, 1962.

18. Brungardt, T. F.: Fluorescein patterns: they are accurate and they can be mastered, *J. Am. Optom. Assoc.*, *32*(12):973–974, 1961.

19. Goodlaw, E. I.: Use of slit lamp biomicroscopy in the fitting of contact lenses, in *Encyclopedia of Contact Lens Practice*, South Bend, Indiana, International Optics, 1959–1963, vol. 2, Chap. 11, pp. 5–47.

20. Abrams, B. S., and Bailey, N. J.: Contact lens news and views, *J. Am. Optom. Assoc.*, *32*(9):725–726, 1961.

21. Korb, D. R.: Recent developments in the observation of the cornea-lens relationship, in *Encyclopedia of Contact Lens Practice*, South Bend, Indiana, International Optics, 1959–1963, vol. 3, App. B, pp. 98–101.

22. Goodlaw, E. I.: The biomicroscope, *J. Calif. Optom. Assoc.*, *27*(2):58–67, 76, 1959.

23. Baldwin, W. R., and Shick, C. R.: *Corneal Contact Lenses: Fitting Procedures*, Philadelphia, Chilton, 1962.

ADDITIONAL READINGS

Brungardt, T. F.: Contact lens clinic (fluorescein and stain), *Optom. Weekly*, *59*(27):42–43, 1968.

Brungardt, T. F.: Contact lens clinic (fluorescein pattern study), *Optom. Weekly*, *59*(32):38–39, 1968.

Brungardt, T. F.: Contact lens clinic (specific diag-

nostic lenses), *Optom. Weekly*, *59*(39):40–41, 1968.

Brungardt, T. F.: Contact lens clinic—fluorescein stain: central corneal abrasion, *Optom. Weekly*, *60*(7):50–51, 1969.

Brungardt, T. F.: Contact lens clinic—fluorescein

stain: central corneal abrasion, *Optom. Weekly*, 60(3):46–47, 1969.

Brungardt, T. F.: Fluorescein: pattern analysis and staining, *J. Am. Optom. Assoc.*, 47(3):333, 1976.

Conlon, J. R., Jr.: Use of a trial set in patient screening, *Contacto*, 3(7):203, 1959.

Filderman, I. P.: Principles of the contact lens "pupilens," *Optom. Weekly*, 53:2389–2396, 1962.

Gamboney, E.: Use of trial lenses in contact lens fitting, *Contacto*, 5(2):63, 1961.

Goldberg, J. B.: Mini-thin contact lenses—a new method for fitting small, thin corneal lenses, *Optom. Weekly*, 60(7):31–38, 1969.

Jenkin, L.: The very small corneal lens, *The Optician*, 154(3998):495–496, 1967.

Lecoeur, G.: Fitting, fluoroscopy, general rules, spherical corneae, *Cah. Verres Contact*, 14:41–48, 1967.

Mandell, R. B.: It's a perfect fit . . . why does he still have problems?, *Int. Cont. Lens Clin.*, 1(3):28–29, 1974.

Chapter 9

ASTIGMATISM

MORTON D. SARVER

THE ULTIMATE OBJECTIVE in the design of a corneal contact lens is to provide a lens whose physical properties are compatible with the physical and physiological characteristics of the eye and whose optical properties provide the necessary visual correction. The toric cornea and the astigmatic refractive error may provide a challenge when designing a lens to meet this objective. The reader must, at the outset, clearly distinguish between the terms *toric cornea* and *astigmatism*. The former is a physical description of corneal curvature, while the latter describes one property of the light rays that have passed through the eye's various refractive interfaces to form an image upon the retina.

Corneal toricity is generally the prime contributor to an astigmatic refractive error, but when the toricity is not too great, it may be present without producing an astigmatism, because of the influence of the other refractive interfaces of the eye.[1] However, an astigmatic refractive error may be present when the cornea is spherical or when the corneal toricity is not in agreement with the astigmatic error produced.[2] These, then, are two separate

considerations in the fitting of corneal contact lenses—corneal toricity (a physical problem) and astigmatism (a refractive or optical problem).

Basic types of contact lenses, made up of spherical surfaces, may or may not satisfy the required optical needs and may or may not provide an acceptable physical fit. More complex lens types, made up of one or more toric surfaces, may be required to achieve an optimum physical fit and/or an optimum correction of the refractive error. Such lenses, however, are more costly, more difficult to manufacture accurately, and more difficult to fit effectively.

This chapter will include a description of the various lens types that may be used to correct an astigmatic refractive error, to fit a toric cornea, to correct a residual astigmatism, and to correct an induced astigmatism. It will include the recommended fitting techniques for each type of lens and a description of the conditions under which each lens type is most useful. Methods of calculating or otherwise determining the required optical specifications will be included where necessary.

CORNEAL TORICITY

Progress has been made in recent years in describing the topography of the human cornea.[3-10] An adequate understanding of corneal toricity is dependent upon a knowledge of the contour of the cornea along each principal meridian—actually, the difference in corneal contour along these meridians. The keratometer provides relatively valid information about the toricity of a small central area of the cornea but very invalid information about the toricity of peripheral corneal regions.

The contour of the cornea, along a single meridian, was described in considerable detail in Chapter 3. It must be pointed out here, however, that the degree of asphericity, or rate of peripheral flattening, may vary in each principal meridian. Since the toricity of a surface is defined as the difference between the radius of curvature of the two principal meridians, the corneal toricity can be said to vary as a function of the corneal annular zone being described. For any such annular zone, the toricity may be greater or less than the central corneal toricity. Korb introduced the term *true toricity* to describe this characteristic of corneal toricity.[11] He points out that, for purposes of obtaining a uniform lens-cornea bearing relationship, the corneal toricity must be evaluated in terms of the optical zone diameter of the contact lens being fitted. This concept is simply an extension of Moss and Bier's contour fit principle to two meridians whose aspherical properties differ. To the same extent that the central keratometer reading of the flatter principal meridian does not fully describe the contour of the cornea in that meridian, so the difference in keratometer readings does not fully describe the toricity of the corneal surface. Clinical observation with contact lenses indicates that, in general, the peripheral areas of the cornea are more toric in the direction of with the rule than are the central areas.[12] These observations and concepts must be borne in mind when consideration is given to the various techniques that may be employed to fit the toric cornea.

THE SPHERICAL LENS

The spherical corneal contact lens is justifiably the lens of choice for fitting the toric cornea and for correcting the astigmatism when this lens construction will provide an optimum physical fit, physiological response, and optical result. Fortunately, this is possible when the corneal toricity is not too great and when this toricity is largely responsible for the astigmatic refractive error. The spherical lens is easier to fit, manufacture, modify, and duplicate than lenses of more complex construction. The various techniques that may be used to fit such a lens have been described in other chapters and will not be repeated here. There are, however, a number of additional considerations that are unique to the fitting of toric corneas with spherical lenses which should be discussed.

A spherical lens fitted exactly parallel to a spherical cornea results in a lens-cornea bearing relationship that might be described as exhibiting a perfect physical fit. The bearing is uniformly distributed over the surface of the cornea. It has long been observed, however, that such a bearing relationship often produces an interference with the adequate interchange of precorneal fluid beneath the lens. The result is a disturbance to the normal metabolism of the cornea and subsequent inability of the patient to tolerate the lens for but brief periods of wear. The problem is resolved by reducing the lens diameter and/or optic zone diameter, increasing the optic zone radius, or increasing the radius of the secondary curve and peripheral curve to obtain a more efficient interchange of precorneal fluid. A spherical lens cannot, on the other hand, be fitted parallel to a toric corneal surface. When, as is common practice, the lens is fitted near parallel to the flatter principal meridian of a toric cornea, it will be flat in relation to the steeper principal meridian of this cornea. Providing the corneal toricity is not so great as to preclude an acceptable physical bearing relationship between the lens and cornea, this kind of fit permits a more efficient interchange of precorneal fluid and results in less disturbance to the normal physiochemistry of the cornea. A small or moderate degree of corneal toricity is, therefore, a desirable characteristic for the fitting of spherical corneal contact lenses.

When the corneal toricity is not too great, a satisfactory lens-cornea bearing relationship can be obtained by fitting the spherical lens essentially parallel to the flatter principal meridian of the cornea. The procedures employed are described in Chapter 8. The limiting corneal toricity that permits use of these procedures is stated by some to be as low as 0.50 D.[13] and by others to be as high as 4.00 D.[14] The limit is best determined by employing spherical diagnostic lenses to evaluate the fit of a spherical lens on the toric cornea in question. Observations should include lens position, lens movement, the fluorescein pattern, and the patient's physical and physiological response when wearing the lens for a period of time. As the toricity of the cornea increases, it becomes more difficult to obtain a satisfactory lens-cornea bearing relationship with a spherical lens. It may sometimes be obtained by using a lens whose base curve is steeper than the flatter principal meridian of the cornea. This is sometimes possible with corneas whose toricity is as great as 6.00 D. *K* reading.

A procedure referred to as splitting *K* has been employed by some fitters to fit a spherical lens to a toric cornea. The base curve of the contact lens has a radius of curvature that is halfway between that of the steeper and flatter meridians of the cornea. The lens diameter must be relatively small (8.0 mm. to 9.0 mm.) to prevent excessive peripheral bearing in the flatter meridian of the cornea. The author prefers a less severe approach. A base curve is selected that permits proper lens performance for the lens design being used without regard to the amount of corneal toricity. When a base curve is selected that is steeper than the flatter principal meridian of

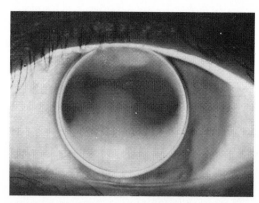

Figure 9.1. The typical dumbbell-shaped fluorescein pattern that is observed when a spherical corneal contact lens is fitted on K to a cornea having a with-the-rule toricity.

the cornea, the resulting fluorescein pattern has the characteristic dumbbell shape (Figure 9.1).

For those fitters who prefer to select or specify the posterior central curve radius (base curve) of the *initial* lens on the basis of the keratometer readings, Table 9.1 is offered as a guide.

A few examples will serve to illustrate the use of this table.

TABLE 9.1

A Guide for Selecting the Optical Zone Curvature (in Diopters *K* Reading) of the Initial Spherical Corneal Contact Lens. ΔK Is the Difference Between the Central Keratometer Readings of the Cornea. *K* Is the Keratometer Reading of the Flatter Principal Corneal Meridian.

Corneal Toricity ΔK	Base Curve
0 to 0.25 D.	K − 0.25 D.
0.50 to 2.00 D.	K
2.00 to 4.00 D.	$K + \dfrac{\Delta K}{4}$
> 4.00 D.	Toric or bitoric

EXAMPLE 1. Keratometer readings are 45.00/90 and 44.00/180; therefore, *ΔK* is 1.00 D., and the base curve is specified as 44.00 D. *K* reading or 7.67 mm. radius.

EXAMPLE 2. Keratometer readings are 47.00/90 and 44.00/180; therefore *ΔK* is 3.00 D., and the base curve is specified as 44.00 + (3.00/4) = 44.75 D. *K* reading or 7.54 mm. radius.

When the toricity of the cornea becomes too great, it is not possible to obtain a satisfactory bearing relationship with a spherical lens. The characteristic observations and patient response to a spherical lens under these conditions include lens decentration, eccentric pooling of the precorneal fluid, superior or lateral dimple veiling, visual disturbance caused by a flare effect, lens rocking, peripheral corneal staining in the flatter meridian, spectacle blur, and physical discomfort. Alleviation of these problems lies in the use of a lens having a toric base curve and/or toric secondary curves. The problems and benefits of such lenses will be described later in this chapter.

RESIDUAL ASTIGMATISM

The term *residual astigmatism*, as used in the contact lens field, must be given an operational definition. This is necessary in order to include within the definition the numerous factors that can contribute to the presence of an astigmatic refractive error with contact lenses. Residual astigmatism will be defined as *the astigmatic refractive error that is present when a contact lens is placed upon the cornea to correct the existing ametropia.* Note that the type of lens, i.e. spherical, toric, is not contained in the definition. This is most consistent with the general use of the term in the contact lens field. It is therefore necessary to qualify the term when it is used descriptively. For example, one may wish to describe the residual astigmatism that is present with a spherical contact lens or the residual astigmatism that is present with a toric base contact lens. Normally, when the term is not qualified, it is understood that reference is being made to the residual astigmatism with a spherical contact lens.

PHYSIOLOGICAL AND INDUCED RESIDUAL ASTIGMATISM

Residual astigmatism, as defined previously, may be subdivided into *physiological residual astigmatism and induced residual astigmatism.* Physiological residual astigmatism is the residual astigmatism that is contributed to the eye's refractive system by any or all of the following:[1,15]

1. That portion of the anterior corneal surface cylinder which is not neutralized by the fluid lens
2. The difference in curvature of the principal meridians of the posterior corneal surface
3. The difference in curvature of the principal meridians at interfaces of the crystalline lens
4. Tilt of the crystalline lens
5. Variability of the refractive index of the cornea, crystalline lens, or vitreous
6. The oblique incidence of light upon the cornea
7. An eccentric position of the fovea in relation to the visual axis
8. Misalignment of the various elements that constitute the optical system of the eye
9. Some irregularity in the shape of macular area

Which of these physiological factors is most responsible for residual astigmatism is not definitely known. Those who feel that the crystalline lens is responsible will often refer to residual astigmatism as *lenticular astigmatism*. Obviously, this is an improper synonym, since it implies knowledge of the anatomical site of the cause of residual astigmatism. Actually it is of little consequence whether the site is lenticular, posterior corneal, or retinal. The contact lens practitioner can do nothing to alter the source of physiological residual astigmatism.

Induced residual astigmatism is the astigmatism that is introduced into the contact lens–eye system by the contact lens itself. Possible causes of induced residual astigmatism are the following:

1. Tilt or decentration of the contact lens.[16-18]
2. Toric anterior and/or posterior surface of the contact lens.[19]
3. Warping or flexure of a very thin contact lens.[20-22]

These factors will be discussed in some detail later in this chapter.

CALCULATED RESIDUAL ASTIGMATISM

The residual astigmatism present with a hard spherical contact lens is calculated by applying the familiar equations of geometrical optics that describe the path of paraxial rays having normal incidence upon a centered optical system. The calculation necessitates certain assumptions that may not be justified for the system being described. The limitations that are imposed upon the accuracy of the calculation, by these assumptions, should be understood by the reader. It is assumed that the keratometer reading of corneal curvature accurately describes the radius of curvature, in each principal meridian, of that portion of the cornea that contributes to the formation of an image upon the fovea. Although the corneal cap has been reported to be spherical along any given meridian,[6,9] more recent research has demonstrated that most of the corneal topography is aspherical.[10] The accuracy with which the keratometer readings will describe the anterior corneal cylinder is a function of the aspherical properties of that part of the cornea through which the line of sight passes. If the keratometer readings do not give a valid description of the anterior corneal cylinder, the calculated residual astigmatism will be in error.

It is assumed that all the astigmatism

resulting from the incidence of light upon the anterior corneal surface is due to the difference in curvature between the two principal meridians of this surface. If the line of sight is oblique to this surface, an additional astigmatic error is imposed upon the refractive state of the eye. If the angle between the line of sight and the normal to the cornea at the point where the line of sight passes through the cornea is about 5°, and if this angle lies in a horizontal plane, an against-the-rule astigmatism of one-half diopter is introduced into the refractive system of the eye.[16,23,24] One study of a small sample of subjects ($N = 9$) demonstrated that the mean value of this angle is about 3°, with a range of from 0.8 to 7.4°.[16] This part of the astigmatism that is produced by the anterior corneal surface is not measured with the keratometer. Thus, the calculated residual astigmatism will be in error.

It is further assumed that the chief ray from an object of regard exhibits normal incidence upon the various refracting surfaces of the contact lens–fluid lens system. When this assumption is not justified, the system produces an oblique astigmatism due to the tilt of one or more of its interfaces relative to the line of sight. In the study previously cited,[16] in which corneal lenses of about 9.5 mm. diameter were fitted on *K*, contact lens tilts that produced up to 0.25 D. of oblique astigmatism were measured. Although this amount of astigmatism is not great, it contributes to the discrepancy that can exist between the calculated and measured residual astigmatism.

It is also assumed that the contact lens does not introduce a cylinder by flexing on the eye. It has been shown that a thin contact lens will flex on a toric cornea and introduce 0.25 D. of cylinder for each 0.25 D. *K* of flexure.[22,25]

The cumulative inaccuracies of the preceding assumptions often produce a difference between the calculated and measured residual astigmatism. This difference will be considered shortly.

There are a number of ways to calculate the residual astigmatism.[2,26-29] The method that will be described here is probably the most direct approach. The calculation is made by simply determining the amount of anterior corneal cylinder that is neutralized by the fluid lens and subtracting this value from the total astigmatism of the eye referred to the plane of the cornea. The amount of anterior corneal cylinder that is neutralized by the fluid lens is taken to be given by ΔK, where ΔK is the difference between the keratometer readings of the two principal meridians of the cornea and is also *the power, in air, of the fluid lens cylinder that is formed by the corneal curves.* Since the keratometer is calibrated for an index of refraction that is equal to, or very nearly equal to, that of the fluid lens, the amount of anterior corneal cylinder that is neutralized by the fluid lens is given directly by ΔK. This ΔK is taken to be a minus cylinder, the axis of which is along the flatter principal meridian of the cornea.

The calculated residual astigmatism (C.R.A.) is determined by subtracting ΔK from the total astigmatism of the eye at the corneal plane. The following examples will serve to illustrate these calculations:

EXAMPLE 1. Given:

Spectacle correction	−2.00 −1.00 ax 180
Keratometer readings	44.00/90 43.00/180

Calculation:

$\Delta K = -1.00$ ax 180

C.R.A. $= (-1.00$ ax $180) - (-1.00$ ax $180) = 0$

EXAMPLE 2. Given:

Spectacle correction	−1.00 −2.00 ax 180
Keratometer readings	44.00/90 42.50/180

Calculation:

$\Delta K = -1.50$ ax 180

C.R.A. $= (-2.00$ ax $180) - (-1.50$ ax $180) =$
-0.50 ax 180

Studies have shown that with-the-rule residual astigmatism occurs much less frequently than against-the-rule residual astigmatism.[16,30,31]

EXAMPLE 3. Given:

Spectacle correction	−1.00 −2.00 ax 180
Keratometer readings	45.00/90 42.50/180

Calculation:

$\Delta K = -2.50$ ax 180

C.R.A. $= (-2.00$ ax $180) - (-2.50$ ax $180) =$
$+0.50$ ax 180

This result should be transposed to +0.50 = −0.50 ax 90. The calculated *residual astigmatism* is −0.50 ax 90.

EXAMPLE 4. Given:

Spectacle correction	+1.00 −2.50 ax 90
Keratometer readings	42.00/90 43.50/180

Calculation:

$\Delta K = -1.50$ ax 90

C.R.A. $= (-2.50$ ax $90) - (-1.50$ ax $90) =$
-1.00 ax 90

When the spherical component of the spectacle correction is such that the power in either principal meridian exceeds ±4.00 D., the total astigmatism of the eye at the plane of the cornea (the effective cylinder) may differ significantly from that given by the correction at the spectacle plane.[24] It is necessary to refer the power of each principal meridian of the spectacle correction to the plane of the cornea in order to determine the effective power of the cylinder at this plane. This is readily accomplished by employing Formula 7.1.

The effective cylinder is then given by the difference between the effective powers at the corneal plane in each of the two principal meridians. An example will serve to illustrate this calculation.

EXAMPLE 5. Given:

Spectacle correction	−10.00 −2.00 ax 180
Vertex distance	13 mm.
Keratometer readings	44.00/90 42.00/180

Calculations:

$$F_{e90} = \frac{-12.00}{1 - 0.013\,(-10.00)} = -10.38 \text{ D.}$$

$$F_{e180} = \frac{-10.00}{1 - 0.013\,(-10.00)} = -8.85 \text{ D.}$$

The effective cylinder at the plane of the cornea is given by $F_{e90} - F_{e180}$, which equals −1.53 ax 180. The calculated residual astigmatism is (−1.53 ax 180) − (−2.00 ax 180) = +0.47 ax 180 or +0.47−0.47 ax 90.

Many *effective power* tables (Appendix 2) are readily available to the fitter and can be used to determine the effective cylinder at the corneal plane without resorting to any but the final calculation given here.

It must be pointed out that the axis of the correcting spectacle lens cylinder will not always be the same as the axis of the corneal cylinder. When this situation exists, the calculation that must be performed to subtract the cylinder given by ΔK from the total astigmatic correction is more complex. It is accomplished by changing the axis of the ΔK cylinder by 90° and *adding* this cylinder to the effective cylinder determined from the spectacle correction. The two cylinders are combined by employing conventional crossed cylinder equations or by using a graphical solution. The resultant cylinder represents the power and axis of the lens that would be calculated to correct the residual astigmatism. This procedure involves a more tedious calculation and is seldom worth the time and trouble of the fitter. As long as the axes are within ±20 degrees of each other, it is quite adequate to assume that they are the same. When the difference in axes exceeds this amount, it is best to reserve judgment until a spherical diagnostic contact lens can be used to determine the residual astigmatism by actual refraction.

Several investigators have calculated the residual astigmatism of independent samples of patients with very similar results.[32,33] The mean calculated residual astigmatism was about −0.50 axis 90. The results are summarized in Table 9.2.

MEASURED RESIDUAL ASTIGMATISM

Investigators have found the correlation between calculated and measured residual astigmatism to be statistically significant. Correlations of 0.78[16] and 0.51[34] have been reported. These investigators also agreed, however, that a significant difference exists between the calculated and measured residual astigmatism, with the calculated residual astigmatism being generally higher than the measured residual astigmatism.

The measured residual astigmatism can be predicted from the calculated residual with an accuracy no better than ±0.50 D.[31,34]

TABLE 9.2

DISTRIBUTION OF CALCULATED RESIDUAL ASTIGMATISM REPORTED BY FOUR INVESTIGATORS
(ATR: AGAINST-THE-RULE, WTR: WITH-THE-RULE)

Investigator	N	Mean	Mode	S.D.	Range
Carter[32]	100	0.50 D. atr	0.50 D. atr	±0.41 D.	0.50 wtr 2.00 atr
Kratz & Walton[33]	295		0.50 D. atr		
Sarver[31]	408	0.51 D. atr	0.75 D. atr	±0.45 D.	0.75 wtr 2.00 atr
Dellande[34]	83	.60 D.			? wtr
	8	atr .23 D. wtr			1.25 atr

PREDICTED RESIDUAL ASTIGMATISM (P.R.A.)

Sarver[31] found the measured residual astigmatism to be related to the calculated residual astigmatism by the regression equation $y = 0.274 x + 0.086$ (S.D. $= \pm0.25$ D., $N = 408$ [Figure 9.2]), while Dellande[34] found the relationship to be $y = 0.510 x + 0.026$ (S.D. $= \pm0.26$ D., $N = 83$). The clinical application of these results is embodied in the following equations:

P.R.A. = 0.3 C.R.A. ± 0.50 D.   (Sarver)
P.R.A. = 0.5 C.R.A. ± 0.50 D.   (Dellande)

These equations can be used to predict the limits of the residual astigmatism expected with spherical corneal contact lenses.

EXAMPLE 6. Given:

Spectacle correction	$-1.00 = -0.50$ ax 180
Keratometer readings	45.00/90 43.00/180

Calculation:

$\Delta K = -2.00$ ax 180

C.R.A. $= (-0.50$ ax $180) - (-2.00$ ax $180) =$
          $+ 1.50$ ax 180

P.R.A. $= 0.3$ C.R.A. ± 0.50 D.
     $= 0.3 (+1.50$ ax $180) \pm 0.50$
     $= (+0.50$ ax $180) \pm 0.50$
     $= 0$ to $+ 1.00$ ax 180   (Sarver)

P.R.A. $= 0.5$ C.R.A. ± 0.50 D.
     $= 0.5 (+1.50$ ax $180) \pm 0.50$
     $= (+.75$ ax $180) \pm 0.50$
     $= +0.25$ ax 180 to $+1.25$ ax 180   (Dellande)

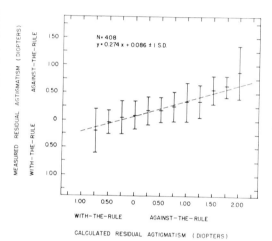

Figure 9.2. Calculated versus measured residual astigmatism with the mean and plus and minus one standard deviation of measured values plotted for each calculated value. The linear regression line y = 0.274x + 0.086 has been plotted to show the goodness of fit. From M. D. Sarver, A Study of Residual Astigmatism, *American Journal of Optometry*, 46(8):578–582, 1969.

In this example the probable limits of the expected residual astigmatism are 0 to 1.25 D. against the rule. A refraction over diagnostic lenses is necessary to determine if a significant residual astigmatism will be present with spherical corneal lenses.

INCIDENCE OF RESIDUAL ASTIGMATISM

Bailey points out that "residual astigmatism (with spherical corneal contact lenses) and a consequent reduction in visual acuity are the rule, rather than the exception, among contact lens wearers."[30] In a study of 105 subjects selected at random from a file of some 2,000 records, he found that 83 percent of the sample showed at least 0.50 D. residual astigmatic error in one or both eyes.

Sarver,[31] in a study of 408 eyes from a total sample of 250 patients, found the mean measured residual astigmatism to be −0.23 D. axis 90° ± 30° (S.D. = ± 0.30 D.). Thirty-four percent of the eyes showed a residual astigmatism of 0.50 D. or more. The distribution of residual astigmatism found in his study is shown in Table 9.3 together with the distribution reported by Bailey in the earlier study.

The residual astigmatism that is present with spherical contact lenses does not disappear as the patient wears the lenses. The magnitude of the required astigmatic correction may vary from one refraction to the next, but this variation is within the range of the error of measurement. The average patient wearing contact lenses is less critical in making acuity judgments with small changes in cylinder power than the same patient without contact lenses, nor do changes in lens centration, which may occur with adaptation or with the use of different base curves, optical zone diameters, or lens diameters, have a significant effect in altering the residual astigmatism. Only in rare instances will the tilt or decentration of a high plus or minus contact lens introduce a measurable amount of astigmatism into the contact lens–fluid lens system.[16]

The fitter can thus determine the final residual astigmatism with a good degree of validity by employing spherical diagnostic contact lenses and refraction. When, in the judgment of the fitter, the residual astigmatism exceeds an acceptable amount, special lens types and fitting procedures are required to obtain adequate correction of the refractive error and good visual acuity.

CORRECTION OF RESIDUAL ASTIGMATISM

It has been clearly established that a very large percentage of those patients fitted with spherical corneal contact lenses manifest a significant residual astigmatic refractive error and that the mean value of this error is 0.25 to 0.50 D. against the rule. This means that most patients fitted with such lenses demonstrate a visual acuity that is less than the optimum acuity that the patient is capable of attaining with full correction. The patient who is capable of 20/20 acuity will, on the average, attain an acuity of 20/20− or 20/25+. It is nonetheless common to hear such a patient say that he sees better with contact lenses than with glasses. A number of reasons can be offered to account for this phenomenon. The contact lenses provide an unobstructed field of view; they do not induce most of the aberrations produced by spectacle lenses;[35] there is a psychological effect resulting from the patient's desire to wear contact lenses. One must also remember that the patient is comparing the acuity obtained with contact lenses to the acuity experienced with spectacle lenses following the removal of the contact lenses. Thus, changes in corneal curvature and/or small degrees of epithelial edema reduce the acuity attained with the spectacle correction. Furthermore, the spectacle lenses are generally a year or two old and do not

TABLE 9.3

MEASURED RESIDUAL ASTIGMATISM IN DIOPTERS

Investigator	With-the-Rule	0-0.24	0.25-0.49	Against-the-Rule 0.50-0.74	0.75-0.99	1.00 or more
Sarver N = 408	4%	42%	20 %	27 %	6%	1%
Bailey N = 208		12%	21.6%	29.4%	24%	13%

provide maximum visual acuity, even under the best of conditions.

When the residual astigmatism is 0.50 D. or less, it will seldom reduce the acuity enough to cause any visual distress[36] or asthenopia. Furthermore, any attempt to provide a contact lens construction that will correct so small an amount of astigmatism may cause more visual problems than it cures, not to mention the additional physical and physiological problems that might be precipitated. When the residual astigmatism exceeds 0.50 D., the fitter must rely upon his experience and professional judgment in reaching a decision on the proper course of action. He must carefully weigh the advantages of fitting a conventional spherical lens, even though residual astigmatism is present, against the disadvantages of fitting a lens of more complex construction, even though the residual astigmatism may be reduced or eliminated.

Thin, Spherical Contact Lenses

One set of circumstances that lends itself well to the use of thin, spherical corneal contact lenses is when the corneal toricity is with the rule and the residual astigmatism present with a hard spherical corneal contact lens of standard thickness is against the rule. A spherical lens with a center thickness of 0.12 mm. or less will flex on a toric cornea.[25] The amount of flexure is greater with thinner lenses and more toric corneas (Figures 9.3 to 9.5). A spherical lens that flexes on a with-the-rule toric cornea will reduce an against-the-rule residual astigmatism.[37] A thin lens can be used to advantage under these conditions. If the residual astigmatism is against the rule and the corneal toricity is also against the rule, a spherical lens thin enough to flex on the eye will increase the residual astigmatism and should not be used (*see* Chapter 7).

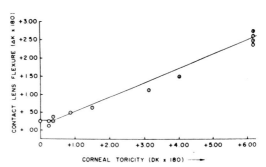

Figure 9.3. Contact lens flexure for a 0.08 mm. center thickness lens on corneas of various toricities. From M. G. Harris and C. S. Chu, The Effect of Contact Lens Thickness and Corneal Toricity on Flexure and Residual Astigmatism, *American Journal of Optometry*, 49(4):304–307, 1972.

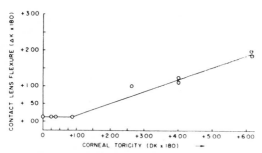

Figure 9.4. Contact lens flexure for a 0.09 mm. center thickness lens on corneas of various toricities. From M. G. Harris and C. S. Chu, The Effect of Contact Lens Thickness and Corneal Toricity on Flexure and Residual Astigmatism, *American Journal of Optometry, 49(4)*:304–307, 1972.

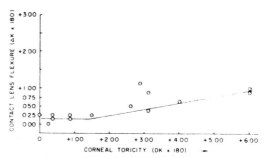

Figure 9.5. Contact lens flexure for a 0.12 mm. center thickness lens on corneas of various toricities. From M. G. Harris and C. S. Chu, The Effect of Contact Lens Thickness and Corneal Toricity on Flexure and Residual Astigmatism, *American Journal of Optometry, 49(4)*:304–307, 1972.

Spherical Lenses with Cylindrical Spectacles

A technique that can be successfully applied for some patients, in the interest of avoiding a more complex lens construction, is simply to provide spherical contact lenses for general wear supplemented by the necessary cylindrical correction in the form of spectacle lenses. The patient needs the added correction only when his visual task demands optimum acuity, i.e. driving at night, movies, etc. The patient whose refractive error is −5.00 −0.25 axis 90 and whose residual refractive error with spherical contact lenses is +0.50 − 1.00 axis 90 might get along fine with 20/30 acuity for most routine seeing tasks. If the spectacle correction of +0.50 −1.00 axis 90 improves the acuity to 20/20, it can be worn when more critical acuity is required. Although this technique is not recommended as a routine procedure and, in fact, will often meet with resistance from the patient, it may be the best solution when the patient wears spherical lenses comfortably but responds poorly to the more complex lens constructions. This procedure is generally more successful with patients having relatively high refractive errors.

Sometimes an acceptable correction can be obtained by increasing the power of the spherical lens by an amount equal to the spherical equivalent of the residual refractive error. For instance, a patient wearing a spherical contact lens, the power of which is −3.00 D., may have a residual refractive error of plano −1.00 D. cyl. axis 90. The equivalent sphere of this residual correction is −0.50 D. sphere. If a −0.50 D. trial lens is placed before the eye and improves the acuity significantly, the power of the spherical contact lens should be increased to −3.50 D.

Nonrotating Lenses

When the decision is in favor of a contact lens that will correct the residual astigmatism, the fitter must select the type of lens that is most likely to produce the desired results. The choice is seldom a simple one, but it is more readily made when the fitter is familiar with the various lens constructions available, their advantages, disadvantages, and fitting characteristics, as well as the usual problems encountered with each type of lens.

To correct a residual astigmatism with contact lenses, it is necessary to either prescribe a lens with one or more toric surfaces or to use a spherical lens that will flex an appropriate amount on the eye. A lens with toric surfaces must also be designed to orient properly when *in situ* and to maintain its meridional orientation, within small tolerance limits, against the forces that will act to rotate the lens.

These forces include lid torque and gravity. The forces acting to maintain the meridional orientation of the lens include surface tension of the precorneal fluid as influenced by the lens-cornea bearing relationship, lid tension or position, and gravity, for certain lens constructions.

Meridional orientation is achieved by incorporating one or more of the following lens design features into the construction of the lens:

1. Prism ballast
2. Peri-ballast
3. Metal disc ballast
4. Single truncation
5. Double truncation
6. Some form of scleral flange
7. Spherical lens with toric peripheral curves*
8. Toric base curves*

These lens design features are assembled in various combinations depending upon the physical characteristics of the patient's cornea and lids and the experience and judg-

---

*Toric base curve lenses, bitoric lenses, and spherical lenses with toric peripheral curves are discussed later in this chapter. Although these lenses are used primarily to obtain an optimum physical fit on a toric cornea, they may, under certain conditions, be used to reduce or correct a residual astigmatism.

ment of the fitter. The competent fitter must understand the design, fitting principles, and specific use of each of the resultant lens types.

The Prism Ballast Lens

When the corneal toricity is not too great, some form of the prism ballast lens is generally the lens of choice for correcting residual astigmatism. This lens has a spherical back surface, a prism base down (90 ±15°), and a toric front surface that provides the necessary correcting cylinder (generally a plus cylinder at or near axis 180°). The lens may be circular in form or may have a bottom truncation (Figure 9.6). Less frequently a top truncation is also incorporated in the lens design. The lens functions in the manner of a pendulum. As the normal blinking action of the lids causes the lens to rotate upward nasally, the force of gravity pulls the heavier prism base edge of the lens to an inferior position.

THE TRUNCATED PRISM BALLAST LENS. Ewell, Gates, and Remba made significant contributions in the development of the prism ballast lens.[38] They recommend a lens whose physical dimensions are illustrated in Figure 9.7. The base curve of the lens is fitted in the manner usually employed for spherical lenses of equivalent diameter and with the same general considerations. The amount of prism generally required to maintain meridional orientation

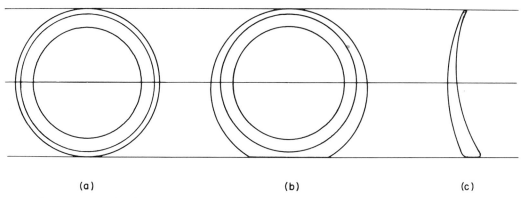

(a)   (b)   (c)

Figure 9.6. (*a*) The circular prism ballast corneal contact lens, (*b*) the truncated prism ballast corneal contact lens, and (*c*) a vertical section through these lenses.

is 1.25 to 1.75 prism diopters. Less prism will not provide the lens with sufficient weight differential to permit it to maintain its meridional orientation against the rotational force of the lids. More prism will result in a heavy lens and in too much difference in thickness between the superior and inferior lens edge* and is likely to cause physical discomfort and physiological distress.

The bottom truncation is designed to conform to, and rest against, the edge of the lower lid. This gives the lens added orientation stability and also serves to keep the lower edge of the lens from impinging upon the inferior limbal region. The vertical diameter of the lens must be large enough to permit the lens to extend about 1 mm. beyond the superior edge of the pupil (under conditions of reduced illumination). An average vertical diameter is 8.9 mm. (range 8.2 to 9.2 mm.). The horizontal diameter is about 0.4 to 0.6 mm. longer than the vertical diameter. The optic zone of the lens is decentered up to provide the best lens-cornea bearing relationship and to obtain better centration of the optic in front of the pupil. The optic zone diameter varies between 7.0 and 7.8 mm.

Finally, the base of the prism is displaced nasally so that the base-apex line is rotated

---

*For a 10 mm. diameter lens, each prism diopter produces a difference of about 0.2 mm. between the base and apex edge thickness of the prism lens,[39]

10° to 15° from the vertical meridian. This places the base-apex line of the right lens at an axis of 100° to 105° and the base-apex line of the left lens at an axis of 75° to 80° (Figure 9.8). The purpose of this displacement is to increase the rotational moment of the lens so that it will resist the rotational forces exerted by the lids and will recover its orientation quickly following a blink. The bottom truncation prevents the lens from rotating back beyond its intended position of orientation.

Although the power of the lens can be determined from keratometer readings and refractive error information, there are too many variables to make this an accurate procedure. A more accurate method is to perform a spherocylindrical refraction through a spherical diagnostic contact lens whose base curve is the same as that of the prism ballast lens to be fitted. The lens power ordered from the laboratory will be equal to the sum of the powers of the spherical diagnostic contact lens and the spherocylindrical correction lens determined by refracting over the lens. Although the latter procedure increases accuracy, it still does not insure a precise correction of the refractive error because information about lens orientation will not be available until the finished lens is actually placed on the eye. This suggests a third refinement that does increase the accuracy of the correction. The refraction is performed through a spherical prism ballast trial lens whose base curve

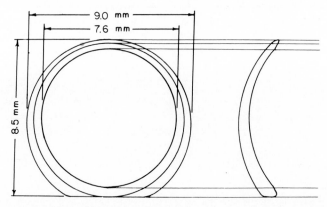

Figure 9.7. The truncated prism ballast corneal contact lens showing typical average dimensions.

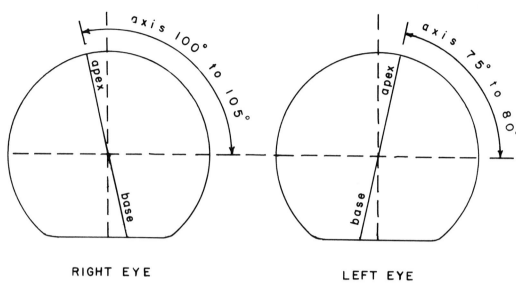

RIGHT EYE   LEFT EYE

Figure 9.8. Orientation of the base-apex line of truncated prism ballast corneal contact lenses.

and other dimensions closely approximate those of the finished lens. Lens orientation can be determined by marking the base-apex line with a sharp grease marking pencil and observing the axis of this line when the lens is *in situ*. Goldberg suggests the use of a trial frame containing a plano lens across which a line has been drawn.[40] The lens cell of the trial frame is rotated until the line on the plano lens lines up with the line on the prism ballast lens. This gives the orientation axis of the base-apex line of the prism ballast lens and permits a more accurate placement of the axis of the front surface cylinder.

This form of the prism ballast lens performs best on eyes having normal to high inferior lids and slightly high superior lids of moderate to loose tension. Ideally, the lens does not contact the superior lid except during a blink. The thin upper lens edge must be well rounded and polished to a relatively uniform thickness. If flare becomes a problem, the vertical diameter must be increased. If upper lid irritation is present, it may be necessary to increase the vertical lens diameter so that the lens positions beneath the upper lid. The lower, truncated edge must be

relatively square to prevent the lens from slipping beneath the lower lid. It is sometimes necessary to alter the axis of truncation because the bottom edge of the lens does not bear evenly upon the lower lid. A top truncation may be added if the upper lid is too tight or the palpebral aperture is small. It may be curved rather than straight.

Typical problems encountered with this lens design include the following:

1. Blurred vision immediately following each blink as the lens undergoes rotation. This rotation produces a pair of obliquely crossed cylinders (the contact lens front surface cylinder and the residual astigmatism) changing both the spherical and the cylindrical correction.

2. Physical disturbance to the corneal epithelium in the region of the corneal apex due to the low riding position of the lens. It may occur even though most of the lens weight is supported by the lower lid.

3. Physiological disturbance of the cornea due to the pooling of fluid beneath the lens in the inferior corneal region.

4. Lower lid or inferior limbal irritation due to the weight and bumping action of the

lens.

5. Inadequate correction of the residual astigmatism even though the lens cylinder, as measured with a lensometer, appears to be proper.

THE CIRCULAR PRISM BALLAST LENS. Many fitters and laboratories prefer the circular prism ballast lens over the truncated design for correcting residual astigmatism.[39,41] There are fewer variables to control. The optical zone is centered. The lens is easier to manufacture and easier to duplicate.

The base curve, diameter, and other lens variables are selected by observing the performance of spherical diagnostic contact lenses on the eye, keeping in mind that the lens will probably position low on the cornea when prism is added. The spherocylindrical power required to correct the refractive error is determined by refracting over the diagnostic lens. The amount of prism should be kept to a minimum consistent with acceptable rotational stability. The lens is generally ordered with 1.25 base down (range 1Δ to 1.5Δ base down).[42] The cylinder axis must be corrected to compensate for the rotation of the lens on the eye. A rule often used is to subtract 15° from the axis of the right lens and add 15° to the axis of the left lens. Thus, if refraction over a spherical diagnostic contact lens results in cylinders at an axis of 90° O.U., the prism ballast lenses would be ordered with base down prism and a cylindrical axis of 75° for the right lens and 105° for the left lens. A small error in lens orientation seldom causes any difficulty.

Borish controls the cylinder axis and power by fitting a spherical ballasted lens to the eye and determining the power and axis of the cylinder after lens orientation stabilizes following patient adaptation.[43,44] The cylinder is placed on the spherical ballasted lenses when possible or when new lenses are ordered. Prism ballast ranging from 0.75Δ to 1.5Δ is used. The amount of prism ballast used is a function of lens diameter and lens power.

Korb points out that the lens can often be fitted to maintain a centered position on the cornea rather than riding on the lower lid.[45] This is accomplished by carefully selecting the base curve, lens diameter, and amount of prism ballast. The base curve is selected to give a minimal apical clearance fit. The diameter must be relatively small, varying from 8.4 mm. to 9.3 mm. The amount of prism required to maintain lens orientation is 0.75Δ $\pm$ 0.37. The greater the lens diameter, the greater must be the prism. The maximum prism that will permit lens centration is 1.5Δ. The amount of prism selected should be the minimum amount that will provide lens orientation and stability, for any more may destroy centration. The optical zone diameter varies from 6.8 mm. to 7.4 mm.

When this lens centers and maintains its orientation and stability, it is preferred over the truncated design because it produces less physical and physiological distress. When, however, adequate meridional orientation cannot be achieved together with centration, the truncated design offers the greatest chance for success.

Prism ballast lenses must perform on the eye in a specific manner to provide a good visual and physiological result. A centered to low centered position on the cornea with adequate coverage of the pupil will contribute to a good visual response. Meridional orientation within ±5° will permit stable vision. Adequate vertical lens movement during each blink prevents an adverse physiological response. A low riding lens that impinges upon the sclera and/or does not exhibit adequate blink lags will generally precipitate a corneal edema after a brief period of lens wear.

THE BT PRISM BALLAST LENS. Good meridional orientation and rotational stability have been reported with a prism ballast BT lens construction.[46] The lens is circular in shape and requires about one diopter of prism to maintain its meridional orientation. The necessary front surface cylinder is determined by refracting through a spherical BT diagnostic contact lens.

CONOCOID PRISM BALLAST LENS. The conocoid lens has a truly aspheric posterior surface that is available in eccentricities ranging from 0.6 to 1.1. The lens is fitted to obtain slight apical pooling (0.50 D. to 0.75 D. steeper than *K*). Conner states that this lens can be fitted with 1.25 Δ of ballast to provide a lens with good rotational stability and 'that it is not necessary to allow for rotation in ordering the axis of the front surface cylinder.[47]

BINOCULAR CONSIDERATIONS. Although the prismatic component of a prism ballast lens is intended only to weight the lens for orientation purposes, its effect upon binocular vision cannot be disregarded. If the lens is used to correct the residual astigmatism of one eye, it is generally necessary to fit the other eye with a prism ballast lens also to avoid inducing a vertical phoria. Fortunately, a high bilateral correlation of residual astigmatism has been demonstrated[48] so that when residual astigmatism must be corrected the need generally is bilateral.

VERIFICATION OF LENS POWER. The power of a toric front surface prism ballast contact lens is verified with the lensometer by placing the lens with its back surface against the lensometer lens stop and rotating the lens until the position of the target image indicates the prism base is down (axis 90°). The cylinder axis can then be related to the base-apex line of the prism, and in turn to the eye, depending upon the meridional orientation of the lens *in situ*.

Generally, the image of the lensometer target is not sharply defined when measuring the power of any prism ballast contact lens. This is especially true when the lens contains a cylinder. Numerous aberrations are responsible, including spherical aberration, variation in spherical power from apex to base of the lens (the lens increases in plus power at the rate of about 0.25 D. per 0.1 mm. increase in lens thickness), and perhaps a less than optimum quality toric surface due to technical difficulties associated with manufacturing such surfaces.

The quality of the lensometer image can be improved by masking out some of the peripheral rays that create these aberrations. The lens stop aperture can be reduced to 3 or 4 mm. by drilling a hole through a thin piece of opaque plastic and attaching the plastic to the face of the lensometer lens stop.

An alternate method for obtaining the cylinder power is to measure the front sur-

TABLE 9.4

TABLE OF OPTICAL CONSTANTS FOR CONVERTING THE SURFACE VALUE OF A PLASTIC CONTACT LENS
(n = 1.490)

To Convert from	to	Multiply by
Contact lens surface power in air	Contact lens surface power in fluid	$C_1 = 0.314$
K reading of contact lens surface	Contact lens surface power in air	$C_2 = 1.452$
K reading of contact lens surface	Contact lens surface power in fluid	$C_3 = 0.452$

Derivation:

$$C_1 = \frac{^{n}\text{fluid} - {^{n}}\text{plastic}}{^{n}\text{air} - {^{n}}\text{plastic}} = \frac{1.336 - 1.490}{1 - 1.490} = 0.314$$

$$C_2 = \frac{^{n}\text{air} - {^{n}}\text{plastic}}{^{n}\text{air} - {^{n}}\text{keratometer}} = \frac{1 - 1.490}{1 - 1.3375} = 1.452$$

$$C_3 = \frac{^{n}\text{fluid} - {^{n}}\text{plastic}}{^{n}\text{air} - {^{n}}\text{keratometer}} = \frac{1.336 - 1.490}{1 - 1.3375} = 0.452$$

face radii of curvature with a keratometer. The cylinder is equal to the difference in K readings times a constant. For lenses whose index of refraction is 1.490, the value of this constant is 1.452[27] (*see* Table 9.4). Thus, if the keratometer readings of such a toric surface are 43.00 D. and 45.00 D., the cylinder power is $(45.00 - 43.00) \times 1.45$ or 2.90 D.

The same procedure can be employed with a radiuscope. The radius values of the two principal meridians are easily converted to K readings and their difference is multiplied by the constant given previously.

The Peri-Ballast Lens

The peri-ballast lens has an advantage over the prism ballast lens in that the optical portion of the lens contains none of the prism that reduces the optical quality of prism ballasted lenses.[49] Since prism is absent in the optical portion of the lens, it is useful for correcting residual astigmatism that is limited to one eye.

The lens is of lenticular design with a high minus carrier. Removal of all but a portion of the high minus carrier during the manufacturing process produces a lens with a ballasted lens periphery, which is only a portion of the original high minus carrier (Figure 9.9).

Spherical Base Curve with Double Truncation

Although prism ballast is generally favored as a means for orienting a spherical base lens so that the residual astigmatism can be corrected by applying a front surface cylinder, some prefer to employ a double truncation to achieve meridional orientation (Figure 9.10). Fairmaid describes the use of lenses having a horizontal diameter of 9.0 to 9.6 mm. and a vertical diameter of 7.7 to 8.2 mm. that varies with the size of the palpebral aperture and the pupil.[50] The base curve is selected to provide bare apical clearance. No allowance need be made for cylinder axis rotation as the lenses orient within a few degrees of horizontal. He reports that 82 percent of a sample of fifty-three patients fitted with double truncated front surface toric lenses were wearing their lenses throughout their waking hours with acuity equal to their spectacle acuity.

The Semisclerocorneal Flange Lens

Moss has described the use of a corneal lens with a narrow scleral flange extending approximately halfway around the circumference of the lens (Figure 9.11).[51] The scleral flange section is 0.5 mm. wide and makes an angle of from 15° to 25° with a line perpendicular to the axis of the lens. The flatter flange positions above the superior limbus, while the heavier section opposite the flange helps keep the lens stabilized.

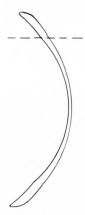

Figure 9.9. Peri-ballast contact lens is formed from a minus-carrier lens.

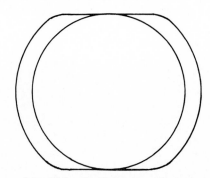

Figure 9.10. The spherical lens with double truncation.

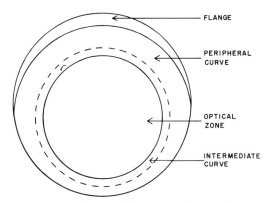

FLANGE

PERIPHERAL
CURVE

OPTICAL
ZONE

INTERMEDIATE
CURVE

Figure 9.11. The semisclerocorneal flange lens.

The optical zone radius is generally fitted 0.05 mm. to 0.15 mm. flatter than *K*. The pressure of the upper lid holds the lens in position. In the absence of adequate lid tension, the lens will sag and rotate. When properly fitted, the lens will stabilize well and permit the addition of a front surface cylinder to correct the residual astigmatism.

The Haptic Lens

The fitting of haptic lenses is covered in detail in Chapter 32. Here it is only necessary to describe how and why these lenses can be used to correct residual astigmatism. One of the major advantages of the haptic lens is its orientational stability.[52] It is this fact that makes this type of lens an excellent choice for correcting residual astigmatism.[53,54] A grease marking pencil is used to place a horizontal working axis on the lens while the eye is in the primary position. The line is applied with short, gentle strokes to avoid rotating the lens. This should not be done until all fitting procedures have been completed and the lens has settled into its final orientation. The cylindrical correction can then be determined by refracting through the lens. It is applied to the front surface of the optic by the laboratory, using the marked working axis as the necessary reference for the cylinder axis.

TORIC CORNEAL CONTACT LENSES

Noel Stimson introduced toric corneal lenses in 1950. Schapero[55,56] and Baglien[57] described the toric base corneal contact lens and its use in 1952 and 1953. Interest in the lens was relatively dormant until Wesley,[13,58] Korb,[11,12,19] and others revived it through clinical and laboratory research. Lens manufacturing techniques were crude and inaccurate and the proper use of the lens was not completely understood. The calculation of bitoric lenses was hit or miss,[59] and the optics remained somewhat mysterious. Today, however, the lens is manufactured with greater accuracy and fitted with a fuller understanding of the physical and physiological principles involved.[11,12] The optics of the various toric lens forms have been explored and described in considerable detail[26,27,60-66] and provide the information needed to understand the proper

use of the lens for correcting refractive errors.

The toric back surface corneal contact lens is used to obtain an optimum lens-cornea bearing relationship when the toricity of the cornea precludes the use of a spherical back surface lens. Thus, its principal use is to fit a toric cornea and *not* to correct an astigmatic refractive error or residual astigmatism. When, however, it is necessary to use a toric back surface lens to fit a given cornea and residual astigmatism is present, the meridional orientation properties of the lens can be used to orient the cylinder that is required to correct the astigmatism. For the moment, the power effect of this lens will be disregarded and only the principles and methods of obtaining a proper physical fit and physiological result will be discussed.

INDICATIONS FOR FITTING THE BACK SURFACE TORIC LENS

Wesley feels there are advantages to fitting toric base lenses to corneas having even small amounts of corneal toricity—as low as a half diopter.[67] Grosvenor prefers to use toric base lenses only if spherical lenses prove to be uncomfortable.[68] Remba suggests that toric base lenses are indicated when a minimum acceptable bearing relationship between the cornea and a spherical lens cannot be achieved, but he agrees that the most familiar and uncomplicated fitting approach should be tried first.[69]

It is most difficult to state a limiting value of corneal toricity, in terms of keratometer readings, beyond which a toric lens should be fitted. Central keratometer readings do not provide a valid description of corneal toricity,[19] but they do alert the fitter to the possible need to fit a toric base lens. Toric lenses should be used when the application of spherical lenses clearly demonstrates their need. An unacceptable fluorescein pattern with spherical lenses (Figure 9.12), poor lens centration, excessive lens movement, and rocking all suggest the possible need for a toric lens construction.

The results of a spherical diagnostic lens fitting procedure are not always conclusive, and it is frequently necessary to further evaluate the need for a toric back surface lens by having the patient wear carefully fitted spherical lenses for a number of weeks. The decision to fit the toric lens is thus reserved until an evaluation of the patient's response to the spherical lenses has been made. If the response is not a favorable one, the fitter will have gained additional information that will help him do a better job in fitting the toric lens.

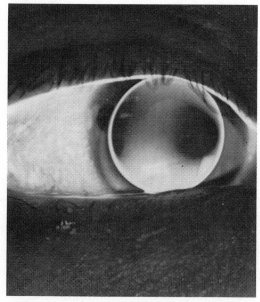

Figure 9.12. An unacceptable fluorescein pattern formed by a spherical lens on a with-the-rule toric cornea.

The symptomatology of an inadequate fit of a spherical lens on a toric cornea has already been described.

In the final analysis, it may be stated that a toric back surface contact lens is fitted to a toric cornea when, at any stage of the fitting procedure, it is determined that an acceptable physical and physiological result *cannot be attained with a spherical lens.* This may be apparent as soon as keratometer readings are taken, after fitting with spherical diagnostic lenses, or not until an evaluation is made of the patient's response to wearing carefully fitted spherical lenses over a period of time.

SPHERICAL BASE CURVE LENS WITH TORIC PERIPHERAL CURVES

This lens design is used to improve the fit of a spherical lens on a toric cornea. Its use may permit the fitter to avoid the more complex procedures associated with the fitting of a toric base lens but must be limited to corneas in which the toricity is not too great.

It is the lens of choice when the cornea is relatively spherical centrally but becomes increasingly toric peripherally. Such a corneal contour should be suspected when an oval-shaped cornea (significantly less diameter vertically) has near spherical central *K* readings. This type of corneal topography must be verified with spherical diagnostic lenses. Peripheral keratometry is not accurate or adequate for this purpose.[10]

The base curve is typically fitted steeper than the flattest corneal curvature and flatter than the steepest corneal curvature.[70] This reduces edge stand-off in the steeper corneal meridian and produces a lens in which the optical zone is oval in shape (Figure 9.13). The lens will orient so that the smaller optical zone diameter is along the flatter principal meridian of the cornea. If the peripheral

corneal toricity is sufficiently great and if the peripheral curve radii are carefully chosen, the lens will maintain its meridional orientation.

Greeman recommends the use of toric periphery lenses to control lens rotation and to improve lens centration.[71] He suggests the use of a toric periphery diagnostic lens set having five amounts of peripheral toricity and suggests fitting lenses about 9.6 mm. in diameter and about 7.0 mm. in optic zone diameter.

Brucker recommends the use of small, thin lenses with peripheral toric curves selected by central keratometry.[72]

Selection of the proper peripheral curve radii is at best not a simple task. Central keratometer readings will serve as a guide for the fabrication of the initial lens, the secondary curves being made 0.8 mm. to 1.2 mm. flatter than the respective central corneal

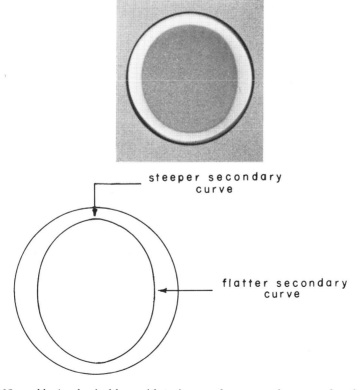

Figure 9.13a and b. A spherical lens with toric secondary curves has an oval optical zone.

curves. This lens must be viewed as a trial lens that leads to the final lens specifications. The fluorescein pattern demonstrated with spherical diagnostic lenses will help the fitter select the necessary curves for the flatter principal meridian of the cornea. The use of a precision set of toric peripheral curve diagnostic lenses is best for evaluating the bearing and venting relationships. Such a set is seldom available to the average fitter. Spherical lenses with toric peripheral curves are difficult to verify in the office, and the fitter loses a degree of control in the fitting of his patient.

When the optimum peripheral lens toricity produces a lens that maintains its meridional orientation, a toric front surface may be incorporated into the lens design for the correction of residual astigmatism. This generally requires ordering a new lens. Lens orientation and cylinder correction must be included in the final lens specifications.

FITTING THE BACK SURFACE TORIC LENS

An optimum lens-cornea bearing relationship and adequate venting is achieved with the back surface toric lens by employing the same general methods and principles as those used in fitting spherical lenses, except that attention must be given to a greater number of variables. To obtain a good physical fit, the toric back surface of the lens must be aligned with the toric surface of the cornea. However, just as a precise alignment of a spherical lens on a spherical cornea interferes with the fluid and gaseous interchange, so a precise alignment of a toric lens on a toric cornea produces the same result. Careful attention must thus be given to the selection of the radii, lens diameter, and optic zone diameter so that a proper balance between an ideal physical bearing relationship and one that permits the cornea to maintain its normal physiological state will be achieved. It must be kept in mind that a lens of this construction will not undergo rotation or lag to the same extent as a spherical lens and will thus present greater venting problems. It is more difficult to maintain a normal corneal metabolism with toric base lenses than with spherical lenses.[12]

Peripheral curves may be either spherical or toric. Some fitters prefer the optimum bearing afforded by the use of toric peripheral curves.[12,73] A major problem in the author's experience with the use of toric peripheral curves has been the limitations imposed upon the accurate office verification and modification of such curves. The greater complexity of these curves makes their modification an extremely difficult task and one that should not be attempted by any but the most experienced fitters. This poses additional problem for the average fitter who encounters the need to change the peripheral curves or reduce the optical zone diameter. Many feel that spherical peripheral curves are quite acceptable.[69,74,75]

The Keratometer Method

Remba has described a procedure for selecting the initial base curve specifications for a toric lens from the keratometer readings (Table 9.5).[60,69]

Note that the base curve radii are flatter than the respective keratometer readings of both principal corneal meridians. This is done to prevent a tight mechanical fit and the attendant physiological distress. Remba states, however, that "the use of a trial toric lens is highly advisable, if not imperative, to check the meridional orientation of the lens, its base curve-cornea relationships, its centering

TABLE 9.5

A Guide for Selecting the Initial Base Curve
Specifications of a Toric Lens from the
Keratometer Readings

Corneal Toricity (Keratometric Difference)	*Flattest Meridian Should Be Flatter Than Flattest Corneal Meridian by*	*Steeper Meridian Should Be Flatter Than Steepest Corneal Meridian by*
2.00 D.	0.25 D.	0.25 D.
3.00 D.	0.25 D.	0.50 D.
4.00 D.	0.25 D.	0.75 D.
5.00 D.	0.50 D.	0.75 D.

and riding properties, and also allow a refraction through the lens." He suggests a lens diameter that is generally 0.5 mm. to 1.0 mm. smaller than a conventional spherical contact lens, the mean being 8.8 mm. The mean optical zone diameter suggested is 7.5 mm. This lens design generally centers well and, where the corneal toricity is great enough (at least 2.00 D.), maintains its meridional orientation.

Goldberg offers a table (Table 9.6) that can be used to select the initial lens diameter and optic zone diameter for each base curve and base curve cylinder.[76] He suggests the

use of somewhat larger lens diameters.

The larger diameter lens permits more stable meridional orientation and less lens rotation. Optic zone diameters must be made relatively small to permit adequate venting of the retro-lens space. Secondary venting techniques (fenestration and trunctation) may become necessary when the larger lens is used.

Goldberg has also offered an emperical method for selecting the toric base curves such that they are respectively steeper than the flat corneal *K* reading and flatter than the steep corneal *K* reading.[77] Specific values are based on corneal *K* readings and are determined by the use of an empirical formula.

As has been stated, Korb feels that the toric base lens cannot be fitted on the basis of keratometer readings.[19] However, he does offer the fitter some general statements about the relationship between the keratometer readings and the final lens design. On the basis of his observations in fitting 218 toric lenses to seventy-three eyes, he reports the following:

1. The flatter corneal meridian in all cases required a radius flatter than the *K* reading in that meridian if the optic zone diameter of the contact lens exceeded 7.0 mm. The average degree of flatness was 0.75 D. with a 7.5 mm. optic zone diameter.

2. The steeper meridian of the cornea, if it was the vertical, could be fitted in closer proximity to the *K* reading of that meridian

TABLE 9.6
A Guide for Selecting the Initial Lens Diameter and Optical Zone Diameter for Each
Flatter Optical Zone Radius and Cylinder. Dioptric Values Are Given in K Readings.

Corneal Lens Base Curve	Lens Design	Amount of Base Curve Cylinder		
		2.00 D.	*3.00 D.*	*4.00 D.–6.00 D.*
40.00 D. to 41.75 D.	Diam.	9.4 mm.	9.2 mm.	9.0 mm.
	O.Z.D.	8.0 mm.	7.8 mm.	7.6 mm.
42.00 D. to 43.75 D.	Diam.	9.2 mm.	9.0 mm.	8.8 mm.
	O.Z.D.	8.0 mm.	7.8 mm.	7.6 mm.
44.00 D. to 45.75 D.	Diam.	9.0 mm.	8.8 mm.	8.6 mm.
	O.Z.D.	7.6 mm.	7.4 mm.	7.2 mm.

than could the flatter meridian. The average was 0.37 D. flatter with a 7.5 mm. optic zone diameter.

3. In approximately one-half of the cases, the *K* readings were of no value. Several cases with spherical *K* readings required toricities of 0.40 mm. (2.00 D.).

4. The majority of corneas manifesting with-the-rule astigmia required greater toricity on the lens than evidenced by the keratometer.

5. The majority of against-the-rule corneas required less toricity on the lens than evidenced by the keratometer.

The fitter will do better in arriving at the proper toric lens dimensions by employing spherical diagnostic lenses to evaluate the toricity of the cornea. The first toric lens fitted may have to be viewed as a diagnostic lens.

The Diagnostic Lens Method

The ideally fitting toric back surface lens is not nearly as difficult to describe as it is to fit. It maintains its meridional orientation and has a symmetrical fluorescein pattern of central alignment and distinct, but not excessive, peripheral clearance (Figure 9.14). The necessary lens dimensions are best determined by employing spherical and toric diagnostic lenses to evaluate the lens-cornea bearing relationships both centrally and peripherally. The proper lens dimensions for the flatter principal corneal meridian are determined first by observing the fluorescein pattern formed in this meridian with spherical diagnostic lenses.[11] The corneal toricity can be judged at the same time.

With the information thus gained, an initial toric lens can be ordered or selected from a toric diagnostic fitting set with some assurance that at least the specifications of the lens in the flatter meridian are already known. The overall bearing relationship of the toric lens may then be studied to ascertain the final toric base specifications. Many laboratories will supply the fitter with two or

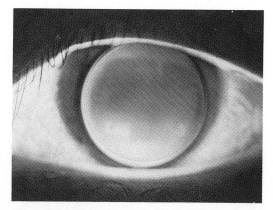

Figure 9.14. The fluorescein pattern obtained with an ideally fitting toric back surface lens on a toric cornea.

three lenses "on memorandum" to permit him to make these observations prior to ordering the lenses.

Sellers employs a toric base, spherical front surface diagnostic lens fitting set to achieve an acceptable bearing relationship and attempts to select the amount of lens toricity to correct the refractive error simultaneously.[75] His lens diameters range from 8.4 mm. to 9.0 mm., and optic zone diameters average 7.0 mm. He reports being able to fit 82 percent of those patients requiring a toric lens with a seven lens diagnostic lens set containing the following base curves:

    7.75 mm./7.25 mm.
    7.95 mm./7.25 mm.
    7.95 mm./7.42 mm.
    7.95 mm./7.58 mm.
    8.15 mm./7.60 mm.
    8.15 mm./7.95 mm.
    8.25 mm./7.60 mm.

He employs additional toric base, diagnostic lenses as needed.

Of the 120 patients in his sample fitted with toric lenses, 20 percent required a toric lens for one eye only, 40 percent required a compensating oblique front surface cylinder, and 60 percent were corrected optically with a back-surface toric lens with a spherical front surface.

Bayshore describes the fitting of palpebral

aperture lenses of multitoric constructions.[73] The lens is designed with a toric base curve, toric peripheral curve, toric bevel, and, if necessary, toric anterior curve to correct any induced or residual astigmatism.

An acceptable bearing relationship can be obtained with either a small, thin lens design or a larger diameter modified contour lens construction. When the meridional orientation of the lens is an important consideration, the base curves must be selected to provide a closer corneal alignment. This may produce corneal edema. Prism ballast can be added to a toric base or bitoric lens to help control meridional orientation.[42] Lens fenestration can be added as needed to combat corneal edema (*see* Chapter 15).

Optical Considerations

One of the most perplexing problems associated with the fitting of toric lenses is that of correcting the refractive error. Although the back toric surface is designed to provide a proper physical fit and physiological result, it also has certain optical properties that cannot be ignored if the fitter expects to give the patient good visual acuity. It is not unusual to obtain a good physical and physiological result after exerting considerable effort, only to find that the refractive error has not been adequately corrected—the primary reason for prescribing and fitting a contact lens. Thus, it is necessary to understand the application, advantages and disadvantages of the several *optical forms* of the toric base lens in order to achieve a proper correction of the refractive error.

The Toric Base, Spherical Front Surface Lens

When a toric base, spherical front surface lens is applied to the cornea, a cylinder is introduced into the refractive system because of the difference in refractive index between the plastic contact lens and the precorneal fluid lens. The resultant cylinder

thus formed seldom corrects the astigmatic refractive error[19,78,79] and, in point of fact, frequently increases it by inducing additional residual astigmatism.[27] The toric base of the contact lens forms a minus cylinder, the axis of which is along the flatter principal meridian of the toric contact lens surface and the power of which, *in situ*, is equal to 0.314 times the power of the cylinder in air or 0.452 times the K value of the back surface cylinder (*see* Table 9.4). If the radii of the toric back surface of the contact lens are 7.85 mm. (43.00 D. K reading) at 180° and 7.50 mm. (45.00 D. K reading) at 90°, the power of this cylinder is -2.90 D. axis 180° in air* and -0.90 D. axis 180° when *in situ*.†

It can be seen from this example that when a toric back surface contact lens orients properly on a cornea having a with-the-rule toricity, a minus cylinder is induced at axis 180°. This would correct a physiological residual astigmatism that is with the rule. Most such residual astigmatism, however, is against the rule. Thus, a toric base, spherical front surface contact lens will generally increase the total residual astigmatism under these conditions. Korb states that the application of a toric lens compounds whatever astigmia is residual.[19]

Wesley has observed that this lens construction frequently does *not* increase the residual astigmatism, even though the laws of optics would predict such an increase.[58] Some fitters support his views[75] and report good clinical results in correcting refractive errors with toric base lenses having spherical front surfaces. The author has had an opportunity to order and inspect many such lenses and finds they invariably contain an unordered front surface cylinder that is a byproduct of the manufacturing process. The amount of this front surface cylinder is fre-

---

*Power of cylinder in air equals $(43.00 - 45.00) \times C_2 = -2.00 \times 1.452 = -2.90$ D. axis 180°.

†Power of cylinder *in situ* (fluid) equals $(43.00 - 45.00) \times C_3 = -2.00 \times 0.452 = -0.90$ D. axis 180° or $-2.90 \times 0.314 = -0.90$ D. axis 180°.

quently of sufficient magnitude to neutralize the cylinder induced by the back surface cylinder when the lens is *in situ*.

There is, however, one set of circumstances when a toric base, spherical front surface lens construction is the one of choice, namely, when the corneal toricity is against the rule and the physiological residual astigmatism is equal to, or nearly to, 0.452 times the K value of the back surface lens toricity. Then, providing the lens maintains its meridional orientation, the minus cylinder present at the contact lens–fluid lens interface will correct the physiological residual astigmatism. This is the one condition under which the toric fitting qualities of the lens does assist in correcting the astigmatic refractive error.

If the lens does not orient so that its flat meridian is aligned with the axis of the physiological residual astigmatism or if it does not retain its meridional orientation due to lid torque, an astigmatism is formed that is the oblique resultant of the physiological residual astigmatism and the induced cylinder.

The Bitoric Corneal Contact Lens

Since the toric base, spherical front surface lens will likely fail to correct the residual astigmatism and, as pointed out, will frequently increase it, it is generally necessary to add an additional toric surface to the front of the lens to correct both the physiological residual astigmatism and the residual astigmatism induced by the back toric surface of the lens. This produces a bitoric lens.

PRINCIPAL MERIDIAN CALCULATION METHOD. Calculating the optical specifications of a bitoric lens is theoretically a straightforward and easy task. If the lens is fitted on K in both principal meridians, its power is equal to the power of the correcting spectacle prescription referred to the corneal plane. If the lens is fitted flatter than K in either principal meridian, +0.25 D. is added to the meridional power of the contact lens for each 0.25 D. K

reading that the base curve is flatter than the cornea in that meridian. This calculation is readily made by placing the meridian powers of the spectacle correcting lens (referred to the corneal plane) on an optical cross[80] and adding +0.25 D. for each 0.25 D. K reading that the base curve is flatter than the corneal K reading of that meridian.

EXAMPLE.

Spectacle correction $-1.00\ -2.00$ axis 180
Keratometer readings   43.00 at 180 and 44.00 at 90

If the lens is fitted on K in both meridians, the power is simply $-1.00 = -2.00$ axis 180° (Figure 9.15a). If the toric base curve is specified as 42.75 at 180 and 43.50 at 90, that is 0.25 flatter than K at 180° and 0.50 flatter than K at 90°, +0.25 and +0.50 D. respectively must be added to the optical cross of 9.15a. The resulting lens power is $-0.75\ -1.75$ axis 180° (Figure 9.15b).*

This lens will fully correct the refractive error, providing the following: (1) the axis of corneal toricity is the same as the axis of the spectacle correction; (2) the lens orients properly; (3) the lens maintains its meridional orientation against the forces of gravity and lid torque; and (4) all of the assumptions made in calculating the residual astigmatism (p. 248) are justified. In addition, the front and back toric curves must be accurately manufactured and must have the same axis. All of these conditions are seldom met, and therefore, it is unusual for a bitoric lens to correct the refractive error fully. Generally an oblique residual astigmatism is present. It may vary as the lens undergoes rotation. If its magnitude is small, it will not cause any significant visual distress. If large, a new lens will have to be made.

When the axis of the corneal toricity, the axis of the correcting spectacle lens cylinder, and/or the axis of the residual astigmatism

---

*For a detailed explanation of the optics of this system, refer to reference 27.

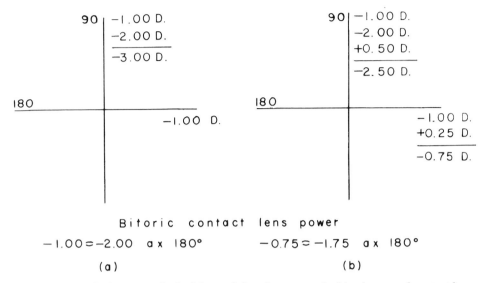

Figure 9.15. Optical cross method of determining the power of a bitoric corneal contact lens: (*a*) fitted on K, and (*b*) fitted 0.25 D. flatter than K in the horizontal meridian and 0.50 D. flatter than K in the vertical meridian.

are not in agreement (differ by more than ±15°), the power of the toric lens has to be calculated by employing crossed cylinder equations. This procedure is too complex for clinical application and, in addition, the results are generally disappointing.

REFRACTION METHOD. Because of the many errors associated with calculating the power of a bitoric lens, a recommended alternative suggested by several authors[75,81-83] is to first fit the patient with toric base, *spherical front surface lenses*. The meridional orientation of the lens is carefully measured (as previously described for prism ballast lenses) and a spherocylindrical refraction is performed with the contact lens *in situ*. The result of this refraction is conveyed to the laboratory together with the toric base lens specifications and its meridional orientation. The laboratory will fabricate a lens whose toric back surface is the same as that of the diagnostic lens used and whose toric front surface

is designed to provide the necessary additional refractive correction.

TORIC BACK SURFACE WITH SPHERICAL POWER EFFECT[62] The procedures and calculations thus far described for determining the power of a bitoric lens, are necessary *only when a significant amount of physiological residual astigmatism is present*, that is to say, when the lens is used not only to fit a toric cornea but also to correct a residual refractive error. When, however, a spherical lens provides a satisfactory correction of the refractive error but the toric base lens is necessary to obtain a proper fit, the bitoric lens power can be calculated so as to provide the power effect of a spherical lens when it is on the eye. This lens has several optical advantages.

1. Its power can be calculated without regard to the accuracy of corneal *K* readings or the meridional orientation of the lens.

2. The lens can rotate on the cornea without producing the visual effects characteris-

tic of other toric base lens types.

The lens design is basically quite simple. A plus cylinder is applied to the front surface of the lens. This cylinder is equal, but opposite, in power to the minus cylinder that is present at the contact lens–fluid lens interface. The axes of the two cylinders are the same. Thus, the front surface cylinder precisely neutralizes the back surface cylinder *when the lens is on the eye.* Under these design conditions the lens has the power effect of a spherical contact lens when it is on the eye but is actually a bitoric spherocylindrical lens when it is measured in air.*

An example will serve to illustrate how the power of this lens is determined:

A lens whose toric back surface radii are 8.04 mm. and 7.50 mm. (42.00 D. and 45.00 D. *K* reading respectively) gives an optimum lens-cornea bearing relationship and permits proper venting. A *spherical* diagnostic contact lens whose base curve is 8.04 mm. (42.00 D.) and whose power is −3.00 D. corrects the refractive error with a negligible residual astigmatism remaining. The bitoric lens that will have the same power effect as the spherical lens will have a power of −3.00 D. in the flatter principal meridian and −6.00 D. in the steeper principal meridian, as will be shown. The power in the flatter principal meridian is determined by doing a spherical refraction through a spherical trial contact lens whose base curve is equal to that of the flatter radius of curvature of the toric base lens. The power in the steeper principal meridian of the lens is calculated by using the equation

$$F'_s = F'_f + K_f - K_s \quad \text{(Formula 9.1)}$$

where

F'_s = the back vertex power of the contact lens in the steeper principal meridian (in air)

---

*The front surface cylinder will be 0.314 times the magnitude of the back surface cylinder for lenses whose refractive index is 1.490.

F'_f = the back vertex power of the contact lens in the flatter principal meridian (in air)

K_f = the base curve of the contact lens in the ~~steeper~~ *flatter* principal lens meridian (in air)

K_s = the base curve of the contact lens in the flatter principal lens meridian (expressed in diopters *K* reading)

In this example, the power in the steeper (90°) meridian is as follows:

$$F'_s = -3.00 + 42.00 - 45.00 = -6.00 \text{ D.}$$

When measured with the lensometer, this lens will read −3.00 −3.00 axis 180°. When on the eye it will have the power effect of a −3.00 D. sphere *regardless of its meridional orientation.*

The sequence of procedures for ordering this type of lens may be briefly summarized as follows:

1. Select the base curve radii (K_f and K_s), lens diameter, optic zone diameter, and secondary curve radii that provide an optimum physical fit.

2. Using a spherical trial lens whose base curve is the same as the flatter base curve, K_f, of the toric lens selected in   Step 1 above, do a spherical refraction to determine the required power of this spherical trial lens. This power is F'_f.

3. Calculate the power, F'_s, of the steeper meridian of the toric base lens by using Step 1.

4. Order the lens by specifying all necessary dimensions and including the base curve and power in each of the two principal lens meridians.

(e.g. B.C. 42.00   Power −3.00 D.
      B.C. 45.00   Power −6.00 D.)

Verification of Toric Base Contact Lenses

The practitioner cannot hope to master the fitting of contact lenses until he becomes skilled at determining the precise specifications of the lenses with which he is working. This is especially true with toric base lenses. To understand both the fitting and power characteristics of such a lens, the fitter must have accurate information about the optic zone radii of curvature, the axis of the back surface cylinder, the power of the lens in air (including cylinder axis), and the cylindrical power of the lens when *in situ*. All of these parameters can be measured with a good degree of accuracy.

The base curve radii are measured with the radiuscope, the keratometer, or the R-C device. The procedure is the same as with a spherical lens, except that readings are taken of both principal meridians. The lens is rotated until its principal meridians of curvature are at 90° and 180°. With the keratometer, the procedure is the same as for measurement of the cornea. For the radiuscope and R-C device, it must be remembered that the horizontal radius of curvature is determined when the vertical image of the target is sharp, and vice versa. The axis of the lens (flatter principal meridian) is gently and carefully marked with a sharp grease marking pencil by placing a light stroke on each edge of the lens along this meridian. A heavier line is then made on the front sur-

face of the lens after which the lens is oriented and remeasured to check both curvature and axis.

The power of the lens in air is measured by placing the concave surface of the lens against the lensometer lens stop and rotating the lens until the marked axis is horizontal. One thus obtains both the lens power (sphere and cylinder) and the axis of the cylinder in reference to the axis of the back toric surface.

The cylindrical power that is of even greater significance to the fitter is the one that is present when the lens is *in situ*. This can be measured directly with the lensometer. The technique, developed by the author, is illustrated in Figure 9.16a. An annulus of double-sided tape is applied to both surfaces of a plastic washer. A spherical contact lens of good optical quality and about 0.3 mm. center thickness is attached to the double-sided tape as illustrated. The surfaces of this lens must be measured with a radiuscope or keratometer to make certain that the pressure of applying the lens to the tape did not distort them into toric curves (*they must be spherical*). The device is attached to the lens

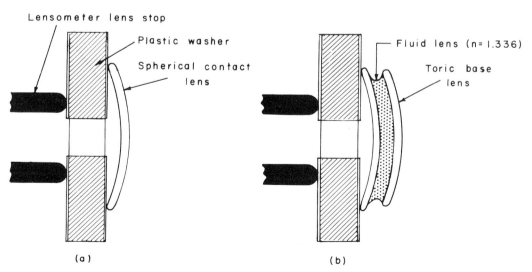

Figure 9.16. A device for measuring the cylindrical power that will be present when a toric back surface or bitoric corneal contact lens is *in situ*.

stop of a lensometer by means of the double-sided tape on the opposite side of the washer.

A small drop of ophthalmic irrigating solution (n = 1.336, the same as tear fluid) is placed in the concavity of the toric base lens, and the lens is placed piggyback upon the spherical lens of the device (Figure 9.16b). The lens is gently rotated until the back surface axis is oriented as it would be expected to orient on the eye. During measurement the lens is held in place only by the surface tension of the fluid. The spherical power measured has no meaning and must be ignored, but the cylinder power and axis are those which will be induced by the contact lens *when it is on the eye.*

This technique provides a most convenient means for verifying the accuracy of the toric base, spherical power lens. No cylinder should be found when this measurement is made, even though a significant cylinder might be present when the lens is measured in air.

Finally, it should be pointed out that a toric lens surface is difficult to produce accurately. To manufacture two accurate toric surfaces on the same lens is an extremely difficult task. Even though the fitter may recognize this, he must nonetheless place himself in the position of critically evaluating the finished product that he receives from the laboratory. Accurate information about the lens dimensions will help him understand his patients' response to the lens and to order any necessary modifications intelligently.

REFERENCES

1. Borish, I. M.: *Clinical Refraction*, 2nd ed., Chicago, Professional Press, 1954, pp. 46–47.

2. Bailey, N. J.: Residual astigmatism with contact lenses, Part 2, Predictability, *Opt. J. Rev. Optom.*, 98(2):40–45, 1961.

3. Bonnet, R., and Cochet, P.: New method of topographical ophthalmometry, *Bull. Soc. Ophthalmol. Fr.* 73:688–716, 1960, translation by E. Eagle, *Am. J. Optom.*, 39(5):227–251, 1962.

4. Ellerbrock, V. J.: Variables in corneal topography, *Am. J. Optom.*, 38(10):556–562, 1961.

5. Grosvenor, T.: Clinical use of the keratometer in evaluating the corneal contour, *Am. J. Optom.*, 38(5):237–246, 1961.

6. Jenkins, T. C. A.: Aberrations of the eye and their effects on vision—Part 1, *Br. J. Physiol. Opt.*, 20(2):59–91, 1963.

7. Knoll, H. A.: Corneal contours in the general population as revealed by the photokeratoscope, *Am. J. Optom.*, 38(7):389–397, 1961.

8. Mandell, R. B.: Methods to measure the peripheral corneal curvature, *J. Am. Optom. Assoc.*—Part 1, Photokeratoscopy, 33(2):137–139, 1961; Part 2, Geometric construction and "computers," 33(8):585–589, 1962;

Part 3, Ophthalmometry, 33(12):889–892, 1962

9. Mandell, R. B.: Reflection point ophthalmometry, *Am. J. Optom.*, 39(10):513–537, 1962.

10. Mandell, R. B.: *Corneal Contour and Contact Lenses.* Paper read before the annual meeting of the American Academy of Optometry, Chicago, Dec., 1963.

11. Korb, D. R.: Corneal contact lenses with toric optical zones and spherical or toric peripheral zones, in *Encyclopedia of Contact Lens Practice*, South Bend, Indiana, International Optics, 1959–1963, vol. 2, Chap. 9, pp. 16–64.

12. Korb, D. R.: A preliminary report of continuing performance of toric inner surface contact lenses, *Contacto*, 5(10):317–323, 1961.

13. Wesley, N. K.: Inside toric curve contact lens fitting, *Contacto*, 5(1):31–45, 1961.

14. Grosvenor, T. P.: *Contact Lens Theory and Practice*, Chicago, Professional Press, 1963, pp. 270, 283.

15. Duke-Elder, W. S.: *Textbook of Ophthalmology*, St. Louis, C. V. Mosby, 1949, vol. 4.

16. Sarver, M. D.: The effect of contact lens tilt upon residual astigmatism, *Am. J. Optom.*, 40(12):730–744, 1963.

17. Tocher, R. B.: Astigmatism due to the tilt of a

contact lens, *Am. J. Optom.*, *39(1)*:3–16, 1962.

18. Wesley, N. K.: Residual astigmatism, *Contacto*, *3(9)*:369–375, 1959.

19. Korb, D. R.: A preliminary report on toric contact lenses, *Optom. Weekly*, *51(48)*:2501–2505, 1960.

20. Bailey, N. J.: Residual astigmatism with contact lenses—Part 3, Possible sites, *Opt. J. Rev. Optom.*, *98(3)*:31–32, 1961.

21. Marano, J. A.: Front surface cylindrical contact lenses, *Optom. Weekly*, *53(37)*:1803–1804, 1962.

22. Harris, M. G.: Contact lens flexure and residual astigmatism on toric corneas, *J. Am. Optom. Assoc.*, *41(3)*:247–248, 1970.

23. Bailey, N. J.: Residual astigmatism with contact lenses, *Arch. Soc. Am. Ophthalmol. Opt.*, *11(1)*:37–41, 1959.

24. Mote, H. G., and Fry, G. A.: The relation of the keratometric findings to the total astigmatism of the eye, *Am. J. Optom.*, *16(11)*:402–409, 1939.

25. Harris, M. G., and Chu, C. S.: The effect of contact lens thickness and corneal toricity on flexure and residual astigmatism, *Am. J. Optom.*, *49(4)*:304–307, 1972.

26. Gordon, S.: The correction of residual astigmatism through toric inside contact lenses, *Optom. Weekly*, *52(4)*:186–192, 1961.

27. Sarver, M. D.: Calculation of the optical specifications of contact lenses, *Am. J. Optom.*, *40(1)*:20–28, 1963.

28. Kaplan, M. M.: Residual astigma and the precorneal fluid, *Optom. Weekly*, *53(43)*:2138–2141, 1962.

29. Brungardt, T. F.: Predicting residual astigmatism, *Optom. Weekly*, *62(22)*:521–522, 1971.

30. Bailey, N. J.: Residual astigmatism with contact lenses—Part 1, Incidence, *Opt. J. Rev. Optom.*, *98(1)*:30–31, 1961.

31. Sarver, M. D.: A study of residual astigmatism, *Am. J. Optom.*, *46(8)*:578–582, 1969.

32. Carter, J. H.: Residual astigmatism of the human eye, *Optom. Weekly*, *54(27)*:1271–1272, 1963.

33. Kratz, J. D., and Walton, W. G.: A modification of Javal's Rule for the correction of astigmatism, *Am. J. Optom.*, *26(7)*:295–306, 1949.

34. Dellande, W. D.: A comparison of predicted and measured residual astigmatism in corneal contact lens wearers, *Am. J. Optom.*, *47(6)*:459–463, 1970.

35. Westheimer, G.: Aberrations of contact lenses, *Am. J. Optom.*, *38(8)*:445–448, 1961.

36. Sarver, M. D.: Vision with hydrophilic contact lenses, *J. Am. Optom. Assoc.*, *43(3)*:316–320, 1972.

37. Harris, M. G.: The effect of contact lens thickness and diameter on residual astigmatism: a preliminary study, *Am. J. Optom.*, *47(6)*:442–444, 1970.

38. Ewell, D. G., Gates, H., and Remba, M. J.: The prism ballast contact lens principle, in *Encyclopedia of Contact Lens Practice*, South Bend, Indiana, International Optics, 1959–1963, vol. 2, Chap. 16, pp. 31–38.

39. Korb, D. R.: A survey of current fitting techniques for prism ballast corneal contact lenses, in *Encyclopedia of Contact Lens Practice*, South Bend, Indiana, International Optics, 1959–1963, vol. 3, App. B, pp. 88–97.

40. Goldberg, J. B.: A clinical procedure to determine the effective cylinder axis for prism ballast lenses, in *Encyclopedia of Contact Lens Practice*, South Bend, Indiana, International Optics, 1959–1963, vol. 3, Chap. 16, pp. 31–38.

41. Goldberg, J. B.: Correction of residual astigmatism with corneal contact lenses, *Br. J. Physiol. Opt.*, *21(3)*:169–1973, 1964.

42. Sutton, R. T.: Toric lens survey, *J. Contact Lens Soc. Am.*, *4(3)*:17–19, 1970.

43. Borish, I. M.: Cylinder lenses, Bulletin #4, Indiana Contact Lens Co., Marion, Indiana, 1960.

44. Borish, I. M.: *Review of 500 Cases of Residual Astigmatism Corrected by Front-surface Ballasted Contact Lenses.* Paper presented at 1st annual symposium on contact lenses, Ohio State University, 1963.

45. Korb, D. R.: Technique to achieve centration with prism corneal contact lenses, in *Encyclopedia of Contact Lens Practice*, South Bend, Indiana, International Optics, 1959–1963, vol. 4, App. B, pp. 117–123.

46. Bayshore, C. A.: Corneal contact lenses, postgraduate course, Chicago, American Academy of Optometry, Dec. 4–6, 1963.

47. Connor, J. J.: Prism ballast front surface toric

contact lenses, *Austr. J. Optom.*, *55(10)*:403–404, 1972.

48. Hofstetter, H. W., and Baldwin, W.: Bilateral correlation of residual astigmatism, *Am. J. Optom.*, *34(7)*:388–391, 1957.

49. Braff, S. M.: A new corneal contact lens design for the correction of residual astigmatism, *Optom. Weekly*, *61(1)*:24–25, 1970.

50. Fairmaid, J. A.: The correction of residual astigmatism with double truncated front surface toric micro-lenses: a report of 50 cases, *Austr. J. Optom.*, *50*:33–38, 1967.

51. Moss, H. L.: Semi-sclero-corneal flange lens for correcting residual astigmatism, *J. Am. Optom. Assoc.*, *31(1)*:57–58, 1959.

52. Nissel, G.: Correction of residual astigmatism with contact lenses, *The Optician*, *137(3552)*:407–408, 1959.

53. McKellen, G. D.: Corneal lenses and residual astigmatism, *The Ophthalmic Optician*, *7(2)*:60, 1967.

54. Labandz, A. R.: The anterior toric contact lens: a helpful contact lens for the correction of residual astigmatism, *J. Contact Lens Soc. Am.*, *3*:17–20, 1969.

55. Schapero, M.: A review of a new corneal contact lens, *Optom. Weekly*, *43(18)*:713–716, 1952.

56. Schapero, M.: The fitting of highly toric corneas with toric corneal contact lenses, *Am. J. Optom.*, *30(3)*:157–160, 1953.

57. Baglien, J. W.: The use of toric corneal contact lenses, *Optom. Weekly*, *44(4)*:129–130, 1953.

58. Wesley, N. K.: A new contact lens for toroidal eyes, *Opt. J. Rev. Optom.*, *97(20)*:39–43, 1960.

59. Kaplan, M. M.: Residual astigmatism and the bitoric lens, *Optom. Weekly*, *54(3)*:99–105, 1963.

60. Remba, M. J.: The A.B.C.'s of toric contact lens fitting, *Opt. J. Rev. Optom.*, *99(24)*:25–30, 1962.

61. Ellerbrock, V. J.: The role of toric surfaces in contact lens practice, *Am. J. Optom.*, *40(8)*:439–446, 1963.

62. Sarver, M. D.: A toric base corneal contact lens with spherical power effect, *J. Am. Optom. Assoc.*, *34(14)*:1136–1137, 1963.

63. Schapero, M.: Bitoric corneal lenses, *J. Calif. Optom. Assoc.*, *30(3)*:188–191, 1962.

64. West, D. C.: Method for predicting subjec-tive cylinder when using toric base contact lenses, *J. Am. Optom. Assoc.*, *36(3)*:231–234, 1965.

65. Koetting, J. F.: Optical considerations in fitting toroidal back surface lenses and the management of residual astigmatism, *Contacto*, *9(1)*:14–22, 1965.

66. Ellerbrock, V. J.: The role of toric surfaces in contact lens practice, *Am. J. Optom.*, *40(8)*:439–446, 1963.

67. Wesley, N. K.: More facts about toric base curve lenses, *Contacto*, *61(1)*:28–30, 1962.

68. Grosvenor, T. P.: *Contemporary Contact Lens Practice*, Chicago, Professional Press, 1972, p. 57.

69. Remba, M. J.: Contact lenses and the astig-matic cornea, *Contacto*, *11(2)*:38–43, 1967.

70. Haynes, P. R.: Corneal contact lenses with toric peripheral curves, in *Encyclopedia of Contact Lens Practice*, South Bend, Indiana, International Optics, 1959–1963, vol. 1, App. B, pp. 26–32.

71. Greeman, N., Jr.: Toric periphery lens fitting, *Contacto*, *11(1)*:9–15, 1967.

72. Brucker, D.: Personal communication, 1973.

73. Bayshore, C. A.: Toric contact lens fitting, *Contacto*, *11(2)*:35–36, 1967.

74. Blackstone, M. R.: Toroidal micro-corneal lenses, *The Optician*, *155(4014)*:235–238, 1968.

75. Sellers, F. J. E.: Fitting of toric corneal contact lenses, *Am. J. Optom.*, *46(2)*:127–130, 1969.

76. Goldberg, J. B.: Clinical application of toric base curve contact lenses, *Optom. Weekly*, *53(39)*:1911–1915, 1962.

77. Goldberg, J. B.: Toroidal cornea lens design-ing, *J. Am. Optom. Assoc.*, *38(3)*:213–216, 1967.

78. Brungardt, T. F.: The case against toric base curve contact lens construction, *J. Am. Optom. Assoc.*, *33(11)*:830–832, 1962.

79. Kaplan, M. M.: Residual astigmia and the toric concavity, *Optom. Weekly*, *53(27)*:1339–1343, 1962.

80. Borish, I. M.: *Clinical Refraction*, 2nd ed., Chicago, Professional Press, 1954, pp. 412–413.

81. Wilhelm, D.: Use of bitoric contact lenses: a case report, *Contacto*, *5(5)*:175–176, 1961.

82. Morrison, R. J., Kaufman, K. J., and Seruly,

E.: Oblique bitorics: a method to calculate and/or check prescriptions as indicated on the lensometer, *J. Am. Optom. Assoc.*, *36*(*12*):1068–1069, 1965.

83. Cappelli, Q. A.: Determining the final power of bitoric lenses, *Br. J. Physiol. Opt.*, *21*(*4*): 356–263,1964.

ADDITIONAL READINGS

Abdulla, N.: Full back toric contact lens fitting: optical principles, *The Disp. Opt.*, *29*(*18*):69–70, 1977.

Borish, I. M.: Specialized procedure for fitting ballasted corneal contact lenses, *Int. Cont. Lens Clin.*, *1*(*4*):56–64, 1974.

Borish, I. M.: Ballasted cylindrical lenses, *J. Am. Optom. Assoc.*, *47*(*3*):318, 1976.

Cohen, A. L.: Role of gravity in prism ballasting, *Am. J. Optom. Physiol. Opt.*, *53*(*5*):229, 1976.

Dickson, D. P.: A toric alternative, *Cont. Lens Forum*, *3*(*5*):39, 1978.

Goldberg, J. B.: The corneal astigmatic bearing area, *Optom. Weekly*, *65*(*40*):27–28, 1974.

Grosvenor, T.: What causes astigmatism?, *J. Am. Optom. Assoc.*, *47*(*7*):926–933, 1976.

Grosvenor, T. P.: Optical principles of toric contact lenses, *Optom. Weekly*, *67*(*2*):37–39, 1976.

Inman, O. R.: Peripheral design of toric corneal lenses, *The Optician*, *167*(*4318*):13–17, 1974.

Jackson, W. R.: Control residual astigmatism through special design contact lenses, *Contacto*, *19*(*4*):10–11, 1975.

Janoff, L. E.: A pilot study of the comparison of validity and reliability between the Radiuscope and Toposcope, *Int. Cont. Lens Clin.*, *4*(*2*):68–73, 1977.

Kemmetmuller, H.: Improving vision by means of contact lenses in cases of astigmatism, *The Ophthalmic Optician*, *16*(*16*):676–678, 1976.

Keyser, L. J.: Optical principles of spherical and bitoric hard contact lenses, *Optom. Weekly*, *67*(*34*):915–918, 1976.

King, B.: Astigmatism: alternatives with contact lenses, *Optom. Monthly*, p. 89, Feb. 1980.

Lee, W. C.: Bitorics for the toric cornea, *Cont. Lens Forum*, *4*(*12*):37, 1979.

Lee, W. C.: Practical notes on bitorics, *Cont. Lens Forum*, *5*(*2*):41, 1980.

Neefe, C. W.: Toric base and bitorics calculated by 1,2,3, *Optom. World*, *64*(*12*):5–6, 1977.

Paige, N.: Formula fitting of toric lenses, *Cont. Lens Forum*, *4*(*1*):39, 1979.

Chapter 10

GAS–PERMEABLE LENSES

One of the primary requisites for contact lens success is to provide sufficient oxygen to satisfy the basic needs of the cornea.[1] For hard contact lenses of standard P.M.M.A. material, this oxygen must be supplied by the tear pump mechanism as described in Chapter 6. Other contact lenses are available, however, in materials that can allow oxygen to pass directly through the lens itself. Unfortunately, it is often found that these materials suffer from other deficiencies, which seriously limit their application.

PERMEABILITY OF LENS MATERIALS

Examples of hard permeable plastics that have been used for contact lenses are as follow: cellulose acetate butyrate (C.A.B.), various silicon-P.M.M.A. combinations, 4-methyl-pentene-1, and others. Unfortunately, several of these materials have been found to present other properties that make them unsuitable for contact lenses. The most notable of these is poor wettability, which often seems to accompany the property of good oxygen permeability in plastics. Other characteristics that are unfavorable for contact lens use and that are often found in gas-permeable materials are a tendency to accumulate deposits of proteins, lipids, or inorganic compounds; poor physical stability of the contact lens shape; and poor machining characteristics.

MECHANISM OF PERMEABILITY

Hard permeable plastics transmit oxygen by a mechanism that differs from that of hydrogel contact lenses.[2] A hydrogel lens transmits oxygen primarily through the water phase of its structure, and the water percentage usually determines its permeability. A hard plastic, however, transmits oxygen directly through the molecular structure, and its makeup determines the permeability. The hydration of hard plastics may in fact reduce the permeability in some cases.

NEED FOR GAS–PERMEABLE LENSES

It is obvious from an examination of the P.M.M.A. contact lens wearing population that the tear pump alone is not sufficient to provide the corneal oxygen needs of many patients. Studies by Korb[3] and others[4,5] have shown that the incidence of edema in the typical clinical population of P.M.M.A. contact lens wearers is significant. Low amounts of corneal edema were detected in about 40 percent of the patients. This edema is not likely to have significant clinical effects and may be ignored. However, moderate or severe edema was present in another 30 percent of the cases. This edema is known to cause significant clinical effects and may lead in the long run to lens intolerance. In these cases, there is little question of a need for an additional oxygen supply to the cornea. Some practitioners argue that even a low amount of edema is significant and indicates most contact lens patients should be fitted with a gas-permeable material.[6]

OXYGEN PERMEABILITY REQUIREMENT

Hard permeable contact lenses may provide oxygen to the cornea either by the tear pumping mechanism or by direct transmission through the lens material.[7,8] It is not necessary to depend upon permeability itself to provide the entire oxygen supply. Consequently, even low permeabilities may be significant in contributing to the success of the lens.

From the discussion of the oxygen need in Chapter 6, it may be concluded that

1. the minimum corneal oxygen need varies between 2 and 5 percent (equivalent atmospheric) depending on the individual characteristics.[9,10]

2. P.M.M.A. contact lenses usually supply between 1 and 3 percent oxygen at the corneal surface.[7] Therefore, a significant proportion of the contact lens wearing population has a partial oxygen deficit at the corneal surface.

From Figure 10.1 it may be seen that

3. an oxygen level at the corneal surface of 1 percent will cause between 3 and 8 percent corneal swelling.

4. an oxygen level at the corneal surface of 2 percent will cause from 0 to 6 percent corneal swelling.

5. an oxygen level at the corneal surface of 3 percent will cause from 0 to 4 percent corneal swelling.

Figure 10.2 shows the relationship between the various oxygen-permeable hard materials and the oxygen level produced at the corneal surface. As is characteristic of all contact lens materials, the oxygen level increases as the lens thickness is reduced. A comparison can also be made of the thicknesses required by different materials to produce the same oxygen concentration at the cornea. For example, a lens made of the flex material, which is 0.32 mm. thick, would produce an oxygen level at the corneal surface of 2 percent. To produce the same oxygen level at the cornea with a lens made of C.A.B. material would require that the thickness be re-

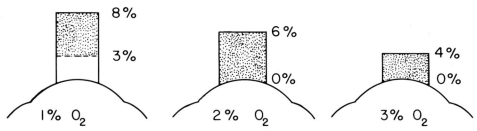

Figure 10.1 Corneal swelling caused by oxygen levels at the corneal surface of 1, 2, and 3 percent.

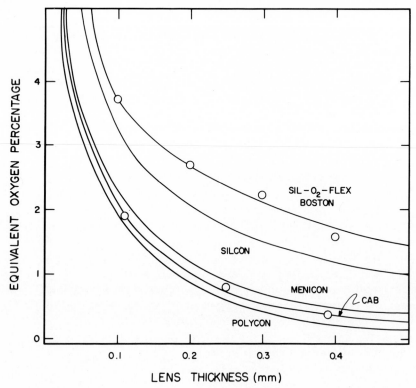

Figure 10.2 Relationship between various oxygen-permeable hard materials and the equivalent oxygen percentage that is produced at the corneal surface.

duced to 0.1 mm.

Since most patients who wear P.M.M.A. contact lenses probably have at least a partial oxygen deficiency, this indicates that either

1. a poor pump mechanism exists because of an improper blink pattern or a lens-cornea relationship with poor pump efficiency.

2. the cornea has a high oxygen requirement.

Unfortunately, in a clinical setting it is impossible to say whether a patient exhibits corneal edema because of a high oxygen need or because of an inefficient lens-tear pump. Both of these factors may also contribute to the problem simultaneously. For some patients who exhibit corneal edema with a P.M.M.A. lens, a simple modification can improve the tear pump, such as flattening the peripheral curve or reducing the diameter, and this will eliminate the edema. Such a result indicates

that the lens did not provide an adequate tear pump. However, patients are commonly seen clinically for whom no amount of lens modification seems to improve the fit in terms of reducing edema. These patients likely have a high oxygen need and are good candidates for contact lenses made of an oxygen-permeable material. Unfortunately, in the clinical setting neither the oxygen need of the individual nor the efficiency of the tear pump mechanism can be easily determined. Hence, there is a trend towards a selection of the highest permeability material that can be obtained so that all patients will be provided with a maximum oxygen supply.

The question arises as to what level of permeability is needed for clinical success (Figure 10.3). Any level of permeability will be helpful but may not be sufficient for some patients. For example, a patient who has an oxygen need of 3 percent and a tear exchange

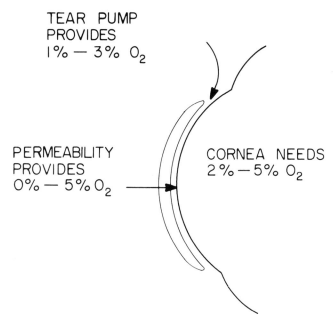

TEAR PUMP
PROVIDES
$1\% - 3\%$ O_2

PERMEABILITY
PROVIDES
$0\% - 5\%$ O_2

CORNEA NEEDS
$2\% - 5\%$ O_2

Figure 10.3 The individual corneal oxygen need varies between 2 and 5 percent. This requirement may be fulfilled by tear pumping action, lens permeability, or both. Since tear pumping
provides a limit of 3 percent oxygen, it cannot satisfy the requirements of all corneas. Contact
lens permeability varies from 0 percent for polymethyl methacrylate lenses to at least 5
percent for high permeability materials.

of 14 percent with each blink will benefit by
wearing a C.A.B. lens 0.22 mm. thick. This
lens is capable of producing an oxygen level
of 1 percent, which, when added to that
provided by the pumping mechanism, satisfies the patient's individual oxygen requirement. However, if the patient had less than a
14 percent mixing efficiency, the C.A.B. lens
would not completely eliminate the edema
(Figure 10.4).

OTHER FACTORS

Factors other than oxygen supply may
influence corneal hydration. Pressure has been
discussed as having a possible effect in producing corneal edema in contact lens wearers.[11]
There is no question that undue pressure
from a contact lens is capable of producing
damage to the corneal epithelial cells and is
responsible for some staining.

However, it is unlikely that pressure plays
a primary role in the production of the mild
to moderate corneal edema commonly seen
in contact lens wearers. The effect of pressure and other factors were tested by Polse
and Mandell,[12] who fitted a patient with a
very tight P.M.M.A. contact lens and produced central corneal clouding and corneal
edema. After the edema was present, and without removing the contact lens, the patient
was provided with a pair of goggles through
which 80 percent oxygen was pumped across
the cornea. The oxygen supply, which was
reduced by wearing the contact lens, was now
increased by four times. Under this condition, the patient's central corneal clouding
disappeared, and the corneal edema was
reduced. This demonstrated that the corneal

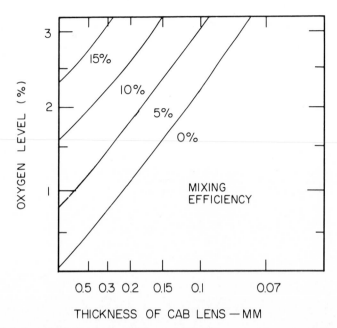

Figure 10.4 Relationship between the thickness of C.A.B. contact lenses and the oxygen level that is produced at the anterior corneal surface. The curves represent the mixing efficiency or the percent of tears that are exchanged during each blink. From I. Fatt, Oxygen Supply under a Gas Permeable Hard Lens, *Contact Lens Forum*, 4(4):57–61, 1979.

edema could be eliminated simply by the addition of oxygen, even when the pressure effects of the lens remained constant.

Although excess carbon dioxide is certainly a potential problem to the cornea, Fatt has shown that when carbon dioxide is formed in the cornea as a product of metabolism and cannot be discharged to the tears from the epithelium, it is forced backwards through the cornea and discharged into the aqueous humor.[13] This movement of carbon dioxide would occur at such a rapid rate that it could never reach a very significant concentration at the epithelium. Hence, it would appear that carbon dioxide presents very little difficulty with a tight contact lens.

There are many other aspects of the tear exchange problem that are known, and perhaps several that are unknown. The most important consideration is preservation of the normal tear constituents on the external cornea. It has been shown in a number of experiments that the precorneal film contains numerous substances that are vital for a healthy epithelium. Probably the most important of these is mucus, which is found on the exterior surface of the cornea but is not produced there. Rather, it is produced in the goblet cells of the palpebral portion of the conjunctiva. The mucus is dissolved in the tears and is deposited or rubbed onto the external corneal surface.[14] Mucus is necessary in order to prevent drying of tears on the cornea. The mucus has the effect of making the cornea hydrophilic rather than hydrophobic, as it would be otherwise.

There are many other substances in the tears that may be vital to corneal health over a long period of time, including sodium and potassium ions, immunoglobulins, etc.

The author's experience with various experimental hard permeable lenses shows that when the lens is fitted tightly on the eye, there is a disturbance to the normal appearance of the external corneal surface. Examination with fluorescein under the biomicroscope shows numerous areas of poor wetting and some light punctate staining. Hence, it would appear that at least some tears need to be exchanged beneath the contact lens in order to provide at least a minimum supply of the other corneal necessities. Some researchers have tried to develop contact lens materials that are so oxygen permeable that they will provide all of the needs of the cornea. It is then felt that the lens might be fitted in any way possible and still not cause any corneal disturbance. Such a goal may not even be desirable. If a lens provided all the corneal oxygen need, the fitter might be tempted to choose a design that would result in a very tight fit. Such a design would likely disturb a cornea in other ways, even though an adequate oxygen supply was available.

FITTING OF GAS–PERMEABLE LENSES

For most patients, gas-permeable lenses should be fitted according to the same guidelines and procedures used for P.M.M.A. lenses. However, several differences in lens construction may be employed to advantage in some patients:

1. Larger lens diameters may be used to aid in lens centration.

2. Larger optic zone diameters may be used to avoid flare problems.

3. Steeper peripheral curves may be used to improve lens comfort by keeping the lens periphery close to the cornea and away from the lids.

CELLULOSE ACETATE BUTYRATE

Of the various gas-permeable hard materials, C.A.B. was one of the earliest to be recognized as having properties that would be useful for contact lenses.[15-18] There are many different types of C.A.B. materials and its properties can be varied over a wide range. However, most of the C.A.B. materials that have been used for contact lenses have nearly the same oxygen permeability and suffer the same deficiencies.

CHEMISTRY OF CELLULOSE

Cellulose is a very large molecular weight substance, which is the major constituent of the woody fibers of plants, occurring in widely diffuse forms such as wood, which contains about 60 percent cellulose, and cotton fibers, which are nearly pure cellulose. Regardless of the source, the cellulose structure is that of a linear polymer composed of glucose units linked end to end. Some 2,000 to 3,000 glucose units comprise the basic cellulose chain.

When cellulose is combined with acetic acid and butyric acid, it forms cellulose acetate butyrate, which has many useful properties for a wide variety of applications. Only a limited number of formulations of C.A.B. are suitable for contact lenses. In these formulations, C.A.B. can be molded to produce either finished or semifinished lenses or buttons, from which lenses can be fabricated on lathes.[19] In using C.A.B. for contact lenses, some trade-off must be made between the most desirable properties for manufacturing purposes and those which enhance the physiological tolerance to the lens. Individual manufacturers will vary as to their preference of formula, and consequently, the properties of their various products will also vary slightly.

Cellulose acetate butyrate material has a relatively low oxygen permeability but has a good wetting angle. Its greatest disadvantage is a lack of dimensional stability. This gives C.A.B. contact lenses a greater tendency to warp compared to P.M.M.A. lenses. In order to compensate for this lower stability, contact lenses of C.A.B. are usually made about 0.06 mm. thicker than P.M.M.A. lenses in the low minus power range.[20] Increasing the lens center thickness does tend to stabilize the lens dimensions. However, the problem is still clinically significant, especially for high power minus lenses.[21-23] The greater thickness of this lens negates some of the advantages of the oxygen permeability of the C.A.B. material. Nevertheless, lenses of C.A.B. material are successful in reducing corneal edema in many contact lens patients. Several studies have shown that corneal edema was reduced when patients wore C.A.B. contact lenses as compared to P.M.M.A. lenses.[24-33] However, a small percentage of patients continued to show minor amounts of edema. This is consistent with the results by Mandell,[34] in which nine patients who were wearing P.M.M.A. contact lenses unsuccessfully were refitted with C.A.B. contact lenses. In each case, the original fitter had made one or more attempts to alleviate the edema by modifications or change of P.M.M.A. lenses. The C.A.B. lenses were chosen according to the judgment of the fitter to achieve the best possible fit. They were fitted on K and between 8.8 and 9.2 mm. in diameter. In addition to the usual clinical observations for edema, the subjects were measured by pachymetry, both with their P.M.M.A. lenses and their C.A.B. lenses, after a wearing period of between seven and eight hours. All of the nine patients who were given C.A.B. lenses to replace their P.M.M.A. lenses showed reduced corneal swelling (Figure 10.5). The average corneal swelling was 6.65 percent with P.M.M.A. lenses and 2.35 percent with C.A.B. lenses. These results are consistent with the theoretical conclusion that C.A.B. contact lenses in the thickness range of 0.16 to 0.20 mm. are capable of supplying a significant portion of the minimum corneal oxygen needed to prevent edema.

Fatt has predicted this relationship on a theoretical basis by showing the relative contributions to be expected from C.A.B. permeability combined with the pump mechanism.[35] Hence, there is considerable evidence, both clinical and theoretical, that C.A.B. contact lenses of 0.2 mm. thickness supply about 1 percent oxygen at the corneal surface.[36-40] Additional oxygen must be provided by the pump mechanism to reach a level that satisfies the cornea's individual oxygen need.

This conclusion was also supported in an experimental study by the author of four subjects who wore both P.M.M.A. and C.A.B. lenses of the same dimensions. It was found that less corneal swelling (Figure 10.6) and keratometer changes (Table 10.1) were found when C.A.B. lenses were worn.

LENS DESIGNS

Lenses of C.A.B. materials may be custom designed, but some laboratories provide them only in standard designs. In general, C.A.B. lenses are made thicker than P.M.M.A. lenses. The following are examples of standard lenses that are available.

Meso® Lens

The Meso lens is made by Danker & Wohlk, Inc. The lens diameter varies with the base curve as in Table 10.2. A second series is available for high plus powers with larger diameters (Table 10.3). The thickness of the lens varies with the power (Table 10.4).

CABCURVE® Lens

CABCURVE contact lenses (made by Soft Lenses, Inc.) are available in the following

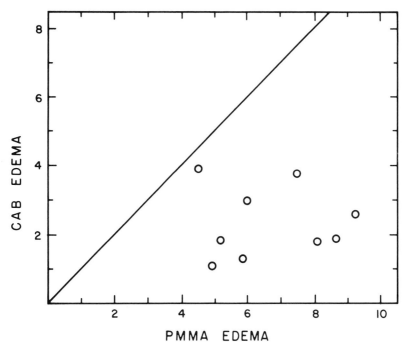

Figure 10.5 Corneal pachymetry measurements of edema in nine patients who were given C.A.B. lenses to replace their P.M.M.A. lenses. In each case the amount of corneal edema was reduced.

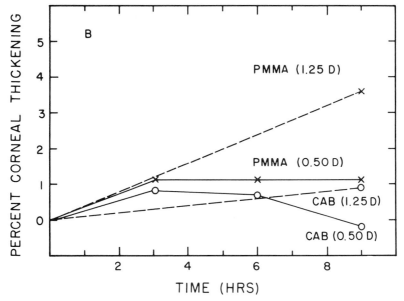

Figure 10.6 Corneal swelling that was produced when a subject wore P.M.M.A. and C.A.B. lenses which were fitted 1.25 D. and 0.5 D. steeper than the cornea edema.

TABLE 10.1
KERATOMETRY INCREASES WITH
C.A.B. AND P.M.M.A. LENSES

Subject	C.A.B.		P.M.M.A.	
	Horiz.	*Vert.*	*Horiz.*	*Vert.*
P	.25	.25	.75	.95
L	.37	.25	.63	.38
M	.50	.50	1.12	.87
B	.37	0	1.00	0
Average	.37	.25	.86	.52

TABLE 10.2
MESO MINUS POWER LENSES

Base Curve		Recommended Diameter
52.00	6.49	8.4
50.00	6.75	8.5
48.00	7.03	8.7
46.00	7.34	8.8
45.00	7.50	8.9
44.00	7.67	9.0
43.00	7.85	9.1
42.00	8.04	9.2
40.00	8.44	9.3
39.00	8.65	9.4

specifications:

1. Diameter: 8.8, 9.2, and 9.6 mm.
2. Base Curve: 41.00 D. to 47.00 D. steps
3. Power range: plano to −8.00 D. in 0.25 D. steps

A recommended trial set is given in Table 10.5.

FITTING

Cellulose acetate butyrate contact lenses may be fitted either by the method of direct ordering or by trial lenses. When trial lenses are used, it is not necessary to have a trial set made from C.A.B. material. In fact, a trial set with similar dimensions may be more useful if it is constructed of P.M.M.A. material, which is more stable.

Base Curve

The base curve is usually selected to provide slight apical clearance. In comparison to lenses designed of P.M.M.A., the fit is generally 0.25 to 0.50 D. steeper. This fit is recommended to achieve better centering with lenses that are usually thicker, and thus heavier, than average.

Power

The calculation of the correct power for a given patient is exactly the same procedure that is used for other hard contact lenses.

Evaluation of the Fit

A properly fitted C.A.B. lens may be evaluated in the same way as P.M.M.A. contact lenses. The fit is usually slightly steep, as shown by the fluorescein test. If a lens shows central touch, or there is excessive movement, it should be verified that lens flattening has not occurred. The most common problem found in wearers of C.A.B. contact lenses is reduced visual acuity. This usually indicates that the lens has become warped. It should be removed and checked on the radiuscope.

SOLUTIONS AND LENS CARE

Cellulose acetate butyrate contact lenses are attacked by many organic solvents that do not affect P.M.M.A. lenses. Recommended solutions and lens care are given in Chapter 12.

EXTENDED WEAR

Contact lenses of C.A.B. material have occasionally been recommended for extended wear. The relatively low oxygen permeability of this material would not appear to provide sufficient oxygen to satisfy the minimum corneal need under conditions of eye closure. Thus, this lens should not be recommended for extended-wear patients.

LENS MODIFICATIONS

Care must be exercised in carrying out modifications on C.A.B. lenses. The material has a lower melting temperature than P.M.M.A. and can be melted on the surface by the heat of polishing. All procedures must be carried out at slow speeds and with caution.

Cellulose acetate butyrate is attacked by polishing compounds with ammonia (such as Silvo®) and some organic solvents.

SILOXANE–P.M.M.A. COMBINATION LENSES

Silicon is one of the most common substances on the earth, yet its broad use in a variety of chemical compounds has only recently been expanded. Silicon has the property of joining with oxygen to produce long chain length molecules, which form the well-known substance silicone rubber. This substance, with only minor modifications, has been used to make a flexible contact lens,• which has undergone investigation since about 1960. More recently, however, it has been found that siloxanes (monomers of silicon, oxygen, and a radical), in combination with methacrylates, can produce substances that are used to form hard contact lenses. Such substances may have a variety of properties, depending upon the siloxane monomers used and the way they are joined together, but generally they are permeable to oxygen and carbon dioxide.[41]

Siloxane-P.M.M.A. combination contact lenses vary greatly in their wetting properties according to the structure of the compound. Some lenses are extremely hydrophobic and must be coated with hydrophilic

TABLE 10.3
HIGH PLUS POWER* MESO LENSES

Base Curve		Diameter
41.00	8.23	9.7
41.50	8.13	9.7
42.00	8.04	9.6
42.50	7.94	9.6
43.00	7.85	9.5
43.50	7.76	9.5
44.00	7.67	9.5
44.50	7.58	9.4
45.00	7.50	9.4

*Power range: +11.00 to +16.00 D.

TABLE 10.4
MESO LENS THICKNESS

Power	Thickness
−1.00 to −1.75	0.22
−2.00 to −2.75	0.20
−3.00 to −3.75	0.18
−4.00 to −5.75	0.16
+0.50	0.22
+1.00	0.24
+1.50	0.26
+2.00	0.28
+2.50	0.30
+3.00	0.32
+3.50	0.34
+11.00 to +11.50	0.41
+12.00 to +12.50	0.43
+13.00 to +13.50	0.44
+14.00 to +14.50	0.46
+15.00 to +15.50	0.48
+16.00	0.50

TABLE 10.5
RECOMMENDED TRIAL SET FOR CABCURVE LENSES

Diameter	Base Curve		Power
8.8	46.00	7.34	−3.00
8.8	45.50	7.42	−3.00
8.8	45.00	7.50	−3.00
8.8	44.50	7.59	−3.00
9.2	44.50	7.59	−3.00
9.2	44.00	7.67	−3.00
9.2	43.50	7.76	−3.00
9.2	43.00	7.85	−3.00
9.2	42.50	7.94	−3.00
9.2	42.00	8.04	−3.00
9.6	42.50	7.94	−3.00
9.6	41.50	8.13	−3.00

materials or have surface treatments to make them suitable for contact lenses.[42] Other materials, however, have been produced that have inherent properties of hydrophilicity.

Siloxane-P.M.M.A. contact lenses usually have high dimensional stability and hence can be made in minimum thickness, which enhances their oxygen transmission.[43] In addition, the material usually has good machining properties and hence may be formed into a contact lens by ordinary lathing methods. Consequently, all of the lens types that can be produced in P.M.M.A. material can also be produced with siloxane-P.M.M.A. Molding has also been used to produce contact lenses of this material.

Siloxane-P.M.M.A. contact lenses may be divided into two types, those with low permeability and those with high permeability.

LOW PERMEABILITY SILOXANE–P.M.M.A.

The first contact lens to be produced from a siloxane-P.M.M.A. combination was the Polycon® lens (made by Syntex Laboratories). This lens has a permeability that is nearly equal to C.A.B. but is more dimensionally stable and, hence, can be made thinner to allow a greater transmission of oxygen. The lens is generally successful as a replacement for P.M.M.A. contact lenses.

The Polycon contact lens is capable of providing the cornea with a significant portion of its oxygen supply, although some oxygen must also be supplied by the tear pump.[44,45] Nevertheless, in most clinical situations the Polycon contact lens will eliminate corneal edema. The exceptions occur for lenses of thicknesses greater than 0.20 mm., where significant oxygen deprivation may be present. The theoretical expectation of minimum edema is supported by several clinical studies in which it was shown that the Polycon lens eliminates significant corneal edema. Sarver et al. reported forty-six patients who had experienced failure with small, thin P.M.M.A. lenses, primarily due to excessive edema.[46] When the lenses were replaced with Polycon lenses, no significant edema was observed (Figure 10.7). Of the forty-six previous P.M.M.A. lens failures refitted with Polycon lenses, thirty-one (67%) wore the Polycon lenses successfully. The remaining thirteen patients (28%) could not wear Polycon lenses because of discomfort, but no significant edema was present.

Sarver et al., in another study, compared P.M.M.A., BPFlex®, and Polycon lenses of small diameter and concluded that the patients developed less edema with the Polycon lenses.[47]

Finnamore and Korb evaluated 100 patients from their contact lens practice, 50 of whom had no contact lens experience and 50 who were failures with P.M.M.A. lenses.[48] The incidence of higher grades of edema was significant in the P.M.M.A. lens wearers (55%), but no severe edema was present in wearers of the Polycon lens. A higher incidence of low grade edema was also found among the P.M.M.A. wearers.

Other clinical reports have supported the efficacy of Polycon lenses in relieving edema and its complications. Kame reported that, in fifty-two eyes of long-term P.M.M.A.

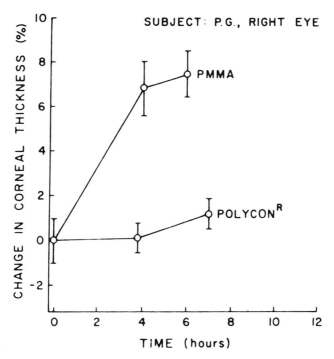

Figure 10.7 Change in corneal thickness (±S.D.) for the right eye of one adapted patient wearing a P.M.M.A. lens and a Polycon lens during eight-hour periods. From M. D. Sarver, K. A. Polse, and M. G. Harris, Patient Responses to Gas-permeable Hard (Polycon) Contact Lenses, *American Journal of Optometry and Physiological Optics, 54(4)*:195–200, 1977.

wearers, the edematous corneal formations that had been produced were relieved when the patients were refitted with Polycon lenses of the same base curve–cornea relationship.[49] Other authors have found similar results and have recommended the use of Polycon lenses for any P.M.M.A. lens wearer who showed edema or related corneal changes.[50]

Fitting

The fitting of Polycon lenses generally follows the same procedures used for P.M.M.A. lenses. Polycon lenses are available in standard lenses and may also be ordered by custom design. Minus lenses that are standard are available in two diameters, 9.5 and 8.5 mm. The principles followed in fitting the 9.5 lens are essentially those of the lid attachment philosophy described in Chapter 7. The

principles involved in fitting the 8.5 lens are similar to the small, thin lens philosophy described in Chapter 7.

Fitting of 9.5 Polycon Lens

The 9.5 mm. diameter Polycon lens is designed to position in the superior quadrant of the cornea.[50] In most cases, the upper edge of the lens is beneath the upper lid. The lens is generally fitted approximately 0.1 to 0.2 mm. flatter than the average K. However, the exact specification should be determined by a trial lens procedure.

After the initial trial lens is selected and placed on the eye, the following criteria should be evaluated:

POSITION. After the blink, the lens should position so that the upper edge is near the superior limbus.

Lens Movement. After completion of the blink, the lens should move to a superior position. It should not drop down to a centered position on the eye after each blink (*see* lid attachment philosophy, Chapter 7).

Comfort. The patient should be asked to compare comfort from one trial lens to the next. A lens that is not comfortable generally is not moving with the lid.

Fluorescein Pattern. The pattern for fluorescein should appear to be slightly flat by the usual criteria. The pattern should be evaluated with the lens in the superior riding position. If the lens moves to a centered position on the cornea, it should have the appearance of a lens that is too flat (Figure 10.8).

Changes in Trial Lenses. If the initial diagnostic lens does not satisfy the criteria of position, movement, and comfort, it is usually because the lens is too flat. The next steeper base curve should be tried. The optimal base curve is the steepest of the equally comfortable lenses that satisfies the other criteria of position and movement. If the criteria of position and movement are satisfied but sensation or discomfort are present, the next flatter base curve should be tried.

If the initial diagnostic lens position is too low, a lens with the next flatter base curve should be used. If the lens drops rapidly to a low position after insertion, it may indicate an incomplete blinking pattern, or simply that excess tearing is present.

Fitting Set. A trial set of standard lenses of 9.5 mm. diameter is given in Table 10.6.

Refraction. The Polycon lens may be considered a hard lens and follows the usual rules for determination of the refraction and lens power.

The 8.5 and 9.0 Polycon Lenses

The 8.5 mm. diameter lens is designed to position centrally on the cornea, although in some cases the upper edge of the lens may be

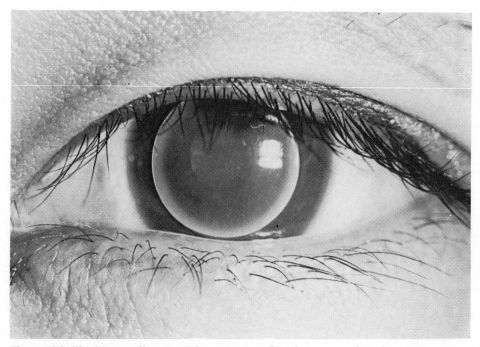

Figure 10.8. The 9.5 mm. diameter Polycon appears flat when centered on the cornea.

TABLE 10.6
9.5 MM. POLYCON TRIAL SET

Base Curve	Power	O.Z.D.	I.C.R.	I.C.W.	P.C.R.	P.C.W.	tc	te	Edge Lift
7.20	−3.00	8.4	9.0	.35	10.5	0.2	.11	.08	.11
7.30	−3.00	8.4	9.1	.35	10.5	0.2	.11	.08	.10
7.40	−3.00	8.4	9.1	.35	10.5	0.2	.11	.09	.10
7.50	−3.00	8.4	9.3	.35	11.0	0.2	.11	.09	.10
7.60	−3.00	8.4	9.3	.35	11.0	0.2	.11	.09	.10
7.70	−3.00	8.4	9.5	.35	11.0	0.2	.11	.10	.09
7.80	−3.00	8.4	9.7	.35	11.5	0.2	.11	.09	.10
7.90	−3.00	8.4	9.9	.35	12.0	0.2	.11	.09	.10
8.00	−3.00	8.4	10.0	.35	12.0	0.2	.11	.09	.09
8.10	−3.00	8.4	10.1	.35	12.0	0.2	.11	.10	.09
8.20	−3.00	8.4	10.2	.35	12.5	0.2	.11	.10	.09
8.30	−3.00	8.4	10.4	.35	13.0	0.2	.11	.09	.09
8.40	−3.00	8.4	10.6	.35	13.0	0.2	.11	.10	.09
8.50	−3.00	8.4	10.6	.35	13.0	0.2	.11	.10	.09
8.60	−3.00	8.4	10.8	.35	13.0	0.2	.11	.10	.09

slightly beneath the upper lid. The lens is generally designed to be very thin. It has the advantage of maximizing the oxygen transmission both through its permeability and pumping action. The lens suffers from the disadvantage that it has a small optic zone and often gives rise to flare problems or visual acuity disturbances.

FITTING PROCEDURE. The fitting procedure generally follows that of the small, thin lens. The lens is usually fitted on K or slightly steeper than K. On a toric cornea, it is not usually necessary to fit the lens steeper than K by more than one-third the difference in K

readings. A trial lens procedure is recommended. The manufacturer's recommended trial set is given in Table 10.7.

The Polycon 9.0 lens generally performs in the same way as an ultrathin lens design of P.M.M.A. material. In some cases, even greater flexing of the Polycon lens will occur due to its higher flexibility. This must be accounted for in predicting residual astigmatism. As a general guide, the procedures that were outlined for ultrathin lenses may be followed, but it should be recognized that an allowance may need to be made for the greater flexing (Table 10.8).

TABLE 10.7
8.5 MM. POLYCON TRIAL SET

Base Curve	Power	O.Z.D.	I.C.R.	I.C.W.	P.C.R.	P.C.W.	tc	te	Edge Lift
7.20	−3.00	7.0	7.7	0.65	17.0	0.1	.08	.08	.07
7.30	−3.00	7.0	7.8	0.65	17.0	0.1	.08	.08	.06
7.40	−3.00	7.0	7.9	0.65	17.0	0.1	.08	.08	.06
7.50	−3.00	7.0	8.0	0.65	17.0	0.1	.08	.08	.06
7.60	−3.00	7.0	8.1	0.65	17.0	0.1	.08	.09	.06
7.70	−3.00	7.0	8.2	0.65	17.0	0.1	.08	.09	.06
7.80	−3.00	7.0	8.3	0.65	17.0	0.1	.08	.09	.06
7.90	−3.00	7.0	8.4	0.65	17.0	0.1	.08	.09	.05
8.00	−3.00	7.0	8.5	0.65	17.0	0.1	.08	.09	.05
8.10	−3.00	7.0	8.6	0.65	17.0	0.1	.08	.09	.05
8.20	−3.00	7.0	8.7	0.65	17.0	0.1	.08	.09	.05

TABLE 10.8
9.0 MM. POLYCON TRIAL SET

Base Curve	Power	O.Z.D.	I.C.R.	I.C.W.	P.C.R.	P.C.W.	tc	te	Edge Lift
7.20	−3.00	7.8	8.10	.40	10.20	0.2	.12	.10	.09
7.30	−3.00	7.8	8.30	.40	10.40	0.2	.12	.10	.09
7.40	−3.00	7.8	8.40	.40	10.70	0.2	.12	.10	.09
7.50	−3.00	7.8	8.60	.40	10.90	0.2	.12	.10	.09
7.60	−3.00	7.8	8.70	.40	11.20	0.2	.12	.10	.09
7.70	−3.00	7.8	8.80	.40	11.50	0.2	.12	.10	.09
7.80	−3.00	7.8	9.00	.40	11.70	0.2	.12	.10	.09
7.90	−3.00	7.8	9.10	.40	12.00	0.2	.12	.10	.09
8.00	−3.00	7.8	9.30	.40	12.30	0.2	.12	.10	.09
8.10	−3.00	7.8	9.40	.40	12.60	0.2	.12	.10	.09
8.20	−3.00	7.8	9.60	.40	12.90	0.2	.12	.10	.09
8.30	−3.00	7.8	9.70	.40	13.20	0.2	.12	.10	.09

Polycon Lens Availability

In addition to the various standard lenses that are available in minus powers, it is possible to obtain Polycon lenses in low plus and aphakic series. The general outline of lens availability is described in Table 10.9. In addition, any lens dimensions may be ordered on a custom basis.

Extended Wear

Because the Polycon lens allows some oxygen transmission, a few fitters have attempted to allow patients to wear the lens on an extended basis. The oxygen permeability of the Polycon material is not sufficient to allow a safe extended wear procedure.

HIGH PERMEABILITY SILOXANE–P.M.M.A.

Several lenses have been made with siloxane-P.M.M.A. copolymers, which have high oxygen permeability. Some are hydrophobic and require special coating to render their surfaces hydrophilic. For other lenses, however, there is good wettability, and in at least one case it is greater than that of P.M.M.A. Two lenses that have high oxygen permeability (Dk = 10.5) and other similarities are the Boston lens and the flex lens. They differ only in that the flex lens has better wetting properties and is more easily machined. Hence, there are fewer manufacturing problems and generally fewer defects in the final lenses.

Fitting

In general, the high permeability lenses may be fitted larger and tighter than any of the other hard permeable lenses and still not precipitate corneal edema. This is possible because the material passes large amounts of oxygen to the cornea as shown in Figure 10.2. This high oxygen permeability has been verified both in animal studies and in measurements with an oxygen electrode. It indicates that lenses that are 0.1 mm. thick transmit about a 3.7 percent oxygen equivalent to the corneal surface. Hence, even without the additional oxygen supply from the lens-tear pump, it is possible to supply nearly all corneas with their full oxygen requirement. The addition of any reasonable lens pump produces an oxygen level at the corneal surface that is above the minimum for all patients.

The higher permeability of these materi-

TABLE 10.9

POLYCON (SILAFOCON A) LENS AVAILABILITY

LENS	INVENTORY		NON-INVENTORY	
	BASE CURVE	POWER	BASE CURVE	POWER
STANDARD 9.5 Dia.	7.20 to 8.60 .05 increments	+5.00D to −10.00D in .25D increments	Steeper than 7.20 & flatter than 8.60 in .05 increments	+5.25D to +8.00D & −10.25D to −20.00D in .25D increments
APHAKIC 9.5 Dia.	7.40 to 8.50 .05 increments	+13.25D to +15.50D Front Vertex .25 D increments	Steeper than 7.40 & flatter than 8.50 in .05 increments	+8.25D to +13.00D & +15.75D to +20.00D Front Vertex .25 increments
APHAKIC 10.0 Dia.	7.60 to 8.65 .05 increments	+13.25D to +15.50D Front Vertex .25D increments	Steeper than 7.60 & flatter than 8.65 in .05 increments	+8.25 to +13.00D & +15.75D to +20.00D Front Vertex .25 increments
STANDARD 8.5 Dia.	7.10 to 8.35 .05 increments	Plano to −6.00D .25D increments		
KERATOCONUS			7.35 & Steeper in .05 increments (Lenses made to	All Powers specifications)
DIAGNOSTIC SETS 9.5	7.40 to 8.40 or 7.45 to 8.45 .10 increments	−8.00D −2.75, −3.00 or −3.25D −1.25D single cut −1.25D minus carrier +2.75, +3.00 or +3.25D		
DIAGNOSTIC SETS APHAKIC 9.5 & 10.0 Dia.	7.60 to 8.60 7.55 to 8.55 7.65 to 8.65 .10 increments Mixed Diameters	+13.25 to +14.75D Mixed Powers		
DIAGNOSTIC SETS 8.5	7.20 to 8.20 7.25 to 8.25 .10 increments	−2.75, −3.00 or −3.25D		
DIAGNOSTIC SETS KERATOCONUS			[11 or more lenses made to specifications]	

TABLE 10.10
AUTHOR'S HIGH-PERMEABILITY TRIAL SET (8.9 DIAMETER)

Base Curve		Power	O.Z.D.	I.C.R.	I.C.W.	P.C.R.	P.C.W.	tc	te	Edge Lift
46.00	7.34	−3.00	7.7	8.4	0.2	10.2	0.4	.13	.10	.10
45.50	7.42	−3.00	7.7	8.4	0.2	10.2	0.4	.13	.10	.09
45.00	7.50	−3.00	7.7	8.7	0.2	10.2	0.4	.13	.11	.09
44.50	7.58	−3.00	7.7	8.7	0.2	10.5	0.4	.13	.10	.09
44.00	7.67	−3.00	7.7	8.7	0.2	10.8	0.4	.13	.10	.09
43.50	7.76	−3.00	7.7	9.0	0.2	10.8	0.4	.13	.11	.09
43.00	7.85	−3.00	7.7	9.0	0.2	11.1	0.4	.13	.11	.09
42.50	7.94	−3.00	7.7	9.3	0.2	11.1	0.4	.13	.11	.09
42.00	8.04	−3.00	7.7	9.3	0.2	11.1	0.4	.12	.10	.08
41.50	8.13	−3.00	7.7	9.6	0.2	11.1	0.4	.12	.10	.08
41.00	8.23	−3.00	7.7	9.6	0.2	11.1	0.4	.12	.11	.08
40.50	8.33	−3.00	7.7	9.6	0.2	11.1	0.4	.12	.11	.08

als is particularly valuable in plus lenses having thicknesses of greater than 0.2 mm. From Figure 10.2 it may be seen that lenses that are 0.32 mm. thick still provide a 2 percent oxygen level at the corneal surface, which, when added to the expected oxygenation from the lens-tear pump, should supply from 3 to 5 percent oxygen equivalent at the corneal surface. Hence, it may be seen that the flex lens and Boston lens provide sufficient oxygen permeability to insure that the cornea receives an adequate oxygen supply, regardless of the lens design or power that is used.

Trial Set

A recommended trial set is shown in Table 10.10. All lenses in the trial set are 8.9 mm. in diameter with a 7.7 mm. optic zone diameter. The lenses are designed with a 0.12 or 0.13 mm. center thickness in order to resist lens flexing while on the eye. If additional oxygen is required at the corneal surface, it may be obtained by using a lens with ultrathin dimensions (*see* Chapter 7). Such a lens will have flexing on the eye that is comparable to that of the Polycon lens.

REFERENCES

1. Smelser, G. K., and Ozanics, V.: Importance of atmospheric oxygen for maintenance of the optical properties of the human cornea, *Science, 115*:40, 1952.

2. Refojo, M. F.: Mechanism of gas transport through contact lenses, *J. Am. Optom. Assoc., 50*(3):285–287, 1979.

3. Korb, D. R., and Exford, J. M.: The phenomenon of central corneal clouding, *J. Am. Optom. Assoc., 39*(3):223–230, 1968.

4. Hazlett, R. D.: Central circular clouding, *J. Am. Optom. Assoc., 40*(3):268–275, 1969.

5. Kerns, R.: Research in orthokeratology, Part IV: results and observations, *J. Am. Optom. Assoc., 48*(2):227–238, 1977.

6. Finnemore, V. A., and Korb, J. E.: Corneal edema with polymethylmethacrylate versus gas-permeable rigid polymer contact lenses of identical design, *J. Am. Optom. Assoc., 51*(3):271–272, 1980.

7. Fatt, I., and Hill, R. M.: Oxygen tension under a contact lens during blinking: a comparison of theory and experimental observation, *Am. J. Optom., 47*(1):50–55, 1970.

8. Fatt, I., and Lin, D.: Oxygen tension under a soft or hard gas-permeable contact lens in the presence of tear pumping, *Am. J. Optom. Physiol. Opt., 53*(4):104–111, 1976.

9. Polse, K. A., and Mandell, R. B.: Critical oxygen tension at the corneal surface, *Arch. Ophthalmol., 84*:505–508, 1970.

10. Mandell, R. B., and Farrell, R.: Corneal swelling at low atmospheric oxygen pressures, *Invest. Ophthalmol., 19*(6):697–702, 1980.

11. Thoft, R. A., and Friend, J.: Biochemical aspects of contact lens wear, *Am. J. Ophthalmol. , 80*(1):139–145, 1975.

12. Polse, K. A., and Mandell, R. B.: Hyperbaric oxygen effect on corneal edema caused by a contact lens, *Am. J. Optom., 48*(3): 197–200, 1971.

13. Fatt, I.: Gas transmission properties of soft contact lenses, in Ruben, M. (Ed.): *Soft Contact Lenses*, New York, Wiley, 1978, p. 108.

14. Holly, F. J., and Lemp, M. A.: Wettability and wetting of corneal epithelium, *Exp. Eye Res., 11*:239–250, 1971.

15. Stahl, N. O., Reich, L. A., and Ivani, E.: Report on laboratory studies and preliminary clinical application of a gas-permeable plastic contact lens, *J. Am. Optom. Assoc., 45*(3):302–307, 1974.

16. Rosenthal, I.: A clinical evaluation of the Rx56 contact lens, *Contact Lens, 2*(3):20–25, 1976.

17. Reich, L. A.: The Rx-56 gas permeable hard contct lens, *Contacto, 19*(1):12–18, 1975.

18. Gellman, M., Barker, K., and Foyle, M.: A comparative study of Rx-56 gas permeable and PMMA contact lenses with respect to corneal edema inducement, *Rev. Opt., 113*(7):44–48, 1976.

19. Feldman, G. L.: Chemical and physical properties of cellulose acetate butyrate as

related to contact lenses, *Cont. Lens J.*, 11(1):25–31, 1977.

20. *Thickness Guide*, Danker & Wohlk "MESO" CAB 500 Lens Inventory System.

21. Pearson, R. M.: Dimensional stability of lathe cut C.A.B. lenses, *J. Am. Optom. Assoc.*, 49(8):927–929, 1978.

22. Stone, J.: Changes in curvature of cellulose acetate butyrate lenses during hydration and dehydration, *J. Br. Contact Lens Assoc.*, 1(1):22–35, 1978.

23. Sarver, M. D., Gold, G., Trezza, J., and Lopez, D.: Stability of CAB contact lenses with hydration, *J. Am. Optom. Assoc.*, 49(12):1377–1380, 1978.

24. Hales, R. H.: Gas-permeable cellulose acetate butyrate (CAB) contact lenses, *Cont. Lens J.*, 11(3):17–22, 1978.

25. Wyckoff, P.: Experience with new hard contact lens materials, *Contacto*, 24(2):16–19, 1980.

26. Garnett, B.: Gas permeable hard contact lenses, *Can. J. Optom.*, 42(1):45–49, 1980.

27. Blake, R. F., and Pearlstone, A. D.: Clinical experience and fitting characteristics of gas permeable lenses, *Int. Cont. Lens Clin.*, 6(6):246–249, 1979.

28. Stranch, L. A. W.: Problem solving with a new F.D.A.-approved rigid contact lens material, *Technology*, pp. 33–36.

29. Kline, L. N., and De Luca, T. J.: A clinical study of CAB lens wear, *J. Am. Optom. Assoc.*, 49(3):299–302, 1978.

30. Hodd, N. F. B.: Further experience with CAB materials, *The Optician*, 175(4538):11–15, 1978.

31. Kame, R.: Clinical management of edematous corneal formations, *Rev. Opt.*, 116(4):69–71, 1979.

32. Lee, J. M.: Regression of induced, irregular astigmatism in hard lens wearers refit with CAB lenses, *Rev. Opt.*, 116(6):54–56, 1979.

33. Katz, K., and Miller, S. B.: Corneal rehabilitation with CAB lenses, *Rev. Opt.*, 117(1):44–45, 1980.

34. Mandell, R. B.: Oxygen-transmitting hard contact lenses, *J. Am. Optom. Assoc.*, 50(3):323–324, 1979.

35. Fatt, I.: Oxygen supply under a gas permeable hard lens, *Cont. Lens Forum*, 4(4):57–61, 1979.

36. Morris, J. A., and Fatt, I.: A survey of gas-permeable contact lenses, *The Optician*, Nov. 4, 1977.

37. Mandell, R. B.: Oxygen permeability of hard contact lenses, *Cont. Lens Forum*, 2(9):35–43, 1977.

38. Stranch, L. A. Q.: Relative oxygen permeability of rigid contact lens materials related to center thickness: a preliminary report, *Int. Cont. Lens Clin.*, 5(1):24–28, 1978.

39. Refojo, M. R., Holly, F. J., and Leong, F.: Permeability of dissolved oxygen through contact lenses, I. Cellulose Acetate Butyrate, *Contact Lens*, 3(4):28–33, 1977.

40. Gasson, A.: Hartflex CAB lenses, *Optician*, 175(4521):20–22, 1978.

41. Fatt, I.: Gas transmission properties of soft contact lenses, in Ruben, M. (Ed.): *Soft Contact Lenses*, New York, Wiley, 1978, p. 99.

42. Tsuda, S., Tanaka, K., and Hirano, J.: A report on experiments with Toyo's super gas-permeable hard contact lens, *Austr. J. Optom.*, 62(2):55–72, 1979.

43. Williams, C. E.: Curvature stability of Polycon contact lenses, *Rev. Opt.*, 117(5):31–85, 1980.

44. Fatt, I., and Lin, D.: Oxygen tension under a soft or hard gas-permeable contact lens in the presence of tear pumping, *Am. J. Optom. Physiol. Opt.*, 53(4):104–111, 1976.

45. Mandell, R. B.: Oxygen permeability of hard contact lenses, *Cont. Lens Forum*, 2(9):35–43, 1977.

46. Sarver, M. D., Polse, K. A., and Harris, M. G.: Patient responses to gas-permeable hard (Polycon) contact lenses, *Am. J. Optom. Physiol. Opt.*, 54(4):195–200, 1977.

47. Sarver, M. D., Brown, L. R., and Riggert, R. H.: Corneal edema with several hard corneal contact lenses, *Am. J. Optom. Physiol. Opt.*, 56(4):231–235, 1979.

48. Finnemore, V. M., and Korb, J. E.: Corneal edema with polymethylmethacrylate versus gas-permeable rigid polymer contact lenses of identical design, *J. Am. Optom. Assoc.*, 51(3):271–274, 1980.

49. Kame, T.: Clinical management of edematous corneal formations, *Rev. Opt.*, 116(4):69–72, 1980.

50. Williams, C. E.: New design concepts for permeable rigid contact lenses, *J. Am. Optom. Assoc.*, 50(3):331–336, 1979.

ADDITIONAL READINGS

Anan, N., Ando, N., and Tsuda, S.: Fitting and analysis of the Menicon soft lens—Part I, *Int. Cont. Lens Clin.*, 4(4):55, 1977.

Anan, N., Ando, N., and Tsuda, S.: Fitting and analysis of the Menicon soft lens—Part II, *Int. Cont. Lens Clin.*, 4(5):24, 1977.

Bailey, N.: Syntex Ophthalmics: the new name in contact lenses, *Cont. Lens Forum*, 4(4):17, 1979.

Bailey, N. J., and Hill, R. M.: An oxygen permeable PMMA?, *Cont. Lens Forum*, 2(9):45, 1977.

Bailey, N. J., and Hill, R. M.: Can oxygen pass through PMMA?, *Int. Cont. Lens Clin.*, 5(1):48, 1978.

Blume, A. J.: Clinical study of Air-Thru PMMA contact lenses, *The Eye Opener*, 1(1):1977.

Brannen, R. D.: Clinical comparison of PMMA and BPFlex lenses, *Rev. Opt.*, 115(4):57, 1978.

Breger, J. L.: Macromolecular structure of thermoplastic polymers, *Cont. Lens Forum*, 1(6):39–41, 1976.

Clarke, A. F.: Cellulose acetate butyrate: an industrial plastic, *The Optician*, 176(4564):18, 1978.

Danker, F.: Progress with cellulose acetate butyrate contact lenses (tape talk), *The Ophthalmic Optician*, 17(22):828, 1977.

Dickinson, F.: A new hydrophilic hard contact lens, *J. Optom. (NZ)*, 5(1):6–8, 1973.

Dickinson, F.: There's a lot of mileage in the hard lens yet, *Cont. Lens J.*, 6(3):13, 1977.

Dickinson, F.: Corneal respiration: some observations on the comparative performance of PMMA and CAB materials, *Cont. Lens J.*, 6(5):16, 1978.

Eschmann, R.: Clinical experience with CAB lenses, *Contacto*, 23(5):24–30, 1979.

Espy, J.: A new gas permeable hard contact lens, *Ann. Ophthalmol.*, 10(6):761, 1978.

Fatt, I.: A rational method for the design of gas-permeable soft contact lenses, *The Optician*, 173(4470):12–15, 1977.

Fatt, I., and Lin, D.: Oxygen tension under a hard, gas-permeable contact lens, *Am. J. Optom. Physiol. Opt.*, 54(3):146–148, 1977.

Fatt, I., and St. Helen, R.: Oxygen tension under an oxygen-permeable contact lens, *Am. J. Optom. Arch. Am. Acad. Optom.*, 48(7):545–555, 1971.

Garcia, G. E.: Initial experience with RX56 gas permeable lenses, *Cont. Lens Med. Bull.*, 6(4):27–29, 1973.

Gasson, A.: An appraisal of corneal lens designs: fitting parabolar and CAB lenses, *Cont. Lens J.*, 8(3):5–8, 1979.

Gasson, A.: Oxygen permeable contact lenses: thin HEMA, CAB and silicone, *The Ophthalmic Optician*, 19(22):840, 1979.

Gaston, D. C., and Gustason, G.: The evaluation of a cold solution maintenance procedure for Polymacon contact lenses, *Cont. Lens J.*, 12(1):29, 1978.

Goldberg, J.: Gas-permeable contact lenses—how good are they?, *Int. Cont. Lens Clin.*, 6(6):281, 1979.

Goldberg, J. B.: Must the gas go through?, *Optom. Weekly*, 66(34):938–939, 1975.

Hales, R. H.: Gas-permeable cellulose acetate butyrate (CAB) contact lenses, *Ann. Ophthalmol.*, 9(9):1085, 1977.

Hill, R. M.: Can a "hard" contact lens material transmit adequate oxygen?, *Am. J. Optom. Arch. Am. Acad. Optom.*, 50(12):949–951, 1973.

Hill, R. M.: The rigid lens: an exhausted option?, *Contacto*, 18(6):33–35, 1974.

Hill, R. M.: Osmotic edema associated with contact lens adaptation, *J. Am. Optom. Assoc.*, 46(9):897–899, 1975.

Hill, R. M.: Anoxia: the ultimate debt, *Int. Cont. Lens Clin.*, 4(5):32, 1977.

Hill, R. M.: C.A.B.: a practical contact lens option?, *J. Am. Optom. Assoc.*, 48(3):387, 1977.

Hill, R. M., and Terry, J. E.: The importance of osmotic equilibration, *Cont. Lens Forum*, 1(7):57–59, 1976.

Hirano, J.: A new gas-permeable hard contact lens I. Physico-chemical properties, *J. Jap. Cont. Lens Soc.*, 20(4):61, 1978.

Hodd, N. F. B.: The permeable hard option, *The Optician*, pp. 17–19, Sept. 7, 1979.

Hubben, H. H.: Why are CAB lense often more successful than PMMA lenses?, *The Ophthalmic Optician*, 19(17):646–650, 1979.

Kline, L., and DeLuca, T. J.: A clinical study of CAB lens wear, *J. Am. Optom. Assoc.*, 49(3):299–302, 1978.

Lees, M. E.: Polycon-CAB a clinical comparison, *The Ophthalmic Optician*, 18(22):186, 1978.

Lippman, J. I.: Current status of gas permeable lenses, *Cont. Intraoc. Lens Med. J.*, 3(2):37–39, 1977.

Masnick, K.: Newer hard contact lens materials, *Austr. J. Optom.*, 62(4):138–142, 1979.

Montlake, E.: A new oxygen permeable hard contact lens, *The Disp. Opt.*, 31(6):169–171, 1979.

Newlove, D. B.: Development of a new hard lens material, *Contacto*, 18(6):11–16, 1974.

Nintcheff, P.: Three year implementation of RX 56 lenses, *Cont. Intraoc. Lens Med. J.*, 4(4):53–57, 1978.

Chapter 11

CLINICAL PROCEDURES

OFFICE PROCEDURES for the care of a contact lens patient are subject to considerable variation depending upon the preferences of the fitter. It is difficult to give a representative technique that would be acceptable to all practitioners. The author favors the technique described in this chapter because it allows complete control over the patient during all phases of the fitting procedure and utilizes a minimum amount of the fitter's time.

METHOD OF DIRECT ORDERING

FIRST VISIT

During the first visit the patient is interviewed, his history is ascertained, and, if time permits, the examination is performed. Some practitioners prefer to have the patient return for the examination so that the patient will be more relaxed and perhaps less apprehensive about the fitting procedure.

Following the examination, the contact lenses are ordered. They are inspected upon arrival and if they are satisfactory, the patient is notified to come in for the training session. The lenses usually arrive about one week after ordering.

SECOND VISIT

The patient is introduced to lens handling procedures, and the fitter receives his first opportunity to evaluate the lenses on the patient's eyes. Very little can be determined about the fit at this time. If the patient shows complete ability to handle the lenses, he may be allowed to take them home. Another visit is scheduled within two or three days. If the patient is unable to demonstrate an ability to handle the lenses, another visit should be scheduled the following day for further training.

THIRD VISIT

The patient should be able to wear his contact lenses for several hours before the third visit is scheduled. He will then be reasonably adapted to the lenses during the examination.

A complete refraction and examination should be performed (*see* Chapter 14).

296

SUBSEQUENT VISITS

The number of additional visits will depend upon the progress of the patient. Weekly visits are often necessary for the first few months of wear. When the fitting has been completed, the visits may be reduced to two a year.

TRIAL LENS METHOD

If the trial lens fitting method is used, the examination is ordinarily extended to two visits. The first part of the procedure is essentially the same as with direct ordering.

It is preferable for the lenses to be inserted first by the fitter rather than by the patient. In this way a minimum of time is lost in placing the lens on the patient's eye, and the lens is inserted with less irritation than the patient would inflict upon himself. The fitter should avoid making a preliminary ritual of lens cleaning or prolonging discussion once the patient is aware that the lens is to be placed on his eye. The lens should be cleaned and ready for insertion when the fitter enters the room; it may be shown briefly to the patient. He should be reassured that there will be no pain but only minor discomfort when the lens is inserted. It is most important to keep positive control of the patient at this point. While the instructions are being given, the patient should be repeatedly encouraged to relax. The lens should then be inserted gently and quickly, and the patient should be told to keep his eyes open and to look down to the floor. If the lens is quickly placed on the eye, the patient's apprehension will be relieved, and he may be more easily controlled from that point. A few patients will have a blepharospasm because of their fear. They should be instructed to *open their eyes* and look down, thereby relaxing the tension on the orbicularis muscles.

Usually the patient will find the contact lenses much more comfortable than he had anticipated.

LENS HANDLING PROCEDURES

INSERTION BY PRACTITIONER

The initial insertion should be done by the practitioner rather than by an assistant to maintain the confidence of the patient. The patient should be instructed to fixate on an object in his lower field of view. The practitioner then balances the contact lens on his index finger and places it on the patient's cornea. Care should be taken to avoid blocking the patient's vision until the lens is placed on the cornea. This is possible if the practitioner approaches the cornea either from the side or above (Figure 11.1). The lens should be allowed to remain on the eye about twenty minutes for the patient to adapt to the initial sensation. The symptoms will gradually subside, and the patient will find the lenses reasonably comfortable. He may then be allowed to remove the lenses himself; removal is usually easier than insertion for the new wearer. By being allowed to remove his lenses, the patient gains confidence in his ability to handle them. If he has extreme difficulty in removing his lenses, the fitter should remove them before the patient irritates his eyes.

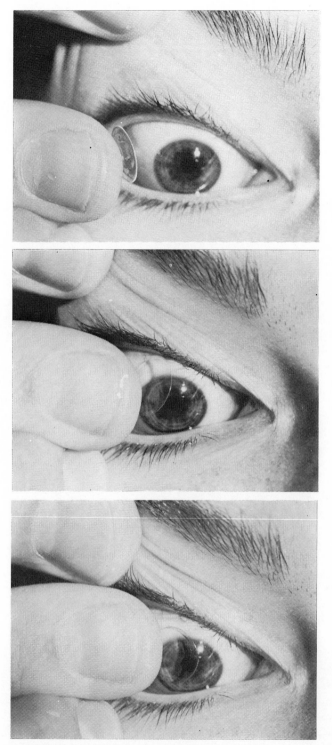

Figure 11.1. Lens insertion by the practitioner. The patient's line of sight is not blocked until the lens is placed on the cornea.

REMOVAL BY PRACTITIONER

The patient should be told to open his eyes widely. The contact lens is then removed by placing the index fingers at the outer canthus of the eye (Figure 11.2). The lower lid should be manipulated into a scissors position by gently pulling the outer canthus. The lens will be caught and ejected by the lid margins (Figure 11.2).

If the patient is in a state of discomfort due to a bad edge or foreign body, removal is usually easier and less traumatic with the aid of a suction cup (Figure 11.3).

INSTRUCTION FOR LENS INSERTION BY PATIENT

1. Wash and dry hands.
2. Using the forefinger and the thumb, distribute wetting solution evenly on both surfaces of the lens.

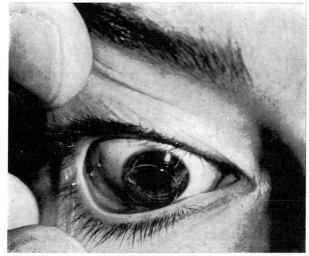
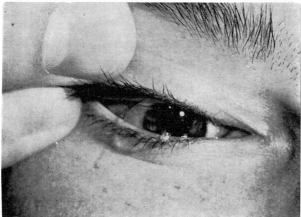

Figure 11.2. Lens removal by the practitioner.

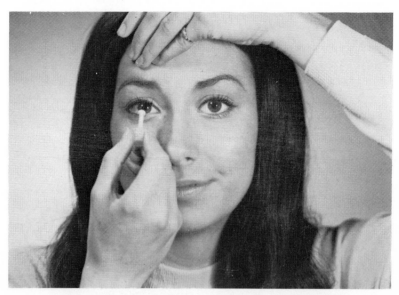

Figure 11.3. Removal of lens with DMV suction cup.

3. Rinse the lens with cold or lukewarm water (but never with hot water); keep the lens moist.

4. Moisten the forefinger of the right hand and place the clean, moist lens, concave surface upward, on the tip of that finger (Figure 11.4a).

5. Bend the head down so that the eyes will be fixating straight down and looking at the working surface (table surface, for example).

6. Keep both eyes open all the time during insertion.

7. Place the left middle finger at the margin of the upper right eyelid; grasp the lashes and pull the lid up. (This should be done in such a way that the lens will not touch the lashes during the insertion.)

8. Place the right middle finger at the margin of the lower lid and pull it down (Figure 11.4b).

9. Slowly bring the right forefinger with the lens toward the cornea; look straight through the lens so that the lens can be seen as a blurred circle. It is important to keep the eyes straight.

10. Gently place the lens on the cornea and release the lower lid first, and then upper lid slowly.

11. Straighten the head, look down, and blink several times.

12. Repeat the same procedure for the left eye.

Some alternative methods of insertion are listed below.

1. a. Place the lens on the tip of the right middle finger (Figure 11.4c).

   b. Hold the upper lid with the left forefinger and the lower lid with the left middle finger

   c. The rest of the procedure is the same as before.

2. a. Place the lens on the tip of the right forefinger.

   b. Place the left forefinger at the right upper lid margin, and the left thumb on the lower lid mergin and pull the lids apart.

   c. The rest of the procedure is the same as before.

3. a. If it is impossible to "look through the lens" as it approaches the eye, put a

mirror on the working surface in front of the face and place the lens right on the cornea by looking into the mirror.

b. Learn not to use the mirror as soon as possible.

RECENTERING THE LENS

If not inserted correctly, the lens may be off center. In this case any of the following methods may be used to recenter the lens.
1. One-finger method
   a. Locate the lens by closing the eye and feeling over the lid with the forefinger.
   b. When located, massage gently toward the center, looking at the direction of the lens until it slips back into proper position.
2. Five-finger method
   a. Instead of the forefinger, all five fingers may be placed over the lid (Figure 11.5).
   b. Locate the lens first, and then gently massage it back to the center, looking toward the direction of the lens.
3. Mirror method
   a. Place the left middle finger on the margin of the upper lid and the right middle finger on the margin of the lower lid, and pull the lids apart.

b. Looking into the mirror, locate the lens; it may be necessary to move the eye around slowly
c. When the lens is located, slide the lens back to the center by pushing it with lower or upper lid margin (Figure 11.6).

4. a. Locate the lens first by using a mirror or by feeling with the fingers.
   b. When located, open the eyes and move the eyeball horizontally away from the lens position. Thus, the lens is now at the central region of the lid opening.
   c. Place the left middle finger on the upper lid margin and the right middle finger on the lower lid margin, and gently squeeze the lids so that the lens is kept in this central position.
   d. Now move the eyeball to the straight ahead position. The lens should slip back to the center of the eye.

REMOVAL OF THE LENS

Remember that removal is easier if the lens is on the center of the eye; therefore, recenter the lens before removal, if it is off center.
1. a. Bend the head down so that it is parallel to the working surface.
   b. Place the left hand, palm up beneath the lens that is being removed so that the lens is caught as soon as it falls out of the eye.
   c. Place the right middle finger at the outer canthus of the right eye.
   d. Keep both eyes wide open, and look straight ahead at the palm of the left hand.

e. Exert a pull at the outer canthus in the up and outward direction.
f. The lens should slip out easily only by applying the pull (Figure 11.7), but it may be helpful to blink hard a few times while pulling the eyelids.

2. a. Bend the head down so that it is parallel to the working surface.
   b. Place the right thumb at the outer canthus of the right eye.
   c. Open the right hand palm in front of the right eye to receive the lens when it falls out of the eye.
   d. Exert a push in an outward and upward direction. The lens should easily drop

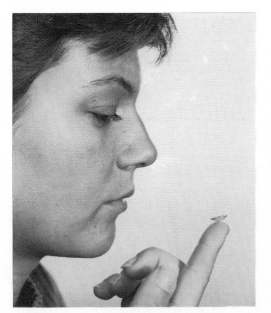 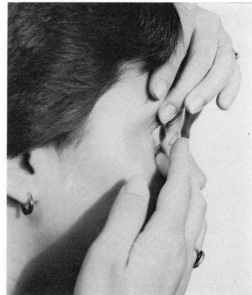

Figure 11.4a and 11.4b. Lens insertion by patient.

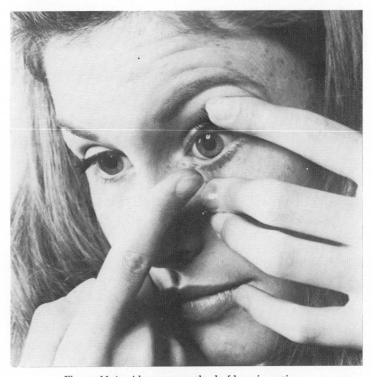

Figure 11.4c. Alternate method of lens insertion.

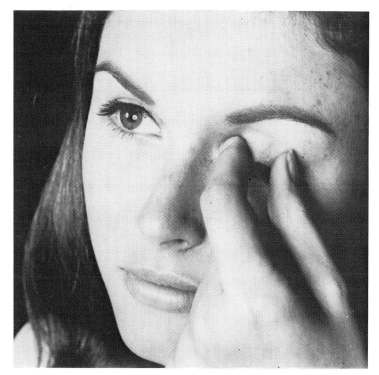

Figure 11.5. Location of displaced lens by feeling through lid.

into the palm of the hand.

e. For the left eye, use the left hand.

3. a. Place the right forefinger at the right upper lid margin and the right middle finger at the right lower lid margin.

b. Keep both eyes wide open.

c. Gently move both lids in scissors motion by bringing the fingers together and then apart.

d. The lens should drop into the palm of the left hand, which has been placed beneath that eye.

OFFICE CONTAMINATION

Cross contamination in the office may be reduced by the use of a clean contact lens container for each patient. Kramb describes the development of a disposable sterile container to prevent cross contamination between patients.[1] Another disposable container is used by Sarver in the Contact Lens Clinic of the University of California School of Optometry. The container consists of a permanent acrylic plastic holder and two disposable paper cups. The holder is marked with an R and an L to identify the lenses. The cups are one-half ounce No. 050 Portion Control Cups (normally used to dispense medication in a clinic or hospital) (Figure 11.8).

When the patient removes his lenses, he drops them into the respective cups. A distinct advantage is their generous size. The patient with poor vision seldom misses the cup openings. The plastic lenses are easily heard as they fall into the cups and strike the stiff paper. The hazard of lost lenses that is

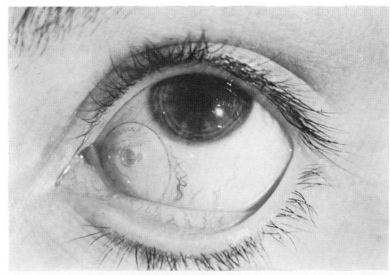

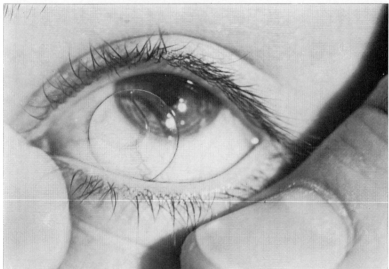

Figure 11.6. (*top*) Locating a displaced contact lens and (*bottom*) recentering the lens.

present with the usual flat acrylic lens tray is thus eliminated.

The lenses may be taken to the laboratory for inspection, polishing, or modification. They are cleaned with a full strength contact lens cleaner and rinsed with water prior to being returned to the paper cups. Although neither the portion cups nor the lenses are sterile, the bacterial contamination has been minimized. Soaking solution is added to the cups, and the lenses remain immersed until returned to the patient. The paper cups are then discarded.

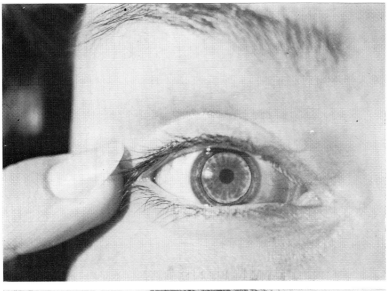

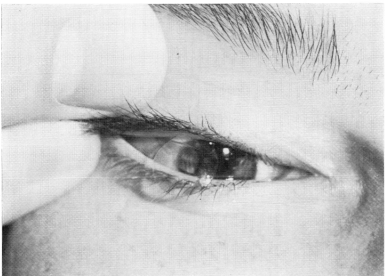

Figure 11.7. Lens removal by patient.

ADAPTIVE SYMPTOMS

During the first few days of contact lens wear, the patient experiences a number of subjective symptoms that are normal reactions to the lenses. A contact lens is a foreign body in the eye, and reactions occur as they would to any foreign body. These adaptation symptoms normally diminish greatly in a few hours and are nearly gone by the time the patient has reached full wearing time. Persistence of the symptoms usually indicates an improper fit.

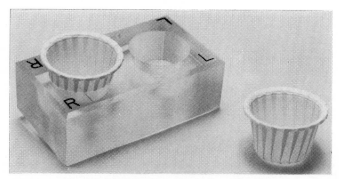

Figure 11.8. Sarver holder for contact lenses.

TEARING

The first time contact lenses are placed on the eye, profuse tearing usually results, which subsides greatly after about ten minutes. As the wearing time is increased, the amount of tearing rapidly decreases to a nearly normal amount. It may be noted, however, that a slightly greater than normal tearing persists for several weeks. Tearing is increased by any factor that tends to irritate the lids.

Tearing that persists beyond the normal time may be caused by a bad lens edge or by a flat-fitting lens. If the tearing subsides in a normal manner but later recurs, the cornea has probably been irritated by the lens or by the presence of a foreign body.

LID IRRITATION

One of the most sensitive areas stimulated by the contact lens is the lid margin. A tickling sensation is often evoked, which can usually be eliminated temporarily by holding back the patient's lids so that they do not touch the lens.

DIFFICULTY IN LOOKING UP

When the patient attempts to look up, the lens may be drawn upward and then drop and strike the lower lid, initiating a blink reaction and tearing. This can be observed by watching the patient closely and noting whether a blink is instigated when the lens touches the lower lid. By directing the gaze downward, the lens is moved less by the upper lid and less sensation is felt.

INTERMITTENT VISUAL BLURRING

The patient may note that when the contact lenses are first worn he is able to see very well initially but then periods occur when his vision blurs or becomes misty. Part of this problem is caused by the excessive tears under the lens, which cause a pooling effect and do not present an even optical surface. A second contributing factor is that, due to the large amount of tearing, the lens has a tendency to move around on the cornea, and very often the optical zone is displaced from in front of the pupil.

DIFFICULTY IN MOVING EYES

Some patients fear losing the lens, and they attempt to move the eyes as little as possible. This fear is usually unwarranted, and the patient's apprehension can be relieved by purposely directing him to roll his eyes.

REFLECTIONS

In the early stages of wear, the patient may report that he is bothered by the shimmering appearance of objects. This is caused by the pooling of excessive tears on the lens and at the lens edge. It will subside after the patient has adapted to the lens.

HEAD TILT

In an effort to reduce lens movement and the resultant lid sensation, the patient may tilt his head backward and appear to be in a rather awkward position. A few patients continue to do this after the period of adaptation simply from habit, and they will stop if a conscious effort is made to keep the head in the normal position.

EXCESSIVE BLINKING

An increased blink rate is caused by the lens irritation of the lid margins. Blinking that persists after the normal period of adaptation usually indicates a lens with a bad edge or a loose fit.

PHOTOPHOBIA

In the initial period of contact lens wear, photophobia can be considered a normal symptom, resulting from lens irritation of the cornea and lids. Bailey demonstrated that anesthetizing the corneas of contact lens wearers relieved the photophobia.[2] With normal adaptation, the photophobia will diminish.

It is recommended that the patient wear spectacle sunglasses for the outdoors during the adaptation period. Lightly tinted contact lenses usually are not absorptive enough to be effective against photophobia, and darker shades are inconvenient for night wear. The spectacle sunglasses must be dark shades. Tinted spectacles also offer some protection against wind and dust.

Since it is normal for the patient to experience a number of adaptive symptoms, he should be forewarned of their probable occurrence. Written instructions are often helpful in this regard. The following instructions are

issued to patients of the School of Optometry, University of California.*

WEARING YOUR LENSES

Every contact lens wearer experiences a few annoying sensations, brief periods of discomfort or
other minor problems. These occur most often
during the first few weeks of wear when the eyes
are adapting to the lenses. In addition to these
more-or-less normal consequences of wearing contact lenses, other problems may arise that are more
significant. At first, it may not be obvious to you
which problems are important and which ones
are not. If you have any doubt about what you
should do when a problem arises, call your
optometrist for advice. Even when minor problems
occur, mention them to your doctor during the
next office visit. This will help in evaluating your
progress. The following outline gives most of the
problems that are apt to occur and instructions
on how to react to them.

Normal Experiences:

1. **Lenses Off Center.** Your lenses may not remain
exactly centered on the corneas. They may ride a
little high or to one side due to the shape of the
eyes.

2. **Lens Movement.** Contact lenses are designed to
move on the eye. This permits a normal flow of
tears under the lenses. Movement may be excessive
during the first few days of wear because of increased
tear flow and tight lids.

3. **Edge Reflections.** You may be aware of the lens
edges under certain conditions during the first few
weeks. If this interferes with your vision, advise
your optometrist.

4. **Tearing.** During the first days of wear, increased
tear flow normally occurs. Later on, excessive tear
flow, after the first minutes of wear, usually indicates the lenses need cleaning.

5. **Minor Irritation or Discomfort.** When you first
begin to wear your lenses, you will be aware of
them on your eyes and in contact with your lids.
This will gradually disappear. Irritation also may
occur if the lenses need cleaning, if they have
been worn too long, or if you have been in a
smoke filled room, riding in an open car or exposed

*Compiled by Doctors H. S. Player, M. D. Sarver, and
K. E. Kerr.

to dry wind. If cleaning the lenses does not correct
the problem, remove the lenses until the eyes feel
normal. Call your optometrist if discomfort persists.

6. **Light Sensitivity.** Almost all contact lens wearers
are more sensitive to bright light. If this is bothersome, a good pair of "plain" sunglasses is recommended for outdoor wear. Sensitivity to light that
is not eliminated by sunglasses should be reported
to your optometrist immediately.

7. **Morning Wear.** Morning wear is generally more
uncomfortable and should be avoided during the
first weeks.

8. **Burning.** You may experience a mild burning or
warm sensation when reading, watching TV or
movies, or when in a closed room. Avoid keeping
your eyes fixed in one position too long because
this may interfere with normal tear flow around
the lenses. Keeping your lenses clean will also
help insure normal tear flow and decrease heat
buildup.

9. **Blurring.** Some of the natural oils secreted by the
lid glands may accumulate on the lenses and cause
vision to blur. Remove, clean, wet, and replace the
lenses. Use a contact lens cleaner if this is a frequent problem. If cleaning your lenses does not
eliminate the blurring, call your optometrist for
advice.

10. **Spectacle Blur.** Blurred or distorted vision immediately after changing from contact lenses to spectacles is not uncommon. Notice how much time is
required for vision to clear and mention this to
your optometrist. This will help in evaluating the
fit of your lenses.

11. **Foreign Body Reaction.** A sudden sharp pain is
usually caused by a bit of dirt being trapped under
the edge of the lens. Remove, clean, wet, and replace
the lens.

12. **Lenses Becoming Dislodged.** During the first
weeks, the lenses may have a tendency to move off
the cornea or even fall out because of increased
tear flow and tight lids. Advise your optometrist if
this happens.

13. **Blinking.** Excessive blinking during the early
weeks of wear is not uncommon. If excessive
blinking occurs mainly when looking up or to the
side, practice this simple exercise: Extend your
arm fully and hold your forefinger up before your

eyes. Look steadily at the fingertip as you slowly trace a large figure eight. Concentrate on not blinking until you have completed the figure and are looking straight ahead again. After a bit of practice, you will be able to look easily in any direction without blinking.

Inadequate blinking is a common cause of failure to wear contact lenses successfully. Practice blinking fully and naturally. If necessary, your optometrist will prescribe blinking exercises.

14. **Itching.** Your eyes may itch while wearing your lenses or after they are removed. Never rub your eyes; instead use a cold cloth or cold water to soothe them.

15. **Dizziness or Headache.** You may experience lightheadedness or a slight headache for a few days, especially if you wear a complex spectacle prescription.

16. **Haze or Fog.** Vision may fog toward the end of the wearing period until the eyes adapt to the lenses. If fog persists or recurs after removing and cleaning the lenses, discontinue wear and report this to your optometrist.

Abnormal Experiences:

If any of the following problems occur, discontinue wearing your lenses and call your optometrist for advice.

1. Pain when placing the lenses on the eyes, while wearing the lenses, or after removing them.

2. Burning or hot feeling that causes excessive tearing of the eyes.

3. Inability to keep your eyes open.

4. Severe or persisting haze, fog, or halos while wearing the lenses.

GENERAL INSTRUCTIONS

In order to wear your lenses properly, you must develop the skills and habits of lens use that have been described. Learn to place, remove and recenter a lens promptly, easily, gently, anytime, anywhere. Avoid squinting, raising your head or exhibiting other conspicuous mannerisms. Maintain a consistent pattern of daily lens use and follow your optometrist's instructions for hygienic cleaning, wetting and soaking of lenses.

Learn to remove a lens on the first try. Repeated attempts may irritate the eye and lids or move the lens off the cornea. Know how to recenter a lens without hesitation in a confident and relaxed manner. Learn to do every step without a mirror as soon as possible so that you can remove, clean and replace a lens that is uncomfortable without delay. Wearers who are unsure of their abilities are likely to put off removing an uncomfortable lens that may cause needless eye irritation.

Do not wear your lenses immediately upon arising. Take time to thoroughly awaken; wash your face and eyelids before wearing your lenses.

Never wear your lenses when sleeping. Remove them about one-half hour before going to bed. If you accidently fall asleep while wearing the lenses, remove them as soon as you awaken and leave them off until your eyes feel normal.

Do not wear your lenses in severe dust, near chemical fumes, during serious illness or when your eyes are red and irritated.

Never wear a lens if your eye is blurred or uncomfortable. If such trouble occurs, remove the offending lens and clean it. If the problem continues after the lens has been replaced, leave the lens off for awhile. If trouble still continues, consult your optometrist.

If you do not wear your lenses for a day or more, it is necessary to rebuild the wearing time gradually. This is especially important if you have been ill. Call your optometrist for a new wearing schedule.

Don't wear your lenses while swimming unless you have your doctor's consent. You may lose the lenses.

Never wear a cracked, scratched or otherwise damaged lens.

Keep a pair of eyeglasses available for use during a part of each day and for use during emergencies when contact lenses cannot be worn. Use "plain" sunglasses of good quality when wearing contact lenses outdoors on sunny days. The "wrap-around" styles are especially helpful for protecting the eyes from the wind as well as excess light.

Keep an identification card in your wallet that states you wear contact lenses and requests that the lenses be removed in case of accident or other emergency.

Many doctors also recommend you obtain a Medic Alert emblem to call attention to the fact that you are wearing contact lenses. It alerts emergency personnel to remove your lenses should you be unconscious or unable to communicate. Ask your doctor for information regarding this matter, or write directly to Medic Alert Foundation, P. O. Box 1009, Turlock, CA 95380.

If you move to another city or plan a vacation far from home, contact your optometrist before you leave. He/she may recommend another doctor or advise you about emergency eyecare while you are away.

Know what to expect if a lens is damaged, lost or needs to be replaced for other reasons. Your optome-trist will discuss the fees for replacing your lenses or providing a spare pair. This information may be recorded below.

Remember that regular eye examinations are essential for prolonged and comfortable wear of contact lenses, for continued good vision and for the safety of your eyes. Both your eyes and your contact lenses are subject to change, so don't wait until you have trouble before seeking help. Have your eyes examined every six months, or more often if advised by your optometrist.

WEARING SCHEDULES

Various specific wearing schedules have been proposed as guides for the patient on the length of tolerable wearing time for the first few weeks of contact lens wear. It must be remembered that people vary in the time necessary for adaptation to contact lenses and that one schedule is not necessarily ideal for all patients. If the wearing time is either increased too rapidly or is sporadic and the lens does not fit well, corneal abrasions may result; the patient suffers considerable discomfort, and further wearing must be postponed until the cornea heals.

Unless the patient is to be monitored carefully in the office, the maximum tolerable wearing time on the first day is four hours. The lenses may feel very comfortable at the end of this period, but the patient should be cautioned against continued wear, since the aftereffects of overwearing are not felt sometimes for several hours. The most rapid increase in wearing time that can be safely prescribed is one additional hour per day. With this schedule it is possible for the patient to achieve full-time day wear (considered as fifteen hours) in only eleven days. Many practitioners prefer a slower schedule, which gives the patient some leeway for overwearing and allows for possible adjustments needed in the fit. Patients, especially the young, cannot always be depended upon to remove their lenses at the specified time.

The minimum wearing time schedule suggests that the patient begin with one hour of wear on the first day and increase the time by thirty minutes on each additional day. If the wearing time is increased more slowly, adaptation to the lenses is prolonged, and the patient may lose his motivation due to the discomfort.

In a comparison of six groups of patients who followed various wearing schedules, Bier found the optimum adaptation period to be three to four weeks.[3] One group started with daily one-hour wearing periods and gradually built up their tolerance by an increase of half an hour daily or an increase of one hour every third day. Another group, which adapted at the rate of two hours on the first day and an additional two hours daily, experienced more adaptation problems. The optimum wearing schedule would appear to be between these two schedules. Other groups that progressed at faster or slower rates showed definite adaptation difficulties.

Most fitters prefer a wearing schedule for the patient that begins on the first day with two to three hours of wear and increases by an additional thirty minutes to one hour every day. The exact time for the period of wear should be told to the patient, and the dangers of overwear emphasized.

The most frequent instance of overwear occurs with young people when they are dating. They are overly anxious to demonstrate their new contact lenses, and since no discomfort is felt, the lenses are not removed. The patient may also find no convenient opportunity to remove the lenses, or they are forgotten. The reckoning does not usually occur until several hours after the patient removes his lenses when he experiences excruciating pain. The discomfort is so great that the patient rarely repeats the carelessness.

It is best to advise the patient to wear the lenses only at home for the early part of the adaptation period. This diminishes the probability of overwearing and decreases the chance of losing the lenses, which is greatest during the first few days of wear. During the first days of adaptation, any attempt to wear the lenses while working will usually fail, and driving a vehicle should be strictly prohibited because of the possibility of accidental lens ejection. For the first few days, the lenses may be worn in the evening, and activities such as watching television are advisable. Extended reading should not be attempted until the patient is well adapted to the lenses.

The patient can be advised of the possibility of dividing the wearing period into parts, distributed throughout the day. The total wearing time should not be altered, however.

Elaborate wearing schedules by which the patient may or may not wear his lenses during certain periods are too involved to expect him to follow.

Some practitioners prefer to write the wearing schedule so that the patient will not be confused about the instructions.

The wearing schedule may be altered at each visit if the patient is slow in adapting or if the lens appears to be fitting improperly. It is only necessary to advise the patient of the wearing time to be followed until his next visit.

After full-time day wear has been achieved, the patient should be instructed to avoid large variations in the daily wearing schedule. If the lenses are not worn for several days, the wearing time should be shortened to eight hours and gradually built up again to full day wear.

ONE DAY ADAPTATION

If care is exercised, it is possible to exceed the normal wearing schedule without difficulty. This should only be done, however, when it is possible to maintain close control over the patient, if adverse responses are to be avoided

It is possible for a patient to wear contact lenses all day on the first day of lens wear providing that an adequate tear pump is present, i.e. the lens does not have a tight fit. Unfortunately, this can only be evaluated after a period of lens wear. In Chapter 6 it was shown that excess tearing on the first day of lens wear produced a maximum edematous response at three hours following lens insertion. This presents an optimum time to perform a first evaluation of the patient's response

to new contact lenses. If a careful biomicroscopic examination shows that no edema is present, the patient may be allowed to continue lens wear until the end of the day. A second biomicroscopic examination should be performed at eight to ten hours following insertion. If no edema is detected at this time, the patient may be assigned a wearing schedule that begins at ten hours on the following day. If edema is present at either the three or eight hour examination, appropriate adjustments must be made to the lenses in order to increase tear pumping. The patient may then be reevaluated in the same way with the modified lens design at the next available opportunity.

CONTINUOUS DAY AND NIGHT WEAR

A few practitioners tell their patients that P.M.M.A. contact lenses can be worn while sleeping and that they never need be removed. Although it is claimed that this can be done without apparent harm,[4-8] there is little justification for the procedure.[9-10] If an abrasion occurs while the contact lens is being worn, removal at night allows an opportunity for the abrasion to heal. This procedure also exposes the cornea to a greater chance of infection. In studies of animals fitted with contact lenses, it was found that continuous wear was invariably associated with corneal complications.[11]*

It also has been occasionally recommended that, instead of removing the contact lenses from the eye, they may be pushed onto the sclera when they are not needed. While this procedure appears convenient, it is often found that the lenses have a tendency to become heavily coated with secretions and must be removed anyway for cleaning. It is convenient for brief periods, such as when taking a nap.

REFERENCES

1. Kramb, R. A.: Bacterial cross-contamination in the contact lens office, *Am. J. Optom.,* 44(3):162–167, 1967.
2. Bailey, N. J.: Photophobia and contact lenses, *Contacto,* 2(3):79–81, 1958.
3. Bier, N.: Rate of adaptation with corneal lenses, in *Transactions of the International Ophthalmology and Optomology Congress,* London, Lockwood, 1962, pp. 125–135.
4. Dick, R. B.: Contact lenses in constant use for a three month period: a case report, *Am. J. Optom.,* 35(2):248–250, 1958.
5. Sato, T., and Saito, N.: Contact lenses for babies and children, *Contacto,* 3(12):419, 421–424, 1959.
6. Magatani, H.: Limitless wearing of the contact lenses without interruption, *Contacto,* 4(3):81–82, 84, 86–87, 1960.
7. Sloan, D. P.: A report on continuous contact lens wearing, *Contacto,* 4(4):117–122, 1960.
8. Sloan, D. P.: A further report on continuous contact lens wearing, *Contacto,* 5(1):13–18, 1961.
9. Carlson, A. G.: Sleep and corneal type contact lens, *Optom. Weekly,* 50(4):159–161, 1959.
10. Portfolio, A. G.: Continuous contact lens wear, *Arch. Ophthalmol.,* 70(3):443, 1963.
11. Dixon, J. M., and Lawaczeck, E.: Corneal vascularization due to contact lenses, *Arch. Ophthalmol.,* 69(1):72–75, 1963.

ADDITIONAL READINGS

Atkinson, T. C. O.: Economic aspects of contact lens practice, *The Ophthalmic Optician,* 15(22): 1012–1017, 1975.
Maberley, A. L., Tuffnel, P. G., and Hill, J. C.: Contamination of trial contact lenses, *Can. J. Ophthalmol.,* 5(1):46–54, 1970.

McEachern, C. L.: Handling your soft contact lens patients, *Optom. Weekly,* 67(39):38–44, 1976.
McEachern, C. L.: The role of patient education in contact lens practice and as a factor in the successful use of contact lenses, *Contacto,* 23(6): 30–33, 1979.

---

*It should be noted, however, that it is unlikely the animals received the same care in fitting the lenses as is given to humans. In addition, the animals are incapable of telling the experimenter when painful sensations occur.

Chapter 12

LENS CARE AND STORAGE

VARIOUS SOLUTIONS are available for making contact lenses safer, more comfortable, and easier to wear.[1-17] They include *wetting solution*, which facilitates wetting of the lens; *soaking solution*, which serves as an antimicrobial storage medium and prevents dehydration and distortion of the lens; *cleaning solution*, which removes accumulated eye secretions and other foreign contaminants; *combination solution*, which combines the functions of two or more of the preceding; and various other *accessory solutions*. The number of solutions has increased to the point where the patient may be confused as to their function.[18-21]

WETTING SOLUTION

The principal functions of a wetting solution are as follows:

1. It converts the hydrophobic surface of the contact lens to a temporarily hydrophilic one.[22]
2. It helps to keep the lens clean during insertion.
3. It helps to hold the lens on the fingertip during the insertion procedure.
4. It acts as a mechanical buffer between the lens and the surface of the cornea.

In addition to the specific wetting agent for plastic contact lenses, most wetting solutions contain some or all of the following ingredients:

1. Self-sterilizing agent
2. Methylcellulose, polyvinylpyrrolidone, sodium alginate, or gelatin (which acts as a viscosity-building agent)
3. Coloring agents
4. Distilled water
5. Perfume, which is occasionally added for aesthetic purposes

Many wetting solutions also contain sodium chloride and/or potassium chloride to control tonicity.

WETTING

If a clean, dry piece of plastic is dipped in water and then removed, very little water will cling to its surface. This is because the plastic is *hydrophobic*, or water repellent. Certain compounds known as *wetting agents* are able to convert the dry plastic surface into one that is *hydrophilic*, that is, one which will spread the fluid over the lens surface. Figure 12.1a shows how water falling on a hydrophobic surface tends to form beads, whereas water on a hydrophilic surface spreads in a uniform film. The advantage of contact lenses having a hydrophilic surface is obvious, since for purposes of optical clarity it is important that the tears spread evenly over the surfaces of the lens (Figure 12.1b).

The force of attraction between molecules of one substance for those of another sub-

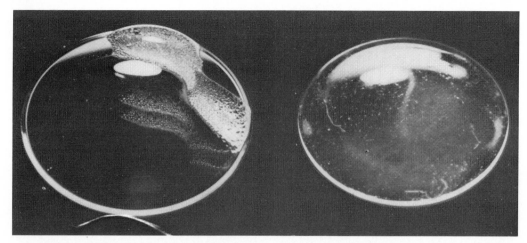

Figure 12.1a. Water on a hydrophobic surface will form beads (*left*), but water spreads uniformly on a hydrophilic surface (*right*).

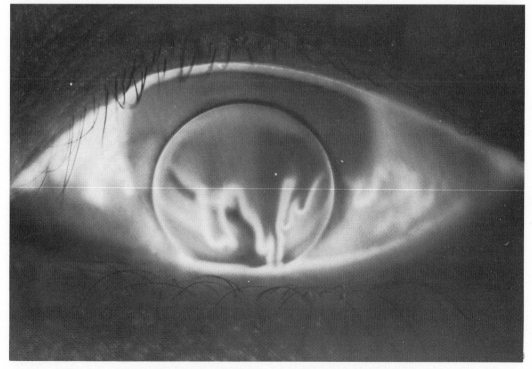

Figure 12.1b. Lens with a hydrophobic surface.

stance is defined as *adhesion*. If a clean glass capillary tube is placed in a container of pure water, the level of water in the tube is higher than the level inside the larger jar (Figure 12.2).

In addition, the surface of the water in the tube is concave. The molecules of water are attracted to the molecules of glass more than to the neighboring water molecules.

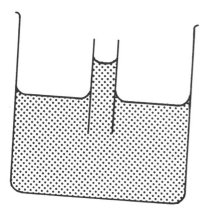

Figure 12.2. Level of water in tube is higher than level inside beaker due to adhesion.

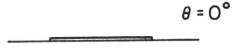

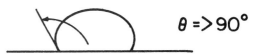

Figure 12.3. Contact angle.

A drop of liquid placed on a solid may spread out to cover the whole surface of the solid, or it may stay "bunched up" in the form of a drop. Whether the liquid spreads is decided by the relationship of the force of cohesion (attraction of molecules in the liquid for each other) and adhesion. The angle between the liquid surface and the solid surface is an indication of the relative values of the force of adhesion and cohesion. This is known as the angle of contact, θ (theta) (Figure 12.3).

Contact angle can be measured in degrees of arc, and the value obtained is an index of the ability of a liquid to wet a solid. An angle of contact, θ, of 0° implies complete wetting of the solid by the liquid. When the attraction of the liquid for itself (cohesion) is maximal, there is no attraction for the solid, so the contact angle is 180°. This indicates absolute nonwetting.

Polymethyl methacrylate is a relatively hydrophobic solid, with a contact angle of 60°. Thus, wetting solutions are needed to increase the wettability of the contact lens.

POLYVINYL ALCOHOL

Many wetting solutions utilize polyvinyl alcohol (P.V.A.) as a wetting agent.[23,24] Polyvinyl alcohol is a long-chain polymer with the general chemical structure shown in Figure 12.4. It possesses a number of properties that make it particularly useful with contact lenses. Polyvinyl alcohol is water soluble and relatively nonviscous. It is colorless, and its solution has a refractive index (1.336) that approximates natural tears. It forms a clear solution in water with a pH of approximately 7 and will not settle on standing.

One theory of wetting by P.V.A. is as follows. Plastic contact lenses are lipophilic (fat loving) in nature, and their surfaces are therefore not wettable with water. The polyvinyl alcohol molecule has both lipophilic groups and hydrophilic groups. When applied to the lens, the lipophilic groups bind to the plastic lens surface, forming a monomolecular layer of P.V.A. molecules oriented such that their hydrophilic groups are exposed. This new surface is readily wettable with water (Figure 12.5). An alternate theory explains wetting as a simple process of lowering the surface tension of tears.

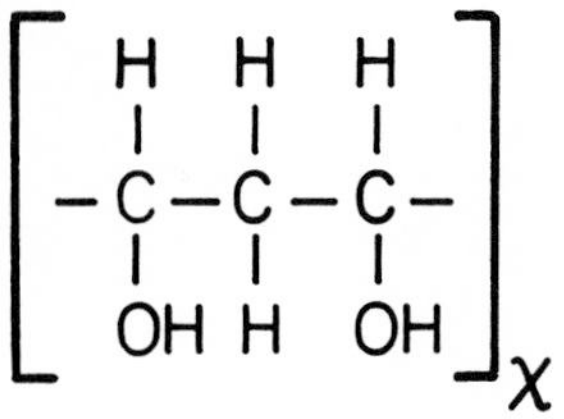

$$\begin{bmatrix} \overset{\displaystyle H}{\underset{\displaystyle OH}{-C}} & \overset{\displaystyle H}{\underset{\displaystyle H}{-C}} & \overset{\displaystyle H}{\underset{\displaystyle OH}{-C}} - \end{bmatrix}_X$$

Figure 12.4. Polyvinyl alcohol.

Polyvinyl alcohol can be regarded as non-toxic to ocular tissues, even when inadvertently introduced into the anterior chamber through an ocular injury or damaged tissue.[24] This is important, since components of wetting solutions should not interfere with corneal healing.[25]

Some patients are able to insert their contact lenses without using a wetting agent and to wear them comfortably. However, because the use of a good wetting solution does have several practical advantages (as outlined previously), current opinion is in favor of wet insertion.

STERILITY OF WETTING SOLUTIONS

Initial sterility of wetting solutions is achieved during manufacture, usually by gas sterilization. Once the bottle is opened, sterility should be maintained so the eye is not inoculated with a contaminant or potentially dangerous microorganisms via the wetting solution.[26] This is known as the *resterilizing*, or self-sterilizing, ability. Once the initial seal of sterility is broken, the wetting solution must not become a breeding ground for bacteria. To overcome this, bactericidal agents are used to preserve sterility.

Wetting solutions are sometimes erroneously considered to have germicidal activity when used on the contact lens. It is doubtful that the contact time between a wetting solution and the contact lens is sufficient to allow a significant germicidal action to overcome a contaminated lens.[27] This is the function of a soaking solution.

MAINTAINING LENS CLEANLINESS

The wetting solution plays a role in maintaining the cleanliness of the contact lens during the insertion process. It tends to prevent smudging of the lens by the fingers and helps to prevent contamination.

LUBRICANT AND MECHANICAL BUFFER

It has been proposed that using a wetting solution prevents the initial irritation reported by some patients after inserting their lenses and that a wetting solution may have some cushioning effect due to the viscosity of the fluid. However, since incorrect insertion may lead to discomfort, even when wetting solution is used, emphasis on prevention of insertion irritation probably should be directed towards the technique of insertion rather than towards the mechanical means of completely eradicating irritation.

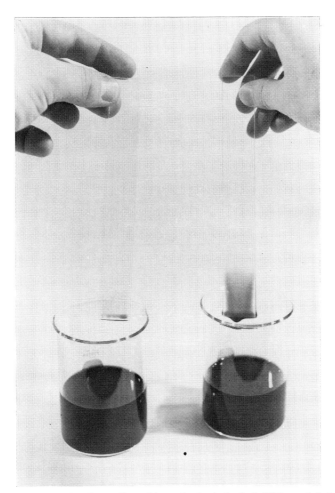

Figure 12.5. Slide on right has been dipped in polyvinyl alcohol. Slide on left is clean. When two slides are dipped into colored water, the water clings to the slide on right.

PHYSICAL CHARACTERISTICS

Wetting solutions of various manufacturers differ greatly in their pH and buffer capacity, osmolality solids value, and surface tension.

pH and Buffer Capacity

There is considerable variation in the pH and buffer capacities of the various wetting solutions.[28-31] This has given rise to considerable argument and controversy among various solution manufacturers and contact lens practitioners. It has been shown that the pH of commonly used (wetting) solutions varies from about 4 to 8.5[32] It is also known that when the eye is exposed for extended periods to solutions of either high or low pH irritation occurs. The usual range of comfort for the average eye is considered to be within a pH of about 6.6 to 7.8. A pH value of 7.4 is usually considered to be average for tears. Values higher than 7.4 are considered *relatively* alkaline, whereas values lower than 7.4

are considered *relatively* acidic. The approximate limits outside which tissue epithelial damage occurs are 4.0 and 10.0 (*see* Chapter 2).

Neither pH nor buffer strength alone uniquely influences eye stinging or irritation upon installation, but rather the improper combination of both. For example, if the solution has an extreme pH that is either high or low but has very low buffering capacity, one will find the following: When a drop of the solution is placed in the eye, because the solution has low buffering capacity, the pH is quickly diluted by the tears, and the pH is modified to within the normal range.

A contact lens manufacturer usually formulates his wetting solution first to achieve the properties of wetting and self-sterilization. Depending upon the components that are used, it may be found advantageous to keep the solution at either low or high pH in order to achieve stability. In this case, the solution should also have low buffering capacity so that the pH will be changed quickly as the solution is introduced into the eye. If, on the other hand, the solution is formulated to have a pH similar to that of the tears (7.4), then it is possible to utilize high buffering in order to retain the solution at a constant pH.[31]

Hill and Young have found in studying a variety of wetting solutions that those having the most alkaline values initially tended also to be the best buffered and changed the least over a period of one year in which they measured the change in pH.[32] Conversely, wetting solutions that were initially more acid in most instances had low buffering capacity and tended to become more acidic with time.

Osmolality

The osmotic pressure of a solution is commonly expressed in terms of the equivalent solution of NaCl. The normal osmolality of the tears is considered to be 0.9 percent sodium chloride equivalent. Bathing the eye with solutions that differ from this as little as 0.2 percent can have an effect on the corneal thickness (Chapter 2). However, a drop or two of a solution added to the tears is quickly diluted by tears and has little effect on the cornea. Osmotic solutions of low value seldom have any effect on eye comfort, but a drop of a solution with osmolality above 1.8 percent NaCl equivalent will usually cause some discomfort.

Hill and Young found a wide range of initial osmolality values from 0.14 percent NaCl equivalent to 1.4 percent NaCl equivalent in a sample of ophthalmic solutions.[32] In testing these solutions over a period of one year, they found a slight shift towards the hypertonic direction. This shift was accentuated if the bottle was left uncapped.

Solids Value

The solids value refers to the percent of total dissolved solids in the solution. If too high, it may lead to a gumming effect of the solution.

Surface Tension

A wide range of initial surface tension values can be found among contact lens solutions that are currently available. Hill and Young found that a great majority of solutions had values below that of tears.[32] Over the course of a year, every solution, capped or open, fell somewhat in value, but none appeared to increase significantly.

SUBSTITUTES FOR WETTING SOLUTION

Unsuccessful attempts have been made to use common household substances, such as soaps and detergents, as substitutes for commercially formulated wetting solutions. These substances are usually inadequate as wetting agents for contact lenses and are often irritating to the eyes. A further disadvantage is that they often tend to produce fogging by leaving a tenacious film on the lenses.

Some patients have used saliva as a wetting agent for their lenses under the mistaken impression that it contains antibacterial enzymes. Although it is true that saliva may be an effective wetting agent, it is also a potential source of ocular infections, and this practice should be condemned.[33,34]

SOAKING SOLUTION

Whenever the contact lens is removed from the eye, it should be placed in a soaking solution (Figure 12.6) until it is worn again. Soaking solutions have the following functions as outlined by Szekely:[19,35]

1. To aid in cleaning the lens of ocular secretions after the lens is removed from the eye

2. To prevent eye infection by a contaminated lens

3. To maintain the state of hydrated equilibrium, which the lens achieves while it is being worn[36]

CLEANING THE LENS

While the lens is being worn, it is exposed to and collects the oily and sebaceous secretion of the eye and surrounding structures. If these secretions are not removed from the lens, they will accumulate over a period of time and will eventually impair the optical clarity and wettability of the lens surface. Usually, these secretions can be removed by cleaning the lens with cleaning solution as soon as it is taken from the eye. (Wetting solutions have been used for this purpose in the past, but they clean primarily by their viscous action. A cleaning solution is much more effective in removing foreign debris.) Placing the lens in a soaking solution that contains agents capable of removing these secretions also helps to prevent their accumulation.

Water is an inadequate substitute for soaking solution both because it will not cleanse away oily secretions and because it almost always contains microbial and mineral contaminants.[34,35] Distilled water contains no minerals but is not sterile; even boiled or triple-distilled water, though initially sterile, is a good culture medium for many species of ocular pathogens, including *Pseudomonas aeruginosa*.[37]

If the lens is allowed to dry between wearing periods, the secretions remaining on it will eventually form a hard film, which can only be removed by polishing and refinishing. Bailey reported on a series of patients who complained of discomfort upon inserting their lenses.[38] In two cases a hardened spot of mucus on the concave surface of the lens was sufficiently large and firm to prevent lens rotation and to produce corneal abrasions.

STERILIZING THE LENS

Probably the most important function of the soaking solution is to sterilize the contact lens. Although the external eye is commonly exposed to various microbiological organisms, even when a contact lens is not worn, every effort must be made to avoid further contamination of the eye via the contact lens. Admittedly, the introduction of a contaminated lens to the eye will, in most cases, not result in an ocular infection. This fact has caused some to assume a rather casual attitude about contact lens asepsis. This approach must be condemned and every effort made to use the best available means to achieve contact lens sterility.

Ocular Infection

The microbial hazards from bacterial and fungal infections and parasitic infestation during contact lens fitting can be conveniently discussed under the categories of conjunctivitis and corneal ulcers.[39-43]

Conjunctivitis

Conjunctivitis is the most common of all eye diseases in the Western Hemisphere. Most cases are caused by pyogenic bacteria, which produce a copious discharge. Other causes are viral infection, allergy, and parasitic infestations. The majority are exogenous, but conjunctivitis may be endogenous, as in conjunctival tuberculosis. Bacterial conjunctivitis, the most frequent type, is usually self-limited, lasting about ten to fourteen days untreated. Treatment with one of the many available antibacterial agents usually clears the condition in about three days.

The conjunctiva contains many blood vessels and mucus-producing cells, but few pain fibers. This accounts for the marked inflammatory response without pain, which is characteristic of conjunctivitis. When the lids are closed, as in sleeping, the temperature of the conjunctival sac is elevated. The incubating effect of this increase in temperature promotes the growth of invading bacteria, and this in turn promotes the production of pus cells, thus sticking the lids together in the morning.

When the eyes become inflamed, the patient usually seeks treatment early. A diagnosis of conjunctivitis is suggested by a history

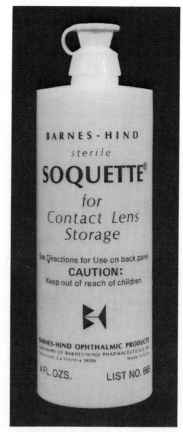

Figure 12.6. Example of a soaking solution.

of red eye of short duration, without pain or photophobia, and by the inflamed appearance of the conjunctiva and the presence of a conjunctival exudate.[44] The diagnosis may be confirmed and specific pathogens identified by immediate microscopic examination of stained material from the conjunctival surface. It is always well to rule out keratitis, glaucoma, and iritis, particularly in the earliest stages of conjunctivitis when inflammation and discharge are not marked.

Corneal Ulcers

Scarring or perforation due to corneal ulceration is a significant cause of blindness throughout the world. The normal cornea is devoid of any direct vascularization and depends on diffusion for its metabolites. Invasion of this tissue by microorganisms is more serious than when other tissues are invaded. The inflammatory response to corneal infections is usually localized in the conjunctiva, and the direct effect of tissue defenses is not experienced within the cornea. The environmental conditions for microbial growth are actually enhanced by increased filtration flow into the diseased cornea. Due to the lack of phagocytosis and other local body defense mechanisms, microbial growth continues uninhibited. Most forms are amenable to therapy. Visual impairment can be avoided only if appropriate treatment is instituted promptly; in some cases this means within a matter of hours after onset.

Sources of Pathogens

Because of its exposed position, the eye comes in contact with more microorganisms than any other mucous membrane. The conjunctiva offers luxuriant living conditions for certain types of organisms, whereas some of those which grow abundantly on the nasal and other mucosa fail to multiply in the conjunctival sac. Few, if any, organisms can directly invade the corneal epithelium due to its intrinsic resistance when intact. Once the epithelial layer is broken, however, the resistance is broken, and the organism may enter the cornea and cause infection.

Bacteria, fungi, and parasites can be transferred into the eye by the patient from his hands, hair, nails, clothes, family towels, and even dandruff via his pillow.

The manner of dissemination of viral infections is not clearly understood in all instances. Some viruses require the transfer of cellular debris, such as could be transferred with a tonometer used in testing for intraocular pressure. Some viruses are quite seasonal, being more prevalent in hot weather while others are believed to be airborne.

The most dangerous and opportunistic organism is *Pseudomonas aeruginosa*.[45,46] This organism actually grows better in the cornea than in any other known medium, even syn-

thetically prepared, and has been found as a contaminant of many commonly used eye solutions, particularly, sodium fluorescein solutions. During the fitting of patients, the contact lens practitioner may come in contact with a number of potential sources of the organism. It is a common inhabitant of the human skin, is an air contaminant, and can survive in water with minimal nutrient material, such as dust or inorganic salts. Its ability to thrive and multiply in sodium fluorescein solutions is well known (*see* Chapter 7).

The organism is extremely resistant to many antibacterial agents. Once in the stroma, the residual traces of antibacterial agents are neutralized by tissue components, and the organisms find an excellent culture medium for rapid growth and dissemination throughout the cornea and anterior segment of the eye.[47] *P. aeruginosa* infections progress so rapidly that the loss of the eye can occur in as short a period as twenty-four hours after onset. Under optimal conditions, where the eye is saved, marked or complete impairment of vision usually results. The greatest potential hazard in contact lens practice is this microorganism because of the intrinsic dangers of the use of a contaminated solution of fluorescein. If the contact lens practitioner sees a patient with a corneal abrasion, the transfer of the *P. aeruginosa* organism into the abrasion could be tragic.

Antimicrobial Agents

Among the preservatives used in ophthalmology, and of equal importance as additives in contact lens solutions, the following have been studied extensively: polymyxin B sulfate, quaternary ammonium compounds, chlorobutanol, organic mercurials, *p*-hydroxybenzoic acid esters, and certain phenols and substituted alcohols.

Polymyxin B Sulfate

Polymyxin B sulfate was found to be the most active agent known when tested against a group of strains of *P. aeruginosa*.[39] However, the drug lacks adequate activity against gram-positive organisms. Since this agent is an indispensable tool in drug treatment of pseudomonal ulcers, it has been suggested the drug be restricted to the treatment of known pseudomonal and other potentially dangerous infections, rather than to be used as a preservative agent.

Quaternary Ammonium Compounds

Benzalkonium chloride, in concentrations ranging from 1:10,000 to 1:100,000, is used as a preservative in ophthalmic and contact lens solutions.[48-51] Benzalkonium chloride has a broad antibacterial and antifungal activity. However, benzalkonium chloride *alone* would not appear satisfactory for soaking solution. For example, Riegelman and associates reported on a strain of *P. aeruginosa* that multiplies in a 1:5,000 concentration of benzalkonium chloride.[52]

Benzalkonium chloride is an effective germicide, however, when it is used in combination with other compounds. MacGregor et al. demonstrated that disodium ethylenediaminotetraacetate (EDTA) enhanced the bactericidal action of a quaternary ammonium compound related to benzalkonium chloride on *P. aeruginosa*.[53] The EDTA was thought to disrupt the integrity of the cell wall and so accelerate the action of benzalkonium chloride by increasing the permeability of the cell to benzalkonium chloride. In the presence of EDTA 0.1 percent, *Pseudomonas* is killed in 1:10,000 benzalkonium chloride.[53]

Careful formulation of solutions can result in a synergistic system possessing a capacity to resterilize a heavily contaminated solution, even when benzalkonium chloride resistant pseudomonal organisms are used.

Caution must be used in determining the optimal concentration of this quaternary compound to be used in contact lens solutions.[54] If used repeatedly in concentrations of 1:5,000 or stronger, benzalkonium chloride can denature the corneal protein causing irreversible

damage. Swan noted that 0.04% (1:2,500) to 0.05% (1:2,0000) solutions of benzalkonium chloride produced superficial punctate disturbance of the corneal epithelium.[55] Swan performed further experiments with a very strong solution, i.e. 0.1% (1:1,000).[55] He observed both conjunctival and corneal lesions. The *conjunctival* reaction consisted of hyperemia, edema, and sometimes strands of pseudomembranes (due to desquamation of conjunctival epithelium). The *corneal* lesions began within ninety seconds, and consisted of multiple punctate gray areas in the corneal epithelium as seen with the biomicroscope. The tiny areas gradually became confluent and within ten minutes could be seen with the naked eye. Similar, but less severe, reactions were seen in several patients instilling 0.03% (1:3,500) and 0.04% (1:2,500) benzalkonium chloride into the conjunctival sac three to four times daily over periods of two to eight weeks. The patients frequently complained of a sensation of sand in their eyes. The effects were cumulative. A single instillation was often well tolerated, whereas a second or third instillation at short intervals produced discomfort and objective signs of irritation. On discontinuance of the benzalkonium chloride instillation, recovery was rapid (conjunctiva and cornea returned to normal in twelve hours).

A degree of confusion exists as to the desired activity of benzalkonium chloride in contact lens solutions. It is added to a wetting solution only for its antimicrobial activity. It is not an active wetting ingredient.

Benzalkonium chloride is cationic in character and is avidly adsorbed by cotton, protein, and other negatively charged molecules. The antibacterial effectiveness of benzalkonium chloride and other quaternaries can be interfered with by the improper formulation of a solution, such as the wetting agent where an interaction with thickening or lubricating agents added to the formulation can occur.[56,57] It is inactivated by many other compounds.[56] The final solution must be tested not only for its sterility, but also for its antimicrobial activity by a resterilizing test. (Disposable capsules have been tried to increase sterility.)[58]

Other quaternary ammonium compounds are qualitatively similar in their antimicrobial activity, including cetylpyridinium chloride, Phemerol® (diisobutylphenoxyethoxyethyl dimethyl benzyl ammonium chloride), myristyl Γ-picolinium chloride, cetyltrimethylammonium bromide, and others. Most, or all, of these do not equal benzalkonium chloride in their antipseudomonal activity and, therefore, are not considered good preservatives for ophthalmic solutions.

Chlorobutanol

Chlorobutanol is a relatively slow bactericide and fungicide at concentrations greater than 0.35%. It appears to possess synergistic activity when combined with phenols and quaternaries, such as benzalkonium chloride.

Chlorobutanol has the advantage of acting on bacteria by a mechanism unique to this chemical type. It is believed to be converted to an epitoxoid by the bacteria after penetration and thereby becomes lethal to the organism. It is a valuable compound to use in conjunction with other antimicrobial agents.

Chlorobutanol has several disadvantages, especially when used in wetting solution.

1. Chlorobutanol is volatile, and its concentration can fall below the effective level. However, a solutions manufacturer states that the soaking solution they manufacture meets the label claim for a period exceeding two years.

2. In preparation of solutions, care must be taken to maintain a temperature high enough to dissolve the drug but not high enough to destroy it. However, this is not a serious drawback.

3. There is evidence that it causes stinging.

Organic Mercurials

Phenylmercuric nitrate or acetate in concentrations from 1:25,000 to 1:100,000 have been commonly used as an antibacterial agent for ophthalmic solutions and has been proposed for use in certain solutions to be used in contact lens fitting. Mercurials in general are well known for their bacteriostatic activity but are notoriously slow acting in their germicidal activity.[59,60] Pseudomonal organisms survive exposure to 1:25,000 concentrations longer than one week. After this period, the organisms are still capable of causing corneal infection on injection into the rabbit's cornea. Phenylmercuric nitrate is nearly completely hydrolyzed in aqueous solution and exists predominantly as the poorly ionized hydroxide at pHs greater than 3. It therefore differs from other common organic mercurials in that it is not precipitated in slightly acid pHs. The phenyl mercuric ion reacts with halide ions to form insoluble salts. Phenylmercuric nitrate is commonly used as a preservative for sodium fluorescein solution as an antifungal and gram-positive bacteriostatic agent. However, this system should be packaged in sterile single-patient-use containers to reduce the hazard of transmittal of gram-negative organisms such as *P. aeruginosa*.

Other organic mercurial germicides have been used in the eye: nitromerosal (Metaphen®) 1:2,500 and thimerosal (Merthiolate®) 1:5,000 to 1:20,000. Both compounds are basic salts of weak organic acids and have to be restricted to alkaline solutions. The compounds are slowly acting germicides and can easily be inactivated by corneal fluids.

p-Hydroxybenzoic Acid Esters

The *p*-hydroxybenzoic acid esters, the parabens, particularly the methyl, propyl, and butyl esters, have been used in pharmaceutical products for two decades as fungicides and in higher concentrations as antibacterial agents. The British Pharmacopoeia Code, 1954, recommended the use of 0.0229% of the methyl ester combined with 0.0114% of the propyl ester. However, it has been shown that these concentrations are completely ineffective against many strains of *P. aeruginosa*.

A 0.1% solution has been used in England as an ophthalmic preservative. This concentration definitely produces ocular irritation. Furthermore, to qualify as an ideal ocular solution preservative, the agent should possess rapidly resterilizing activity for contaminated solutions. Critical evidence on this aspect is lacking for the parabens.

Phenols and Substituted Alcohols

The following compounds have been reported to be bactericidal against gram-positive and most gram-negative organisms and only slightly irritating upon instillation into the eye: *p*-chlorometacresol, 0.05%; *p*-chlorometaxylenol, 0.03%; phenylethyl alcohol, 0.5%; phenoxyethanol, 0.3%; phenylethyl alcohol, 0.1%, plus phenol, 0.25%; phenyl alcohol plus chlorobutanol, 0.5%. None of these systems has been intensively studied for its use as rapidly resterilizing germicides for pathogenic organisms.

A summary of the composition of various solutions used in contact lens care is presented in Appendix 14.[61]

Compatibility

A few solutions have been found to be incompatible when mixed.[62,63] This may be due to the formation of a precipitate or to a neutralization of one component. This can usually be avoided if the patient uses all products from the same manufacturer.

Wet Versus Dry Storage

Whether a soaking solution is the most favorable storage method has been challenged by Allen[64] and others[65-68] who prefer dry storage. Current opinion appears to be in favor of using commercial soaking solution with antimicrobial additives.[69-74]

The studies of Clifton and Hall established that a soaking solution containing benzalkonium chloride and chlorobutanol killed a variety of microorganisms within five to ten minutes.[69] Hall and Krezanoski examined the

TABLE 12.1

SURVIVAL OF ORGANISMS ON DRIED LENS

Organisms	Day					
	1	2	5	6	7	8
Staphylococcus aureus	+	+	+	+	+	+
Escherichia coli	+	+	+	+	+	+
Proteus vulgaris	0	+	+	+	0	0
Pseudomonas aeruginosa	+	+	+	+	+	+
Bacillus subtilis	+	+	+	+	+	+
Candida albicans	+	+	+	+	+	+

survival of organisms on dried lenses. Table 12.1 shows that with the exception of *Proteus vulgaris*, which gave somewhat inconsistent results, all the organisms tested survived desiccation for the length of the experiment. It is quite obvious that desiccation does not protect the patient from eye infections. Table 12.2 gives the levels of antimicrobial activity of the active ingredients contained in a soaking solution.

Evidence for the value of the commerical soaking solution was presented in a study by Bettman.[75] Bettman's study was in two parts. In Part 1 the subjects' conjunctival fornices and contact lens cases were examined for bacteria. In Part 2 various methods of lens storage were evaluated for their effectiveness in eliminating known concentrations of bacterial contaminants from contact lenses. The results of the first part of the study showed that in cultures taken from sixty-three contact lens cases—some containing soaking solution, some containing water, and some dry—a significantly higher number of those which contained soaking solution were sterile than of the others. Almost twice as many sterile cultures were taken from the fornices of subjects using soaking solution (82%) as from those using dry storage (42%). These data are summarized in Figure 12.7.

As can be seen in Figure 12.7, the species of bacteria encountered varied considerably. Three of them are common causes of corneal ulcer: *Pseudomonas aeruginosa, Streptococcus hemolyticus,* and *Klebsiella pneumoniae. P. aeru-*

TABLE 12.2

MICROBIAL KILL OF DRIED BUT VIABLE ORGANISMS VS. CONTACT TIME BY A
SOAKING SOLUTION IN A SOAKING CASE

Organism		*1*	*3*	*5*	*10*	*15*	*30*
Staphylococcus aureus	lens	0	+	0	0	0	0
	soaking solution	+	+	0	0	0	0
Escherichia coli	lens	+	+	0	0	0	0
	soaking solution	0	0	0	0	0	0
Proteus vulgaris	lens	+	0	0	0	0	0
	soaking solution	0	0	0	0	0	0
Pseudomonas aeruginosa	lens	0	+	+	0	0	0
	soaking solution	0	+	+	0	0	0
Bacillus subtilis	lens	+	0	0	0	0	0
	soaking solution	+	0	0	0	0	0
Candida albicans	lens	0	0	0	0	0	0
	soaking solution	+	+	+	0	0	0

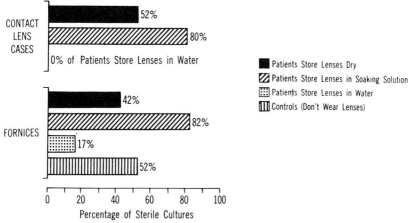

Figure 12.7. Data of Bettman.[75]

ginosa is the most pathogenic and destructive to corneal tissue.

Out of 156 cultures from the fornices and storage cases of the patients in Bettman's study, 5 (3.2%) contained *P. aeruginosa*. One of the five was from a carrying case containing soaking solution, but the case had never been cleaned and was fitted with sponge rubber, against which many manufacturers of soaking solution specifically warn. A second culture of *P. aeruginosa* was taken from the conjunctival fornix of the patient who was using the contaminated storage case. A third was taken from a dry case. The other two were taken from cases containing tap water.

In the second part of the Bettman study, it was shown that lenses deliberately contaminated with high concentrations of bacteria could be sterilized by overnight soaking in soaking solution. This was not true of lenses stored dry or in water. Bettman concluded that storing the lenses in soaking solution was bacteriologically safer than dry storage and that a greater percentage of patients using soaking solution had bacteriologically sterile fornices and cases than those who did not use soaking solution.

A study by Dabezies supports and extends

the results by Bettman.[72] Dabezies instructed a group of thirty patients who wore contact lenses to use wet storage for one lens and dry storage for the other. He found that, in general, considerable bacterial contamination was associated with both the dry lens and the wet lens, but contamination was more frequent with the dry lens (67.5%) than with the wet lens (40.5%). Potential pathogens were relatively more frequent with the dry lens (61%) than with the wet lens (33.5%).

Kapetansky et al., on the other hand, found pathogenic organisms in the cul-de-sacs of 4 percent of individuals wearing contact lenses.[65] It was also found that 10 percent of the patients had pathogens in their carrying cases, and 8 percent had pathogens in their wetting or soaking solutions. Kapetansky et al. recommend that lenses should be stored dry.[65] Their conclusion is supported by the results of Obear and Winter, who tested the cases of eighty consecutive contact lens patients.[66] They found that bacterial cultures were positive in 90 percent or more of both the wet and the dry cases, but isolation of pathogens was twice as frequent from wet as from dry cases. *Pseudomonas* was recovered from seventeen of thirty-nine wet cases (44%) and from nine of forty-one dry cases (22%). Other pathogens were removed from four of the thirty-nine wet cases. None was found in the dry cases.

Volume of Storage Fluid

There does not appear to be any universally accepted specification regarding the ideal volume of storage fluid that should be used for the storage of contact lenses.[76] Values ranging from a minimum of 3 ml. to a maximum of 8 ml. have been proposed (Tables 12.3 and 12.4).

TABLE 12.3

	Volume Fluid Two Lenses	*Compartment Letter Coding*	*Compartment Color Coding*	*Patient Identification*	*Lens Cleaning Provision*	*Lens Rinsing Provision*	*Complete Lens Submersion*	*Mirror*	*Absence of Metal Components*	*Boilability*	*Light Background Color*
1. Kelley-Hueber Mailer	(1.8 ml) 0	1	0	0	0	0	0	0	1	0	1
2. Multi-Pack	(0.8 ml) 0	1	1	1	0	0	0	1	1	0	1
3. W/J B-Lens Mailer	(2.8 ml) 0	1	0	0	0	0	0	0	1	0	1
4. Slim Jim	(0.8 ml) 0	1	1	1	0	0	0	0	1	0	1
5. Hydra-Kit	(5.0 ml) 1	1	1	0	0	0	1	0	0	0	1
6. Aquacell Mates	(6.5 ml) 0	1	1	1	0	1	1	0	1	0	1
7. Antisept Jeweled	(1.2 ml) 0	1	0	0	0	0	0	0	1	0	0
8. Guardian	(6.0 ml) 0	1	0	1	0	0	1	0	1	0	1
9. Ideal	(5.6 ml) 0	1	0	1	0	0	1	0	1	0	1
10. Multimaster	(7.7 ml) 0	1	0	0	0	0	1	0	1	0	1
11. Comfort Case	(6.0 ml) 0	0	1	0	0	0	1	0	1	0	1
12. Sentinal	(7.4 ml) 0	1	1	1	0	0	1	1	1	0	1
13. Clean-N-Stow	(8.0 ml) 0	1	1	0	0	1	1	0	1	1	1
14. Clean-N-Soakit	(4.7 ml) 1	1	1	0	0	1	0	0	1	1	1
15. porta-FLOW	(4.0 ml) 1	1	1	1	1	1	1	1	1	1	1
16. Una-Pac	(6.5 ml) 0	1	1	0	0	1	0	0	0	1	1
17. Hydra-Mat	(30 ml) 0	1	0	0	1	1	1	0	1	0	1
18. Tote and Soak	(8.0 ml) 0	0	1	0	0	1	0	0	1	1	1
19. Lensine	(1.8 ml) 0	1	0	0	0	0.	0	0	1	1	1
20. Dispos-A-Kit	(7.0 ml) 0	1	0	0	0	0	0	0	1	0	1

TABLE 12.4

MANUFACTURERS OF THE POPULAR CONTACT LENS
CASES IN TABLE 12.3

1. Kelley & Hueber, Inc., Philadelphia, Pennsylvania 19143
2. Kelley & Hueber, Inc., Philadelphia, Pennsylvania 19143
3. Wesley Jessen, Inc., Chicago, Illinois 60603
4. Kelley & Hueber, Inc., Philadelphia, Pennsylvania 19143
5. Barnes-Hind Ophthalmics, Inc., Sunnyvale, California 94086
6. Barnes-Hind Ophthalmics, Inc., Sunnyvale, California 94086
7. Wesley Jessen, Inc., Chicago, Illinois 60603
8. Kelley & Hueber, Inc., Philadelphia, Pennsylvania 19143
9. R & F Products, Inc., Englewood, Colorado 80110
10. R & F Products, Inc., Englewood, Colorado 80110
11. H & W Optical Products, Hazel Park, Michigan 48030
12. Kelley & Hueber, Inc., Philadelphia, Pennsylvania 19143
13. Allergan Pharmaceuticals, Inc., Irvine, California 92664
14. Allergan Pharmaceuticals, Inc., Irvine, California 92664
15. Flow Pharmaceuticals, Inc., Palo Alto, California 94303
16. Kelley & Hueber, Inc., Philadelphia, Pennsylvania 19143
17. Barnes-Hind Ophthalmics, Inc., Sunnyvale, California 94086
18. Kelley & Hueber, Inc., Philadelphia, Pennsylvania 19143
19. The Murine Company, North Chicago, Illinois 60064
20. Barnes-Hind Ophthalmics, Inc., Sunnyvale, California 94086

Because the commonly recommended storage solutions differ as to their germicidal composition and potency, one might expect that, in fact, different volumes might be required to achieve contact lens disinfection in a reasonable period of time.

All of the preservatives commonly incorporated in solutions formulated for storage purposes are adversely affected by many environmental agents encountered by the contact lens wearers. Proteins, mucin, fatty acids, and anionic detergents are classic examples of substances that may precipitate or destroy the activity of otherwise effective germicides.

The following studies were conducted by Krezanoski and Lowry: Three problem-free contact lens wearers used storage solution containing 0.0133% benzalkonium chloride along with other active ingredients.[76]

In the first phase of the study, the contact lens wearers were asked to put their lenses away for overnight storage in their storage solution at the end of the day without cleaning their lenses. In the second phase of the study, the contact lens wearers were asked to put their lenses away for overnight storage in their storage solution without cleaning their lenses or changing the storage solution for two consecutive days. In the third phase of the study the two contact lens wearers who showed the greatest benzalkonium loss were asked to clean their lenses prior to putting their lenses away for overnight storage. The storage solutions from all three phases of the study were collected from each of the three contact lens wearers and analyzed in duplicate. The resulting average benzalkonium chloride depletions are presented in Table 12.5.

The data presented in Table 12.5 were used to produce Table 12.6, in which a relationship between the resulting percentage benzalkonium chloride concentration loss and volume of storage solution is expressed. It was assumed that the total amount of benzalkonium chloride lost in the tests performed would have been the same irrespective of the volume of the storage solution used. Only the data on contact lens wearers JBL (showing the greatest depletion) and TAO (showing the least depletion) after one day storage were used.

Having collected these in-use data, Krezanoski and Lowry draw the following conclusions.[76]

1. Dirty lenses removed from the cornea are coated with tear constituents consisting of proteins, mucopolysaccharides, oils, as well as many other complex components that inac-

Contact Lens Practice

TABLE 12.5

DEPLETION OF BENZALKONIUM CHLORIDE IN STORAGE CASE

Patient Code	Occupation	Percent Benzalkonium Chloride Lost		
		One Day No Cleaning	Two Days No Cleaning No Fresh Solution	One Day With Cleaning Prior to Storage
JBL	Chemist	23.1	31.2	4.9
JLM	Student	13.3	37.8	0.0
TAO	Secretary	9.1	12.6	

TABLE 12.6

RELATIONSHIP BETWEEN BENZALKONIUM CHLORIDE DEPLETION AND VOLUME OF SOAKING SOLUTION

Volume Storage Solution	1 ml	2 ml	3 ml	4 ml	5 ml	6 ml	7 ml	8 ml
JBL (highest loss) benzalkonium chloride	92.5	46.2	36.3	23.1	18.5	15.4	13.2	11.5
TAO (lowest loss) benzalkonium chloride	36.4	18.2	14.3	9.1	7.3	6.1	5.2	4.6

tivate preservatives, e.g. benzalkonium chloride or thimerosal. Different contact lens wearers vary widely in the amount of preservative that they inactivate in their storage solution by introducing their lenses into storage solution. The amount of preservative inactivation varies widely from day to day with any given patient.

2. There is wide variation in the amount and probably the type of preservative inactivating principles transferred to the lens surface by the patients' fingers. These agents generally consist of organic salts, soap residues, oily sebum, and cosmetics.

3. The prophylactic daily use of an effective cleaner prior to lens storage in a storage solution curtails the loss of active disinfectant ingredients very markedly. This beneficial effect is, of course, in addition to the well-known improved physical cleanliness, clarity, and the better comfort associated with clean lenses.

4. Many patients fail to realize the significance of daily cleaning before storing their lenses. The storage solution should be designed so that even if 25 percent of the active disinfectant concentration is depleted because of their failing to clean their lenses, there is an adequate amount of disinfectant still remaining to disinfect the lenses.

5. The hazard of not replacing the storage solution with fresh solution on a daily basis is evident. Only two-thirds of the original disinfectant agent may remain active during the second day's storage in the same solution. This could be even less with very sloppy patients.

6. The data presented in Table 12.6 indicate that the use of less than 3 ml. solution may not be adequate to achieve sterility.

The variety of results found by different investigators who have studied the bacteriology of contact lens storage has led to considerable confusion in the field. The following conclusions seem warranted:

The studies that show the worst results with the use of storage solutions were those in which cultures were taken from the cases of patients who were already established in their storage routine. No special instructions were given to these patients, and they came from a variety of sources with the past history unknown. Better results were obtained in studies where the investigator instructed the patient as to the proper use of the soaking solution. In this case, the results were usually much better than could be achieved by means of dry storage. Hence, storage solutions are only effective if the patient follows the recommended regimen.

The most common reason for a failure of the storage solution to produce a sterile storage medium is that the patient did not change the storage medium at frequent intervals or did not clean his case. It is not uncommon to find patients with cases that are never cleaned and some are so dirty as to defy any reasonable amount of judgment. The patient must be instructed as to proper cleaning procedures for the case and must follow recommended procedures for changing soaking solution.

Under the worst conditions of patient care, the use of storage solution does not present much advantage over dry storage when only sterility is considered. Even so, the other advantages of a storage solution, which accrue from maintaining a constant environment, would certainly tip the scale in favor of the use of a soaking solution.

One factor that has not been discussed is the method by which data are obtained in the bacteriological studies. For the study of lenses in soaking solutions, cultures are usually taken from the contact lens cases. It must be considered that the patient is removing the lens from the case, rinsing it, adding wetting solution, and then placing the lens on the eye. It is very likely that the latter regimen serves to reduce or eliminate any bacteriological contamination that may have occurred in the case. This is not to excuse the poor results that have been found as a result of storage in a soaking solution in some studies but rather to point out the limitations of some of their results when applied to the practical situation of the contact lens wearer. It might be more realistic to culture the contact lens after it has been put through the preinsertion regimen and just before it is placed on the eye.

It must be concluded that if dry storage is to be followed, the case should be left open or a case used in which air is free to circulate over the lens. A dry storage technique in which the lens is placed in a closed container cannot be recommended under any circumstances. It is very likely that enough moisture will be contained inside the container to support bacterial growth.

HYDRATION OF THE LENS

Plastic contact lenses absorb significant amounts of water, achieving their maximum point of hydration in forty-eight hours and drying out, if stored dry, in twelve hours (Figure 12.8). This is an important observation because the "natural state" of the contact lens is submersion, i.e. in tear fluid, while the lens is on the eye. As the lenses are worn for longer and longer periods, they take up more and more water. Most lenses, because of strains in the plastic stock used or strains introduced in the manufacture, will flatten as water is absorbed.[77-78] This variation in the curvature of the lens may cause irritation and/or visual disturbances. One function of the contact lens soaking solution is to maintain the lens at a constant level of hydration when out of the eye so that fluctuations in curvatures will not occur (*see* Chapter 13).

COMFORT

Soaking of the contact lens has been shown to aid in preventing foreign material from drying on the lens, to help the wetting properties of the lens, and to stabilize the lens cur-

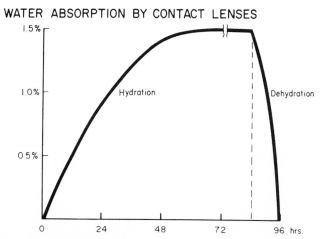

Figure 12.8. Water absorption by contact lenses. From H. W. Hind and I. J. Szekely, Wetting and Hydration of Contact Lenses, *Contacto*, *3*(3):65–68, 1959.

vature when it is out of the eye. All of these factors help to increase the comfort of the wearer.[72]

Dabezies found the following in questioning fifty patients who used wet storage on only one eye: Of 281 evaluations of the "dry storage" eye, no discomfort was reported in 18.2 percent; initial discomfort (temporary discomfort immediately following insertion of the lens, which lasted one to fifteen minutes) was reported in 63.3 percent; and intermittent discomfort throughout the day was reported in 14.2 percent.[72]

Of 281 evaluations of the wet eye, no discomfort was reported in 92 percent, and initial discomfort was reported in 8.0 percent.

VISION

Dabezies found that a better visual performance, especially from a subjective viewpoint, was recorded with the wet lens.[72] However, the subjective visual disturbance associated with the dry lens was also not too severe in most instances. Out of 273 examinations of the dry lens eye, no visual disturbance was recorded in 75.9 percent, mild visual disturbance in 21.9 percent, and a severe visual disturbance in 2.2 percent. Six of the fifty patients (12%) experienced such severe visual disturbance with the dry lens that they wished to discontinue the study.

STORAGE CASES

Many types of storage cases are available (Figure 12.9), which have the following features (Table 12.3):

COMPARTMENT CODING

Most kits designed for lens storage are adequately coded with large elevated letters R and L for the right and left lenses. In addition, some kits contain an elevation over

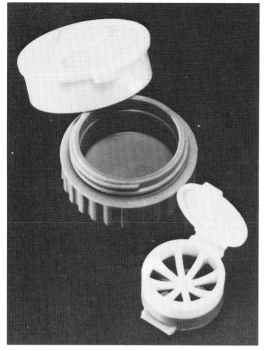
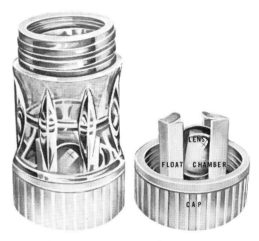

Figure 12.9. Examples of storage cases. *Left*, Porta-Flow® and *right*, HydraKit®. Courtesy of Flow Pharmaceuticals and Barnes-Hind, Inc.

the right compartment for easy tactile identification for those patients who are visually handicapped without their lenses on.[79]

Through generally accepted convention those manufacturers who color code lens compartments use white for the right lens and some other color of their choosing for the left.

LEAKPROOF FEATURE

A leakproof case design is the objective of all manufacturers and contact lens specialists, as well as patients. Unfortunately, this is very difficult to achieve with plastics and design alone.

PATIENT IDENTIFICATION

Many cases have identification tags. Some also make provision for recording the fitter's name and telephone number.

CLEANING

Two basic approaches have been taken to incorporate cleaning. In both instances the lenses are retained in perforated compartments. In the first instance the lens compartments are forced up and down in a cleaning fluid (Figure 12.10). In the second design the perforated transfer unit is held against the water faucet to promote cleaning with a hydrostatic spray of fresh water (Figure 12.11).

Low power ultrasonic devices for cleaning have not been shown to provide any significant cleaning action. Shaking a lens in storage fluid is only minimally effective.

PROVISION FOR LENS RINSING

Exposed or removable perforated lens compartments permit rinsing to be performed by running tap water over the unit.

COMPLETE LENS SUBMERSION

It is readily apparent that if a storage kit is to perform its function in accordance with the specialist's assumptions and the patient's expectations, it must provide for complete lens submersion in storage solution irrespective of the position of the kit.

MIRROR

Most contact lens specialists prefer that their patients learn to insert and remove their lenses without the aid of a mirror. There are, however, many occasions when it is essential for the patient to view an uncomfortable eye, to check whether it is red or severely inflamed and irritated, in order that appropriate corrective measures may be taken.

METAL COMPONENTS

Occasionally patients are still presented storage kits that contain metal springs. There is conclusive information regarding the interaction of metals with chelating agents such as disodium edetate commonly contained in most storage solutions. Chelating agents corrode these springs, mobilizing undesirable metals into the storage solution at the expense and loss of activity ascribed to them.

CLEANING ACCESSIBILITY

An important requirement for accessory devices should include easy cleaning.[79] Smooth, exposed surfaces should lend themselves readily to wiping or periodic scrubbing with a clean toothbrush. Most contact lens specialists instruct their patients to clean their cases thoroughly at least once a week. Accumulated debris or foreign matter collected in a hidden or inaccessible device compartment may readily deplete the active germicidal agents contained in an otherwise safe and effective storage solution and promote patient hazard.

Cleaning of the Case

Ideally, accessory devices should be made of materials that permit periodic boiling for purposes of cleaning and disinfection. The

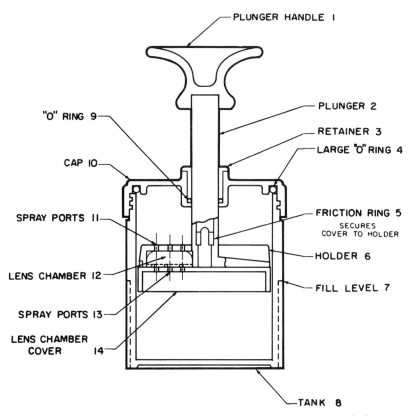

PLUNGER HANDLE 1

"O" RING 9

PLUNGER 2

RETAINER 3

CAP 10

LARGE "O" RING 4

SPRAY PORTS 11

FRICTION RING 5
SECURES
COVER TO HOLDER

LENS CHAMBER 12

HOLDER 6

FILL LEVEL 7

SPRAY PORTS 13

LENS CHAMBER
COVER   14

TANK 8

Figure 12.10. Hydromat hydraulic cleaning. Courtesy of Barnes-Hind, Inc.

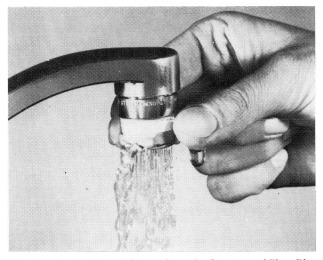

Figure 12.11. Hydraulic cleaning with transfer unit. Courtesy of Flow Pharmaceuticals.

patient may be instructed to throw the empty case in boiling water for fifteen to twenty minutes to clean and disinfect it at least once a month. The merit of this feature is obvious. Polypropylene is one plastic that makes this possible. Unfortunately, polyethylene and polystyrene cannot tolerate boiling.

Finally, it is most important that the device components do not deplete active ingredients contained in storage solutions and do not leach dyes or other deleterious extractives into storage solutions during normal patient use. All responsible manufacturers adhere to this self-imposed and rational specification.

CLASSIFICATION OF ACCESSORY CONTACT LENS DEVICES

1. *Mailing devices* are flat polyethylene plastic units with small cavities and snap closures designed for mailing dry lenses. When labeled, they are also useful for lens identification during manufacture and dry storage of stock lenses in the specialist's office. These devices are not intended for distribution to patients for effective wet lens storage.

2. *Soaking kits* are available in a variety of shapes and sizes for wet storage of contact lenses.

3. *Cleaning and storage devices* are designed to provide effective wet storage and effective spray cleaning for contact lenses.

4. *Cleaning units* are devices designed for cleaning of contact lenses.

5. *Disposable soaking kits* are economically constructed devices designed for use for approximately thirty days, after which time they are to be discarded. It is the manufacturer's intent that they be discarded with

every bottle of solution used.

6. *Lens holder* is an open holder used in the office to reduce contamination.[80]

It is readily apparent that mailing containers designed for dry storage should not be dispensed along with storage solutions. A device that is designed to hold less than 3 ml. of storage solution may be seriously deficient insofar as providing adequately disinfected lenses on a routine basis. The efficacy of the best storage solutions may be destroyed by using an inadequate volume of solution, improper provision for cleaning of the case, lack of daily use of fresh solution, or improper lens cleaning and handling prior to storage.

Devices that lack the leakproof features are often responsible for avoidable ocular discomfort upon lens insertion. This is due to the fluid evaporating and thereby increasing the salt and preservative concentration to an intolerable level.

CLEANING SOLUTIONS

Various commercial cleaning solutions are available.[81-83] It is important that the patient never be allowed to resort to household products for use with his lenses.[84] These products can cause problems for the wearer as well as damage to the lens. The psychological effect of permitting the patient to experiment with these various items leads to poor control of the patient as well as carelessness and sloppiness in handling the lens. Patients must understand the following points:

1. When the lens is removed from the cornea, it will be covered with ocular secretions of oil, mucus, crystalline deposits, etc.

2. These contaminants must be removed prior to lens storage.

3. It is not sufficient to clean the lens by rinsing with water, for not only do the deposits adhere tenaciously to the surface but also oil and mucus are not soluble in water and, therefore, are not adequately removed by rinsing or by storage in the soaking solution.

4. In order to solubilize these films and deposits to permit their removal, a detergent must be used.

5. Household detergents often leave a film on the lens surfaces and in many instances are damaging to the eye.

6. Wetting solutions cannot be expected to contain adequate detergent activity, for they must adhere to the lens surfaces for mechanical cushioning effect and, therefore, would be too irritating with a high detergent content.

7. A separate cleaning solution must be used daily in addition to soaking or wetting solutions.[85]

8. Patients should clean the lens by applying three or four drops of a cleaning solution or a small dab of gel cleaner (Figure 12.12) and by rubbing the lens between thumb and forefinger or in the palm of the hand for approximately ten seconds; then he should thoroughly rinse the lens in lukewarm water. The patient should then hold the lens by the edge between the thumb and forefinger and examine to determine cleanliness. If the lens does not appear clean, the procedure should be repeated until a properly clean lens is obtained. Cleaning in this manner helps materially to remove contamination from the patient's fingers, thereby avoiding transference of the finger contaminants to the soaking solution. Lutes recommends the use of a cotton swab for cleaning the lens.[86]

Various contact lens cleaning solutions are available for use in the office by the fitter. Ordinary benzine (*not* benzene) is an effective solvent for this purpose; it is harmless to plastic and leaves virtually no residual film. Fine abrasives such as calamine lotion and some silver polishes can be rubbed on the lenses without scratching. Kerosene and lighter fluid should not be used. Alcohol should never be used because it damages the surfaces of some types of plastic lenses. Acetone will dissolve the lenses.

Various cleaning devices are available to eliminate the need for lens cleaning with the fingers.[87-90]

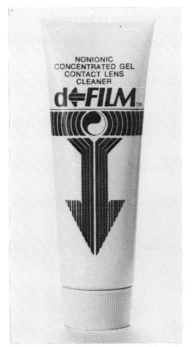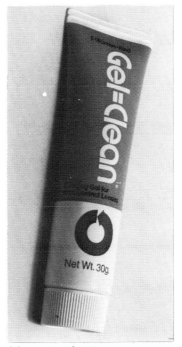

Figure 12.12. Cleaning gel for contact lenses.

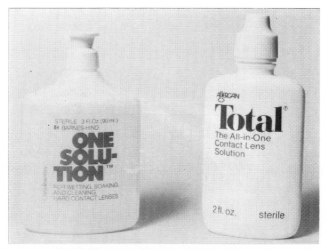

Figure 12.13. Combination solutions.

COMBINATION SOLUTIONS

Various combinations of wetting, soaking, and cleaning solutions are available as all purpose solutions. In some cases all three of these functions are combined whereas in others only the soaking and cleaning functions are combined (Figure 12.13).

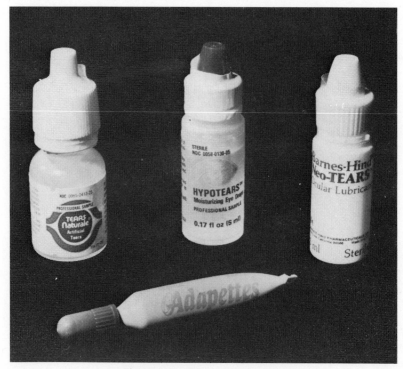

Figure 12.14. Ocular lubricants.

ACCESSORY SOLUTIONS

OCULAR LUBRICANTS

Many contact lens wearers with excellent fits experience some discomfort after several hours of wearing their lenses. The causes may vary from personal idiosyncrasies and heightened touch perception levels to inadequate tear formation.

To overcome this problem, many patients remove their contacts temporarily and instill an ocular lubricant (Figure 12.14). Others go through the complete rewetting cycle again.

Some fitters recommend that patients instill a solution that cleans the ocular surfaces and rewets the contact lens without removing the lens from the eye (Figure 12.15).

INSERTION SOLUTION

Some solutions are formulated to reduce lens sensation upon insertion. They usually have higher viscosity than wetting solution.

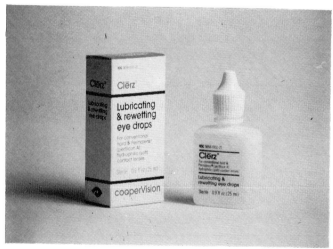

Figure 12.15. Lubricating and rewetting eye drop. Courtesy of Cooper Laboratories, Inc.

REFERENCES

1. Krezanoski, J. Z., Hind, H. W., and Szekely, I. J.: Pharmaceutical aspects of contact lenses and their solutions, *J. Am. Pharm. Assoc.*, NS2(7):417–422, 438, 1962.
2. Rankin, R.: Suggested considerations for contact lens solutions, *Contacto*, 6(5):137, 1962.
3. Richard, J. P.: Antibacterial properties of contact lens wetting and storage solutions, *Br. J. Physiol. Opt.*, 21(3):147–156, 1964.
4. Rankin, R.: Method for evaluation of contact lens solution effect on cornea and conjunctiva, *Contacto*, 9(2):9, 1965.
5. Dabezies, O. H.: Contact lenses and their solutions: a review of basic principles—

Part 1, *Eye, Ear, Nose and Throat Mon.*, 45(1):39–44, 1966.

6. Dabezies, O. H.: Contact lenses and their solutions: a review of basic principles— Part 2, *Eye, Ear, Nose and Throat Mon.*, 45(2):68–72, 1966.

7. Dabezies, O. H.: Contact lenses and their solutions: a review of basic principles— Part 3, *Eye, Ear, Nose and Throat Mon.*, 45(3):82–84, 1966.

8. Dabezies, O. H.: Contact lenses and their solutions: a review of basic principles, *J. La. State Med. Soc.*, 119.

9. Blaug, S. M.: Contact lenses and their solutions, *J. Am. Pharm. Assoc.*, NS31(1):74–80, 1967.

10. Phillips, A. J.: Contact lens plastics, solutions, and storage—some implications—Part 1, *The Ophthalmic Optician*, 8(19):1058, 1075–1076, 1968.

11. Phillips, A. J.: Contact lens plastics, solutions, and storage—some implications—Part 2, *The Ophthalmic Optician*, 8(20):1134–1136, 1143, 1968.

12. Phillips, A. J.: Contact lens plastics, solutions, and storage—some implications—Part 3, *The Ophthalmic Optician*, 8(21):1190–1192, 1203–1205, 1968.

13. Phillips, A. J.: Contact lens plastics, solutions, and storage—some implications—Part 4, *The Ophthalmic Optician*, 8(22):1234–1238, 1968.

14. Phillips, A. J.: Contact lens plastics, solutions, and storage—some implications—Part 5, *The Ophthalmic Optician*, 8(23):1312–1315, 1968.

15. Phillips, A. J.: Contact lens plastics, solutions, and storage—some implications—Part 6, *The Ophthalmic Optician*, 8(25):1405–1408, 1413, 1968.

16. Krezanoski, J. Z., and Petricciani, J. C.: Simplifying contact lens care, *Contacto*, 13(1): 48–50, 1969.

17. Krezanoski, J. Z., and Petricciani, J. C.: Changing concepts on patient contact lens care, *Eye, Ear, Nose and Throat Mon.*, 48(8): 459–464, 1969.

18. Rankin, F.: Contact lens solutions: a pharmacist's approach, *Optom. Weekly*, 1961.

19. Szekely, I. J.: The eye, the contact lens, and the contact lens solution: the role of

adjunctive preparation in contact lens practice and wear, in *Transactions of the International Ophthalmologic and Optometry Congress*, London, Lockwood, 1962, pp. 136–147.

20. Player, H. S.: Solutions used in contact lens practice management, *Second AOA Cont. Lens Symposium*, 44–54, 1965.

21. Pigeon, R. J.: The patient's dilemma about contact lens solutions, *South J. Optom.*, 13(9):3, 12, 1971.

22. Krezanoski, J. Z.: What is wetting, *Contacto*, 7(4):20–22, 1963.

23. Krishna, N., and Brow, F.: Polyvinyl alcohol as an ophthalmic vehicle; effect on regeneration of corneal epithelium, *Am. J. Ophthalmol.*, 57(1):99–106, 1964.

24. Krishna, N., and Mitchell, B.: Polyvinyl alcohol as an ophthalmic vehicle; effect on ocular structure, *Am. J. Ophthalmol.*, 59(5): 860–864, 1965.

25. Rucker, I. et al.: A safety test for contact lens wetting solutions, *Ann. Ophthalmol.*, 1972.

26. Klein, M., Millwood, E. G., and Walther, W. W.: On the maintenance of sterility in eye drops, *J. Pharm. Pharmacol.*, 6:725, 1954.

27. Newton, N. L., and Garner, H.: Contact lens and storage, *Eye, Ear, Nose and Throat Mon.*, 45(8):59–62, 1966.

28. Hind, H. W., and Goyan, F. M.: A new concept of the role of hydrogen ion concentration and buffer systems in the preparation of ophthalmic solutions, *J. Am. Pharm. Assoc.*, 36:33–41, 1947.

29. Gould, H. L., and Inglima, R.: Corneal contact lens solutions, *Eye, Ear, Nose and Throat Mon.*, 43(4):39–49, 1964.

30. Adler, I. N., Wlodyga, R. J., and Rope, S. J.: The effects of pH on contact lens wearing, *J. Am. Optom. Assoc.*, 39(11):1000–1001, 1968.

31. Panel discussion: Effects of pH on contact lens wearing, *J. Am. Optom. Assoc.*, 40(7): 719–722, 1969.

32. Hill, R. M., and Young, W. H.: Ophthalmic solutions, *J. Am. Optom. Assoc.*, 44(3):263–270, 1973.

33. Ostrolenk, M. et al.: Numbers of bacteria removed from the mouth as measured by rinse method, *J. Am. Pharm Assoc.*, 41: 89–93, 1952.

34. Hind, H. W., and Szekely, I. J.: Wetting and hydration of contact lenses, *Contacto*, *3(3)*: 65–68, 1959.

35. Szekely, I. J.: The eye, the contact lens, and the contact lens solutions, *Contacto*, *6(12)*: 347, 1962.

36. Kokoski, C. S., and Schwartz, S. M.: A study of the effects of various soaking solutions on the wettability of plastic lens surfaces, *Contacto*, *7*:15–21, 1963.

37. Favero, M. S. et al.: *Pseudomonas aerugenosa*: growth in distilled water from hospitals, *Science*, *173(3999)*:836–838, 1971.

38. Bailey, N. J.: Contact lenses must be kept wet, *J. Am. Optom. Assoc.*, *31(12)*:985, 1960.

39. Szekely, I. J., Riegelman, S., and Petricciani, J. C.: World contact lens St. Comm. report—Part 3, Ophthalmic microbial hazards, antimicrobial agents, and use of contact lens solutions, *Contacto*, 1959.

40. Bitonte, J. L., Kopetansky, F., and Suie, T.: Bacteriological studies, *Contacto*, *9(1)*:6, 1965.

41. Bixler, D. P.: Bacterial decontamination and cleaning of contact lenses, *Am. J. Ophthalmol.*, *62(2)*:324–329, 1966.

42. Szekely, I. S., and Krezanoski, J. Z.: Hygienic contact lens care and patient comfort, *Am. J. Optom.*, *37(11)*:572–579, 1960.

43. Bixler, D. P.: Bacterial testing of contact lens solution, *Am. J. Ophthalmol.*, *65(1)*:122, 1968.

44. Allen, J. H.: Staphylococci ocular inflamation, *Lancet*, *62*:20–21, 1942.

45. Dixon, J. M., Lawaczeck, E., and Winkler, C. H., Jr.: Pseudomonas contamination of contact lens containers: preliminary report, *Am. J. Ophthalmol.*, *54(3)*:461, 1962.

46. Theodore, F. H.: Microbiology in relation to contact lenses, *Eye, Ear, Nose and Throat Mon.*, *46(3)*:354, 383, 1967.

47. Kohn, S. R., Gershinfield, L., and Barr, M.: Effectiveness of antibacterial agents presently employed in ophthalmic preparations as preservatives against *Pseudomonas aeruginosa*, *J. Pharm. Sci.*, *52(10)*:967–974, 1963.

48. A new medium for study of quarternary bactericides, *Soap and Sanitary Chemicals*, *23*: 119–122, 1947.

49. Lawrence, C. A.: Inactivation of the germicidal action of quarternary ammonium compounds, *J. Am. Pharm. Assoc.*, *37*:57–61, 1948.

50. Lawrence, C. A.: Quaternary ammonium compounds, in Reddish, G. R. (Ed.): *Antiseptics, Disinfectants, Fungicides, and Sterilization*, 2nd ed., Philadelphia, Lea and Febiger, p. 581.

51. Black, L. A.: Factors to be considered in testing quaternary ammonium compounds, *J. Milk-Food Tech.*, *12(4)*:224–229, 1949.

52. Riegelman, S., Vaughn, D. G. and Okumoto, M.: Antibacterial agents in *Pseudomonas aeruginosa* contaminated ophthalmic solutions, *J. Am. Pharm. Assoc.*, *45*:93, 1956.

53. MacGregor, D. R., and Elliker, P. R.: A comparison of some properties of strains of *Pseudomonas aeruginosa* sensitive and resistant to quaternary ammonium compounds, *Can. J. Microbiol.*, *4*:449–503, 1958.

54. Dabezies, O. H. et al.: Evaluation of a stronger concentration of preservative (benzalkonium chloride) in contact lens soaking solution, *Eye, Ear, Nose and Throat Mon.*, *45*:78, 1966.

55. Swan, K. C.: Reactivity of the ocular tissues to wetting agents, *Am. J. Ophthalmol.*, *27*:118, 1944.

56. Myers, G. E., and Lefebure, C.: Antibacterial activity of benzalkonium chloride in the presence of cotton and nylon fibers, *Can. Pharm. J.*, *94(7)*:55–57, 1961.

57. Lee, J. C., and Fialkow, P. J.: Benzalkonium chloride—source of hospital infection with gram negative bacteria, *J.A.M.A.*, *177*:144, 1961.

58. Krishna, N.: Wet storage of contact lenses; disposable soaking solution capsules and semidisposable lens cases, *Am. J. Ophthalmol.*, *61(6)*:1538–1541, 1966.

59. Lawrence, C. A.: An evaluation of chemical preservatives for ophthalmic solutions, *J. Am. Pharm. Assoc., Sci. Ed.*, *44*:457, 1955.

60. Eriksen, S. et al.: Suitability of thimerisol as a preservative in soft lens soaking solutions, in Bitonte, J. L., and Keates, R. H. (Eds.): *Symposium on The Flexible Lens*, St. Louis, Mosby, 1972.

61. Krezanoski, J. Z.: Contact lens products, *J. Am. Pharm. Assoc.*, *NS10(1)*:13–18, 1970.

62. Vodnoy, B. E.: Contact lens cleanliness and proper patient control—a grave responsi-

bility, *Optom. Weekly,* 56(27):23–31, 1965.

63. Jimison, R. E.: Compatibility of contact lens solutions, *Opt. J. Rev. Optom.,* 102(11):46–51, 1965.

64. Allen, H. F.: To wet or not to wet (editorials), *Arch. Ophthalmol.,* 67(2):119–120, 1962.

65. Kapetansky, F. M. et al.: Bacteriologic studies of patients who wear contact lenses, *Am. J. Ophthalmol.,* 57(2):255–258, 1964.

66. Obear, M. F., and Winter, F. C.: Bacteriologic culture of wet and dry contact lens storage cases, *Am. J. Ophthalmol.,* 57(3):441–443, 1964.

67. Winkler, C. H., and Dixon, J. M.: Bacteriology of the eye: IIIA. Effect of contact lenses on the normal flora; B. Flora of the contact lens case, *Arch. Ophthalmol.,* 72(6):817–819, 1964.

68. Rubin, M. L.: Optics and visual physiology, *Arch. Ophthalmol.,* 73(6):863–889, 1965.

69. Clifton, C. E., and Hall, N. C.: Re-sterilizing activity of certain contact lens solutions, *Contacto,* 3(10):301–302, 1959.

70. Gould, H. L.: Rationale in the use of contact lens solutions, *Eye, Ear, Nose and Throat Mon.,* 41:359–360, 1962.

71. Szekely, I. J., and Riegelman, S.: Corneal lens storage: a critical appraisal, *Br. J. Physiol. Opt.,* 21(4):239–249, 1964.

72. Dabezies, O. H.: Wet vs dry storage of corneal contact lenses: a statistical evaluation, *Am. J. Ophthalmol.,* 54(4):684–696, 1965.

73. Magoon, R. C., and Sexton, R.: Wet or dry contact lens storage, *Arch. Ophthalmol.,* 77(2):197–199, 1967.

74. Magoon, R. C., and Sexton, R.: Contact lens storage, *Modern Medicine,* 35(10):140, 1967.

75. Bettman, J. W.: Contact lens storage, wet or dry? A bacterial analysis, *Am. J. Ophthalmol.,* 56(1):77–84, 1963.

76. Krezanoski, J., and Lowry, J. B.: Accessory contact lens cases and devices: a critical review, in press.

77. Salvatori, P.: The effect of hydration upon corneal radius, *J. Am. Optom. Assoc.,* 32(8):644, 1961.

78. Neill, J. C., and Hanna, J. J.: A study of the effect of various media on the radii of micro-corneal contact lenses, *Contacto,* 7(9):10–13, 1963.

79. Lutes, R.: The importance of the storage case for contact lenses, *Optom. Weekly,* 56(35):33–34, 1965.

80. Sarver, M. D.: Minimizing contact lens contamination in the office, *Optom. Weekly,* 59(8):19–20, 1968.

81. Jia-Ruey, L., Silverman, H. I., and Korb, D. R.: Studies on cleaning solutions for contact lenses, *J. Am. Optom. Assoc.,* 40(11):1106–1115, 1969.

82. Lewis, E.: A new method of cleaning contact lenses, *Eye, Ear, Nose and Throat Mon.,* 45(6):43–46, 1966.

83. Baldone, J. A.: Contact lens cleaning: updated, *Contact Lens Med. Bull.,* 4(2):9–12, 1971.

84. Burns, C. A. et al.: Polident as a contact lens cleaning solution, *Am. J. Ophthalmol.,* 65(2):251, 1968.

85. Stager, D. R., Keates, R. H., and Kapetansky, F. M.: Contamination of contact lenses, *Am. J. Ophthalmol.,* 63(1):144–145, 1967.

86. Lutes, H. R.: Care and handling of contact lenses, *Optom. World,* 556(11):6–10, 1968.

87. Krezanoski, J. Z.: New concepts in contact lens cleaning, *N. Engl. J. Optom.,* 15(7), 1964.

88. Hamner, M. E., and Kirkendol, P. L.: A tracer method for determining the cleaning of contact lenses, *Eye, Ear, Nose and Throat Mon.,* 44(5):50–52, 1965.

89. Elstrom, G. P.: What's new—Hydra-mat®, *J. Am. Optom. Assoc.,* 36(5):483, 1965.

90. Hamner, M. E.: Evaluation of a new method for cleaning contact lenses, *Eye, Ear, Nose and Throat Mon.,* 45(4):62–64, 1966.

ADDITIONAL READINGS

Allen, J. H.: Who's afraid of the little green bug, *Cont. Lens Med. Bull.,* 5(1):2–14, 1972.

Applegate, R. A.: Contact lens surface damage related to cases and case removal techniques,

Am. J. Optom. Physiol. Opt., 53(6):305–313, 1976.

Ayotte, R. G.: The how, where and why of storage solutions, *Cont. Lens J.,* 12(4):13, 1979.

Benedetto, D. A., Shah, D. O., and Kaufman, H. E.:

The dynamic film thickness of cushioning agents on contact lens materials, *Ann. Ophthalmol.,* *10*(*4*):437, 1978.

Brigden, B.: A practical approach to the production of contact lens solutions in line with the requirements of the D.H.S.S.: *Cont. Lens J.,* *7*(*4*):25, 1978.

Boyd, J. R.: Real answers to the problems of artificial tears, *Cont. Lens Forum,* *1*(*4*):34–37, 1976.

Bulle, K., and MacKeen, G. D.: Buffers and preservatives in contact lens solutions, *Contacto,* *21*(*6*):33, 1977.

Bulle, K. B.: Solutions and the service life of lenses, *Contacto,* *22*(*1*):23, 1978.

Cason, L., and Winkler, C. H.: Bacteriology of the eye, I. Normal flora, *Arch. Ophthalmol.,* *51*(*2*): 196–199, 1954.

Cureton, G. L. et al.: Development and performance of a triple purpose contact lens solution, *J. Am. Optom. Assoc.,* *46*(*3*):259–267, 1975.

Dabezies, O. H., and Naugle, T.: A new technique of contact lens storage, soaking, and cleaning, *Eye, Ear, Nose, and Throat Mon.,* *50*(*10*):27–34, 1971.

Dickinson, F.: Contact lens containers, *The Optician,* *173*(*4466*):21–25, 1977.

Duncan, A. J.: Some preservatives in eyedrop preparations hasten the formation of dry spots in the rabbit cornea, *Proc. B.P.S.,* p. 359, 17–19 Dec., 1975.

Gasson, A.: Aspects of hard lens aftercare, *Cont. Lens J.,* *8*(*6*):4, 1979.

Gesser, H. D.: The wettability of contact lenses by hydroxyl free radicals, *J. Am. Optom. Assoc.,* *38*(*3*):191, 1967.

Gesser, H. D., Funt, B. L., and Warriner, R. E.: A method of improving the wettability of contact lenses by free radical treatment, *Am. J. Optom. Arch. Am. Acad. Optom.,* *42*:321–324, 1965.

Gold, R. M.: Reducing failure in cold disinfection systems, *Cont. Lens Forum,* *4*(*12*):57, 1979.

Goodlaw, E.: Contact lens solutions, *J. Am. Optom. Assoc.,* *47*(*3*):367, 1976.

Gourley, D. R.: Contact lenses, contact lens solutions and the eye, *U.S. Pharm.,* *2*(*2*):40, 1977.

Hall, N. C.: Antimicrobial synergism in a contact lens soaking solution, *N. Engl. J. Optom.,* *14*(*9*): 229–233, 1963.

Hardberger, R., Hanna, C., and Boyd, C. M.: Effects of drug vehicles on ocular contact time, *Arch. Ophthalmol.,* *93*(*1*):42–45, 1975.

Hill, R. M.: How wet are your patient's tears?, *Int. Cont. Lens Clin.,* *4*(*6*):46, 1977.

Hill, R. M.: Aging ophthalmic solutions, *Int. Cont. Lens Clin.,* *5*(*3*):51, 1978.

Hill, R. M., and Terry, J. E.: Viscosity: the "staying power" of ophthalmic solutions, *J. Am. Optom. Assoc.,* *46*(*3*):239–241, 1975.

Hind, H. W.: Contact lens solutions: questions and answers, *The Optician,* *169*(*4381*):27–30, 1975.

Hind, H. W.: Aspects of contact lens solutions, *The Optician,* *169*(*4380*):13–29, 1975.

Holden, B.: Contact lens care and maintenance—2 "soaking" solutions, *Austr. J. Optom.,* *56*(*6*):219–233, 1973.

Houston, J. C.: Effect of various solvents on five contact lens plastics, *Cont. Lens J.,* *12*(*2*):18, 1978.

Koetting, R. A.: Interpreting corneal contact lens base curve changes, *Opt. Weekly,* pp. 9–12, Dec. 29, 1966.

Kokoski, C. S., and Schwartz, S. M.: A study of the effects of various soaking solutions on the wettability of plastic lens surfaces, *Contacto,* *7*(*5*):15–21, 1963.

Kurz, G. H.: Contact lens remover adherent to cornea, *Am. J. Ophthalmol.,* *82*(*2*):317–318, 1976.

Norton, D. A. et al.: The antimicrobial efficiencies of contact lens solutions, *The Optician,* *168* (*4360*):14–21, 1974.

Chapter 13

INSPECTION AND VERIFICATION

A LTHOUGH STANDARDS in the manufacture of contact lenses have greatly improved during the last decade, many lenses do not fulfill the specifications of the order sent to the laboratory. Practitioners are often too willing to accept the manufacturer's assurance of good quality and correct physical characteristics of contact lenses that should be rejected.[1]

RESPONSIBILITY OF PRACTITIONER

Much of the reason for poor quality in the manufacture of contact lenses is due to laxity on the part of the practitioner, who very often has not taken the trouble to learn how to evaluate the quality of lenses and who often accepts lenses that should be rejected. The practitioner has found from experience that the standards and quality of spectacle lenses are very high. He assumes that contact lenses will have even higher standards. Unfortunately, only a few contact lens laboratories have succeeded in maintaining a quality control that can compete with spectacle lens standards. Since the fitter has often not been able to differentiate between good and poor lenses, there has been little reason for the laboratories to concentrate on producing quality products. It costs considerably more to produce a high quality lens than a poor quality lens.

The inability to evaluate a lens adequately has been the cause of considerable frustration to the practitioner during the fitting of contact lenses. A large variety of symptoms can be attributed to faulty lens construction. These symptoms are not always easily differentiated from those which are due to an improper fit. Undoubtedly, many unnecessary lens modifications could have been prevented if only a proper lens inspection had been made.

FAIRNESS TO LABORATORY

Although it is mandatory that only high quality lenses be accepted from laboratories, the fitter also has a responsibility not to make outrageous demands for his lenses. Certain lens dimensions can be measured to an accuracy that is greater than is necessary to be clinically significant. For example, it is possible to measure the lens thickness to an accuracy of 0.01 mm. It is doubtful if a variation of 0.02 mm. in thickness will have any material effect on the fit of the lens. A lens that fails to meet its thickness specification by 0.02 mm. is therefore acceptable. Standards for lens quality should be based upon a clinical evaluation of the variation that will cause a significant change in the manner in

342

which the lens fits, reasonable product control in manufacturing, and the limitations of verification procedures.[2] These standards should not simply reflect how well each particular dimension can be measured.

INSPECTION ROUTINE

Twelve variables and characteristics must be inspected or verified:

1. Total diameter
2. Optical zone diameter
3. Peripheral curve width
4. Blend
5. Base curve
6. Peripheral curve radius
7. Power
8. Center thickness
9. Edge
10. Surface quality
11. Optical quality
12. Color

Many of the lens dimensions may be verified by using equipment that is already available in the practitioner's office. Other dimensions must be checked by using equipment specifically designed for this purpose.

Care should be taken to record the specifications of the lens received from the laboratory accurately. The record form should have a space below each lens variable to indicate any discrepancy between lens dimensions that are ordered and those which are received (*see* Figure 4.6). If there is then a need to duplicate the lens at a later date, it can be based on the actual specifications of the lens that was worn by the patient. Numerous problems occur after a lens has been lost and replaced because the original lens did not comply with the actual specifications that were ordered. Often the lens is given to the patient anyway. It is worn comfortably, and no substitute lens is ordered. Later, if the lens is lost and a second lens is ordered from the original specifications, the lenses may vary enough to cause a difference in the fit.

Proper recording will also insure that all characteristics of the lens have been checked.

TOTAL DIAMETER

Measuring Magnifier

The total diameter is most easily verified with a measuring magnifier, which has the advantage that other lens dimensions can also be measured with the same device. A measuring magnifier simply consists of a graticule or scale against which the lens is held so that both the lens and scale can be viewed through a plus lens, which provides magnification (Figure 13.1). The contact lens is held by the index finger, with its concave surface directly against the scale and moved until the edge is aligned with the zero position. The diameter can then be read directly from the scale. The contact lens should be rotated and measured in various meridians to check for roundness; occasionally a lens will not be cut properly and will have a slightly oval shape. Some caution should be taken so that the contact lens is perfectly dry when it is measured, since a wet lens will have a miniscus formed at the edge and will give a reading that is too large.

Alternate Methods to Measure Total Diameter

A V-channel gauge, which is designed specifically for use with contact lenses, provides a very rapid method for measuring total diameter. It consists of a V-shaped groove, which has been cut into a plastic or metal bar and

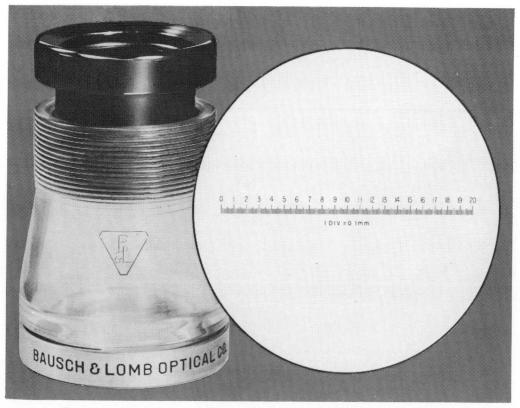

Figure 13.1. Measuring magnifier and scale. Courtesy of Bausch and Lomb, Inc.

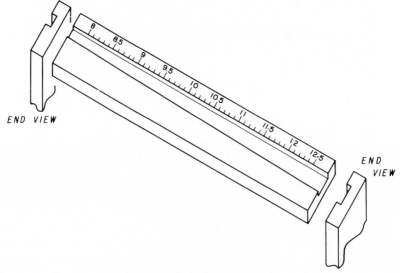

Figure 13.2. V-channel gauge.

into which the lens is placed, concave side down, and allowed to slide by its own weight and gravity until it is stopped by the sides of the groove (Figure 13.2). The diameter is read from a scale on the edge of the groove at the point where the lens touches the side. The lens must be dry, and the gauge must be clean for best results; otherwise, the lens will be restricted from moving as it should, and the reading will be too large. Care must be taken that the lens is not forced into the gauge. In such a case, the lens may warp and cause a reading that is too small. If the gauge is made from metal, there is also danger of scratching the edge of the lens. The test should be repeated with the lens rotated in different positions to check for roundness.

V-channel gauges are occasionally inaccurate. They may be checked with precision diameter buttons, which are manufactured for this purpose.[3]

Other possible methods to check total diameter include the use of a "go or no-go gauge" and alternately a projection magnifier, but these are infrequently used for this measurement. Another type of gauge is needed for lenses that are mounted on modification equipment and which cannot be conveniently removed. This gauge is made by cutting a series of open rectangular slots of varying widths in the sides of a bar of metal or plastic so that the bar can be slipped over the lens while it is in place on the mounting.[4]

Since the total diameter is the sum of the optical zone diameter and the width of the peripheral curve(s), it is axiomatic that a lens having an incorrect diameter must also have an error in the width of one or more of its zones.

Tolerance for Total Diameter

A tolerance of less than ±0.05 mm. from the size ordered is adequate for the total diameter.[5] Most laboratories have little difficulty in producing lenses that are within 0.05 mm. of the requested diameter, and few lenses need be rejected for an inaccuracy of this dimension. Some laboratories purposely send lenses that are slightly larger than the diameter requested and point out that the size can be reduced if necessary but can never be made larger. Although this is true, the decision as to whether an allowance is necessary should be made by the fitter, not the laboratory, and the requested dimensions should be demanded.

OPTICAL ZONE DIAMETER

Measuring Magnifier

Optical zone diameter can most easily be verified by means of the measuring magnifier and is conveniently checked immediately following the measurement of the total diameter. It is much more difficult to determine the limits of the optical zone than it is to measure the total diameter of the lens when viewing with the measuring magnifier. Proper lighting becomes a necessity. The lens should be viewed with the magnifier directed toward a background of variable brightness such as the edge of a fluorescent lamp or a window. The magnifier can then be moved back and forth slightly until the variation in lighting is found that makes the transition at the limit of the optical zone most visible (Figure 13.3).

Measurement of the optical zone diameter is much more difficult if the lens has a very wide blend. Sometimes an attempt is made to estimate the central point of the blend and call this the limit of the optical zone. For practical purposes, however, the diameter of the optical zone includes only that area which has good optical characteristics and which is undistorted by a blend. The author prefers to include any appreciable blend width as a part of the width of the

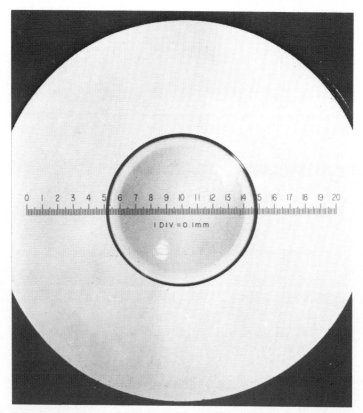

0 I 2 3 4 5 6 7 8 9 10 II 12 13 14 15 16 17 18 19 20

I DIV = 0 I mm

Figure 13.3. Appearance of zones of bicurve lens when viewed through a measuring magnifier. Courtesy of Bausch and Lomb, Inc.

peripheral curve.

Alternate Methods to Measure Optical Zone Diameter

A projection magnifier may also be used to determine optical zone diameter (Figure 13.4), but it is a much more expensive instrument than a measuring magnifier. The projection magnifier offers the advantage that it may also be used for inspection of the edge.

Tolerance for Optical Zone Diameter

Optical zone diameter should be within ±0.1 mm. of the value ordered.* The blend should not be so heavy that the optical zone

---

*If there is a complete blend, it becomes difficult to be accurate within 0.4 mm.

diameter cannot be measured. It is especially important that the optical zone not be too small, since when the lens is worn it may cause subjective sensations from stray light refracted by the peripheral curve. This error cannot be rectified because the optical zone size cannot be increased (on the same lens) once the lens has been ground.

Recommendations

From the results of an experimental study and clinical experience, it is apparent that there is considerable variability in the ability to measure the optic zone diameter. This ability depends mainly upon the type of blend used between the optic zone and the second curve. Lenses with no blends give the highest accuracy (two standard deviations equal about

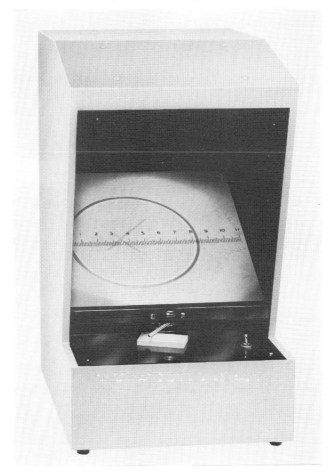

Figure 13.4. Projection magnifier. Courtesy of Plastic Contact Lens Co.

0.2 mm.), whereas lenses with heavy blends give the lowest accuracy (two standard deviations equal about 0.5 mm.). Since there are differences in the preference of blend type by various practitioners and there is no experimental evidence to indicate a superiority of a specific blend type, it is recommended that the optic zone diameter accuracy be related to the blend ordered.

Blend	Optic Zone Diameter Accuracy
None	±0.1 mm
Light (0.1 wide)	±0.2 mm
Medium (0.3 wide)	±0.3 mm
Heavy (0.5 wide)	±0.4 mm

PERIPHERAL CURVE WIDTH

Measuring Magnifier

The width of the peripheral curve may also be verified by means of the measuring magnifier. Like the optical zone diameter, it is much more easily measured when there is no blend. If a blend is present, the peripheral curve width is usually measured from the outer border of the optical zone to the edge of the lens.

As an alternative to measuring the peripheral curve width directly, a simple calculation may be made from the values found for the optical zone diameter and the total diameter. The optical zone diameter is subtracted from the total diameter, and the remainder divided by two to give the width of the peripheral curve. This calculation has the advantage that the sum of the widths of the zones will automatically equal the total diameter. When each zone is measured separately, it often happens that the total diameter does not appear to equal the sum of its zones. This discrepancy is usually caused by the difficulty of selecting the transition points of the zones when they have been blurred by blending. If more than one peripheral curve is present, the widths of all peripheral curves must then be measured separately. Care should be taken that the sum of the widths of all the zones is equal to the total diameter.

Tolerance for Peripheral Curve Width

The ability to measure the peripheral curve(s) width depends upon the type of blend used between its adjacent curves. It is recommended that the peripheral curve width accuracy be related to the blend ordered.

Blend	Peripheral Curve Width Accuracy
None	±0.1 mm
Light	±0.2 mm
Medium	±0.3 mm
Heavy	±0.4 mm

BLEND

Blends are commonly designated as light, medium, or heavy.[6] Exact measurement of the blend width is not possible, but it can usually be estimated with a fair degree of accuracy.[7] When viewed through the measuring magnifier, the blend appears as a zone of brightness, or dullness, depending upon whether the background is light or dark, and the optics appear irregular. Its visibility is enhanced by moving the measuring magnifier back and forth slightly to vary the brightness of the background.

Since the blend is not usually a true curve, there is no method by which its radius can be verified. The specification of the tool used to produce the blend may be given by the laboratory, but there is no way to verify if this is correct. In any case, it is doubtful whether the exact radius of the tool is of material importance, since it is not touched to the lens long enough to actually impart its radius.

The width of the blend should be less than 0.2 mm. for a touch blend and within 0.2 mm. of the specified value for a heavy blend. Considerable caution should be taken that the blend is not too wide. The most serious problem caused by excessively heavy blends occurs when the blend between the optical zone and peripheral curve is so wide that it effectively reduces the diameter of the optical zone. Such a blend may cause optical distortion. It may also cause stray light and other optical disturbances.

It should be remembered that heavy blending makes it possible for the laboratory to compensate for an error in making an optical zone of incorrect diameter.

OPTICAL ZONE RADIUS (BASE CURVE)

Various instruments can be used to measure the radius of the optical zone.[8-22]

Keratometer

Although the keratometer was originally designed for use in measuring the radius of the cornea, which is of convex curvature, it may be used equally well for measuring the radius of a concave surface, such as the optical zone of a contact lens. The measurement of optical zone radius requires that an appropriate holder be attached to the keratometer to support the lens.

Some holders are designed to position the lens so that it is perpendicular to the optic axis of the instrument (Figure 13.5). The lens must be attached to a depression in the holder with some adhesive substance, such as toothpaste, clay, or one of various creams. Care must be taken in mounting the lens, as there is considerable likelihood that the pressure on the lens may cause warping and distortion of its surface. In one of the better holders, the lens is held in position only by water.[23]

A favored holder for measuring the optical zone radius with the keratometer allows the lens to be placed with its surfaces horizontal, while the keratometer remains in its normal position.[24,25] A front surface mirror, which is oriented at a 45° angle to the optic axis of the keratometer, reflects light from the mires to the contact lens (Figure 13.6). For optical purposes, the lens is the same as if it were placed in front of the keratometer (Figure 13.7). By allowing the lens to lie flat, no adhesive substance is needed, and distortion ceases to be a problem. The section of the holder upon which the lens rests has a depression that can be filled with fluid. With the lens in place, the fluid is in contact with the convex surface of the lens. Since the refractive index of the fluid is very near to the index of the lens, it tends to cancel the reflective property of the convex surface. Hence, light from the mires is imaged by only the posterior surface of the lens. Various fluids can be used to fill the space. It has sometimes been recommended that glycerine is best, since its refractive index (1.47) is so near to that of plastic (1.49), but it has been found that water or wetting solution works equally well.

Before the lens is placed on the holder, it should be cleaned and dried carefully. If any fluid remains on the optical zone of the lens or if fluid is accidentally spilled on the lens during mounting, it will cause a distortion of the mire images, and a reading will not be possible. If there is not enough fluid in the holder, the front surface of the lens will reflect light, and the mire image will appear doubled.

Conversion

Values for keratometer measurements actually represent radius values but are given on the instrument in terms of diopters of refracting power, based on a refractive index for tears of 1.3375. Since a radius value is desired for the base curve, the power reading must be converted to its corresponding radius by using tables (Appendix 1) based upon this index.

Since the keratometer is usually calibrated for a convex surface, some error will be present on a purely optical basis when a concave surface is measured. Conversion tables designed to correct for this error are available (Appendix 5). For example, if the keratometer reading for a concave surface is 42.00 D. the radius of the surface will be 8.07 mm.

Warpage

A lens that is warped shows surface distortions which give the optical zone an appearance of regular or irregular toricity. A lens can be checked for warpage by measuring the optical zone radius in more than one meridian. This may be done with the keratometer by measuring the lens with both the horizontal and vertical power drums. If the two powers are different, indicating warpage, it must be determined first that the warpage is not caused by the lens holder. The lens should be remounted and measured again. If warpage is then verified, the lens should be rejected. A variation of ± 0.12 D. in any two meridians is cause for rejection. A lens that is warped is easily differentiated from a lens which has an astigmatic component. Warping a lens affects both surfaces equally and does not affect the total power. The lens will have its original power when measured in the

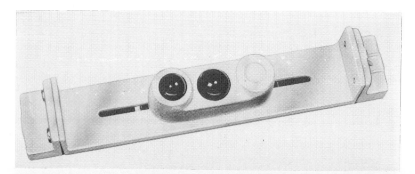

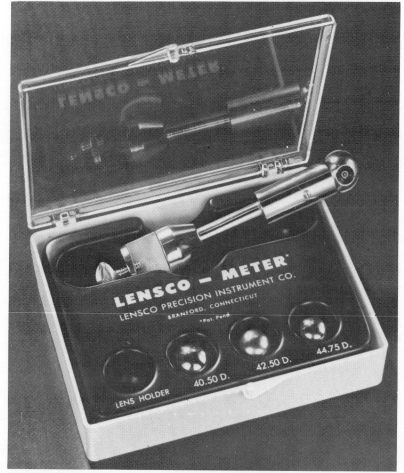

Figure 13.5. Lens holders for measuring radius of the optical zone. *Top*, courtesy of Plastic Contact Lens Co.; *bottom*, courtesy of Bausch and Lomb, Inc.

lensometer.

If the lens is lathe cut from solid heat-treated plastic, it can be placed in boiling water for one or two minutes.[26] (Hot water should not be used on a pressed or pressure-molded lens.) After heating, gradually allow the water containing the lens to become completely cooled. Some water must be in

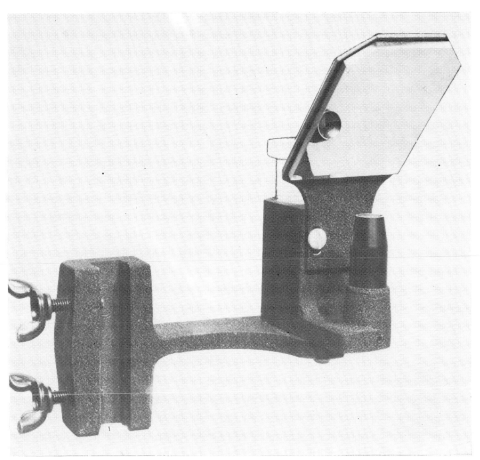

Figure 13.6a. A mirror type of lens holder for measuring the radius of the optical zone. Courtesy of Plastic Contact Lens Co.

the container with the lens until the lens is cold to support the lens. This lens should again be measured with the keratometer; in most instances, it will be found spherical. If this treatment does not produce a spherical base curve or if the lens is pressed (deformation process) or pressure molded, it should be rejected.

Alternate Methods to Measure Optical Zone Radius

Optical Spherometers

Various optical spherometers have been produced (American Optical Radiuscope[27] and The Microspherometer[28]) that are designed specifically for the measurement of optical zone radius and, if desired, front surface radius of contact lenses. The instruments are accurate and rapid and are used by many practitioners and laboratories. They have not received wider usage simply because the same measurements can be made with the keratometer, which most practitioners already have in the office. However, many practitioners find it convenient to have a separate instrument for the measurement of optical zone radius, since it is more convenient than using the keratometer for a dual purpose. The optical spherometer is described in Chapter 33.

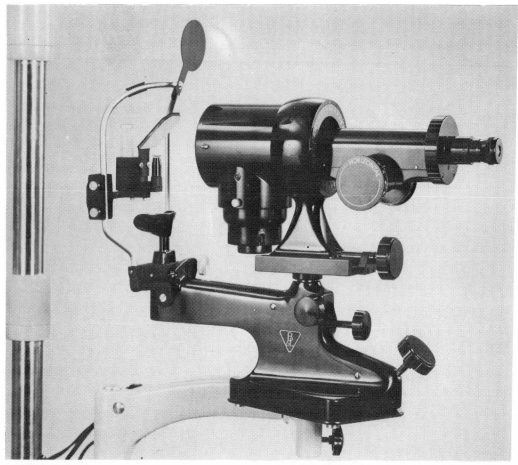

Figure 13.6b. Mirror type of lens holder mounted on a keratometer. Courtesy of Bausch and Lomb, Inc.

Mechanical Spherometers

Various mechanical spherometers are also available for use with contact lenses but are only accurate for curves at least 9 mm. in diameter (Obrig Radius Dial Gauge[29]). Templates can also be used to check large diameter curves but are somewhat inconvenient.[30] Tests such as the Newton ring principle with test spheres are theoretically possible but too impractical to merit discussion.

R-C Device

Sarver and Kerr made a device that can be used in conjunction with a lensometer to determine the optical zone radius of a contact lens.[12] This radius of curvature measuring device (R-C device) consists of a standard lens with known surface curvatures. It is mounted on the lensometer so that the front surface of the standard lens is in the plane of the lensometer lens stop. The back surface of the standard lens is wetted with a fluid having an index of 1.490. The contact lens with unknown base curve is placed against the back surface of the standard lens so that the fluid fills the space between the standard lens and the front surface of the contact lens (Figure 13.8a). Since the fluid has the same index of refraction as the contact lens, the powers of

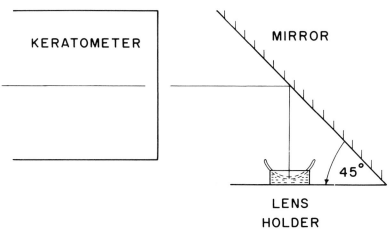

Figure 13.7. Contact lens position for measurement of optical zone radius with mirror type of lens holder.

both the front surface of the contact lens and the back surface of the standard lens are effectively cancelled (Figure 13.8b). The power of the lens system, which is read from the lensometer, will now be a function of the front surface of the standard lens, the back surface of the contact lens, and the thickness of the elements separating these two surfaces (Figure 13.8c). The front surface of the standard lens and the thickness of the system (contact lens–standard lens) are determined by the construction of the R-C device so only the optical zone radius is unknown. The optical zone radius is a function of the power measured on the lensometer and the thickness of the system and, with these dimensions known, can be found from tables.

Tolerance for Optical Zone Radius

The optical zone radius should be accurate within ± 0.025 mm. of the specified value. It is difficult to be certain of the accuracy for optical zone radius measurements within ± 0.025 mm., and great care must be taken that the instrument used is in good order. Attention to the procedures necessary to obtain maximum accuracy with these instruments cannot be overemphasized (*see* Chapter 33).

Effect of Hydration

Plastic corneal contact lenses absorb a small amount of water when kept in an aqueous environment, and this absorption is accompanied by a measurable amount of lens flattening (lengthening of the base curve radius).[32-41] When removed from the wet environment and permitted to dry out thoroughly, the lenses return to their original curvature. In practical terms, this means that a lens absorbs water from the tears as it is being worn and also from the soaking solution if stored wet when not in use. On the other hand, if stored dry overnight, the lens will go through a daily cycle of hydration and dehydration, and it will undergo all the base curve changes inherent in these processes. Since any variation in base curve can affect changes in the relationship of the lens to the corneal surface on which it is worn, it is evident that a thorough knowledge of lens behavior during wetting and drying is of value to the practitioner in helping him achieve the best possible results in fitting each patient.

All minus lenses and the lower powered plus lenses achieve a stability of base curve readings at the end of twenty-four hours of continuous wetting, whereas the higher

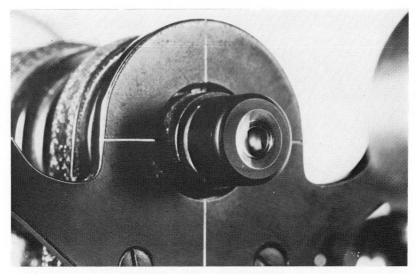

Figure 13.8a. The R-C device.

powered plus lenses require up to forty-eight hours.

Gordon ran a study in which the tested lenses were kept wet for a month and checked for any further evidences of base curve changes at the end of seventy-two hours, one week, and four weeks.[35] No significant variations in curvature were observed as compared with the values found at twenty-four hours for minus lenses and forty-eight hours for plus lenses. Therefore, for all practical purposes, these figures represent the duration of wetting required to reach a state of maximum or total hydration.

The amounts of base curve flattening observed in groups of lenses of various powers, when maximum or total hydration had been achieved, are shown in Table 13.1. The follow-

ing can be seen: (1) some flattening occurs, (2) the amount of flattening is greater for minus lenses than for plus lenses, and (3) there is an orderly progression in the amount of flattening that occurs, in going from high plus to plano and then continuing on to low minus, moderate minus, and finally high minus.

Effects of Center Thickness

In the groups of lenses listed in Table 13.1, it was observed that the thinner lenses generally flattened slightly more than the thicker lenses of the same power. For all plus lenses, and the lower powers of minus lenses, the difference in flattening between the thickest and thinnest lenses of the same power category was approximately 0.005 mm., but

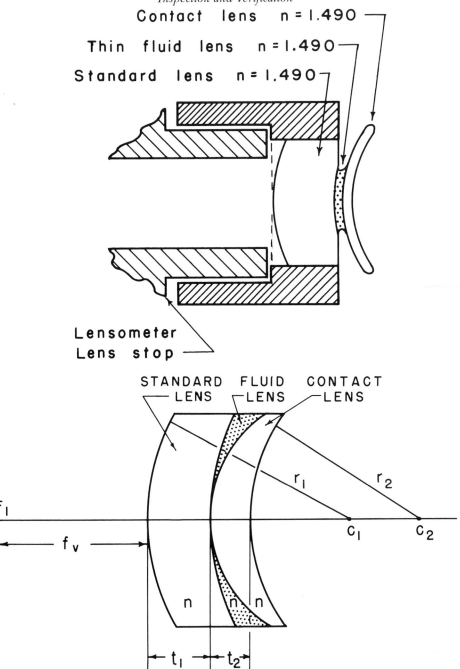

Figure 13.8b and c. Optical components of the R-C device.

for the higher powers of minus, it was found that the thinner lenses flattened as much as 0.010 to 0.020 mm. more than did the thicker lenses.

Effects of Lens Color

The tests included both clear and "through

TABLE 13.1

FLATTENING OF LENS BASE CURVES AT MAXIMUM HYDRATION
(Increase in Radius as Compared With Dry Lenses)

Test Group No.†	Range of Powers of Lenses (Diopters)	Lens Center Thickness (mm's.)	Flattening at Maximum Hydration Group Flattening, Range* (millimeters)	Mean Value of Lens Flattening
I	Semi-finished lens blanks	2.00	.015 to .030	.022 mm.
II	+10.00 to +20.00	.40 to .60	.020 to .035	.028 mm.
III	+ 5.00 to + 9.00	.25 to .40	.020 to .035	.030 mm.
IV	+ 1.00 to + 3.00	.20 to .28	.025 to .040	.033 mm.
V	− 1.00 to − 3.00	.12 to .22	.030 to .045	.038 mm.
VI	− 4.00 to − 6.00	.10 to .20	.030 to .050	.042 mm.
VII	− 7.00 to − 9.00	.08 to .18	.035 to .060	.047 mm.
VIII	−10.00 to −13.00	.08 to .17	.035 to .065	.052 mm.
IX	−14.00 to −18.00	.08 to .16	.040 to .070	.058 mm.
X	−19.00 to −22.00	.07 to .15	.045 to .080	.065 mm.

* More than 90% of the findings fell within this range.

† The first group consisted of 50 lens blanks, ½″ dia., with inside surfaces only finished. The other nine groups contained 20 completely finished lenses each. Thus, a total of 230 lens blanks and lenses comprised the ten groups tested.

and-through" colored lenses in the light shades of blue, green, gray, and brown. No significant differences in flattening were observed among them.

Effects of Lens Manufacture and Material

No significant differences in flattening were observed among the machined, cast, and compression molded lenses made of the various plastic formulations used with each of these production techniques.

Effects of Lens Diameter

Variations in diameter had absolutely no observable effect upon the amounts of flattening. This was double-checked by taking another group of lenses (not listed in Table 13.1), consisting of "uncut" lenses all 12.0 mm. in diameter, hydrating them, and measuring their base curves, then thoroughly drying them and reducing their size to 8.0 mm., whereupon they were again hydrated and checked. This experiment confirmed the earlier observations that variations in lens diameter had no effect on lens flattening.

Effects of Peripheral Curves

The presence or absence of peripheral curves was found to have no effect upon the amounts of base curve flattening observed.

Effects of Power

Figure 13.9 is a graph of the base curve changes observed in the various groups of lenses having average powers ranging from +15.00 to −16.00 D., plotted as a function of time during a forty-eight hour wetting-drying cycle. Starting with totally dehydrated lenses, they were thoroughly soaked for twenty-four hours, with base curve readings taken at frequent intervals and the variations from the original (dry) readings recorded and plotted. At the end of the twenty-four-hour soaking period, the lenses were removed from the liquid and allowed to dry for twenty-four hours, with base curve readings again being taken at frequent intervals and the changes recorded and plotted. As can be seen from the graph, the base curve changes of plus lenses differ markedly from those of minus lenses, both during hydration and during

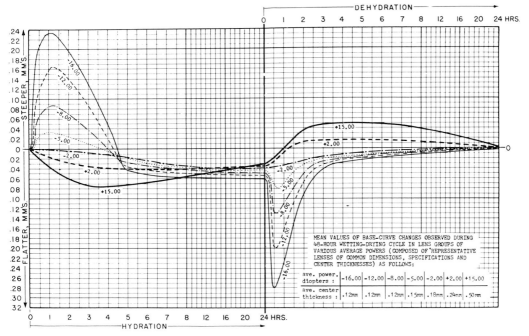

Figure 13.9. The wetting-drying cycle. From S. Gordon, Contact Lens Hydration: A Study of the Wetting-Drying Cycle, *Optometry Weekly*, 56(*14*):55–62, 1965.

dehydration.

In examining Figure 13.9, the following will be noted:

1. Minus lenses of low power flatten slowly.

2. Plus lenses of low power flatten rapidly, reaching their maximum flattening in about four hours and maintaining this curvature with only a slight retreat from this maximum value during the remainder of the hydration period.

3. Plus lenses of moderate and high power begin flattening rapidly during the first hour of hydration and reach maximum flattening in about four hours; then, they slowly reverse the direction of change and begin to steepen moderately until, at full hydration, they have recovered more than halfway from their flattest values.

4. Minus lenses of moderate and high power behave in an opposite manner to plus lenses, steepening almost immediately upon being exposed to an aqueous environment.

The maximum steepening is reached in about one hour, after which the lenses reverse their direction of change and begin to flatten until, in three or four more hours, they have completely retreated from their initial (first hours) steepening. Then they continue flattening at a decreasing rate of speed until maximum flattening is reached at full hydration.

Effects of Power and Thickness Increments in Higher Powered Lenses

Among the higher powered plus lenses, there was little difference in performance between a +10.00 and a +20.00 D. lens. Also, only slight differences were observed as the center thicknesses of the high plus lenses were varied within the commonly used range of 0.40 to 0.60 mm. Among the higher powered minus lenses, however, it was found that (1) an increase in lens power for a given center thickness magnifies the initial steepening, as is clearly seen in Figure 13.9, and (2) a decrease

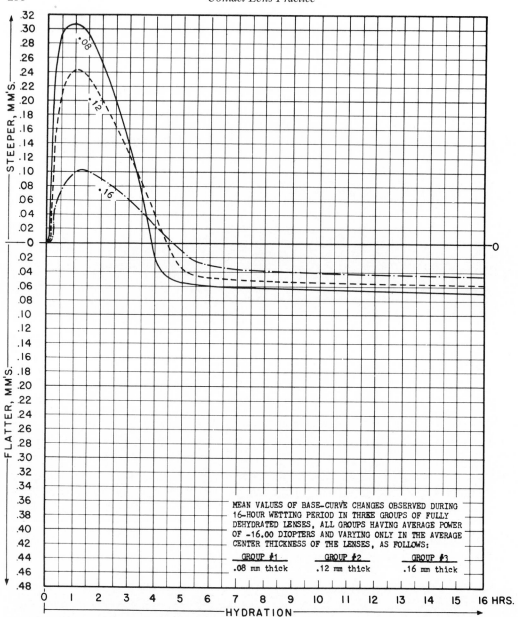

Figure 13.10. Influence of lens thickness during hydration period. From S. Gordon, Contact Lens Hydration: A Study of the Wetting-Drying Cycle, *Optometry Weekly*, *56*(*14*):55–62, 1965.

in center thickness for a given power also has the effect of greatly increasing the initial lens steepening, as shown in Figure 13.10. This graph also shows that the thinner the minus lens, the more rapidly it retreats from its initial great steepening and the sooner it arrives at its maximum flattening.

Dehydration Observations

In examining Figure 13.9, the following will be noted:

1. Minus lenses of low power slowly and steadily return, during the dehydration period, to their original dry base curve radii.

2. Plus lenses of low power rapidly return

to their original curvatures as they dehydrate, and then they actually steepen slightly, this steepening being maintained for many hours, after which the lenses finally return, slowly, to their original dry base curve radii.

3. Higher powered plus lenses rapidly return to their original dry curvatures as they begin to dehydrate, and then they continue to steepen until they are about 0.05 mm. steeper. After maintaining this steepness for several hours, the lenses slowly return to their true base curves as they become completely dehydrated.

4. Moderate and high powered minus lenses behave just the opposite of plus lenses at the start of the dehydration period (Figure 13.11). Instead of returning to normal curvature from their state of maximum flattening at full hydration, they almost immediately and very rapidly begin to flatten still further as they begin drying out. This extreme and sudden flattening reaches a maximum within a period of thirty to sixty minutes from the start of drying; then, the lenses reverse their behavior and rapidly start to steepen, con-

tinuing to do so at a gradually decelerating pace until they finally return to their original dry base curvatures when total dehydration is accomplished.

In the case of a patient who stores his lenses dry each night, there will be alternating periods of hydration (when the lens is worn) and dehydration (when not being worn). It is apparent that the lenses are never permitted to hydrate or dehydrate completely, for normally there is no continuous period of twenty-four or more hours during which the lenses are steadily wetting or steadily drying.

Inspection of Ultrathin Lenses

The extreme flexibility of the ultrathin lens makes some additional care and allowances necessary during the inspection procedure. If the lens is simply held between the fingers, it may be flexed enough to induce a cylinder during the measurement of the base curve. The practitioner should not be alarmed when this occurs, as it has no effect on the shape of the lens after it is placed on the eye.

PERIPHERAL CURVE RADIUS

Difficulties in measuring a peripheral curve radius are so great that this measurement is seldom attempted, even though various methods are available. The measurement problem occurs because the peripheral curve is very often not a true curve and cannot be specified in terms of a single radius. It is frequently irregular and poor in optical quality. If a blend has been added to the lens, there is often very little area remaining on the peripheral curve that can be used for a measurement.

Since the laboratory is in no better position to measure the peripheral curve than the practitioner, the radius that the laboratory specifies for a lens is simply the radius of the tool which was used to grind and polish the peripheral curve. Although it is usually assumed that the peripheral curve has

the same radius as the tool by which it has been polished, it has been shown that this is not necessarily true (*see* Chapter 16).

If verification of the radius of the peripheral curve of a new lens is desired, the lens should be ordered without any blend. This will leave the peripheral curve with the maximum width possible and the best optical quality. The blend, if desired, can be added later by the practitioner. If the peripheral curve is at least 0.7 mm. wide and of good optical quality, it can be measured by one of the following methods:

Lensometer

Brungardt has described a technique of using the lensometer for measurements of the peripheral curve radius, which is based upon finding the power of the part of the

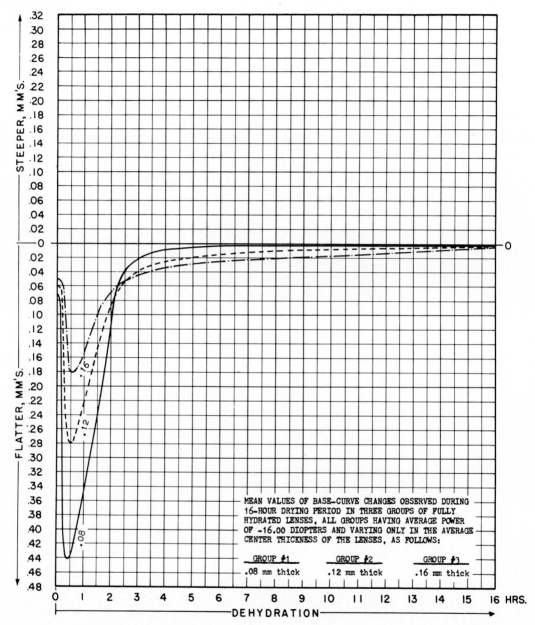

Figure 13.11. Influence of lens thickness during dehydration period. From S. Gordon, Contact Lens Hydration: A Study of the Wetting-Drying Cycle, *Optometry Weekly*, 56(14):55–62, 1965.

lens formed by the peripheral curve and the anterior surface.[42,43] The method is limited to lenses in which the front surface has a single curve that does not have a wide front bevel and in which the peripheral curve is 0.7 mm. or more in width. The peripheral

curve must also have a true spherical surface and high optical quality.

Measurement of the peripheral curve with a lensometer is conveniently explained by considering a bicurve contact lens as though it were composed of two imaginary lenses having different powers. The first imaginary lens consists of the section of the contact lens corresponding to the optical zone, and its power is determined in the usual way from the lensometer (Figure 13.12a and b horizontal lines). A second imaginary lens consists of the peripheral curve for its back surface together with the front surface of the contact lens (Figure 13.12c, hashed area). The power of the second imaginary lens can be read from the lensometer just as though the peripheral curve extended over the optical zone. The reading is most conveniently found after the measurement has been taken of the power of the optical zone in the usual way. The power wheel should be turned in the direction of more plus, or less minus. It will be found that the target image will soon reappear in its original form, though somewhat dimmer than usual. The power is read again, and its difference in diopters is noted from the first reading. The curvature of the peripheral curve is determined from the difference in powers of the first and second readings. For each 0.75 D. of power difference, there is approximately 0.1 mm. difference between the curvature of the central and peripheral curves. For example, given a lens having a

base curve of 7.6 mm. and a power of −5.00 D., the second focus in the lensometer occurs at +1.00 D., so the difference is 6 D. Therefore, the peripheral curve has a radius that is flatter than the base curve by the following:

$$\frac{6.00}{0.75} \times 0.1 = 0.8 \text{ mm.}$$

The radius of the peripheral curve is 8.4 mm. (7.6 mm. + 0.8 mm.).

Some error occurs in this formula due to differences in various optical zone radii and lens thicknesses. The formula has not been corrected for spherical aberration, which could cause considerable error in some circumstances. The formula should therefore not be considered to give an accuracy of better than 0.2 mm.

When taking the measurement with a lensometer, the practitioner should expose the entire lens to the aperture of the lensometer. If the aperture is smaller than the lens, light will be prevented from passing through the peripheral curve, and the second focus will not be seen. In this event, the lens should be moved sideways, until the peripheral curve definetly covers the aperture, before the second reading is attempted.

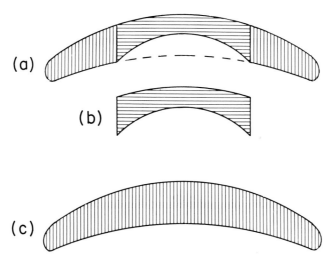

Figure 13.12. Measurement of peripheral curve radius with a lensometer. (a) Bicurve lens considered as two imaginary lenses (b and c).

Optical Spherometer

Most types of optical spherometers have a lens holder that can be tilted and moved to allow a measurement of the radius of the peripheral curve of a contact lens.[27] An aperture within the instrument is used to limit the size of the ray bundle that reflects from the lens so that a small area can be measured. By reducing the size of the ray bundle, some accuracy is lost in the measurement.

Polishing Tools

It is possible to use polishing tools of known radii for a gross measurement of the peripheral curve radius.[4] The tools must be covered with nonwaterproof tape or some other hard material that is not compressible. Felt or moleskin pads are not acceptable. The lens is first covered with a waterproof coating material such as Carter's Marks-a-Lot® (Figure 13.13) and then touched lightly to a polishing tool. The tool should be spinning in the same way as would occur when modifying the radius of the peripheral curve of a lens. Only a brief contact of the lens to the tool is necessary for this test. Afterwards, the lens is inspected to see what area of the coating has been removed. If the coating has been removed from the inner border of the peripheral curve but not the outer border, it indicates that the peripheral curve of the lens has a longer radius of curvature than the tool. This occurs because the outer portion of the peripheral curve tends to have greater clearance than the inner portion when the lens is placed against the tool (Figure 13.14). Hence, the coating is removed from only the inner border. If the coating has been removed from the outer border of the peripheral curve but not the inner border, it indicates that the peripheral curve of the lens has a shorter radius of curvature than the tool. If the coating is removed from the entire peripheral curve it indicates that the lens and tool are of nearly the same radius. By a systematic process of trial and error, using various polishing tools of different radii, the radius of the peripheral curve can be determined. With some practice, it is usually possible to make a fair estimate of the radius of the peripheral curve by using only three tools, and the procedure is not as lengthy as it might appear. This method is particularly useful for lenses that have been heavily blended and which cannot be measured in any other way.

POWER

The power of a contact lens can be measured with a lensometer (vertometer or any comparable instrument) in the same way as this instrument is used with spectacle lenses.[44] Since the lensometer is not designed for use with contact lenses, however, it suffers several shortcomings that have caused considerable disagreement in terms of the procedure to be followed for accurate contact lens power measurements.[45] The principal disagreement is the way in which a contact lens should be held in the lensometer for a measurement, that is, with its front or back surface against the stop. Actually, it makes little difference how the lens is held, so long as the measurement is interpreted correctly, and that depends upon a simple knowledge of lens powers.

The power of a contact lens, like a spectacle lens, is most conveniently measured with reference to one of its surfaces. If the back surface is the reference point, then the lens power is the reciprocal of the distance from the back surface of the lens to the secondary focal point, or *back vertex power.* This will not be equal to the *front vertex power*, which is the reciprocal of the distance from the front lens surface to the primary focal point. A difference in front and back vertex powers occurs when the lens is bent into a meniscus form (Figure 13.15). Symmetrical biconvex and

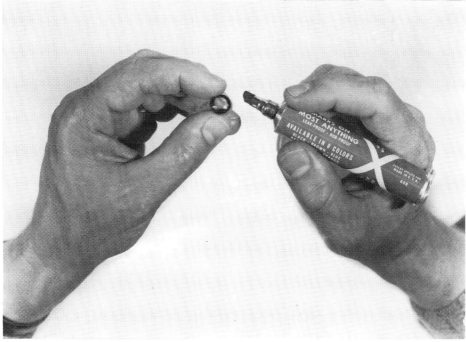

Figure 13.13. Coating the back surface of a contact lens.

biconcave lenses (such as most spectacle trial lenses) do not have differences in their front and back vertex powers. Spectacle lenses are not bent to the same extent as contact lenses and do not commonly have large differences in their front and back vertex powers, though a small difference does exist. A contact lens is bent a considerable amount, and significant differences may exist between its front and back vertex powers.

The differences in the front and back vertex powers will vary with the power of the contact lens. Positive power lenses will always show less plus for their front vertex powers than their back vertex powers. Negative power lenses will always show less minus for their front vertex powers than their back vertex powers.

When the lensometer is used to measure the power of a spectacle lens, the lens is placed with its posterior surface against the *lens stop* of the instrument. The position of the lens stop is very important, since it is assumed that the posterior surface of the lens is at that position, and the power read from the instrument is based upon that assumption. If the lens is held away from the stop, the power reading will be in error. This occurs because the instrument determines the power of the lens by finding the distance of its focal point from the stop. If the back surface of the lens is in the plane of the stop, the power will be determined by the distance of the focal point from the posterior surface of the lens or back vertex power. If the lens is now turned around so that the front surface is against the stop, the power measured is front vertex power. When a contact lens is measured with a lensometer, it is considerably more difficult to make either of its surfaces coincide with the plane of the stop in order to achieve an accurate reading. When the lens is placed against the stop, the high curvatures of the surfaces make the following: (1) the posterior surface falls in front of the stop if the back vertex power is being measured; and (2) the

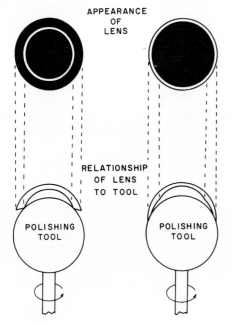

APPEARANCE
OF
LENS

RELATIONSHIP
OF LENS
TO TOOL

POLISHING
TOOL

POLISHING
TOOL

PERIPHERAL CURVE
FLATTER THAN TOOL

PERIPHERAL CURVE
STEEPER THAN TOOL

Figure 13.14. Measurement of the peripheral curve radius by briefly touching coated lens to a polishing tool.

anterior surface falls behind the stop if the front vertex power is being measured (Figure 13.16). Consequently, a discrepancy will occur in the power measurements of a contact lens with a lensometer for two reasons:

1. Actual differences in front and back vertex power
2. Error caused by the lens surface not being in the plane of the lensometer stop

An error caused by the lens position, relative to the lensometer stop, will increase the back vertex power of plus lenses and decrease the back vertex power of minus lenses. The net effect, therefore, is for the lens position to accentuate the difference in vertex power measurements for plus lenses and to diminish the difference for minus lenses.

There is yet another variable factor in lensometer measurements that influences the distance between the surface of the lens and the plane of the lensometer stop.[46] This variable is the diameter of the lens stop itself. In some instances, older models of one lensometer type will have a different aperture diameter from current models. Thus, a practitioner measuring high plus contact lenses on an older instrument may find a power that is slightly different from that found by the laboratory, which usually has the latest equipment.

In the early days of corneal contact lens manufacture, all contact lenses were specified in terms of front vertex power. This probably was due to the ease with which the front vertex power could be measured during the manufacture of the lens.[45] It was also found by the practitioner that the lens could be held against the lensometer much more easily when the convex side of the lens was placed against the lensometer stop.

In terms of accuracy for measurements with the lensometer, it cannot be said that either front or back surface power is correct. They are simply powers with different reference points, and one can easily be converted to the other.

Since the power of the lens is useful only in terms of its relationship to the eye, however, the back vertex power becomes of fundamental importance. Refractors, corrected curve trial lenses, and spectacle lenses are all specified in terms of back vertex power. Calculations for lens effectivity in determining the difference in lens power when changing from spectacles to contact lenses are given in terms of back vertex powers. In order to make the contact lens power correspond to the ametropia at the corneal plane, it must be expressed in terms of back vertex power. From a refractive standpoint, the front surface power is valueless.

Unfortunately there is still considerable confusion and disagreement among manufacturers and practitioners as to whether front or back vertex power should be measured. In a survey of nineteen laboratories by Ullen,[46] eight specified power in terms of front vertex power and eleven in terms of back vertex power. His sampling of practitioners (number not specified) showed that 80 percent checked front vertex power on the lensometer.

Sarver has made the necessary calculations relating the front and back vertex powers for various types of contact lenses.[47] These are plotted on graphs that allow the conversion of front vertex powers, which are measured on a lensometer, to back vertex power (Figures 13.17 and 13.18). The calculations that were made consider both the true differences in front and back vertex power and also the effect of the contact lens being out of the plane of the lensometer stop. The aperture stop was considered to be 6.5 mm. in diameter.

One may note from the graphs that minus power lenses have only small differences in their front and back vertex powers as read from the lensometer. Positive power lenses, however, have considerable difference between their front and back vertex powers. For example, a lens that has a 43.00 D. base curve and which is 0.60 mm. in thickness measures +20.00 D. for the front vertex power. The back vertex power as determined from the table would be +21.50 D., which is a significant difference. Bailey has illustrated the need to specify which vertex power is measured by comparing the measurements of front and

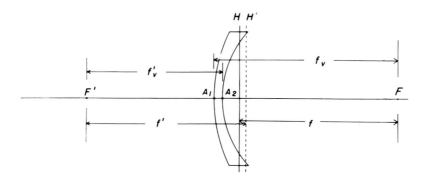

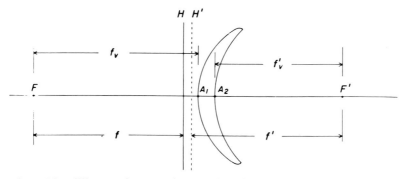

Figure 13.15. The difference between front and back vertex powers. From M. D. Sarver, Verification of Contact Lens Power, *Journal of the American Optometric Association, 34(16)*:1304–1306, 1963.

back vertex powers for a number of contact lenses used in his practice.[45]

Table 13.2 shows a series of minus lenses, the front and back vertex powers of which were measured by Bailey on a Bausch and Lomb Vertometer. As can be seen, only small differences are evident, even in the rather high powers.

In Table 13.3, however, the refractive powers of a number of plus contact lenses that were worn by Bailey's patients are shown. As the refractive power and the thickness of the plus lenses are increased, the discrepancy between front and back vertex power increases sharply, as would be predicted by the graphs of Sarver. This would mean that high hyper-

opes or aphakic patients may be properly refracted and the correct vertex distance calculations made, but still the selection of the proper lens power cannot be made with certainty unless the back vertex power of the lens is used.

Special Apertures

A number of special aperture devices have been made that may be attached to the lensometer and used as aids for positioning the back surface of a contact lens in the plane of the lensometer stop. One such device consists of an insert that fits inside the lensometer stop and reduces its effective aperture to 4 mm.

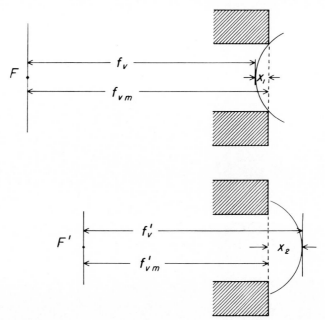

Figure 13.16. When a contact lens is placed against a lensometer stop to measure back vertex power, the back surface of the lens should be towards and in the plane of the stop. Under usual conditions the high curvatures of the lens surfaces make the front surface fall behind the stop if the front vertex power is being measured (*top*), and the posterior surface falls in front of the stop if the back vertex power is being measured (*bottom*); x_1 and x_2 are the distances from the convex and concave surfaces, respectively, to the plane of the stop; f_v is actual front vertex power; f_v is actual back vertex power; f_{vm} is measured front vertex power; f_{vm} is measured back vertex power. From M. D. Sarver, Verification of Contact Lens Power, *Journal of the American Optometric Association, 34(16):*1304–1306, 1963.

in diameter.[23] The face of the insert is curved to conform approximately to the curvatures found on the concave surfaces of contact lenses. It should be noted that when any aperture device is added to the lensometer, the face of aperture device against which the lens is

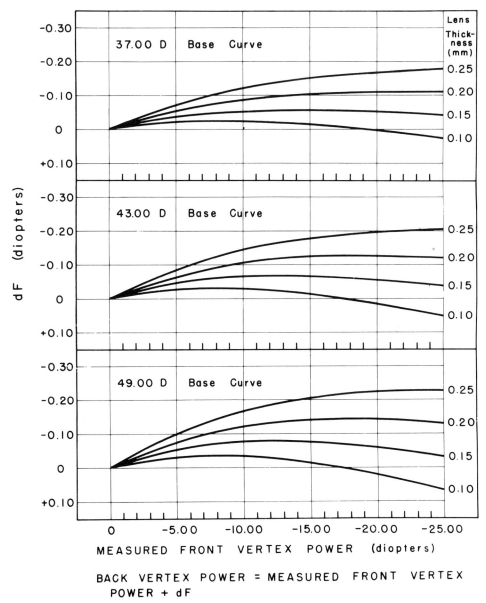

BACK VERTEX POWER = MEASURED FRONT VERTEX
POWER + dF

Figure 13.17. The back vertex power for various base curves and lens thicknesses for a minus lens when the front vertex power is measured by placing the front surface of the contact lens against the aperture stop of a lensometer or vertometer. From M. D. Sarver, Verification of Contact Lens Power, *Journal of the American Optometric Association, 34(16)*:1304–1306, 1963.

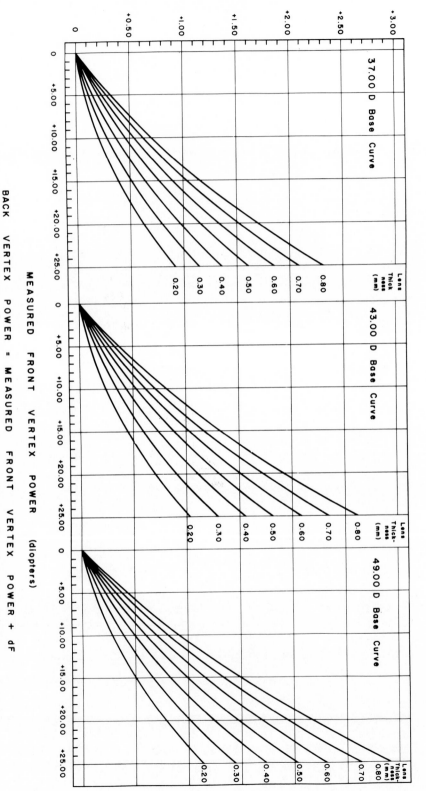

BACK VERTEX POWER = MEASURED FRONT VERTEX POWER + dF

Figure 13.18. The back vertex power for various base curves and lens thicknesses for a plus lens when the front vertex power is measured by placing the front surface of the contact lens against the aperture stop of a lensometer or vertometer. From M. D. Sarver, Verification of Contact Lens Power, *Journal of the American Optometric Association, 34*(16):1304–1306, 1963.

placed must be adjusted so that it is in the same position as the original lensometer stop.

Recent models of the American Optical Lensometer are equipped with a special lens holder, which allows a direct measurement to be made of the back vertex power of contact lenses.

Lens Prism

Unwanted prism is sometimes present in a contact lens as a result of faulty manufacturing method. The prism may be detected with the lensometer. If the contact lens is centered in front of the lensometer stop, the prism can be read directly by noting the displacement of the target image seen in the instrument. An alternate method is to move the contact lens across the stop until the target image is centered, then spot the lens with the marking pin of the lensometer. The spot should be centered with respect to the geometric center of the lens. If this is not the case, it indicates that prism is present. The prism power may be determined by measuring the distance of the spot from the geometric center of the lens, using a measuring magnifier and calculating the prism from Prentice's rule.

Tolerances for Power and Prism

Lens power should be correct within ± 0.25 D. of the power ordered, with less than ± 0.12 D. of unwanted cylinder. There should be less than the following prism power limitations:

Power of Lens	Acceptable Prism
Less than ± 10.00 D.	$<0.25\Delta$
More than ± 10.00 D.	$<0.50\Delta$

CENTER THICKNESS

Thickness Gauge

Various gauges are available for the measurement of center thickness of contact lenses.[48] The usual type is a dial gauge, which has a rounded base, upon which the lens is placed with the convex side down. A spring-loaded plunger is then slowly lowered until it touches against the convex side of the lens (Figure 13.19). The amount by which the plunger is separated from the base, which can be read from the dial scale, will determine the lens thickness. Care should be taken not to scratch the lens with either the plunger or base.

The thickness gauges recommended for use with contact lenses are usually calibrated in tenths of a millimeter, which are preferred to gauges calibrated in thousandths of an inch. Some laboratories have advocated that con-

TABLE 13.2

VERTEX POWER

Lens	Base Curve	Thickness	Front Vertex Power	Back Vertex Power
1	7.30	.17	− 4.75	− 4.75
2	8.30	.33	− 5.37	− 5.37
3	7.85	.21	− 8.00	− 8.00
4	7.45	.15	−11.90	−12.10
5	8.10	.23	−15.87	−15.75

TABLE 13.3

VERTEX POWER

Lens	Base Curve	Thickness	Front Vertex Power	Back Vertex Power
1	7.80	0.51	+ 4.50	+ 4.70
2	7.67	0.70	+ 7.00	+ 7.50
3	7.95	0.89	+11.00	+12.00
4	8.33	0.55	+14.25	+15.25
5	8.20	1.34	+18.50	+22.37

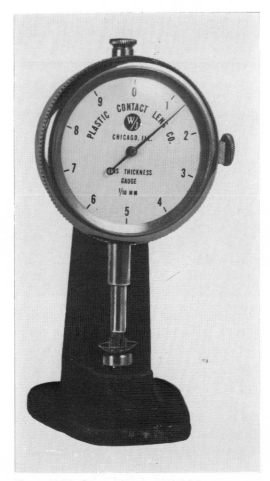

Figure 13.19. Contact lens center thickness gauge.

tact lens thickness should be specified in terms of thousandths of an inch. This recommendation is given because the machines (lathes) they used to cut the contact lens curves are equipped with English rather than metric scales.

A scale for converting thousandths of an inch to millimeters is given in Appendix 3. It may be noted that 0.001 inch is equivalent to more than 0.02 mm. Consequently, if contact lens thickness is expressed in steps of thousandths of an inch, less accuracy will be obtained than if it is expressed in terms of hundredths of a millimeter.

Thickness gauges will frequently lose their accuracy with use and should be checked often with a standard thickness template. A simple adjustment can be made on the gauge to compensate for any error.

Alternate Method to Measure Center Thickness

It is possible to use an ordinary "lens clock" or Geneva lens measure in a modified way to determine center thickness of a contact lens.[49-51] The following method is used:

1. Check the accuracy of the clock by touching the three pins against a flat plane of

glass. The dial reading should be zero.

2. Place the contact lens on the plane of glass with the concave side up.

3. Align the clock so that the middle pin is over the center of the contact lens and gently press down until the two outside pins make contact with the glass.

4. Note the dioptric reading on the scale. Each diopter will be approximately equal to 0.10 mm. of thickness.

The exact conversion will vary somewhat with the particular lens clock that is used and depends upon the separation of its pins. An accurate scale can be made by checking the clock on a series of metal strips of known thickness or on a feeler gauge.

The disadvantage of using a lens clock to measure center thickness is that the pins are usually very sharp and can easily scratch the plastic lens. If the clock is to be converted exclusively to a thickness gauge, the points may be blunted slightly by polishing with fine emery.

Tolerance for Center Thickness.

The thickness of a contact lens should vary no more than ±0.02 mm. from the value ordered. Laboratories usually have little difficulty in making lenses of the correct thickness.

Thickness of a contact lens is most important when there is some basis for comparison by the patient between one lens and another. When the two lenses worn by a patient differ in thickness, one eye may be uncomfortable. It is also frequently found that, to be comfortable, a second pair of lenses must have the same thickness as the original pair and that replacement lenses must have the same thickness as those lenses they replace.

EDGE

Evaluation of the contact lens edge represents the most difficult but most important part of the inspection routine.[52] Various instruments may be used for this purpose with good results, but each demands a high degree of training and practice before any proficiency is possible.[53] The edge must usually be viewed with some type of magnification device, which distorts the viewer's perception of dimensions and limits the area of the lens that may be seen at one time. Even with magnification, the edge imperfections that must be detected appear small, and it is difficult to relate the appearance of one lens to another that has been seen previously.

A major difficulty in learning to identify a good contact lens edge occurs because its contour is so difficult to describe. Edge contour has not been commonly expressed in any quantitative terms and is usually referred to by qualitative descriptions such as rounded, blunt, sharp, knife edge, square, or tapered. It is therefore not surprising that there is disagreement among fitters as to the optimum edge contour. Each fitter has a concept based on his experience of what the edge contour should be, and one practitioner cannot communicate effectively to another to determine whether they are actually in agreement or not. An edge that one fitter calls thin may be called sharp by another and perfect by a third. Past descriptions of the optimum edge thickness provide little information, since it is usually not specified where and how the measurements were taken. Values given for the optimum edge thickness by various authors vary from 0.13 to 0.20 mm.,[51-54] but because of the differences in the positions where the thickness measurements were taken, they may not actually refer to any real difference in the edges.

In an experiment by the author, an attempt

was made to determine what the optimum contact lens edge should be. This study also presented an opportunity to gather information about the quality and uniformity of edges on the lenses from various manufacturers. A contact lens was solicited and contributed from each of twenty-six leading manufacturers, which had the following specifications:

B.C.R.	OZ.D.	P.C.R.	P.C.W.	T.D.	T	Power
7.85	7.5	8.85	1.0	9.5	0.18	−3.00

Each manufacturer was told that his contact lens was to be used in a study of edges and was instructed to produce a lens having the best edge he could possibly make.

During the course of the experiment, the lenses were worn for short periods of time by a group of twenty-six students. These subjects were selected from approximately 700 university students on the basis that they had *K* readings of 43 D. and close similarity between their two eyes so that all could wear the same lenses. None of the subjects had worn contact lenses prior to the time of the experiment. For a period of four months the students attended short sessions each week in which they wore the lenses in different combinations and gradually eliminated those which did not feel comfortable.

Figure 13.20 shows replicas of the edge contours from twenty of the twenty-six lenses used in the experiment. The dashed line represents the optimum edge contour (lens e), which is included with each lens for comparative purposes. These replicas were made at the termination of the experiment by cutting the lenses in half along a diameter and photographing the sectional view of the edges through a microscope. As can be seen, considerable variability was found to exist in the edges of the various lenses used in the experiment. Finishing the edge properly requires considerable time, and for some laboratories the economic considerations may outweigh the desire for perfection. Because of this, the lens edge often serves as a good index of the quality of the entire lens and the care that

has gone into its manufacture. There should be no doubt as to the need for careful inspection of the edge by the fitter.

The following conclusions were made from the experiment:

1. Lenses with edges represented as a through e in Figure 13.20 were preferred by the subjects; lenses with edges represented as f through p were generally uncomfortable, with those represented as q through u causing the greatest discomfort.

2. Most subjects preferred lenses with the same type of edge. Their preferences were not materially affected by the eye in which the lens was worn.

Some caution must be exercised in interpreting the results of this experiment. Although it clearly shows preference by the subjects for certain types of edges, it does not demonstrate that any of the less-preferred edges could not be worn successfully. It is likely that lenses with the less-preferred edges could be worn comfortably by some people, as evidenced by many patients who have been wearing lenses with edges similar to the less-preferred types having no subjective problems. It is also likely, however, that a much larger proportion of patients will be more comfortable with lenses having edges of the type found in a through e of Figure 13.20.

The results are also limited by conducting the experiment with only one lens construction, and the conclusions are not necessarily applicable to lenses of other construction. Many authors feel that a custom edge design is necessary for each patient, thus attempting to meet the requirements for individual eye variations.[54] This view is not supported by the results of this experiment. The subjects all had *K* readings of 43 D., but they varied greatly in terms of astigmatism, corneal diameter, peripheral corneal flattening, angles between the cornea and sclera, and lids. Yet, they generally preferred edges of the same type. It would appear that, at least with this particular lens construction, the variations

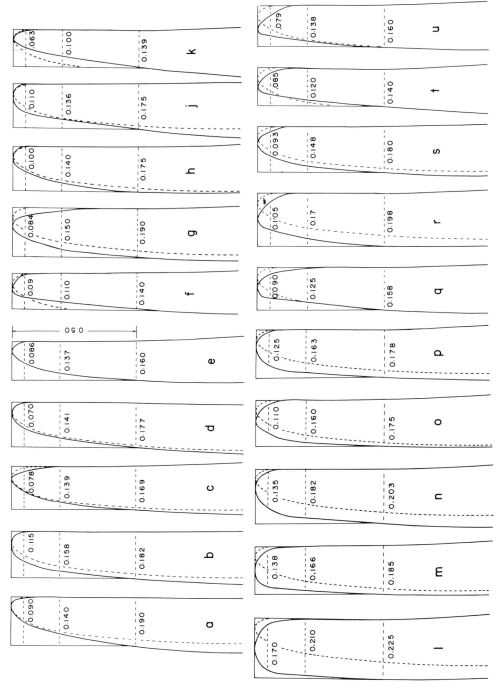

Figure 13.20. Replicas of edge contours from twenty lenses used in experiment on edge preference.

in design of the edges themselves contributed far more to the degree of comfort than did the variation of the subjects' eyes.

What then can be said about the edges of lenses with other dimensions? It is probable that their optimum edge is very nearly the same, at least for lenses that tend to ride partly beneath the upper lid. Many think that small lenses, which ride within the palpebral fissure, are most comfortable when the edge is thicker and more rounded. This aids in keeping the lens centered and is purposely designed to help prevent the lens from passing beneath the lower lid. Various other special lens designs may also require variations in the edge contour.

Other Considerations

When inspecting the contact lens edge, it is important to consider the clinical circumstances of the patient. New patients will probably be less critical of the edges than experienced patients, but the edge may well be a factor in determining the success of the new patient. If an experienced patient has been wearing lenses with bad edges, he is usually pleasantly surprised at the improvement when he receives new lenses with better edges or has his old lenses modified. One of the most difficult problems associated with the replacement of lost lenses is with patients who are accustomed to wearing lenses with good edges and are not able to tolerate replacement lenses with bad edges.

The most critical situation in which a patient can make a judgment of a bad edge is when a difference exists in the edges of the lenses worn on his two eyes. Consequently, it is most important that the edges for a pair of lenses be as much alike as possible. Patients are also very critical of edges that are not uniform around their entire circumference. It is therefore necessary to check edges closely for consistency.

Optimum Edge Contour

The replica of the contact lens edge may be characterized by thickness at various positions and by the location of the apex. The author uses a boxing system similar to that used with spectacle lens shapes. The box has one standard dimension of 0.50 mm. for its width. Its height must be determined by a systematic application of the following procedure:

1. A template is constructed with an L shape, the longer leg having a length that is equivalent to 0.50 mm. at the same magnification as the edge.

2. The template is adjusted on the replica of the edge contour so that end A touches the lens, the short leg touches the apex, and the long leg touches at one additional point (Figure 13.21).

3. At point A, a line is drawn through the lens perpendicular to the long leg. At the point where this line intersects with the front edge, another line is drawn parallel to the long leg of the template to complete the box.

The position at which the template's short leg touches the lens determines the apex, which is specified by its distance from the base line. Thicknesses are given at 0.05, 0.2, and 0.5 mm. from the apex and are measured along lines parallel to the height of the box. The optimal dimensions are as follows:

1. Apex—0.03 mm. from base line
2. Thickness at 0.05 mm. from apex— 0.08 mm.
3. Thickness at 0.2 mm. from apex— 0.14 mm.
4. Thickness at 0.5 mm. from apex— 0.16 mm.

The variations of the edge thickness in these positions illustrate the need for a specific reference to the position at which edge thickness is measured.

The most common fault of uncomfortable edges is that they are too thick and present too much resistance to the lid. Thick edges are represented in Figure 13.20 by 1 to p. Fewer edges are found that are too sharp

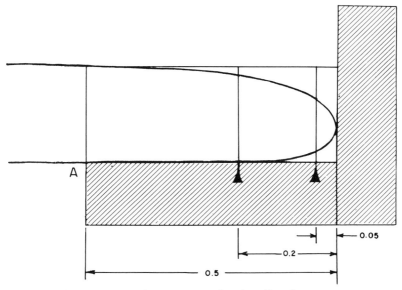

Figure 13.21. Boxing system used to describe edge contour.

because these are more easily detected by the manufacturer.

The apex of the lens must be near to the posterior surface. If the apex is too far forward, the lid will catch and cause uncomfortable sensations. Edges q to u illustrate this condition.

Unfortunately, with the usual inspection devices, it is not possible to measure directly the dimensions of the contact lens edge, and it is necessary to estimate them. The simplest method for an inexperienced fitter is to make a direct comparison to a standard lens with an ideal edge, which is kept for this purpose. The two lenses can be held side by side and compared directly by any of the inspection methods that follow.

Methods of Inspection

The various methods that can be employed to inspect the contact lens edge are using the stereomicroscope, hand loupe, and projection magnifier, rubbing on the wrist or fingers, wearing in the fitter's eye, and molding.

Stereomicroscope

The stereomicroscope provides one of the best methods for checking the edge but represents the most difficult technique to master.[55] The microscope should have a low magnification that ranges between ×20 and ×40, with ×25 being about the best.[26] The light source should produce a focused illumination and is nearly as important as the quality of the microscope itself.

Although many lens holders are available, lenses can be inspected best when they are held in the hands so that they can be moved to take best advantage of the lighting. The hands should be washed in order to avoid smudging the lens; smudges are sometimes difficult to tell from a lens imperfection.

The most difficult problem for the novice using the stereomicroscope is holding the lens steadily in the correct position for viewing. It is sometimes difficult even to find the lens when it is first viewed through the microscope. To help in orienting the lens, the microscope stage should be marked at the position where the lens is to be held. This position is located by focusing the microscope on the stage and observing while a pencil is moved about on the stage until it is seen to be in the center of the field of view. This position is then marked on the stage for future reference. It is best to place a piece of tape at this position so that it can be easily located for all future use of this microscope. The scope is now ready for use.

1. Hold the lens between the thumb and forefinger of the left hand, and place it on the tape that has been placed on the stage. Adjust the lamp so that maximum illumination is cast on the top edge of the lens (Figure 13.22). Most right-handed people prefer to have the illumination come from the right side.

2. Look through the microscope. Raise the microscope with the adjustment knob until the top edge of the lens is in focus (Figure 13.23). Steady the lens with the thumb and finger of the right hand, but avoid interfering with the illumination on the lens.

3. View only the top area of the lens at one time. Tilt the lens back and forth slightly towards the front and back to appreciate the contour better (Figure 13.24).

4. Rotate the lens about 40° to bring another section of the edge into view (Figure 13.25). Keep the lower edge in contact with the stage to maintain the upper edge in focus. The edge cannot be viewed while the lens is being rotated.

5. Continue to rotate the lens to different positions to examine the entire edge.

Hand Loupe

The use of a small hand loupe with a power of between ×7 and ×10 allows the fitter to make a reasonably accurate inspection of the lens edge. The loupe has the advantage of being portable and available at minimum cost.

Projection Magnifier

With the projection magnifier it is possible to obtain a greatly magnified profile image of the lens edge. This method suffers the disadvantage of not allowing an adequate evaluation of the polish of the lens edge or of the lens surface. Projection magnifiers are of greater use to the manufacturer than the practitioner because of the ease with which they may be used. It is possible to use some types of slit lamps as projection magnifiers.[56]

Rubbing on the Wrist or Fingers

It is possible with some practice to detect certain defects in the edge by rubbing the lens across the wrist or fingers. The easiest defect to detect by this method is a sharp edge, but it is also possible to feel sharp ridges and unpolished corners. There is a tendency not to notice edges that are excessively thick, and since this appears to be the most common defect of lenses received from the laboratories, the method cannot be considered satisfactory.

Wearing in the Fitter's Eye

Even though the lens may not fit well on the practitioner's eye, it is possible to make a reasonably accurate appraisal of the edge quality by wearing the lens for only a few minutes. It is necessary, however, that the practitioner be experienced in wearing contact lenses.

Lensometer

It is somewhat possible to observe the contact lens edge contour with a lensometer,[57] but this technique is not commonly used.

Molding

Various pliable plastic compounds have been used to mold the edge of the contact lens.[58] The mold is then sectioned to provide a profile view of the edge. The technique is accurate and provides a convenient method to maintain a permanent record of the edge contour on any lens. Molding is not generally used, however, because it is a lengthy procedure; it does not reveal the quality of the edge polish; it must be repeated at various positions on the edge to insure that there is uniformity of the contour.

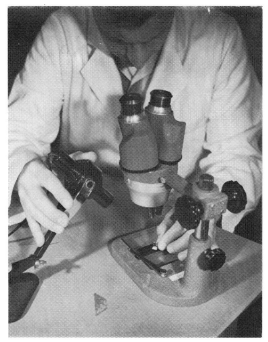

Figure 13.22

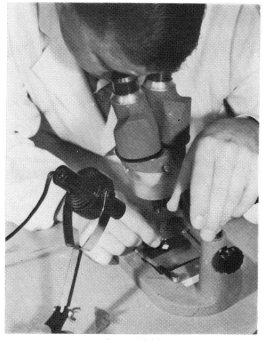

Figure 13.23

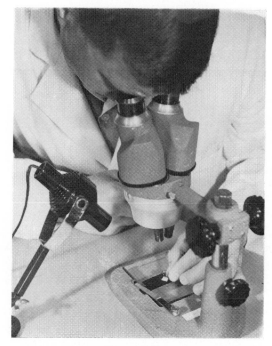

Figure 13.24

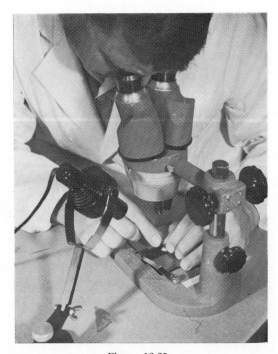

Figure 13.25

SURFACE AND OPTICAL QUALITY

Much information can be obtained about the surface and optical qualities of a contact lens by a simple visual inspection with the unaided eye. The edge of a fluorescent lamp is viewed through the lens, and the lens is moved back and forth with a motion similar to that used in hand neutralization of spectacle lenses. As the lens is rotated, the edge of the fluorescent lamp should remain straight. A discontinuity will be visible at the various zones of the lens, which is due to their difference in powers. It is also possible to detect internal defects such as bubbles and striae.

To inspect surface quality, the lens should be held so that the light from the fluorescent lamp is reflected from the lens to the eye. The light reflex from the lens surface should appear bright and sharp and should not become distorted as the lens is tilted back and forth. No scratches or lathe marks should be visible. A closer inspection can be made of the lens surface quality by using a hand loupe or stereomicroscope. This procedure should follow that used in edge inspection. It simply involves tilting the lens to various positions so that the light source is seen in specular reflection. Under magnification it is possible to see much finer scratches, burrs, gouges, or bumps on the lens than can be seen with the naked eye. (A few fine line scratches can hardly be avoided in a lens and do no harm.) Care should be taken that the lens is clean and dirt is not mistaken for poor surface quality.

One of the most important clues to the optical quality of a lens is found during the measurement of the lens power with the lensometer. The image of the target, when focused, should appear as sharp and clear as it does with a spectacle lens. A target image that is blurred or dim may indicate a poor polish or a nonspherical surface on the lens.

COLOR

The specification of color in a contact lens is not standard,[59,60] and such lenses can only be checked by making visual comparison to a set of test lenses in the various colors. These are available from the contact lens company from which the lenses are purchased.

Care should be taken in duplicating a single lens from a pair of tinted lenses. If the laboratory does not maintain rigid standards for the colored plastic, the replacement lens may have a slightly different darkness or even a variation in hue.

Variation in Thickness

Small variations in lens thickness can cause considerable difference in the color intensity and, thus, the transmission of light through the lens. Hence, if the lens ordered is thicker than the test sample, it will appear much darker, even though it was cut from the same type of plastic.

Tolerance for Color

Lens color can be checked by comparing the lens to a standard sample when both lenses are placed on a white piece of paper. A visual inspection in this manner can be very sensitive, and any noticeable difference in the hue or darkness of the color should be cause for rejection.

SUMMARY OF INSPECTION ROUTINE

It is possible to inspect contact lenses accurately and quickly if a definite routine is followed. This routine should be designed to involve the fewest steps possible and to use the fewest instruments. The routine should also be such that the lens is cleaned a minimum number of times. Such a routine can be accomplished in five steps, using the following instruments:

1. Lensometer
2. Measuring magnifier
3. Radiuscope
4. Binocular microscope
5. Thickness gauge

When the lens is first removed from the mailing container, it is usually very clean and can be placed on the lensometer for a power reading. Care should be taken not to touch the surface of the lens as it is removed from the mailing container of the laboratory. After the lensometer reading is completed, the lens is placed against the measuring magnifier. During this procedure, it is necessary to touch the convex surface of the lens with your finger. Measurements should now be made of the total diameter, optic zone diameter, and peripheral curve widths. The lens may now be removed and placed on the radiuscope. The concave surface should still be clean for a reading. After the radius measurement is taken, the lens can be dried off for inspection under a binocular microscope. Following this, thickness is measured with a thickness gauge.

REFERENCES

1. Brown, H.: Contact lens inspection techniques, *Contacto, 5(10)*:335–337, 1961.
2. Elmstrom, G. P.: Contact lens standards, *Contacto, 6(11)*:332–334, 1962.
3. Manufactured by the Plastic Contact Lens Company, Chicago, Illinois.
4. Haynes, P. R.: Quality control and inspection of contact lenses, in *Encyclopedia of Contact Lens Practice*, South Bend, Indiana, International Optics, 1959–1963, vol. 1, Chap. 23, pp. 8–64.
5. Contact Lens Committee of N.Y. State Optom. Assoc.: Contact lens tolerances, *Opt. J. Rev Optom., 94(12)*:46, 1957.
6. Tahler, Z.: Modified method for curvature width measurement in corneal lenses, *Contacto, 8(2)*:11, 1964.
7. Stewart, C. R.: Blending corneal lenses, *Optom. Weekly, 54(51)*:2359, 1963.
8. Baldwin, W. R., and Shick, C. R.: *Corneal Contact Lenses: Fitting Procedures.* Philadelphia, Chilton, 1962.
9. Grosvenor, T. T.: *Contact Lens Theory and Practice.* Chicago, Professional, 1963.
10. Brown, W.: Minimum standards of contact lens practice, *Optom. Weekly, 56(36)*:57–60, 1965.
11. Girard, L. J.: *Corneal Contact Lenses*, St. Louis, Mosby, 1964.
12. Kienst, E. J.: Contact lens inspection, *Optom.*

Weekly, 51(26):1347–1349, 1960.
13. Shick, C.: A simple mire modification to improve keratometer efficiency, *J. Am. Optom. Assoc., 34(5)*:388–390, 1962.
14. Isen, A.: Methods that help achieve accurate ophthalmometry, *J. Am. Optom. Assoc., 30(10)*:723–724, 1959.
15. Tannehill, J. C., and Sampson, W.: Extended use of the radiuscope in contact lens inspection, *Am. J. Ophthalmol., (1)*:132–139, 1966.
16. Bailey, N. J.: The examination and verification of a contact lens, *J. Am. Optom. Assoc., 30(8)*:557–560, 1959.
17. Freeman, M. H.: Measurement of contact lens curvatures, *Am. J. Optom., 42(11)*:693–701, 1965.
18. Huang, D. T.: Technique of contact lens inspection, *Optom. Weekly, 52(10)*:459–564, 1961.
19. Dickins, R.: Investigation into the accuracy of the radius checking device, *The Optician, 151(3911)*:265–269, 1966.
20. Bennett, A. G.: Calibration of keratometers, *The Optician, 151(3913)*:317–322 1966.
21. Fletcher, R.: Contact lens standards, *The Ophthalmic Optician, 6(4)*:177–179, 1966.
22. Koetting, R. A.: Minimizing problems resulting from changes in contact lens radius, *Optom. Weekly, 54(43)*:1999–2002, 1963.

23. Manufactured by Kontur Kontact Lens Company, Richmond, California.

24. Laycock, D. E.: A microlens measuring aid, *Am. J. Optom.*, 34(10):538–539, 1957.

25. Brezel, D.: An instrument for measuring the base curves of contact lenses, *J. Am. Optom. Assoc.*, 31(5):379–380, 1959.

26. Bailey, N. J.: Inspection of a contact lens with the stereomicroscope, *Optom. Weekly*, 50(47):2317–2319, 1959.

27. Manufactured by American Optical Company, Southbridge, Massachusetts.

28. Bier, N.: Two new contact lens instruments, *Optom. Weekly*, 49(43):2032–2033, 1958.

29. Manufactured by Obrig Laboratories, Sarasota, Florida.

30. Manufactured by George Nissel, Inc.

31. Sarver, M. D., and Kerr, K.: A radius of curvature measuring device for contact lenses, *Am. J. Optom.*, 41(8):481–489, 1964.

32. Andrews, R., and Bord, S.: An investigation into the alteration in curvature of corneal lenses, *The Optician*, 143:276–278, 1962.

33. Arner, R. S.: The dimensional stability of corneal contact lenses as a function of fabrication technique, *J. Am. Optom. Assoc.*, 38:202–207, 1967.

34. Estevez, J. M. J.: Poly(methyl methacrylate) for use in contact lenses, *Contact Lens*, 1:19–21, 26, 1967.

35. Gordon, S.: Contact lens hydration: A study of the wetting-drying cycle, *Optom. Weekly*, 56(14):55–62, 1965.

36. American Optometric Association Contact Lens Standards, American Optometric Association, 7000 Chippewa Street, St. Louis, Mo., June 25, 1968.

37. Morrison, R. J., Kaufman, K. J., and Cerulli, E.: Base curve of polymethyl methacrylate contact lens, *Am. J. Optom.*, 42(1):17–20, 1965.

38. Neill, J. C., and Hanna, J. J.: A study of the effect of various media on the radii of microcorneal contact lenses, *Contacto*, 7:10–13, 1963.

39. Phillips, A. J.: Contact lens plastics, solutions, and storage—some implications, *The Ophthalmic Optician*, 8(19):1058, 1075–1076; 8(20):1134–1136, 1143; 8(2):1190–1192, 1203–1205; 8(22):1234–1238; 8(23):1312–1315; 8(25):1405–1508, 1413; 9(1):19–20, 25–27; 9(2):65–66, 75–79, 1968–1969.

40. Salvatori, P. L.: The effect of hydration upon corneal radius, *J. Am. Optom. Assoc.*, 32:644, 1961.

41. West, D. C.: A preliminary report on a comparative study of two methods for evaluating contact lens ocular zone radius, *J. Am. Optom. Assoc.*, 35:1065–1066, 1963.

42. Brungardt, T. F.: A fast, accurate and practical measurement of the secondary curve radius, *J. Am. Optom. Assoc.*, 34(2):131–134, 1962.

43. Brungardt, T. F.: The secondary curve radius, *J. Calif. Optom. Assoc.*, 31(3):184, 186, 191, 1963.

44. Bennett, A. G.: *Optics of Contact Lenses*, 3rd ed. London, Association of Dispensing Opticians, 1963.

45. Bailey, N. J.: The refractive power of a contact lens, *Optom. Weekly*, 51(21):1071–1074, 1960.

46. Ullen, R.: Front versus back vertex power readings on contact lenses, *J. Am. Optom. Assoc.*, 34(4):307–309, 1962.

47. Sarver, M. D.: Verification of contact lens power, *J. Am. Optom. Assoc.*, 34(16):1304–1306, 1963.

48. Cappelli, P. A.: Thickness of contact lenses, *The Dispensing Optician*, May, 1964.

49. Lester, R. W.: Contact lens checking in the office, *Contacto*, 1(3):44, 1957.

50. Lester, R. W.: The full circle of contact lens care, *J. Am. Optom. Assoc.*, 29(7):442–444, 1958.

• 51. Huang, D. T.: Technique of contact lens inspection, *Optom. Weekly*, 52(10):459–464; 52(12):565–569, 1961.

52. Swanson, W. L.: Results of edge contouring of contact lenses, *Optom. Weekly*, 51(43):2255–2257, 1960.

53. Shanks, K. R.: Subjective comparison of corneal lens edges, *Br. J. Physiol. Opt.*, 23(1):50–54, 1966.

54. Isen, A. A.: The relationship of edge thickness to center thickness of a contact lens, *Optom. Weekly*, 50(53):2581–2582, 1959.

55. Elmstrom, G. P.: Contact lens standards, *Contacto*, 6(11):332–334, 1962.

56. Lester, R. W.: Contact lens inspection using the slit lamp as a projection magnifier, *J. Calif. Optom. Assoc.*, 30(3):194–196, 1962.

57. Langsen, A. L.: Contact lens lensometer inspection, *Optom. Weekly, 52(19)*:923–924, 1961.

58. Tajiri, A.: Impression technique to determine edge contour of contact lenses, *Contacto, 4(9)*:391–397, 1960.

59. American Standards Association: *The Special Transmissive Properties of Plastics for Use in Eye Protection*, New York, 1955.

60. Glatt, L. D.: Effects of tinted contact lenses—a rebuttal, *Opt. J. Rev. Optom., 103(16)*:42, 45–46, 1966.

ADDITIONAL READINGS

Chaston, J.: Hard lens verification—an appreciation of errors, *The Optician, 170(4389)*:12–15, 1975.

Egan, D.: Toric base curves: lensometer vs. radiuscope, *Cont. Lens Forum, 4(7)*:55–59, 1979.

Gordon, S.: *Contact Lens Hydration: New Facts for the Fitter*, Gordon Contact Lenses, Inc.

Gordon, S.: Dimensional stability of contact lenses, *J. Am. Optom. Assoc., 42(3)*:239, 1971.

Gordon, S.: Dimensional stability of contact lenses—update 1976, *J. Am. Optom. Assoc., 47(3)*:336, 1976.

Hill, R. M.: PMMA and its environmental variations, *Int. Cont. Lens Clin., 5(1)*:63, 1978.

Lin, W. H., and Pinkus, A. G.: Assessment of hydrophilicity by contact angle measurement, *Optom. Weekly, 64(3)*:33–36, 1973.

Mandell, R. B.: Front vs. back power, *Int. Cont. Lens Clin., 2(2)*:24–25, 1975.

Ostrich, A. D., and Pailet, E.: Hydration of contact lenses, *Optom. Weekly, 51(27)*:1408–1409, 1960.

Pearson, R. M.: Dimensional stability of several hard contact lens materials, *Am. J. Optom. Physiol. Opt., 54(12)*:826–833, 1977.

Chapter 14

SYMPTOMATOLOGY AND REFITTING

SYMPTOMS

IN THE FIRST WEEK of contact lens wear, it is not anticipated that a patient will have normal, comfortable vision (Chapter 11). The patient will probably experience various adaptive symptoms that are later expected to diminish greatly or completely subside. If the adaptive symptoms persist beyond their expected duration, they are classed as abnormal symptoms, and steps must be taken for their correction.

In addition to the persistent adaptive symptoms, other abnormal symptoms may arise during the adaptive period. These may be masked by the adaptive symptoms and thus may not be recognized until the fourth or fifth day of contact lens wear. In general, abnormal and adaptive symptoms can be differentiated by observing the progress of the symptoms; abnormal symptoms persist and become worse, whereas adaptive symptoms diminish with each day of contact lens wear.

Some types of abnormal symptoms may not occur until months or even years after contact lenses are fitted.

Usually, a symptom has a physical or physiological basis. In a few instances, a symptom may have a psychological basis. If the symptom can be correlated with some physical cause, the source can usually be determined and corrected.[1,2] This may involve making a modification of the lens, changing the lens, removing an extraneous irritant, or correcting a faulty wearing procedure. If the symptom cannot be correlated with a physical cause,

the fitter should hesitate to make extensive corrections. During the first weeks of wear, it is especially important that the fitter does not interpret every symptom as a mandate for a lens change. One very often makes a premature decision of improper lens fit, and the lenses are modified or replaced when the adaptive process had actually not been completed and the change was not necessary.

There are six possible causes of an early symptom, only two of which require a lens change.

1. Adaptive problems
2. Procedural error by patient
3. Extraneous sources of irritation
4. Psychological problems of patient
5. Fitting error ⎫ Require lens
6. Faulty lens ⎬ modification
   construction ⎭

An abnormal symptom that occurs in the first few weeks of contact lens wear may be dismissed by the fitter as an adaptive symptom. If the patient is told that he is experiencing a normal adaptation, he may feel that the discomfort is too great and give up wearing the lenses.[3]

Some symptoms are related to ocular tissue changes. When the symptom and ocular tissue changes are related, the source may be obvious. At other times the defensive mechanism of the eye does not issue warning of the impending danger, and ocular changes occur without any symptoms. This may happen in two situations.

1. When the ocular change is insidious, so few symptoms occur. In this event symptoms may occur later. Detection of the ocular effect may allow its correction before any symptom occurs.

2. When the symptom occurred briefly but was ignored, and the patient adapted to its source.

Thus a routine examination is necessary for all contact lens patients, whether or not subjective discomfort is present.

EXAMINATION

With various tests it is possible to detect the sources of symptoms and also the ocular changes that may occur without symptoms. These tests should be performed during the examination and are given in their recommended order.

Interview

Considerable information about the source of a symptom can be determined from the patient's case history.[4] Sometimes a definite diagnosis can be made on this basis, but usually one or more tests are necessary for confirmation. If the patient is given sufficient opportunity to describe his symptom and is asked the proper questions, his statements will provide a clue to what the practitioner is likely to find in his other tests and, in addition, which tests are most needed. The discussion of differential diagnosis of symptoms from the history will be presented later in this chapter.

Visual Acuity

The patient's visual acuity with contact lenses should be measured before any other tests are given. This is advisable for the fitter's legal protection as well as for the diagnostic information provided. The patient's eyes may also become irritated during one of the other tests, thus invalidating a visual acuity measurement made later in the examination.

Examination of Lens *in situ* with White Light

A white light may be used to detect errors in riding position and movement of the lens. The specific characteristic for each lens depends upon the fitting philosophy that is being followed.

During the examination with white light, it should also be noted whether the appearance of the eyes is normal. A gross inspection can be made of the conjunctiva and lids for injection and other signs of irritation.

Observation of Blink

The patient's blinking characteristics and head and eye position should be noted during the interview without drawing attention that the observation is being made. A backward head tilt, downward gaze, squint, or partial blink will indicate an incomplete or abnormal adaptation (Figure 14.1).

Refraction

A routine refraction should be performed while the patient wears his contact lenses, using both retinoscopy and subjective tests. The subjective examination is usually composed of two parts. First, the correction that gives the maximum visual acuity is obtained by using only changes in spherical lenses. Second, if a satisfactory acuity is not achieved with the first method, the subjective test is extended using both spherical and cylindrical lenses.

Some practitioners prefer not to use any cylindrical lenses during the subjective examination. They point out that a patient who manifests 0.25 to 0.50 D. of astigmatism through his contact lenses may be satisfied

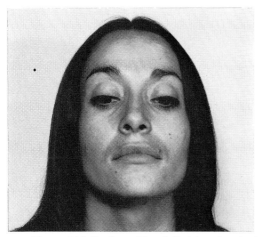 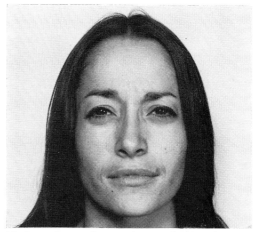

Figure 14.1. Backward head tilt (*a*) and squinting (*b*) due to incomplete or abnormal adaptation to contact lenses.

until he is shown that better correction is possible. If a residual astigmatic error remains when the patient wears his contact lenses, it can only be corrected by switching from one of the basic lens types to one of the special lens types (*see* Chapter 9). The special lenses are usually more difficult to fit and often cause more wearing problems than do the basic lens types. Their use may cause more difficulty than the slight residual refractive error present with spherical lenses. Consequently, the spherical lenses are preferred as long as the residual astigmatic error is low (as determined by the retinoscopy test) and as long as the patient has no blurring of his vision or subjective discomfort. If the patient feels that his vision is blurred through his contact lenses, and if the blurring cannot be cleared by spherical lens changes during the subjective examination, cylindrical lenses must be used.

Occasionally during the subjective examination in which only spherical lenses are used, the patient's visual acuity does not appear to be affected by large changes in either plus or minus power lenses. The small magnification effects of a contact lens as compared to a spectacle lens have sometimes been cited as the cause of this phenomenon. However, Abrams and Bailey have shown that, for the low powers involved, the difference in the magnification of spectacles and contact lenses is insignificant and cannot adequately explain this phenomenon.[5] They point out that it is most often due to the existence of residual astigmatism.

Biomicroscopy with White Light

The biomicroscope may be used to examine certain physical aspects of the contact lens fit, as described in Chapter 8. It may also be used to examine the appearance of the cornea, sclera, and lids to see if there are any signs of irritation by the contact lens. In addition, the contact lens front surface may be examined for coating and scratches.

The biomicroscope is most important because it is the only method by which corneal edema can be detected. Corneal edema may be caused by an improper bearing relationship of the contact lens.

Fluorescein Test with Lens *in situ*

The fluorescein test is conducted as it was described in the trial lens fitting method (Chapter 8). The criteria for its evaluation vary with the fitting philosophy used. Many practitioners make a brief sketch of the fluorescein pattern, indicating the areas of possible excessive bearing. (A space for this is provided in the record form [Chapter 4].) The drawing provides a quick reference for comparison during the other tests or at a later date.

The Contact Lens May Now Be Removed.

Fluorescein Test Without Contact Lens

Aside from providing a test to determine the bearing relationship between the contact lens and the cornea, fluorescein may also be used to evaluate the integrity of the corneal epithelium.[6-11] Epithelial injury may be caused by the chemical and physical changes that occur in the cornea when a contact lens is worn or by direct trauma. The fluorescein dye will collect or stain where destructive changes have occurred in the corneal epithelial tissue. A clear outline of the injured area may then be seen.

Detection of Abrasions

Abrasion refers to an actual mechanical injury to the cornea that removes tissue. Minor abrasions will only remove the epithelial layer, but more severe abrasions may remove parts of the deeper corneal layers. Illustrations of various abrasions when stained with fluorescein are given in Figure 14.2.

The term *erosion* is sometimes used to indicate an abrasion of the cornea caused by the continual rubbing of the cornea by a contact lens that has an incorrect bearing relationship. This will be discussed later.

Detection of Other Tissue Injury

If the corneal tissue is disrupted either by foreign chemical (or gaseous) substances, by inflammation, or by the accumulation of the products of metabolism in abnormal quantities, chemical destruction may occur. The areas of cornea disturbances will also collect the fluorescein stain and have certain charac-

teristic appearances, which are shown in Figure 14.2 and described later.

Viewing Aids for Fluorescein Test

Very large corneal abrasions usually can be seen with ultraviolet light and the naked eye. Smaller abrasions and other corneal injury can only be observed with the assistance of some type of hand magnifier. Very minor corneal injuries can only be detected with the aid of a biomicroscope that is equipped with a source of ultraviolet illumination. Such a biomicroscope is necessary to detect the minute early changes of disturbances in corneal metabolism.[12] Its use has been found to be nearly indispensable in contact lens practice.

Keratometry

The standard technique for keratometry measurements should be used to determine the corneal curvature. The measurement is conducted to detect any changes in the power or toricity of the cornea that have occurred since the lenses were fitted. In addition, the mire images should be observed during the measurement. If they are irregular, it indicates the corneal shape has been distorted. It is sometimes found that the focusing circles on the Bausch & Lomb keratometer mire image cannot be made to coincide. This is also an indication of corneal distortion.

Inspection of the Lens

Lens inspection is described in Chapter 13.

Recording Test Results

The results of the diagnostic tests can be better organized and interpreted if the record form contains specific spaces for their recording. (*See* record form, Figures 4.6 to 4.8.)

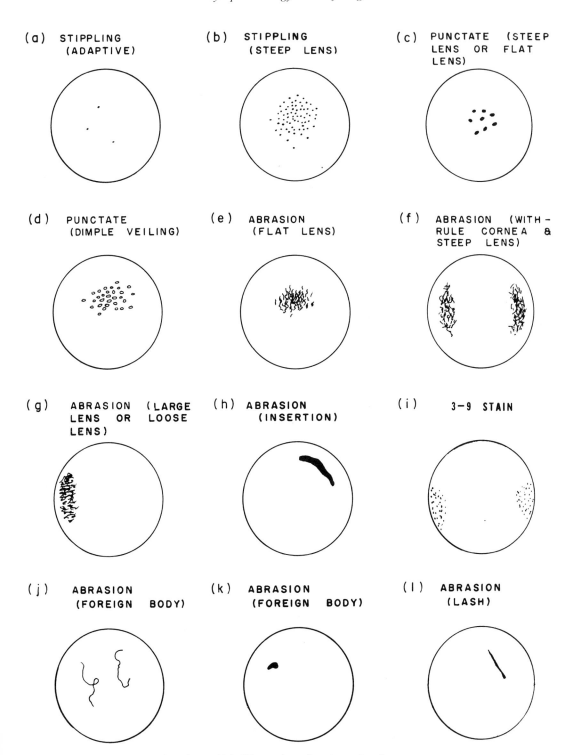

Figure 14.2. Illustration of various abrasions.

ORIGINS OF ABNORMAL SYMPTOMS AND OCULAR CHANGES

In Chapter 5 it was stated that a contact lens must fulfill various optical and physiological requisites to be worn comfortably. When these requisites are not fulfilled, abnormal signs and symptoms occur.

If an optical requisite of the lens fit has not been fulfilled, some type of visual disturbance will usually result. If a physiological requisite of the lens fit has not been fulfilled, some type of discomfort will usually result. The latter symptom is usually accompanied by tissue changes that may be detected by objective tests. If the condition is allowed to progress, it may eventually cause visual disturbances, too.

When the symptoms and signs of visual or physiological interference are correlated with observation of an apparent error in the physical lens fit, it is usually possible to determine the changes that are needed in the contact lens.

In analyzing the patient's wearing problems, the fitter should consider possible changes to be made in the contact lenses. If only a minor change needs to be made, the fitter (or his technician) may prefer to do this in his own laboratory. At other times the change will require that a new lens be ordered from the manufacturer. When possible, the fitter will usually prefer to modify the original lens rather than order a new one. The fitter will thus be concerned with which changes can be made on the lens and which will require a new lens (Table 7.4).

After the adaptation period there are five possible causes of symptoms and/or ocular change: fitting problems, faulty lens construction, procedural error, extraneous sources, and psychogenic factors.

FITTING PROBLEMS

Residual Refractive Error

A residual refractive error may occur even though every effort was made to obtain the correct power in the contact lenses during the fitting. The residual error may be spherical or astigmatic.

A residual spherical refractive error may be due to a lens that does not have the correct power or optical zone radius. The error may also be due to an incorrect determination of the original power needed for the contact lens. Possible sources are an incorrect refraction, failure to allow for working distance, and a mistake in converting from spectacle lens power to contact lens power. Also, a common power error occurs from an inaccurate measurement of the corneal power. This creates a different relationship between the optical zone radius of the contact lens and the cornea than is thought to exist. For example, if the cornea were measured as 43.00 D. and

it was really 44.00 D. and if the lens is thought to be fitted on *K*, it is really being fitted flatter than *K*, and the refractive error through the lens will be +1.00 D. The same type of error may be due to a cornea that is of such a shape that the keratometer does not give a valid reading. Haynes has pointed out that because of the many factors contributing to residual refractive error, small errors within the working tolerances may combine to produce a significant total error.[13]

A residual refractive error may occur because of the normal predictable condition when a contact lens is present, because of unwanted astigmatic power in the contact lens, or because of many factors that contribute to the total astigmatism of the eye (Chapter 9).

Symptoms

If the contact lens is made with (or when worn produces) excessive minus power to correct the patient's refractive error, it is often found that the overcorrection goes unnoticed by the patient and no symptoms are reported. An overcorrection in minus power of -2.00 D. was noted in one patient. She had apparently been wearing the lenses for some time with no symptoms. This of course was an unusual case, but patients are often seen whose lenses are 0.50 D. overcorrected in minus power and who have no symptoms. Toleration of an overcorrection in minus power in contact lenses when the same overcorrection in spectacle lenses would probably be intolerable is difficult to explain.

An excessive plus power or deficiency of minus power in the contact lens will usually be detected immediately by the patient as a constant blur. Any significant astigmatic error that occurs when the lenses are worn may prompt a report of blur by the patient or may cause asthenopic symptoms which are described by the patient as a vague discomfort.

Signs

The first indication of a residual refractive error may be a decrease in the visual acuity. Residual refractive error is confirmed by conducting a refraction while the contact lenses are worn by the patient. If a residual refractive error is present, the power and optical zone radius of the contact lens should be checked to determine whether the lens is in error or whether there was an error in the original order.

Alleviation

When the subjective part of the refraction is performed with only spherical lens changes and the patient's visual acuity is improved, the spherical power should be changed in the contact lenses. A power change up to ±0.75 D. can be made on the original contact lenses.[14] Larger power changes require that new lenses be made.

If the patient's visual acuity can only be improved by using both cylindrical and spher-

ical lenses, a full spherocylindrical correction is necessary. The question now arises whether the reduced visual acuity is bothersome enough to the patient to warrant the additional time, expense, and inconvenience of fitting a special contact lens with a spherocylindrical power. The patient must make this decision with the guidance of the fitter.

Lens Does Not Cover Sufficient Pupil Area

Sometimes the original measurement or estimate of the maximum pupil size was too small, and the optical zone diameter of the final lens is not large enough to cover the pupil. Also the final lens may not ride in a centered position before the pupil, so even though the optical zone diameter is large enough, it does not cover sufficient pupillary area.

Symptoms

Two possible symptoms may be reported: (1) intermittent blurring of vision or (2) reflection and fluttering of lights (flare). Blurring occurs because at times the pupil is partially covered by the peripheral curve of the contact lens, which does not give the proper correction for the patient's refractive error. Flare occurs because the peripheral curve of the lens causes a prismatic displacement of the light that passes through it.[15] Flare may also be due to pooling of tears at the edge of the lens, which has a prismatic effect on the light (Figure 14.3).[16] Tears at the lens edge form a meniscus, which has the shape of a prism with its base towards the geometric center of the lens. Flare from the peripheral curve is probably responsible for the fringes on lights, whereas the tear layer is usually responsible for the flare in which the light appears in long streaks. The patient may use any number of terms to describe the flare such as fringe, flashing light, glare, halo, ghost image, or even doubling. In the last case the patient is usually referring to the appearance of lights. He may see the light

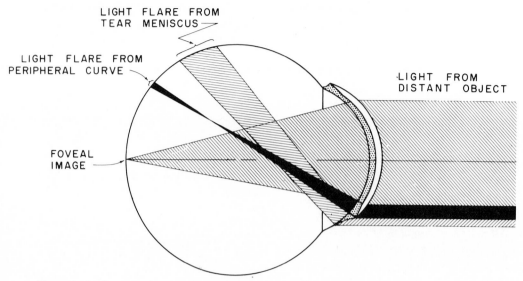

LIGHT FLARE FROM
TEAR MENISCUS

LIGHT FLARE FROM
PERIPHERAL CURVE

·LIGHT FROM
DISTANT OBJECT

FOVEAL
IMAGE

Figure 14.3. Flare may be caused either by the peripheral curve or by the tear meniscus at the lens edge.

itself as being separate from the blurred fringe, which he interprets as a second image.

If it is reported that the blur or flare occurs constantly and the lens is centered on the eye, it is likely that the optical zone is too small. If the patient reports that the blur or flare fluctuates, the lens is probably changing position. The patient may report that when he looks to the side his vision is improved. Usually this occurs because with the eyes turned to the side, the lens is trapped between the lids and centered before the pupil. The patient may also report that in looking to the side his vision becomes blurred. This is usually due to a lens that is loose and becomes displaced by the lids during lateral gaze.

Signs

The lens should be observed closely as the patient views an acuity chart. Ask the patient to report when his vision appears to be good or bad or when flare occurs. It can usually be noted that the best vision (or least flare) is obtained when the lens is centered. It is sometimes useful for the fitter to manipulate the

patient's lids to center the contact lens and then to note the changes in visual acuity.

Flare may be detected with a simple clinical test (Figure 14.4).[17] A square of light is projected on the acuity chart. The patient is then informed that the light should be in the shape of a perfect square and asked if there appears to be any fringes around the light and in which direction they are. The fringe of light that the patient sees will always be in the opposite direction of the decentration of his lens if the lens is off center. If the lens rides in a low position, the fringe of light will be seen on the top border of the square of light, and it will be seen to the left or right if the lens is decentered to the right or left, respectively (Figure 14.4). The direction of the flare can usually be confirmed by observing the lens position while the patient views the square. If the patient reports that there appears to be a flare around the entire square, it indicates that the optical zone is too small in proportion to the pupil size.

If changing the lens position does not eliminate the blur or flare, it may be concluded that the optical zone diameter is too

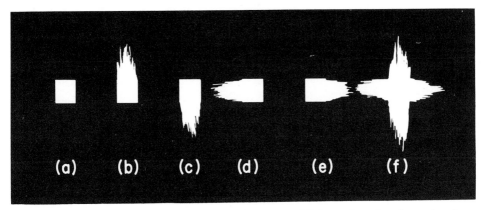

Figure 14.4. Detection of flare by observation of a square of light projected on the acuity chart.

small.

Alleviation

In only a few cases can a modification be made in the original lenses when the optical zone diameter is small. One instance is when a lens rides in a decentered position. This lens may be made to center better by thinning the edge or by reducing the total diameter so that less influence is imparted by the lid.

The method of correction for a decentered lens will depend on the direction of the decentration.

The displacement of lenses that ride nasally or temporally may be due to asymmetry of the cornea. Either the corneal apex is decentered or one-half of the cornea flattens more rapidly than the other. This has often been confirmed by the author in studies of the corneal topography of these patients, using the small mire keratometer (Chapter 3).

As a general rule, lenses that ride nasally or temporally should be replaced by lenses with larger optical zones and/or larger total diameters. Even when the corneal contour is known, it is not always possible to predict the effects of changes in the lens dimensions. Trial lenses should be used.

Occasionally, lateral displacement is caused by the lid configuration. This fitting problem can be corrected by using a small, steep lens, which rides within the palpebral fissure.

Lenses that ride high are most often those with minus power. It is extremely rare to see a lens with plus power that rides in a high position. Lenses with minus power present several characteristics that contribute to a high riding position.

1. *Center of gravity* for a lens of minus power tends toward the posterior side of the lens (*see* Chapter 5). The lens weight is easily supported by the cornea when the lens is in a high position.

2. *Edge thickness* of a minus lens presents a prominence that can be easily gripped by the lid. However, this is not the only force contributing to the faulty riding position.

3. *Corneal Contour* is often suspected as at least a contributing factor in high riding lenses. While there has been considerable speculation on this point, a valid study is lacking that shows a definite relationship between a given corneal topography and high riding lenses.

The first modification that should be made to a high riding lens is to make the lens edge as thin as possible. A lenticular lens may be necessary. If this is unsuccessful, the total diameter may be reduced. Unfortunately, the effect of the latter modification is unpredictable and may cause the lens to ride even higher. Usually, the lens is too thick for the smaller diameter, which results in excess movement. If the previous modifications do not correct for the high riding positions, the lens should be replaced by another. Modifications of the lens dimensions should be those which tend to make a lens fit tighter (Chapter 5). Special lens designs may be necessary (*see* Chapter 15).

The change that will most often center the lens is an increase of the optical zone diameter. This will give greater pupillary coverage and will often help to center the lens. An increase of 0.4 mm. will usually be sufficient.

Accommodation and Convergence

A myope must accommodate more through his refractive correction if it is in contact lenses than if it is in spectacles. If his accommodative amplitude is insufficient, it may be found that with contact lenses he develops symptoms when doing close work. In addition, a myope must converge more through his contact lenses, which may place new stress on his fusional convergence.

Hyperopes usually are not bothered by the switch from spectacles to contact lenses. They are then required to accommodate less and converge less.

Symptoms

The symptom of accommodative and convergence problems is usually one of vague discomfort after a period of wear. If the accommodative amplitude is low, there may be blurring after a period of sustained near work.

Signs

Accommodation and convergence problems may be detected by phorometry while the contact lenses are worn.

Alleviation

If the symptoms are due to an accommodative insufficiency through the contact lenses and the patient is young, he may eventually adapt to the condition. If he does not adapt, then visual training may be in order. As a last resort, it may be necessary to supply plus lenses in spectacle form as a supplementary correction to be worn for near work. For older patients plus lenses are the only possible correction.

If the symptoms are due to a convergence problem, they may be alleviated by visual training. If this is not possible, then a scleral contact lens may be used into which it is possible to incorporate prism. If a vertical phoria is present, it may be corrected up to two prism diopters by a prism ballast lens of proper prism power used in only the hyperphoric eye (*see* Chapter 15).

Tear Fluid Exchange

When the tear fluid behind the contact lens is not renewed periodically, the cornea is deprived of oxygen, and its metabolic products are not removed. This disruption of the normal corneal metabolism causes certain corneal effects and symptoms.

Tear fluid exchange behind the lens may be hampered by five conditions, which impede the contact lens pump (Chapter 5): (1) The lens may conform so closely to the corneal contour that little or no channel is present that will allow the lens to rock or in which fluid flow may take place. This condition most often occurs when a spherical cornea is fitted with a contact lens having a base curve of the same radius as the cornea. (2) The lens may have excessive apical corneal clearance because it either has a short radius of curvature or a large optical zone. Such a lens tends to bear heavily on the cornea at the border of the optical zone, and fluid is thus prevented from passing either into or out of the area behind the optical zone of the lens. (3) Lens rides in a decentered or low position onto a flatter peripheral part of the cornea, which gives the effect of a steep lens. (4) Inadequate peripheral curve, which interferes with the lens pump. (5) The lid may exert excessive force upon the lens. This condition is usually caused by a superior lid that covers too large an area of the lens (as may occur when a lens rides high), when a lens is too large, or when the superior lid is abnormally low. It may also be due to a superior lid that is excessively tight.

Impedance of tear exchange may be localized to one corneal area. Very often it is the corneal area behind the optical zone of the lens, but occasionally it may be the corneal area behind the peripheral zone of the lens, especially if the latter is covered by the lid.

Symptoms

Symptoms of metabolic interference do not ordinarily occur until some period of time after the contact lenses are inserted. The delay of onset is apparently directly related to the amount of tear exchange. With most corneal lenses there is a likelihood that tears will only be partially blocked; thus, symptoms of metabolic interference would not usually occur until two to five hours after the lenses are inserted. The symptoms are most often described as a hot, dry, or burning sensation, which is intensified with continued lens wear.* If, when the symptoms occur, the lenses are removed for a few hours and then worn again, the symptoms will at first be relieved but will latter reappear. If the patient continues to wear his lenses when discomfort persists, his vision is usually affected. The patient then reports that everything has a misty appearance, or, in some severe cases, that there are

halos around lights.†

It is sometimes found that the symptoms of metabolic interference may persist up to several hours after the contact lenses are removed. This interference with visual acuity, which has been called *spectacle blur*, may also be caused by other factors.

Signs

EXTERNAL EXAMINATION. Lenses that prevent adequate tear exchange are referred to as tight lenses, since in many cases they move very little and appear to be tightly held on the cornea. However, the appearance of inadequate movement does not necessarily prove that tear exchange is not taking place. Some lenses center well and apparently have little movement but are rocked sufficiently during blinking to provide adequate tear exchange.

FLUORESCEIN TEST. The amount of tear exchange may be estimated by the fluorescein test. However, this test is not conclusive, as most of the tear exchange takes place during blinking and occurs too rapidly to be observed. A steep fluorescein pattern may indicate that tear exchange is impeded. If, however, in spite of such a test result, the patient reports continuous comfortable lens wear and no edema is detected, the fitter may conclude that the fluorescein pattern was misleading. The fluorescein pattern interpretation may have been correct, but the test simply was not adequate to evaluate tear exchange.‡

---

*Smelser found that when experimental subjects had their corneas bathed in an increased CO_2 concentration, smarting or stinging sensations were caused.[18] It is not definitely known, however, whether this is the clinical cause of these sensations, though it is known that CO_2 is a waste product of corneal metabolism. Smelser also concluded that increased CO_2 concentration did not cause corneal edema and subjective symptoms of halos; these can be attributed to oxygen deprivation.

†The symptoms of misty vision and halos around lights often occur when haptic lenses are worn; they are associated with the lack of a tear-fluid exchange and are caused by corneal edema. These symptoms were described early by Fick and Sattler and have since become known as *Fick's phenomenon* or *Sattler's veil*.[19] These names, however, are seldom used to describe what are apparently the same symptoms (with the same cause) with corneal lenses.

‡The low correlation between the static fluorescein pattern and the performance of a contact lens is apparently what caused Mazow[20] and others to reject the fluorescein test. As the author has implied throughout this text, it is usually not the fluorescein test but the assumptions made on the basis of the test that are faulty.

A steeply fitted lens does not necessarily hamper tear exchange beneath the lens.[21] It is possible in some cases for a steep lens to be rocked and manipulated by the lids in such a way that adequate tear exchange is accomplished; however, it is also possible that a lens can have considerable movement on the cornea and still not provide adequate tear exchange. This most frequently occurs when a lens does not ride at a central position but is displaced to a high, low, or lateral position most of the time.

CENTRAL CORNEAL CLOUDING. When there is inadequate exchange of tears behind a contact lens, the oxygen level between the lens and cornea drops below the minimum level needed at the corneal surface to maintain normal corneal physiology. The cell walls on the outer corneal surface are disrupted and begin to allow water from the tear layer to pass into the epithelium. As the water collects in the cells, two effects occur: the cornea thickens,[22] and there is a disruption of the normal corneal transparency.

The edematous area scatters light in all directions (Figure 14.5a) and has the appearance of a hazy or cloudy area, which is usually light grey but may have a slight tint from the iris.[23] (The process is analogous to the formation of clouds in the sky from water droplets.)

The detection of this unique corneal edema, which is only found in hard contact lens wearers, can be achieved by using a specific observation procedure as follows:

1. The patient is seated at the slit-lamp biomicroscope, and the usual adjustments made.

2. The room is darkened completely.

3. A slit beam about 2 to 3 mm. in width is focused at the limbus from an angle of 45° to 60°.[23] A slight oscillation of the beam may be necessary to enhance the appearance of the edema.

4. The cornea is observed from a side position without the aid of the microscope. This may be accomplished by leaving the microscope in a centered position and observing from the sides or by swinging the biomicroscope out of the way. The observer must move his head back and forth slightly to obtain the best position for observation. The edema is detectable primarily by the contrast of its border against the dark background of the pupil, and the observer must find the proper viewing angle to accomplish this (Figure 14.5b). If the edema is viewed from a frontal position, the border may be superimposed on the iris and impossible to detect.

The edema can be observed with the lens in place but is somewhat easier to observe immediately after the lens is removed. If the observation is made properly, a round or oval cloudy area of 2 to 5 mm. diameter should be visible in the central region of the cornea.

The exact size depends upon the number of hours that the lenses have been worn and the magnitude of the tear exchange interference. The position is usually central but may be slightly off center corresponding to the riding position of the lens.

This type of edema has had various names,* but the author prefers that of *central corneal clouding* (abbreviated C.C.C.).

Onset. A contact lens wearer who has a deficient tear interchange begins to get corneal edema shortly after the lens is inserted. However, a period of one to three hours is necessary before the edema progresses enough that the C.C.C. is visible. The C.C.C. first becomes detectable when swelling reaches 4 to 7 percent (*see* Figure 14.7a). This level may be reached, and the C.C.C. may be visible earlier in an unadapted wearer because of the additional edema caused by the excess tearing effect. With the adapted wearer, the C.C.C. may appear at anytime from about two hours until the end of the wearing period, depending on the severity of the edema. An earlier appearance of C.C.C. indicates greater interfer-

---

*Central circular clouding; large, round edema; small, round edema; gross, circumscribed edema; disc edema.

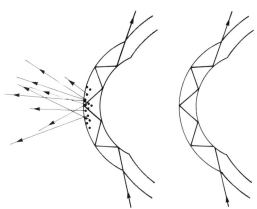

Figure 14.5a. Edematous area (*left*) scatters more light than normal (*right*).

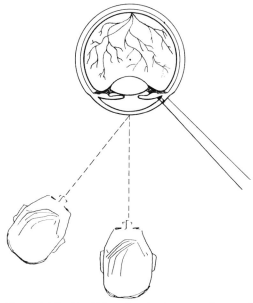

Figure 14.5b. Conditions for viewing central corneal clouding. The slit beam is focused at the limbus from an angle of 45° to 60°. The head is moved from a central to lateral position to aid the observation.

ence with the tear exchange. In order to detect mild cases of C.C.C., the adapted contact lens wearer should be examined after as many hours of wear as possible.

Grading C.C.C.. It is convenient for clinical purposes to grade C.C.C. according to degree (Table 14.1).

Observation Time. The density of the C.C.C. begins to fall immediately upon lens removal as shown in Figure 14.6. A grade two or three C.C.C. is usually not visible five to eight minutes after lens removal.

Incidence. Differences in the reported incidence of C.C.C. occur and are probably at least partly accountable for differences in observation technique. The two most common reasons for failure to detect C.C.C. are failure to observe immediately after the lens is removed and failure to use a completely dark room for the examination. The incidence of C.C.C. on the first day of lens wear and after adaptation is given in Figure 14.7b.

BIOMICROSCOPY. When corneal edema occurs as a result of contact lens wear, it is usually the milder type, confined to the epithelium. Epithelial edema, or *bedewing*, may sometimes be seen with direct illumination, although it is usually more clearly seen by using indirect or retroillumination. If the epithelial edema persists, the stroma eventually becomes involved.[24] This represents a more advanced edema.

Interference with corneal metabolism can lead to staining, which is best observed with a biomicroscope. Even before subjective symptoms appear, small, scattered pinpoint staining (from 1 to 20, round and discrete) may be

TABLE 14.1

0. No C.C.C.
1. Just detectable corneal haze without distinct borders.
2. Borders distinct but visible only against pupil background. Light density.
3. Borders very distinct. Area of clouding visible against iris and in dimly lighted room.

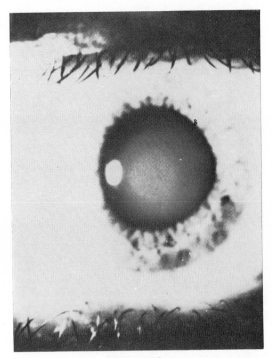

Figure 14.6a

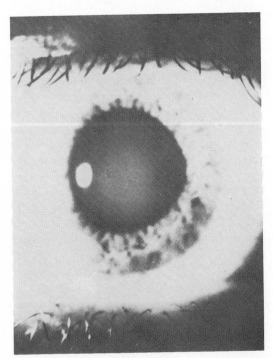

Figure 14.6b

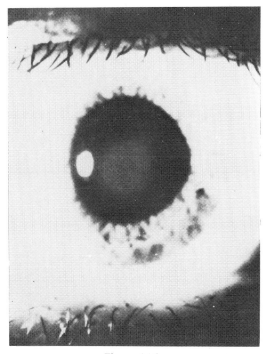

Figure 14.6c

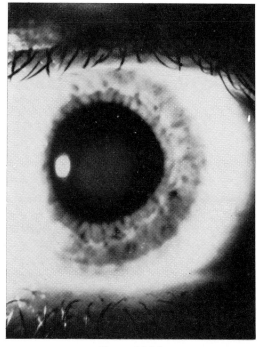

Figure 14.6d

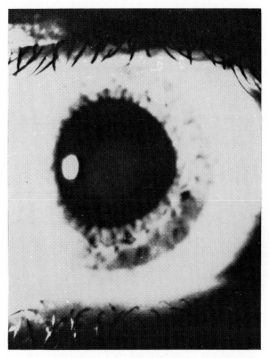

Figure 14.6e

Figure 14.6. The density of C.C.C. begins to fall immediately upon lens removal. Time in minutes after lens removal: (*a*) zero, (*b*) one, (*c*) two, (*d*) three, (*e*) five.

noted in the central corneal area. The staining is visible with direct or indirect illumination and is often termed *stippling*. If the condition is not corrected, the pinpoint stainings increase in number and size and coalesce into large areas of staining, which are visible with ultraviolet light and little or no magnification. When stippling becomes visible to the naked eye, it is distinguished as *punctate stains*.

The cornea must be examined for stippling immediately following a period of several hours of contact lens wear. If the lenses have been worn less than an hour, it is unlikely that any evidence of stippling will be present. If the cornea is examined several hours after the contact lenses have been removed, the rapid repair of corneal tissue may erase any evidence of stippling that occurred.

If the patient experiences symptoms similar to those associated with metabolic disturbance, the maximum observable effects will usually be seen coincident with or following the time of onset for the symptoms.[25]

KERATOMETRY. In addition to its direct observation with the biomicroscope, corneal edema may also be indicated by changes in the corneal curvature, which may be detected by keratometry. Any change of more than 0.25 D. from the original reading before contact lenses were fitted is significant. Unfortunately, keratometry is less reliable for the detection of corneal edema than the observation of C.C.C.[26] Although there is usually an increase in the keratometer power reading (Figure 14.8a), there may be no change or occasionally even a decrease, although corneal thickening has taken place (Figure 14.8b). This paradox occurs because the edema may or may not affect the areas of the cornea from which the keratometer mires are reflected (Figure 14.9a). This also causes distortion or

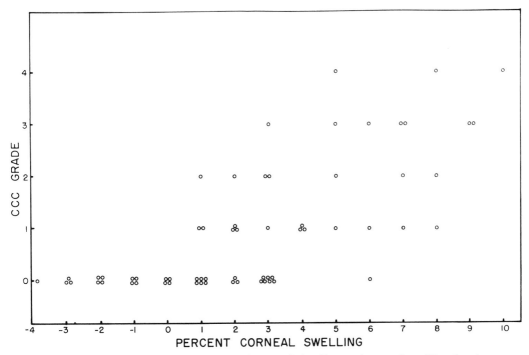

Figure 14.7a. Relationship between central corneal clouding and corneal swelling for sixty-four patients on first day of lens wear.

a change in clarity of the corneal mire images (Figure 14.9b). In addition, the size of the edematous area has more effect on changes in the keratometer reading than does the amount of corneal thickening (Figure 14.10).

REFRACTION. The corneal curvature increase that results from edema raises the refractive power of the cornea and, thus, the total refractive power of the eye. The net effect is an apparent change towards myopia. This change is only detectable by performing a refraction after the contact lenses have been removed. The technique is more reliable than keratometry but is used less because of the time involved.

SPECTACLE BLUR. A patient may report that vision is excellent with contact lenses, but after removing the lenses and resuming spectacle wear, his vision is blurred.

Differential Diagnosis

It must first be definitely established that

spectacle blur is actually present. Usually the patient's spectacles are not changed at the time contact lenses are given and do not have the correct prescription; thus, by contrast with the vision obtained with contact lenses, the patient may feel that the spectacle lenses give worse vision. A careful visual acuity measurement will enable the fitter to determine whether visual acuity has actually decreased with the spectacles.

Blur from corneal edema that follows a period of contact lens wear has two origins: the haze caused by the fluid and the temporary myopia collection caused by the corneal curvature increase. Depending on the grade of the edema, the blur may persist from a few minutes up to hours after the lenses are removed.

Alleviation

Metabolic disturbances of all types, which are caused by inadequate tear exchange, may

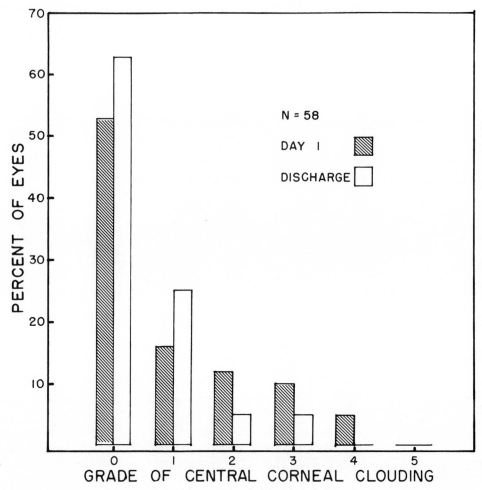

Figure 14.7b. Distribution of central corneal clouding by grade after first day of contact lens wear and discharge for sixty-four patients.

be corrected by the same modifications. If centrally located on the cornea, the occurrence of punctate staining or dimpling is often due to a steep optical zone on the lens. This can usually be eliminated by flattening the optical zone.

There are four possible modifications which can be made to the original lens, which may assist the tear exchange:

1. Flattening the peripheral curve
2. Reducing the total diameter
3. Reducing the optical zone diameter

4. Blending

Flattening the optical zone of the lens is a desirable method to increase tear exchange, but it requires that a new lens be made. Increasing lens thickness also requires a new lens and is not always effective in increasing tear exchange.

The simplest modification that can be made is to flatten the radius of the peripheral curve. This increases the rocking action of the lens on the cornea, thus providing a more effective pump mechanism.

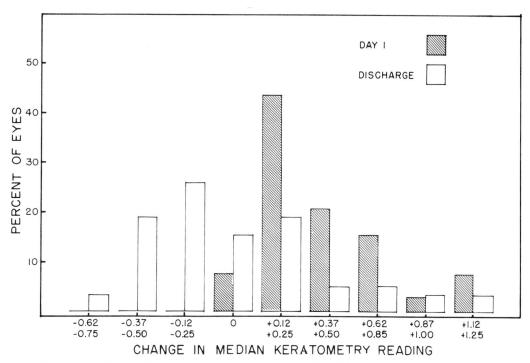

Figure 14.8a. Change in keratometry reading on first day of lens wear and at discharge for sixty-four patients.

The radius of the peripheral curve should be flattened until adequate circulation is achieved.

The diameter of the optical zone may be reduced by increasing the width of the peripheral curve, keeping its radius constant. This has the same effect as both flattening the optical zone and giving greater clearance to the peripheral curve. Reducing the optical zone diameter, however, introduces a chance that the optical zone may then only partially cover the pupil and result in reflections and flare. Hence, if the original lens has been selected with the minimum optical zone diameter for the pupil diameter, this modification will not be possible.

Blending the junction between the optical zone and the peripheral curve will have the same adverse effect as decreasing the optical zone diameter. Occasionally, blending will make the lens conform more closely to the corneal contour and thus make the lens fit tighter rather than looser on the cornea. A tool that is closer to the peripheral curve radius than the optical zone radius should be used.

If the corneal changes occur at the superior portion of the cornea, they may be caused by one of two factors, which will determine the lens changes to be made.

1. The lens may ride high so that the optical zone traps tear fluid at a superior position. The optical zone in this case is not necessarily steep, and if the optical zone is flattened, the lens will still ride high and cause the same problem. The lens must therefore be made to ride lower by decreasing the total diameter (which will also aid the tear circulation) or, paradoxically, by making the optical zone steeper.

2. The peripheral curve may be too steep. This may be detected from the fluo-

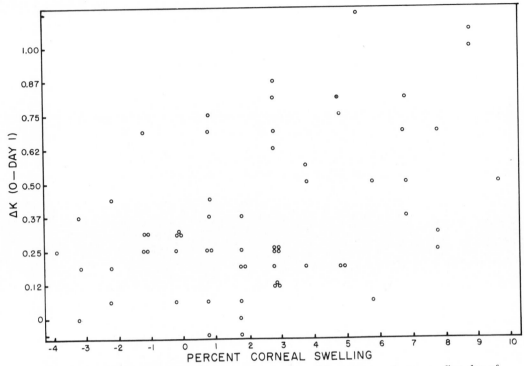

Figure 14.8b. Relationship between corneal swelling and keratometer change on first day of lens wear for sixty-four patients.

rescein pattern and corrected by flattening the peripheral curve.

Mechanical Pressure on Cornea

Intolerable mechanical pressure is exerted on the cornea whenever the contact lens bears on only a few small areas. The pressure may be caused by a lens that is too flat, in which case corneal trauma occurs in the central region; by a lens that is too steep, in which case corneal trauma occurs at the optical zone junction; or by a spherical optical zone on a highly astigmatic cornea. Since these three causes have varying effects, they will be discussed separately.

If the optical zone of the contact lenses is flatter than the cornea, the lens will rest on the central cornea and abrade only that area (*see* Figure 14.2). The lens may also be loose, since it does not conform to the cornea.

Symptoms

The patient may build up his wearing time with normal progress and then find that, following a few months of comfortable wear, his lenses become extremely painful and cause a stinging sensation. This pain may persist for several hours, even after the lenses have been removed.

Signs

The earliest signs of central corneal trauma are only visible with the biomicroscope.

Epithelial edema is often the first sign but may be confused with the edema of normal adaptation or with an interference in tear exchange.[27]

If the corneal clouding is due to exces-

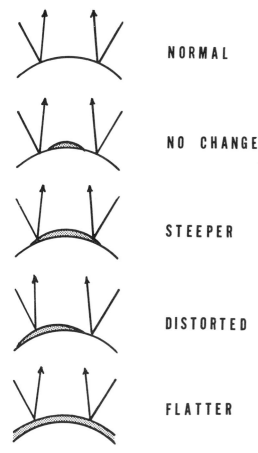

NORMAL

NO CHANGE

STEEPER

DISTORTED

FLATTER

Figure 14.9a. The area of corneal edema affects the keratometer reading.

bearing relationship. If, however, edema is present, the pattern may be misleading. If any abrasion is present excessive tearing may be caused, which interferes with a correct interpretation of the fluorescein pattern. The most accurate fluorescein pattern may be obtained when the patient has not worn his lenses for a day, or until no corneal stain is present.

Alleviation

The central corneal trauma usually results from both a flat lens and from excessive lens movement on the cornea. The first step in correction should be the reduction of the excess lens movement by one of the following methods:

1. Increasing total lens diameter
2. Increasing optical zone diameter
3. Decreasing lens thickness
4. Reducing edge thickness
5. Blending
6. Steepening optical zone
7. Steepening peripheral curve

Most of the changes suggested for making a lens fit tighter require the manufacture of a new lens. If the old lens is modified, it is only possible to blend the optical zone and reduce the edge thickness to tighten the lens. If the junction at the periphery of the optical zone is blended, it may increase the optical zone diameter. The radius of the blend curve should be as near as possible to the radius of the optical zone. The radius of the blend will ordinarily need to be at least 0.8 mm. longer than the optical zone radius to avoid damage to the optical zone during manufacture.

Reducing the edge thickness will reduce lens movement, which is caused by lid forces on the contact lens. A thinner edge provides less resistance to the lid and allows it to slide more easily over the lens.

If a new lens is to be ordered, the first consideration should be that the optical zone may be made steeper. The amount of change

sive apical bearing, the following usually happens:

1. The area of clouding usually corresponds roughly to the bearing area of the contact lenses.

2. At very early stages no changes or effects can be seen on the corneal epithelium. Later the epithelium will show minute erosion abrasion. If the condition is allowed to continue, the cornea will show edema with droplet formation and extensive central staining.

Fluorescein Pattern. The fluorescein pattern may provide evidence of an improper

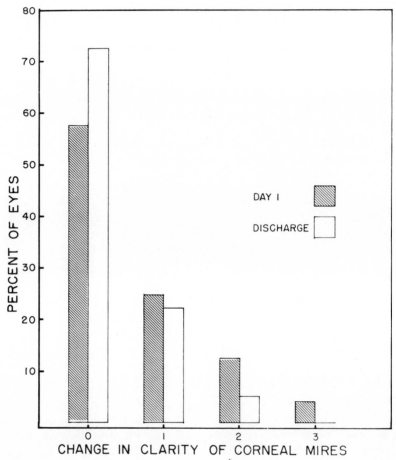

Figure 14.9b. Change in clarity of corneal mires on first day of lens wear and at discharge for sixty-four patients.

necessary may be determined by the fluorescein patterns of trial lenses and will usually be about 0.50 D. If considerable tightening of the lens is necessary, the total lens diameter or optical zone diameter may be increased. Steepening the peripheral curve and decreasing the lens thickness are less effective measures for reducing lens movement and may affect the lens pump.

Dimple Veiling

Occasionally, a small area of dimples or spherical pits appear in the corneal epithe-lium after contact lenses are worn.[28] Dixon and Lawazeck found corneal dimples in 65 of 353 patients wearing corneal lenses.[29] However, they are more common with the earlier fitting methods with flat lenses. The dimples can be seen with the biomicroscope as small depressions in the epithelium. Fluorescein will collect in the depressions, but most of it can be flushed out with irrigation fluid. The dimples may distort the image of the mires seen through a keratometer. One to four hours after the contact lenses are removed, the dimples usually disappear.

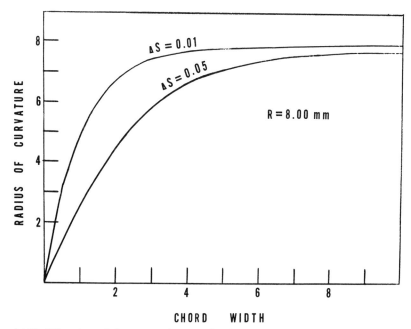

Figure 14.10. The size of the area of corneal edema has more effect on changes in the keratometer reading than does the amount of corneal thickening. Shown is the radius change for corneal thickening of 0.01 mm. and 0.05 mm.

Corneal dimples are not usually associated with any symptoms unless they are centrally located, and then they may cause a slight blurring. The appearance of corneal dimples, however, may be an indication that the fit of the lens is incorrect, and this may eventually cause other symptoms and effects to the corneal tissue.

The exact cause of corneal dimples is not known, but they appear to be associated with impaired tear flow in a space where there is excessive lens clearance in the post-lens area. Some authors attribute their occurrence to the presence of air bubbles that have been trapped behind the lens and impressed into the cornea (Figure 14.11).[30,31] Dixon and Lawazeck feel, however, that the dimples occur before the bubbles.[29] They observed on several occasions with a biomicroscope that a patient who had just put on his contact lenses had bubbles in the post-lens area and that the bubbles did

not remain stationary. After the lenses had been worn sixty to ninety minutes, they detected a few punctate stains. Thirty to sixty minutes later the punctate stain areas had increased in size to form the dimples, and the bubbles collected in them. The bubbles would not collect unless dimples were present. The bubbles remained trapped and stationary in the dimples while the lens and the post-lens fluid were moving.

Dixon and Lawazeck further attempted to determine the contents of the bubbles that remained in the dimples, and which had been collected with mercury-filled micropipettes and analyzed by spectroscopy.[29] They were found to contain air saturated with water vapor.

Excessive Lens Movement—Lid Irritation

Usually, if the lids are bothered by the contact lenses and the lenses have a normal

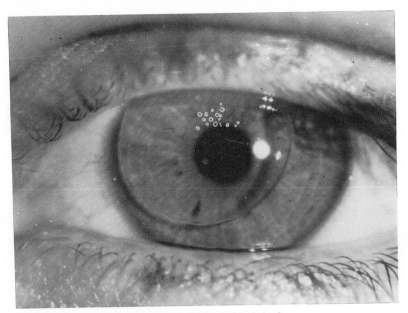

Figure 14.11. Bubbles behind the lens.

fitting relationship, the edges of the lenses have not been properly finished.

Symptoms

The lenses are uncomfortable as soon as they are put on the eye and become more uncomfortable the longer they are worn. Occasionally photophobia, excess lens movement, and difficulty in eye movement are present. The sensation may be described as a scratchy feeling, an itch, or mild pain. Relief is normally immediate upon removal of the contact lenses.

Signs

The lenses ride off center or fall out. Hyperemia at the lid margins may or may not be present. Hindered passage of the lids over the lens may be observed with a biomicroscope.

Alleviation

The lens edge should be modified to con-

form to "acceptable" contour.

Other Causes of Lid Irritation

Occasionally a lens that is exceptionally loose will strike the lower lid repeatedly and create symptoms of discomfort even though the edge contour is acceptable. Such a lens can only be corrected by reducing lens movement. Patients vary considerably in their ability to tolerate a lens that rides downward and touches the lower lid.

Poorly Fitted Lenses That Cause No Problems

Normally, if the physical criteria of the contact lens fit are fulfilled, a minimum of symptoms can be expected. This usually proves to be true. If the physical criteria are not fulfilled, symptoms are expected to occur. This is often, but not always, true. What constitutes an optimally fitting lens for one eye may be inadequate for another eye. For example, though a near parallel relationship between the optical zone and the central cornea is ideal for most eyes, for some eyes this relationship is not ideal. Sometimes the optical zone must be flatter to allow sufficient tear circulation behind the lens. At other times the optical zone must be steeper to eliminate improper bearing.

It may not be possible to determine what the best characteristics of a lens are for an individual eye until a lens has been worn. Consequently, it is not usually advisable to change the lens characteristics on the basis of the fit alone. Fitting characteristics that are only slightly in error may still be adequate. Of course, if the fit is obviously wrong, a change should be made immediately, but this should only be done if there is a good chance that the lens will eventually cause symptoms or tissue change. For example, if a lens rides high and there is obvious blanching of the vessels at the superior limbus, it is wise to take steps to center the lens because tissue damage is likely to occur eventually. However, if the lens rides low

and bumps against the lower lid, there is no need to change the lens unless symptoms occur. It may be that the lower lid is insensitive and no harm is done by having lens touch.

In certain instances the lenses may appear to be fitted poorly, but the patient experiences no subjective symptoms, and there is no evidence of ocular tissue change. Whether the lenses should be changed to produce a better fit will depend on the nature of the "fitting error" and on whether it is likely to produce symptoms or tissue changes at a later date. It also depends upon whether there will only be visual effects or whether tissue effects are also to be expected.

Three and Nine O'Clock Staining

Three and nine o'clock staining refers to a characteristic peripheral form of corneal staining associated with contact lens wear.[32] It is usually confined to those areas of the cornea at the three and nine o'clock positions which are not covered by the contact lens or the upper lid.[33] The staining appears as an area of arcuate shape, which is composed of small, punctate stains (Figure 14.12).

Although the stain is commonly found at the three and nine o'clock positions on the cornea, it also may be found at a lower corneal position and may extend around the entire inferior corneal area. The exact shape and area of staining is determined by the lens design and riding position.

Three and nine o'clock staining may result from wearing all types of contact lenses,[34] but it is felt that the incidence is usually greater for the interpalpebral fitting philosophy.[35] With larger contact lenses the staining may be confined to the extreme periphery, while a smaller lens may have a broader area of stain. It is usually bilateral.[36]

There have been various causes and solutions offered for this problem, but the results are indefinite.

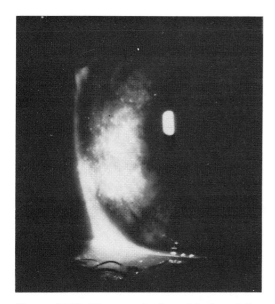

Figure 14.12. Three and nine o'clock staining appears as an area of arcuate shape. Courtesy of D. Korb.

Peripheral staining may occur during the first few days of lens wear but usually requires weeks of all-day wear. It rarely disappears spontaneously after its first occurence and usually continues to increase in severity.

The consensus of most authorities is that the staining is caused by a disturbance of the normal tear layer. This disturbance is thought to occur as a result of inadequate blinking. It is felt that the contact lens presents enough irritation to the lid that the normal blinking process is inhibited and gives rise to partial blinks. Hence, the lid only occasionally covers the lower corneal area completely. This effect is sometimes detectable as "prow lines" on the contact lens at the lid closure position (Figure 14.13). The area immediately below the lens is not commonly affected because a partial blink is sufficient to move the lens across this area. Hence, the only corneal area that is not covered at any time by either the lid or the contact lens is the three and nine o'clock area (Figure 14.14).

A possible mechanism by which the inhibition of blinking leads to three and nine o'clock staining has been given by Lemp et al.[37,38] They feel that the blinking process is necessary in order to massage mucus, formed on the palpebral conjunctiva, onto the cornea. The cornea itself has no goblet cells and must receive its mucus supply by this indirect route.

An alternate theory proposes that the edge of the lens holds the lid away from the cornea and produces a lid gap.[33]

For most patients, three and nine o'clock staining is minimal and rarely leads to complications. However, a few patients have a progression of this condition, which leads to an infiltrated lesion affecting the stroma and which may ulcerate.[34]

Various techniques have been attempted to eliminate three and nine o'clock staining, including artificial mucus substitutes, artificial tears, various lens modifications, and blinking exercises. None of these is totally successful in eliminating this condition. The most effective treatment would appear to be making whatever changes are necessary in the lens design that will allow the patient to

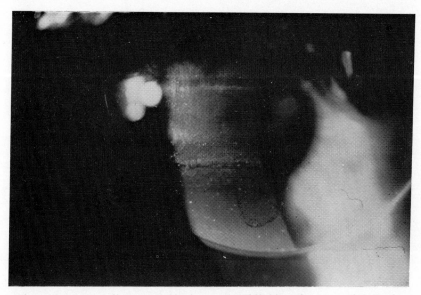

Figure 14.13. Prow lines caused by incomplete blinking. Courtesy of D. Korb.

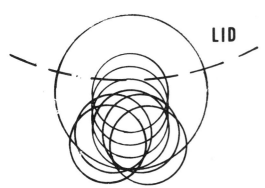

LID

Figure 14.14. Corneal areas that are not covered by the lid or the contact lens correspond to the area of three and nine o'clock staining.

adopt a more normal blink pattern.

Recurrent Corneal Erosion

It is occasionally found that following trauma to the cornea, healing appears to be complete but that subsequently new abrasions continue to form in the same area. Typically the patient will report that upon arising in the morning he feels a sudden pain in the eye, which is accompanied by tearing and photophobia. The symptoms usually persist for several hours and then are relieved only to be repeated again the following day. The patient may go for a period of weeks with no further symptoms and then experience the same phenomenon again.

When the patient is first examined, it may be felt that there is no apparent problem with the cornea. However, a careful examination may reveal a slight epithelial edema or an abnormally short tear breakup time.

This condition may occur in either a patient who is wearing or not wearing contact lenses. The contact lens wearer may have had his lenses for some time with absolutely no wearing problem. Then following a corneal abrasion due to a foreign body or some other cause, the sequence described occurs.

This condition results because the basal membrane of the epithelium requires considerably longer healing time than does the epithelium and leaves the epithelium with a weak adherence to the underlying tissue.[39-42] Any mild trauma is then sufficient to detach the epithelium once again from Bowman's membrane. This detachment may be caused simply by an adherence of the lid to the epithelium during sleep so that upon opening the eyes in the morning, the epithelium is pulled from its base.

When this condition occurs in a hard contact lens wearer, there is no solution other than to remove the lenses for a period of two to three months to allow the cornea sufficient time for complete healing. Alternately, the patient may be switched to a hydrogel contact lens, which is purported to cause less traumatic effect in these cases.

Conjunctival Xerosis

Occasionally a contact lens wearer develops a perilimbal xerosis, localized most frequently along the 180° meridian on the nasal and/or temporal bulbar conjunctiva.[43] The slightly elevated, pearly surface gives these areas much the same appearance as the classical Bitot spot.

The presence or absence of a contact lens can influence the level of development of these xerosis lesions to a point of stability (full development or complete absence) within a few days. They all appear to subside, regardless of how long they are established. Such a time course of days would not be expected if this is, in fact, a typical xerosis, incorporating epidermidalization and keratinization of the conjunctival epithelium.

There is yet no obvious lens design or physiological factor that appears reliably correlated with the xerosis condition.[43]

PROCEDURAL ERRORS

Faulty Insertion

A few patients have more than usual difficulty inserting a contact lens, and sometimes a lens may be inserted so poorly that corneal abrasion results.

Symptoms

The patient usually reports that he felt immediate and intense pain upon inserting the lenses. The pain may last for several hours and is often accompanied by blepharospasm and profuse lacrimation. If the abrasion is large, the patient may be unable to wear his lenses.

Signs

An abrasion from faulty insertion procedure usually, but not always, has a crescent-shaped appearance. When stained with fluorescein and observed under ultraviolet light, it can usually be seen even without the assistance of a magnifier.

Alleviation

To insure that the abrasion is not repeated, the patient should practice insertion under the guidance of the fitter until his technique is perfected.

Wearing Time Changes and Rapid Increases

When the patient first begins to wear contact lenses, he is limited to only a few hours of wear. Various physiological adaptations take place in the cornea that may not be completed for several weeks.

Even for patients who are fully adapted, it is found that if the contact lenses are not worn for several days, it is not possible to resume full wearing time without a risk of irritation to the cornea. It is usually advisable for the patient to limit his wear to six hours on the first day of resumed lens wear.

He may then increase his wearing time a few hours each day.

Some people appear to be extremely sensitive to any changes in their wearing schedule. Others find they can wear their lenses full time one day, a few hours the next day, and full time again on the third day without any discomfort. However, if a patient exceeds his recommended wearing time by three or more hours, there is always a danger that the cornea will be irritated.

Symptoms

If the lenses are worn only a slightly longer time than advisable, there may be a mild reaction of discomfort and slight blur.

If the lenses are worn much too long, the reaction is often one of extreme pain. The patient will tear profusely and have severe photophobia with blepharospasm.

Frequently, a patient who overextends his wearing period does not experience any immediate effects of discomfort upon removal of the lenses. The patient may retire, only to be awakened a few hours later by ocular pain of a most severe type. The delay of symptoms is due to corneal anesthesia, which is produced by a lack of oxygen and by the accumulation of metabolic by-products when the contact lenses are worn.[44] Later, when the anesthesia diminishes, symptoms caused by the corneal disturbance are experienced.

Signs

Mild reactions to overwear are usually due to corneal edema, which may be seen with the biomicroscope.

If the symptom is pain, a central corneal abrasion is probably present. The abrasion appears very much like that caused by a lens with a flat bearing relationship. If the patient is not seen until several hours after the abrasion occurs, it is unlikely that evidence of the abrasion will be seen.

Alleviation

The patient should be told the reason for his painful reaction and instructed on proper wearing procedures.

Switched Lenses

Cause

Lenses are usually switched when both lenses are removed from the eye before one lens has been placed in the storage case.

Symptom

The symptom will depend upon the difference in construction and power of the two lenses. If the lenses vary in power considerably, the patient may have blurred vision in one eye and realize his error immediately. Occasionally one eye has more minus power but a steeper corneal curvature than the fellow eye, and when the lenses are switched there may be little effect on visual acuity, so the patient is unaware of the switch. However, the fit would probably be incorrect for both eyes and cause enough irritation to indicate to the patient that something is wrong.

Sign

Any sign that corresponds to incorrect fit will be present. The practitioner should check the lens specifications.

Prevention

The patient should be taught to remove one lens and place it in the case before removing the lens from the other eye.

Incorrect Lens Storage

If the lens is not cleaned when it is removed from the eye, sebum and mucus may coat the lens. If it is then allowed to dry between wearing periods, the secretions may form a hard coating on the lens surface that is not easily removed. The lens may have a tendency to flatten if allowed to dry between wearing periods (Chapter 13).

Symptoms

The coating on the lens may interfere with vision or (rarely) cause corneal abrasions.

Signs

An abrasion may be present. If the lens flattens, it may show an incorrect fitting relationship.

Alleviation

The patient should be made to understand the value of cleaning his lenses upon the removal from the eyes and the necessity of storing the lenses in a soaking solution.

EXTRANEOUS SOURCES

Foreign Bodies

Numerous foreign bodies present an occasional menace to contact lens wear. Foreign bodies may be in the form of a solid, gas, or liquid.

Solid Foreign Bodies

These are particularly hazardous for a patient wearing contact lenses because the foreign body may become trapped behind the lens and cause considerably more corneal damage than would occur if the contact lens were not present. It is also more likely that the foreign body will actually become embedded in the cornea if the contact lens remains in position. Usually foreign bodies consist of dirt or sand, but they may be any fine piece of solid material that is introduced into the eye. Usually a foreign body that is embedded in the cornea behind a contact lens is smaller than that which is likely to become embedded when no contact lens is worn. If the patient is constantly exposed to small particles, scleral lenses may be needed.[45]

Signs

The appearance of the corneal abrasions caused by a solid foreign body is quite variable. It may have a spiral appearance, which is caused by the movement of the foreign body from the periphery of the lens toward the center while the lens shifts up and down (Figure 14.15a). The foreign body may also have a single, discrete area of abrasion if it has not been moved around significantly by the lens (Figure 14.2).

For women, cosmetics and the various applicators for their use present potential hazards. It is not uncommon to see an abrasion of several vertical lines at the superior portion of the cornea. The abrasion may be thought to be caused by faulty insertion procedures or a bad lens edge, but it is often caused by striking the cornea with a mascara brush. It is possible to produce this type of abrasion even while the contact lenses are being worn. If the cornea is relatively insensitive, due to contact lens wear, the pain may not be felt until a much later period. The delay of symptoms often makes the diagnosis of this type of abrasion difficult.

It is possible that pieces of the mascara or eye shadow may enter the eye. These may be irritating but rarely cause abrasions.

Symptoms

A foreign body that does not cause corneal abrasion will still produce discomfort. The contact lens should be removed immediately to prevent the possible entrapment of the foreign body behind the lens.

Immediate pain accompanied by profuse lacrimation and photophobia is usually experienced when an abrasion is produced by a contact lens. Usually the extreme severity of the pain will force the wearer to remove his contact lens. It is particularly dangerous, however, if a patient does not remove his lenses when pain is experienced, as he may adapt to the pain and feel that the irritation has been removed.

Thermal, Chemical, and Irradiative Injuries

There are various irritants that may harm the cornea either with or without the contact lens, but the presence of the contact lens may intensify the symptoms. Thermal injuries of the cornea commonly occur from flames, hot fluids, or various gases. Patients who must work in smoky rooms may find it impossible to wear their lenses. Aerosol sprays, e.g. hair spray, may be accidently directed into the eyes (Figure 14.15b). The corneal effects will depend upon the extent of the exposure and may vary from mild stippling to complete denudation.

WETTING SOLUTION. It is occasionally proposed that various wetting solutions can themselves cause irritation to the eye. It is thought that factors may be responsible, such as high pH. Other sources may be responsible such as soap on the hands, any number of chemicals, or the condensation of tobacco smoke on

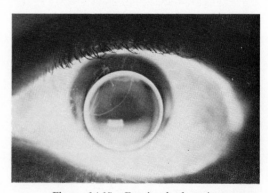

Figure 14.15a. Foreign body stain.

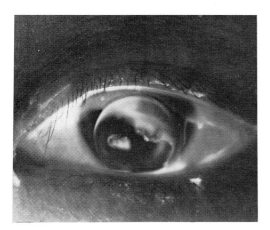

Figure 14.15b. Lens coated with aerosol spray.

the fingers.

SYMPTOM. A stinging or burning sensation may occur immediately after the lens is inserted. It may diminish with time or may be so severe that the patient removes and reinserts his lenses, starting the cycle over again.

SIGN. None.

ALLEVIATION. Switch wetting solution brand or improve hygiene.

Pathology

Various pathological conditions of the body may affect the ocular tissue. If contact lenses are worn, these conditions may need to be alleviated, especially if there is an infectious agent present. These conditions have been discussed in Chapter 4.

General metabolism may be affected by various endocrine disturbances, pregnancy, or menopause. These may produce changes in the tear volume and cause varying degrees of discomfort when contact lenses are worn.

Birth Control Pills

There has been considerable publicity with respect to ocular side effects that are caused by various birth control pills.[46-50] These medications may upset the normal tear supply or cause corneal edema and lead to a temporary inability to wear contact lenses.[51-56]

Vitamin Deficiency

It is entirely possible that deficiencies of the various vitamins could predispose the cornea to tissue damage by a contact lens. This is probably extremely rare in the United States.

Vitamin A deficiency could produce dryness of the conjunctiva or corneal xerosis or possible keratomalacia. Vitamin B complex deficiency could cause corneal vascularization. McLaren,[57] however, feels that invasion of the cornea by capillaries is more likely due to other causes than nutritional deficiency. Unless there is other confirming evidence of vitamin deficiency, ocular effects that occur when wearing contact lenses should not be attributed to this source.

Psychological

Symptoms that do not follow any definite pattern and which are not accompanied by any objective signs of ocular irritation may have a psychological origin.

DIFFERENTIAL DIAGNOSIS OF SYMPTOMS AND SIGNS

Very often information can be gained from the case history to determine the cause of a patient's symptom. The patient should be allowed to explain his problem in detail, and the practitioner should learn to extract the maximum information by asking pertinent questions. In this way he can more easily effect a differential diagnosis.

Symptoms are most easily differentiated on the basis of their type, time of onset, and course following onset.

TYPE OF SYMPTOM

Symptoms may be divided broadly into two types, visual interference and discomfort. Within these types, the divisions become less distinct. It becomes increasingly difficult to interpret exactly the terms that the patient uses to describe the visual symptom or discomfort he is experiencing. The sensations that are described are subjective evaluations of experiences that are interpreted quite differently by one patient in comparison to another, e.g. what one patient calls discomfort, another may call stinging. Consequently, some latitude must be given to the interpretation of any term used by the patient to describe his experience.

Visual

A visual anomaly that an experienced observer would call blur will most likely be called a blur by a patient. He may, however, use terms such as fogging or hazing. These must be differentiated from the hazing that is sometimes reported by the patient when the cornea is edematous, from the halo effect that is only seen in connection with lights, and from the flare or "fluttering" appearance of lights.

When the visual sensation is clarified, the time of onset should be ascertained. It is most important to know if the symptom begins immediately upon insertion of the lenses or if it is delayed until after some period of comfortable wear. If the symptom has a delayed onset, the time of onset should be determined, but this usually tells only the degree of effect and is not very informative for differential

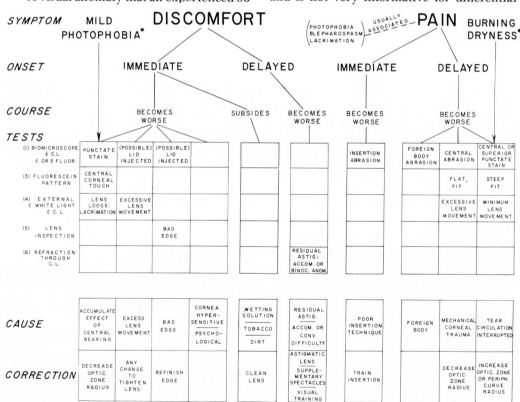

Figure 14.16. Scheme for differential diagnosis of symptoms and signs.

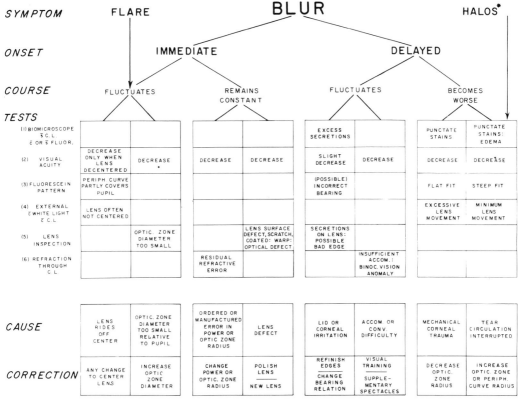

Figure 14.16a.

diagnosis.

Once the time of onset is determined, the course of the symptom should be established. Whether the symptom fluctuates, remains relatively constant, or diminishes or increases in intensity should be considered.

When all the information about the symptom has been gathered, the practitioner is ready to perform the tests. If he is concerned only with the immediate symptom, he may use only those tests which will in all likelihood verify the tentative diagnosis made from observation of the symptom. This course of events is presented in schemative form in Figure 14.16. Beginning at the top, the type of visual symptom present is selected. The procedure is determined by the time of onset, which is illustrated on the step below symptom types. On the third step down, the possible symptom courses are illustrated; the appropriate one should be isolated. At this point the number of possible sources for the symptom will have been greatly reduced. Further differentiation is now possible by various specific tests.

Discomfort

If the symptom is of some type of discomfort, the same analysis procedure may be used as was applied to the visual symptom.

Usually it is fairly easy for the patient to differentiate between two types of discomfort, a mild feeling of "hurt" or a more severe pain. The time of onset and the course that the symptom follows are then determined. A series of tests are used for the final differentiation. In some cases only a visual or discomfort symptom will be present; at other times both will be present. In the latter case, it should be possible to analyze the disturbance from either the visual or discomfort symptom. The same analysis from each of the symptoms will usually confirm the correct analysis.

No symptoms may be present, but during the examination abnormal signs may be found and their causes may also be differentiated by Figure 14.16. One only needs to compare the results of the appropriate tests (given in the respective rows) until the cause is found. If the same result is found in more than one vertical column, further differentiation may be possible by testing for the other results found in the corresponding vertical columns.

All the information that is necessary to diagnose the multitude of signs and symptoms which sometimes accompany contact lens wear cannot be presented in a table, no matter how complex. However, this schema does indicate the most probable cause of any symptom or sign, and it may be used as a *general* guide for the procedure of differential diagnosis.

Ocular Problems Not in Schema

In addition to the causes of signs and symptoms on the schema, there are a few problems that cause such definite symptoms or signs that they can be differentiated on that basis.

Symptoms Associated with Reading

The patient may report that he has difficulty wearing his lenses while reading but is comfortable at all other times. The symptoms may have various causes, which are differentiated by their type and time of onset.

BLUR. If blurring is experienced as soon as the lenses are worn, the lens is probably no longer centered before the pupil. The patient should be observed while he reads to see if the lenses center correctly. Very often a lens may strike the margin of the lower lid and be displaced upward while reading. This difficulty may be corrected by reducing the total diameter of the lens.

In a few few cases of myopia, immediate blur with reading may be caused by an insufficient amplitude of accommodation. The myope is unable to meet the increased accommodative stimulus produced by the substitution of contact lens correction for spectacles (*see* Chapter 4). This may be corrected by visual training or supplementary spectacles.

If blur does not occur until an hour or more after the lenses are inserted, discomfort will usually accompany it. The blur and discomfort are occasionally due to an accommodative insufficiency or binocular imbalance. More often, however, delayed blur and discomfort result from an inadequate tear exchange. During reading, the gaze is lowered with an accompanying drop in the position of the superior lid. The lid covers a larger than normal area of the lens and exerts greater force on the lens. During blinking the lid travels less distance than normal and produces less rocking of the lens. The net effect of the lid relationship to the lens during reading is a less efficient lens pump. The symptoms are typical of those associated with any condition of tear exchange interference.

Inadequate tear exchange during reading is usually best corrected by reducing the total diameter of the lens. An alternate correction of flattening the peripheral curve may be tried if it is felt that a smaller lens may not fit correctly for distance vision, but this is usually less effective in relieving the symptoms.

Secretions

The tear fluid contains appreciable quantities of mucoid and sebaceous secretions, which, in excessive amounts, may cause difficulties for the contact lens wearer. The exudate sometimes becomes so thick that it covers the lens and interferes with vision (Figure 14.17). If allowed to dry on the lens, the deposits may act as an abrasive and irritate the cornea. A lens coated with dry deposits will not wet properly and may cause a slight blurring of vision. The poor wetting properties may be observed with the biomicroscope when the lens is *in situ*.

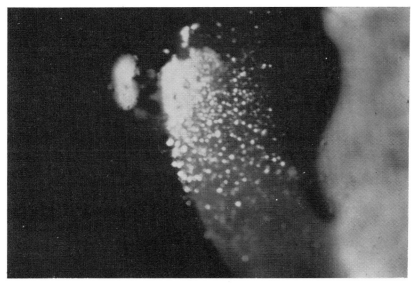

Figure 14.17. Lens coated with excess eye secretions.

Excessive secretions may occur as a result of the normal reaction to a contact lens, just as secretions increase in the presence of other foreign bodies. Excessive secretions may also indicate that the lens is causing abnormal irritation to the cornea or lids. The exact cause may be difficult to locate, as it may be nearly anything that will irritate the eye. Bad edges, loose lenses, and improper bearing relationships are common causes.

Occasionally it is found that excessive secretions suddenly begin after months of comfortable wear. These may be due to defects that have been imparted to the lens, such as edge roughness or warping. It is often found, however, that the secretions are only transitory and are probably caused by allergic reactions, foreign bodies, or systemic factors. The only treatment is frequent cleaning of the lenses.

Accumulation of the exudate during sleep is largely responsible for the discomfort experienced upon inserting the contact lenses in the morning.

Frothing

Frothing is occasionally seen around cor-neal contact lens edges but is more often a problem associated with haptic lens wear. It has the appearence of foam, which, with the biomicroscope, may be seen as composed of tiny bubbles.

Froth in contact lens wear is apparently due to the same causes that produce excessive secretions. Froth is simply the product of a mechanical whipping of the excessive seba-ceous secretions by the lids[58] and contact lens. Froth is present in smaller quantities for most people who do not wear contact lenses. It is often seen at the outer canthus and along the palpebral borders. In such cases froth may be increased by rapid blinking for about a minute.

Persistent Photophobia

In a few patients the photophobia that has been considered to be normal in the early stages of wear will continue to persist for several months. This must then be considered as an abnormal symptom, and an attempt should be made to locate its cause.

The explanation that photophobia is due to the greater light transmission of contact lenses as compared to spectacle lenses was proved inadequate by Bailey.[59] Nevertheless, it is still appalling how often this reason is given as the explanation for photophobia. Bailey points out that transmission data and the simple experiment of having the patient wear plano glass spectacle lenses over his contact lenses both indicate that the transmission difference is negligible. It might also be considered that patients with low refractive errors who have photophobia with their contact lenses do not have photophobia when no correction at all is worn.[60]

Braff and others have suggested that prolonged photophobia is very often associated with a contact lens that bears on the central cornea.[61] Since this area is the most abundantly supplied with pain receptors, the explanation has some physiological basis. Braff

recommends that apical clearance lenses be prescribed. Bailey lists several possible causes for photophobia with contact lenses, including uncorrected refractive errors, residual astigmatism, and dirty lenses. He points out that tinted contact lenses seldom are effective in eliminating photophobia, since they seldom provide sufficient absorption to be physiologically effective. An absorption of 50 percent is considered necessary to be effective.

Care must be taken to differentiate between true photophobia, which is characterized by pain and lacrimation, and the dazzling effects that are caused by a poorly fitted contact lens.[62] Normally, the dazzling and reflection effects are greater in the nighttime, when photophobia tends to be lessened.

LOST LENSES

When a patient has lost one or both lenses, the practitioner must take certain precautions in supplying a new lens. It should first be determined that the lens is definitely lost. Occasionally lenses that were reported lost were actually displaced into the fornix and only thought to be lost.[63,64] In two cases lenses lodged in the fornix were not found for over a year.[65,66] In one case the lens had actually become embedded in the conjunctival tissue

and was not even seen by the fitter who performed an internal inspection of the eye (Figure 14.18).

The author saw one patient who thought he had lost a lens but had actually placed both lenses in one side of his carrying case. The lenses were allowed to dry in the case and had become stuck to each other. When the patient opened the case he thought only one lens was present.

REEXAMINATION

When the patient loses a lens and has not been to see his practitioner for some time, this presents an ideal occasion to reexamine

the patient. If any visual changes have taken place, they can be corrected in the new lens.

WEARING TIME

It is often necessary to remind the patient who must wait a week or so for his new lens that he should shorten his normal wearing

time for a few days when beginning to wear the new lens.

LONG–TERM REFRACTIVE CHANGES

Sometimes significant corneal and refractive changes occur in patients who have worn contact lenses for long periods.[67-72] These changes are closely related to the fit of the lens and the period of time they have been worn.[73] The refractive change may be spherical, but more often it takes the form of a with-the-rule astigmatism.[74] This is usually roughly correlated with a with-the-rule corneal toricity that is measureable with the keratometer.

When the contact lenses are removed and an attempt is made to do a refraction, it may be impossible to achieve an expected visual acuity with any correction.[75] The acuity is commonly reduced from 20/15 to between 20/20 and 20/30. The acuity is usually normal when the contact lenses are being worn, but in more severe cases a slight decrease in acuity with lenses may also occur.

The decrease in acuity may be due to either a mechanical distortion of the cornea by the contact lens or to corneal reactions to lenses that do not allow proper tear exchange. Corneal distortion most often occurs when the posterior surface of the lens varies significantly from the curvature of the cornea. For example, corneal distortion was com-

monly caused by early types of contact lenses, which were fitted much flatter than the cornea. For myopic patients it was common to find that after the lens was worn and removed, the flattened cornea reduced the total refractive power of the eye and partially or fully corrected the myopia. The patient then obtained better vision with no correction rather than with his spectacles, which then gave an overcorrection. Within a few hours, however, the cornea resumed its normal shape, although in a few cases normal curvature was not restored for several days.

Modern types of corneal lenses are seldom fitted with bearing relationships limited to small areas, though there are some exceptions. A lens that is too steep or flat, for example, will commonly distort the cornea because of an inherently small bearing area. Also, corneal distortion commonly occurs when there is corneal toricity of greater than 1.00 D. with a spherical optical zone on the lens, because this lens, since it cannot conform well to the cornea, necessarily has small areas of bearing.

Any lens with a faulty bearing relationship will likely cause not only direct corneal distortion but corneal trauma as well. This may disturb the metabolic activity of the cornea and create edema. The edema may be a secondary factor in producing corneal distortion.

In milder cases the corneal integrity may appear normal with the biomicroscope. In more advanced cases, severe corneal edema may be present and perhaps also a diffuse punctate stain.

This condition is usually discovered when the patient presents himself either to obtain a pair of spectacle lenses for part-time wear or to be refitted with contact lenses. The return of the patient for an examination is often prompted by his experiencing wearing problems.

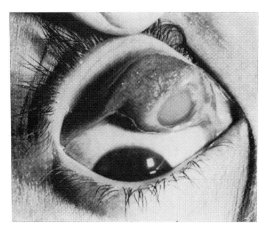

Figure 14.18. Contact lens that became embedded in the conjunctival tissue.

PROVIDING SPECTACLES FOR PART-TIME WEAR

Very often the patient is getting along reasonably well with his contact lenses but wishes to obtain a pair of spectacles for use in the evening or other periods. An examination may be conducted and glasses prescribed. The patient may later return complaining that the glasses do not provide adequate vision. A subsequent refraction at that time shows a major change from the first refraction. If an additional refraction is done at a later time, it may be found that still another correction is found. This difficulty in stabilizing the refractive correction is a major problem in providing spectacles for intermittent wear.[76]

The patient should first be evaluated in the morning before contact lenses are worn to determine if refitting is necessary. Corneal distortion may have occurred as a result of a poor bearing relationship, and the lens may need to be changed. A second examination should be made late in the day when the patient has had an opportunity to wear the lenses for a long period so that possible corneal edema may be detected. Edema may be diagnosed from direct observation or by a sig-nificant difference between the morning and afternoon refractions. If edema is present, an attempt should be made to eliminate it before the glasses are given.

The best time in which to do an examination for the purpose of providing spectacles to be used in the evening is near the end of the day.[77] The prescription will then be suited to this time in the wearing schedule. However, if significant corneal edema is present, the prescription may be adequate when the contact lenses are first removed, but after a few hours, the vision becomes disturbed.

An exception to the preceding problems may occur for a patient who wishes to have a pair of spectacles to be used only for reading. This is often the case for a student who wishes to wear his contact lenses during the day but finds he is more comfortable in the evening during long periods of study if he wears his glasses. In this case the patient may have a perfectly adequate fit for normal wearing conditions. However, the conditions during reading present an added problem in terms of tear pumping.

REFITTING

The patient who is being considered for refitting of contact lenses must first be evaluated for the condition of his cornea. If the cornea exhibits mild edema and/or mild distortion, the condition is not considered serious and a new fitting may proceed immediately. However, if the cornea shows extensive staining, the lenses should be removed for a period of one week and a reevaluation of the corneal condition made. The patient should be followed until the corneal health is restored. As an interim measure, a pair of temporary spherical spectacle lenses may have to be provided for the patient. This procedure usually results in considerable inconvenience to the patient and may require strong control of the patient.

Patients who have no corneal staining and only mild edema may be fitted immediately with contact lenses. There is no need to force the patient to suffer through a period of weeks without contact lenses in this situation. If the cornea is refitted with a new contact lens, either edema or distortion will be reduced (Figure 14.19). The patient may be refitted with either a hard lens or a hydrogel lens. Either lens may require a longer period for the cornea to return to normal than if the lenses were removed entirely, but the patient has the advantage of having normal visual acuity during the interim.[78]

Changes in the refractive state under various conditions have been studied extensively by Rengstorff.[69] He found that considerable individual variation existed but that most patients who stopped wearing their contact lenses showed wide fluctuations in both the refractive state and corneal curvature as measured by a keratometer (Figure 14.20). In many cases the direction of change as measured with the keratometer does not correlate closely with the refractive change. This discrepancy is to be expected, considering the condition of the cornea. A small corneal distortion can give rise to a considerable effect on a keratometer reading and the actual value of the change cannot be considered as valid (*see* Figure 14.9). Hence, it is incorrect to feel that the cornea is actually changing in curvature over the wide range corresponding to the change in keratometer readings. Rather, it is simply going through various distortional changes. These effects are usually accentuated if the patient has a large pupil, where the effects of corneal distortion will be even more effective in producing a refractive change.

LOSS OF NORMAL WEARING TIME

It is sometimes found that a patient is able to wear his lenses with apparent comfort for a period of months or even years and then suddenly have decreased wearing time until there is an inability to wear the lenses at all. This situation often occurs in patients who have a significant amount of corneal edema created each day from a tight lens but not enough edema to cause sufficient discomfort that they have the lenses changed. The patient

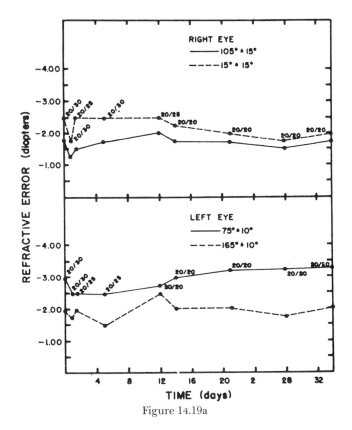

Figure 14.19a

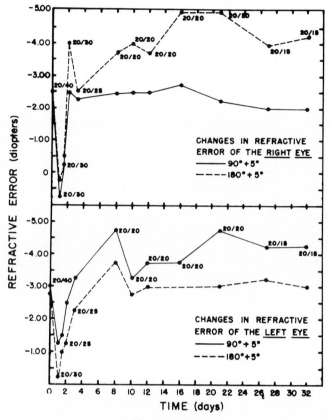

Figure 14.19b

may feel that it is perfectly normal that he experience a slight discomfort with the lenses near the end of the day.

This patient represents a borderline failure, whose symptoms lie below a level that would cause him to seek a correction (*see* Response II in Table 7.12). If any new stress condition is now superimposed on this patient, it will be enough to cause the lenses to become intolerable. The stress situation might be a cold, allergy, hormonal change, change in wearing environment, or one of many unknown causes.

A condition sometimes seen in long-term contact lens wearers is that of edematous corneal lines in the epithelium. These are detectable by the same observation technique as used for central corneal clouding (Figure 14.21).

PATHOLOGICAL COMPLICATIONS

It is fortunate that so few pathological complications occur as a result of wearing contact lenses. This may be credited to the inherent protective mechanism of the cornea. Before any permanent damage is inflicted on the eye, the lenses become so uncomfortable or the vision so affected that the patient usually stops wearing the lenses and seeks care. This does not mean, however, that corneal injury is impossible with contact lenses, and such injury is best prevented by a well-informed and cautious patient. Usually, path-

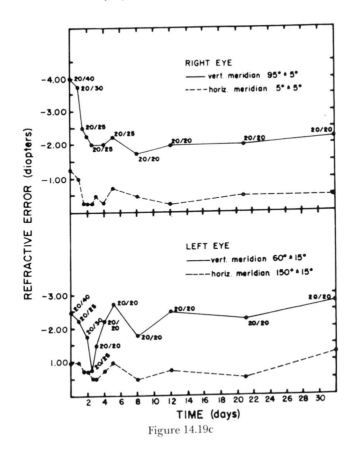

Figure 14.19c

Figure 14.19. Visual acuity and refractive error of patients refitted with (*a*) hard, (*b*) gel, or (*c*) no contact lens. From M. G. Harris, R. J. Blevins, and S. Heiden, Evaluation of Procedures for the Management of Spectacle Blur, *American Journal of Optometry and Archives of American Academy of Optometry,* 50(4): 293–298, 1973.

ological conditions occur only when the patient has not used good judgment in the wearing of his lenses, such as building wearing time too rapidly, wearing the lenses for periods longer than accustomed, wearing the lenses for irregular periods, and sleeping with lenses in place on the corneas. Other complications usually occur because of an improperly fitted lens, which either bears heavily on one portion of the cornea and causes traumatic abrasion or which causes interference with the tear circulation over the cornea.

Valid statistics on the incidence of permanent corneal injury from wearing contact lenses are not available. Surveys of ophthalmologists have produced figures as high as 14 percent who have seen cases of permanent corneal damage associated with contact lenses, but the cases have not been carefully documented.[79] Vidal had only seen one case of permanent scarring.[80]

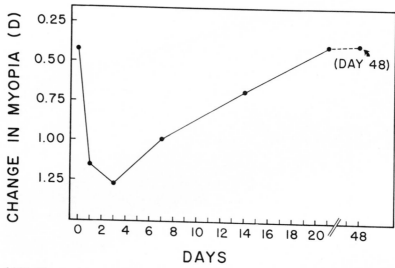

Figure 14.20. Fluctuations in refractive state and corneal curvature after removal of contact lenses. From R. H. Rengstorff, Variations in Myopia Measurements: An After-effect Observed with Habitual Wearers of Contact Lenses, *American Journal of Optometry, 44*(3):149–161, 1967.

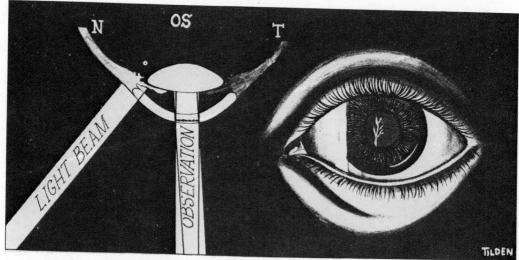

Figure 14.21. Edematous corneal lines. Courtesy of D. Korb.

INFECTION

Infections do not occur often with the wearing of contact lenses, but nonetheless, they must be guarded against closely. Early stages of infection are indicated by a change in the area surrounding the site of the abra-sion; it becomes greyish and may show an exudate. This may be viewed with a biomicro-scope. By the time infection occurs, the sub-jective symptoms are usually pronounced pain, lacrimation, and photophobia. Vision may be blurred due to accompanying edema. Objective signs of conjunctival infection may also be present.

Infections that do occur probably result from improper care after a corneal abrasion has occurred. This could be caused by unclean habits in handling the lens; contaminated cleaning, wetting or fluorescein solutions; or a local or systemic infection that existed concurrently with the abrasion.[81]

In view of the possible consequences, it is doubtful whether there is any justification for the continued wearing of contact lenses when infection is present. A suggestion has been made that properly fitted contact lenses can be worn during a corneal infection if antibiotic solution is inserted in the eye four times daily.[80] It is doubtful if the majority of ophthalmologists would agree on this procedure. If the patient has been given medication in ointment form, the lenses cannot be worn comfortably with the ointment on the eye.

Payrau and Perdriel reported two cases of infected corneal ulcers with hypopyon, which apparently resulted from infectious complications of contact lens abrasions.[82] Evidence of mishandling was present in both cases.

SCARRING

It is very rare to find permanent corneal scarring that is a direct result of contact lens wear. When scarring does occur, it is usually the result of handling difficulties or improper wearing procedures. Occasionally, patients who have various pathological conditions and who also wear contact lenses may blame the contact lenses for scarring, when in reality it was due to another condition.

Even when the cornea has been abraded extensively by an improperly fitted contact lens, scarring seldom occurs unless the patient continues to wear the lens through a period of extreme discomfort. Even abrasions that occur during faulty insertion seldom remove more than the epithelial layer. Most scarring occurs from gouges with the fingernail, injuries when the contact lens was worn, or mishandling of the lens to the point of absurdity.

The greatest danger of scarring occurs when an abrasion is allowed to become infected and cause a corneal ulcer.

CORNEAL VASCULARIZATION

Occasionally, corneal vascularization has been reported to be caused by an improperly fitted contact lens or by complications arising from corneal injury, which was due to wearing contact lenses. The most common instances have been in those cases where the lens rides high and impinges upon the sclera. Very often the lens is held tightly against the superior portion of the limbus by the lid, disrupting the normal tear circulation at this position as well as interfering with the conjunctival circulation. Stagnation of the aqueous veins can sometimes be noted directly with the biomicroscope. The author has seen a few of these cases at the University Clinic. The vessels appear to invade 2 to 3 mm. into the cornea, and corneal edema and opacification also occur. These patients were advised to give up wearing their contact lenses.

It is surprising to note the ability of the cornea to recover from this condition. The vascularization usually is gone in a few days, and the corneal clarity may improve for several weeks. The great improvement that is usually found in these patients suggests that most of the vascularization is not really a new invasion of vessels into the cornea but simply an engorgement of the very tiny vessels of the limbal loops. Under normal conditions these vessels are so small that they may be entirely overlooked. When the cornea has regained its normal appearance, the patients may be safely refitted with new contact lenses. Effort should be made to have the new lens ride in a low or centered position. This may be accomplished by using very small lenses or, if necessary, a prism ballast lens.

Occasionally a lens will ride in a nasal position and apply pressure to the nasal limbus. Engorgement of the limbal loops may occur in the immediate area of the irritation, but no invasion by other vessels into the cornea has been noted. The vessel engorgement is usually accompanied by subjective discomfort. Relief is obtained by refitting with a lens that rides at a central or low position on the cornea.

Corneal vascularization has occasionally been reported as a sequel to corneal abrasion.[83] While there is always a possibility of this occurrence, it only occurs when the abrasion is of long standing. Before the corneal vascularization occurs, the patient will usually experience considerable pain, conjunctival injection, and blurring from corneal edema. If the patient has been properly instructed not to continue wearing his contact lenses under adverse conditions, the likelihood of corneal vascularization following abrasion is very remote.

If the patient had a history of corneal vascularization before the contact lenses were worn, he may show a greater susceptibility to repeated invasion than the average patient. The vessels that were formed in the cornea during the original inflammation may be emptied of their blood, but the vessels remain and refill during subsequent irritation. Such a patient should be told that recurrence of the vessel invasion may take place, and he should be checked routinely at frequent intervals.

If corneal vascularization occurs when the patient is wearing contact lenses, it should not necessarily be assumed that the vascularization is directly due to the contact lenses. Many other pathological conditions may occur, which are unrelated to the wearing of contact lenses and which cause corneal vascularization.

Dixon and Lawaczeck fitted corneal contact lenses on thirty-one rabbits and ten dogs and then studied the ensuing pathological corneal complications.[84] All subjects developed extensive corneal vascularization of both the superficial and deep stroma. The conditions of the experiment, however, would make this result appear inevitable. The animals were not given an opportunity to adapt to the lenses properly and wore them continuously for both day and night in spite of obvious corneal damage. The experiment does reveal the possible consequences of contact lens wear but under conditions that are not likely to be duplicated with human patients.

ULCERATION

When an abrasion is allowed to become infected, a corneal ulcer or progressive loss of corneal tissue may result. Ulcers arising as a complication of corneal damage from contact lens wear are extremely rare; but nonetheless, care must be taken to guard against their occurrence. Ulceration is best prevented by judicious care of any corneal abrasion and by cessation of contact lens wear when signs of corneal abrasion are present.

A case of corneal ulcer caused by an infection following an abrasion due to contact lenses was reported by Fitzgerald et al.[85] Visual acuity was reduced to 20/200, and keratoplasty was necessary.

REFERENCES

1. Wesley, N. K., and Jessen, G. N.: Symptoms and corrections in fitting contact lenses, *Optom. Weekly*, *42*(*44*):1713–1717, 1951.

2. Poster, M.: Symptomology as related to the structural nature of a contact lens, *Contacto*, *4*(*10*):477–479, 1960.

3. Giraldi, O. T.: Dresser drawer wearing, *Contacto*, *4*(*3*):93–94, 1960.

4. Abrams, B. S.: Subjective symptom evaluation, *Optom. World*, *48*(*8*):23–24, 1960.

5. Abrams, B. S., and Bailey, N. J.: Contact lens news and views, *J. Am. Optom. Assoc.*, *32*(*4*): 322–323, 1960.

6. Black, C. J.: Corneal staining, *Contacto*, *1*(*1*): 3–6, 1957.

7. Ackerly, E.: Effects of contact lenses on the cornea, *Contacto*, *3*(*6*):145–152, 1959.

8. Tortolero, J., Wesley, N. K., and Bronstein, L.: *Fluorescein Staining*, Chicago, The Plastic Contact Lens Co., 1959.

9. Passmore, C.: Abrasions from corneal contact lenses, *Contacto*, *4*(*11*):489–491, 1960.

10. Tortolero, J.: Corneal tissue changes following corneal contact lens wear, *Contacto*, *5*(*5*): 161–173, 1961.

11. Dick, R. B.: The incidence and classification of corneal lesions in beginning contact lens wearers, *J. Am. Optom. Assoc.*, *33*(*3*): 219–221, 1961.

12. Dick, R. B.: Incidence of corneal insult in contact lens wearers—a preliminary report, *J. Am. Optom. Assoc.*, *32*(*8*):632–634, 1961.

13. Haynes, P. R.: Comments on factors which must be considered in the fitting of contact lenses, *J. Am. Optom. Assoc.*, *32*(*4*):299–302, 1960.

14. Marano, J. A.: Office procedure for adding plus and minus power to contact lenses, *Optom. Weekly*, *52*(*36*):1735–1737, 1961.

15. Haynes, P. R.: The physical and physiological basis of edge reflections and marginal confusion with clinical comments on their correction, in *Encyclopedia of Contact Lens Practice*, South Bend, Indiana, International Optics, 1959–1963, vol. 1, pp. 6–12.

16. Dixon, J. M., and Lawaczeck, E.: A mechanism of glare due to corneal lenses, *Am. J. Ophthalmol.*, *54*(*6*):1135–1137, 1962.

17. Farnum, F. E.: Causes and correction of light dispersion, *Contacto*, *3*(*10*):298–300, 1959.

18. Smelser, G. K.: Relation of factors involved in maintenance of optical properties of cornea to contact lens wear, *Arch. Ophthalmol.*, *47*(*3*):328–343, 1952.

19. Bier, N.: *Contact Lens Routine and Practice*, 2nd ed., London, Butterworths, 1957, p. 3.

20. Mazow, B.: *Synopsis of Corneal Contact Lens Fitting for Optometrists*, Amer. Acad. Optom. Ser., vol. 2, Minneapolis, Burgess, 1962.

21. Goldberg, J. B.: Transition zone between optic diameter and bevel, *Contacto*, *6*(*3*):79–80, 1962.

22. Mandell, R. B., and Polse, K. A.: Corneal thickness changes accompanying central corneal clouding, *Am. J. Optom.*, *48*(*2*): 129–132, 1971.

23. Korb, D. R., and Exford, J. M.: The phenomenon of central circular clouding, *J. Am. Optom. Assoc.*, *39*(*3*):223–230, 1968.

24. Sarwar, M.: Corneal veiling, *Br. J. Physiol. Opt.*, *11*(*3*):167–169, 1954.

25. Baldwin, W. R., and Shick, C.: *Corneal Contact Lenses*, Philadelphia, Chilton, 1962, p. 81.

26. Hazlett, R. D.: Central circular clouding, *J. Am. Optom. Assoc.*, *40*(*3*):268–275, 1969.

27. Korb, D. R.: Corneal transparency with emphasis on the phenomenon of central circular clouding, in *Encyclopedia of Contact Lens Practice*, South Bend, Indiana, International Optics, 1959–1963, vol. 4, pp. 106–116.

28. Bier, N.: *Contact Lens Routine and Practice*, 2nd ed., London, Butterworths, 1957, pp. 107, 211.

29. Dixon, J. M., and Lawaczeck, E.: Corneal vascularization due to contact lenses, *Trans. Sec. Ophthalmol.*, *A.M.A.*, pp. 60–65, 1962.

30. Mazow, B.: *Synopsis of Corneal Contact Lens Fitting for Optometrists*, Am. Acad. Optom. Ser., Minneapolis, Burgess, 1962, vol. 2, p. 55.

31. Grosvenor, T. P.: *Contact Lens Theory and Practice*, Chicago, Professional Press, 1963, p. 66.

32. Barabas, R. J., and Fontana, A. A.: Juxtaposi-

tion staining, *Contacto*, *11(4)*:3–5, 1967.

33. Korb, D. R., and Exford, J. M.: A study of three and nine o'clock staining after unilateral lens removal, *J. Am. Optom. Assoc.*, *41(3)*: 7–10, 1970.

34. Mackie, I. A.: *Contact Lenses*, Symposium, Munich-Feldafing, S. Karger, Basel/New York, 1967, pp. 66–73.

35. Arner, R. S.: Corneal contact lens design by minimal corneal insult, *J. Am. Optom. Assoc.*, *40(3)*:308, 1969.

36. Sarver, M. D., Nelson, J. L., and Polse, K. A.: Peripheral corneal staining accompanying contact lens wear, *J. Am. Optom. Assoc.*, *40(3)*: 310, 1969.

37. Lemp, M. A. et al.: The precorneal film. I. Factors in spreading and maintaining a continuous tear film over the corneal surface, *Arch. Ophthalmol.*, *83(1)*:89–94, 1970.

38. Lemp, M. A., Holly, F. J., and Dohlman, C. H.: Corneal desiccation despite normal tear volume, *Ann. Ophthalmol.*, *2(3)*: 258–261, 284, 1970.

39. Boruchoff, S. A.: Recurrent corneal erosions, *Am. J. Optom.*, *47(5)*:413–414, 1970.

40. Roseborough, G. F.: Traumatic recurrent corneal erosion or aseptic corneal inflammation, *Can. J. Ophthalmol.*, *5(4)*:348–352, 1970.

41. Lowe, R. F.: Recurrent erosion of the cornea, *Br. J. Ophthalmol.*, *54(12)*:805–809, 1970.

42. Tripathi, R. C., and Bron, A. J.: Ultrastructural study of non-traumatic recurrent corneal erosion, *Br. J. Ophthalmol.*, *56(2)*: 73–85, 1972.

43. Lowther, G. E., Bailey, N. J., and Hill, R. M.: Conjunctival xerosis associated with contact lenses, *Am. J. Optom.*, *48(9)*:754–758, 1971.

44. Krezanoski, J. Z.: Physiology and biochemistry of contact lens wearing, in *Encyclopedia of Contact Lens Practice*, South Bend, Indiana, International Optic, 1959–1963, vol. 4, pp. 18–26.

45. Dickinson, F.: Heat, sunglare and dust are factors in contact lens fitting in South Africa, *Am. J. Optom.*, *37(4)*:201–209, 1960.

46. Eye damage from oral contraceptives? *J.A.M.A.*, *204(5)*:19, 1968.

47. Behrman, S.: Homonymous hemianopia after oral contraceptives, *Br. Med. J.*, *4*:684, 1967.

48. Cogan, D. G.: Do oral contraceptives have neuro-ophthalmic complications? *Arch. Ophthalmol.*, *73(4)*:461, 1965.

49. Connel, E. B., and Kelman, C. D.: Ophthalmologic findings with oral contraceptives, *Obstet. Gynecol.*, *31(4)*:446–460, 1968.

50. Elliott, F. A.: Contraceptive pills, *J.A.M.A.*, *206(1)*:2742, 1968.

51. Caron, G. A.: Contact lenses and oral contraceptives, *Br. Med. J.*, *1(5493)*:980, 1966.

52. Koetting, R. A.: The influence of oral contraceptives on contact lens wear, *Am. J. Optom.*, *43*:268–274, 1966.

53. Ruben, M.: Contact lenses and oral contraceptives, *Br. Med. J.*, *1(5495)*:1110, 1966.

54. Sarwar, M.: Contact lenses and oral contraceptives, *Br. Med. J.*, *1(5497)*:1235, 1966.

55. Parsons, C. P., and Peter, P. A.: Observations in some contact lens wearers using oral contraceptives, *Contacto*, *22(3)*:3–11, 1967.

56. Peter, P. A., and Parsons, C. P.: Observations of some contact lens wearers using oral contraceptives, *J. Contact Lens Soc. Am.*, *1*: 9–14, 1967.

57. McLaren, D. S.: *Malnutrition and the Eye*, New York, Academic, 1963, p. 237.

58. Norn, M. S.: Foam at outer palpebral canthus, *Acta Ophthalmol.*, *41(5)*:531–537, 1963.

59. Bailey, N. J.: Photophobia and contact lenses, *Contacto*, *2(3)*:79–81, 1958.

60. Enoch, J. M., and McGraw, J. L.: Contact lenses: some aspects of visual acuity and photophobia, *Am. J. Optom.*, *31(2)*:78–87, 1954.

61. Braff, S. M.: Scleral lenses in contact lens practice, *Am. J. Optom.*, *39(4)*:195–202, 1962.

62. Lebensohn, J. E.: Photophobia: mechanism and implications, *Am. J. Ophthalmol.*, *34(9)*: 1294–1300, 1951.

63. Green, W. R.: An embedded—"lost"—contact lens, *Arch. Ophthalmol.*, *69(1)*:23–24, 1963.

64. Manchester, T. P., Jr.: Use of cul-de-sacs in contact lens wear, *Am. J. Ophthalmol.*, *55(5)*: 1056–1057, 1963.

65. Long, J. C.: Retention of contact lens in upper fornix, *Am. J. Ophthalmol.*, *56(2)*:309, 1963.

66. Michaels, D. D., and Zugsmith, G. S.: An unusual contact lens complication, *Am. J. Ophthalmol.*, *55(5)*:1057–1058, 1963.

67. Rengstorff, R. H.: The Fort Dix Report—a

longitudinal study of the effects of contact lenses, *Am. J. Optom.*, *42(3)*:153–163, 1965.

68. Rengstorff, R. H.: Corneal curvature and astigmatic changes subsequent to contact lens wear, *J. Am. Optom. Assoc.*, *36(11)*:996–1000, 1965.

69. Rengstorff, R. H.: Variations in myopia measurements: an after-effect observed with habitual wearers of contact lenses, *Am. J. Optom.*, *44(3)*:149–161, 1967.

70. Ruben, M.: Corneal changes in contact lens wear, *Trans. Ophthalmol. Soc. U.K.*, *87*:27–43, 1967.

71. Miller, D.: Contact lens-induced corneal curvature and thickness changes, *Arch. Ophthalmol.*, *80(4)*:430–432, 1968.

72. Pratt-Johnson, J. A., and Warner, D. M.: Contact lenses and corneal curvature changes, *Am. J. Ophthalmol.*, *60*:852–855, 1965.

73. Rengstorff, R. H.: The relationship between contact lens base curve and corneal curvature, *J. Am. Optom. Assoc.*, *44(3)*:291–293, 1973.

74. Rengstorff, R. H.: Contact lenses and aftereffects: some temporal factors which influence myopia and astigmatism variations, *Am. J. Optom.*, *45(6)*:364–373, 1968.

75. Rengstorff, R. H.: A study of visual acuity loss after contact lens wear, *Am. J. Optom.*, *43(7)*:431–440, 1966.

76. Rengstorff, R. H.: Diurnal•variations in corneal curvature measurements after wearing contact lenses, *Am. J. Optom.*, *48(3)*:239–244, 1971.

77. Rengstorff, R. H.: Overnight myopia changes induced by contact lenses, *J. Am. Optom. Assoc.*, *41(3)*:249–252, 1970.

78. Harris, M. G., Blevins, R. J., and Heiden, S.: Evaluation of procedures for the management of spectacle blur, *Am. J. Optom. Arch. Am. Acad. Optom. 50(4)*:293–298, 1973.

79. Jaeckle, C. E.: Discussion of paper: acute complications from present day corneal contact lenses, *Trans. Sec. Ophthalmol.*, A.M.A., p. 161, 1960.

80. Vidal, F. L.: Medical complications of contact lenses, *Int. Ophthalmol. Clin.*, *1(2)*:495–504, 1961.

81. Lansche, R. K., and Lee, R. C.: Acute complications from present day corneal contact lenses, *Arch. Ophthalmol.*, *64(2)*:275–285, 1960.

82. Payrau, P., and Perdriel, G.: Bilateral hypopyon ulcer of the cornea following the continuous wearing of contact lenses, *Bull. Soc. Ophthalmol. Fr.*, *9*:852–854, 1956.

83. Ullen, R. L.: Corneal vascularization in the wearing of contact lenses, *Precision-Cosmet Digest*, Precision-Cosmet Company, Minneapolis, June, 1963.

84. Dixon, J. M., and Lawaczeck, E.: Corneal vascularization due to contact lenses, *Arch. Ophthalmol.*, *69(1)*:72–75, 1963.

85. Fitzgerald, J. R., Kapustiak, W., and McCarthy, J. L.: Contact lens corneal ulcer, *Am. J. Ophthalmol.*, *54(2)*:307–308, 1962.

ADDITIONAL READINGS

Arakia, A. et al.: Detection and measurement of corneal alterations due to conventional contact lens wear, *J. Am. Optom. Assoc.*, *48(3)*:327, 1977.

Arner, R. S.: Corneal deadaptation—the case against abrupt cessation of contact lens wear, *J. Am. Optom. Assoc.*, *48(3)*:339, 1977.

Avisar, R.: Tear secretion in patients with non-specific eye complaints, *Israel J. Med. Sci.*, *14(3)*:339, 1978.

Bailey, I. L., and Carney, L. G.: A survey of corneal curvature changes from corneal lens wear, *Cont. Lens J.*, *6(1)*:3, 1977.

Bayshore, C. A.: Flare, *J. Am. Optom. Assoc.*, *47(3)*:354, 1976.

Bowman, K. J., Smith, G., and Carney, L. G.: Corneal topography and monocular diplopia following near work, *Am. J. Optom. Physiol. Opt.*, *55(12)*:818–823, 1978.

Brannen, R. D.: Incidence of central edema and peripheral staining as a function of contact lens fitting philosophy, *J. Am. Optom. Assoc.*, *48(3)*:391, 1977.

Breger, J.: Why K's change and what you can do about it, *Cont. Lens Forum*, *2(7)*:23–25, 1977.

Brown, F. G.: Refractive changes induced by corneal contact lenses, *The Optician*, *156(4031)*:1–5, 1968.

Brown, S. I.: The tear film alteration associated with dellen, *Ann. Ophthalmol.*, *6(8)*:757–761, 1974.

Brungardt, T. F.: Contact lens clinic—superior corneal periphery stain, *Optom. Weekly, 59*(*51*): 29–30, 1968.

Collins, I. W.: Symptomatology, *J. Am. Optom. Assoc., 47*(*3*):352, 1976.

Dickinson, F.: The "overwear" syndrome, *The Optician, 167*(*4325*):15–17, 1974.

Dixon, J. M.: Ocular changes due to contact lenses, *Am. J. Ophthalmol., 58*(*3*):424–443, 1964.

Dixon, J. M.: Corneal vascularization due to corneal contact lenses: the clinical picture, *Trans. Am. Ophthalmol. Soc., 65*:333–340, 1967.

Dixon, J. M. et al.: Complications associated with the wearing of contact lenses, *Opt. J. Rev. Optom., 103*:13–16, 1966.

Dixon, J. M., and Lawaczeck, E.: Corneal dimples and bubbles, *Am. J. Ophthalmol., 54*(*5*):827–831, 1962.

Dixon, W. S., and Bron, A. J.: Fluorescein angiographic demonstration of corneal vascularization in contact lens wearers, *Am. J. Ophthalmol., 75*(*6*):1010–1015, 1973.

Egan, D. J.: Differential staining in contact lens practice, *Int. Cont. Lens Clin., 5*(*4*):54, 1978.

Farris, R. L., Kubota, Z., and Mishima, S.: Epithelial decompensation with contact lens wear, *Arch. Ophthalmol.,* pp. 651–660, June 1971.

Figazolo, J. F.: The case of the mysterious edema, *Cont. Lens Forum, 5*(*2*):67, 1980.

Friedberg, M. A.: Spectacle blur, *J. Am. Optom. Assoc., 47*(*3*):355, 1976.

Galin, M. A., and Morrison, R.: Side effects of corneal contact lenses, *Int. Cont. Lens Clin., 1*(*2*): 88–93, 1974.

Grant, A. H.: Flare reduction and elimination, *J. Am. Optom. Assoc., 39*(*3*):255–258, 1968.

Greenberg, M. H., and Hill, R. M.: The physiology of contact lens imprints, *Am. J. Optom. Arch. Am. Acad. Optom., 50*(*9*):699–702, 1973.

Harris, M. G.: Prescribing spectacles for hard contact lens wearers, *Int. Cont. Lens Clin., 2*(*3*):25–27, 1975.

Harris, M. G., Wong, N. H., and Low, A. W.: Patient response to PMMA contact lenses, *J. Am. Optom. Assoc., 46*(*11*):1184–1187, 1975.

Haynes, P. R.: Refitting the contact lens patient, *J. Am. Optom. Assoc., 47*(*3*):289, 1976.

Hess, R. F., and Garner, L. F.: The effect of corneal edema on visual function, *Invest. Ophthalmol. Vis. Sci., 16*(*1*):5–13, 1977.

Hunter, J. E.: Suggested clinical classification of diffuse corneal edema, *Int. Cont. Lens Clin., 5*(*3*): 31, 1978.

Janoff, L. E.: Hard contacts: some problem cases, *Cont. Lens Forum, 1*(*7*):46–53, 1976.

Kerns, R. L.: Prescribing spectacles for the existing contact lens wearer, *Int. Cont. Lens Clin., 3*(*2*): 47–51, 1976.

Korb, D.: The role of blinking in successful contact lens wear, *Int. Cont. Lens Clin., 1*(*2*):59–71, 1974.

Korb, D. R., and Herman, J. P.: Corneal staining subsequent to sequential fluorescein instillations, *J. Am. Optom. Assoc., 50*(*3*):361, 1979.

Mandell, R. B.: The problem patient, what causes central corneal clouding?, *Int. Cont. Lens Clin., 1*(*2*):26–29, 1974.

Mandell, R. B.: The problem patient: what causes three and nine o'clock staining?, *Int. Cont. Lens Clin., 1*(*2*):30–33, 1974.

Mandell, R. B.: The problem patient: what is a tight lens?, *Int. Cont. Lens Clin., 1*(*2*):34–40, 1974.

Mandell, R. B.: May I get my contacts polished?, *Int. Cont. Lens Clin., 1*(*4*):21, 1974.

Marisi, A., and Aquavella, J. V.: Hypertonic saline solution in corneal edema, *Ann. Ophthalmol., 7*(*2*):229–233, 1975.

Polse, K. A.: Observation of corneal dry spots, *Optom. Weekly, 66*(*19*):498–499, 1975.

Chapter 15

OPTIONAL LENS FEATURES

COLORED CONTACT LENSES

CONTACT LENSES may be tinted for light absorption, cosmetic appearance, or ease of location and identification. They are usually available in the following colors:[1]

Gray	Blue	Brown	Green	Pink
Light	Light	Light	Light	Light
Medium	Medium	Medium	Medium	Medium
Dark	Dark	Dark	Dark	Dark

Also available, but rarely used, are additional shades of red, lavender, blue, and amber. The colors may be given different names by various contact lens companies.

ABSORPTION OF LIGHT

Colored contact lenses offer a variety of possibilities for selectively filtering the light that strikes the eye.

Lenses that are colored one of the lighter shades have only a minimum of absorption, and the wearer is hardly aware of a reduction in the apparent brightness of his environment. Medium shades provide a definite light reduction but somewhat less than is generally preferred for a sunglass lens. Dark shades offer approximately the same amount of absorption as spectacle sunglasses.

For the most part, tinted contact lenses provide less ultraviolet radiation absorption in the critical range between 250 nm and 380 nm than do spectacle lenses (Figures 15.1 to 15.3). Nearly all tinted contact lenses cut off the significant ultraviolet transmission at approximately 300 nm, whereas ordinary spectacle crown has a cutoff at approximately 320 nm. Contact lenses can be made with increased ultraviolet absorption, but it is questionable whether this is actually of benefit. The detrimental physiological effects of radiation upon the eyes would be less with a colored spectacle lens than with a colored corneal lens, even when both absorb identical radiant energy.[2] More protection would be obtained by the colored spectacle lens because more of the eye would be shielded. A colored corneal contact lens only protects the corneal surface and the media behind the cornea. Exposure to ultraviolet rays by intense reflections from snow, sand, or water could still cause inflammation of the conjunctiva and of the limbal area of the cornea. Hence, skiers and others who are exposed to considerable ultraviolet radiation should not be made to feel that they are protected by even the darkest of contact lenses.

Tinted contact lenses can provide good protection against infrared light, but they are rarely used for this purpose.

Obrig and Salvatori make the following

431

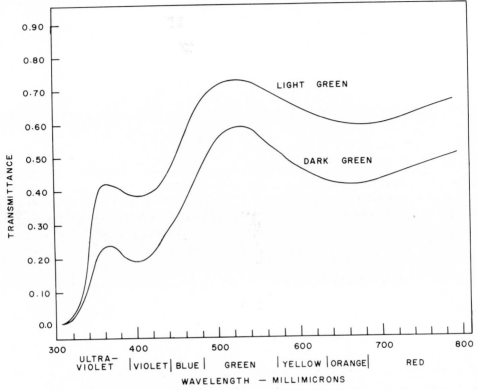

Figure 15.1. Transmission of colored contact lenses.

recommendations for choosing a colored lens that is to absorb either ultraviolet or infrared radiation. The ultraviolet absorption in the spectrum from 300 to 400 nm, of several of the colored lenses is as follows:

Dark Green	75% at 370 nm	85% at 400 nm	(Figure 15.1)
Dark Brown	75% at 370 nm	86% at 400 nm	(Figure 15.2)
Light Green	58% at 370 nm	62% at 400 nm	(Figure 15.1)
Gray	50% at 370 nm	42% at 400 nm	(Figure 15.2)
Smokey Black	48% at 370 nm	65% at 400 nm	(Figure 15.2)
Smoky Brown	40% at 370 nm	45% at 400 nm	(Figure 15.2)

If ultraviolet absorption were the only factor to be considered, the first three lenses would be the logical choices.

When it is desired that a colored corneal lens be used to reduce the total amount of light entering the eye and diminish the total amount of the visible spectrum in an approximately even proportion, the following lenses should be considered:

Light Blue	absorbs 15% of visible spectrum	(Figure 15.3)
Gray	absorbs 25% of visible spectrum	(Figure 15.2)

| Smoky Brown | absorbs 40% of visible spectrum | (Figure 15.2) |
| Smoky Black | absorbs 55% of visible spectrum | (Figure 15.2) |

When it is desired that a colored plastic lens be used to absorb both the ultraviolet radiation and the short infrared radiation, the lens of choice is

| Dark Green | absorbs 75% at 370 nm and 50% at 800 nm | (Figure 15.1) |

It is sometimes stated that a contact lens is too thin to be of much value as an absorptive lens. Actually, thickness is only one factor contributing to the potential absorptive properties of a lens. The quantity of colorant materials added to the plastic during its manufacture determines the degree of absorption, and enough colorant can provide the contact lens with the same absorption as is found in the much thicker spectacle glass.

The human eye is actually a good judge of the relative amounts of light that are transmitted by filters. If a contact lens and a spectacle lens are held side by side and appear to have the same degree of darkness, it is likely that they transmit approximately the same amount of light.*

---

*This, of course, does not hold true for the nonvisible forms of radiation.

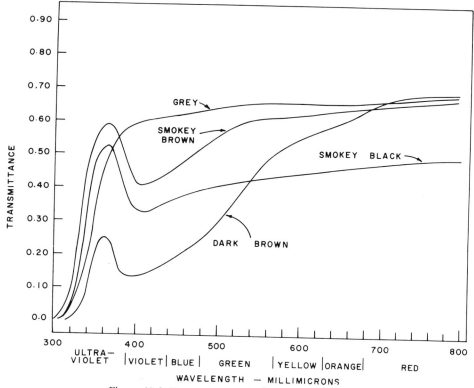

Figure 15.2. Transmission of colored contact lenses.

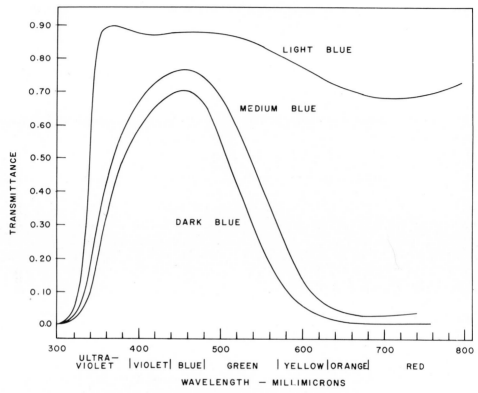

Figure 15.3. Transmission of colored contact lenses.

"Matrix Lenses"
Dark Irides as well

CHANGING THE EYE COLOR

If the eye is of a light color, it is usually possible to alter the color in a variety of ways by wearing tinted contact lenses. This may be done purposely for cosmetic appearance, or it may be a necessary but unwanted accompaniment for light absorption.

The appearance of some iris colors may be easily changed. For example, a grey iris can be made to appear the color of nearly any contact lens tint. Darker irises are seldom changed in appearance by wearing any but the darkest of contact lens tints. They can be made to appear darker but not lighter.

An attractive cosmetic appearance is usually obtained when a contact lens is tinted the same color as the iris. Care should be taken with the moderate and dark shades of blue and green, however, as they tend to give an artificial appearance to the eyes, which is very conspicuous. The exact effect of a colored lens on changing the eye color is not always predictable, and it is usually best to have the patient wear a colored trial lens before a decision is made to tint the final lenses.

It is not necessary to have a separate trial lens set of colored lenses. The regular trial fitting set can include lenses in various colors. This also makes it possible to identify the lenses in the set easily.

If a significant change is produced by the color of the contact lens, it may be necessary to make the lens larger in diameter than usual. A small, dark lens on a large, lightly colored eye is very noticeable and may give a rather grotesque appearance.

Many people are surprised to find that when the colored lens is on the eye it appears to have a much richer (saturated) color than when held in the hand. The same effect is achieved by looking through the lens and then laying it on a piece of white paper; the color effect is much more vivid on the paper.

This occurs because light must pass through the lens twice before it is seen by an observer. Outside light passes through the lens to the iris, which absorbs a certain amount of this light; the remainder is reflected and passes through the lens again.

EASE IN LOCATING LENSES

Contact lenses are often tinted for easy locating, both off and on the eye. Even the lightest tints in nearly any color will greatly enhance the visibility of a lens that has been displaced onto the sclera or "lost" in the fornix. If the lens should fall on a lightly colored surface, its tint will also lend contrast from the background, but lightly tinted lenses on dark backgrounds are still difficult to locate. Tinted lenses are of considerable aid to patients who are not correctible to normal acuity with spectacles and who have great difficulty finding misplaced contact lenses.

ORDERING

Contact lens colors are usually selected on a cosmetic basis from a trial set containing lenses of various colors.

The final lens color will only appear the same as the trial lens color if the ordered lens is the same thickness as the trial lens. Dou-

bling the thickness of a lens produces a color that appears as dark as that of a lens with the next darker shade in the original thickness. Because of the relative differences in thickness, positive power lenses will normally appear darker than negative power lenses.

DUPLICATING TINTED LENSES

Occasionally, some variation occurs in the coloring of the contact lens plastic. If one lens from a pair must be replaced, some slight variation may be noted in the second lens. If an exact match is needed, it is best to return the remaining lens to the laboratory so it can be matched.

TINTED LENSES AT NIGHT

One of the disadvantages of tinted contact lenses is that it may not be convenient to remove them in the evening, as can easily be done with sunglasses. Various authors have cautioned against wearing tinted lenses for night driving. The lens absorption data used to support this claim is not valid, however, since it refers to extreme thicknesses, which are *never* encountered in present-day lenses.[3] It is doubtful whether contact lenses with light tints will have any appreciable effect on night visibility, but medium and dark colored lenses should not be worn.

LENTICULAR CONSTRUCTION

Various types of lenticular constructions are available for contact lenses of both high positive or negative powers. These construc- tions are normally used either to reduce the weight of the lens or to modify the edge thickness.

STANDARD LENTICULAR

The usual lenticular construction for a positive power contact lens is similar to that for a positive power spectacle lens. The optical portion of the front surface of the lens is restricted to the central area, and the peripheral portion is given much less curvature (Figure 15.4a and b). In this way the center thickness, and consequently the weight, can be reduced considerably. A minus power len- ticular lens is constructed by adding a second curve to the periphery of the front surface; this has the effect of creating a front bevel (Figure 15.5a and b). A reverse effect can be obtained by adding a minus bevel known as a minus carrier. This option is normally used for low-power lenses that ride low, to give extra lens lift (Figure 15.5c).

MINUS CARRIER

It is possible to curve the surfaces of the carrier portion of high positive power contact lenses in a way that would ordinarily produce a minus lens power. In using a minus carrier, the center thickness and the lens weight can be even less than is possible with the standard lenticular (Figure 15.6a and b).

The minus carrier contact lens, due to its design, gives the practitioner many variables that can alter the performance of the lens on the eye (Figure 15.6c and d). The base curve, optic zone, total lens diameter, and lens power are all determined by normal fitting procedures. The secondary and peripheral curves of the minus carrier lens are likewise ordered in a customary manner. The center thickness of the lens, which is one of the most important variables of the lens, is dependent on the total lens diameter, base curve, power, and junction thickness of the lens.

The junction thickness has been found in most cases to be optimal at a thickness of 0.13 mm. Using this optimum junction thickness of 0.13 mm., a graph can be used to find the minimum center thickness of any plus lenticular lens, once the other variables are selected (Figure 15.7).

Two important variables that the practi- tioner must determine in designing his lenticular lens are the anterior optic cap size and the anterior peripheral radius. The anterior optic cap is usually determined by the patient's pupil size and is kept to a minimum in order to reduce the center thickness and weight. The anterior peripheral radius of the carrier portion of the lenticular contact lens can be made any desirable radius. It is usually specified relative to the base curve.

For an average lens of +13.00 D., Nelson and Mandell[4] found the following:

In Figure 15.8 the average lens position is plotted against the value of the anterior peripheral radius. The flatter the carrier, the higher the lens will position itself. A 9.0 mm. carrier invariably positions itself too low on the subject. It is characteristic for this lens to be picked up just momentarily by the lid and then is dropped to the lower lid. A 13.0 mm. carrier is usually too flat when combined with the other parameters of the lenses. It invariably positions quite high on the patient. The 10.0 mm., 11.0 mm., and 12.0 mm. carriers center well, for 90 percent of the patients have good movement and an excellent subjective response.

The second variable to consider is the

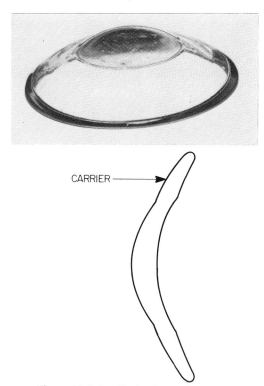

CARRIER ──────▶

Figure 15.4. Lenticular lens: plus power.

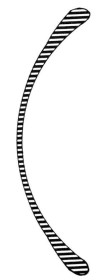

Figure 15.5c. A minus carrier can be used in conjunction with a minus power lens to achieve greater lift.

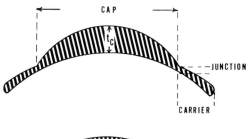

CAP

t_c

──JUNCTION

CARRIER

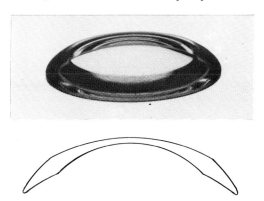

Figure 15.5. Lenticular lens: minus power.

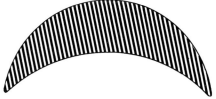

Figure 15.6a. Minus carrier contact lens with standard junction thickness of 0.13 compared to a single-cut lens of equal power.

anterior optic cap diameter and its relationship to lens position, which can be found in Figure 15.9. The relationship found was linear, with the smallest cap size riding in the highest position and the largest cap size the lowest position. This is exactly what one would predict. For instance, the larger the cap size, the thicker the lens, and, thus, a heavier lens

that drops. This might be due to the increased lens thickness and weight or the decreased width of the carrier.

The third variable that can be varied is the overall lens diameter. In Figure 15.10, average lens position is plotted against total lens diameter. It is found that all the lenses, except the 8.6 mm. diameter, center very well.

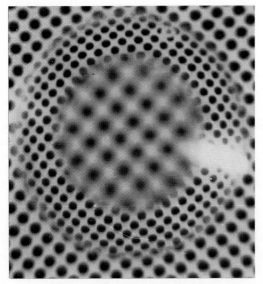

Figure 15.6b. Minus carrier lens.

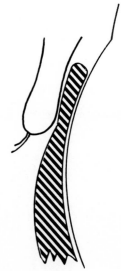

Figure 15.6c. Minus carrier lens is pulled by lid to a high position.

The latter lens usually rides low on the cornea and does not seem to cover the surface

area necessary to promote lens stability. However, increasing the diameter just 0.4 mm. to

LID-LENS FIT
Minus and Lenticulars

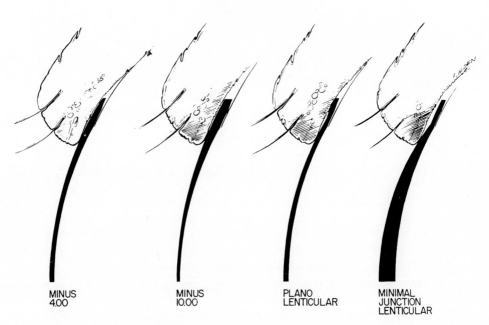

MINUS 4.00   MINUS 10.00   PLANO LENTICULAR   MINIMAL JUNCTION LENTICULAR

(all lenses 9.0 diameter, 7.70 base)

Figure 15.6d. Comparison of edge configuration for different lens powers. Courtesy of D. Korb.

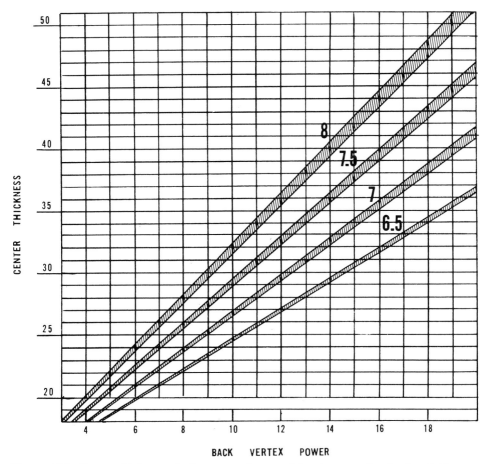

Figure 15.7. Center thickness of plus power lenses with minus carrier, having 0.13 mm. junction thickness. Each hatched band represents a cap diameter of 6.5, 7.0, 7.5, or 8.0 mm. The lower boundary of each band represents a base curve of 40.00 D and the upper boundary represents a base curve of 45.00 D. From R. B. Mandell, *J. Am. Optom. Assoc.*, July, 1968.

a 9.0 value gives the lens the stability and lid action necessary for a central position in 90 percent of the cases. Increasing the total diameter to 9.4 or 9.8 mm. does not improve the positioning of the lens.

Edge Taper

Even when the best carrier curve is used, the effect on lens performance is modified or even nullified by the edge taper. For example, in the lens design illustrated in Figure 15.11a, the radius for the carrier portion is constant but has three possible edge tapers. The lenses *theoretically have the same minus carrier* but in fact will perform quite differently on the eye.

TANGENT PERIPHERY

A special type of lenticular design can be produced by making the peripheral portions of both the front and back lens surfaces straight rather than curved (Figure 15.11b). The tran-

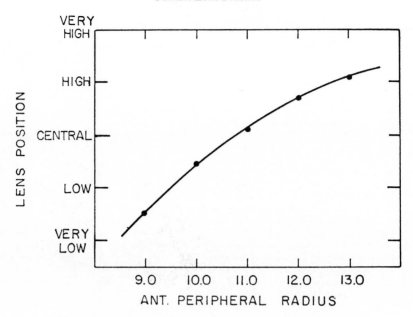

Figure 15.8. Lens position versus anterior peripheral radius.

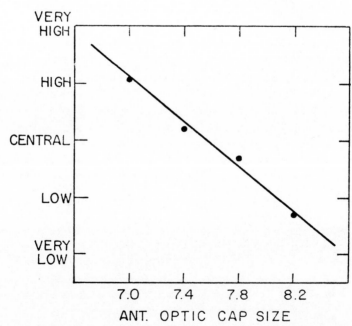

Figure 15.9. Relation between anterior optic cap diameter and lens riding position.

sitions to the straight peripheral portions are smooth. This design has the disadvantage of not allowing control of the peripheral curves for fitting.[5]

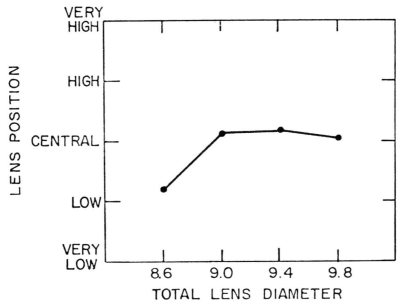

Figure 15.10. Relation between total lens diameter and average lens riding position.

POSITIVE CARRIER FOR MINUS LENSES

It is possible to curve the surfaces of the carrier portion of high minus lenses in a way that would ordinarily produce a lens of positive power. In this way it is possible to reduce the edge to any thickness desired (Figure 15.12a).[6] This design is often called a *myolenticular* lens.

It is sometimes difficult for the fitter to decide when a lenticular design is desirable. No decision is needed when high-minus-power lenses are considered, such as −10.00 D. or higher. The manufacturing laboratory will usually assume that these lenses should be in lenticular form whether or not it is ordered.

The decision is more difficult for a minus lens in the medium power range. Rules such as all minus lenses higher than −6.00 D. power should be myolenticular are not sufficient if the fitter really wants to achieve the best lens design. The problem becomes even more critical when working with ultrathin lenses.

In designing a contact lens having a given diameter, center thickness, and set of poste-

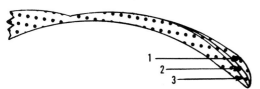

Figure 15.11a. Effect of edge taper on shape of minus carrier. The lenses have the same carrier front radius but in fact will perform quite differently on the eye. 1. Taper is too narrow—lens is less comfortable and moved excessively by the lids. 2. Optimal. 3. Taper is too great—loses the advantage (lift) of a minus carrier.

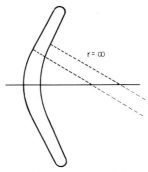

Figure 15.11b. Tangent periphery lens.

rior curves, the front curve radius will be fixed by the lens power and will determine the edge thickness. Lenses of higher minus power will have thicker edges, and vice versa. If 0.08 mm. is adopted as the optimum edge thickness, it will be found that for one power, the *critical edge power*; the front curve will be exactly right to produce this edge thickness (Figure 15.12b). The critical edge power varies with the lens design but is usually about −4.00 D. At the critical edge power, no front periphery tapering is needed, and all that must be done to finish the edge is simply to round it off and polish. Every lens that is of higher power than the critical edge power must have some process to reduce the edge thickness. If the lens power is only slightly higher than the critical edge power, a front taper is all that is necessary. A front peripheral curve could be cut, but it cannot be given a good optical polish.

An optical cut and polish of the front peripheral curve is that factor which distinguishes the myolenticular design from a simple front bevel. For manufacturing purposes, the radius of the front peripheral curve must be at least 1 mm. shorter than the radius of the front central curve. Otherwise, when the front peripheral curve is polished, there is a likelihood of running the polisher onto the central curve and distorting the lens optics. In addition, the junction between the front central and peripheral curves is smeared and may produce light scattering or flare.

Figure 15.12c shows that for ultrathin lenses of 8.2 and 8.7 mm. diameters, a front peripheral curve is needed for minus powers greater than about −5.00 D., when the base curve is flat, and −7.00 D., when the base curve is steep. Powers for other base curves may be obtained from the chart.

Upper Limit of Myolenticular Designs

For higher minus power lenses, even a myolenticular design may not eliminate the edge discomfort problem if the lens is not designed properly. For example, Figure 15.12d shows two lenses, −8.00 and −12.00 D., of 8.2 mm. diameter. The higher minus lens would not be very comfortable to wear for two reasons. First, the slope of the front peripheral curve would be too steep and would produce resistance when the lid moves across it during a blink. Second, the junction angle between the central and peripheral front curves would be too sharp and also could be felt by the lid.

This problem can be solved in two ways. First, the front optical zone diameter can be reduced, which allows a more gradual slope to the front peripheral curve. Unfortunately, for a lens diameter of 8.2 mm. with a 7.0 mm. optical zone diameter, a reduction in optical zone diameter is likely to produce flare problems. The alternative solution is to increase the lens diameter. It is critical, however, to maintain the same optic zone diameter, for if it is also increased the edge problem will be made even worse. Figure 15.12c illustrates this by showing that myolenticulars in the 8.2 mm. diameter and higher powers should be changed to an 8.7 mm. diameter. Myolenticulars of 8.7 mm. diameter and higher powers should be changed to a 9.2 mm. diameter.

NONROTATIONAL LENSES

Lenses may be modified in various ways to reduce their radial movement on the cornea. Such designs are used principally for certain types of bifocal contact lenses, for lenses with astigmatic powers, and for lenses with a prism component. They are occasionally used to provide better centration or to improve the bearing relationship of conventional lenses. Nonrotational lenses are typically more difficult to fit than conventional lenses, but they have been refined to such an extent that they are now used in a significant percentage of cases.

The clinical success of nonrotational lenses has demonstrated that lens rotation is not necessary for proper tear exchange beneath the lens. On the contrary, in some cases the reduced motion of a nonrotational lens produced less corneal trauma than did conventional lenses.

Many attempts have been made to design various types of nonrotational lenses, and their success has varied considerably. The following descriptions will introduce the general lens types, which are available, and discuss their applications, but detailed fitting procedures will be discussed separately. There are four general types of nonrotational lenses: noncircular lenses, toric surface lenses, ballast lenses, and corneal flange lenses.

NONCIRCULAR SHAPES

Lenses have been cut in various asymmetrical shapes in an attempt to stabilize their rotation. Most commonly, a straight cut is made across the top and/or bottom of a circular lens. If only one cut is made, the lens has a single truncation (corresponding to a truncation of any geometric figure). If both the top and bottom of the lens are cut, the lens has a double truncation (Figure 15.13). The corners at the end of each truncation are usually rounded to provide a smooth transition to the rounded portions of the lens.

A lens with a single truncation will tend to ride on the cornea with the truncated area in a downward position, but this is difficult to control. With blinking and eye movements, the lens may be rotated to a reverse position in which the truncation is at the top. These changes in position usually produce considerable discomfort for the wearer, and consequently, a single truncation is seldom used as the only means of avoiding rotation.

A lens with double truncation will have greater radial stability than one with a single truncation, but the former lens construction has only met with limited success. It tends to ride on the cornea with the long axis horizontal and is stabilized chiefly by the lids. With each blink, however, the lid raises the nasal side of the lens further than the temporal side, and the lens rotates. When the lens drops back in place after the blink it tends to assume a compensatory rotation to bring it

once again to its original position. Occasionally the lens will rotate a full 90° during blinking and ride momentarily with its longer axis in a vertical position. This causes considerable discomfort for the wearer.

The amount of rotation by a double truncated lens varies considerably with the bearing relationship, but rotation is seldom adequately controlled without the aid of additional lens designs.

Consistently, the most difficult problem

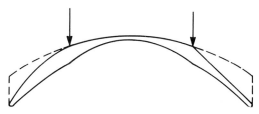

Figure 15.12a. Methods for thinning the edge of a high-minus power lens. Left side illustrates a front peripheral curve, or myolenticular, and the right side illustrates a front taper.

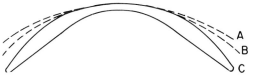

Figure 15.12b. The critical edge power occurs when the front curve C, together with the other lens parameters, produces the edge thickness desired. Front curves A and B, for higher minus powers, require a front peripheral curve or bevel.

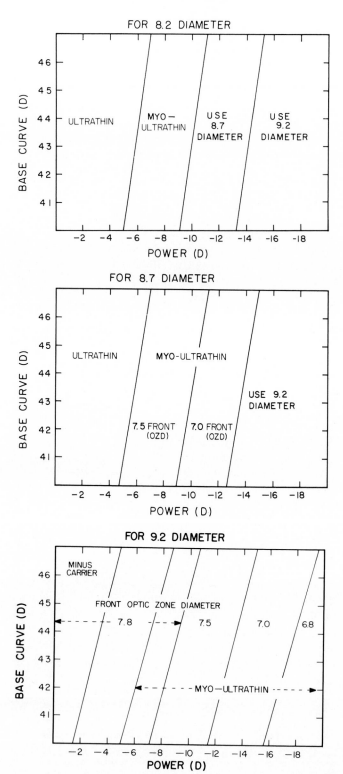

Figure 15.12c. Guide to optimal lens design for three diameters, given base curve and power. Low powers allow single cut, medium powers require myolenticular, and high powers need larger diameters.

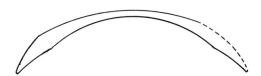

Figure 15.12d. As the minus power is increased, the junction becomes sharper and may lead to discomfort. Reducing the front optical zone diameter (right side) improves the lens design.

in manufacturing a double truncated lens is producing a comfortable edge. The area along the truncation is usually considerably thicker than the rounded portion, and proper edge finishing is difficult.

Oval Lenses

If a double truncated lens is rounded at the corners, it begins to assume an oval shape (Figure 15.13). Oval lenses suffer from the same disadvantages as other double truncated lenses, and they are difficult to manufacture. Hence, they are seldom used.

Square Lenses

A double truncated lens may also have two additional cuts on each side, thus producing a lens that is nearly rectangular; only the corners would be rounded. This lens is difficult to manufacture and provides no advantages over other nonrotational lenses (Figure 15.13).

Triangular Lenses

Lenses made in triangular form usually produce considerable irritation to the upper lid and offer no advantages in terms of radial stability (Figure 15.13).

OTHER NONROTATIONAL LENSES

Toric Base Curve

The toric base curve lens is one of the earliest attempted for stabilizing the rotation of corneal lenses.[7,8,9] Generally, a surface is ground that is very nearly the same toricity as the cornea to which it will be fitted. When the lens is placed on the eye, it tends to align its curvature with that of the cornea. Lens movement is principally in the direction of the steeper corneal meridian so that vertical motion usually dominates. The relationship between a toric base curve lens and the cornea is analogous to the fit of a saddle to the horse's back before it is cinched. The saddle may slip from side to side or forward and back, but rotation is difficult.

The disadvantage of a toric base curve for lens stabilization is that it is only effective when the corneal toricity is greater than 2.00 D. These lenses have been used for less toricity, but they usually continue to rotate and produce intolerable optical effects.

The toric optical zone is selected primarily on the basis of the bearing relationship. This zone modifies the necessary optical correction, and this modification must be taken into account when computing the optical power of the lens. A toric optical zone can seldom adequately correct an astigmatic re-

 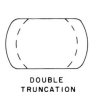 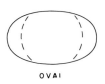 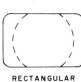

SINGLE TRUNCATION   DOUBLE TRUNCATION   OVAL   RECTANGULAR   TRIANGULAR

Figure 15.13. Various optional lens shapes.

fractive error if the anterior surface of the lens is spherical. Consequently, the appropriate toric surface is usually needed for the front surface of the lens as well. Such a lens is known as a bitoric lens (*see* Chapter 9).

Toric Peripheral Curve

A toric peripheral curve may be used alone or in conjunction with a toric base curve to reduce lens rotation. However, this has not proved very successful and is seldom used.

Prism Ballast

If sufficient prism is ground in a contact lens, the lens will tend to ride with the base of the prism at the inferior position, and thus, rotation is nearly eliminated. This occurs because the lens is much thicker and heavier at the prism base position; consequently, this point is attracted downward by the force of gravity. In comparison with the other forms of nonrotational lenses, the prism ballast lens has the advantage of independence from the anatomical configuration of the cornea or the lids to maintain its orientation. Greater freedom is possible in selecting the lens characteristics, and fitting is usually on less of a trial and error basis.

The prism ballast may be combined with most other lens designs that reduce rotation and provide further stability, or it may be used alone. However, the two lenses must have a prism of the same power so that the apparent displacement of the visual field is the same for both eyes.

The amount of prism that must be incorporated into a lens to provide sufficient ballast varies with the lens construction, but it is generally between 1.5 and 2 Δ.[10] Prism power is directly related to the base and apex lens thicknesses, and the difference between these increases with the diameter of the lens. If the prism power is too low, the lens will not stabilize, and if it is too high, the lens becomes uncomfortable.

The prism ballast principle was used by Black and Cinefro in 1957 and mentioned later by others.[9] Its acceptance has been rather slow, but recent interest has been high, since the technique was tested and proved clinically feasible.

In addition to the usual applications of nonrotational lenses, the prism ballast lens can be used in spherical power form to position the lens low on the cornea and thus aid in the following circumstances:

1. Lowering the riding position of a lens that is consistently too high on the cornea

2. Avoiding structures that may be irritated by the lens such as pingueculas, scars, superior lid growths

3. Alleviating excessive lens movement

MODIFICATIONS TO INCREASE TEAR EXCHANGE

In an attempt to increase tear exchange, it has occasionally been proposed that apertures be placed in the lens[11-15] or that facets or channels be ground at the periphery of the back surface.[16,17] The apertures may be produced by drilling or by laser burning.

APERTURES

The value of apertures in scleral lenses to provide tear exchange has been demonstrated conclusively.[18,19] Their value in corneal lenses is less definite. Most practitioners do not place apertures in the lenses unless other methods to produce tear exchange are inadequate.

Often there is difficulty in producing an aperture that will not cause various wearing problems. Corneal lens apertures have been known to cause corneal abrasions, visual disturbances, and lens warpage. Korb states that the lens apertures must conform to the following conditions:[14]

1. The diameter of the aperture should not exceed 0.40 mm. As the diameter of the aperture increases, there is an increase in the frequency of corneal irritation and abrasion. In addition, the frequency of lens warpage increases with larger diameters.

2. A straight bore is indicated. Although some success has been achieved with tapered designs, they have not proved as satisfactory as the straight bore.

3. The juncture of the hole at either lens surface should present a right angle to the surface and should be free of any irregularities as observed under a minimum magnification of 35×.

4. The interior walls of the aperture must be highly polished, comparable in quality to the finish of the lens surfaces. If this requirement is not met, fluid transfer through the opening is not optimum, and in daily use, the aperture is prone to clog with secretions.

5. The direction of the aperture should be along a normal to the ocular surface of the lens. (The projection of any aperture should intersect the center of curvature of the base curve of the lens.) Thus, in the case of multiple applications, no two apertures would be parallel.

Korb prefers the use of three fenestrations placed 1.75 mm. from the center of the lens in a triangular pattern (Figure 15.14a). Many others prefer a larger number of apertures in various patterns (Figure 15.14b).

Korb has shown that a fenestration may be effective for only a small corneal area around the fenestration position (Figure 15.15).

KORB FENESTRATIONS

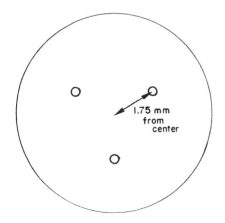

Figure 15.14a. Three fenestrations placed in center of the lens.

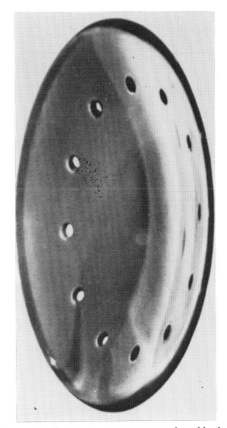

Figure 15.14b. Aperture pattern produced by laser burning. Courtesy of Continuous Curve contact lenses.

FACETS AND CHANNELS

An attempt has been made to increase tear exchange by adding four small facets to the periphery of the posterior lens surface. Other modifications for the same purpose are made by grinding channels of various shapes into the periphery of the posterior lens surface (Figure 15.16). These lens modifications have not been adequately evaluated, but generally they have not been regarded as very helpful.

SPORTS LENS

Various lenses have been produced under the name "Sports lens." Usually these lenses are tricurve or multicurve lenses and are relatively large (total diameter > 10 mm.). They are fitted very tight and cannot be easily removed; thus, they are not easily dislodged during contact sports.[20,21] Some types may be used for swimming.[22] They are meant to be worn for only a few hours, so the patient must have a second pair of conventional lenses.

One "sports lens" is a scleral lens with a narrow haptic portion.[23]

UNDERWATER LENS

Two types of lenses have been developed that enable the wearer to see clearly when under water. They are used primarily by skin divers.

Jessen has made a lens with a tiny button on the front surface.[24] The button has a power of approximately +150 D. in air and +50 D. when immersed in water. It effectively replaces the corneal power when the eye is under water.

Nagle and Monical devised an underwater contact lens with a flat front surface and an air cell.[25,26] Use of this lens construction has also been reported by Grant.[27,28]

COATING TO PRODUCE WETTABLE SURFACES

Largely through the work of Erb,[29] methods have been developed to coat contact lenses with a thin film of titanium dioxide.[30] When properly coated, the lens becomes more wettable, that is, fluid on the lens is more uniformly distributed. Clinically, however, the effect has been shown to be of short duration and of little practical value.

WETTABLE PLASTICS

By adding small quantities of hydrogel to P.M.M.A. polymer, it is possible to produce a hard lens with higher than usual wettability.

PINHOLE CONTACT LENS

A pinhole lens can be used to improve visual acuity in cases of regular ametropia and of other anomalies not correctible by ordinary spectacles, such as irregular astig-

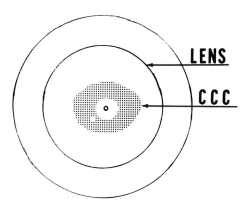

Figure 15.15. Effect of fenestration on corneal edema only occurs for small areas surrounding the fenestration (Korb).

matism and corneal distortion.[31,32] It can often be used to restrict the light bundle entering the eye to a particular area, thus avoiding the opacities that scatter light and reduce visual acuity.

The general principle of pinhole correction on simple myopia is illustrated in Figure 15.17. Limiting the diameter of the bundle of light rays that enter the eye reduces the blur circle diameter.

The chief attribute of the pinhole lens is that it tends to improve the image of any type of refractive irregularity. It is mainly used in conditions of irregular eye surfaces.

The pinhole principle has a number of limitations when attempted in spectacle lenses. Central vision is only possible when the line of sight is directed through the pinhole so that peripheral objects can be viewed only by turning the head. This problem is sometimes solved by using a multiple pinhole device, but each time the fixation is changed, a realignment must be made with one of the other pinholes contained in the spectacle. Also, since the pinhole limits the ray bundle entering the eye, the pupil becomes the field stop, and changes in pupil size therefore limit the field of view.

A pinhole contact lens is highly preferable to a pinhole spectacle lens for several reasons. Since the contact lens rides on the cornea, no realignment of sight through the pinhole is necessary. Also, there is considerable gain in the field of view, as shown in Figure 15.18.

If a pinhole is moved closer to the eye, there is little effect on the image, but the field of view is increased. If the pinhole is placed in a contact lens, the field of view will be of almost normal limits.

The illuminance of the retinal image is greatly reduced by any reduction in pupil diameter. If the pupil diameter is cut in half, the retinal image is dimmed by a factor of four. A pupil diameter reduction of 8 mm. to 2 mm. would cut the retinal illuminance by a factor of sixteen. This calculation is based on the relationship of the illuminance to the area of the pupil, which in turn is a function of the square of the pupil diameter. The relative change in retinal illuminance can be

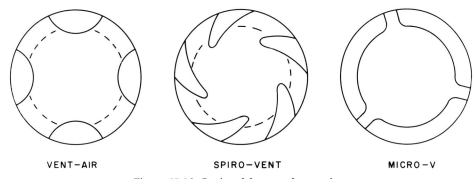

VENT–AIR   SPIRO–VENT   MICRO–V

Figure 15.16. Optional features for venting.

MYOPIC   EYE

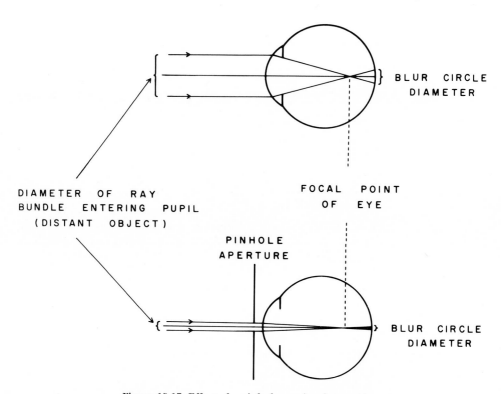

Figure 15.17. Effect of a pinhole on simple myopia.

found very simply by comparing the relative sizes of the pupil diameters squared.

$$\text{Rel. Ret. illuminance} = \frac{d_1^2}{d_2^2}$$

Loss of retinal illuminance is rarely of concern under daylight illumination, but in dim lighting it may tend to lower acuity enough to offset any benefit of the pinhole. Pinhole lenses are therefore of little value at night.

PINHOLE POSITION

If a pinhole is placed before an emmetropic eye, the position of the retinal image is not affected, even if the pinhole is not before the center of the pupil. This is illustrated in Figure 15.19, where rays from three positions are shown to focus at the same retinal position. Should the eye be out of focus, however, the retinal image position will vary with the location of the pinhole. It therefore follows that as long as an eye is emmetropic, or made so by correction, the position of the retinal image will remain constant; consequently, movement of the pinhole contact lens will not result in an apparent movement of the field of view. It may also be noted that a pinhole can be placed at any position in a

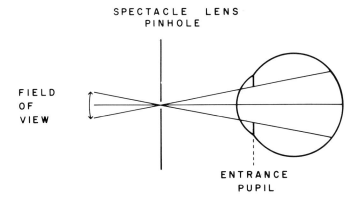

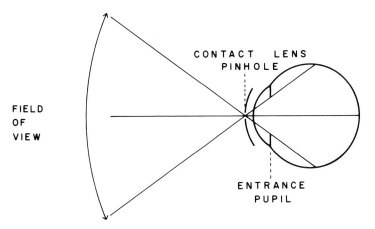

Figure 15.18. Field of view with pinhole in spectacle lens (*top*) and contact lens (*bottom*).

contact lens, providing the lens does not rotate, and work equally well. This can be of value in certain cases, such as partial subluxation of the crystalline lens. In this case only a small peripheral section of the lens is exposed to the pupil, but after the eye is corrected (as in aphakia), the exposed section of the lens is large enough to cause a second image to be formed, which is out of focus but which casts a light glare on the retina and which can be extremely annoying to the patient. Since the crystalline lens is in an inferior position, the pinhole should be decentered superiorly in the contact lens.

The actual shape of the pinhole is not important. It should always be as large as possible so that a maximum degree of light enters the eye. The pinhole in a contact lens used for a subluxation case could well have a moon shape. However, pinhole shapes other than round call for special manufacturing procedures.

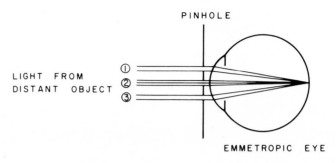

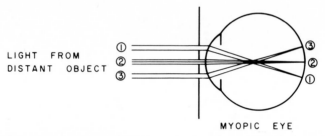

Figure 15.19. The position of a pinhole before the pupil does not affect the position of the retinal image if the eye is emmetropic.

TYPES OF PINHOLE LENSES

Pinhole aperture corneal lenses are of several types. The simplest and least expensive is a lens consisting of a transparent center of given diameter and a dense black periphery. This lens is made from black plastic stock, in which a hole has been drilled and then filled with clear plastic. When the lens is cut, the curves are smooth and no line of demarcation is noted between the two colors of plastic. The lens can be made in any power. The disadvantage of this type of lens is a cosmetic one, but it does provide an inexpensive trial lens and can occasionally be used on patients with very dark irises.

Another pinhole aperture corneal lens contains an opaque lamination that limits the transmissible area to a small hole, which is filled with clear plastic. The opaque area is often colored to make an artificial iris (Figure 15.20).

The Multi-Range contact lens (originally called the Cosmetic Bifocal) has a pinhole in the center, which is surrounded by six radial slits placed in three meridians (Figure 15.21). These slits serve to increase the field of view and act as stenopeic slits when the lens is decentered on the eye. The principle of fitting the Multi-Range contact lens is similar to that of fitting a single vision lens, with a few additional measurements necessary for ordering the lens.

Standard values for the lens dimensions

PINHOLE LENS TYPES

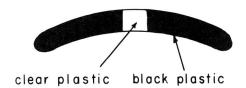

clear plastic   black plastic

coating

lamination

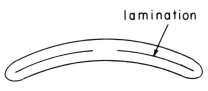

Figure 15.20. Pinhole lenses.

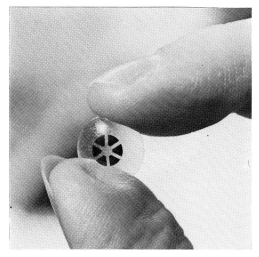

Figure 15.21. Multi-Range contact lens.

have been established by the laboratory, but other values are available:

1. Inside diameter (I.D. or pinhole)   1.5 mm
2. Outside diameter (O.D. or opaque area)   4.5 mm
3. Number of slits   6
4. Slit widths   0.4 mm

A measuring magnifier can be used to verify the various specifications of the multi-range contact lens. Other lens parameters can be inspected in the normal manner.

If a patient's pupil is small, a multi-range contact lens may be ordered with a smaller I.D. of 1.0 mm., with six slits, and a width of 0.4 mm. per slit.

The Multi-Range contact lens should be fitted so that the lens is centered over the pupil with minimal vertical movement.

It is recommended that single vision lenses be prescribed first in order to determine the centering and positioning of the lens and to establish wearing time. The same specifications should then be used in fitting the Multi-Range contact lens.

GRAVITYLENS ®

One of the most difficult problems for the contact lens fitter is the patient with a high-riding lens. Lenses that ride high are usually those with minus power. It is fairly rare to see a lens with plus power that rides in a high position.

Lenses with minus power have several characteristics that predispose the lens to a high-riding position: (1) The center of gravity for a lens of minus power tends to be displaced towards the posterior side of the lens. This causes the lens to be more easily supported by the cornea when the lens is in a high position. (2) The increased edge thickness of a minus lens presents a prominence that can be easily gripped by the lids. (3) A displaced corneal apex may be at least a contributing factor in high-riding lenses. While there has been considerable speculation on this point, a valid study is lacking, which shows a definite relationship between a given corneal topography and high-riding lenses.

PROBLEMS CAUSED BY THE HIGH-RIDING LENS

The problems caused by a high-riding lens may be visual, physiological, or both. With a lens in a high position, the optical zone diameter may not be large enough to cover the pupillary area, and hence, light enters through the peripheral curve and causes flare and blur or a reduction in visual acuity. Blurring occurs because at times the pupil is partially covered by the peripheral curve of the contact lens, which does not give the proper correction for the patient's refractive error. Flare occurs because the peripheral curve of the lenses causes a prismatic displacement of the light that passes through it. Flare may also be due to pooling of tears at the edge of the lens, which also has a prismatic effect on the light.

A lens that rides in a high position may be tolerated for a short period of time or even for a period of a year. Eventually, however, the poor positioning of this lens will cause physiological problems. There is usually undue pressure applied in the superior limbal region of the eye, which, in extreme cases, induces neovascularization. This condition is also made worse by the stagnation of tears beneath the contact lens as it is held in the high position. If the tear stagnation is great, the lens may cause tight symptoms, even though the base curve of the lens is on K or flatter than K.

SOLUTIONS TO HIGH-RIDING LENSES

Many attempts have been made to find various lens forms that will correct the high-riding lens. The only modification that can be made on the existing lens which rides high is to make it smaller. Usually when this is done, the lens still rides high and only increases the flare problem because the lower edge of the smaller lens is higher.

If a new lens is made, which is larger, it produces a thicker edge, which causes it to be carried to a higher position. Sometimes the visual problem is solved in this way, but the physiological problems are increased, and the lenses can only be tolerated for short wearing periods.

The next solution that is often tried is to make the lens much thicker. This increases the weight of the lens (and the edge thickness) and shifts the center of gravity forward so that the lens will drop to a low position. However, this solution is seldom satisfactory because the lens now drops with an intolerable force to the lower lid—with a "bang" effect, which is exceedingly uncomfortable for the patient. In some cases, these lenses shift from a high position to a low position from time to time and never occupy a proper position near the center of the cornea. This same effect can be produced by using a prism ballast lens, but there is seldom acceptable comfort on the lower lid because a much higher than normal prism power is usually necessary.

Probably the best solution to date has been the use of a myodisc or minus-power lenticular, which has a large taper or bevel on the peripheral portion of the front surface. In a few cases, this will solve the problem, but most often, the lens still continues to ride high.

LENS DESIGN

The Gravitylens (made by Concise Contact Lens Co.) is designed to maximize the forces that will push the lens away from a high position. In some ways, the lens resembles a plus lens lenticular, which actually inspired this design. There are three zones to the lens. The central zone contains the optical portion of the lens. Surrounding this is a second, or intermediate, zone, which is really a continuation of the central zone into an aspherical curve designed to minimize the weight factor in the peripheral portion of the lens. The third, or outer, zone consists of a carrier of minimum thickness, which is similar to that found on a plus lenticular lens (Figure 15.22).

The success of this lens depends on a precise design of the intermediate zone front curve. This is produced by cutting essentially three curves to form a continuous and smoothly flowing junction. When the lens is worn, the intermediate curve, in conjunction with the carrier, is acted upon by the lid in such a way that as the lid pulls the lens upward, the lens moves up with the lid until a high position has been reached, at which time the lid touches the intermediate zone of the lens and exerts a pushing force similar to that created on a plus lenticular. This tends to push the lens downward and create the desired result (Figure 15.23).

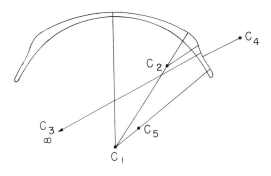

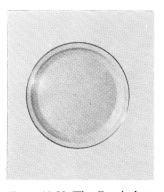

Figure 15.22. The Gravitylens.

HOW TO ORDER

Generally speaking, just as with a plus lenticular lens, the Gravitylens must be larger than the average contact lens. Most lenses that have been fitted are between 9.2 and 9.4 mm. Hence, unless there is a good reason, this diameter range should be used. Many fitters normally prefer a small diameter for regular lenses, but when it is considered that the circulation is increased greatly when the larger diameter Gravitylens is used, there is usually not a tear circulation problem.

Front Optical Zone Diameter. The average front optical zone diameter is 7.8 mm.

Back Optical Zone Diameter. Follow the usual

fitting dimensions preferred by the fitter. The average is 7.6 mm.

Peripheral Curves. Use a standard peripheral curve. Very flat peripheral curves may be used only if a special design is put onto the lenses.

Thickness. The center thickness will be greater than normal by 0.06 to 0.08 mm. The thickness is determined by all the usual lens parameters and, in addition, by the design of the intermediate zone of the lens. Hence, the exact thickness must be determined by the laboratory to correspond to the lens design. The edge thickness will be the same as a much thinner conventional lens.

ANTICIPATED DIFFICULTIES

The Gravitylens is similar to a minus carrier lenticular plus lens in the types of problems that may be encountered. Problems occur when the desired effect is either over– or underaccentuated.

1. Lens drops too fast or stays in a low position. In this case, the gravity effect has been overdone and must be reduced. This may be accomplished by ordering a lens that is thinner by 0.04 mm.

2. Lens still remains in high position. Here the gravity effect is not great enough, and lens thickness should be increased by 0.04 mm.

3. Patient notes flare or halos. If the lens rides in a high position, then more gravity effect must be added. If the lens now rides in a centered position, it indicates that the front optical zone is too small and must be increased in diameter by 0.4 mm. This may also necessitate an increase in the total diameter of the lens.

4. Patient is comfortable for a period from one to five hours but then begins to get a hot, uncomfortable sensation. If the lens rides in a high position, once again this problem, which is physiological, may be solved by adding more of the gravity effect to pull the lens down. If the lens is riding in the centered position, it indicates there is a need for more peripheral curve clearance. The peripheral curve should be flattened by 1 mm.

For many patients, this lens requires a trial-and-error fitting to achieve the proper balance between the high lens position and the gravity principle. This may be best accomplished with the use of trial lenses.

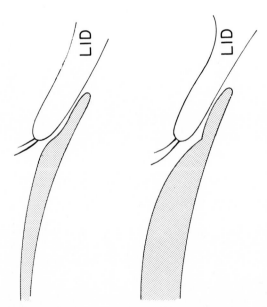

Figure 15.23. Design of Gravitylens (*left*) tends to lower the lens on the cornea, as does a plus lenticular (*right*).

ASPHERIC LENSES

Various lens designs have been produced in which the posterior surface is given the shape of an aspheric curve.[33-37] This has the advantage of eliminating any junction and producing one continuous curve. An aspheric lens construction is said to have the advantage of eliminating flare from the usual peripheral curve. In addition, there is some evidence that it allows better lens centration for some eyes and may be helpful in rare cases when corneal abrasion occurs from the junction of regular lenses.

The main disadvantage of the aspheric lens and the reason that it has not received wider acceptance is that they are somewhat difficult to understand, and the advantages presented have not been accepted. They are difficult or impossible to verify.

Most aspheric lenses are made in the form of one of the conical curves (Figure 15.24).[38]

This is usually an ellipse.[39] The other conical curves that are sometimes used are a parabola or a hyperbola. There is no need to have an exhaustive understanding of these curves in order to fit this general lens type. Much confusion has resulted from the description of these lenses in terms of various mathematical formulas which are taken from analytical geometry. These descriptions are not necessary.

Figure 15.25 shows how the corneal contour can be represented approximately by an ellipse. Although no corneal contour will ever be exactly an ellipse, the approximation is close enough for practical purposes. Different corneas, which have different rates of peripheral flattening, can each be represented by different ellipses with different rates of flattening. This is shown in Figure 15.26, where various conic curves are shown in

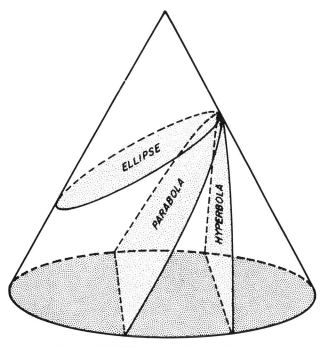

Figure 15.24. The family of conical curves.

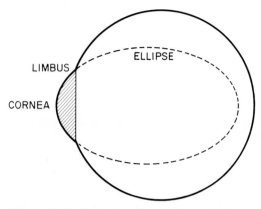

Figure 15.25. Representation of the corneal contour as an ellipse.

relation to a circle. Each of these curves has the same radius of curvature at the apex, or point where they touch the circle; however, each curve flattens at a different rate, just as the various corneas flatten toward the periphery.

The only difference between the ellipse, the parabola, and the hyperbola is in the rate in which they flatten. Hence, if the cornea is found to be nearly spherical, that is, not flattening very much, it will be more like an ellipse. If the cornea flattens a great deal, it will be more like a hyperbola. There is another similar curve, the parabola, which cannot represent all corneas because the parabola has only one rate of flattening for a given apex radius, and it is known that corneas of different patients differ in their rates of peripheral flattening.

In fitting an aspheric curve, the task is simply to find the conic that has a rate of flattening slightly greater than that of the cornea in order to allow tear interchange. This rate of flattening is usually specified as the edge lift or standoff.[40,41]

CON–O–COID LENSES

The most successful method in determining the lens design for the patient is with the use of fitting or trial lenses.

Con–o–coid lenses are designated by two numbers: apical radius of curvature (r), which specifies magnitude, and conicity (c), which indicates the degree of flattening in the peripheral area.[42]

The complete fitting trial set contains thirty lenses in three conicity values, .5, .6,

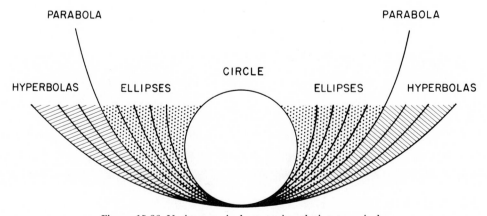

Figure 15.26. Various conical curves in relation to a circle.

and .7. Base curves are from 7.30 to 8.10 in steps of 0.10 mm., and the sizes are 9.0, 9.3, and 9.6.

1. Measure the two principal corneal meridians with a keratometer.

2. Convert the readings to radius of curvature.

3. Transpose the spectacle prescription to minus cylinders, then disregard the cylinders.

4. If the difference in the corneal readings is less than 0.20 mm., select a lens with a base curve .10 steeper than the flattest meridian and as close to the patient's prescription as possible and with a .6 conicity value.

5. If the corneal readings differ by 0.20 mm. or more, select a lens using the following table as a guide:

When the Principal Meridians Differ by	Steepen Flatter Reading by
0.20 mm.	0.15 mm.
0.30 mm.	0.20 mm.
0.40 mm.	0.25 mm.

0.50 mm.	0.30 mm.
0.60 mm.	0.35 mm.

6. To determine the size of a lens, measure the horizontal visible iris. The following guide is the relationship of overall size to corneal diameter.

For Corneal Diameter of	Use Lens Diameter of
11.0 mm.	8.7 mm.
11.5 mm.	9.0 mm.
12.0 mm.	9.3 mm.
12.5 mm.	9.6 mm.

A basic method of determining the relationship of the diameter of a lens to the base curve is that the steeper the base curve, the smaller the lens diameter.

Base Curve Indications of	Use Lens Diameter of
7.20 mm.	8.4 mm.
7.35 mm.	8.6 mm.
7.50 mm.	8.8 mm.
7.65 mm.	9.0 mm.
7.80 mm.	9.2 mm.
7.95 mm.	9.4 mm.
8.10 mm.	9.6 mm.

CONOID LENS

The conoid lens, as it has been named, can be best described by visualizing a cone with the upper two-thirds cut off and replaced by a sphere.[43]

The back optic radii are varied in steps of 0.1 mm. from 5.0 mm. radius to 8.5 mm. The cone angle is tangential to the optic, from 6.9 mm. upwards, and is generally nontangential below 6.8 mm., as this series is designed for the keratoconic cornea.

All standard diagnostic lenses have the following specifications:

Overall diameter 9.0 mm.

Optic diameter 6.5 mm.

All lenses are fenestrated with one hole 2 mm. in from the lens edge, 0.25 mm. in diameter.

All lens designs fall into two main classifications:

1. Optic fitting
2. Peripheral fitting

The optic fitting group has back optic radii selected to conform to the corneal curve, and the base curve is critical to the fitting. The peripheral zones are essentially clearance zones, to facilitate circulation beneath the lens. The fitting is determined by variations in back optic radii, optic zone diameter, peripheral curves, and overall diameter. Such lens designs rarely locate centrally on the cornea, being designed to float over the corneal area, to facilitate circulation. Relatively large optic zone diameters are required so that the pupil is adequately covered by the lens, in all positions.

Peripheral fitting lenses are designed to fit the peripheral corneal zones with central apical clearance. The base curve is not critical to the fitting, as the peripheral fitting is determined by the slope or contour of the peripheral flange.

The fitting of the conoid lens is made up of two main zones:

1. Central spherical area, referred to as the back optic radii
2. Tangential cone periphery

The basic lens design of the diagnostic lenses can be varied by altering the cone of the cone periphery, back optic radii, and the overall diameter. The optic diameter is increased as the size of the spherical corneal cap increases and is closely related to the cone angle selected in the fitting procedure. The steeper the cone angle required, the larger the optic diameter necessary to maintain the tangential form. Therefore, it is not necessary to specify this component of the lens.

The principle of fitting conoid lenses is as follows:

1. To provide adequate apical clearance beneath the lens in order to facilitate flow of tears over the corneal surface from the fenestration
2. To select a peripheral cone angle that tangentially contacts the cornea beneath it around the whole conoid periphery
3. To use an overall diameter of minimum size, which will adequately locate the lens over the pupil

Optimum Fitting

The optic zone radius is 0.3 mm. steeper than K of the flattest corneal meridian. Back optic radii steeper than 0.3 should not be prescribed, as there is a danger of frothing occurring beneath the lens, over the apical zone, when the initial lid pressure is relaxed.

The cone angle is selected by direct observation of the fluorescein pattern of the diagnostic lenses. The angle is selected so that a clearance around the lens edge of approximately 0.3 mm. wide is achieved. This may readily be estimated by comparing the width of the fluorescein glow around the lens edge with the diameter of the fenestration, which is 0.25 mm. diameter.

Cone Angle Too Steep

If the cone angle is too steep, the edge clearance will be less than 0.3 mm. In general practice, only keratoconic corneas require flatter than tangential cone angles.

If the apical clearance is excessive and the "bubble point" is exceeded, a small bubble will be observed over the apical zone. This bubble will break down into a fine froth and produce multiple corneal indentations simulating corneal stippling. A flatter back optic radius should be prescribed to reduce the apical clearance.

Cone Angle Too Flat

When the cone angle is too flat to contact the cornea tangentially, the edge clearance will be wider than 0.3 mm. This is usually accompanied by lens instability, which increases proportionately to the degree of flatness of the cone angle. The corneal contour determines the cone angle. The larger the optic cap, the steeper the cone angle required.

Lens Diameter

The optimum lens diameter is controlled by the size of the cornea. Generally speaking, the larger the cornea, the larger is the lens diameter required. As most corneas are oval, with the horizontal meridian the longest, the vertical diameter is taken as a guide to corneal size.

On a 11.0 mm. vertical diameter cornea, the optimum overall lens diameter has been found to be 9.00 mm. For each 0.5 mm. corneal diameter increase or decrease, the lens diameter is correspondingly increased or decreased by 0.25 mm.

A 12 mm. diameter cornea would therefore require a 9.5 mm. diameter lens, and a 10 mm. cornea an 8.5 mm. diameter lens.

When lens centration occurs with the standard trial lens, the overall diameter should not be increased.

When the lens diameter is increased, an adjustment must be made to the cone angle to compensate for the outward movement of the tangential contact band. Should this not be done, the edge clearance will be excessive and the lens fitting unstable.

For each 0.25 mm. increase in diameter, the cone angle must be that of a lens 0.2 mm. steeper than the diagnostic lens, e.g. 7.6 (9.0) Conoid 64.7° lens fitting would be adjusted to 7.6 (9.5) Conoid 63.2°. That is the tangen-tial cone angle on the diagnostic lens with a back optic radius of 7.2 mm.

If lenses are made too large in diameter, the wearing time will be limited because of excessive corneal coverage. Diameter alterations of 0.25 mm. are necessary to have a significant effect with conoid lenses.

Fenestration

For the fenestration to be effective, it must pass into the apical pool. Should it be located over a contact zone, it will be sealed off and circulation will stop. When this occurs, the cornea will become edematous.

OFFSET CONTACT LENSES

Offset contact lenses differ slightly from true aspheric lenses in that they are composed of several spherical curves. They differ from usual lenses because the peripheral curve has a center of curvature that is displaced from the axis of symmetry in the same way as occurs for the peripheral cornea. This displacement or offset makes the peripheral curve join the base curve without a junction and hence has the general appearance of the aspheric lens.

REFERENCES

1. Glasflex, Inc.
2. Obrig, T., and Salvatori, P.: *Colored Contact Lenses*, Obrig Laboratories, Inc.
3. Richards, O. W., and Grolman, B.: Avoid tinted contact lenses when driving at night, *J. Am. Optom. Assoc.*, 34(1):53–55, 1962.
4. Nelson, G., and Mandell, R. B.: The relationship between minus carrier design and performance, *Int. Cont. Lens Clin.*, 2(2): 75–81, 1975.
5. Sanning, F.: Edge treatment of high minus lenses, *Contacts*, 16(4):6–9, 1961. (Publication by Obrig Laboratories, Inc., N.Y.)
6. Gordon, S., and Masling, B.: Minimized lens "settling," *Opt. J. Rev. Optom.*, 97(16):39–40, 1960.
7. Schapero, M.: A review of a new corneal contact lens, *Optom. Weekly*, 43(18):713–716, 1952.
8. Schapero, M.: The fitting of highly toric corneae with toric corneal contact lenses, *Am. J. Optom.*, 30(3):157–160, 1953.
9. Bailey, N. J.: Special contact lenses and their applications—prism contact lenses, *Opt. J. Rev. Optom.*, 97(2):54–56, 1960.
10. Brucker, D.: Prisms and contact lenses, *Optom. Weekly*, 52(29):1428–1429, 1961.
11. Korb, D. R., and Filderman, I. P.: A new approach to contact lens ventilation, *Optom. Weekly*, 52(49):2375–2380, 1961.
12. Friedberg, M. A.: Contact lens apertures and toric curve designs, *J. Am. Optom. Assoc.*, 32(8):642–644, 1961.
13. Korb, D. R.: Application of multiple micro holes, *J. Am. Optom. Assoc.*, 32(11):891–892, 1961.
14. Korb, D. R.: Recent advances in corneal lens fenestration, in *Encyclopedia of Contact Lens Practice*, South Bend, Indiana, International Optics, 1959–1963, vol. 3, pp. 58–66.

15. Haynes, P. R.: Aperture venting techniques in corneal contact lenses, in *Encyclopedia of Contact Lens Practice*, South Bend, Indiana, International Optics, 1959–1963, vol. 1, pp. 9–13.

16. Elmstrom, G. P.: Case history—facet corneal contact lenses, *Optom. Weekly*, *44(37)*:1528, 1953.

17. Lewison, L., and Hollander, H.: The "vent-air" corneal lens, *Opt. J. Rev. Optom.*, *92(7)*:34, 41, 1955.

18. Bier, N.: The tolerance factor and Sattler's veil as influenced by a new development of contact lens making, *Am. J. Optom.*, *24(12)*:611–615, 1947.

19. Bier, N.: The practice of ventilated contact lenses, *Am. J. Optom.*, *26(3)*:120–127, 1949.

20. Yarwood, R. A.: The use of contact lenses in all kinds of sports, *J. Am. Optom. Assoc.*, *31(8)*:633–635, 1960.

21. Gyorffy, I.: Sports and contact lenses—observation of four hundred cases, *Contacto*, *4(11)*:495–498, 1960.

22. Dickinson, F.: Adaptation of corneal lens design for swimming, *Contacto*, *8(1)*:4–5, 1964.

23. Silbert, M.: The corneo-limbus-scleral lens, *Opt. J. Rev. Optom.*, *99(9)*:35–36, 1962.

24. Jessen, G.: Personal demonstration, 1963.

25. Nagel, C. F., and Monical, J. B.: The design and development of a contact lens for underwater seeing, *Am. J. Optom.*, *31(9)*: 468–472, 1954.

26. Gregg, J.: Visual effects of skin diving, *Skin Diver*, April, 1961.

27. Grant, A.: Vision in sports: contact lenses for diving, *J. Am. Optom. Assoc.*, *35(3)*:220, 1964.

28. Grant, A. H.: SCAL: Skindivers contact air lens, *Opt. J. Rev. Optom.*, *100(21)*:22–24, 1963.

29. Erb, R. A.: Method for producing wettable surfaces on contact lenses by chemical formation of inorganic films. (Report) School of Aviation Medicine, USAF Aerospace Medical Center (ATC), Brooks Air Force Base, Texas, March, 1961.

30. Koven, A. L.: Clinical evaluation of permanent coated contact lenses, *Eye, Ear, Nose and Throat Mon.*, *41*:47–50, 1962.

31. Freeman, E.: Pinhole contact lenses, *Am. J. Optom.*, *29(7)*:347–352, 1952.

32. Mazow, B.: The pupilens—a preliminary report, *Contacto*, *2(5)*:128–131, 1958.

33. Kaplan, M. M.: The aplanatic contact lens, *Optom. Weekly*, *58(6)*:25–29, 1967.

34. Nissel, G.: Aspheric contact lens, *The Ophthalmic Optician*, *7(19)*:1007–1010, 1967.

35. Nissel, G.: Aspheric contact lenses, *Aust. J. Optom.*, *51(2)*:45–48, 1968.

36. Bennet, A. G.: Aspherical contact lens surfaces, *The Ophthalmic Optician*, *8(19)*:1037–1040, 1968.

37. Nissel, G.: Aspheric contact lenses, *Contacto*, *12(1)*:46–49, 1968.

38. Bennet, A. G.: Aspherical contact lens surfaces—Part 2, *The Ophthalmic Optician*, *8(23)*:1297–1300, 1311, 1968.

39. Elliot, D. O.: The "Ellipsoidal" contact lens, *Optom. Weekly*, *58(14)*:25–27, 1967.

40. Steele, E.: The fitting of aspheric corneal contact lenses, *The Ophthalmic Optician*, *9(22)*:1216–1218, 1969.

41. Steele, E.: The fitting of aspheric corneal contact lenses, *Contacto*, *13(4)*:55–57, 1969.

42. Obrig Laboratories Manual: Technique in the fitting of con-o-coid corneal contact lenses.

43. Thomas, P. F.: The prescribing and fitting of "conoid" contact lenses, *Contacto*, *12(1)*: 66–69, 1968.

ADDITIONAL READINGS

Blue, H. D.: Method of producing permanent wettability on plastic contact lenses, *J. Am. Optom. Assoc.*, *37(7)*:678–681, 1966.

Blume, A. J.: Clinical study of Air-Thru PMMA contact lenses, *The Eye Opener*, *1(1)*, 1977.

Elliott, D. O.: Venting and fenestration, *J. Am. Optom. Assoc.*, *47(3)*:339, 1976.

Harris, M. G., Baretto, D. J., and Matthews, M. S.: The effect of peripherally fenestrated contact lenses on corneal edema, *Am. J. Optom. Physiol. Opt.*, *54(1)*:27–30, 1977.

Hirst, G.: The fitting of a true aspheric contact lens, *Contacto*, *18(1)*:15–19, 1974.

Hirst, G.: Recent developments in hard and hydrophilic aspheric contact lenses and the use of toric and bifocal hydrophilic lenses, *Contacto*, 24(*1*):35, 1980.

Jones, A.: Checking the contact lens fenestrations, *Contact Lens*, 3(*7*): 20, 1972.

Kerns, R. L.: Clinical evaluation of the merits of an aspheric front surface contact lens for patients manifesting residual astigmatism, *Am. J. Optom. Physiol. Opt.*, 51(*10*):750–757, 1974.

Lebow, K. A., and Goldberg, J. B.: Aspheric and ellipsoidal corneal lenses, *J. Am. Optom. Assoc.*, 47(*3*):322, 1976.

Mandell, R. B.: What is a gravity lens?, *Int. Cont. Lens Clin.*, 1(*4*):29–35, 1974.

Mandell, R. B.: Do fenestrations really work?, *Int. Cont. Lens Clin.*, 1(*4*):24–28, 1974.

Mandell, R. B.: The design of minus-carrier lenses, *Int. Cont. Lens Clin.*, 2(*2*):35–43, 1975.

Moore, C.: Should every low-plus lens have a minus carrier?, *Int. Cont. Lens Clin.*, 2(*2*):58–61, 1975.

Moore, C.: ELP—a technique for lens centration, *Int. Cont. Lens Clin.*, 3(*2*):42–46, 1976.

Pereira, A.: Cosmetic corneal contact lenses—illustrative cases, *Optom. Weekly*, 64(*49*):63–65, 1973.

Phelps, D. C. L.: Trouble with truncations, *The Optician*, 176(*4551*):23, 1978.

Chapter 16

MODIFICATION PROCEDURES

PHILLIP R. HAYNES

REGARDLESS OF THE excellence of his fitting technique, the contact lens practitioner will invariably find that minor lens modifications are necessary. The practitioner has the choice of making the modifications himself or having them done by his laboratory. Irrespective of his choice, it is recommended that the practitioner do at least part, if not all, of the minor modifications. There are several advantages to this.

1. Lens modifications performed in the office save time for the patient. He is not required to be without his lenses at a time when his motivation is high or his wearing needs are great.

2. The fitter has the opportunity to correlate the applied lens modifications with the fitting results desired.

3. Some finishing techniques are difficult to obtain from the laboratory.

4. The fitter can develop those lens finishing techniques and procedures which give him optimum results.

5. The fitter will be better able to evaluate lenses that are modified by the laboratory.

MANUFACTURE OF CONTACT LENSES

Although few practitioners will become involved in the actual manufacturing of contact lenses, a basic knowledge of the techniques used is helpful in understanding the modifications that may be made on a lens.

The initial contact lens blank, which is to consist of a spherical or toric ocular surface and a spherical or toric front surface can be fabricated by means of (1) lathe cutting both surfaces and polishing, (2) molding, (3) molding one surface and lathe cutting and polishing the opposite surface.[1] The possible molding techniques consist of compression molding, injection molding, and casting. Typically, the molding procedures produce lenses of excellent optical quality with precision curved and highly polished surfaces, but because of the technical problems involved in curing the finished lens, there have been numerous problems of lens warpage. However, recent developments in plastics and curing techniques offer some encouragement for improving casting and injection molding methods. It is conceivable that these methods could eventually replace the conventional cut and polish methods used today.

CUTTING AND POLISHING BACK SURFACE

The majority of contact lens fabricating laboratories use a technique in which a plastic button is placed in an appropriate holder (collet chuck) of a precision instrument lathe or radius generator to have curves generated on it by a diamond cutting tool.[2-9] The depth and radius of the cut are monitored by suitable gauges. Figure 16.1 shows a lathe used in lens fabrication. Figures 16.2 and 16.3 illustrate the cutting, and Figure 16.4, the polishing of the concave surface of the lens. Some laboratories generate the concave surface on the lathe and then transfer the button to an automatic polishing machine, which will polish two or more lenses at the same time (Figure 16.5).

Techniques to Reduce Lens Stress

It has been proposed that there is excessive stress on the lens button when it is placed in a collet chuck. When this stress is released, lens warpage results. To eliminate this problem, some laboratories mount the button on a flat chuck with pitch. With this technique they eliminate the mechanical stress on the button. Other techniques can also be used to reduce lens stress. (1) While generating the surface, a liquid coolant can be sprayed on the plastic surface to eliminate excessive surface heat production; (2) the operator can make very slow and shallow cuts (which also result in a smoother curve); (3) the timing of the polishing operation can be controlled so the surface will not be excessively polished. After these steps, many laboratories cure the button to eliminate any strain remaining in the plastic. The surfaces are checked for quality, and the radii are measured. The back surface buttons are filed in an inventory for future fabrication of lens prescriptions.

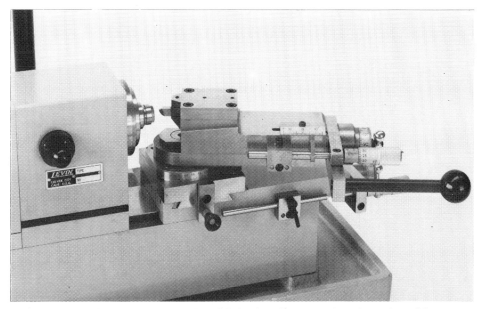

Figure 16.1. Lathe used for contact lens fabrication. Courtesy of Louis Levin and Son, Inc.

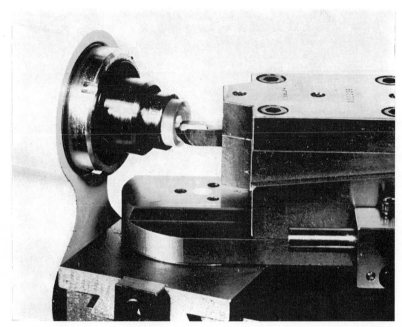

Figure 16.2. Cutting the back surface of a contact lens with a lathe. Courtesy Louis Levin and Son, Inc.

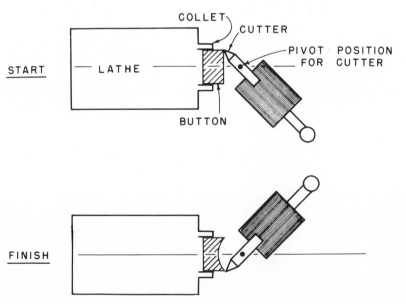

Figure 16.3. Motion of cutter on the lathe for cutting the back surface of a contact lens.

Adding Peripheral Curves

When a contact lens order comes to the laboratory, a finished back surface button with the appropriate back surface radius is selected from stock and verified. One of two procedures can then be followed.[10] In both procedures,

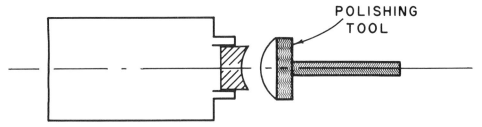

Figure 16.4. Polishing the concave surface of a contact lens.

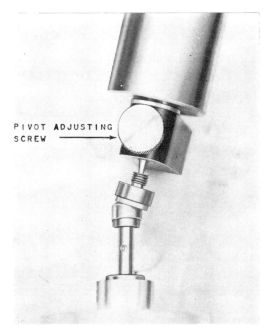

PIVOT ADJUSTING SCREW →

Figure 16.5. Automatic polishing machine. Courtesy Louis Levin and Son, Inc.

the intermediate and peripheral curve are generated and polished on the thick button before the front surface is generated and polished.

In the first procedure, the button is placed in a lathe, and the peripheral curves are generated with a diamond cutting tool. This technique is advantageous because the lens blank is stable and will not flex, thus aiding fabrication of precision peripheral curves. The button is then removed from the lathe, and the curves are polished on peripheral curve laps (described later). In the second procedure, the back surface peripheral curves are generated on the initial button by means of a grinding operation. The back surface of the button is placed directly against precision fine grit grinding spheres (Figure 16.6). After the curve is ground to the appropriate width, it is polished on a peripheral curve lap.

Conical, elliptical, and parabolic peripheral curves can be fabricated on a corneal lens. A conical curve is generated (1) by a precision cutting operation on a lathe or (2) by using a fine grit abrasive cone with the appropriate conical angle. The generated conical flange is polished on a matching conical polishing lap. The generation of parabolic and elliptical curves requires the use of a special lathe technique[11] or a generator that can be suitably programmed. When the back surface is completely fabricated, the button is returned to the lathe for the fabrication of the front surface.

CUTTING AND POLISHING FRONT SURFACE

The cutting of the front surface curve is shown in Figure 16.7. It is possible to generate (1) a single cut, (2) a plus lenticular, (3) a tangent periphery, or (4) a minus lenticular front surface.

Some laboratories generate and polish the back surface on the button and then immediately fabricate the front surface. The peripheral curves are then generated on this lens blank.

OPTIONAL FEATURES

The fabrication of toric surfaces can be carried out in two ways. The simplest approach is to flex (bend) a thin contact lens button to a specified toric surface, place it in a lathe, and generate and polish a spherical surface. When the flexure of the lens is released, the lens surface becomes toric. This technique is advantageous because the surface is easy to polish. A second technique utilizes the same principles as the toric generator for ophthalmic spectacle lenses and produces surfaces of excellent quality.[12]

In the fabrication of prism ballast lenses, the button is "blocked" so that the at front surface is inclined to an axis of the lathe by an angle equal to the amount of prism ballast desired. Then the operator generates the front surface radius in the usual manner.

DIAMETER AND SHAPE

After the front and back surfaces are generated, the manufacturer cuts the lens down to the specified shape and size and then contours and polishes the edges. These procedures are discussed in detail in subsequent sections.

Sometimes the lenses are also sold with only a single front and back curve. The practitioner may obtain these *uncut* lenses and finish the lens himself. As a rule, however, this is not done.

EQUIPMENT FOR LENS MODIFICATION

MODIFICATION UNITS

There are many types of modification units available for use on contact lenses. They fall into two broad categories, the lathe unit and the bucket unit (Figure 16.8). Either unit can be used, but the bucket unit is more popular. It consists of a round or square bucket, or splash pan, within which are mounted one or (usually and preferably) more spindles. The spindles rotate on a vertical axis at various speeds. Tools, grinding stones, and polishing laps can be mounted on the spindles. The splash pan should be easy to remove and clean. Also, a soft plastic splash pan or bowl is better than an aluminum, brass, or hard plastic bowl, since a lens that may accidentally be thrown from the spinning tool will not be as easily fractured or chipped against the soft plastic.

In addition to the modification unit, various accessories are needed such as grinding stones, polishing laps, polish, and lens holders. These normally come with the unit and are designed especially for it. Some of the accessories designed for one unit cannot be used with any other unit. However, many accessories are interchangeable.

Attaching Tools to Spindle

The spherical grinding and polishing tools typically attach to the spinning spindle by one of the following techniques:

1. Jacob's chuck. The shaft of the tool fits in a ¼ inch adjustable precision Jacob's chuck (Figure 16.9). This frequently used technique is advantageous in keeping the tool centered and secure. The main disadvantage is that it is very time-consuming when changing from

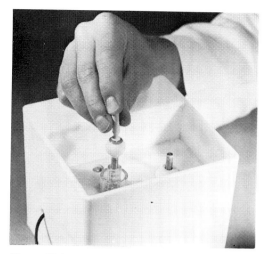

Figure 16.6. Grinding the peripheral curve with a precision grinding sphere.

one tool to another.

2. Form fit on a tapered spindle (Figure 16.10). This technique uses tools with a ¼ inch tapered hole drilled perpendicular to the axis of the tool. These are applied to a tapered spindle head and are held by friction. This technique assures rapid tool changes without resorting to a Jacob's wrench.

Speeds of Spindle

There has been much discussion on the proper speed for grinding, polishing, and edge treatment procedures. One manufacturer has standardized the speed of the major grinding and polishing lathe at 1200 R.P.M. and the edge treatment lathe at 100 R.P.M. Another has chosen 500 R.P.M. for the edge treatment machine, and still another has a variable speed control. The author has a variable speed polishing unit with speeds available up to 3000 R.P.M. While higher speeds (1500 to 1800 R.P.M.) may be desired under certain circumstances, slower speeds (500 to 1000 R.P.M.) are essential for finer abrasive and polishing procedures. Safety of operation and greater accuracy as well as surface perfection are more fully assured by moderate or slow speeds. Higher speeds throw off the grinding and polishing materials very rapidly, requiring constant feeding of the polish or abrasive. At high speeds one is more likely to have a dry tool and burn the surface of the lens. With slow speeds the grinding material is not thrown off, thus producing the most effective work. Foot pedal switches or rheostats enable the operator to monitor the speed of the machine effectively while leaving both hands free for lens, polish, and tool manipulations.

LENS MOUNTINGS

To hold and manipulate a contact lens during the modification procedures, it is necessary for the lens to be fastened to some type of mounting. Most bucket modification units can use two types of mountings, a *mounting tool* or a *lens holder* (Figure 16.11).

1. A mounting tool fits on the spindle of the unit so that the contact lens turns with the spindle. This type of mounting is normally used only for diameter reduction and edge finishing.

2. A lens holder, of which there are various types, is held in the operator's hand. It is used to place the lens in contact with various tools that are turning on the spindles of the unit.

Generally the same methods are used to attach a contact lens to either a lens holder or a mounting tool. The mounting of the contact lens must be done carefully to insure that the lens will not slip or shimmy on the mounting material. The mounting substance should hold the lens securely, be easily cleaned and removed from the contact lens, and not

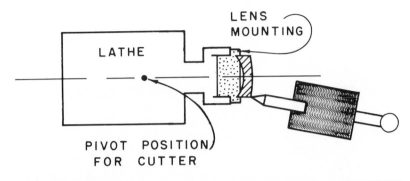

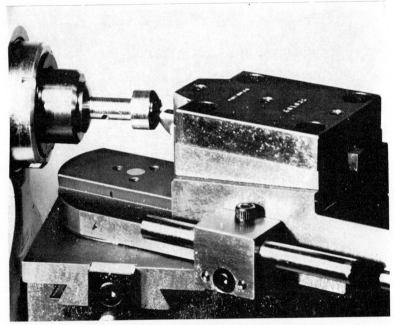

Figure 16.7. Cutting the front surface of a contact lens with a lathe. Courtesy Louis Levin and Son, Inc.

cause any damage to the surface of the lens.

Double-faced Tape

Special tapes are available that have adhesive on both sides. They are commercially called double-faced tapes. These are commonly used to mount the lens on the end of a holder for various fabrication and modification procedures. The double-faced adhesive tape is advantageous in that it is inexpensive, usually holds the lens securely without wobble or shimmy, is quickly applied, and can be easily cleaned from the lens. Its disadvantage is that certain polishing substances interfere with the adhesive characteristics of the tape, causing the lens to be dislodged. This drawback can be easily checked and is not often a practical problem.

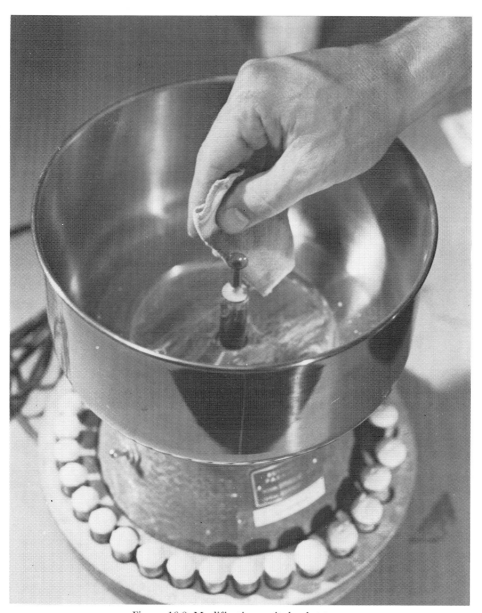

Figure 16.8. Modification unit: bucket type.

Technique for Mounting Tool

A mounting tool is placed on the spindle, and the exposed end is covered with double-faced mounting tape. As the chuck is spinning, a pointed scribe should be placed on the surface of the double-faced tape and moved towards the center of the holder until there is no wobble. This will leave a small indentation in the tape at the geometrical center and the axis of rotation of the lens holder. Now the

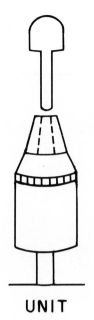

UNIT

Figure 16.9. Jacob's chuck and tool.

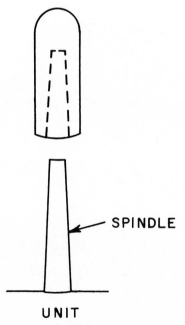

SPINDLE

UNIT

Figure 16.10. Form fit spindle and tool.

spotted optical center of the lens (Chapter 13) should be visually aligned with the axis

of the lens holder and the lens placed lightly onto the holder. If the lens is seated on the lens holder so that the optical axis of a nonprism contact lens is aligned with the central axis of the holder, there will be no oscillation of the image of the light bulb produced from reflection at the surface of the contact lens. However, if the contact lens contains ground prism, one might be led to finish a lens that is not optically centered. To avoid this possibility, one must simultaneously view the reflections of a single light source from both surfaces of the lens when both the light source and the primary line of sight of the observing eye are aligned with the central axis of the lens holder.

Technique for Lens Holder

The face of the holder can be covered with tape and the lens placed on the holder manually or with one of the various centering devices available from laboratories.

Pitch

A contact lens can be attached to the lens holder or mounting tool with pitch.

Technique for Mounting Tool

The tool is heated in a flame produced by an alcohol lamp or Bunsen burner. A small piece of mounting compound should be held and used to test the tool periodically by trying to get the mounting compound to melt on the surface of the lens holder or chuck. As the metal begins to heat, the mounting compound will get tacky when pressed on the metal; it will eventually melt when touched to the metal chuck and flow like heavy oil. It usually takes ten to fifteen seconds exposure to the flame to reach this temperature. This is the proper temperature for applying the mounting compound. Enough compound should be melted on the face of the metal to mount the lens, and then the surface of the lens should be placed onto the metal facing,

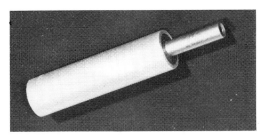

Figure 16.11. Lens holder (spinner).

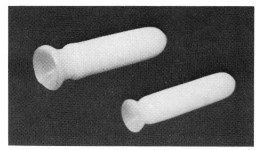

Figure 16.12. Suction cups. Courtesy of Plastic Contact Lens Co.

which is covered with flowing mounting compound. One way to avoid overheating the tool is to hold the metal tool with one hand and heat the tool until it is almost too hot to handle; this is the right temperature.

While the pitch is soft, the lens is placed on the mounting tool and centered as much as possible. Then the spindle is rotated. The lens is centered by spinning and gently pressing a hard object against the edge. A light image reflected from the lens will no longer oscillate when the lens is centered.

Technique for Lens Holder

It is not often that a lens will be fastened to a holder with pitch. However, when it is done, the method used is the same as that employed with a mounting tool.

Suction Cup

A number of small rubber suction cups are available, which need only be wetted and attached to the lens to provide a holder. There is considerable difference in the various brands of suction cups, some being too flexible for use. Suction cups usually come in two sizes (Figure 16.12).

In many instances a suction cup may produce warping of the lens, which, in turn, will affect the accuracy of the grinding of the peripheral curves. If a suction cup is used, a hollow cylindrical plastic tube should be placed in the stem of the suction cup so that the center and intermediate zones of the lens

will be supported during the fabrication or modification procedures. This also makes the holder more rigid, so it is easier to handle the lens. The plastic tube should not touch the lens surface, since it will mar or abrade the front surface. A suction cup should not be used on ultrathin lenses because it causes too much distortion of the surface with resultant errors in the peripheral curves.

Lens flexure by a suction cup can be reduced by careful mounting. The lens should be placed concave side down on the fleshy portion of the index finger. This provides a backing for the lens as the suction cup is pressed against it and attached.

One type of suction cup has no aperture and creates suction from the cup only (Figure 16.13). This cup is too weak for use in making lens modifications but is excellent for removing a lens from the eye.

Checking the Mounting

When the operator is first learning the mounting procedures, it may be helpful to

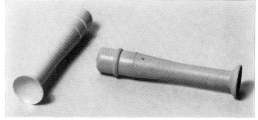

Figure 16.13. DMV lens holder.

check whether the mounting causes distortion or flexure of the lens. After a lens is mounted on a holder, the concave surface of the lens can be observed with a radiuscope or kera-tometer to check for distortion. If the lens surface is distorted or is off radius, there may be errors in the subsequent operations.

SEQUENCE OF MODIFICATIONS

Most modifications will consist of single operations, such as changing the radius of a peripheral curve on the original lens. In a few cases the practitioner may wish to do all finishing on the lens himself. He then begins with an uncut lens that has a specified power, center thickness, single cut back or ocular surface, and a single cut or lenticular construction front surface.

Regardless of whether the entire finishing process is performed or only a few modifications are made, the same sequence of modification must be followed. Otherwise, a subsequent operation may affect the results of a previous operation. The lens should be modified according to the following ranking with operations listed in sequence, from first to last:

·1. Total diameter
2. Intermediate curve radius and width
3. Peripheral curve radius and width
4. Blend
5. Edge contour and polish
6. Surface polish or power change

Following is a list of the interrelationship of individual operations.

Can be done alone

1. Surface polish or power change
2. Edge contour and polish
3. Blend

Affect others

1. Peripheral curve radius and width
2. Intermediate curve radius and width
3. Total diameter

MODIFICATION TECHNIQUES

DIAMETER REDUCTION

There are various methods that may be used to make a diameter reduction. In all methods the diameter should be reduced down to 0.1 to 0.2 mm. over the desired size for the final lens. This leaves sufficient stock for the edge finishing process.

Mounting Tool

With the lens spinning on a mounting tool, a sharp object is used to trim material from the edge. Possible cutting objects are a file, scalpel, razor blade, or emery board.

Conical Abrasive Stones

A commonly used technique for reducing lens diameter employs a special abrasive tool that has a cone-shaped depression. The abrasive cone is fabricated from Crystolon or other suitable hard abrasive material. The lens can be held with a suction cup or fastened onto a holder with pitch or double-faced tape. The lens should be placed in the center of the spinning abrasive cone (Figure 16.14). The cone should be constantly lubricated with cool water so the edge of the lens is not burned.

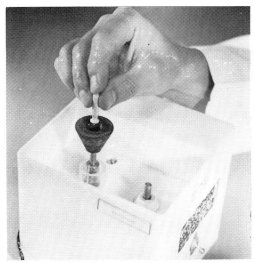

Figure 16.14. Reducing the total lens diameter with an abrasive cone.

It is important that the lens holder be kept vertical and that side pressure be eliminated so the edge stock will be removed concentrically. When using this tool, care should be taken to start with a lens that is free of prism so that the optical center of the finished lens will coincide with the geometrical center of the lens.

If prism ballast lenses are cut down with an abrasive cone, more stock will usually be removed from the thinner side. One of the other cut-down techniques is usually more desirable.

By using a series of special lens holders with diameters ranging in 0.5 mm. steps from 7.0 to 12.0 mm., it is possible to look at the mounted lens and instantly assess if it is edged to a given size. For example, to reduce the diameter of a lens to 10.5 mm., select a 10.5 mm. diameter lens holder.

Punches

Manufacturing laboratories use precision punches to punch out the lens to approximate diameter. The punches are made in 0.1 mm. steps, and the technician merely places the uncut blank in the appropriate punch, applies pressure, and the excess material is removed. The main disadvantage of this process is that the lenses are usually geometrically centered on the punch and if there is a ground prism in the original uncut blank, the final lens will not be optically centered. However, laboratories with precision techniques consistently produce spherical lenses free of ground prism, which enables them to use this system effectively.

Lathe

If the modification unit is of the lathe type, the lens is clamped in place and spun. The edge is contoured with a file or other cutting object.

FABRICATION OF PERIPHERAL CURVES

The first step in fabricating the peripheral curves is to mount the lens on a holder properly so it is not astigmatically or spherically flexed. If this requirement is not met, serious radius errors in the peripheral zones may result.[13]

Both a grinding operation and a polishing operation must be used in the fabrication of the peripheral curves to produce a true spherical curve of desired radius. The grinding operation can be carried out with (1) fine grade Crystolon or emery spherical grinding balls or (2) a grit abrasive on a pad-covered radius lap.

Coating Lens Surface

Before proceeding with the grinding and polishing of the peripheral curves, some technicians prefer to cover the lens with a waterproof protective coating so that the optical zone of the lens will not be damaged during the grinding (or polishing) operations. The coating also leaves a sharp demarcation between the zone being fabricated and the adjacent zone, so one can easily monitor the widths and diameters of the various zones of the lens.

An effective coating is made by dissolving a Blaisdell® wax pencil lead or a Listo® wax pencil lead in 20 cc. of carbon tetrachloride. This solution may then be brushed onto the surface of the lens. After finishing the lapping and polishing operations, the protective coating can be removed by cleaning the lens in benzine or carbontetrachloride. Another equally effective coating is sold by Frontier Contact Lens Company.[14] It is also easily removed by cleaning the lens with carbontetrachloride.

The author frequently uses Carter's Marks-a-Lot as a protective coating for the lens. It comes in a small container and can be easily applied. The coating should be allowed to dry about one minute before making the fabrication. After the lens is finished, the coating can be removed with benzine or carbontetrachloride.

Any of the various protective coatings should be applied only to an area of the lens that is slightly larger than the specified finished optical zone diameter. This procedure will minimize the clogging of the pad or grinding balls with the protective wax or other substances. The heat produced by the friction of the lens against the tool tends to melt the wax coverings, and they will gum up. Therefore, only a very thin layer should be used.

Grinding Peripheral Curve

Grinding Balls

Spherical grinding balls* made from Crys-

---

*Since the abrasive tools are actually spherical balls, they can easily be checked for curvature by measuring the diameter through various planes of the sphere with a micrometer. A watchmaker's micrometer, which is calibrated directly in millimeters, can be used, thus alleviating the necessity of converting inches to millimeters. Another technique for checking the balls is to use female profile gauges or lap gauges, which are available from some laboratories.

tolon (silicon carbide) material are available. They are graded according to their abrasive characteristics.[15-18] If it is desirable to remove large amounts of stock from the surface rapidly, then a coarse grade spherical abrasive ball is used. The balls are designated by number, and a commonly used semicoarse ball is number 70. When a coarser abrasive ball is used, the final curve will not have a high quality spherical surface. For finer work, a less abrasive tool, such as a number 220, may be used. This produces a finely ground surface that is easily polished and which, in turn, offers a higher grade optical surface. The Crystolon abrasive grinding balls can be obtained in any specified radius. A workable set ranges in radii from 7.50 mm. to 9.00 mm. in 0.1 mm. steps, and from 10.00 mm. to 15.00 mm. in 0.25 mm. or 0.50 mm. steps.

In addition to Crystolon abrasive grinding balls, there are emery grinding balls,[19] diamond abrasive balls, and carborundum balls.

Metal tools of any radius or shape may be covered with diamond dust to produce an excellent grinding tool (Figure 16.15).

Surfacing Laps

Spherical surfacing laps are used for grinding (with the aid of an abrasive) and polishing the peripheral curves. For the latter use, they are normally covered with some type of polishing pad (Figure 16.16). The laps are usually obtained from the manufacturer with the curves indicated in terms of diopters or millimeters by numbers engraved or stamped

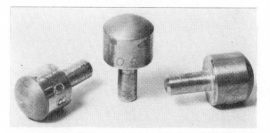

Figure 16.15. Peripheral curve grinding tools with diamond dust surfaces.

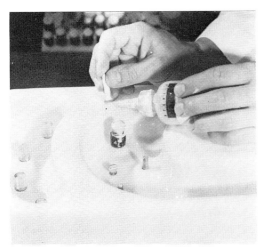

Figure 16.16. Polishing the peripheral curve.

onto the shaft of the lap. They are typically made from brass, steel, aluminum, or plastic stock.

LAP DEFECTS. Alignment. One of the common defects found in the spherical lap is a misaligned hole for fitting the tool on a tapered spindle. When the hole is not properly aligned with the center of rotation of the spherical surface, an aberrated peripheral curve is generated on the contact lens.

WORN LAPS. Through continued use, the originally perfect lap will become worn and will require correction by truing. The curvature may be checked with a female lap, a template, or a profile gauge that has the proper curvature.

LAP MATERIALS. There has been some discussion about which material is best for fabrication of the spherical and toric laps. The following are useful guide rules:

1. If the lens is to be used directly with the grinding abrasive to grind the peripheral curves, a hard metal, such as steel, should be used to fabricate the tool.

2. If the tool is to be used only for holding a polishing pad, then aluminum, brass, plastic, or steel can be used.

Plastic laps are advantageous in that the radius, sphericity, and quality of the curve can be easily checked on the radiuscope. Plastic tools also have the advantage of being easily recut to a new accurate radius value. However, because of the softness of the plastic, the tapered shaft hole tends to wear rapidly, producing a polishing lap that may wobble or become loose on the rotating spindle. The ideal radius lap would have a hard steel shaft or taper hole with a plastic lap surface that was always covered with a pad. Such a tool would be inexpensive, sturdy, easily checked, and easily retrued.

SPECIFICATION OF TOOL CALIBRATION. Several decades ago the laps for glass spectacle lens grinding were based on a standard 1.53 index of refraction. Spectacle lap profile gauges were also based on this index of refraction. However, the index of crown glass used in ophthalmic lenses is 1.523. This slight difference in the index does amount to enough in high powers to become important. Therefore, the index measurements are now differentiated by *optical power* for lenses and *curvature power* for tools.

This same discrepancy was introduced in the manufacture of contact lenses. Most plastic stock for contact lenses has an index of refraction of 1.49, while the spherical laps that are used to grind or polish the peripheral curves are often specified in diopters with a reference index of 1.3375. This is the index of refraction assumed for the cornea. To avoid confusion, many manufacturers specify only the radius of the tool in millimeters, and others specify both the preceding dioptric value and the radius of curvature in millimeters.

Grinding Technique

The desired tool (stone or lap) is placed on the spindle of the unit and rotated at about 1500 R.P.M. The lens, which is mounted on a holder, is placed concave side down on the tool and rocked back and forth (*See* Figure 16.16) The holder should be turned constantly in the hand so that equal pressure is distributed to all meridians of the lens.

As an alternate technique, the lens may be

mounted on a small lens block. The mounted lens and block can then be held against the tool with a stylus, which fits in a small depression on the block. This allows the lens to turn freely on the tool (Figure 16.17). The spinning lens block is moved over the lap surface in a figure-eight motion. The double rotation technique, in which both the tool and the lens rotates, produces a circular optical zone and true spherical peripheral curves. The single rotation technique, in which the tool rotates and the lens is held on a non-rotating lens holder, may cause the rocking in of a toric curve in the lens periphery.

In grinding the peripheral curve, care should be taken that the width be kept 0.10 mm. undersize to allow for the polishing operation, i.e. the optical zone diameter should be somewhat oversized. The peripheral curve width can be checked periodically (during the grinding) with a reticule magnifier, which

can be read to an accuracy of 0.10 mm.

The lens surface should be washed with water before proceeding to the polishing operation.

Polishing Peripheral Curve

Peripheral curves are usually polished by using a lap of the desired curvature. The lap is covered with a polishing pad that has been soaked with polishing compound.

Radius of Lap with Pad

When using a padded lap, one must always allow for the thickness of the pad in specifying the radius of the compensated tool. The pad thickness can be measured with a micrometer or with a standard lens thickness gauge (Figure 16.18). The thickness of the pad must be added to the radius of the lap to determine the compensated radius. For example, if the lap has a radius of 8.7 mm. and the pad is 0.3 mm. thick, the effective radius of the tool with the pad is 9.0 mm. Parke-Davis Tape No. 20-24-2 has a specified thickness of 0.20 mm., which means that the radius of a convex tool is increased by a factor of 0.20 mm.

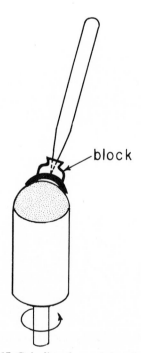

Figure 16.17. Grinding the peripheral curve. Contact lens is mounted on a lens block and turns freely.

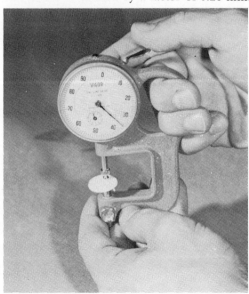

Figure 16.18. Measuring the polishing pad thickness with a thickness gauge.

and is dioptrically flattened by a factor of one diopter (0.05 mm. is approximately equal to a dioptric change of 0.25 D.).

Pad Material

The choice of the polishing pad material, type of polish, and the speed of the polishing operation is important.[20] A thin, hard polishing pad that is noncompressible must be used to obtain a precision spherical curve. Also, the thickness of the pad should not change with the amount of pressure, water, polish, or carrier (which is used to hold the polish in suspension). A thick, compressible pad may cause the generation of an aspheric curve of unknown specifications. Materials such as nonwaterproof adhesive tape, Pellon® fabric, velveteen, and Mystik® tape are satisfactory. Moleskin, velveteen mounted on double-faced tape, and other thick pads are undesirable for this operation. The polishing pad of choice at the present time is a nonwaterproof adhesive tape, Mystik tape, or a thin, closely woven velveteen. The latter is attached to the spherical lap by a thin layer of cement. Some of the commonly used polishing pad materials used in polishing peripheral curves are listed in Table 16.1.

Mystik plastic tape provides one of the most suitable pad materials for the polishing laps. A circular section, the size of a penny, is cut from the roll and applied to the polishing lap. As the tape is applied, it will tend to bunch up in the periphery, resulting in some deep wrinkles. Place the pad covered lap down in the hot beads of a spectacle frame warmer and allow the plastic tape to heat. Then remove the tool and smooth out the wrinkles with your finger. This will result in a uniformly smooth pad that has sufficient friction to polish out a secondary curve rapidly. The pad wears well and can be easily cleaned.

Attaching Pads

Various techniques are used to attach the pad materials to the spherical lap. White

TABLE 1

THICKNESS CHART FOR POLISHING PADS AND DOUBLE FACED TAPE

Pad or Tape Material	Thickness (mm.)	Flattens Tool Dioptrically by a Factor of
Non-waterproof Adhesive Tape (Parke-Davis No. 30-24-2)	0.20	1.00 D.
Velveteen Pad (Plastic Contact Lens Co.)	0.275	1.37 D.
Moleskin	0.625	3.12 D.
Econo-cement for Cementing Pad	0.05 to 0.10	0.25 to 1.50 D.
Double Faced Tape (Minnesota Mining)	0.31	1.50 D.
Double Faced Tape (Precision Cosmet Co.)	0.10	0.50 D.
Double Faced Tape (Plastic Contact Lens Co.)	0.275	1.37 D.
Double Faced Tape (Arno Tape)	0.32	1.62 D.
Double Faced Tape (Permacel Tape)	0.11	0.50 D.
Velveteen and Double Faced Tape Combination (Plastic Contact Lens Co.)	0.55	2.75 D.
Jeweler's Velveteen	0.275	1.37 D.

moleskin, Mystik tape, and non-waterproof adhesive tape are self-adhesive and easily applied to the tool. Velveteen and Sylvet® pads may be applied by using Econo-Pad-Cement®, double-faced tape, or pitch. With the Econo-Pad-Cement, only a very thin layer of cement is required. It has excellent pad retention, and it can easily be removed from the tool with a solvent. Double-faced tapes produce a thick cushion under the pad, thus increasing their compressibility.

Polishing Compounds

There are many commercially available polishing compounds such as tin oxide, precipitated calcium carbonate, and Lustrox®. It is sometimes desirable to mix the compound in water or some other carrier and to pour it through a fine nylon mesh screen just before using it to eliminate any chunks or large particles. The mixture should be thick and creamy so that it will stick to the rotating polishing lap and not be thrown from the rotating tool.

Optical polishing grade tin oxide can be purchased from most contact lens laboratories. It should be mixed in the ratio of one-third water and two-thirds tin oxide. This produces a pastelike preparation, which can be brushed onto the polishing pad. If the preparation is too watery, it will be thrown from the revolving tool and produce little polishing.

To eliminate contamination with foreign material, one should keep the mixture in a plastic bottle with a small nozzle opening. By shaking the bottle, the tin oxide is again put in suspension and ready for use. In selecting the grade of the tin oxide, calcium carbonate precipitate, or other polish, one must not assume that the finer the grade, the easier the polishing operation. A polish that is too fine will tend to foam and is so nonabrasive that it tends to lubricate rather than polish. Commonly used polishing compounds are listed in Table 16.2.

Polishing Procedure

The lens is mounted in the same way as for the grinding operation. The polishing lap

TABLE 16.2

POLISHING COMPOUNDS

1. Tin Oxide (Stannic oxide).
2. Calcium Carbonate Precipitate.
3. Powdered Jeweler's Rouge.
4. Optical Rouge.
5. Stellar Speed Polish.
6. Silvo Silver Polish.
7. Nissel No. 1 First Stage Polishing Powder.
8. Nissel No. 2 Finishing Polishing Powder.
9. Nissel No. 3 Polishing Powder for Peripheral Bands.
10. Pol-Mo Polishing Compound.
11. Pol-Mo Prime Metal Tin Oxide.
12. Pol-Mo "Hi-Gloss" Finishing Polish.
13. Lustrox.

is turned at 500 to 1000 R.P.M., and the lens is applied to the polish-covered lap. The width of the zone and the quality of the surface are periodically checked with a $10 \times$ magnifier. It is sometimes desirable to divide the polishing operation into two steps. In the first step a tin oxide or precipitated calcium carbonate is used on a thin, hard pad such as adhesive tape. In the second step, a very fine polish such as calamine lotion is used on a soft padded lap such as velveteen. The second step removes little or no stock but gives a high lustre polish to the surface.

Additional Curves

In the fabrication of a tertiary curve or other peripheral curve, one recoats the surface with the protective coating substance, selects the appropriate laps, and performs the operation in the same manner as discussed previously.

Toric Peripheral Curves

Toric peripheral curves can be fabricated by several methods. The most direct and accurate technique is with toric tools, as follows. First, the lens should be mounted on a lens holder, marked so that the meridional orientation of the lens can be determined.[20] Second, a toric radius tool is used that has radii r_1 and r_2 as illustrated in Figure 16.19. The lens is then held against this pad-covered tool, and the secondary curve is polished with radii equal to r_1 and r_2. A noncircular toric optical zone is thus produced.

Blend

After the various zones have been fabricated, the junction between two zones can be blended by applying the lens to a polishing lap with a radius between the radii of the two adjacent zones. The choice of pad material for this operation is important. A thick, soft pad will round off the junction, whereas a thin, hard pad will produce an intermediate curve at the junction. The blend is specified

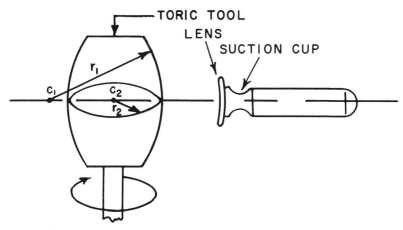

Figure 16.19. Grinding toric peripheral curve on a toric stone.

by the radius of the tool, the desired width of the blend, and the desired visual characteristics of the blend. It is best to first apply a thin, hard protective coating substance on the lens surface. The width of the blend can then be easily specified by measuring the width of the annular zone, which has been polished free of the protective coating. If, after the removal of the protective coating, one can see no sharp demarcation, a well-blended junction has been produced.

EDGE

The contact lens edge must have both a proper shape or contour and a good polish. Fabrication and modification procedures that incorporate a two-step procedure of first contouring the edge to the proper shape and polishing this contour will typically result in the best edges.

Roughing Edge of Unfinished Lens

The condition of the edge immediately after the lens is fabricated to size is dependent upon the procedure used to reduce the diameter of the lens. Punching procedures will typically cause a very ragged edge, while procedures using a conical abrasive cone, cut down with a scalpel, fine file, or abrasive tool and lathe, will typically result in a rough edge free of excessive ragged sections.

After having (1) reduced the lens diameter to approximate size, leaving enough stock for the edge treatment operation, (2) lapped and polished the secondary curves and bevels to their specified widths and radii, and (3) knocked the burrs off the edge, the lens is ready for shaping and polishing.

Edge Method 1: Cut and Polish

Cutting

Precision cutting techniques offer good control over the edge contour and are very rapid and easily performed. The actual cutting may be done with a cutting tool mounted on a lathe and guided by a suitable template[21] or by use of a hand-held scalpel[22] (Figure 16.20). The scalpel blade is curved so that it is possible to cut continuously, moving the blade from the inside edge of the lens around to the outside edge. The lens should be dry while it is being cut so that one can see exactly how much plastic is removed.

The speed of the cutting action is a func-

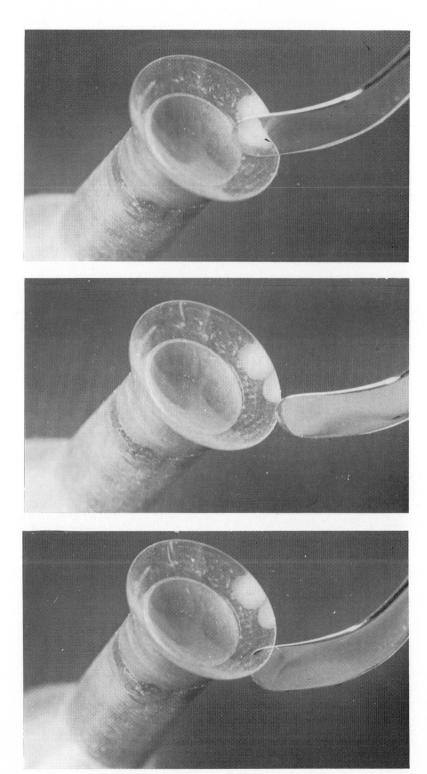

Figure 16.20. Shaping a contact lens edge with a scalpel: (a) starting with the blade on the inside of the lens; (b) shaping with the blade moving around the edge in a continuous motion; (c) finishing the cut on the front of the lens. Courtesy of A. A. Isen.

tion of the force exerted on the scalpel blade. At the end of this stage the lens diameter should be 0.10 mm. to 0.15 mm. over the specified dimension. This leaves enough stock for the shaping and polishing operation. It is possible to add an anterior lenticular bevel, as well as to shape the edge contour in this operation.

Polishing

Some tin oxide should be mixed in a solution approximately the consistency of light cream. Then a small piece of polyester foam (or similar flexible hand polisher) is dipped into this polishing compound. The polyester foam, saturated with tin oxide, is applied to the edge of the lens and rolled from the front surface of the edge to the back surface in a smooth circular motion (Figure 16.21). The lens must remain geometrically centered with respect to the lens holder so that there will be no oscillation or vibration of the lens in the rotating chuck. The polishing lathe motor should be set at high speed. Enough pressure should be applied with the polishing pad against the rotating lens for the motor to be slightly slowed. This will provide sufficient friction for the polishing action. The flexible polyester foam polisher is held between the first finger and the thumb. When it is held properly, one can feel that it is polishing evenly over the entire edge of the lens. The polisher must be kept moist and well soaked with polishing agent. It should take approximately twenty to sixty seconds to completely polish the edge. After the edge has been polished, it should be checked with a magnifier or a binocular stereomicroscope to determine whether the edge is perfectly finished and polished.

A hard felt dental polishing disc, chamois skin, or other suitable polishing pad can be substituted for the polyester foam polishing pad. Many technicians use a hard felt pad

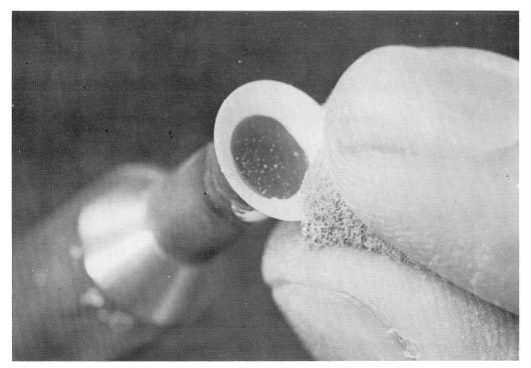

Figure 16.21. Polishing the lens edge. Courtesy of A. A. Isen.

mounted on a flat tool, which enables them to have optimum control over the pressure, position, and motion of the pad. The tool can be easily made by attaching the pad material to a tongue depressor.

Edge Method 2: Buffing

One of the first and still commonly used techniques for finishing an edge of a contact lens is a rag-wheel buff mounted on a polishing lathe. A multilayer rag-wheel should be selected that is sewn so that the rag-wheel has some body. The lens can be mounted on a spinner holder or a brass lens holder. In the choice of the polishing compound, these rules should be followed:

To remove a great deal of plastic, Radoff should be used on the rag-wheel. Radoff is very abrasive and must be used sparingly. Basically, it is used to reduce lens diameter and to shape the edge contour. It is not to be used as a polishing compound but, rather, as an abrasive compound.

In the smoothing and shaping operation and in the initial polishing operation, a rag-wheel impregnated with Moldent or some similar buffing agent can be used. In the final polishing operation, it is best to use a fine grade jeweler's rouge or Bendeck polish when performing a dry buffing operation, or tin oxide in a creamy mixture when performing a wet buffing operation.

The Precision Cosmet Spinner assembly illustrated in Figure 16.22 uses a double rotation principle in which both the lens and the rag-wheel buff spin. This assures even distribution of the buffing action. The three positions of the lens during the buffing operation are illustrated in Figure 16.22. The first position is with the lens holder or spinner pointed upward at approximately 30° to 40° from the horizontal (Figure 16.22a). In the second position, the spinner is pointed downward 30° to 40° from the horizontal (Figure 16.22b). In the third position, the lens holder or spinner is held horizontally (Figure 16.22c). To round the edge of the lens and insure

uniform smoothness, the lens must be buffed at the various angles illustrated. The lens should constantly be moved back and forth across the buff to obtain a better edge and to prevent grooves from forming in the buff.* If one uses a rod lens holder (without spinner) he should rotate the lens holder slowly and steadily to insure even and constant pressure. Speeding up the rotation of the lens holder does not speed up the buffing process. After the lens edge is properly contoured, the final wet polishing operation may be performed. The lens is rolled on a wet tin-oxide-impregnated sponge or pad to achieve a final polish (Figure 16.23).

Edge Method 3: Pad

Several commercially available edgers consist of a flat motor driven disc, 3 to 4 inches in diameter, covered with moleskin or other suitable pad material.[23] The lens is secured to a hand-held spinner with double-faced tape or mounting wax. The spinner is held at a large angle to the pad. The edging process is started by pressing the edge of the lens against the flat, rotating polishing pad. When the edge of the lens touches the rotating flat pad, the lens will start spinning, thus forming a double rotation system. The lens should be moved in the direction shown by the arrow in Figure 16.24. As the lens edge is stroked across the polishing pad, the position of the plane of the lens should be constantly changed so that on finishing the stroke, the plane of the lens is almost vertical. In this way all portions of the edge may be polished. The operator may selectively remove more or less stock from a given part of the edge contour by controlling the time spent and the pressure exerted on that part. This offers excellent control over the shape of the edge.

---

*If the rag-wheel buff starts to fray, it must be trimmed so that the frayed ends do not interfere with the buffing operation. This is done by holding coarse sandpaper mounted on a wood block against the frayed fibers. This technique is safe and can easily be repeated.

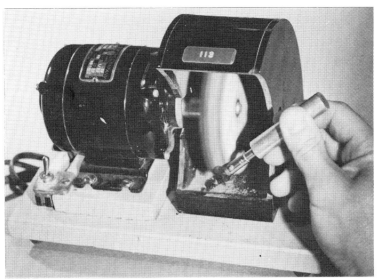

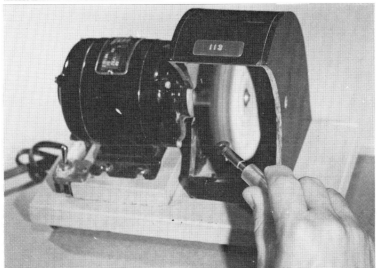

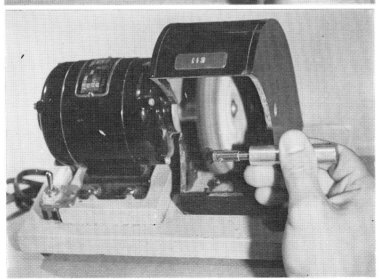

Figure 16.22. Spinner and buff assembly used to shape edge (*see* text).

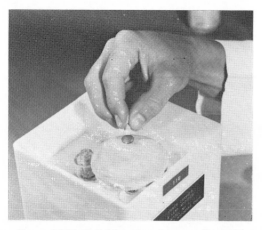

Figure 16.23. Polishing the edge on a flat pad.

The same process should be used for both the convex and concave portion of the edge. The front portion of the edge typically takes less time, since there is less plastic to be removed. By extending the polishing operation onto the front surface of the lens, one can apply an anterior lenticular bevel with this process.

Edge Method 4: Concentric Grind and Polish

Conical and concentric polishing of a contact lens employs a shaping operation to pro-

duce the initial edge contour and a polishing operation to produce a high quality edge polish.[24-27]

The lens is placed on a lens holder with its convex surface exposed. The 90° fine abrasive Crystolon conical stone is placed in the Jacob's chuck and is rotated at a moderately slow speed. (The commonly used vitreous cone is too abrasive and leaves deep scratches, which are difficult to polish.) The lens is now ground, convex side down, on the 90° stone (Figure 16.25). During this grinding operation, it is necessary to keep the tool lubricated with water. The grinding procedure is continued until the diameter on a plus (or low minus) lens has been reduced to within 0.1 mm. of the final diameter or, on a high minus lens, within 0.05 mm. of the final diameter.

Preparing Polishing Tools

With the modification unit there is a set of pads designed to fit into the female cones of the respective tools. Matching angle male tools are used to press the pads into the female tools. Pad cement is used to secure the pad to the tool if the pad does not have its own adhesive surface. A fine velvet or velveteen material is typically used for the polishing

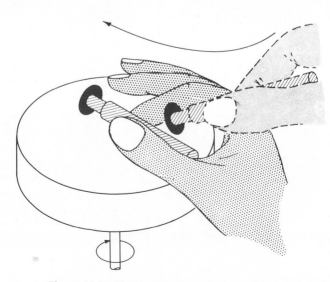

Figure 16.24. Shaping the lens edge on a flat pad.

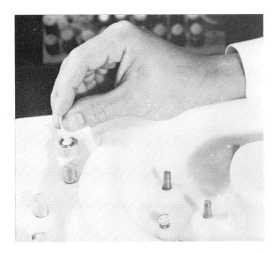

Figure 16.25. Grinding the front bevel with a 90° conical stone.

pad material.

Polishing

The first operation is the polishing of the front of the edge where it has been ground on the 90° abrasive cone.* The polishing operation is performed on a lap that has an inside angle of 90° and which is faced with velveteen. This polishing operation should be continued until there are no hairline scratches under high magnification. This typically takes about three minutes at 100 R.P.M. or one minute at 500 R.P.M. (Figure 16.26).

Figure 16.26 illustrates the finishing of a lens edge in the conical and concentric polishing procedure. In using this technique, it is necessary to modify some of the steps according to the individual lens. When working with a high plus or other lenses with thin edges, it is not necessary to grind the initial 90° cut into the anterior surface of the lens.

---

*There has been some discussion on how fast the tools should rotate for conical and concentric polishing. Cepero,[24] in his original article on concentric polishing, recommended a standard speed of 100 R.P.M. However, recently, several laboratories have switched to 250 R.P.M. and 500 R.P.M. From personal experience 250 R.P.M. seems to be optimum, but 500 R.P.M. is probably not too fast.

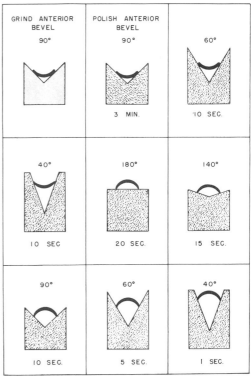

Figure 16.26. Concentric polishing procedure.

Evaluation of Edge Finishing Techniques

1. The shaping operations used in the cutting techniques and with the rotating flat polishing disc are more adaptable to custom fitting procedures than is the conical-concentric polishing method.

2. The shaping operation used in the cutting techniques produces a finer surface for polishing than those produced by the coarse vitreous abrasive cones found in some modification kits.

3. The shaping operation used in the concentric polishing technique is repeatable with minimum training of the technician.

4. The conical-concentric technique, the rag-wheel buffing of a spinning lens, the shaping and polishing of a spinning lens against a rotating flat polishing disc, and the precision cutting and polishing of a rotating lens all employ concentric polishing tech-

niques that tend to produce a uniform edge contour.

5. All techniques produce a high quality surface polish on the edge if done properly.

6. All techniques result in a well-rounded, contoured edge.

7. All techniques can be used to reduce peripheral edge thickness in high minus prescriptions.

8. The precision cut and polish technique, the polishing of a spinning lens against a rotating flat polishing disc, and the rag-wheel buffing of a spinning lens all require fewer fabrication stages and less equipment than the conical concentric technique.

A precision shaped and polished contact lens edge can be produced by any of the preceding methods. However, it is desirable to develop techniques that are automated so that a high quality, precision edge of a desired shape can be easily reproduced without the aid of a highly skilled technician.

POWER CHANGES

Power changes and the removal of scratches from lens surfaces can be accomplished with several different techniques.[28-29] To add plus or decrease minus, the anterior surface of the lens should be pressed and rotated at the center of a polish-impregnated, flexible, flat polyester foam tool (Figure 16.27). The surface of the flexible polisher conforms to the anterior surface of the lens. The portion of the (spinning) tool peripheral to the center of the lens has a greater linear velocity and therefore a greater abrasive and polishing action than the central portions of the tool. Since the abrasive action is greater towards the periphery of the lens, a more convex anterior surface will be produced, which, in turn, will produce less minus or more plus power.

To add minus or reduce plus power, the anterior surface of the lens is pressed at the peripheral zones of the polyester foam tool while the lens is constantly rotated around the axis of the lens holder. Because the lens has a greater force against the center, more

stock is polished from the center of the lens than from the periphery.

A concave polyester foam tool or a hollow drum covered with a stretched velveteen or moleskin pad can also be used for the power-change procedure.

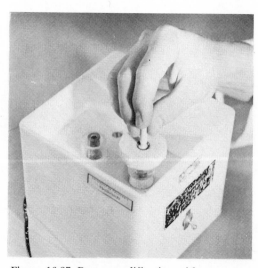

Figure 16.27. Power modification with a sponge.

REMOVING SCRATCHES

Surface scratches can be removed by combining the two techniques for plus and minus power changes to remove stock selectively without changing power. Scratches on the posterior surface can be removed with a convex-shaped polyester foam tool or a suitable pad, mounted on the appropriate radius, convex polishing tool. However, if the scratch is deep, one may remove an excessive amount of plastic, which will cause a change in the physical fit.

A scratch outside of the optical zone of the lens can be removed by polishing with a hard felt polishing ball, cone, or cylinder. This will produce a dip in the surface, but will not produce any disturbance in the optics of the system, since the dip will be located outside of the central optical zone.

TRUNCATION

In the fabrication of a single or double truncated lens one must start with a lens blank with enough center thickness so that the truncated edge will have sufficient stock.[30-33] The stock can be removed with a rotating flat abrasive tool, fine hand file, or a hand-manipulated abrasive stone. Next, the edge of the lens should be contoured with a rag-wheel buff and then hand polished against a wet polyester foam drum tool.

LENS APERTURES

Small precision holes can be drilled through a contact lens to establish venting.[34-37] A vent that is 0.05 to 0.18 mm. in diameter with smooth sides functions best. The lens is mounted on a tool that has a spherical convex surface and a precision guide hole for the drill.[38] The portion of the lens that is to be drilled is aligned with the guide hole, and the lens is mounted to the tool with wax.

Next, fine drilling oil is placed down the guide hole, and then the appropriate drill is placed in the guide and run at high speed to drill the hole. A small twist drill or a watchmaker's pivot drill can be used.

It is very difficult to polish the sides of the aperture. Precision drilling techniques must be used to eliminate the need for polishing.

MODIFICATION OF ULTRATHIN LENSES

Because of the thinness and flexibility of the ultrathin lens, special techniques must be utilized in its manufacture so that a firm backing is provided during all cutting and polishing processes. It is very difficult to finish the peripheral curves or edges when holding the lens with a suction cup. Hence, it is found to be difficult to make in-office modifications. If modifications are made, they are usually easier using a wax mounting rather than a suction cup.

REFERENCES

1. Haynes, P. R.: In *Encyclopedia of Contact Lens Practice*, South Bend, Indiana, International Optics, 1959–1963, vol. 1, Chap. 21, pp. 1–80.
2. *How to Make Contact Lenses with Levins Lens Making Equipment*, Culver City, California, Louis Levin and Son, Inc., 1958.
3. *Radius Turning Machine Model ACEC*, Culver City, California, Louis Levin and Son, Inc., 1963.
4. *Levin Polinex Contact Lens Surfacer*, Culver City, California, Louis Levin and Son, Inc., 1963.
5. *Contact Lens Manufacturing Equipment*,

Waltham, Massachusetts, F. W. Derby-shire, Inc., 1958.

6. *Making Contact Lenses with the Pul-Mo Contact Lens Lathe*, Pontiac, Michigan, Contact Lens Foundation, Ltd., 1958.

7. *The Stellar Parabolic Spherical Lathe*, San Diego, California, American Contact Lens Equipment and Supply Co., 1959.

8. *How to Make Contact Lenses Using the Denbro Contact Lens Lathe*, 2nd ed., Kittanning, Pennsylvania, Denbro Industries, Inc., 1960.

9. *The Nissel System*, Plainfield, New Jersey, George Nissel of America, Inc., 1959.

10. Haynes, P. R.: Comments on the fabrication of peripheral curves, in *Encyclopedia of Contact Lens Practice*, South Bend, Indiana, International Optics, 1959–1963, vol. 2, Chap. 22, pp. 77–80.

11. Obrig Laboratories.

12. Althisar, R.: Fabrication of toric back surfaces with the Nissel toric generator, in *Encyclopedia of Contact Lens Practice*, South Bend, Indiana, International Optics, 1959–1963, vol. 3, Chap. 21, pp. 4–5.

13. *A. O. Radiuscope, Instructions*, Buffalo, New York, American Optical Co., Instrument Division, 1958.

14. Isen, A.: *Supplementary Instruction Bulletin I, Contac-nique Unit*, Buffalo, New York, Frontier Contact Lens Co., 1959.

15. *A Handbook on Abrasives and Grinding Wheels*, Worcester, Massachusetts, Norton Co., 1958.

16. *Abrasives, Their History and Development*, Worcester, Massachusetts, Norton Co., 1958.

17. *Grinding Wheels and Abrasives*, Catalog 1052, Worcester, Massachusetts, Norton Co., 1958.

18. *American Standard Safety Code for the Use, Care and Protection of Abrasives Wheels*, New York, American Standards Assoc., 1956.

19. Isen, A., and Sederle, G.: *Emery Sphere System*, Buffalo, New York, Frontier Contact Lens Co., 1958.

20. Haynes, P. R.: Comments on the fabrication of peripheral curves, in *Encyclopedia of Contact Lens Practice*, South Bend, Indiana, International Optics, 1959–1963, vol. 2, Chap. 22, Supp. 8, pp. 77–80.

21. Braff, S.: Calcon Contact Lens Co., Personal communication.

22. Isen, A.: *Supplementary Instruction Bulletin I, Contac-nique Unit*, Buffalo, New York, Frontier Contact Lens Co., 1959.

23. Isen, A.: *Instructions for Contac-nique No. 2, New Edging System*, Buffalo, New York, Frontier Contact Lens Co., 1961.

24. Cepero, G.: Conical and Concentric Polishing, *Contacto, 3(2)*:28–34, 1959.

25. Cepero, G.: *World Contact Lens Standards Committee Report—Part I, Contact Lens Construction Tolerances, Contacto, 3(9)*:249–251, 1959.

26. Seidner, L.: *Guaranteed Contact Lens Manual*, New York, Guaranteed Contact Lens Co., 1959.

27. Wesley, N. J., and Jessen, G.: *Your Handbook of Instructions for the Procedure of the Conlish Method for Finishing Contact Lenses*. Chicago, The Plastic Contact Lens Co., 1958.

28. Isen, A.: Spherical Power changes in contact lenses, in *Encyclopedia of Contact Lens Practice*, South Bend, Indiana, International Optics, 1959–1963, vol. 1, Chap. 22, pp. 72–74.

29. Gates, H., and Ewell, D.: *Instruction Manual for the Kontur Cut Down and Contour Unit—Model Three*, Richmond, California, Kontur Contact Lens Co., 1959.

30. Haynes, P. R.: Corneal contact lenses with toric peripheral curves, in *Encyclopedia of Contact Lens Practice*, South Bend, Indiana, International Optics, 1959–1963, vol. 1, App. B, Supp. 6, pp. 26–32.

31. Haynes, P. R.: Elliptical double truncated and oval contact lenses, in *Encyclopedia of Contact Lens Practice*, South Bend, Indiana, International Optics, 1959–1963, vol. 2, App. B, Supp. 8, pp. 36–44.

32. Ewell, D., Gates, H., and Remba, M.: The prism ballast contact lens principle, in *Encyclopedia of Contact Lens Practice*, South Bend, Indiana, International Optics, 1959–1963, vol. 2, Chap. 16, pp. 31–54.

33. Ewell, D.: Design and modification of a truncated edge, in *Encyclopedia of Contact Lens Practice*, South Bend, Indiana, International Optics, 1959–1963, vol. 3, Chap. 22, pp. 81–84.

34. Haynes, P. R.: Aperture venting techniques

in corneal contact lenses, in *Encyclopedia of Contact Lens Practice*, South Bend, Indiana, International Optics, 1959–1963, vol. 1, App. B, Supp. 4, pp. 9–13.

35. Gordon, S.: Some aspects of "venting" in corneal contact lenses, in *Encyclopedia of Contact Lens Practice*, South Bend, Indiana, International Optics, 1959–1963, vol. 2, Chap. 6, pp. 6–34.

36. Korb, D. R.: Recent advances in corneal lens fenestration, in *Encyclopedia of Contact Lens Practice*, South Bend, Indiana, International Optics, 1959–1963, vol. 3, App. B, Supp. 14, pp. 58–66.

37. Korb, D. R.: Contact lens news and views, *J. Am. Optom. Assoc.*, *32*(*11*):891, 892, 1961.

38. Policoff, W.: Personal communication.

SECTION III

HYDROGEL LENSES

Chapter 17

BASIC PRINCIPLES OF FLEXIBLE LENSES

FLEXIBLE CONTACT LENSES are lenses that at normal thicknesses will flex and nearly conform to the cornea. They can be folded so that the edges meet and, when released, return immediately to their normal shape without damage (Figure 17.1). An extremely thin P.M.M.A. lens (less than 0.12 mm.) will also flex somewhat, but it is not ordinarily considered a flexible lens because in the usual range of thickness it is rigid and cannot be folded.

Flexible lenses are made from many families of materials, the hydrogel lenses and the silicone lenses providing the two largest classes. Many other materials have been tried,

including vinyls and various other complex polymers.

Flexible lenses have many synonyms, which has led to some confusion. The term *flexible lens* should be applied to the general class of lenses as defined previously. *Hydrogel* (abbreviated gel) lenses are a type of flexible lens that is made from hydrogel plastic, i.e. a polymer which absorbs and binds water into its molecular structure. They should not be called *hydrophilic* lenses, a term meaning only water loving, which is also applied to hard lenses that are treated or coated to give the surface a lower wetting angle. They are sometimes described as *hydroscopic*, meaning that

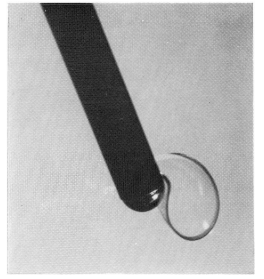

Figure 17.1a. A flexible lens can be folded and immediately returns to its original shape.

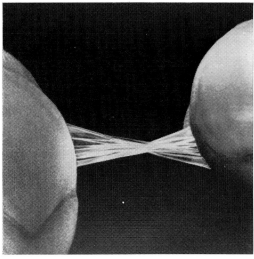

Figure 17.1b. Some gel lenses have high tensile strength and may be stretched. Other lenses will break under stress. Courtesy of Wesley-Jessen.

495

they readily take up moisture.

Hydrogel lenses are also known by the popular name of *soft lenses*. Many other synonyms and also many trade names are used for gel lenses.

Although the hydrogels that have been used for contact lenses are flexible, other types of hydrogels are not. They can be produced with a range of properties that vary from those which are nearly identical to P.M.M.A. to a material so soft it will break at the slightest touch. There are literally hundreds of hydrogels that have been tested for possible contact lens material. Only a few have proven to have a set of properties that can result in an acceptable contact lens.

HYDROGEL CONTACT LENSES

In the late 1950s Professor Otto Wichterle, a polymer chemist, was experimenting with various hydrogels for possible biological applications and conceived of the possibility that this material might be used to form a contact lens.[1] Together with another chemist, D. Lim, and an ophthalmologist, M. Dreifus, some early lenses were produced and fitted, and a report was given in the Czech literature in 1960.[2] Over the next few years, the news of this development began to spread throughout Europe and reached the United States in 1964.[3] During the next few years, the world had a chance to evaluate this unique development.[4-16]

In general, the first results obtained were rather disappointing. It was found that most of the patients were unable to achieve better than 20/40 visual acuity, even with the addition of supplementary trial lenses. All of these patients were able to get 20/20 or better with lenses made of P.M.M.A. There were also reports of patients having scleral injection, lens stability problems, edema, and other difficulties.

The success of the gel lens in Czechoslovakia can only be understood when it is realized that at the time of their introduction, no hard contact lenses were produced or available in that country. When the gel lens was introduced to Western Europe and the United States, it proved to be a poor competitor to the hard contact lens, and they were largely discontinued in the mid-1960s.[17] It was only after a period of research and development that the gel lens was improved to a level where it was accepted by the Western contact lens community.

Nevertheless, it was recognized that the gel lenses represented a potential for comfort that was better than that achieved with hard contact lenses. Hence, a quiet period of development took place in which many investigators made various modifications of these lenses.[18-54] The original Czech inventors also continued to improve the lens.[55-71] First, there were improvements in the material itself. The original Czech material had a yellowish green tinge, was impure, and was inconsistent from batch to batch. The newer material was made much clearer, stronger, and free of defects. At the same time, many lens design improvements took place and new manufacturing techniques were developed.

The first manufacturing technique was that of the original Czech inventor and consisted of spin-casting. The second technique was developed primarily in the United States and involved a lathing method similar to that used for hard contact lenses. Lenses produced by these two methods differ somewhat in their properties and, hence, are conveniently divided on this basis. More recently a casting method has been introduced that does not involve spinning.

WHY ARE GEL LENSES COMFORTABLE?

The principal advantage of a gel lens is its excellent initial comfort. It has been assumed generally that the comfort is related to the softness of the material or to its water content. This is not necessarily true. If a hard contact lens is made in the same dimensions as a gel contact lens and placed on the eye, it will be found that this lens is also very comfortable. Such lenses have been produced for use in special experiments. However, they cannot be tolerated long on the eye because they do not allow any significant tear exchange. When the lens is removed after about an hour of wear, it is invariably found that the cornea exhibits a diffuse punctate stain as a result of interference with the corneal metabolism.

A gel contact lens only has its excellent comfort on the eye under a limited set of conditions. The lens must be nearly as large or larger than the corneal diameter. When hydrogel lenses are made 9 to 10 mm. in diameter and with other dimensions similar to a hard corneal lens, it is found that the lens lags to a low position on the eye and may slide off the cornea. There is considerable lens movement with each blink, and the discomfort is usually much worse than when wearing a hard contact lens. Even a larger gel contact lens that is too loose on the cornea or moves about will be excessively uncomfortable.

The gel contact lens must also have extremely thin edges to achieve the desired comfort. A lens with thick edges is usually felt at the lids and produces extreme discomfort.

Hence, the gel contact lens is only comfortable when it is of large diameter, when it has very thin edges, and when there is limited movement. It is apparent that these conditions serve to produce minimum contact between the lens and the lid margins and in this way reduce lid and eye sensation. Why then is a gel contact lens needed to achieve the extreme comfort on the eye? If a hard contact lens is made in the form of a gel lens, it is not tolerated physiologically. The gel contact lens, however, passes significant oxygen through the lens itself and also allows some tear exchange to take place and thus maintains a normal physiology. It is for this reason that the gel contact lens material can be used to form a successful contact lens.

Another factor to be considered in the comfort of a gel contact lens is the surface quality. Little is understood about the surface characteristics of polymers and their interaction with the eye, but it seems apparent that the gel material offers little resistance to the lid as it glides across the surface of the lens. When other flexible materials are substituted in the same from as a gel lens, it is often found that the comfort is somewhat reduced.

ADVANTAGES AND DISADVANTAGES

In addition to its comfort, the gel lens offers these other advantages:

1. Corneal staining is infrequent.
2. Spectacle blur is minimized.
3. Ejection of the lens from the eye is uncommon.
4. Dislocation of the lens onto the sclera is uncommon.
5. Dust and foreign bodies usually do not get under the lens.
6. Adaptation time is reduced.
7. Some lenses are easy to fit.
8. The lenses can be worn part time or intermittently.
9. They have both cosmetic and therapeutic value.
10. They rarely produce flare.
11. It is rare to have photophobia or ex-

cessive tearing.

Unfortunately, the hydrogel lenses also have the following disadvantages:

1. Often poor visual acuity at far and near distance
2. Unstable visual acuity
3. Limitation of correction
4. Possibility of tearing or splitting
5. Limited durability
6. Difficulty in verification
7. Short life
8. Problems with sterilization
9. Susceptible to contamination by chemicals
10. Cleaning difficulties
11. Manufacturing problems
12. Limitation of types of lenses

Contraindications

Hydrogel contact lenses are contraindicated by the presence of any of the following conditions:

1. Acute and subacute inflammations of the anterior segment of the eye
2. Any eye disease that affects the cornea or conjunctiva
3. Insufficiency of lacrimal secretion
4. Corneal hypoesthesia
5. Any systemic disease that may affect the eye or be exaggerated by wearing contact lenses
6. Early stages of pregnancy

PATIENT SELECTION

The extremely good comfort obtained with the gel contact lens may be so rewarding to the patient that he tends to overlook the other attributes of the gel lens. It is only fair to the patient that a thorough discussion of some of the disadvantages of gel lenses be covered. This should include a discussion of the visual problems that may be encountered, the fragility of the lenses, the need for extra care of the lenses, and the costs involved in replacement or prescription changes.

Success with Hydrogel Lenses

The success with hydrogel contact lenses has been based primarily on their excellent comfort. A new patient who has never worn contact lenses before is usually pleasantly surprised at the degree of comfort experienced with this lens. Comments are often made that the lens cannot even be felt in the eye. However, not every patient experiences this ideal comfort. A few find the lenses even more uncomfortable than hard contact lenses. This may be due to the inability to obtain a good fit on these patients.

A patient who is an experienced wearer of hard contact lenses and who is having no problem may not be overly impressed when he first wears the hydrogel contact lens. However patients who have always reacted poorly to hard contact lenses often find the gel lens is a welcome improvement. Some of the best patients for gel lenses are those who have tried hard lenses and rejected them because they could never adjust to what is apparently edge discomfort. Some patients are so impressed by the extremely good comfort of the hydrogel lens that they are willing to tolerate measurable losses in visual acuity of one to three lines on the Snellen chart.

The degree of success reported for hydrogel contact lenses varies considerably according to the investigator. Reports of success as high as 80 percent and as low as 40 percent may be found in the literature.

PROPERTIES OF HYDROGEL LENSES

Hydrogel material is chemically very similar to polymethyl methacrylate and is named hydroxyethyl methacrylate, or H.E.M.A. (Figure 17.2). However, there is a difference in molecular structure, which allows the H.E.M.A. to bind with water and create a radically different property of this material. Both materials are *polymers*.

Polymer literally means "many parts." The parts are known as monomers and consist of small chemical units that are linked together to form a repeating chain of very high molecular weight. The process of forming this chain is known as polymerization. If more than one type of monomer is used in the chain, the final polymer is known as a copolymer.

The chains of a polymer can be arranged in various configurations. A polymer would be very weak unless the chains were tied together, which is accomplished chemically by the introduction of chemical bonds between the different polymer chains. This is known as cross-linking, which results in a network of chains extending throughout the polymer.

Polymers that are cross-linked vary widely in their reaction to solvents and depend on the frequency of the interchain bonds. If relatively few bonds are present, the polymer may swell to several times its original volume by imbibition of the solvent. If more bonds are present so that it is "tightly" cross-linked, the hydrogel can be essentially unaffected by liquids and does not swell at all. For the hydrogel material used in making some contact lenses, there is only about 1 cross-linking molecule for every 200 monomer units.

DIFFERENCES IN GEL LENS POLYMERS

The original hydrogel contact lenses were made from polyH.E.M.A. (2-hydroxy-ethyl methacrylate, which is lightly cross-linked with ethylene glycol dimethacrylate (E.D.M.A.).

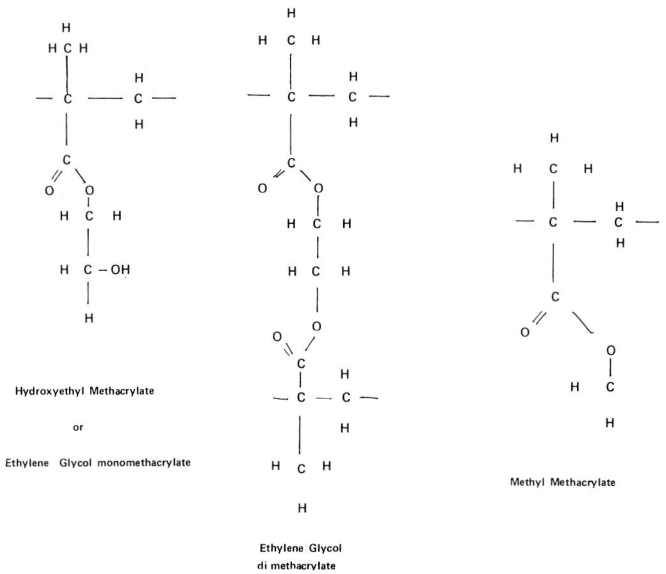

Figure 17.2. Comparison of chemical structure of P.M.M.A. and H.E.M.A.

Considerable improvement has been made in the original polymer material by purification and better polymerization technique. A second group of hydrogels contains poly-H.E.M.A. as one component but adds various other polymers in an attempt to improve the properties of the material. A third group of hydrogel contact lenses contains polymers related to, but different from, H.E.M.A. A list of the hydrogel materials that are available from various manufacturers is given in Appendix 15.

From a clinical standpoint, the exact composition of the polymer is of little interest to the practitioner. In most cases the lens properties depend primarily upon the water content of the material. A few exceptions exist, however, in which the polymer backbone seems to have greater or lesser strength according to its composition. As will be discussed later, the oxygen permeability is dependent primarily upon the water content.

Hence, every hydrogel has two components. There is a stable solid component consisting of the polymer network and a variable component consisting of aqueous or other solution that can exchange with the environment. The spaces between the polymer backbone are full of water and open to the surface of the hydrogel. As the polymer becomes hydrated, the spaces enlarge and can allow water-soluble substances to enter. In most cases, the dimensions of the spaces are too small for the entry of microorganisms, so their presence is generally found only if the polymer structure is cracked or altered in some way. Many ions and water-soluble drugs, such as steroids and antibiotics, can diffuse in and out of a hydrogel lens with relative ease. Estimates of the average pore diameter of various hydrogels ranges from about 0.5 to 3.5 μm. The hydrogels with higher water contents have the largest pores.

WATER CONTENT

Most of the water that is in a hydrogel lens can move easily in or out of the polymer spaces. It may also leave the lens entirely by evaporation. If one part of the lens becomes dehydrated relative to another, then water will move in the direction of the lowest concentration. Hence, a lens that is worn and exposed to the atmosphere may lose water if the evaporation from the front surface occurs at a faster rate than water is restored from the posterior surface. This apparently happens under some conditions of wear. Andrasko and Hill studied a 71 percent water content lens on the eye in various atmospheres.[72] It was found to be at 95 percent or less of its full saturation potential at all times. Under reduced humidity conditions, such as an artificially heated room at 18 percent relative humidity, the hydration level of a lens while being worn dropped to as low as 81 percent of its full saturation. Table 17.1 shows the

difference in hydration levels for four lenses, which were worn for only five minutes on the eye. In every case the hydration level was significantly reduced after lens wear. Such reduction is sufficient to cause a significant change in the oxygen transmission of the lens (Figure 17.3). This could have a significant effect upon the comfort and efficiency of the lenses.

The water content of hydrogel materials varies widely when all the lenses are fully hydrated (Table 17.2).[73] These experimental values vary slightly from the values published by the manufacturers. This is typical of the variation found when various gels are measured[74] and is due to the following conditions:

1. Variation in the water content of batches of gel material manufactured
2. Variation in the testing procedures

TABLE 17.1

OXYGEN PERFORMANCES (EQUIVALENT OXYGEN PERCENTAGES*) IN RELATION
TO THE RELATIVE HYDRATION STATES OF FOUR HYDROPHILIC LENSES

Lens Type	Saturated % Water	Center Thickness (mm.)	Lens Hydration %		EOP* at Removal
			at Start	at Removal	
			100	97	13.1
AO 78	78	0.23	90	94	11.8
			80	88	9.7
			100	90	10.7
Permalens	71	0.23	90	86	9.9
			80	77	8.9
			100	99	6.5
AO 70	70	0.39	90	96	3.7
			80	85	2.0
			100	94	4.1
SOFTCON	53	0.24	90	85	1.7
			80	76	1.3

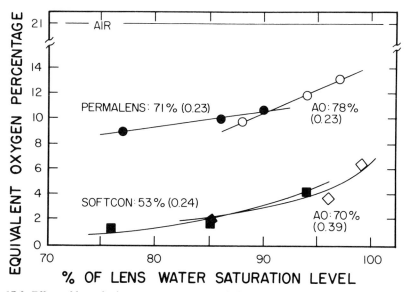

Figure 17.3. Effect of lens drying on oxygen transmission. From G. Andrasko and R. M. Hill, Oxygen and Water Content of Soft Contact Lenses; submitted for publication.

REFRACTIVE INDEX

The refractive index of a hydrogel material is a property of the material plus the water content. The more cross-linking that occurs in a polymer, the less water that is absorbed by the lens and the higher the refractive index of the material. The refractive index is nearly proportional to the water content. Each gel will also have a variable index depending on its state of hydration. As the lens is transformed from a hard to hydrated

TABLE 17.2
HYDROGEL LENSES

Lens Name	Manufacturer	Polymer	Polymer Name	Hydration
Soflens	Bausch & Lomb	HEMA	Polymacon	38.6%
Aquaflex	Union Optics	HEMA/NVP/ MMA	Tetra- filcon A	42.5%
AO-Soft	American Optical	HEMA/NVP/ MMA	Tetra- filcon A	42.5%
Al-47 (Alden)	Alden Labs	HEMA/ MA/NVP	NA	36.5%
Durasoft*	Wesley-Jessen	HEMA/Copolymer	Phemecol	30.0%
Hydron*	National Patent	HEMA	Polymacon	38.6%
Softcon	American Optical	HEMA/PVP	Vifilcon A	57.5%
Sauflon-70*	Medical Optics	NVP/MMA	Lidofilcon A	70.0%
Sauflon PW	Medical Optics	NVP/MMA	Lidofilcon A	79.0%
Hydrocurve II*	Soft Lenses Inc.	HEMA/acrylamide	Bufilcon A	46.0%
Naturvue*	Milton Roy (now B&L)	HEMA/NVP	Hefilcon A	46.0%
Permalens	Cooper	HEMA/NVP MA/NVP	Perfilcon A	71.0%
Soflens	Bausch & Lomb	HEMA	Polymacon	38.6%
N & N* #515	N & N Optical	HEMA polymer	NA (Material by Toyo)	35.6%
N & N* #1500	N & N Optical	HEMA polymer	NA (Material by Toyo)	29.0%
M-79*	N & N Optical	HEMA polymer	NA (Material by Toyo)	37.0%

*Available in toric lenses

state, the index changes continuously. Once the hydrogel has become fully hydrated, the water content remains fairly constant as does the refractive index. When the refractive index is given for a gel material, it usually refers to its fully hydrated state.

The refractive index will also depend upon the type of solvent used to hydrate the gel material.

EFFECTS OF TONICITY AND PH

Normally, gel contact lenses are stored in 0.9 NaCl solution. This tonicity is selected to correspond with the tonicity of the tears so that the lens will be compatible with the cornea.

Aside from its interaction with the tears, the tonicity of the gel lens fluid plays an important role in maintaining the stability of the lens, for if significant changes in tonicity occur, the lens dimensions may be altered.[75]

The diameter change resulting from soaking gel lenses in solutions of different tonicities from 0% to 1.7% sodium chloride for a period of twenty to thirty minutes are presented in Figure 17.4a.[76] The diameters of the lenses were also measured following a thirty-minute soak in acidic or basic solutions of pH from 2.7 to 10.6. These results indicate that the diameter of polyH.E.M.A. lenses remains essentially the same with changes of tonicity of the solution but that Softcon® lenses were very susceptible to tonicity changes.[73] They are larger in hypotonic solution and smaller in hypertonic solution, as compared to the isotonic solution. The diameter changed in one lens from about 14.5 to 12.5 when the sodium chloride concentration was increased from 0.05 percent to 1.5 percent (Figure 17.4a).[76]

There have been reports of significant changes in lens dimensions when some gel lenses were switched from storage solutions of saline to a commercial preparation.[77]

The salt concentration in the saline solution, by its osmotic effect, has considerable influence on the lens adherence to the eye. As the salt content is reduced, the lens movement is reduced (Figure 17.4b). A lens soaked in a 0.3% to 0.5% salt solution will typically show no movement on the cornea for a period of several minutes. After this period, the lens is equilibrated by the patient's tears so that normal movement resumes. A lens that has been soaked in saline solution of less than 0.3% usually sticks tenaciously to the eye and may be difficult to remove. Irrigation of the eye with a normal saline solution will reduce the time for equilibration.

BIOCOMPATIBILITY

There is a large body of literature available on the use of various polymers in contact with body fluids. The hard lens material, polymethyl methacrylate, has been used for many years for bone replacements, dental prosthesis, etc. The hydrogel material has been shown to have a similar inertness in the body tissue.

Although the various plastics used in contact lenses are in themselves inert, they carry the potential that various contaminants may be present which are not compatible with body tissues. These take the form of residual catalysts used in manufacturing, residual monomers, colorants, stabilizers, and other contaminants. These contaminants are not present when careful manufacturing technique is followed.[78,79]

FITTING OF HYDROGEL LENSES

Each of the numerous hydrogel lenses that are available has its own characteristics and recommended fitting procedures. However, every hydrogel lens must satisfy certain basic criteria that are essential to its success. Like the hard contact lens, the gel lens must provide a good optical correction for the eye, the lens must be comfortable, and the lens cannot interfere significantly with the normal ocular physiology. Basically there are six criteria of a good hydrogel lens fit.[80]

1. Good centration. Complete corneal coverage and limbal overlap by at least 0.5 mm. in every direction.

2. Acceptable movement. With normal thickness lenses there should be movement of at least 0.5 mm. to 1 mm. with each blink. Movement may be less with ultrathin lenses.

3. Good quality retinoscopic reflex, which does not vary with the blink.

4. Good visual acuity and overrefraction.

5. Good comfort to the patient for a wear-

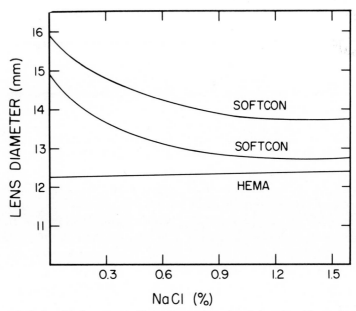

Figure 17.4a. Relationship between gel lens diameter and tonicity of soaking solution. From S. Eriksen, K. Randeri, and J. Ster, Behavior of Hydrophilic Soft Contact Lenses under Stress Conditions of pH and Tonicities, in J. L. Bitonte and R. H. Keates (Eds.), *Symposium on the Flexible Lens*, 1972. Courtesy of C. V. Mosby Co., St. Louis, Missouri.

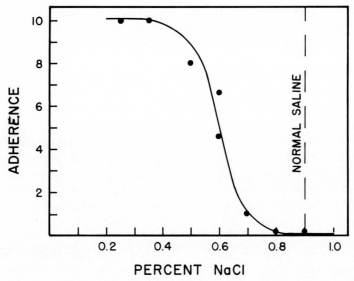

Figure 17.4b. Relationship between salt concentration of lens storage solution and lens adherence.

ing period of at least twelve hours.

6. Normal appearance of the patient, with no outward signs that contact lenses are being worn.

From a clinical standpoint of performance, hydrogel lenses appear to fall into three categories depending upon the water content.

1. Low water content lenses (25% to 35%)
2. Medium water content lenses (35% to 60%)
3. High water content lenses (60% to 85%)

Low water content lenses generally have higher strength and tear less easily. They suffer from lower oxygen permeability and must be made very thin if edema is to be avoided.

Medium water content lenses constitute the largest variety of available hydrogels. Most have water contents between 38 and 45 percent. Hydrogels between 45 and 60 percent begin to assume some of the properties of the higher water content lenses.

Higher water content lenses have significantly greater oxygen permeability compared to other lenses. This occurs because of the logarithmic relationship between oxygen permeability and water content (Figure 17.5). In some cases the high oxygen permeability has been ascribed to some special characteristic of the polymer structure but no such explanation is necessary.

CENTRATION

The mechanism of gel lens centration is complex and not well understood. It has been determined empirically that lenses which are small in diameter, 9 to 11 mm., slide easily off the cornea and do not maintain good centration even when fitted very steeply. Lenses that are approximately equal to the corneal diameter will stay in position, provided that they are thin and have virtually no peripheral curve. A lens that is approximately 1 mm. larger than the cornea will generally remain well centered depending upon the choice of peripheral curve. Large diameter lenses (14 to 16 mm.) were originally found to provide excellent centering characteristics, but as the lens thickness was reduced, it was found that lens diameter could be reduced and still achieve excellent centering.

Centering of hydrogel contact lenses also depends on edge design, but the exact relationship is not well understood. Thicker lens edges tend to cause greater lens movement. This is a special problem in toric gel lens design where there is a significant difference in edge thickness that leads to lens rotation.

A comparison of the lens centering achieved by spin-cast and one lathe-cut design is shown in Figure 17.6. Lens diameter is not the only factor of importance in achieving lens centering.[81] With the spin-cast lenses, however, better centering was achieved, in general, by the

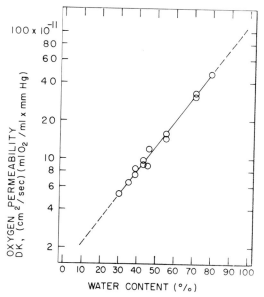

Figure 17.5. Relationship between water content of hydrogel lenses and oxygen permeability.

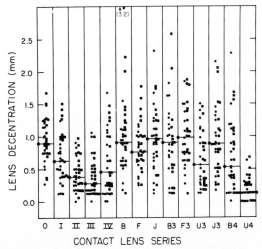

Figure 17.6a. Magnitude of decentration of various spin-cast and lathe-cut lenses for a sample of eighteen patients.

lenses of larger diameter. Thin lenses of the same diameter generally produced better centration than did lenses of greater thickness, however. Centering of lathe-cut lenses is directly related to the base curve–cornea relationship, but once the lens becomes too steep, the centering advantage is lost.

Ideally a gel lens will completely cover the entire corneal area. Corneal exposure ultimately leads to drying effects and punctate staining (*see* Chapter 22). Corneal coverage depends on the corneal diameter, the lens diameter, and the lens centration (Figure 17.7).

Decentration of gel lenses, when it occurs, is generally in a temporal direction, with perhaps a slight upward component. There is considerable difference in the incidence of decentration for different lens designs.

VISION

It was originally thought that hydrogel lenses conformed perfectly to the corneal contour. Later studies showed that this conformation was not complete but instead varied from subject to subject and with the type of lens used.[82] In most cases only a slight tear lens power effect is produced. This tear lens can alter the refractive power effect of the gel lens on the eye, however, and cannot be neglected.

In general, when there is corneal toricity, the gel lens does not conform completely to the toricity and thus tends to reduce the astigmatic error for the eye. This masking effect is generally very small with minus power lenses and only becomes significant for high plus lenses in the power range for aphakic corrections. The presence of residual astigmatism is, therefore, a significant problem for most hydrogel lens wearers. It is responsible for the reduced acuity in a large percentage of gel lens wearers as compared to their potential acuity with spectacles (Table 17.3). Table 17.4 shows the results from a study by Harris et al.[83] in which the corneal toricity was measured in twenty-four patients who were fitted with three types of gel contact lenses. The toricity was transferred to the front of the lens in nearly the same magnitude as the original corneal toricity, but there was a reduction in every case in the final refractive astigmatism achieved on the

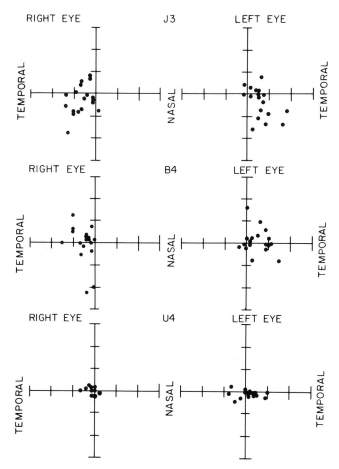

Figure 17.6b. Direction of decentration of various spin-cast and lathe-cut lenses for a sample of eighteen patients.

eye compared to the spectacle correction. No significant differences were found between the individual lenses that were tested (Table 17.5).

Other studies have shown even higher amounts of astigmatism transferred by gel contact lenses.[82] The best prediction for the final residual astigmatism would appear to be between two-thirds and all of the original astigmatism found in the refractive correction. Hence, the best candidates for soft contact lenses are those with low spectacle astigmatic correction. The corneal toricity is generally not a consideration in predicting the residual refractive result. The exception to this rule occurs when the corneal toricity exceeds 2

DK. Then it is generally found that some decentration of the gel lens occurs. This decentration will produce reduced acuity and difficulty in lens wear.

For some patients who are wearing a gel contact lens that rides in a decentered position, an induced astigmatism may be produced by the lens decentration itself (Table 17.6).[84] A change to a different type of lens which achieves better centering may, in fact, reduce the residual astigmatism. This effect has often been confused with the so called "masking" or reduction in residual astigmatism which is thought to occur when a lens change is made. The relationship between lens centration and vision varies with the lens type (Figure 17.8).

FLUOREXON

Hydrogel lenses are susceptible to penetration by fluorescein molecules, and hence this substance cannot be used in the fitting procedure. However, a high molecular weight fluorescein, fluorexon, has been used as a substitute for fluorescein in fitting gel lenses.[85] Its application, however, is extremely limited in a clinical situation. When fluorexon is first applied to a gel contact lens, a pattern is produced that is similar to that which occurs with a hard contact lens fluorescein pattern. However, after a period of several minutes, there is some penetration of the lens by fluorexon. This does not constitute a serious problem because the fluorexon will leach from the lens over a period of time.

The major drawback with fluorexon is that it seems to have little predictive properties in the fitting relationship. There is little or no correlation between the flurexon pattern and the ability to wear a contact lens. It does, however, show variation in the fluid lens characteristics achieved by the various lenses.

Fluorexon may also be used to stain corneas for abrasions or insult, just as in the case of fluorescein. This has the advantage that the gel lens can be reworn on the eye soon after the examination takes place. The disadvantage is that minor corneal insults that would be clearly defined by fluorescein may not be obvious when fluorexon is used.

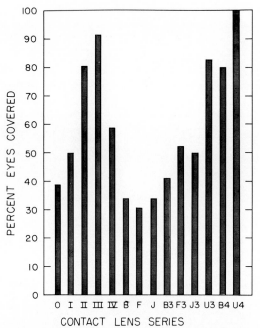

Figure 17.7. Relationship between gel lens type and corneal coverage for a sample of eighteen patients.

TABLE 17.3

Number and Percentages of Eyes That Achieved Indicated Visual Acuity With Best Spectacle Correction and With Three Types of Hydrogel Contact Lenses for 46 Eyes

Visual Acuity	Spectacles		Bausch & Lomb SOFLENS® Contact Lens		HYDROCURVE® II Contact Lens		AOSOFT™ Hydrophilic Contact Lens	
	# of Eyes	% of Eyes	# of Eyes	% of Eyes	# of Eyes	% of Eyes	# of Eyes	% of Eyes
20/15	27	58.7	24	52.2	19	41.3	22	47.8
20/20	19	41.3	16	34.8	21	45.7	18	39.1
20/25-20/30	0	0	5	10.9	5	10.9	5	10.9
20/40-20/50	0	0	1	2.2	1	2.2	1	2.2

TABLE 17.4

Mean Base Line Corneal Toricity and Mean Transferred Corneal Toricity for Three Types of Hydrogel Lenses for 46 Eyes

	Mean	Standard Deviation	Range
Baseline Corneal Toricity (D.K.)	0.80	± 0.44	0-2.00
Bausch and Lomb SOFLENS® Contact Lens (D.K.)	0.76	± 0.50	0-1.87
HYDROCURVE® II Contact Lens (D.K.)	0.84	± 0.51	0-2.12
AOSOFT™ Hydrophilic Contact Lens (D.K.)	0.86	± 0.58	0-2.87

TABLE 17.5

Mean Refractive Astigmatism (Spectacle Cylinder) and Mean Residual Astigmatism With Three Types of Lenses for 46 Eyes

	Mean	Standard Deviation	Range
Spectacle (D.C.)	0.58	± 0.45	0-1.50
Bausch and Lomb SOFLENS® Contact Lens (D.C.)	0.40	± 0.40	0-1.50
HYDROCURVE® II Contact Lens (D.C.)	0.41	± 0.40	0-1.50
AOSOFT™ Hydrophilic Contact Lens (D.C.)	0.36	± 0.34	0-1.25

OXYGEN PERMEABILITY OF GEL LENSES

There have been many studies of oxygen permeability of hydrogel contact lenses that show that hydrogel materials vary considerably in their ability to transmit oxygen.[86-93] Lenses of high permeability allow sufficient oxygen to pass to satisfy the minimum oxygen needs of the cornea. Other hydrogels, however, allow some oxygen permeability but do not satisfy the corneal needs. In the latter case, corneal edema is produced in greater or lesser amounts depending upon the individual corneal oxygen need.

Regardless of the chemical structure of the hydrogel material, the oxygen permeability depends primarily upon its water content. This relationship has been shown to be logarithmic (*See* Figure 17.5); consequently, lenses of higher water content transmit significantly higher oxygen to the cornea. Hence, with few exceptions, when the water content of a hydrogel lens has been determined, its equivalent oxygen level may be found from Figure 17.9. A detailed description of the measurement technique for oxygen permeability is given in Chapter 6. A list of the oxygen permeabilities and water contents of some commonly used hydrogel lenses is given in Table 17.7.

As described in Chapter 6, the permeability of each hydrogel material is a fundamental characteristic. The actual flux of oxygen that passes through a given contact lens is a function of both the permeability and the thickness of the lens.[94-97] Hence, a lens of high permeability may be much thicker than a lens of low permeability, and both transmit the same oxygen to the cornea. A lens of very low permeability that is made extremely thin may be capable of passing large amounts of oxygen to the cornea. Usually lenses made of materials with high permeabilities have greater fragility. To compensate for this, the lenses are made thicker; therefore, some oxygen transmission is sacrificed. Lenses of lower permeability are typically stronger and can be made thinner, which increases the oxygen transmission. Thus, the final oxygen transmission to the cornea is a result of several factors that must be considered in the lens design.

Lens power indirectly affects the oxygen transmission, since high power lenses have significant variation from the center thickness. An average lens thickness may be substituted for center thickness in order to increase the accuracy of the oxygen transmission value.

When a hydrogel contact lens does not provide sufficient oxygen to the cornea, edema is produced, which results in corneal thickening. This edema may be detected clinically using the biomicroscope or may be measured accurately with the use of a pachymeter (*see* Chapter 22).[98,99] The magnitude of the edema is usually predictable based upon the known oxygen transmission of the material. For example, the basic H.E.M.A. with 38 percent water content will provide an oxygen level at the cornea of about 2 percent when the lens is 0.15 mm. thick. Measurements of a population wearing these lenses show corneal thickness increases in the range of 3 to 8 percent.[94] In contrast, when the same material is used to make lenses 0.07 to 0.08 thickness, there is little or no corneal swelling produced. Such a lens will provide an oxygen level at the cornea of about 4 percent. The relationship between lens thickness and corneal thickening has also been investigated experimentally (Figure 17.10).[100]

TABLE 17.6

Lens	Decentration (mm.)	Astigmatism (D.)
−4.25F	2.6	0.25
−4.50J	2.0	1.25
−4.25B	2.3	0.75

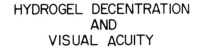

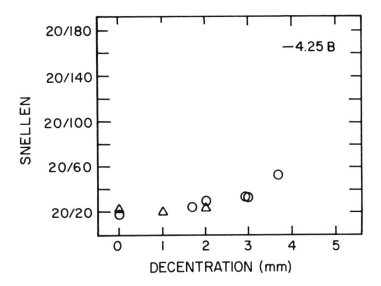

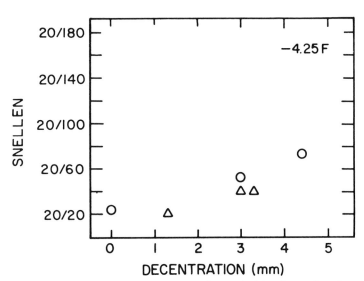

Figure 17.8. Relationship between lens centration and vision for various lens types.

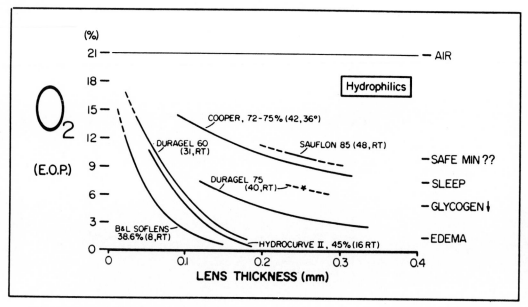

Figure 17.9. Relationship between lens water content and oxygen transmissibility for various lens thicknesses. Courtesy of R. M. Hill.

TEAR PUMPING WITH HYDROGEL LENSES

There has been considerable debate over whether or not hydrogel lenses produce significant tear pumping. Observation of fluorexon patterns under high magnification or with high speed movies often gives the ap-

TABLE 17.7
PERMEABILITY OF GEL MATERIALS

Lens		DK
Hema	Hydron	
	B&L	8.0
Hydrocurve 45		12.0
Hydrocurve 55		16.0
AO soft		8.5
Soflon		16.0
Permalens		34.0
Sauflon 70		30.0
Sauflon 85		48.0
Dow		7.3
Duragel 75		40.0
Durasoft	Wessley	4.0
25°C	Jessen	

pearance that tear interchange takes place with a blink. This appears to be illusory, however, and only indicates that the fluorescein is moved around in the postlenticular space between blinks. Theoretical considerations by Fatt[101] and others predicted that a very small exchange of tears should occur behind a gel lens. This prediction has been substantiated by clinical studies, which show no relationship between the posterior curve of a gel lens and edema produced by tear stagnation.[102] Polse has shown by measurements with a fluorophotometer that tear exchange behind gel contact lenses is of the magnitude of 1 or 2 percent exchange of tears per blink.[103] This may be compared to hard lens tear exchange, which normally occurs at 10 to 20 percent per blink. Hence, gel contact lenses must provide the majority of the oxygen supply of the cornea by their permeability.

ADAPTATION

The gel lens wearer usually has little or no adaptation problems of the type experienced by hard lens wearers. This may be attributed to the minimum touch sensation or irritation to the lids created by this lens.[104] Hence, there is very little or no effect on the subject's blinking or tearing.[105] Since excess tearing is absent, it reduces the corneal edema during the adaptation period due to osmotic changes.

The gel lens wearer can tolerate intermittent wearing periods with little difficulty, which may be explained by the same reasoning.

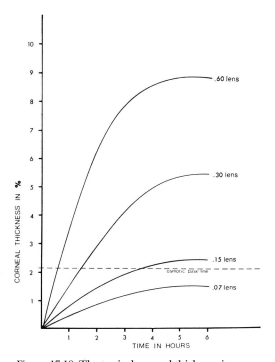

Figure 17.10. The typical corneal thickness increases for hydrogel lenses (40% to 42% hydration) of various thicknesses are illustrated. The data was essentially identical for lenses that would be considered cross-linked H.E.M.A., a graft copolymer of H.E.M.A. onto polyvinylpyrrolidone, and a hydrogel lens of a copolymer not containing H.E.M.A. The conclusion was that the nature of the hydrogel material was not important, provided the water of hydration was similar. The critical factor in maintaining normal corneal thickness and hydration was the thickness of the hydrogel contact lens. Courtesy of M. Refojo and D. Korb.

REFERENCES

1. Wichterle, O., and Lim, D.: Hydrophilic gels for biological uses, *Nature (Lond)*, *185(4706)*:117, 1960.

2. Dreifus, M., Wichterle, O., and Lim, D.: Intracameral lenses of hydrocolloid acrylates, *Cesk. Oftalmol.*, *16*:154–159, 1960.

3. Morrison, R. J.: Hydrophilic contact lenses, *J. Am. Optom. Assoc.*, *37(3)*:211–218, 1966.

4. Rycroft, B. W.: The new hydrophilic gel (soft) contact lens, *Highlights of Ophthalmology*, *7(4)*:252–253, 1964.

5. Turner, R. A.: Hydrophilic contact lenses, *The Ophthalmic Optician*, *4(7)*:343–346, 1964.

6. Turner, R. A.: Hydrophilic contact lenses, *The Ophthalmic Optician*, *4(8)*:404–406, 1964.

7. Rocher, P.: Les lentilles souples gel-kontact, *Les Cahiers de l'Optique de Contact*, *2*:5–6, 1964.

8. "Gel" contact lenses, *Indian J. Optom.*, *35(3)*:23, 1965.

9. Studies with hydrophilic lenses, *The Optician*, *150(3892)*:453, 1965.

10. Blackstone, M. R.: Some questions and answers on hydrophilic contact lenses, *The Optician*, *149*:486–488, 1965.

11. Blackstone, M. R.: Hydrophilic gel lenses, *The Optician*, *150*:388, 1965.

12. Braisbord, M. I.: Hydrophilic lenses, *The Optician*, *150(3892)*:490, 1965.

13. Neill, J. C.: The new gelatin contact lens and its clinical utility in optometric practice, *South. J. Optom.*, *8(5)*:15–17, 25, 1966.

14. Ruben, M.: Preliminary observations of soft (hydrophilic) contact lenses (abridged), *Proc. R. Soc. Med.*, *59(6)*:531–532, 1966.

15. Vesper, G.: Über die korrektur von aphaken mit gelkornealschalen, *Klin Monatsbl Augenheilk under Augenärztliche Fortbildung*, *145(2)*:256–262, 1964.

16. Romani, E.: Considerazioni sull'impiego delle lenti corneali idrofile in glicol metacrilico, *Bolletino d'Oculistica*, *46*:472–478, 1967.

17. Bailey, N. J.: The Bausch and Lomb Soflens: basic concepts and fitting techniques, in Gassett, A. R., and Kaufman, H. E. (Eds.): *Soft Contact Lens*, St. Louis, Mosby, 1972, pp. 61–71.

18. Balík, J. and Kubát, Z.: Excretion of glucose into tears in subjects wearing gel contact lenses, *Sb. Lek.*, *67(6)*:215–218, 1965.

19. Furnal, M. A.: Les lentilles souples on Geltakt, *L'Opticien Belge*, *121*:175–191, 1965.

20. Hart, R. S.: An interesting experience with hydrophilic lenses, *The Optician*, *150*:291, 1965.

21. Jenkins, L.: Problems with hydrophilic contact lenses, *Optom. Weekly*, *56(52)*:11–13, 1965.

22. Naito, Y.: Contact lenses partially made of a soft plastic material, *J. Jap. Contact Lens Soc.*, *7(1)*:2–5, 1965.

23. Turner, R. A.: An appraisal of the problems of hydrophilic contact lenses, *The Ophthalmic Optician*, *4(22)*:1151–1154, 1159, 1964.

24. Blackstone, M.: Hydrophilic lenses: Some practical experiments, *The Optician*, *151*: 56, 1966.

25. Bornschein, H., Wichterle, O., and Windsch, L.: A contact lens electrode for comparative ERG studies, *Vision Res.*, *6*:733–734, 1966.

26. Cochet, P.: Adaptation of soft lenses, *Arch. Ophthalmol.*, *26(3)*:309–312, 1966.

27. Farnik, L.: Clinical experiences with gel contact lenses, *The Optician*, *152*:299–302, 1966.

28. Kaplan, M. M.: Optical considerations of hydrogel contact lenses, *Optom. Weekly*, *57(14)*:29–39, 1966.

29. Magatani, H. et al.: Projection test of gel contact lenses, *J. Jap. Contact Lens Soc.*, *8(6)*:67–71, 1966.

30. Rocher, P.: L'avenir des verres de contact, *Les Cahiers de l'Optique de Contact*, *9*:2–10, 1966.

31. Wajs, G.: Qu'est-ce qu'un gel colloidal?, *Les Cahiers de l'Optique de Contact*, *9*:11–13, 1966.

32. Cochet, P. et al.: Les verres de contact, *Bull. Soc. Belge. Ophthalmol.*, *145*:169–170, 1967.

33. The write-in: thoughts on, and experience with, the gel lens, *Contact Lens*, *1(2)*:10–12, 27–28, 1967.

34. El Hage, S. G.: Les deformations cornéennes

causées par les lentilles souples, *Cah. Verres Contact*, *12*:6–7, 1967.

35. Franklin, J. B.: Hydrophilic corneal contact lens electrode, *Am. J. Ophthalmol.*, *64*: 469–471, 1967.

36. Gregersen, E.: Some experience of flexible and hydrophilic contact lenses, *Acta Ophthalmol.*, *45*(*3*):374–379, 1967.

37. Gyorffy, I.: The role and importance of the contact lens in the up-to-date correction of vision, *Oftalmologia (Bucharest) 11*: 105–114, 1967.

38. Kaplan, M. M.: Optical considerations of hydrophilic lenses—Part 2, Hydration and dehydration, *Optom. Weekly*, *58*(*21*): 19–26, 1967.

39. Kaplan, M. M.: The soft lens centrifuge, *The Optician*, *153*:551–552, 1967.

40. Lecoeur, G.: Nouvelles perspectives pour les lentilles souples, *Cah. Verres Contact*, *16*:30–32, 1968.

41. Blackstone, M., and Blackstone, D.: Hydrophilic lenses, *The Ophthalmic Optician*, *7*(*8*):390–391, 1967.

42. Willis, T. W.: Current reports on the hydrophilic lens, *Austr. J. Optom.*, *50*(*1*):38–45, 1967.

43. Balík, J., and Kubát, Z.: Secretion of potassium in tears with the use of gel contact lenses, *Sb. Lek.*, *70*(*8–9*):254–256, 1968.

44. Gumpelmayer, T. F.: The first decade of hydrophilic contact lenses, *J. Am. Optom. Assoc.*, *43*(*3*):253–255, 1972.

45. Balík, J., and Kubát, Z., and Veprek, L.: Vylucovani sodiku a drasliku do slz pri noseni gelovych kontaktnich cocek, *Sb. Lek.*, *70*(*1*):24–28, 1968.

46. Balík, J., and Kubát, Z.: Changes in tear proteins concentration in patients wearing gel contact lenses, *The Optician*, *155*: 205–207, 1968.

47. Bonnet, R., and El Hage, S. G.: Deformation of the cornea by wearing hard and gel contact lenses, *Am. J. Optom. Arch. Acad. Optom.*, *45*(*5*):309–321, 1968.

48. Dossi, F., and Chiavazza, G.: Prime esperienze sull'uso delle lenti molli nella correzione del cheratocono, *Annali di Ottalmologia e Clinica Oculistica*, *94*(*3*):322–324, 1968.

49. Larke, J. R.: Hydrophilic gel lenses in Czechoslovakia, *Contact Lens*, *1*(*6*):10–13, 1968.

50. Blackstone, M. R.: Hydrophilic contact lenses: 1967, 1968, and outwards, *The Optician*, *155*(*4011*):156–159, 1968.

51. Braun, J.: Symposium on the Czechoslovak gel contact lens, *Manufacturing Opticians International*, *20*(*7*):366–368, 1968.

52. Rocher, P.: Statistical results obtained with geltakt flexible lenses, *Contacto*, *12*(*4*): 44–50, 1968.

53. Nakajima, A., and Magatani, H.: Contact lenses: soft or hard? *South African International Ophthalmology Symposium, First Proceedings*, 1969, pp. 35–40.

54. Vincent, R.: Aspects physiologique et optique de l'adaptation des lentilles souples Spofalens, *Les Cahiers de l'Optique de Contact*, *19*:4–14, 1969.

55. Wichterle, O., Lim, D., and Dreifus, M.: A contribution to the problem of contact lenses, *Cesk. Oftalmol.*, *17*:70–75, 1961.

56. Dreifus, M., Holecková, E., and Wichterle, O.: *Cesk. Oftalmol.*, *18*:268, 1962.

57. Dreifus, M., and Wichterle, O.: Clinical experiences with hydrogel contact lenses, *Cesk. Oftalmol.*, *20*(*5*):393–399, 1964.

58. Wichterle, O.: Les lentilles de contact souples "geltakt" problèmes techniques et chimiques, *Les Cahiers de l'Optique de Contact*, *6*:407, 1965.

59. Dreifus, M.: Experiences cliniques avec les lentilles souples geltakt, *Cah. Verres Contact*, *7*:16–18, 1965.

60. Farnik, L: Czechoslovak work on the new gel contact lenses, *Manufacturing Opticians International*, *19*(*2*):161–163, 1966.

61. Sedlácek, J.: Correction of aphakia with a gel contact lens, *Cesk. Oftalmol.*, *22*(*1*): 76–79, 1966.

62. Wichterle, O.: Mechanical and optical aspects in soft lens fitting, in Dabezies, O. H. (Ed.): *International Symposium on Contact Lenses, 1st*, Munich-Feldafing, 1966, 1967, pp. 133–138.

63. Kamath, P. M.: Physical and chemical attributes of an ideal contact lens, *Contacto*, *13*(*4*):29–34, 1969.

64. Dreifus, M.: Gel contact lenses in clinical practice, in Dabezies, O. H. (Ed.): *International Symposium on Contact Lenses, 1st*, Munich-Feldafing, 1966, 1967, pp. 125–132.

65. Dreifus, M.: Les lentilles Geltakt dans la pratique, *Cah. Verres de Contact*, 14:29–30, 1967.

66. Dreifus, M.: Neue hydrogele Kontaktlinsen aus polyglykollmonomethakryl, *Augenoptik*, 85:36–39, 1968.

67. Dreifus, M.: Experience in the application of gel contact lenses, *J. Jap. Contact Lens Soc.*, 10(3):9–14, 1968.

68. Dreifus, M. et al.: The problems of corneal metabolism with respect to the application of soft gel contact lenses, *Third Congress Eur. Soc. Ophthalmol. (Amsterdam)*, 1968, p. 29.

69. Sedlácek, J., and Vesely, L.: Application of mydriatics by means of a gel contact lens, *Cesk. Oftalmol.*, 24(3):200–202, 1968.

70. Praus, R., Brettschneider, I., and Dreifus, M.: Study of the effect of hydrophilic gel contact lenses on the cornea—Part 1, Lactic acid in the cornea and aqueous humour and cornea hydration after application of contact lenses Geltakt in rabbits, *Ophthalmologica*, 159(4–6):398–406, 1969.

71. Dreifus, M.: Klinische Erfahrungen mit hydrophilen Kontaktlinsen bei einseitig aphaken Kindern, *Ophthalmologica*, 161(2–3):279–285, 1970.

72. Andrasko, G., and Hill, R. M.: Oxygen and water content of soft contact lenses, submitted for publication.

73. Masnick, K. B., and Holden, B. A.: A study of water content and parametric variations of hydrophilic contact lenses, *Austr. J. Optom.*, 55(12):481–487, 1972.

74. Gumpelmayer, T. F.: Dimensional stability of contact lens materials, *Contacto*, 13(4):24–27, 1969.

75. Rocher, P., Moreau, A., and Wajs, G.: Differences in characteristics of various gel hydrophilic contact lenses in function of the hydrating medium, *Contacto*, 17(1):4–11, 1973.

76. Eriksen, S., Randeri, K., and Ster, J.: Behavior of hydrophilic soft contact lenses under stress conditions of pH and tonicities, in Bitonte, J. L., and Keates, R. H. (Eds.): *Symposium on the Flexible Lens*, St. Louis, Mosby, 1972, pp. 213–217.

77. Willis, T. W.: Problem analysis with hydrophilic contact lenses, *Austr. J. Optom.*, 55(10):405–413, 1972.

78. O'Driscoll, K. F.: Polymeric aspects of soft contact lenses, in Gasset, A. R., and Kaufman, H. E. (Eds.): *Soft Contact Lens*, St. Louis, Mosby, 1972, pp. 3–18.

79. Leininger, R.: Plastics for contact lenses (rigid and flexible), in Bitonte, J. L., and Keates, R. H. (Eds.): *Symposium on the Flexible Lens*, St. Louis, Mosby, 1972, pp. 3–10.

80. Mertz, G. W., and Touch, A. J.: Corneal thickness response to the wearing of low minus Soflens contact lenses, *Int. Cont. Lens Clin.*, 4(1):26–35, 1977.

81. Wake, E. et. al.: Centration and coverage of hydrogel contact lenses, *Am. J. Optom. Physiol. Opt.*, to be published.

82. Sarver, D. S.: The gel lens—transferred corneal toricity as a function of lens thickness, *Am. J. Optom. Arch. Am. Acad. Optom.*, Jan. 1972.

83. Harris, M. et. al.: Residual astigmatism and visual acuity with hydrogel contact lenses: a comparative study, *J. Am. Optom. Assoc.*, 50(3):303–306, 1979.

84. Mandell, R. B. et. al.: Vision with decentered gel lenses, submitted for publication.

85. Refojo, M. F.: A new fluorescent stain for soft hydrophilic lens fitting, *Arch. Ophthalmol.*, 87(3):295–277, 1972.

86. Takahashi, G. H., Goldstick, T. K., and Fatt, I.: Physical properties of hydrophilic gel contact lenses, *Br. Med. J.*, 1(5480):143, 1966.

87. Morrison, D. R., and Edelhauser, H. F.: Permeability of hydrophilic contact lenses, *Invest. Ophthalmol.*, 11(1):58–63, 1972.

88. Refojo, M. F.: Physiochemical properties of hydrophilic soft contact lenses and their physiological implications, *J. Am. Optom. Assoc.*, 43(3):262–265, 1972.

89. Fatt, I., and St. Helen, R.: Oxygen tension under an oxygen-permeable contact lens, *Am. J. Optom.*, 48(7):545–555, 1971.

90. Fatt, I., Bieber, M. T., and Pye, S. D.: Steady state distribution of oxygen and carbon dioxide in the *in vivo* cornea of an eye covered by a gas-permeable contact lens, *Am. J. Optom.*, 46(1):3–14, 1969.

91. Peterson, J. F., and Fatt, I.: Oxygen flow through a soft contact lens on a living

eye, *Am. J. Optom.*, *50*(2):91–93, 1973.

92. Holly, F. J., and Refojo, M. F.: Oxygen permeability of hydrogel contact lenses, *43*(*11*):1173–1180, 1972.

93. Hill, R. M., and Fatt, I.: Oxygen uptake from a limited volume reservoir by *in vivo* human cornea, *Science*, *142*:1295, 1963.

94. Fatt, I.: Oxygen supply to the cornea through a hydrogel contact lens, *Contact Lens*, *14*(*1*):3–5, 1972.

95. Jauregui, M. J., and Fatt, I.: Estimation of oxygen tension under a contact lens, *Am. J. Optom.*, *48*(3):210–218, 1971.

96. Fatt, I.: Some effects of the gel contact lens on corneal physiology, *J. Am. Optom. Assoc.*, *43*(3):295–297, 1972.

97. Hill, R. M., and Augsburger, A.: Oxygen tensions at the epithelial surface with a contact lens *in situ*, *Am. J. Optom.*, *48*: 416–418, 1971.

98. Mandell, R. B., and Polse, K. A.: Corneal thickness changes as a contact lens fitting index—experimental results and a proposed model, *Am. J. Optom.*, *46*(7): 479–491, 1969.

99. Mandell, R. B., Polse, K. A., and Fatt, I.: Corneal swelling caused by contact lens wear, *Arch. Ophthalmol.*, *83*:3–9, 1970.

100. Mertz, G.: Corneal thickness response to ultra-thin Bausch and Lomb Soflens (Polymacon) contact lenses, *Am. J. Optom. Physiol. Opt.*, *55*(6):380–383, 1978.

101. Fatt, I., and Lin, D.: Oxygen tension under a soft or hard, gas permeable contact lens in the presence of tear pumping, *Am. J. Optom. Physiol. Opt.*, *53*(3):104–111, 1976.

102. Tomlinson, A., and Soni, P. S.: Peripheral curve design and the tear pump mechanism of soft contact lenses, *Am. J. Optom. Physiol. Opt.*, *57*(6):356–359, 1980.

103. Polse, K. A.: Tear flow under hydrogel contact lenses, *Invest. Ophthalmol. Vis. Sci.*, *18*(4):409–413, 1979.

104. Knoll, H. A., and Williams, J. R.: Effects of hydrophilic contact lenses on corneal sensitivity, *Am. J. Optom.*, *47*(7):561–563, 1970.

105. Brown, M. et al.: The effect of soft and hard contact lenses on blink rate, amplitude and length, *J. Am. Optom. Assoc.*, *44*(3): 254–257, 1973.

ADDITIONAL READINGS

Field, C. L.: Manufacturing problems and clinical performance of hydrophilic materials, *Contacto*, *16*(*1*):12–14, 1972.

Hamano, H., Hori, M., and Hirayama, K.: The effects of hard and soft contact lenses on rabbit cornea, *J. Jap. Contact Lens Soc.*, *14*(2):29–37, 1972.

Hamano, H., Miyabe, K., and Mitsunaga, S.: Thermal constants of hard and soft contact lens materials, *J. Jap. Contact Lens Soc.*, *13*(*10*): 107–109, 1971.

Hamano, H. et al.: Hard and soft contact lenses studied with scanning electron microscopy, *J. Jap. Contact Lens Soc.*, *14*(3):45–54, 1972.

Hill, R. M.: Effects of hydrophilic plastic lenses on corneal respiration, *J. Am. Optom. Assoc.*, *38*:181–184, 1967.

Hill, R. M., and Schoessler, J.: Optical membranes of silicone rubber, *J. Am. Optom. Assoc.*, *38*: 480–483, 1967.

Larke, J. R., Ng, C. O., and Tighe, B. J.: Hydrogel polymers in contact lens applications: a survey of existing literature—Part 1, *The Optician*, *162*(*4206*):12–16, 1971.

Larke, J. R., and Sabell, A. G.: A comparative study of the ocular response to two forms of contact lens—Part 1, *The Optician*, *162*(*4187*):8–12, 1971.

Larke, J. R., and Sabell, A. G.: A comparative study of the ocular response to two forms of contact lenses—Part 2, *The Optician*, *162*(*4188*): 10–14, 1971.

Lindmark, R., Edelhauser, H. F., and McCarey, B. E.: Design and fitting of rabbit hydrophilic contact lenses, *J. Contact Lens Soc. Am.*, *6*(*1*):21–27, 1972.

Masnick, K. B.: Corneal curvature changes using hydrophilic lenses, *Austr. J. Optom.*, *54*(7):240–241, 1971.

Peterson, J. F., and Fatt, I.: Oxygen flow through a soft contact lens in a living eye, *Am. J. Optom.*, *50*(2):91–93, 1973.

Refojo, M. F.: A critical review of properties and applications of soft hydrogel contact lenses, *Survey Ophthalmol., 16(4)*:233–246, 1972.

Refojo, M. F., Korb, D. R., and Silverman, H. I.: Clinical evaluation of a new fluorescent dye for hydrogel lenses, *J. Am. Optom. Assoc., 43(3)*: 321–326, 1972.

Refojo, M. F., Miller, D., and Fiore, A. S.: A new fluorescent stain for soft hydrophilic lens fitting, *Arch. Ophthalmol., 87(3)*:275–277, 1972.

Remba, M. J.: Soft lens fitting observations on rabbits and human subjects, *Contacto, 17(1)*: 15–18, 1973.

Rocher, P.: Optical and metabolic problems with hydrophilic lenses, *The Optician, 162(4209)*:6–8, 1971.

Ruben, M.: The philosophy of soft lenses, *J. Am. Optom. Assoc., 43(3)*:256–258, 1972.

Ruben, M.: Present status of contact lenses, *Practitioner, 209(1249)*:40–46, 1972.

Ruben, M.: Hydrophilic contact lenses, *Br. Orthoptic J., 29*:1–7, 1972.

Swanson, K. V.: Dispensing contact lenses: Hydration and dehydration of the finished corneal lens, *Optical Index, 48(1)*:40, 42, 1973.

Thomson, G.: Complications from wearing soft contact lenses, *Med. J. Austr., 1(1)*:29, 1973.

Tragakis, M. P., and Brown, S. I.: Hydrophilic contact lenses for correcting irregular and high astigmatism, *Arch. Ophthalmol., 88(6)*:596–601, 1972.

Turner, R. A.: The future of contact lenses and the development of new materials, *Dispensing Optician, 26(6)*:192–198, 1971.

Chapter 18

MOLDED LENSES

Spin-casting of contact lenses was the first technique used to make hydrogel contact lenses and is the present manufacturing method for the Bausch and Lomb Soflens® gel lens.[1]

Spin-casting is not a new technique in the field of polymer technology, as it was used before in the production of thin films. The procedure is very simply accomplished by placing a small quantity of the unpolymerized material on a flat platform that can be spun. As the rate of spinning is increased, the centrifugal force causes the material to move towards the periphery and results in the formation of a flat film. If one now places the unpolymerized material in a curved bowl instead of a flat platform and spins the bowl, the material is moved towards the periphery, but no longer is a thin, uniform film produced; rather, a body of variable thickness that assumes the necessary configuration for an optical lens is formed.

The lens is formed from a mixture of two liquid monomers, ethylene glycol monomethacrylate and ethylene glycol dimethacrylate (the cross-linker), with a catalyst. A carefully measured portion is injected onto a spinning mold (Figure 18.1), where it spreads to the edges and reaches a state of equilibrium (Figure 18.2). Polymerization is completed while the mold is spinning (Figure 18.3). The lens is then hydrated, which frees it of the

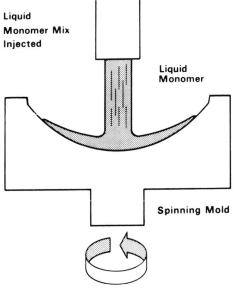

Figure 18.1. In the first phase, the monomer mixture is injected into the spinning mold.

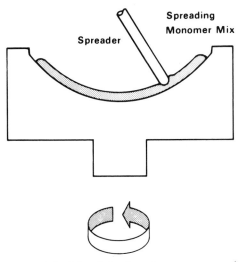

Figure 18.2. After injection, the monomer mixture is distributed by a spreader until it reaches equilibrium. Courtesy of Bausch & Lomb.

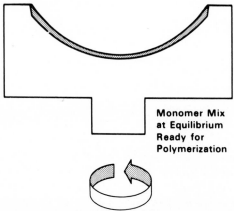

Figure 18.3. Monomer mixture at equilibrium. The polymerization phase can now commence.

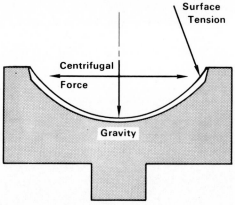

Figure 18.4. The forces of gravity, centrifugal force, and surface tension acting on the fluid polymer form the free spin surface.

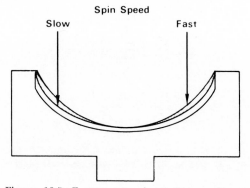

Figure 18.5. Fast speeds of rotation produce a steeper back curvature as opposed to slow speeds for flatter curves.

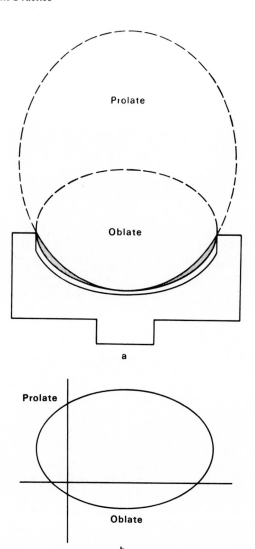

Figure 18.6. (*a*) The back curvature is closer to the oblate curve of an ellipse than the prolate. (*b*) The relationship between oblate and prolate is shown by the two chords.

mold, and then extracted of impurities by boiling at 190° F.

Consequently, the final lens design depends upon the following characteristics:

1. Curvature of the female mold
2. Rate of spin (fast for minus lenses and slow for plus lenses)
3. Amount of monomer mixture used

4. Physical properties of the monomers used
5. Rate of polymerization
6. Time of polymerization[2]

The posterior, or free-flowing aspherical surface of the lens will have characteristics determined by the interaction of several forces (Figure 18.4). Gravity acts to force the liquid into the center of the mold concavity. Centrifugal force acts to force the liquid in the direction 90° from the axis of the mold's rotation. Surface tension acts to hold the monomer mixture together in a meniscus form within the mold aperture. In order to produce different posterior lens curvatures, the mold is spun on its central axis at different speeds. A slower spin speed will produce a flatter curve, and a faster spin speed will produce a steeper curve (Figure 18.5). Hence, the central radius, chord diameter, and sagittal depth of the posterior lens surface are, for all practical purposes, independent variables.

The posterior lens surface approximates a conical curve so that no single radius describes its curvature. The radius is, therefore, specified in terms of the apical curvature, which is known as the posterior apical radius (P.A.R.). Within any given lens series, the conical curve will shift from that resembling the end of an ellipse, a prolate curve, to that resembling the side of an ellipse, an oblate spheroid (Figure 18.6). Thus, within any given lens series, one posterior curve

will be spherical. For example, in the F lens series, the sphere occurs at the 8.10 mm. posterior apical radius.

Lenses with shorter P.A.R. (higher minus powers) still retain the same sagitta and chord and therefore must be aspherical curves of the type that flattens in the periphery (Figure 18.7). This corresponds to the family of ellipses that have a constant apical radius. The prolate or steep end of the ellipse has a shorter radius at its apex and a lengthening radius towards the periphery. The oblate or flat side of the ellipse has a longer radius at its center and shorter radius towards the periphery. Variations in the eccentricity of the curvature is not usually considered in the fitting of soft contact lenses. It may, however, affect the spherical aberration induced by the contact lens and in some cases affect the visual acuity obtained with the lenses.

All lenses that are made from the same mold will have the same diameter. If they also have the same thickness, they will, therefore, have the same sagittal depth. The B, F, and J series all have a sagittal depth of 2.91 mm., whereas the N series lens has a sagittal depth of 3.06 mm. This would only be possible if there were a variation in the eccentricity value for a series of lenses having different powers. Figure 18.8 shows how it is possible to make two lenses of the same thickness in one diameter and yet have different powers.

BAUSCH AND LOMB SOFLENS

The gel material used in the Soflens has the properties described in Table 18.1. Compared to other gel materials, it has a relatively low saline absorption capacity of approximately 38 percent.

All of the lenses that are made from the same mold constitute a lens series, and Soflenses are usually identified by their series letter (Table 18.2). Within a series of lenses, the front radius of curvature remains con-

stant, whereas the back radius of curvature decreases (curvature increases) proportionally to the negative power of the lens. For a positive power lens, the radius of curvature of the posterior surface increases with increasing power of the lens (Figure 18.9).

The lenses for the various series fall in order according to their posterior apical radii, with the radius decreasing as a progression is made through the alphabet (Table 18.3). Some

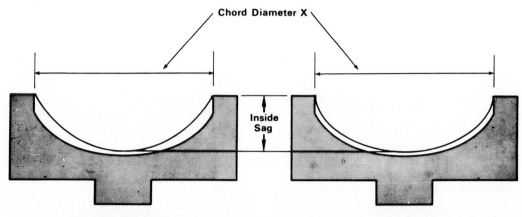

Flattening in the Periphery   **Steepening in the Periphery**

Figure 18.7. Independent of the power and central back curvature, control of the peripheral curvatures is also possible.

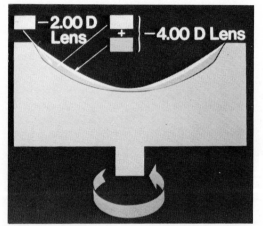

Figure 18.8. It is possible to make two lenses of the same thickness and diameter and yet have different powers. Courtesy of Bausch and Lomb, Inc.

TABLE 18.1

PHYSICAL PROPERTIES OF HEMA POLYMER

Refractive index	
(n_D 20° C equilibrated in H_2O)	1.43
Softening point	120°C
Visible light transmission sample	
thickness 0.75 mm.	>97%
Water content by weight:	
Equilibrated in H_2O	41.7%
Equilibrated in 0.9% NaCl	38.6%
Water content by volume equilibrated in H_2O	47%
Linear swell:	
Equilibrated in 0.9% NaCl	18%

of the series have now been discontinued because their fitting characteristics were found to be insignificantly different from the remaining series. These lenses may still be worn by some patients, however, and a knowledge of their characteristics is needed. In addition to the varying posterior apical radii, the Soflens minus series lenses are available in three different diameters. The smallest lens

has a chord diameter of 12.5 mm. and is identified on the bottle by the power and series only, e.g. −2.00 B; the middle diameter is 13.6 mm. and is identified by adding a 3 to the label, e.g. −2.00 B3. The largest lens, the 14.5 mm. diameter, incorporates the number 4 on the label, e.g. −2.00 B4. A discontinued series, the C series, has a diameter of 13.5 mm.

There are two exceptions to the rule that all lenses in the same series have the same front curve. The B3 and F3 series each have two different anterior curves.

The ultrathin lenses, designated the U series, and the superthin lenses, designated the O series, do not follow the general rule for posterior apical radii. These lenses are so thin that the fitting characteristics differ significantly from the other lens series. (*See* discussion of fitting.)

A principal difference in the fitting characteristics of the lens series is produced by variations in their anterior bevel design (Figure 18.10). Obviously, the bevel width, together with the diameter, will determine the front optical zone diameter. In addition, the front bevel will influence the centering characteristics of the lens and the amount of movement that occurs following a blink.

FITTING OF SOFLENSES

The fitting procedure for Soflenses is designed to arrive at the smallest lens that will fulfill the criteria of good vision, good comfort, and satisfactory physiological response.[3] To

TABLE 18.2

DESIGN DIMENSIONS OF BAUSCH AND LOMB SOFLENS CONTACT LENSES*

Series	Diameter (mm)	Posterior Saggital (mm)	Anterior Radius (mm)	Center Thickness (mm)	Power (D)
C	13.5	3.26 to 3.48	8.24	.09 to .36	-1.00 to -20.00
N	12.5	2.97	8.14	0.14	-0.25 to - 6.00
J	12.5	2.84	8.44	0.11	-0.25 to - 7.50
F	12.5	2.84	8.76	0.14	-0.25 to - 9.50
B	12.5	2.84	9.08	0.11	-0.25 to - 9.00
U	12.5	2.89	8.59	0.07	-0.25 to - 9.00
J3	13.6	3.11	9.02	0.15	-0.25 to - 6.00
F3	13.6	3.06	9.34	0.14	-0.25 to -20.00
B3	13.6	3.10	9.67	0.11	-0.25 to -20.00
U3	13.6	3.09	9.15	0.07	-0.25 to - 9.00
B4	14.5	3.60	10.08	0.12	-0.25 to - 9.00
U4	14.5	4.05	9.07	0.08	-0.25 to - 9.00
			Cntrl/Periph		
low + N	12.5	2.96 to 2.68	8.14	0.19 to 0.47	+0.25 to+ 6.00
		3.09	8.30 / 9.35	0.30	+0.25 to+ 6.00
low + F3	13.6	3.17	7.50 / 9.10	0.42	+6.50 to+10.50
high + N	13.5	3.62 to 3.41	6.40 / 8.28	0.54 to 0.75	+11.00 to+17.50
high + U3	13.6	3.38	6.20 / 8.75	0.57	+11.00 to+20.00
high + F3	13.6	3.37	6.40 / 8.75	0.57	+11.00 to+20.00
high + B3	13.6	3.38	6.60 / 8.75	0.57	+11.00 to+20.00
bandage T	14.7	4.34	8.14 / 8.76	.20	plano

*From information provided by Bausch and Lomb, Inc.

TABLE 18.3a

P.A.R.* OF BAUSCH & LOMB SOFLENSES—MINUS SERIES

POWER D	B MM	B D	F MM	F D	J MM	J D	N MM	N D	S3 MM	S3 D	F3 MM	F3 D	J3 MM	J3 D
-0.25	9.00	37.50	8.65	39.00	8.35	40.50	8.05	42.00	9.60	35.25	9.25	36.50	8.95	37.75
-0.50	8.95	37.75	8.65	39.00	8.30	40.75	8.00	42.25	9.55	35.25	9.20	36.75	8.90	38.00
-0.75	8.90	38.00	8.60	39.25	8.25	41.00	8.00	42.25	9.45	35.75	9.15	37.00	8.85	38.25
-1.00	8.85	38.25	8.55	39.50	8.25	41.00	7.95	42.50	9.40	36.00	9.10	37.00	8.80	38.25
-1.25	8.80	38.25	8.50	39.75	8.20	41.25	7.90	42.75	9.35	36.00	9.05	37.25	8.75	38.50
-1.50	8.75	38.50	8.45	40.00	8.15	41.50	7.85	43.00	9.30	36.25	9.00	37.50	8.70	38.75
-1.75	8.70	38.75	8.40	40.25	8.10	41.75	7.85	43.00	9.25	36.50	8.95	37.75	8.65	39.00
-2.00	8.65	39.00	8.40	40.25	8.10	41.75	7.80	43.25	9.20	36.75	8.90	38.00	8.60	39.25
-2.25	8.65	39.00	8.35	40.50	8.05	42.00	7.75	43.50	9.15	37.00	8.85	38.25	8.60	39.25
-2.50	8.60	39.25	8.30	40.75	8.00	42.25	7.75	43.50	9.15	37.00	8.85	38.25	8.55	39.50
-2.75	8.55	39.50	8.25	41.00	7.95	42.50	7.70	43.75	9.10	37.00	8.80	38.25	8.50	39.75
-3.00	8.50	39.75	8.20	41.25	7.95	42.50	7.65	44.00	9.05	37.25	8.75	38.50	8.45	40.00
-3.25	8.45	40.00	8.20	41.25	7.90	42.75	7.65	44.00	9.00	37.50	8.70	38.75	8.40	40.25
-3.50	8.40	40.25	8.15	41.50	7.85	43.00	7.60	44.50	8.95	37.75	8.65	39.00	8.40	40.25
-3.75	8.40	40.25	8.10	41.75	7.85	43.00	7.55	44.75	8.90	38.00	8.60	39.25	8.35	40.50
-4.00	8.35	40.50	8.05	42.00	7.80	43.25	7.55	44.75	8.85	38.25	8.55	39.50	8.30	40.75
-4.25	8.30	40.75	8.05	42.00	7.75	43.50	7.50	45.00	8.80	38.25	8.55	39.50	8.25	41.00
-4.50	8.25	41.00	8.00	42.25	7.70	43.75	7.45	45.25	8.75	38.50	8.50	39.75	8.20	41.25
-4.75	8.20	41.25	7.95	42.50	7.70	43.75	7.45	45.25	8.70	38.75	8.45	40.00	8.20	41.25
-5.00	8.20	41.25	7.90	42.75	7.65	44.00	7.40	46.00	8.65	39.00	8.40	40.25	8.15	41.50
-5.50	8.10	41.75	7.85	43.00	7.60	44.50	7.35	46.00	8.60	39.25	8.30	40.75	8.05	42.00
-6.00	8.05	42.00	7.80	43.25	7.50	45.00	7.30	46.25	8.50	39.75	8.25	41.00	8.00	42.25
-6.50	7.95	42.50	7.70	43.75	7.45	45.25			8.40	40.25	8.15	41.50		
-7.00	7.90	42.75	7.65	44.00	7.40	45.50			8.35	40.50	8.10	41.75		
-7.50	7.80	43.25	7.60	44.50	7.35	46.00			8.25	41.00	8.00	42.25		
-8.00	7.75	43.50	7.50	45.00					8.20	41.25	7.95	42.50		
-8.50	7.70	43.75	7.45	45.25					8.10	41.75	7.85	43.00		
-9.00	7.60	44.50	7.40	45.50					8.05	42.00	7.80	43.25		
-9.50			7.30	46.25					7.95	42.50	7.75	43.50		
-10.00									7.90	42.75	7.65	44.00		
-10.50									7.80	43.25	7.60	44.50		
-11.00									7.75	43.50	7.55	44.75		
-11.50									7.70	43.75	7.45	45.25		
-12.00									7.60	44.50	7.40	45.50		
-12.50									9.55	35.25	9.20	36.75		
-13.00									9.45	35.75	9.10	37.00		
-13.50									9.35	36.00	9.00	37.50		
-14.00									9.25	36.50	8.90	38.00		
-14.50									9.15	37.00	8.85	38.25		
-15.00									9.05	37.25	8.75	38.50		
-15.50									8.95	37.75	8.65	39.00		
-16.00									8.85	38.25	8.55	39.50		
-16.50									8.75	38.50	8.50	39.75		
-17.00									8.70	38.75	8.40	40.25		
-17.50									8.60	39.25	8.30	40.75		
-18.00									8.50	39.75	8.25	41.00		
-18.50									8.45	40.00	8.15	41.50		
-19.00									8.35	40.50	8.10	41.75		
-19.50									8.25	41.00	8.00	42.25		
-20.00									8.20	41.25	7.95	42.50		

*calculated

achieve this requires that a lens cover the entire cornea, cause no interference with the corneal metabolism, and correct for the refractive error of the eye.

The proper choice of lens, therefore, requires selecting the optimum lens diameter and the appropriate lens thickness.[4-15] The lens power may be determined using standard optical formulae. The following fitting rules should be followed:

1. Measure the horizontal visible iris diameter with a ruler, template, slit-lamp reticle, pupillometer, or photograph.

2. Select the initial lens diameter from Table 18.4.

3. Select the initial lens thickness after consideration of the guidelines that follow under the section titled "Standard Thickness versus Ultrathin."

4. If the initially selected lens (standard or ultrathin) fails to cover the cornea fully, the next larger lens of the same thickness should be the alternate selection (the one exception—the U4 series lens is the alternative if the B4 series lens fails to cover the cornea fully). Full coverage of the cornea is defined as the lens edge extending about 0.75 mm. beyond the visible iris in all direc-

TABLE 18.3b
P.A.R.* OF BAUSCH & LOMB SOFLENSES— MINUS SERIES ULTRA-THIN

POWER	U		U3	
D	MM	D	MM	D
0.00	8.55	39.50	9.15	37.00
−0.25	8.50	39.75	9.10	37.00
−0.50	8.50	39.75	9.05	37.25
−0.75	8.45	40.00	9.00	37.50
−1.00	8.40	40.25	8.95	37.75
−1.25	8.35	40.50	8.90	38.00
−1.50	8.30	40.75	8.85	38.25
−1.75	8.30	40.75	8.80	38.25
−2.00	8.25	41.00	8.75	38.50
−2.25	8.20	41.25	8.70	38.75
−2.50	8.15	41.50	8.70	38.75
−2.75	8.10	41.75	8.65	39.00
−3.00	8.10	41.75	8.60	39.25
−3.25	8.05	42.00	8.55	39.50
−3.50	8.00	42.25	8.50	39.75
−3.75	8.00	42.25	8.45	40.00
−4.00	7.95	42.50	8.40	40.25
−4.25	7.90	42.75	8.40	40.25
−4.50	7.90	42.75	8.35	40.50
−4.75	7.85	43.00	8.30	40.75
−5.00	7.80	43.25	8.25	41.00
−5.50	7.75	43.50	8.20	41.25
−6.00	7.65	44.00	8.10	41.75

*calculated

tions. Lens evaluation should only be done after at least ten minutes of lens wear to allow the lens to stabilize and any tearing to subside.

5. Final lens selection should *not* be considered complete until the patient's lenses are evaluated at a post-fit progress check (one to four weeks is recommended after initial dispensing) *immediately* after at least four continuous hours of lens wear.

6. When a fully covering, standard thickness lens is evaluated—

a. A change to the same diameter ultra-thin lens is warranted at the initial visit or any post-fit visit if the patient experiences excessive lens awareness or unstable vision with the blink.

b. A change to the same diameter ultra-thin lens is warranted at any post-fit visit if vertical corneal striae are encountered (after at least four hours of lens wear).

c. A change to a larger standard thickness lens is warranted at any post-fit visit if the lens is no longer fully covering the cor-

TABLE 18.3c
P.A.R.* OF BAUSCH & LOMB SOFLENSES—HIGH PLUS SERIES

	B3		F3		J3		N	
+ 11.00	7.70	43.75	7.40	45.50	7.15	47.25	7.45	45.25
+ 11.50	7.75	43.50	7.50	45.00	7.20	47.00	7.50	45.00
+ 12.00	7.80	43.25	7.55	44.75	7.25	46.50	7.55	44.75
+ 12.50	7.90	42.75	7.60	44.50	7.35	46.00	7.60	44.50
+ 13.00	7.95	42.50	7.70	43.75	7.40	45.50	7.65	44.00
+ 13.50	8.05	42.00	7.75	43.50	7.45	45.25	7.70	43.75
+ 14.00	8.10	41.75	7.80	43.25	7.50	45.00	7.75	43.50
+ 14.50	8.20	41.25	7.90	42.75	7.60	44.50	7.80	43.25
+ 15.00	8.25	41.00	7.95	42.50	7.65	44.00	7.90	43.00
+ 15.50	8.35	40.50	8.05	42.00	7.70	43.75	7.95	42.50
+ 16.00	8.45	40.00	8.10	41.75	7.80	43.25	8.00	42.25
+ 16.50	8.50	39.75	8.20	41.25	7.85	43.00	8.05	42.00
+ 17.00	8.60	39.25	8.25	41.00	7.95	42.50	8.10	41.75
+ 17.50	8.70	38.75	8.35	40.50	8.00	42.25	8.15	41.50
+ 18.00	8.75	38.50	8.40	40.25	8.10	41.75		
+ 18.50	8.85	38.25	8.50	39.75	8.15	41.50		
+ 19.00	8.95	37.75	8.60	39.25	8.25	41.00		
+ 19.50	9.05	37.25	8.65	39.00	8.30	40.75		
+ 20.00	9.15	37.00	8.75	38.50	8.40	40.25		

*calculated

TABLE 18.3d

P.A.R.* OF BAUSCH & LOMB SOFLENSES—PLUS SERIES

POWER	N		F3	
D	MM	D	MM	D
+ 0.25	8.15	41.50	8.25	41.00
+ 0.50	8.15	41.50	8.30	40.75
+ 0.75	8.20	41.25	8.35	40.50
+ 1.00	8.25	41.00	8.40	40.25
+ 1.25	8.25	41.00	8.45	40.00
+ 1.50	8.30	40.75	8.45	40.00
+ 1.75	8.35	40.50	8.50	39.75
+ 2.00	8.40	40.25	8.55	39.50
+ 2.25	8.40	40.25	8.60	39.25
+ 2.50	8.45	40.00	8.65	39.00
+ 2.75	8.50	39.75	8.70	38.75
+ 3.00	8.55	39.50	8.70	38.75
+ 3.25	8.55	39.50	8.75	38.50
+ 3.50	8.60	39.25	8.80	38.25
+ 3.75	8.65	39.00	8.85	38.25
+ 4.00	8.70	38.75	8.90	38.00
+ 4.25	8.75	38.50	8.95	37.75
+ 4.50	8.75	38.50	9.00	37.50
+ 4.75	8.80	38.25	9.05	37.25
+ 5.00	8.85	38.25	9.10	37.00
+ 5.50	8.95	37.75	9.20	36.75
+ 6.00	9.05	37.25	9.30	36.25
+ 6.50	7.00	48.00	8.25	41.00
+ 7.00	7.05	47.75	8.35	40.50
+ 7.50	7.10	47.50	8.45	40.00
+ 8.00	7.15	47.25	8.50	39.75
+ 8.50	7.20	47.00	8.60	39.25
+ 9.00	7.25	46.50	8.70	38.75
+ 9.50	7.30	46.25	8.75	38.50
+ 10.00	7.35	46.00	8.85	38.25
+ 10.50	7.40	45.50	8.95	37.75

*calculated

TABLE 18.4

SELECTION OF INITIAL SOFLENS DIAMETER

Horizontal Visible Iris Diameter	Lens Diameter (mm.)	Lens Series
Less than 11.5	12.5	F, U, or 03
11.5 to 12.0	13.6	B3, U3, or 03
Greater than 12.0	14.5	B4, U4, or 04

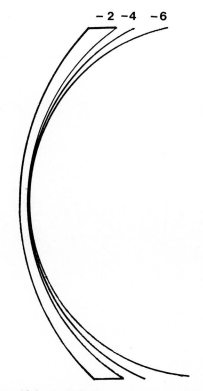

−2 −4 −6

Figure 18.9. A Soflens series has a constant front radius with a variable back radius of curvature to produce different negative power lenses.

a. A change to the same diameter standard thickness lens is warranted at the initial visit or any post-fit visit if the patient is unable to demonstrate the ability to handle properly ultrathin lenses and/or is damaging the lenses at an excessive rate. The patient can always be given ultrathin lenses again at subsequent post-fit visits when handling proficiency has been demonstrated with standard lenses.

b. A change to a larger ultrathin lens is warranted at any post-fit visit if the lens is no longer fully covering the cornea (the obvious exception is the U4 lens, for which there is no alternative within the Bausch and Lomb lens system. This is a rare event.)

In many cases, the choice between a lens of regular center thickness (0.12 mm.) and an ultrathin lens (0.07 mm. center thickness) is

nea (again, the exception is the B4 lens, which would require a change to a U4 lens).

7. When a fully covering, ultrathin lens is evaluated—

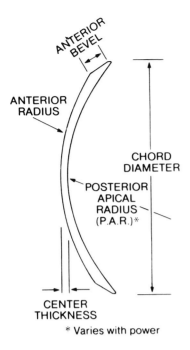

ANTERIOR BEVEL

ANTERIOR RADIUS

CHORD DIAMETER

POSTERIOR APICAL RADIUS (P.A.R.)*

CENTER THICKNESS

* Varies with power

Typical Lens Configuration
Minus Series

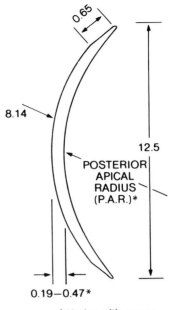

0.65

8.14

12.5

POSTERIOR APICAL RADIUS (P.A.R.)*

0.19–0.47*

* Varies with power

Typical Lens Configuration
Low-Plus Series

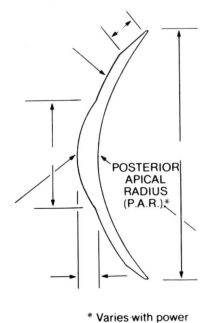

POSTERIOR APICAL RADIUS (P.A.R.)*

* Varies with power

Typical Lens Configuration
High-Plus Series

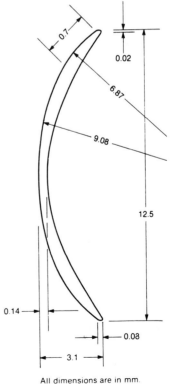

0.7

0.02

6.87

9.08

12.5

0.14

0.08

3.1

All dimensions are in mm.

Figure 18.10. Typical lens configurations for (a) minus series, (b) low-plus series, (c) high-plus series, and (d) average dimensions for B series minus lenses.

arbitrary. This decision should be considered a professional judgment to be made by the practitioner based on the following considerations:

Standard Thickness versus Ultrathin

Ultrathin lenses (U, U3, U4) generally provide superior clinical performance, especially in the areas of comfort and physiological response.[16-19] If it were not for some practitioner's and patient's finding ultrathin lenses difficult to handle, they would always be recommended. Ways of coping with the handling challenge are described in Chapter 21.

Standard thickness lenses (F, B3, B4) are, of course, the alternatives when patient handling is an issue. However, some patients fitted with standard thickness lenses will manifest edema, requiring a change to an ultrathin lens. On the positive side, the patient will generally find the transition to ultrathin series lenses to be relatively easy after his standard lens experience. Some practitioners prefer to dispense standard lenses to patients initially for training purposes and then change to ultrathin lenses later if indicated.

The practitioner may decide between standard thickness lenses and ultrathin lenses by the following guidelines:

1. Unless clinical considerations or practitioner preference dictate otherwise, the fitting of ultrathin lenses is strongly recommended.

2. Refitting patients (who already wear contact lenses and are therefore used to handling them) can be relatively easily accomplished with ultrathin series lenses.

3. Ultrathin lenses of powers greater than −1.50 D are easier to handle (probably because increased peripheral lens thickness reduces the flaccidity). Inexperienced patients requiring lenses of −1.50 D or less should probably be initially fitted with standard thickness lenses.

4. Patients with poor dexterity should probably be fitted initially with standard thickness lenses.

5. In very dry environments, some patients *may* be better fitted with standard thickness lenses.

O Series lenses

The O series lenses are the thinnest of the Bausch and Lomb Soflenses, having a center thickness of only 0.03 mm. In general, they are used less frequently than the other lenses and are usually reserved for patients who exhibit corneal edema with even a U series lens. Unfortunately, the handling properties of the O series lens has interfered significantly with its success.

Power

Bausch and Lomb Soflenses are designated in terms of back vertex power. The lens that corrects the eye properly generally has a power equal to the spherical equivalent of the refraction.[20-23] This power must be modified occasionally because the Soflens does not conform exactly to the corneal contour. A fluid lens is formed, which is similar to that occurring behind a hard lens and which modifies the refractive correction. A change to a lens of a different power can be made following an overrefraction while the lens is on the eye.

Lens Evaluation on the Eye

After the lens has been placed on the patient's eye and a waiting period of ten to fifteen minutes allowed for tearing to subside, an evaluation of the lens fit may be made. Factors to be considered in the lens evaluation are position, movement, tightness, comfort, and visual acuity.

Position

It has been shown in several studies that the cornea must be completely covered by a soft lens in order to avoid long-term drying effects. For many patients, the smaller Bausch and Lomb lenses decenter in a superior and temporal direction so that the lower nasal cornea is exposed. After a period of six to twelve months, it may be observed that staining occurs on the exposed area, which eventually coalesces, whereupon it causes symptoms of discomfort.

Figure 18.11 shows the lens coverage in a sampling of seventeen patients who wore lenses from each of eight Soflens series. The only lens that provided complete corneal coverage in all patients was the U4. However, many patients received complete corneal coverage with each of the other lenses. There does not appear to be any justification for using a lens that is larger than necessary in order to provide corneal coverage. In addition to the adverse physiological effects from corneal exposure due to lens decentration, there is an additional effect on visual acuity. Decentrations of 1 to 2 mm. may degrade the quality of vision, even though there is difficulty in measuring its change on a visual acuity chart. The visual acuity decrement is greater for the F lens than for the B lens series. This result has been predicted by Braun on the basis of differences in the spherical aberration that is produced by these lenses.[24] According to Braun, the lenses that should produce the best visual acuity and also be the least affected by lens decentration are those in the U lens series. Other lenses in order of their optical quality defined in terms of minimum spherical aberration are as follows: U, B, F, J, N.

Movement

It is difficult to assess the magnitude of soft lens movement except with the aid of a biomicroscope.[25-26] The movement is most easily seen when a slit beam is directed towards the lens edge and its movement observed under low power. Following the blink, the lens should appear in downward position and move upward towards centration by 0.5 to 1 mm. This movement should be detectable in all lenses having center thicknesses greater than 0.1 mm. Less movement is generally tolerated by lenses in the ultrathin series.

Lens Tightness

The tightness of a lens is generally inversely

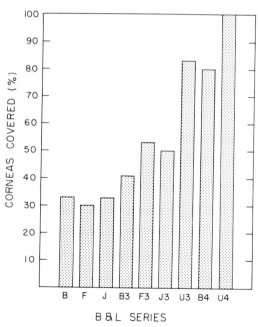

Figure 18.11. Lens coverage in a sampling of seventeen patients who wore lenses from each of eight Soflens series.

related to the lens movement. However, in some cases differences in this relationship are found, and lens tightness should be given greater weight in the lens evaluation. Lens tightness may be judged by one of two signs. Perilimbal vessels should be examined for evidence of blanching in the region just inside the lens edge. In lenses of larger diameters, this blanching may occur farther from the edge and generally is in the region of the limbus. Lens tightness may also be judged by noting a conjunctival drag. Conjunctival drag refers to the movement of the conjunctiva in the direction of the lens movement as it is dragged along by the lid during the blink. It is primarily viewed by noting the movement of the small blood vessels in the conjunctival area just outside the area of the lens.

Comfort

The Soflens is generally very comfortable on most patients, although an extremely loose lens may cause discomfort. Ultrathin lenses present some advantages with respect to comfort, but this is generally significant for only a few patients. Any extreme discomfort will probably indicate that a foreign body is present beneath the lens, and it should be removed, cleaned, and reinserted.

Vision

In addition to the obvious visual decrement that is caused by choosing an incorrect power to correct the refractive error, various fitting factors may lead to poor vision.[27-34] If a lens is fitted so that it is exceptionally steep or flat on a cornea, visual acuity may be reduced. (*See* Chapter 17.) In addition, a lens that decenters on a cornea may cause reduced vision. The most common cause of reduced vision, however, is residual astigmatism.

REFERENCES

1. Alexander-Katz, W.: Experiences of an ophthalmologist in Portugal with hydrophilic contact lenses, *Br. J. Physiol. Opt.*, *25*(1):26–28, 1970.

2. Clements, L. D.: Spin casting Bausch & Lomb Soflens (Polymacon) contact lenses, in Ruben, M. (Ed.): *Soft Contact Lenses*, John Wiley & Sons, 1978.

3. Mertz, G.: A simplified approach to fitting spin-cast hydrogel lenses—Part 1, *Int. Cont. Lens Clin.*, *6*(2):77, 1979.

4. Bartlett, J. D.: A clinical comparison of three high-plus hydrophilic spin-cast contact lens designs, *Int. Cont. Lens Clin.*, *4*(2):28–33, 1977.

5. Baumann, R., and Skolnik, A.: A clinical study in the fitting of the Soflens, *The Oregon Optom.*, *39*(5):8–11, 1972. Part 2, *39*(6):6–11, 1972.

6. Callender, M.: An evaluation of the Bausch and Lomb Soflens "best fit" procedure, *Int. Cont. Lens Clin.*, *3*(3):41–47, 1976.

7. Gasson, A.: Clinical experience with the B&L Soflens, *The Ophthalmic Optician*, *13*(2): 81–84, 1973.

8. Harris, M. G., Sarver, M. D., and Polse, K. A.: Patient responses to 13.6 mm. diameter Bausch and Lomb thin Soflens contact lenses, *Am. J. Optom. Physiol. Opt.*, *54*(10):703, 1977.

9. Hill, J. G.: A clinical comparison of Hydrocurve and Bausch & Lomb thin gel lens systems, *Int. Cont. Lens Clin.*, *4*(6):58–63, 1977.

10. Hodd, N. F. B.: A clinical evaluation of the multi-diameter approach for fitting Bausch and Lomb soft lenses, *Cont. Lens J.*, *6*(4):3, 1977.

11. Janoff, L. E.: Consideration concerning the fitting of the Bausch and Lomb Soflens, *Optom. Weekly*, *64*(33):797–799, 1973.

12. Kolb, E. H.: The Bausch & Lomb Soflens contact lens, *J. Am. Optom. Assoc.*, *47*(3): 301, 1976.

13. Bailey, N. J.: The Soflens: some elementary facts, *Optom. Weekly*, *62*(15):354–356, 1971.

14. Baumann, R., and Skolnik, A.: A clinical study in the fitting of the Soflens—Part 1,

Oregon Optom., *39(5)*:8–11, 1972.

15. Brungardt, T. F.: Flexible lenses: miscellaneous studies and comments, *Optom. Weekly*, *63(27)*:37–38, 1972.

16. Mertz, G. W.: Corneal-thickness response to ultra-thin Bausch & Lomb Soflens (Polymacon) contact lenses, *Am. J. Optom. Physiol. Opt.*, *55(6)*:380–383, 1978.

17. Mertz, G. W., Kissack, B. T., and Walter, H. C.: When and why to use ultra-thin lenses, *Cont. Lens Forum*, *3(7)*:65–72, 1978.

18. Phillips, A. J.: Twelve months with the Bausch & Lomb Ultra-Thin Soflens, *The Ophthalmic Optician*, *19(1)*:10–11, 1979.

19. Gasson, A.: Fitting evaluation of an Ultra-Thin Soflens (Polymacon) contact lens, *The Optician*, supplement, p. 35, Jan. 1976.

20. Coombs, W. F.: Soflens quality assurance, *J. Cont. Lens Soc. Am.*, *5(2)*:17–18, 1971.

21. Farkas, P., and Kassalow, T. W.: Power changes converting aphakics from hard contact lens to the B&L Soflens, *J. Am. Optom. Assoc.*, *46(11)*:1153–1157, 1975.

22. Hutchinson, R. N.: Lacrimal lens effects in Bausch & Lomb Soflens contact lens wear, *J. Am. Optom. Assoc.*, *50(3)*:309, 1979.

23. Mertz, G.: A simplified approach to fitting spin-cast hydrogel lenses—Part 2, *Int. Cont. Lens Clin.*, *6(3)*:39–44, 1979.

24. Elstein, M. V.: Fitting soft lenses: one and a half year's clinical experience, *The Optician*, *163(4224)*:14–15, 1972.

25. Fontana, F. D.: Follow-up routine for the soft lens et rationale, *Optom. Weekly*, *63(26)*:651–652, 1972.

26. Goldberg, J. B.: Current commentary about contact lenses. Reports about soft contact lens fitting, *Optom. Weekly*, *62(41)*:952–954, 1971.

27. Gellman, M., and Hirsch, J.: Comparison of Soflens contact lens (Polymacon) with hard contact lenses and spectacles, *Am. J. Optom. Physiol. Opt.*, *52(2)*:128–133, 1975.

28. Miller, B.: Comparative results in fitting Bausch & Lomb—Soflenses, *Contacto*, *18(1)*:9–12, 1974.

29. Pesner, S.: Corneal astigmatism and the Bausch & Lomb Soflens™ (Polymacon) in aphakia, a case study, *Am. J. Optom. Physiol. Opt.*, *51(1)*:49–50, 1974.

30. Sarver, M. D.: Fitting the Bausch and Lomb Soflens contact lens, *J. Am. Optom. Assoc.*, *44(3)*:258–269, 1973.

31. Wyckoff, P.: Hydrophilic contact lenses, *J. Cont. Lens Soc. Am.*, *6(3)*:12–21, 1972.

32. McMonnies, C. W.: Predicting residual astigmatism with flexible hydrophilic contact lenses, *Austr. J. Optom.*, *55(3)*:106–111, 1972.

33. Sarver, M. D.: Vision with hydrophilic contact lenses, *J. Am. Optom. Assoc.*, *43(3)*:316–320, 1972.

34. Sarver, M. D. et al.: Power of Bausch and Lomb Soflens contact lenses, *Am. J. Optom.*, *50(3)*:195–199, 1973.

Chapter 19

LATHE–CUT LENSES

WHEN HYDROGEL MATERIAL is first formed, it is made without water. As long as it is kept dry, the plastic resembles ordinary polymethyl methacrylate (P.M.M.A.). It can be machined and polished in much the same way as P.M.M.A. with the exception that the usual polishing compounds which are carried in a water base cannot be used. However, this is not a serious drawback, as many of the common polishing compounds can be suspended in an oil base, which provides an adequate substitute. In addition, various organic solvents can be substituted for the usual water-soluble cleaning agents used for P.M.M.A. lenses.

Every aspect of the manufacturing process ·is designed to prevent water from contacting the hydrogel material. In some cases the lens buttons are stored in special containers to withdraw any excessive moisture from the surrounding atmosphere.

When the lens manufacture is complete, the lens is next placed in saline and heated. After a few minutes, the lens undergoes dimensional changes. At first the only evidence of a change is a minor scalloping of the edge, which then appears to coalesce until the entire lens takes on a twisted configuration. After a few more moments, it becomes apparent that an expansion is taking place. Soon the irregularities of the lens disappear, and once again there is a product of perfect geometrical form but larger than the original lens. If the lens is removed from the solution, it is transformed from a hard, inflexible material, to a new, soft and flexible lens.

Unfortunately, the hydration process for a gel lens is not reversible. If the hydrated lens is dried, it will not go back to its original shape, but instead it will shrink and deform into a nondescript entity. At this stage it may appear that the lens has been ruined, but if it is hydrated once again, it will reassume the perfect shape of the hydrated gel lens. Hence, the gel lens only has a regular form in the hard state once—when it is first manufactured—but can always be returned to a regular form in the hydrated stage.

This mode of manufacture makes it possible to produce a wider variey of lathe-cut lens designs than can be created with the spin-casting technique. Any lens that has been formed in the hard lens design can be duplicated in a lathe-cut gel lens.

The expansion properties of the gel lens are interesting to consider and present somewhat of a problem for the manufacturer. During the hydration process, every dimension of the lens changes and also the index of refraction and the refractive power. It is therefore necessary for the manufacturer to machine a lens that is considerably different from the final product. The base curve has a shorter radius, the diameter is smaller, and the power is greater than the final lens. The manufacturer must apply correction factors that will allow him to predict the final dimensions after hydration. This is not always an easy task and leads to some manufacturing difficulties.

Some of the early lathe-cut gel lenses were made to duplicate the specifications of a hard corneal lens, but it was soon found that this lens could not be tolerated on the eye.

LENS SPECIFICATIONS

There are many different lathe-cut designs produced by the various manufacturers, but most can be classified according to the following categories (all specifications are given in the fully hydrated state):

THICKNESS

Regular lenses in minus powers usually have center thicknesses between 0.10 and 0.25 mm. Ultrathin lenses have thicknesses between 0.03 and 0.09 mm. For plus lenses, the thickness usually ranges from 0.25 to 0.70 mm. (Table 19.1).

DIAMETER

Large diameter lathe-cut lenses usually range between 14.0 and 16.0 mm. Small diameter lenses are from 12.0 to 13.5 mm. The lenses are usually manufactured in 0.5 mm. steps, and intermediate diameters have not been found necessary for fitting.

Other parameters that must be considered in the design of lathe-cut gel lenses are the following.

BASE CURVE

The base curve of a lathe-cut gel lens is considered to be the central curve on the posterior surface, just as for a hard lens. The base curves that are usually available range from 7.5 mm. to 9.5 mm. in 0.1, 0.2, or 0.3 mm. steps, depending upon the manufacturer.

PERIPHERAL CURVE

The peripheral curve is usually from 0.5 mm. to 0.9 mm. wide and has a radius of 11.0 mm. to 13.0 mm. (Figure 19.1).

DESIGN CONSIDERATION

A corneal lens, which is 9 mm. in diameter and has an 11 mm. radius peripheral curve of 0.5 width, will have an edge thickness of 0.14 mm. (power −3.00 D., base curve 8.00, and center thickness of 0.14). If it is desired to have the same lens power and base curve in a gel lens, using the same peripheral curve, the edge thickness will be 0.36 mm. This great increase in edge thickness for a gel lens is a consequence of the large diameter (Figure 19.2) and the minus

TABLE 19.1
PLUS LENS THICKNESS

Lens Power	Thickness
+ 2.00	0.20
+ 5.00	0.25
+ 8.00	0.29
+12.00	0.35
+16.00	0.41

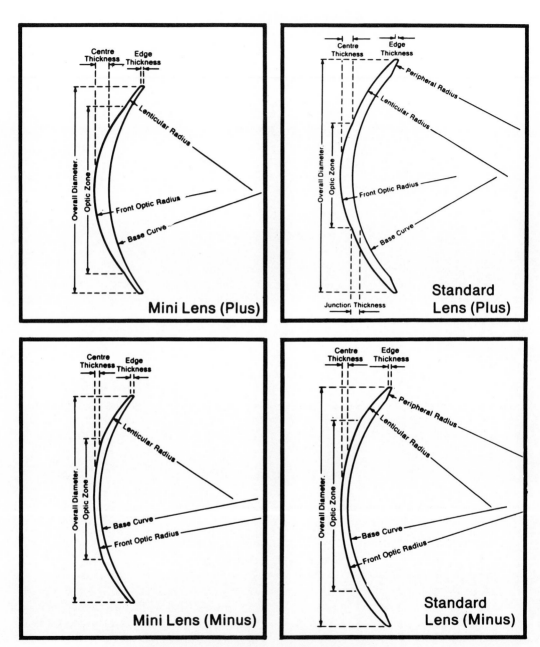

Figure 19.1. Parameters of a lathe-cut contact lens.

power. To alleviate this problem, it has been found necessary to use a second curve on the front surface to produce a myodisc design for most lenses of minus power. In a few lenses of very low minus power, it may suffice to use a wide front bevel. In very high power minus lenses, it has sometimes been found necessary to use several front curves to accomplish the same result. Plus power lenses also present a similar problem and would have very great center thicknesses unless they are constructed in lenticular form (Figure 19.3).

LENSES AVAILABLE

Lathe-cut gel lenses are available from various manufacturers on a worldwide basis[1] but are limited in the United States by F.D.A. requirements. There are differences between the lenses of different manufacturers, which are usually dependent upon the water content and chemical makeup of their material.

FITTING PROCEDURE

The general outline of the fitting procedure for a lathe-cut gel lens is as follows:

1. Refract, measure corneal radii, perform a biomicroscope examination.
2. From this information, select appropriate lens from the trial set.
3. Place the lens on the patient's eye.
4. Check lens size, centering, and movement for a gross misfit. Change lens if necessary.
5. Allow ten to twenty minutes for initial lens adaptation.
6. Recheck lens centering, size, movement, and acuity. Overrefract.
7. Select another trial lens if necessary and repeat steps 4, 5, and 6.
8. Order patient's lenses.

TRIAL LENS PROCEDURE

Lathe-cut gel lenses are fitted from a trial set of ten or more lenses with specifications according to Table 19.2. The trial lens procedure usually follows one of two approaches:

Keratometer Method

The patient's keratometer reading provides

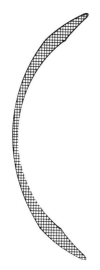

Figure 19.2. Because of the large diameter of a gel contact lens, it is necessary to have a front bevel, even on lenses of low minus power.

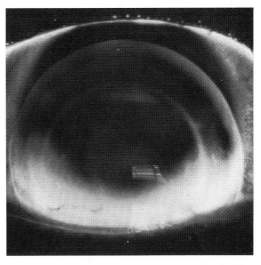

Figure 19.3. Plus power gel contact lenses are always made in lenticular form (fluorexon pattern).

TABLE 19.2
SAMPLE TRIAL SET

Base Curve	Diameter	Power
8.3	13.0	−3.00
8.5	13.0	−3.00
8.3	14.0	−3.00
8.5	14.0	−3.00
8.7	14.0	−3.00
8.9	14.0	−3.00
9.1	14.0	−3.00
9.0	15.0	−3.00
9.3	15.0	−3.00
9.6	15.0	−3.00

a starting point for the trial lens testing.[2] In general, smaller eyes will require both shorter base curve radii and smaller diameters, whereas larger eyes may be fitted with larger lenses and flatter base curves.

Standard Lens Method

Many fitters recommend the use of a standard lens as a starting point in the trial lens procedure.[4] Additional lenses will be tried according to the fitting characteristics of the first trial lens.

EVALUATION OF TRIAL LENS FIT

The evaluation of the fitting characteristics of the lathe-cut lens is somewhat different from that for a hard lens because fluorescein cannot be used in an evaluation of the base curve–cornea relationship. The lens is evaluated primarily by its positioning and movement on the eye.

A well-fitted lathe-cut lens of regular thickness will center well on the cornea, with possibly a small lag of no more than 1 mm. in the downward direction. The large diame-

ter lenses will extend about 2 mm. past the limbus (Figure 19.4). Immediately following the blink, the lens can be seen with the biomicroscope to lag about 1 mm. If the patient moves the eye laterally to the right or left, it will be seen that the lens will lag slightly for a fraction of a second and then recenter on the eye (Figure 19.5). When the patient looks up, the lens will lag down 1 to 2 mm. (Figure 19.6).

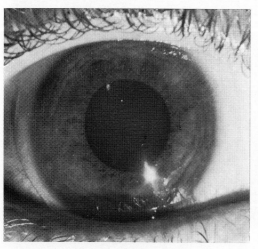

Figure 19.4. A large diameter lathe-cut lens will extend about 2 mm. beyond the limbus.

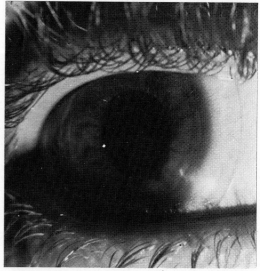

Figure 19.5. With lateral eye movement, the lens will lag slightly.

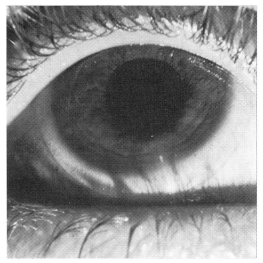

Figure 19.6. When the patient looks up, the lens will lag down 1 to 2 mm.

The fit of the lens may also be too tight or too loose, which is analogous to the same fitting relationship with a corneal lens.

Tight Lens

A tight lens does not appear to have any movement on the cornea following a blink or after eye movements in any direction. It is not uncomfortable to the wearer for short wearing periods. The following tests are diagnostic of a tight lens:

Unstable Vision

With the best subjective overrefraction in place, it is found that vision is slightly blurred. If the patient is asked to blink and observe the visual acuity chart carefully, he will note that immediately following the blink there will be a temporary clearing of vision. This lasts only a fraction of a second, and the patient must observe closely to see it. The vision then returns to its original state, which may be two to three lines poorer on the Snellen chart.

Retinoscopy

The retinoscopic reflex shows a dark, shad-

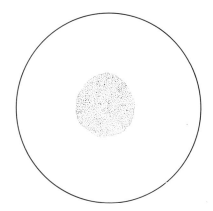

Figure 19.7. Retinoscopic reflex for a steep gel contact lens.

owy area in the central portion of the pupillary area, which has an appearance similar to the dark shadow seen in keratoconus (Figure 19.7). Immediately after a blink, there is sometimes a momentary disappearance of the dark shadow, but it returns again in about a second.

Keratometry

Keratometry is performed with the lens *in situ*, and hence, the measurement is being taken from the front surface of the gel lens. The appearance of the image of the mire seen in the keratometer is usually distorted and appears as irregular or oblique astigmatism (Figure 19.8). The distortion may be reduced immediately following the blink.

The keratometer test is not as reliable as the other tests.

Explanation of the Tight Lens Results

The observations that result from a tight gel lens fit may be attributed to the gel lens being now steeper than the central corneal area and showing apical clearance. The gel lens has assumed a more or less aspherical curve that conforms to the cornea in the peripheral area but deviates from the central cornea to form an aspherical curve in that region (Figure 19.9). This variation in curvature is responsible for the lower visual acuity

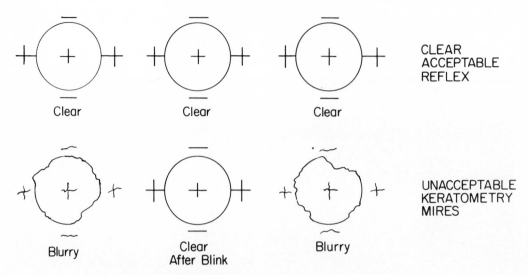

Figure 19.8. Keratometer mire distortion seen in a steep gel contact lens.

with this lens and also the shadow of the retinoscopic reflex and the distorted keratometer image. During the blink, the lid smooths down the lens across the cornea, and there is a temporary adherence of the lens to the central region of the cornea. Following the blink, the lens stays in this position momentarily, but it soon reverts to its previous aspherical curve. During the brief period in which the lens is conforming to the cornea, the subjective visual acuity improves, the spot in the retinoscope reflex disappears, and the keratometer image becomes regular.

These changes in the lens may be demonstrated with the use of fluorexon, which is a modification of fluorescein with high molecular weight. This dye cannot be used clinically because it penetrates some gel lenses after a

few minutes. However, during the first minutes after the dye is introduced, a clear fluorexon pattern is evident (Figure 19.10).

Loose Lens

A loose lens has an excessively flat fit relative to the cornea, analogous to the situation that occurs with a hard corneal lens. With the eyes in the straight-ahead position, the lens will lag downward on the eye from 2 to 4 mm. (Figure 19.11a). In the case of extremely loose lenses, the lens will slide off

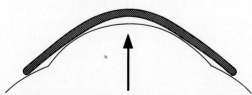

Figure 19.9. A steep gel contact lens tends to form an aspherical curve in the central area. Following the blink, this curve momentarily disappears and then returns.

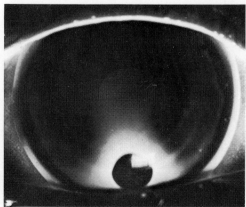

Figure 19.10. A fluorexon pattern for a steep gel contact lens.

the cornea entirely.

When the eyes are moved laterally to the right or left, there is a lag of the lens of 2 to 4 mm. (Figure 19.11b). In extreme cases, the lens may slide off the cornea entirely (Figure 19.11c). After the eyes have moved, the lens will usually slowly recenter itself, which may take three or four seconds. With upward gaze, the lens moves down several millimeters and may slide off the cornea.

A loose lens is also revealed by the following:

Unstable vision

With the best subjective overrefraction in place, as long as the lens centers reasonably well, vision is good in the straight-ahead position. However, immediately following the blink, vision will decrease one to three lines on the visual acuity chart. In a fraction of a second, or in a maximum of one to two seconds, the vision will return to normal.

Retinoscopy

The retinoscopic reflex shows a dark, shadowy area in the inferior portion of the pupil (Figure 19.12). Immediately following the blink, this shadowy area is made worse but in a brief period, returns to its original state.

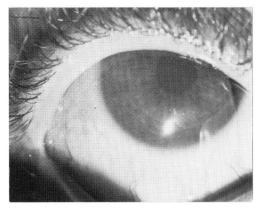

Figure 19.11a. Loose gel lens.

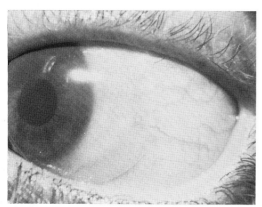

Figure 19.11b. During lateral eye movement, a loose lens lags 2 to 4 mm.

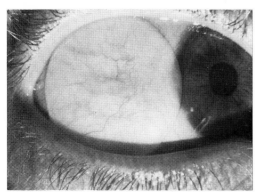

Figure 19.11c. With lateral gaze, a loose gel lens may slide off the cornea.

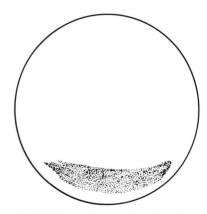

Figure 19.12. The retinoscopic reflex for a loose gel lens shows a dark, shadowy area in the inferior portion of the pupil.

Keratometry

The keratometer image may show slight distortion that is increased momentarily after the blink.

Explanation of Loose Lens Results

These results all occur because the lens is loose on the eye and lags to a low position. The inferior portion of the lens is resting on the inferior sclera and is pushed outward. This creates a distortion effect in the lower region of the lens and an aspherical curvature on its anterior surface (Figure 19.13). During the blink, the lens is pushed further downward. Immediately following the blink, for a brief period the lens remains in an exceptionally low position, and the distortion induced in the lower portion of the gel lens is accentuated. Hence, the vision is lowered momentarily and the distortion effect is seen by retinoscopy and keratometry. In only a fraction of a second or in a maximum of one to two seconds, the lens rises to recenter itself, and the distortion effect and its accom-

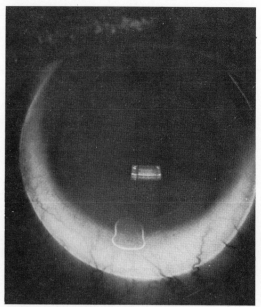

Figure 19.14. Fluorexon pattern of a loose gel lens.

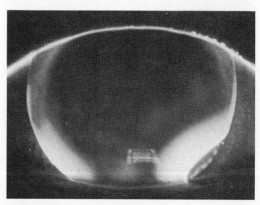

Figure 19.15. A very flat gel contact lens shows air space at edge (Fluorexon pattern).

panying symptoms and signs are reduced or eliminated.

The fitting relationship of a loose lens can also be demonstrated with the use of fluorexon (Figure 19.14).

In an extremely flat fit the edge of the lens may actually stand off the sclera and produce an air space (Figure 19.15).

Criteria for Optimum Fit

The criteria for the optimum fit

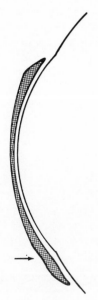

Figure 19.13. A loose gel lens moves onto the inferior sclera and creates a distortion (arrow) which is transferred throughout the lens curvature.

are usually based on visual and physiological considerations. A lens is selected that will give the most stable and best vision and which will be as loose as possible.

A lens that appears to fit well during the trial lens procedure may prove to be somewhat tight at a later period. A lens that has flatter base curve or smaller diameter should be tried. If this lens also appears to fit well, another lens should be tried that is even flatter or smaller.

A judgment should first be made as to whether the lens is the proper diameter. If the diameter is correct, then changes should be made by modifying the base curve. If the lens appears to fit well on the eye, but the diameter is either too small or too large (usually too large), it is possible to change the lens for another of different dimensions without changing the lens fit. This is achieved by changing the diameter and base curve in opposite directions to produce opposite effects on the fit. For example, the diameter can be made smaller, and at the same time, the base curve made steeper. Conversely, the diameter can be made larger, and at the same time the base curve is made flatter. A rule may be used to accomplish this whereby for each

TABLE 19.3

LENSES FALLING ON EACH LINE GIVE BASE CURVES
TO COMPENSATE DIAMETER CHANGE WITH
MINIMUM EFFECT ON FIT

Base	Diameter				
	13	13.5	14	14.5	15
7.8	X	X	X	X	
8.1	X	X	X	X	X
8.4	X	X	X	X	X
8.7	X	X	X	X	X
9.1		X	X	X	X

increase in diameter by 0.5 mm., the base curve is steepened by 0.3 mm. (Table 19.3).

If the lens is tight, a judgment should be made first as to whether the lens is the proper diameter. If the diameter can be reduced, this should be done first. A change is next made to a flatter base curve. Successive changes in diameter and base curve are made until a lens is found that is definitely loose on the eye. A lens that is 0.3 mm. steeper and/or 0.5 mm. larger in diameter will then be the lens to be selected for the patient. A lens that is too small may be uncomfortable for the patient.

ORDERING LENSES

Lenses are ordered by three dimensions only: base curve, diameter, and power. There is usually a limited range of thicknesses available for a given lens due to its complexity.

LIMITATION OF TRIAL LENSES

The standard trial lenses are made in powers of about −3.00 D. The results of testing with this set are not valid for medium plus, high plus, or high minus lenses. The standard set is usable for minus lenses up to about −8.00 D. Lenses outside this range differ significantly in form and thickness to affect their fitting relationship on the eye. Patients with high refractive errors should be tested with trial sets within this high power range.

REFERENCES

1. Larke, J. R., and Sabell, A. G.: Some basic design concepts of hydrophilic gel contact lenses, *Br. J. Physiol. Opt.*, *26(1)*:49–60, 1971.
2. Gasset, A. R., and Uotila, M. H.: Fitting Softcon hydrophilic lenses in normal and diseased eyes. To be published.
3. Aquavella, J. V., Jackson, G. K., and Guy, L.

F.: Bionite hydrophilic contact lenses used as cosmetic devices, *Am. J. Ophthalmol.*, *72(3)*:527–531, 1971.
4. Aquavella, J. V.: Interview: cosmetic fitting of the Griffin Naturalens, *J. Am. Optom. Assoc.*, *43(12)*:1232–1237, 1972.

ADDITIONAL READINGS

ACLP soft lens symposium, *The Ophthalmic Optician*, *12(20)*:1045–1046, 1972.

Agarwal, R. K.: Some thoughts on soft lenses, *Contact Lens*, *14(1)*:28, 1972.

Alexander-Katz, W.: The importance of blinking during the fitting of soft corneal contact lenses, *Contact Lens*, *2(8)*:4–5, 1970.

Aquavella, J. V., Jackson, G. K., and Guy, L. F.: Therapeutic effects of Bionite lenses: mechanisms of action, *Ann. Ophthalmol.*, *3(12)*:1341–1345, 1971.

Aquavella, J. B.: Cosmetic fitting of the Griffin Naturalens, in Gasset, A. R., and Kaufman, H. E. (Eds.): *Soft Contact Lens*, St. Louis, C. V. Mosby, 1972, p. 99.

Bailey, N.: Lasertrace: a soft lens identification system (interview), *Cont. Lens Forum*, *3(7)*:77, 1978.

Bailey, W. R., and Feldman, G. L.: Hydrocurve lens, *Cont. Lens J.*, *8(2)*:17–20, 1974.

Balyeat, H. D.: Hydralens: a new lathe-cut gel lens, *Cont. Intraoc. Lens Med. J.*, *2(1)*:25–26, 1976.

Barbara, G.: Notre expérience en lentilles souples hydrophiles, *L'Optician Lunetier*, *229*:4–8, 1972.

Barbara, G.: Notre expérience en lentilles souples hydrophiles, *L'Optician Lunetier*, *234*:13–17, 1972.

Baronet, P.: Les lentilles flexibles, *Ophthalmologiste Française*, *14*:29–41, 1972.

Baronet, P.: L'adaptation clinique simplifiée des microlentilles flexibles, au service de l'ophalmologiste, *Contact Lens*, *3(7)*:33–38, 1972.

Bayshore, C.: Clinical report on Sof-Form contact lenses, *Cont. Lens Forum*, *4(11)*:31–36, 1979.

Beller, J. J.: The gel lens, *Contact Lens*, *3(4)*:16–18, 1971.

Bernstein, H. N., and Lemp, M. A.: An unusual keratoconjunctivitis occurring after long time wearing of the AO Softcon (formerly Griffing or Bionite) hydrophilic contact lens, *Ann. Ophthalmol.*, *7(1)*:97–106, 1975.

Brucker, D.: The new Hydrocurve contact lens, *Int. Cont. Lens Clin.*, *1(3)*:33–42, 1974.

Brucker, D.: The Hydrocurve lens, *Cont. Intraoc. Lens Med. J.*, *1(3)*:13, 1975.

Brucker, D., and Malin, A. H.: Fitting soft corneoscleral lenses, *J. Am. Optom. Assoc.*, *43(3)*:287–290, 1972.

Brucker, D., and Marano, J. A.: Hydrocurve, *J. Am. Optom. Assoc.*, *47(3)*:306, 1976.

Brucker, D. et al.: An interview with representatives of major manufacturers, *Int. Cont. Lens Clin.*, *1(1)*:41–52, 1974.

Cosenza, D. J., and Blake, R. F.: Utilization of the Hydrocurve soft lens for increasing success in soft lens fitting, *J. Am. Optom. Assoc.*, *49(3)*:293–295, 1978.

Cotte, F.: Bionite-Softcon lenses: handling, cleaning, dimensional stability, visual acuity, *Contacto*, *18(3)*:17–21, 1974.

Davies, M. S., Ruben, M., and Trodd, C.: Experiences with soft lenses, *Contact Lens*, *3(7)*:42–44, 1972.

De Carle, J.: Developing hydrophilic lenses for continuous wearing, *Contacto*, *16(1)*:39–42, 1972.

The development and manufacture of a soft lens, *The Ophthalmic Optician*, *13(11)*:601–602, 1973.

Dickinson, F.: A new American soft contact lens, *The Optician*, *168(4342)*:9–11, 1974.

Dorman-Brailsford, M. I.: The importance of sag heights when fitting Bionite lenses, *The Ophthalmic Optician*, *12(20)*:1047–1048, 1972.

Dupont, G. Z., and Remba, M. J.: Fitting evaluation tests for Tresoft and other lathe-cut semiscleral soft lenses, *Int. Cont. Lens Clin.*, *6(6)*:263, 1979.

Espy, J. W.: Lathe-cut hydrophilic contact lenses:

report of 100 clinical cases, *Ann. Ophthalmol.*, *10(10)*:1337, 1978.

Fanti, P.: Patient response to thin lathe-cut HEMA lenses—fitting results with Hydroflex SD lenses, *The Optician*, July 6, 1979, pp. 23–27.

Friedberg, M. A.: The Griffin Naturalens®: a preliminary report, *J. Am. Optom. Assoc.*, *43(3)*: 334–337, 1972.

Gasson, A.: Hydroflex/SD thin soft lenses, *The Ophthalmic Optician*, *18(22)*:823, 1978.

Greenspoon, M. K.: Aquaflex: the new alternative in soft lens fitting, *Cont. Lens Forum*, *2(11)*:25, 1977.

Grosvenor, T.: Lathe-cut soft contact lens fitting— Part 1: materials and manufacturing process, *Optom. Weekly*, *68(26)*:800, 1977.

Grosvenor, T.: Lathe-cut soft contact lens fitting— Part 2: comparison with conventional "hard" lenses, *Optom. Weekly*, *68(27)*:833, 1977.

Grosvenor, T.: Lathe-cut soft contact lens fitting— Part 6: diagnostic lens procedures, *Optom. Weekly*, *68(31)*:951, 1977.

Grosvenor, T.: Lathe-cut soft contact lens fitting— Part 7: lens ordering, verification and delivery, *Optom. Weekly*, *68(32)*:977, 1977.

Grosvenor, T.: Lathe-cut soft contact lens fitting— Part 9: corneal and refractive changes due to soft lenses, *Optom. Weekly*, *68(34)*:1038, 1977.

Grosvenor, T., and Callender, M.: The N & N soft contact lens, *Am. J. Optom. Arch. Am. Acad. Optom.*, *50(6)*:489–498, 1973.

Gruber, E.: Clinical experience with the hydrophilic contact lens, *Am. J. Ophthalmol.*, *70(5)*:833–842, 1970.

Gruber, E., and Gordon, S.: Low-cost way to fit the Aquaflex lens, *Cont. Lens Forum*, *2(2)*:19–23, 1977.

Gruber, E.: Clinical experiences with the Aquaflex aphakic hydrophilic lens, *Cont. Intraoc. Lens Med. J.*, *6(1)*:22–24, 1980.

Highlights of "An Ophthalmologists' Symposium on the Soft Lens," *Br. J. Ophthalmol.*, *56(12)*:

920–923, 1972.

Hodd, N.G.B.: How to fit Duragel 75 lenses, *The Optician*, March 2, 1979, p. 16.

Janoff, L.: The Softcon lens: its clinical application, *Int. Cont. Lens Clin.*, *6(4)*:18, 1979.

Janoff, L. E.: Fitting the AOSoft lens, *Cont. Lens Forum*, *3(12)*:27, 1978.

Josephson, J. E.: Techniques for determining lens fit acceptability prior to dispensing hydrophilic semi-scleral lathed lenses, *Int. Cont. Lens Clin.*, *4(4)*:52, 1977.

Josephson, J. E.: A report on the refitting of successful Griffin Naturalens wearers with B&L Soflens contact lenses (Polymacon): *Am. J. Optom. Arch. Am. Acad. Optom.*, *50(5)*:416–422, 1973.

Jurkus, J. M.: Problems and opportunities with Durasoft lenses, *Cont. Lens Forum*, *2(11)*:47, 1977.

Kearney, P. F., Jr.: Fitting Hydrocurve lenses without a trial set, *Cont. Lens Forum*, *3(5)*:55, 1978.

Kerr, C.: An appraisal of the Wohlk Hydroflex lens in aphakia, *The Optician*, *174(4500)*:21, 1977.

Kolom, B. M., and Remba, M. J.: Some problems, some solutions, with Tresoft lenses, *Cont. Lens Forum*, *3(5)*:46, 1978.

Lee, A. N., and Sarver, D. S.: The gel lens-transferred corneal toricity as a function of lens thickness, *Am. J. Optom.*, *49(1)*:35–40, 1972.

Malin, A. H.: Fitting small, thin, Hydrocurve lenses, *Cont. Lens Forum*, *4(4)*:27, 1979.

Mandell, R. B.: Lathe-cut hydrogel lenses, *Int. Cont. Lens Clin*, *1(1)*:53–62, 1974.

Passmore, C.: Clinical application of the Aquaflex flexible contact lens, *Can. J. Optom.*, *38(1)*:26–28, 1976.

"Sauflon," *Contact Lens*, *3(3)*:17–22, 1971.

Soft contact lenses, *Br. Med. J.*, *3(5821)*:254, 1972.

Taylor, C. M.: Some suggested fitting techniques for hydrophilic lenses, *The Optician*, *163(4211)*: 10–12, 1972.

Thomas, P. F.: The influence of environment on Bionite Naturalenses, *Austr. J. Optom.*, *55(9)*: 354–357, 1972.

Chapter 20

INSPECTION AND VERIFICATION

It is possible to measure most of the parameters of a gel contact lens.[1] Some of the techniques are somewhat cumbersome, and hence, they may be neglected. However, many unexplained clinical differences in the performance of lenses can be understood if the lens specifications are verified.[2-5] Unfortunately, one of the most difficult dimensions to measure is the width of the front bevel. This parameter can have considerable influence on the movement and centering characteristics of the lens. The lathe-cut gel lens is easier to measure than the spin-cast lens, and more parameters of the lens can be measured.

Several methods are usually available for measuring each of the parameters. The author's preferred method will be presented first, along with alternate methods when they are feasible.

DIAMETER

The diameter of a hydrogel contact lens may be measured using the same measuring magnifier as used with hard contact lenses (Figure 20.1). Care must be taken to place the lens onto the graticule in such a manner that it is not distorted. The lens must be relatively free of any surface water, as this will run onto the graticule and make the edge position difficult to locate. A lens that is allowed to dry too much will tend to shrink and give an error in diameter reading.

An alternate measurement method for lens diameter is with the aid of a wet cell described later for power measurement (Figure 20.2). Some cells have a millimeter scale printed on one side so that a diameter measurement

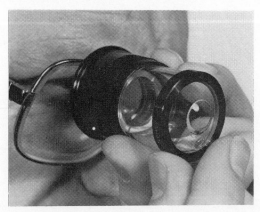

Figure 20.1. Measurement of the diameter of a gel lens with a measuring magnifier.

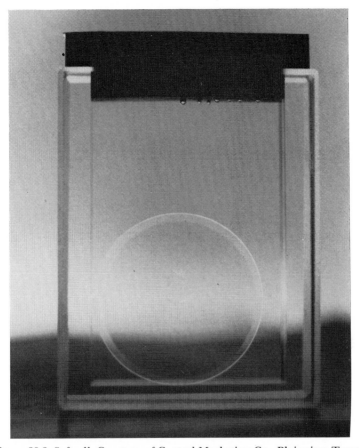

Figure 20.2. Softcell. Courtesy of Central Marketing Co., Plainview, Texas.

can be made at the same time as the power measurement. A diameter measurement can also be made with some of the instruments designed to measure the base curve.

Lens diameter may be measured with a projection comparator,[6] although the other methods are generally more efficient because a second parameter can also be measured using the same device.

POSTERIOR CURVE

There are several methods available to measure the posterior curve of soft contact lenses. Since this curve has such importance in the fitting characteristics of the lens, its measurement is highly desirable.

The Soft Lens Analyzer® (made by Hydro-Vue, Inc.) is a system for comparing the base curve of the lens to a series of spherical templates (Figure 20.3).[7] The templates are im-mersed in a water cell and projected onto a screen for magnified viewing. The space between the lens and the reticule is visible as a light area contrasted against the darker shadows produced by the lens and the reference spheres. The shape of the bright area will then indicate whether the lens is steeper, is flatter, or matches the reference sphere. If the lens is flatter than the test sphere, the

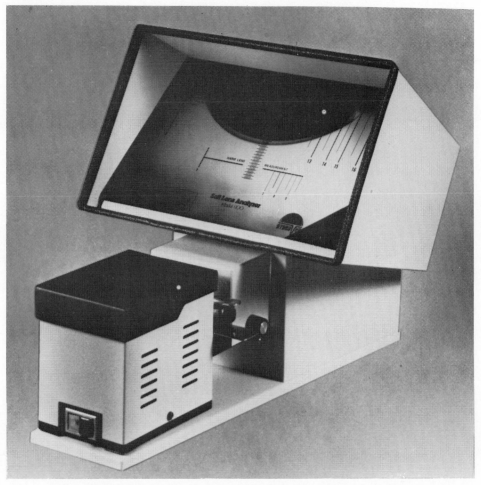

Figure 20.3. Viewer for measuring soft lens base curve (Soft Lens Analyzer).

image will show light passing between the peripheral portion of the lens and the test sphere. If the lens is steeper than the test sphere, light will be passed in the area beneath the center of the lens. On this basis, the spheres are tested in a systematic manner until a match is completed. The base curve of the lens is then assumed to equal the radius of the matching sphere.

A second standard test holder is available to determine the front curve of a Bausch and Lomb Soflens. This is designed to allow the practitioner to determine to which series the lens belongs. Unfortunately, the accuracy of

the technique for this lens is not comparable to its performance with lathe-cut lenses.

The accuracy of the Soft Lens Analyzer is very good, and with some practice, measurements can be made to within 0.15 mm. It is much easier to measure thicker lenses, which have some body and hold their shape easily. Ultrathin lenses are sometimes difficult or impossible to measure. It is also more difficult to measure high plus lenses in lenticular form.

Other methods of measuring the base curve radius include the keratometer,[8,9] radiuscope,[10] spherometer,[11] and various comparators.[12]

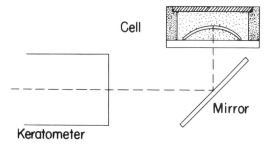

Cell

Mirror

Keratometer

Figure 20.4. Auxiliary keratometer device for measurement of soft lens base curve.

In order to use a keratometer to measure the base curve, it is necessary to have one of the models that is equipped with a high intensity illumination system. The lens must be immersed in a saline solution in a holder for this purpose. The arrangement of the apparatus is similar to that used for measuring hard contact lenses. An auxiliary device must be attached to the keratometer, which consists of a mirror and lens holder (Figure 20.4). The lens holder consists of a liquid-filled cell in which the lens is placed concave side downward to receive the light from the keratometer. It is necessary to multiply the reading by a correction factor in order to arrive at the actual curvature.

A radiuscope can be used to measure the base curve of a soft lens if a proper lens holder is used. The lens must be immersed in saline and held at the correct position beneath the objective lens. Like the kerato-meter, the radiuscope must have high illumination in order to see the reflection from the surface of the lens. Some confusion may result from reflections occurring from both the front and back surfaces. The readings are taken in the usual manner and then multiplied by the refractive index of the medium to obtain the true radius.

Various spherometers are available that consist of a ring which supports the lens and a central moveable post. The lens rests on the ring, and the central post is advanced until contact is made (Figure 20.5). The lens base curve radius may then be calculated using the usual laws for spherometers. Various spherometers have been constructed based on mechanical, electronic, ultrasound, or optical evaluation of the post position.[13] The main drawback of these devices is that when the lens is placed on the support ring, it tends to distort and does not give a true reading.

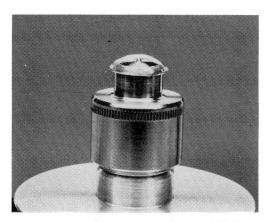

Figure 20.5. Spherometer gauge used to measure the saggital depth of a hydrogel lens.

Projection devices in the form of comparators simply project the magnified image of the lens onto a screen where the base curve may then be compared to a series of reference curves until a match is made. This technique can be very accurate but tends to be time-consuming and, hence, is only rarely used.

The base curve of the lens may also be measured by a system known as optical gauging. A series of spherical templates having graduated curvatures is used for this purpose (Figure 20.6). The radii of the templates usually range between 6.90 and 9.20 mm. The lens is measured while hydrated and without blotting the surface. The lens is simply placed on a template with the radius that is thought to match the base curve. If a perfect match occurs between the base curve and the template, the spacing between the base curve and template is uniform, and no air bubbles will be found under the lens. If the base curve is steeper than the template, the lens will tend to stand off at its center, and a bubble will occur at the middle of the lens. The lens should then be removed and shifted to a template of shorter radius. If the lens is flatter than the template on which it is placed, a space will occur between the edge of the lens and the template and a bubble will be found near the edge. The lens should then be shifted to a template of flatter radius of curvature. The measurement is obtained by systematically shifting the lens back and forth on the templates until an exact match is obtained. If it is not possible to obtain an exact match between the base curve and the template, some interpolation may be necessary.

THICKNESS

Thickness of the lens can be measured using a technique based on the toolmaker's application of the measuring microscope.[14,15] The lens is blotted dry and placed on a flat platform on a radiuscope (*see* Chapter 33). The radiuscope is focused on the upper (back) surface of the lens. The lens is then removed, and the radiuscope focused on the platform surface. The distance between the lens surface and platform is equal to the thickness of the lens.

Gel contact lens thickness may also be measured very accurately using a modification of an ordinary thickness gauge principle. For a soft lens, the gauge is modified so that the contacts consist of plastic hemispheres in which have been embedded wires exposed to the surface (Figure 20.7). When the two contacts are pressed together, the wires complete an electronic circuit, and a light is flashed. One contact is moveable and attached to a gauge. The lens is placed on the stationary contact, and the moveable ball is advanced until touch is indicated by the light. At this point, the lens thickness may be read directly from the dial gauge.

REFRACTIVE POWER

The power of a gel lens can be measured with a lensometer.[16-18] The lens is removed from the bottle and blotted dry carefully (Figure 20.8). Some practice may be necessary to achieve this. The lens should be placed on a lint-free tissue, and the tissue folded over so that both surfaces are blotted (Figure 20.9). The lens is then moved to a dry position on the tissue and blotted gently again. Only handle the lenses with forceps, since touching the lens with the fingers will smudge the surface and make a reading impossible. After the lens has been blotted dry, it should be lifted carefully with forceps and held in

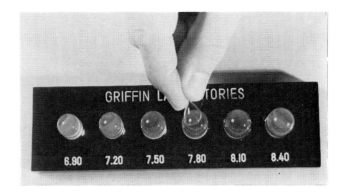

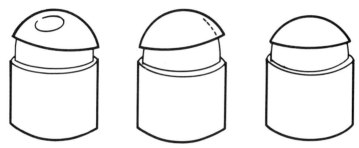

Figure 20.6. Spherical template used for measuring base curve of lathe-cut gel lenses.

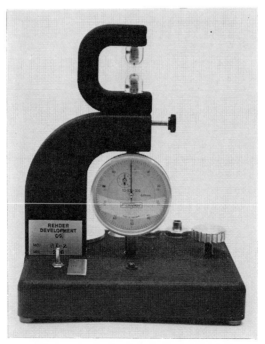

Figure 20.7. Thickness gauge with electrical contacts imbedded in the convex platform and plunger. Courtesy of Rehder Development Co.

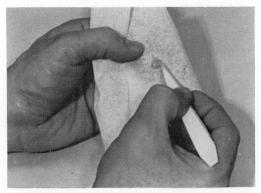

Figure 20.8. Measurement of refractive power of a gel lens. Blotting the lens dry.

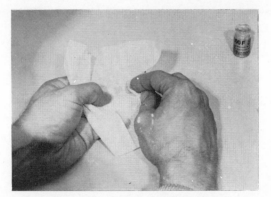

Figure 20.9. Blotting the lens dry.

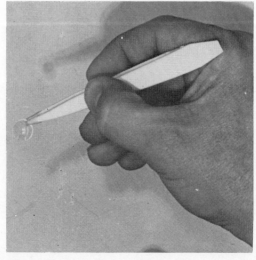

Figure 20.10. Air drying the lens for ten seconds.

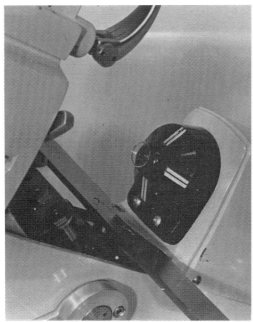

Figure 20.11. Gel lens on lensometer stop.

the air for about ten seconds (Figure 20.10). This allows any additional surface water to dry. The lens is then placed against the stop of a lensometer. It is usually necessary to place the lens with the convex side towards the lensometer stop so that a measurement is made of front vertex power (Figure 20.11). If the lens is dried the proper amount of time, it will remain supported on the lensometer by the small amount of moisture remaining on the surface. If the lens is held too long to dry in the air, it will not stick to the lensometer stop.

A power reading can now be taken in the usual way. If the target image appears blurred in the lensometer, it probably indicates that this procedure was not carried out properly, and the lens should be immersed again in saline and the procedure done over. If the target is blurred on repeated measurement, it indicates that the optical quality of the lens is bad.

There is an insignificant power change over a period of about four minutes after the gel lens is removed from the bottle; however, it should not take more than thirty seconds to take a measurement of the lens.[18]

There has been some question as to whether or not the power reading obtained in this manner is a true measurement of the lens power. Figure 20.12 is an illustration of the lens power measured as a function of time. There is no power change occurring over the first four minutes that the lens is measured, after which it tends to increase in power.[18] The stability of the curve for this period would indicate that it is unlikely that a significant change has taken place within the time that the lens is removed from the bottle and the measurements begun.

The second method of determining hydrogel lens power is with a water cell.[19-21] The lens is placed in a small chamber with parallel glass surfaces, which is filled with saline (Figure 20.13), and the lens system is measured in the lensometer. The dioptric value that is measured is multiplied by a correction factor or multiplier to compensate for the lens's being in saline rather than air. Unfor-

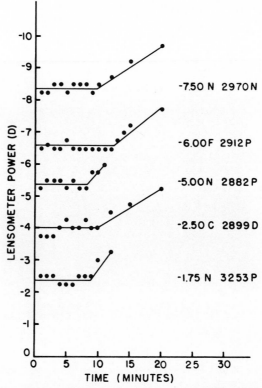

Figure 20.12. Lens power measured as a function of time. From M. D. Sarver et al., Power of Bausch and Lomb Soflens Contact Lenses, *American Journal of Optometry*, *50*(3):195–199, 1973.

tunately, this method of measurement has never gained widespread use due to the error in the correction factor that is commonly advocated for the lens system. The error occurs

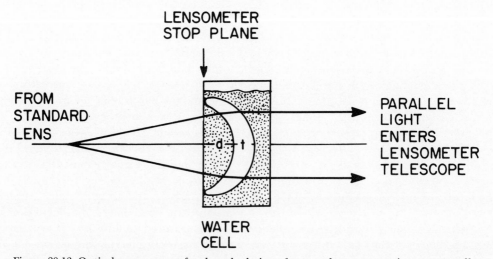

Figure 20.13. Optical arrangement for the calculation of contact lens power using a water cell.

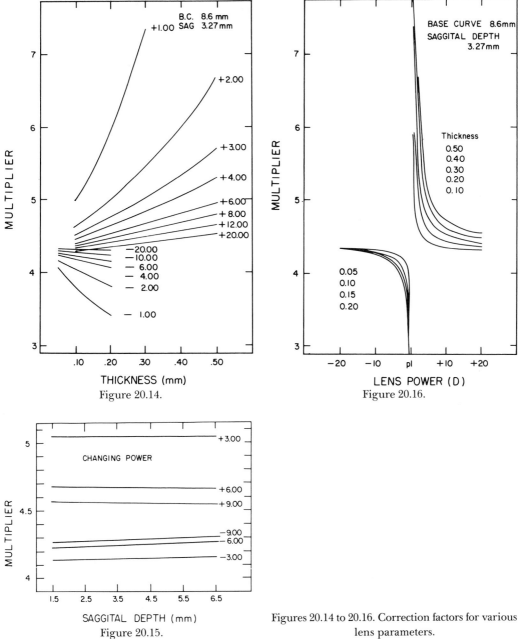

THICKNESS (mm)

Figure 20.14.

SAGGITAL DEPTH (mm)

Figure 20.15.

LENS POWER (D)

Figure 20.16.

Figures 20.14 to 20.16. Correction factors for various lens parameters.

because of an oversimplification in the contact lens optics involved in the problem.

The common method advocated for using a water cell is to place the lens in the water cell and measure the system with a lensometer.

The power reading that is read is then multiplied by a correction factor, which is derived in the following way:

If a contact lens is considered as optically thin, all the power may be considered to occur at one surface. The power of the surface in air would be as follows:

$$F = \frac{1.43 - 1}{R} = \frac{0.43}{R}$$

The same lens in water would have the following power:

$$F = \frac{1.43 - 1.33}{R} = \frac{0.10}{R}$$

The ratio between the power of the lens in air and the power of the lens in water would simply equal 0.43/0.1 = 4.3, the correction factor.

An exact calculation of the lensometer power reading was obtained by Yumori and Mandell[22] by ray tracing through the entire system for a variety of lens designs.

Figures 20.14 to 20.16 show the correction factors, or multipliers, to be used for the calculation of true lens power for a variety of lenses. It may be seen from the figures that the multiplier usually varies between 4 and 6, and that in some cases the use of the standard 4.3× multiplier would result in large errors. The multiplier varies with each parameter of the lens but, interestingly, is not affected significantly by changes in the position of the lens from the surface of the water cell. This occurs because the lens in the cell acts as though its power is reduced by dividing by the correction factor. For a lens of 20.00 D, the power in the water cell is of the order of 4.00 D. Therefore, the lens position within the water cell is not critical for most lenses, and it is possible to use a water cell for making an accurate measurement of back vertex power, which is not easily accomplished otherwise.

Although the graphs shown in Figures 20.14 to 20.16 provide a more accurate method for determining the true lens power using a water cell, there still remains a potential measurement error in this technique. Whenever a lens is measured in the lensometer, the error read is also increased by the multiplying factor. Hence, an error of ⅛ D. in measuring a lens requiring a multiplier of 5 will give a final error for the lens power of ⅝ D., a significant value. Nevertheless, the ease of this method as compared to blotting the lens for a lensometer measurement will probably offset the disadvantages. It is possible to take several lensometer measurements rapidly and average them to give a more accurate reading.

SURFACE INSPECTION

The surfaces of the lenses should be inspected for defects with a biomicroscope or a stereomicroscope, using approximately 15× to 20× magnification. The lens may be either held in the hand or placed on a clean glass slide.

The lens should also be viewed against a clean, white paper to see if any abnormal coloration is present.

REFERENCES

1. Harris, G., Hall, K., and Oye, R.: The measurement and stability of hydrophilic lens dimensions, *Am. J. Optom. Arch. Am. Acad. Optom.*, 50(7):546–552, 1973.
2. Koetting, R. A.: Comparison of the expected anterior curve radius in soft lens fitting, *Contacto*, 18(3):25–30, 1974.
3. Cotti, F.: Bionite–Sofcon lenses: handling, cleaning, dimensional stability, visual acuity, *Contacto*, 18(3):17–21, 1974.
4. Dorman-Brailsford, M. I.: Considerations in the checking and predictability of hydrophilic lenses, *Contacto*, 18(4):13–18, 1974.
5. Brown, S. R.: Drying, opacities, tightening

and warping of the therapeutic soft lens, *Cont. Intraoc. Lens Med. J.*, *21(1)*:22–23, 1976.

6. Sohnges, C. P.: A Sohnges control and measuring unit for hard and soft contact lenses, *Contacto*, *18(5)*:31–33, 1974.

7. Elmstrom, G.: Hydrophilic lens analyzer, *J. Am. Optom. Assoc.*, *50(6)*:757, 1979.

8. Chaston, J.: In-office measurements of soft contact lenses, *Am. J. Optom. Physiol. Opt.*, *54(5)*:286–291, 1977.

9. Holden, B. A.: An accurate and reliable method of measuring soft contact lens curvatures, *Austr. J. Optom.*, *58(12)*:443–449, 1975.

10. Chaston, J.: A method of measuring the radius of curvature of a soft contact lens, *Austr. J. Optom.*, *56(5)*:214–216, 1973.

11. Sarver, M. D.: *Contact Lens Syllabus*, 5th ed., UC Berkeley School of Optometry, Berkeley, Calif., 1979.

12. Ruben, M.: Some physical measurements of soft hydrophilic lenses, *Cont. Lens Med. Bull.*, *7(1–2)*:31–35, 1974.

13. Hamano, H., and Kawabe, H.: Method of measuring radii of a soft lens with an electronic device, *Contacto*, *22(1)*:4–8, 1978.

14. Paramore, J., and Wechsler, S.: Reliability and repeatability study of a technique for measuring the center thickness of a hydrogel lens, *J. Am. Optom. Assoc.*, *49(3)*:272–274, 1978.

15. Barr, J. T., and Lowther, G. E.: Measured and laboratory stated parameters of hydrophilic contact lenses, *Am. J. Optom. Physiol. Opt.*, *54(12)*:809–820, 1977.

16. Grosvenor, T.: Evaluation of soft contact lens use in Canada, *Can. J. Optom.*, *33(3)*:56–63, 1971.

17. Kennedy, J. R.: On the threshold of a miracle, *Optom. Weekly*, *64(12)*:278–282, 1973.

18. Sarver, M. D. et al.: Power of Bausch and Lomb Soflens contact lenses, *Am. J. Optom.*, *50(3)*:195–199, 1973.

19. Poster, M. G.: Hydrated method of determining dioptral power of a hydrophilic lens, *J. Am. Optom. Assoc.*, *42(4)*:369, 1971.

20. Wray, L.: The measurement of hydrophilic contact lenses—Part 1, *The Ophthalmic Optician*, *12(7)*:256, 261–264, 1972.

21. Wray, L.: The measurement of hydrophilic contact lenses—Part 2, *The Ophthalmic Optician*, *12(8)*:301–305, 209–311, 1972.

22. Yumori, R. W., and Mandell, R. B.: Optical power calculation for contact lens water cells, accepted for publication by *Am. J. Optom. Physiol. Opt.*

ADDITIONAL READINGS

Anderson, D. J., and Davis, H. E.: An investigation of the reliability of hydrogel lens parameters, *Int. Cont. Lens Clin.*, *6(3)*:136–142, 1979.

Appelquist, T. D., and Harris, M. G.: The effect of contact lens diameter and power on flexure and residual astigmatism, *Am. J. Optom. Physiol. Opt.*, *51(4)*:266–270, 1974.

Bailey, N. J.: Inspection of hydrogel lenses, *Int. Cont. Lens Clin.*, *2(1)*:42–47, 1975.

Chaston, J.: A method of measuring the radius of curvature of a soft contact lens, *The Optician*, *165(4271)*:8–10, 1973.

Chaston, J.: Measuring the posterior curve radius of a hydrogel lens, *Int. Cont. Lens Clin.*, *3(2)*:87–90, 1976.

Chaston, J. M.: The reliability and reproducibility of soft lens parameters, *Contacto*, *19(4)*:33–38, 1975.

Cochet, P.: Microscopical changes in soft contact lenses, *Trans. Ophthalmol. Soc. U.K.*, *97*:157, 1977.

Davis, H. E., and Anderson, D. J.: An investigation of the reliability of hydrogel lens parameters, *Int. Cont. Lens Clin.*, *6(3)*:65–71, 1979.

Dixon, J. M.: A device for holding hydrophilic contact lenses to measure optical power and thickness, *Trans. Am. Ophthalmol. Soc.*, *70*:357–358, 1972.

El-Nashar, N. F., Larke, J. R., and Brookes, C. J.: The measurement of the Bausch & Lomb Soflens contact lens by interferometry, *Am. J. Optom. Physiol. Opt.*, *56(1)*:10–15, 1979.

Fatt, I.: A simple electrical device for measuring thickness and sagittal height of gel contact lenses, *The Optician*, *173(4474)*:23–24, 1977.

Forst, G.: Measurement of the radii of curvature of soft lenses—a simple method for the practitioner (in German), *Sudd. Optik.*, *28(1)*:7–9, 1973.

Forst, G.: New methods of measurement for controlling soft lens quality, *Contacto*, *18*(6):6–10, 1974.

Hamano, H., and Kawabe, H.: Variation of base curve of soft lens during wearing, *Contacto*, *22*(1):10, 1978.

Hampson, R. M.: Considerations in the checking and predictability of hydrophilic lenses, *The Optician*, *165*(*4283*):4–16, 1973.

Hanks, A.: A study of the reproducibility of spin-cast hydrophilic contact lenses, *Int. Cont. Lens Clin.*, *4*(3):31, 1977.

Hanks, A. J.: A study of the reproducibility of spin cast hydrophilic contact lenses, *Austr. J. Optom.*, *59*(*10*):341–347, 1976.

Holden, B. A.: The accuracy and variability of measurement of the BCOR of hydrated soft lenses using a Zeiss keratometer and Holden wet cell, *Austr. J. Optom.*, *60*(*8*):46–50, 1977.

Holden, B. A.: Checking soft lens parameters, *Austr. J. Optom.*, *60*(5):175, 1977.

Holden, B. A.: Check soft lens parameters, *Cont. Lens Forum*, *3*(6):33, 1978.

Koetting, R. A.: Why not use the radiuscope to measure soft lenses, *Opt. J. Rev. Optom.*, *110*(*20*): 34–35, 1973.

Koetting, R. A.: Soft lens power and curvature: a comparison of "label" and observed measurements, *Am. J. Optom. Physiol. Opt.*, *52*(7):485–492, 1975.

Koetting, R. A.: Surface artifacts found on unboiled hydrophilic lenses, *Int. Cont. Lens Clin.*, *3*(4): 37–41, 1976.

Loran, D. F. C.: Determination of hydrogel contact lens radii by projection, *The Ophthalmic Optician*, *14*(*19*):980–985, 1974.

Masnick, K. B., and Holden, B. A.: A study of water content and parametric variations of hydrophilic contact lenses, *Austr. J. Optom.*, *55*(*12*):481–487, 1972.

Miller, B.: Observations of contact lens surfaces by interference contrast microscopy, *Cont. Lens J.*, *5*(5):17–20, 1976.

Paramore, J., and Wechsler, S.: Reliability and repeatability study of a technique for measuring the center thickness of a hydrogel lens, *J. Am. Optom. Assoc.*, *49*(3):272–274, 1978.

Chapter 21

LENS CARE AND STORAGE

SOFT LENS SOLUTIONS

Various solutions are available for use with soft contact lenses. They generally consist of rinsing, cleaning, and storage solutions. Caution must be taken that only solutions specifically designed for soft con-tact lenses be recommended to patients. Patients should be told that solutions for hard contact lenses contain ingredients that can be injurious to the eye.

SALINE SOLUTION

Saline solutions are generally found in one of three forms. The saline may be pre-mixed, buffered, and distributed in a small container, usually less than 200 ml. This saline is usually buffered with either sodium or potassium borate. It is usually preserved by 0.001% thimerosal and 0.01% disodium edetate.

Nonpreserved Saline

This saline is usually packaged in small units designed for a single use by the patient. The saline may be buffered to raise the pH from that which is normally found in salt solution.

Salt Tablets

Various salt tablets have been used that are designed to be dissolved in a quantity of distilled water to produce a 0.9% saline solution.

The safest and most problem-free solution is that of prepackaged unpreserved saline. Unfortunately, the extra expense of this product prevents its universal use. All chemically preserved salines present a potential irritation problem to some patients. Generally, the concentration of the preservative is so low that the irritation is minor.

The use of salt tablets has been controversial. Reports have occurred in the literature of patient problems with various distilled waters that have been used for mixing the saline solution. Generally, these problems have been minor, however, and the low cost of this technique has encouraged its continued use.

SURFACTANTS

Various surfactants are available that can be used to remove the deposits and coat-ings which commonly occur on soft lenses. These cleaners should be used on a daily

557

basis after the lenses are removed from the patient's eye and before the disinfecting process is undertaken. Generally, the surfactant cleaners contain a nonionic detergent, buffers, sodium chloride, hydroxyethyl cellulose, and polyvinyl alcohol. The cleaners are usually preserved with 0.004% thimerosal and 0.2% disodium edetate. An exception is Pliagel®, which is preserved with 0.1% sorbic acid and 0.5% disodium edetate.

RINSING SOLUTIONS

Various rinsing solutions which usually contain sodium chloride and buffers, are available. They are generally preserved with 0.001% thimerosal, 0.1% disodium edetate, and 0.005% chlorhexidine. Patients are sometimes confused by this solution and attempt to use it as a substitute for a saline boiling solution. Unfortunately, when this is done, the chlorhexidine in the solution causes the lenses to turn a cloudy white.

COLD DISINFECTION SOLUTIONS

Various storage solutions are used as an alternative for heating the lenses in saline. The solutions generally consist of sodium chloride, buffers, and various wetting agents and are preserved with 0.001% thimerosal and 0.005% chlorhexidine. The preservatives have been thought to be the cause of many red eye syndromes, which occur in contact lens patients. Various reports from clinical studies have indicated that approximately 30 percent of patients who use the solutions develop mild injection and slight discomfort. Probably 5 to 10 percent of the patients who use these cold storage solutions develop reactions severe enough to interfere with successful wear of their contact lenses.

ENZYMATIC CLEANER

This cleaner consists of a proteolytic enzyme, papain, which is effective in removing proteinaceous deposits from contact lens surfaces. It should generally be used one time each week, but this varies with the rate at which the deposits form on the lens surfaces for the individual patient. The enzyme is provided in a kit with vials, into which are placed the enzyme tablets. They are dissolved in distilled water, and the lenses are soaked from two to six hours. After the treatment with the enzymatic cleaner, it is necessary to disinfect the lenses.

HYDROGEN PEROXIDE

A 3% solution of hydrogen peroxide is very effective in destroying most of the microorganisms found in soft contact lenses. In addition, the peroxide tends to clean various materials from the lens surfaces and sometimes to remove lens discoloration. A 3% peroxide solution is sometimes used for an in-office disinfecting procedure, since it provides the quickest method for effectively disinfecting a soft contact lens. This is generally accomplished by soaking the lens first in the hydrogen peroxide for five minutes, which is followed by two soakings in regular buffered sodium chloride solution. Caution should be taken in the use of peroxide, since it should not be placed on the eye.

ACCESSORY SOFT LENS SOLUTIONS

Various solutions are available that are designed to be used as eye drops while the lenses are being worn. Their purpose is generally to lubricate and rehydrate the lenses and make them more comfortable on the eye. In some cases, these solutions contain mild cleaners in the form of nonionic detergents. The solutions are usually preserved with 0.1% disodium edetate and 0.004% thimerosal.

INSERTION AND REMOVAL

The large diameter of a gel contact lens might seem to make insertion and removal more difficult than with the smaller corneal lens. Such is not the case; many patients and fitters find the gel lens is indeed easier to handle than the corneal contact lens, although this viewpoint is not universal.

LENS INSERTION BY FITTER

1. Remove the lens from the vial with the aid of tweezers (Figure 21.1). To remove the lens, insert one prong inside the vial and trap the lens between the side of the vial and the prong. Gently slide the lens upward to the mouth of the vial and remove by holding

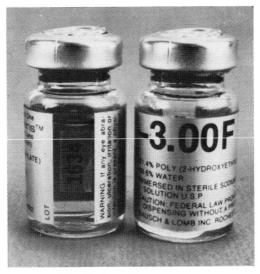

Figure 21.1a. Soft lens in vial.

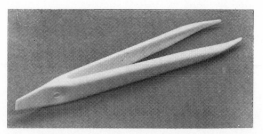

Figure 21.1b. Tweezers for soft lens.

the lens with both prongs of the tweezers. Occasionally when the vial is opened the lens will stick to the stopper. (It may be folded and very difficult to see.)

The lens may also be removed by dumping the entire contents of the vial into the palm of the hand. This is facilitated if the vial is held upside down and shaken vigorously before opening.

Examine the lens for clarity and cleanliness and to be sure it is not turned inside out (Figure 21.2). This may be done simply by flexing the lens between the thumb and index finger. If, upon flexing, the edge is erect and pointing slightly inward, it is in its correct position. If the edge turns outward, folding back on the fingers, it is inside out and must be reversed.

2. Place the lens on the outer edge of the index fingertip, concave side up (Figure 21.3). Have the patient hold his head erect and look straight ahead. Retract his upper lid with your middle finger (Figure 21.4).

3. Have the patient look up and stare at a point on the ceiling. Rest the inner edge of the index fingertip on the patient's lower lid. Roll the lens onto the sclera, moving it about slowly to expel trapped air bubbles.

4. Have the patient close his eyes. Lightly massage through the closed lid to help center the lens on the cornea.

Lens Removal

1. Place your fingertips on the lens while retracting the patient's lower lid, with the patient staring straight ahead.

2. Have the patient look up. This slides the lens down to the sclera.

3. Flex the lens lightly between your thumb and index finger and remove it from the eye. (*See* Figure 21.5.)

INSERTION BY THE PATIENT

There are two general methods for insertion by the patient: the scleral method and the corneal method.

Scleral Method of Insertion

The scleral method of insertion is recommended by many practitioners and manufacturers. Bausch and Lomb recommends the following instructions for the use of the patient (Figures 21.6 to 21.9):

In placing and removing the lenses, the patient should wash his hands thoroughly and work over a clean, dark surface so that he may easily retrieve the lens if he drops it. Placement and removal require only one hand and no mirror. The right lens is always placed and removed first to avoid reversal of lenses. Before removing a lens, the patient should always check his vision to make certain the lens is on the eye.

CORRECT INSIDE – OUT

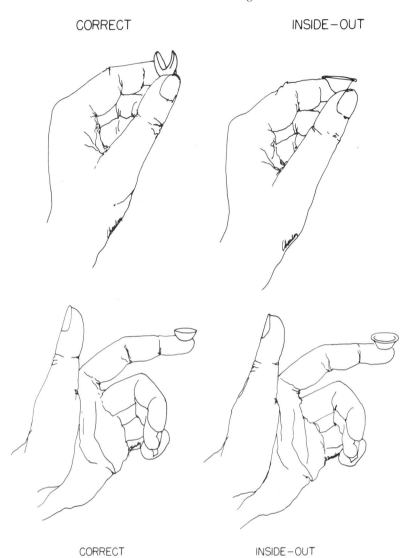

CORRECT INSIDE – OUT

Figure 21.2. Examination to see whether the lens is turned inside out: (*a*) "taco test" — lens that is right side out has the edges pulled in when squeezed. Lens turned wrong side out has the edges pulled away. (*b*) Held on the end of the finger, a right-side-out lens looks like a bowl, with edges erect. An inside-out lens appears to have a lip formed by the edges' bending downward.

Lens Placement

Wash hands thoroughly, making certain that all soap residue has been washed away. Work with the right lens first in order to avoid confusing the lenses. After removing the lens from the case (*see* Figure 21.6), examine it to be sure that it is moist, clean, and clear (*see* Figure 21.7). Be careful not to touch the inside surface of the lens.

1. Place the lens on the outer edge of the index finger of your dominant hand.

2. With your head erect and gazing straight ahead, retract the lower lid with your middle finger (*See* Figure 21.8).

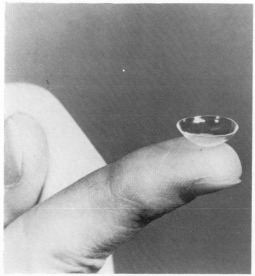

Figure 21.3. Correct way to hold the lens for insertion.

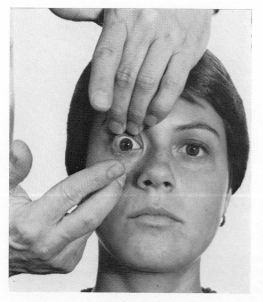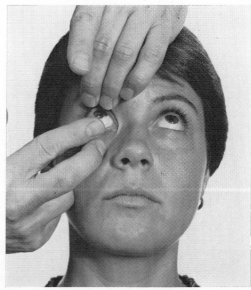

Figure 21.4. Insertion by fitter: (*a*) preparation to place lens on eye, (b) lens placed on lower sclera.

3. Look up and fix your gaze on a point above you. Then roll the lens onto the white part of the eye (*See* Figure 21.9).

4. Remove your index finger and slowly release the lid.

5. Close your eyes momentarily and lightly massage the lids to help center the lens.

One of the unique characteristics of the gel contact lens is the ability of the lens to center itself on the cornea once the lens has been placed on the sclera. This centering may take place with no eye movement what-

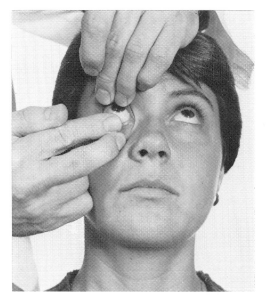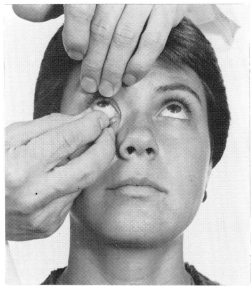

Figure 21.5. Lens removal by fitter: (*a*) place fingertip on lens while retracting the patient's lower lid; have the patient look up, sliding lens down onto sclera. (*b*) Remove lens from eye.

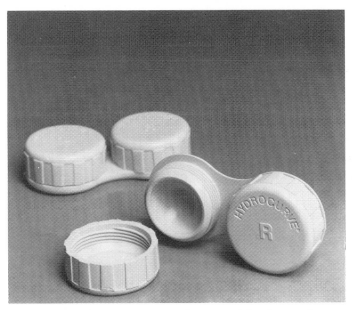

Figure 21.6. Gel lens storage case. Courtesy of Continuous Curve.

soever, but if this does not occur, a simple gaze in the direction of the lens will almost always center the lens on the cornea.

Alternate Method

A gel contact lens may be inserted by the same techniques used for hard contact

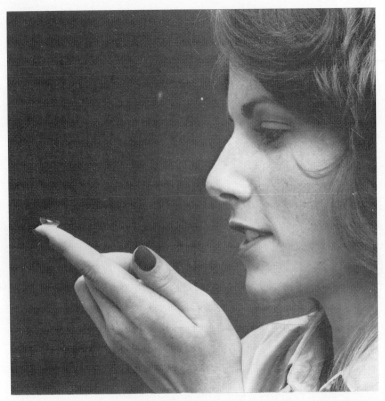

Figure 21.7. Examining lens.

lenses (Figure 21.10a). These techniques are usually preferred by experienced hard contact lens wearers and may be preferred by some new wearers. However, after the lens is in place, a large bubble is often formed under the central portion of the lens (Figure 21.10b). This bubble may take from one to four minutes to disappear, and the patient will note that there is a severe decrement in the visual acuity while the bubble exists. A lathe-cut lens is somewhat more prone to this problem than a spin-cast lens, since lathe-cut lenses generally have a little less flexibility.

Lens Removal

1. Always be sure the lens is in the correct position on your eye before attempting to remove it. A simple check of your vision with each eye separately will tell if a lens is in the correct position. If vision is poor, it is likely that the lens has been lost from the eye. If vision is poor, yet you feel certain that the lens is still in your eye, you should obtain professional assistance for removal of the lens.

2. Having washed your hands and rinsed them thoroughly, begin the removal procedure by holding your head erect and turning your eyes upward. Retract the lower lid with the middle finger and place the index fingertip on the lower edge of the lens. Slide the lens down to the white part of the eye (Figure 21.11).

3. Compress the lens lightly between the thumb and index finger. Rolling the thumb and index finger together causes the lens to double up between the fingers, allowing air underneath. Remove the lens from the eye (Figure 21.12).

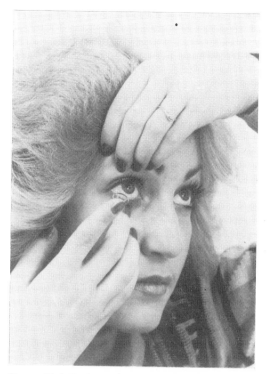

Figure 21.8. Patient ready to place lens. Courtesy of Bausch & Lomb, Inc.

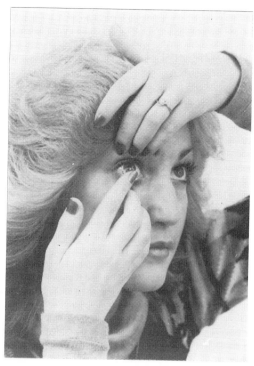

Figure 21.9. Placing the lens on the lower sclera. Courtesy of Bausch & Lomb, Inc.

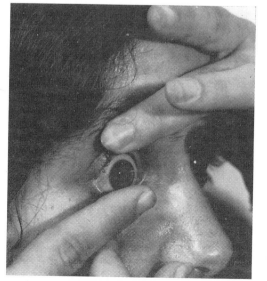

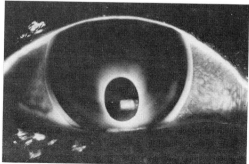

Figure 21.10. Insertion of the gel lens by the hard lens technique (*a*), often leaves a large bubble (*b*) which takes from one to four minutes to disappear.

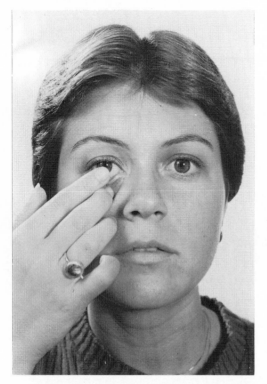 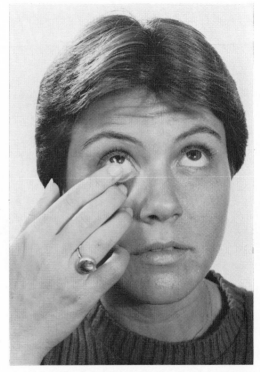

Figure 21.11. Lens removal by patient. (*a*) Patient places fingertip on lower edge of lens. (*b*) Sliding the lens onto the lower sclera.

4. Clean the lens with cleaner, rinse with saline, and replace it in the carrying case. Fill with saline.

An alternate method of removal, which is similar to that used for hard corneal lenses, can be used with a large proportion of patients who wear lathe-cut lenses. This technique can also be used occasionally for Soflens wearers, but most patients prefer the previous technique.

If the patient has a very large palpebral fissure, it may be possible for him simply to open the eye and pull at the outer canthus and blink as with a hard corneal lens. How-ever, most patients do not find that this technique will be effective. An alternate technique, which works for the majority of patients, is to use a two-finger squeezing technique similar to that used with a hard corneal lens. In this technique the first and second fingers are placed against the upper and lower lids respectively. The lids are spread apart to increase the size of the palpebral aperture, and then the fingers are drawn laterally to exert pressure on the lens margins. This motion is followed by a squeezing together of the lid, which acts to eject the lens (Figure 21.13).

COPING WITH THE ULTRATHIN HANDLING PROBLEM

The following tips are offered by Bausch and Lomb for handling the ultrathin lens series.

Check To Be Sure the Lens Is Not Turned Inside Out

A simple, visual inspection will help determine this. Do *not* check by flexing the lens between the thumb and index finger as in Figure 21.2a. That action may cause the lens to fold and stick together. Instead, put the lens on the index finger and allow a few seconds for the lens to dehydrate slightly. Next, inspect the lens closely to see whether the edges turn up (Figure 21.2b). If not, the lens is probably inside out.

If the lens should accidentally be placed inside out on the eye, one of the following signs should be a signal to remove it and reinsert it correctly:

1. It will be less comfortable, and edge sensation may be apparent.

2. The lens may tend to fold on the eye.

3. The lens may drop to a lower position on the eye.

4. The lens may move excessively with the blink.

Be Sure the Lens Rests Correctly on the Fingertip Prior to Insertion

Balancing the lens in an upright position will make it easier to place on the eye. The lens should rest parallel with the fingertip, with all edges up and toward the eye. The lens should not rock forward or sideways so that one edge touches the fingertip. (*See* Figure 21.3).

Keep the Insertion Hand and Fingers Dry

Soft contact lenses have a natural attraction to wet surfaces. Therefore, it is important that your index finger on which the lens rests be kept relatively dry in order to assure a quick and easy placement onto the naturally moist eye. This handling problem is easily solved by using the other hand to remove the lenses from the saline-filled carrying case.

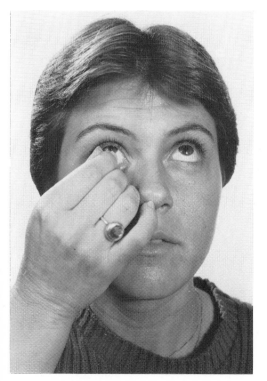

Figure 21.12. Pinching the lens from the sclera.

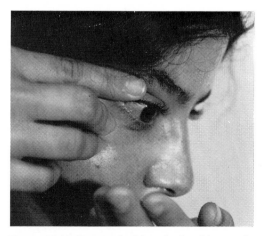

Figure 21.13. Removal of lens by hard lens technique.

What To Do If the Lens Curls and the Edges Stick Together

Place the lens in the palm of the hand and wet thoroughly with fresh saline solution. Then gently slide the edges apart with the thumb and index finger. If this gentle rubbing does not work, soak the lens in saline solution in the storage case until the lens has resumed its normal shape.

What To Do If the Lens Flattens or Drapes Across the Finger

The finger or the lens may be too wet. Transfer the lens to the palm of the opposite hand. Dry the finger, and let the lens dry in the air for a few seconds. (Check to see that the lens is not turned inside out.) Replace the lens on the index finger to see whether the situation has been corrected.

What To Do If the Lens Wrinkles When Placed on the Eye

If the lens is wrinkled, vision will not be as clear, and the lens may feel uncomfortable. Remove the lens, wet it with fresh saline solution, and replace it on the eye.

Lens Removal

Always slide the lens open with the thumb and index finger *immediately* upon removal from the eye to keep the edges from sticking together.

CLEANING

After the lenses have been removed from the eye, and before they are placed in storage, they should be cleaned. Several cleaners have been produced by various companies.

Wet the lens thoroughly in the palm of the hand with cleaner, and rub it with the fingertip (Figure 21.14), or alternately, rub the lenses between the thumb and index finger (Figure 21.15). Rinse thoroughly with normal saline. For very dirty lenses, first clean them with enzyme cleaner, prior to using a surfactant cleaner. If the lens has a soap residue causing it to burn, boil it in distilled water for at least one hour. Equilibrate the lens in normal saline solution before replacing it on the eye.

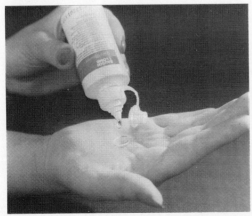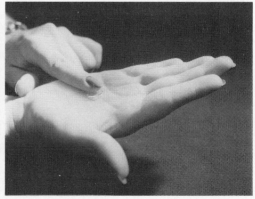

Figure 21.14. Cleaning the gel lens. Courtesy of Bausch & Lomb, Inc.

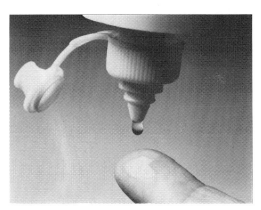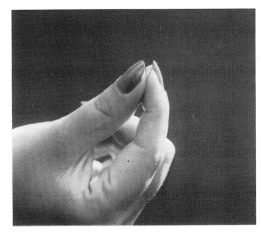

Figure 21.15. Alternate method to clean the gel lens. Courtesy of Bausch & Lomb, Inc.

LENS STORAGE

There are two available techniques for storage of gel lenses: heating and chemical disinfection.

HEATING

Gel lenses can be decontaminated by heating in normal saline solution in a heat disinfection unit (Figure 21.16). This device heats the lenses while in their carrying case. Soft contact lenses are stored and disinfected in normal saline solution (0.9% sodium chloride in distilled water). No unapproved solutions may be used, for they may be absorbed or adsorbed by the lens and cause damage to the eyes. When handling the lenses, hands must be free of any soap residue, which may cause the lenses to sting.

Disinfecting Lenses Daily

In disinfecting the lenses daily, the patient should perform the following routine:

1. Fill the carrying case with normal saline solution.
2. Clamp the carrying case into the heat disinfection unit.
3. Press the activating switch until the light goes on. When the light goes out, the lenses are aseptic and ready for wear.

If a disinfection unit is not available, the lens may be placed in its carrying case with saline, and the entire case boiled in a pan of water for fifteen minutes. Care must be taken, however, that the pan is not allowed to dry, else the case and perhaps its contents will be ruined.

Efficacy of the Heating Technique

There has been considerable controversy over the efficacy of the heating technique. There have been three principal objections to the technique: First, the temperature is said to be inadequate to produce complete sterility of the lenses. Second, the heating effect supposedly tends to break down the hydrogel polymer. Third, boiling presumably tends to make any contaminants on the lens adhere to the surface tenaciously.

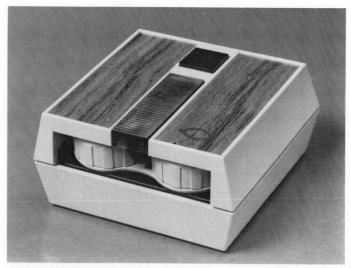

Figure 21.16. The hydrocurve deluxe thermal unit. Courtesy of Hydrocurve.

The heat disinfection unit does not provide complete sterility (total destruction of all microorganisms). It does kill all bacteria, including *Pseudomonas aeruginosa*, but it is not effective against a few spores that are not pathogens to the eye. The conditions to achieve total sterility are usually considered to be autoclaving for fifteen minutes at 120° C and 15 pounds per square inch pressure.

The variation in temperature inside the asepticizer is shown in Figure 21.17 and was measured by placing a thermocouple in the storage case during disinfection. The total time involved in disinfection is over an hour. There is initially a period in which the temperature is rising until it reaches its maximum in about fifteen minutes. The unit then boils for about twenty minutes and shuts itself off. It then requires about forty-five minutes more for the case to cool to room temperature. The total boiling time is dependent on how much water is placed in the heating unit and varies from about eighteen to twenty-six minutes.[1] Knoll reported that the efficacy of the heating process was tested with five organisms, which included three bacteria (*Staphylococcus aureus*, *Pseudomonas aeruginosa*, and *Bacillus subtilis*), one fungus (*Candida albicans*), and one virus (*Herpes simplex*.)[2] These organisms were inoculated into the patient's carrying case and allowed to stand for six hours. They were then subjected to the heating procedure and cultured. In all cases the results of the cultures were negative.

Some practitioners have argued that it is not necessary to heat the lenses every night, and there is some evidence to support this.[2] Tests have shown that there is probably little harm in having the patient skip the disinfection process for a day or two. However, this instruction should never be told to the patient, since it violates the FDA requirements of the lens as a drug and also because any indication that the disinfection procedure can be skipped would probably encourage the patient to skip the procedure for longer periods.

Degradation by Boiling

Since the polyH.E.M.A. material is a plastic, it can be expected that a molecular breakdown will occur as a result of higher temperatures. However, a temperature at which this occurs rapidly is probably about 30° higher than that normally used in the process. Hence, any breakdown of the molecular structure of the material probably occurs at a very slow rate.

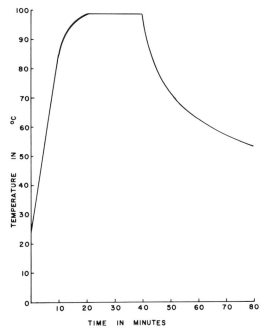

Figure 21.17. Variation of temperature inside the asepticizer. Courtesy of Barnes-Hind, Inc.

Office Aseptor Unit®

A large unit capable of disinfecting seventy-two lenses at a time is available for office use (made by Bausch and Lomb, Inc.) (Figure 21.18). Fitting set lenses should be disinfected each time they are used, but in addition, the entire fitting set should be disinfected about once every two months:

1. Fill the Soflens aseptor-professional unit with 3 quarts of distilled water and place the entire fitting set in the unit.

2. Replace the cover and plug the unit into a 110-volt A.C. outlet. Turn the dial clockwise all the way to the right. The water will remain at 80° C. for at least fifteen minutes during the hour the unit is activated, after which it will turn itself off automatically. The fitting set rack may be removed fifteen minutes after the unit shuts off. Note that the proper temperatures will not be reached unless the cover is on the unit.

CHEMICAL DISINFECTION

The development of a safe and effective disinfecting storage solution has been made difficult because of the property of gel lenses known as their *ad*sorptive, or binding, ability, which is commonly confused with *ab*sorptive properties. Since the hydrophilic lens has the ability to absorb water, it will by necessity *ab*sorb a solution of any chemical that might be presented to it.[3] This should not create a problems if the solution itself is safe in the eye. A potential problem arises, however, if the soft lens can *ad*sorb or concentrate chemicals. When this happens, a wearer can be putting more than a safe concentration of the chemical into his eye.[4] An area of concern are those chemicals which are used as antimicrobial agents. These materials are harmful to living bacterial cells and will generally be damaging to the cells of the eye if they are present in higher than normal concentrations.

Of the materials tested, benzalkonium chloride exhibited the greatest amount of binding, but all of the materials seem to bind to some extent.[5] Some of the materials that bind only slightly, such as the mercurials, may still be unsatisfactory for actual use, since a prolonged contact might be detrimental to the eye. There is some documentation of mercurial sensitization with commonly used mercurial solutions.

The efficacy of the solutions as a disinfecting system has also been challenged. There are reports that the cold storage systems are ineffective against several common viruses.

The recommendation is made that lenses be stored in the cold solution for a minimum of four hours. This slow kill time is attributed to the slow action of the thimerosal.

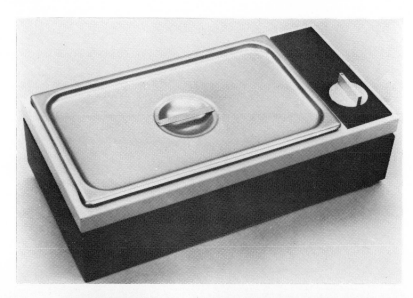

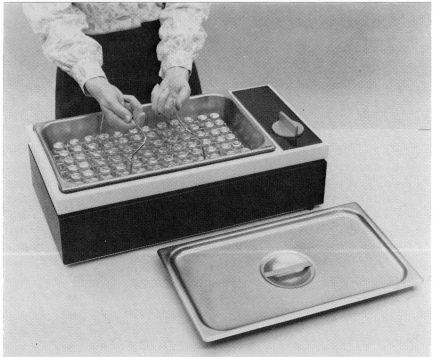

Figure 21.18. Bausch & Lomb office asepticizer unit (*a*), with rack of seventy-two lenses (*b*).

WARNINGS

The following warnings apply to all soft lenses:

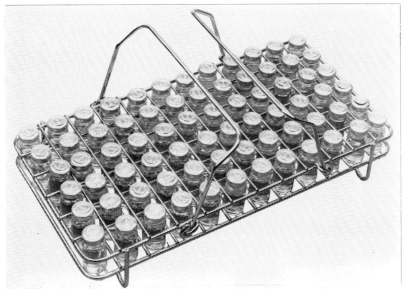

Figure 21.18c. Carrying rack containing seventy-two vials (*c*).

MEDICATIONS AND EYE DROPS

Hydrogel lenses must be stored *only* in normal saline solution. No ophthalmic solutions or medications, including hard contact lens solutions, can be used by gel lens wearers prior to or while the lens is in place on the eye. Also, no solutions, other than normal saline, may be used on a gel lens while the lens is off the eye.

ABRASIONS AND INFECTION

If the lenses become less comfortable to the wearer than when they were first placed on the wearer's corneas, this may indicate the presence of a foreign body. The lens should be removed immediately, and the patient should be examined. If any eye abrasion, irritation, or infection is present, a physician should be consulted immediately.

WEARING RESTRICTIONS

Gel lenses should be removed before sleeping or swimming and in the presence of noxious and irritating vapors.

VISUAL BLURRING

When visual blurring occurs, the lens must be removed until the condition subsides.

LENS SANITATION

Patients who would not or could not adhere to recommended daily sanitary care of gel contact lenses should not be provided with them.

STORAGE

Gel lenses must be stored *only* in normal saline solution. If left exposed to air, the lenses will dehydrate, become brittle, and break readily. If a lens dehydrates, it should be soaked in normal saline solution until it returns to a soft, supple state.

CLEANING AND DISINFECTING

Gel lenses must be *both* cleaned and disinfected daily. One procedure does not replace the other. Cleaning is necessary to remove mucus and film from the lens surface. Disinfecting has been shown to prevent the growth of certain organisms, namely, *Staphylococcus aureus*, *Pseudomonas aeruginosa*, *Bacillus subtilis*, *Candida albicans*, and *Herpes simplex*, on the lens and the carrying case.

If one is using salt tablets, one must prepare fresh saline daily for cleaning and storing the lenses. The carrying case must be emptied and refilled with fresh normal saline solution just before disinfecting the lenses.

If a heating unit is not available for disinfecting the lenses, the lenses must be boiled in their carrying case in a pan of water for fifteen minutes.

HYGIENE

Hands must be washed, rinsed thoroughly, and dried with a lint-free towel before handling the lenses.

Cosmetics, lotions, soaps, and creams must not come in contact with the lenses, since eye irritation may result. If hair spray is used while the lenses are being worn, the eyes must be kept closed until the hair spray has settled.

FLUORESCEIN

Never use fluorescein while the patient is wearing the lenses, because the lenses will become discolored. Whenever fluorescein is used, flush the eyes with normal saline solution and wait at least one hour before reinserting the lenses. Too early reinsertion may allow the lenses to absorb residual fluorescein irreversibly.

REFERENCES

1. Phares, R. E., Jr., and Hall, N. C.: Microbiology of soft and hard contact lens care, in Bitonte, J. L., and Keates, R. H. (Eds.): *Symposium on the Flexible Lens*, St. Louis, Mosby, 1972, pp. 205–212.
2. Panel discussion on cleaning and sterilizing rigid and flexible lenses, in Bitonte, J. L., and Keates, R. H. (Eds.): *Symposium on the Flexible Lens*, St. Louis, Mosby, 1972, pp. 222–234.
3. Phares, R. E.: Pharmaceutical aspects of soft contact lenses, *Optom. Weekly*, 62(16):357–359, 1971.
4. Phares, R. E.: Pharmaceutical aspects of soft contact lenses, *J. Optom.*, 3(4):11–13, 1971.
5. Phares, R. E.: Soft lens care, *J. Am. Optom. Assoc.*, 43(3):308–313, 1972.

ADDITIONAL READINGS

Anderson, A. N. II, and Browne, R. K.: Ophthalmic responses to chlorhexidine digluconate in rabbits, *Toxicol. Appl. Pharmacol.*,32:62, 1975.
Arons, I. J.: Soft lens coating—and what can be done about it, *Rev. Opt.*, 115(4):35, 1978.
Bailey, N. J.: Contact lens storage: a bacteriological study, *Am. J. Optom. Am. Acad. Optom.*, 43(4):244–248, 1966.

Bailey, N. J.: Cleaning of coated soft lenses, *J. Am. Optom. Assoc.*, *45*(9):1049–1052, 1974.

Bailey, N. J.: Contact lens coating: the effect on service life, *J. Am. Optom. Assoc.*, *46*(3):214–218, 1975.

Bailey, N. J.: Microscopic photography, *J. Am. Optom. Assoc.*, *46*(2):142–144, 1975.

Bailey, W. R.: Preservatives for contact lens solutions, *J. Contact Lens Soc. Am.*, *6*(3):33–39, 1972.

Bailey, W. R., Jr., and Feldman, G. L.: Clinical experiences with chemical vs. thermal disinfection of hydrophilic lenses, *Cont. Lens J.*, *8*(4):20–24, 1975.

Baker, S. R.: Developing an eye drop for soft lens wearers, *Cont. Lens Forum*, *2*(9):25, 1977.

Baker, S. R., and Remington, J. S.: Contamination of soft gel lenses, *Contacto*, *16*(3):4–6, 1972.

Baker, V. V., Fichman, S., and Horton, H. R.: Iatrogenic red eyes in soft contact lens wearers, *Int. Cont. Lens Clin.*, *5*(5):20–24, 1978.

Bedding, P.: Deposits on soft contact lenses, *The Optician*, *175*(4538):21, 1978.

Bellemare, F.: Compatibility of enzymatic cleaning with cold contact lens disinfection, *Int. Cont. Lens Clin.*, *6*(5):40, 1979.

Bernstein, H. N.: Evaluation of the "aseptization" procedure for the soflens hydrophilic contact lens, *Can. J. Ophthalmol.*, *8*(4):575–576, 1973.

Blanco, M., Curry, B., and Boghosian, M. P.: Studies of the effect of enzymatic cleaning on the physical structure of hydrophilic lenses, *Contacto*, *19*(5):17–20, 1975.

Bownman, J., Bayeat, H. D., and Rowsy, J. J.: Adenoviral keratoconjunctivitis associated with chemical disinfection of a flexible lens, *Cont. Intraoc. Lens Med. J.*, *4*(4):68, 1978.

Boyd, H. H.: Soaking of soft contact lenses, *Cont. Lens Med. Bull.*, *1*(1–2):192–197, 1975.

Brown, S. I., Traggkis, M. P., and Pearce, D. B.: Bacteriologic studies of contamination associated with soft contact lenses, *Am. J. Optom.*, *75*(3):496–499, 1973.

Browne, R. K., Anderson, A. N., Charvez, B. W., and Azzarello, R. J.: Ophthalmic response to chlorhexidine digluconate in rabbits, *Toxicol. Appl. Pharmacol.*, *32*:621, 1975.

Browne, R. K., Cureton, G. L., Hall, N. C., and Lauck, D. E.: Development and performance of a triple purpose contact lens solution, *see* Cureton, G. L., *J. Am. Optom. Assoc.*, *46*(3):259–267, 1975.

Bruner, B., and Piper, V. M.: Soft lens chemical disinfection, *Cont. Lens Forum*, *3*(10):27–32, 1978.

Bultman, A. T., McEachern, C. L., Cannon, W. M.: Handling your soft contact lens patients, *see* McEachern, C. L., *Optom. Weekly*, *67*(39):1048–1054, 1976.

Burstein, N.: Preservative cytotoxic threshold for benzalkonium chloride and chlorhexidine digluconate in cat and rabbit corneas, *Invest. Ophthalmol.*, *19*(3):308–313, 1980.

Callender, M.: A comparison of soflens (polymacon) wearer sensitivity to thermal or cold disinfecting systems, *Cont. Lens J.*, *7*(3):2, 1978.

Callender, M., and Lutzi, D.: Comparing the clinical findings of soflens wearers using thermal and cold disinfecting procedures, *Int. Cont. Lens Clin.*, *5*(3):46, 1978.

Callender, M., and Lutzi, D.: The incidence of adverse ocular reactions among soft contact lens wearers using chemical disinfection procedures, *Can. J. Optom.*, *41*(3):138–140, 1979.

Cannon, W. M.: A storage and aseptic technique for tweezer, *Int. Cont. Lens Clin.*, *3*(3):71–72, 1976.

Chang, F. W.: The possible adverse effects of over-the-counter medications on the contact lens wearer, *J. Am. Optom. Assoc.*, *48*(3):319, 1977.

Charles, M. A.: Techniques for the isolation of micro-organisms from contact lenses, *J. Am. Optom. Assoc.*, *43*(6):661–662, 1972.

Charles, M. A.: A test system for evaluating bactericidal activity of hydrogel lens solutions, *Contacto*, *18*(5):5–10, 1974.

Cureton, G. L.: New perspectives on solutions for hard and soft contact lenses, *Man. Optom. Int.*, *26*(10):503–511, 1973.

Cureton, G. L., and Sibley, M. J.: Soft contact lens solutions: past, present and future, *J. Am. Optom. Assoc.*, *45*(3):285–291, 1974.

Dabezies, O. H., Jr.: Soft contact lens hygiene, *Cont. Intraoc. Lens Med. J.*, *1*(1–2):103–108, 1975.

Dallos, J., and Houghes, W. H.: Sterilization of hydrophilic contact lenses, *Br. J. Ophthalmol.*, *56*(2):114–119, 1972.

Davies, D. J. G.: Agents as preservative in eyedrops and contact lens solutions, *J. Appl. Bact.*, *44*:19, 1978.

Davies, M. S., Ruben, M., and Trodd, C.: Experiences with soft lenses, *Contact Lens*, *3*(7):42–44, 1972.

De Brabander, J.: Cleaning and disinfecting of hydrophilic contact lenses, *The Optician*, *174*(4513):

29, 1977.

Dixon, J. M., and Winkler, C. H.: Bacteriology of the eye, III. A. Effect of contact lenses on normal flora. B. Flora of the contact lens case, *Arch. Ophthalmol.*, 72(6):817–819, 1974.

Dixon, W. S., Penner, J. L., Jackson, D.: Inhibition of pseudomonas strains in two soft contact lens soaking solutions, *Can. J. Ophthalmol.*, 11(4): 323–326, 1976.

Dyer, J. A., Feldman, G. L., and Black, C. J.: A lubricating solution for flexible contact lenses: a preliminary report, *Cont. Lens J.*, 7(2):27–29, 1973.

Eriksen, S.: Cleaning hydrophilic contact lenses: an overview, *Cont. Lens J.*, 9(2):13–20, 1975.

Eriksen, S.: The storage of hydrophilic lenses. Criteria and test models for solution testing, *Cont. Lens J.*, 5(7):11–14, 1976.

Eriksen, S.: A rational comparison of heat vs. cold disinfection of hydrophilic lenses, *Cont. Lens J.*, 7(4):18, 1978.

Eriksen, S.: Heat compared with cold disinfection of hydrophilic lenses, *The Optician*, 176(4551):10, 1978.

Fatt, H. V.: Chemical disinfection of soft contact lenses: is it safe? *The Optician*, 176(4556):18, 1978.

Feldman, G. L.: The soft lens situation: solutions, sterilization and contamination, *Contacto*, 17(4): 8–32, 1973.

Feldman, G. L., and Bailey, W. R.: Clinical experiences with chemical vs. thermal disinfection of hydrophilic lenses, *Cont. Lens J.*, 8(2):17–20, 1974.

Feldman, G. L., Dyer, J. A., and Black, C. J.: A lubricating solution for flexible contact lenses: a preliminary report, *Cont. Lens. Soc. Am. J.*, 7(2):27–29, 1973.

Fichman, S. H.: Consideration of a soft lens chemical disinfecting solution under field conditions, *Can. J. Ophthalmol.*, 10(1):51–55, 1975.

Filppi, J. A., Pfister, R. M., and Hill, R. M.: Penetration of hydrophilic contact lenses by aspergillus fumagatus, *Am. J. Optom. Arch. Am. Acad. Optom.*, 50(7):553–557, 1973.

Fowler, S., and Allansmith, M. R.: Evolution of soft contact lens coatings, *Arch. Ophthalmol.*, 98:95, 1980.

Fowler, S., Greiner, J. V., and Allansmith, M. R.: Attachment of bacteria to soft contact lenses, *Arch. Ophthalmol.*, 97(4):659, 1979.

Freedman, H., and Suear, J.: Pseudomonas keratitis

following cosmetic soft lens wear, *Cont. Lens J.*, 10(1):21–25, 1976.

Freiberg, J.: Deposition of calcium carbonate and calcium phosphate on hydrophilic contact lenses, *Int. Cont. Lens Clin.*, 4(3):63, 1977.

Galin, M., and Turkish, L.: Sodium hydroxide sterilization of intraocular lenses, *Am. J. Ophthalmol.*, 88:560–564, 1979.

Ganju, S. N.: Antimicrobial efficiency of preservatives in sterile pharmaceuticals, *The Ophthalmic Optician*, 17(22):838, 1977.

Ganju, S. N., and Cordrey, P.: U. V. spectrophotometry study of hydrophilic lenses with new cleaning agent, *Cont. Lens J.*, 5(1):8–14, 1974.

Ganju, S. N., and Cordrey, P.: The physical contamination of hydrophilic contact lenses and their restoration, *The Optician*, 170(4398):19–25, 1975.

Ganju, S. N., and Cordrey, P.: A study of deposits on extended wear soft contact lenses made from sauflon 85+, *The Optician*, 173(4466):8–16, 1977.

Ganju, S. N., and Cordrey, P.: Absorbance studies on sauflon extended wear lenses, *Dis. Optom.*, 29(18):46–49, 1977.

Ganju, S. N., and Cordrey, P.: Control of contact lenses and contact lens solutions, *Ophthalmic Optician*, 18(24):92, 1978.

Gasset, A.: Benzalkonium chloride toxicity to the human cornea, *Am. J. Ophthalmol.*, 84(2):169, 1977.

Gasset, A., Mattingly, T. P., and Hood, I.: Source of fungus contamination of hydrophilic soft contact lenses, *Ann. Ophthalmol*, 11(a):1295, Sept., 1979.

Gasset, A. R., Ishi, Y., Kaufman, H. E., and Miller, T.: Cytotoxicity of ophthalmic preservatives, *Am. J. Ophthalmol.*, 78(1):98–105, 1974.

Gasset, A. R., Lobo, L., and Houde, W.: Spot formation and other abnormalities in hydrogel contact lenses, *Int. Cont. Lens Clin.*, 2(2):64–68, 1975.

Gasset, A. R., Ramer, R. A., and Katzin, D.: Hydrogen peroxide sterilization of hydrophilic contact lens, *Arch. Ophthalmol.*, 93(6):412–415, 1975.

Gellman, M., Nakauchi, S., and Kimmel, E.: Clinical study of hydrophilic contact lens cleaning solutions, *Opt. J. Rev. Optom.*, 113(8):50–56, 1976.

Gold, R. M., and Orenstein, J.: Surfactant cleaners vs. the enzyme cleaner, *Cont. Lens Forum*, 5(1):39, 1980.

Green, H.: The adverse effect of drugs on the

eyes, *The Optician*, *170*(*4389*):19–20, 1975.

Greene, T.: Allergic reaction to soft lens solution preservatives, *Rev. Opt.*, *115*(*12*):14, 1978.

Grosvenor, T. et al.: Soft contact lens bacteriological study: a progress report, *Can. J. Optom.*, *34*(*1*): 11–18, 1972.

Gruber, E.: What's new with the soflens (polymacon) contact lens and accessories 1975, *Cont. Intraoc. Lens Med. J.*, *3*(*1*):608, 1977.

Guthrie, J. W.: An investigation of the chemical contact lens problem, *J. Occ. Med.*, *17*(*3*):163–166, 1975.

Herbst, R. W.: Herellea corneal ulcer associated with the use of soft contact lenses, *Br. J. Oph-thalmol.*,*56*(*11*):848–850, 1972.

Highgate, D.: Physical properties of solutions for hard and soft contact lenses, *The Optician*, *167*(*4329*): 2–25, 1974.

Hill, R.: To pasteurize, sanitize, asepticize, steril-ize . . . or just disinfect?, *Int. Cont. Lens Clin.*, *4*(*3*):39, 1977.

Hill, R. M., and Young, B. H.: Ophthalmological solutions part I – pH and buffer capacity, *J. Am. Optom. Assoc.*, *44*(*3*):263–270, 1973.

Holden, B. A., Contact lens care and maintenance, *Austr. J. Optom.*, *56*(*2*):57–62, 1973.

Holden, B. A., and Markides, A. J.: On the desira-bility and efficacy of chemical "sterilization" of hydrophilic contact lenses, *Austr. J. Optom.*, *54*(*10*):325–336, 1971.

Holden, B. A., and Markides, A. J.: On the desira-bility and efficacy of chemical "sterilization" of hydrophilic contact lenses – Part 1, *Precision-Cosmet. Digest*, *12*(*1*):1–6, 1972.

Holden, B. A., and Markides, A. J.: On the desira-bility and efficacy of chemical "sterilization" of hydrophilic contact lenses – Part 2, *Precision-Cosmet. Digest*, *12*(*2*):1–4, 1972.

Hubbard, W.: Chlorhexidine uptake and release during simulated lens maintenance conditions a preliminary study, *Contact Lens*, *9*(*2*):39–42, 1975.

Inns, H. D.: The septicon system, *Can. J. Optom.*, *41*(*3*):144–146, 1979.

Iverson, G.: Soft lenses: how long a life expectan-cy?, *Cont. Lens Forum*, *1*(*3*):55–63, 1976.

Janoff, L. E.: The effective disinfection of soft con-tact lenses using hydrogen peroxide, *The Opti-cian*, *177*:24, 1979.

Johnson, J., Nygren, B., and Sjogren, E.: Disin-fection of soft contact lenses in liquid – a method

that has been questioned, *Cont. Lens J.*, *6*(*5*):3, 1978.

Josephson, J.: The "multi-purge procedure" and its application for hydrophilic lens wearers uti-lizing preserved solutions, *J. Am. Optom. Assoc.*, *49*(*3*):280–281, 1978.

Karageozian, H. L., Walden, F., and Boghosian, M. P.: Cleaning soft contact lenses, *Int. Cont. Lens Clin.*, *3*(*2*):78–86, 1976.

Kaspar, H. H.: Contact lens solutions binding char-acteristics and microbiological effectiveness of preservatives, *J. Optom. (New Zealand)*, p. 6, 1975.

Keates, R. H.: Sonic sterilization of contact lenses, *Am. J. Ophthalmol.*, *66*(*6*):1175–1176, 1968.

Kleist, F. D.: How effective are soft lens cleaners? *Rev. Opt.*, *115*(*4*):43, 1978.

Kline, L. N., and DeLuca, T. J.: Thermal vs. chem-ical disinfection, *Cont. Lens Forum*, *4*(*2*):28, 1979.

Knoll, H. A.: Microbiology and hydrophilic con-tact lenses, *Am. J. Opt. Arch. Am. Acad. Optom.*, *48*(*10*):840–844, 1971.

Kreiner, C.: Why are questions asked about chlor-hexidine? *The Optician*, Sept. 7, 1979, pp. 29–31.

Krezanoski, J. Z.: The significance of cleaning hydrophilic contact lens, *J. Am. Optom. Assoc.*, *43*(*3*):305–307, 1972.

Krezanoski, J. Z.: Pharmaceutical aspects of clean-ing and sterilizing flexible contact lenses, *The Ophthalmic Optician*, *12*(*20*):1035–1037, 1972.

Krezanoski, J. Z.: Diversos aspects farmaceuticos de limpieza y esterilizacion de lentes de con-tact flexibles, *Revista de la Sociedad Mexicana de Optometria*, *1*(*1*):15–22, 1972.

Krezanoski, J. Z.: Water and the care of soft con-tact lenses, *Int. Cont. Lens Clin.*, *2*(*1*):48–55, 1975.

Krezanoski, J. Z.: New hydrophilic contact lenses and their pharmaceutical accessories, *J. Am. Pharm. Assoc.*, *15*(*10*):578–580, 1975.

Larke, J. R.: Storage of hydrophilic lenses, *The Ophthalmic Optician*, *7*(*14*):751, 1967.

Lieblein, J.: How important is enzymatic cleaning? An in-office evaluation, *Int. Cont. Lens Clin.*, *6*(*3*):80–82, 1979.

Litvin, M. W.: The cleaning of soft contact lenses, *The Optician*, *170*(*4398*):31–32, 1975.

Lo Cascio, G.: Soft contact lens care, *Contacto*, *21*(*4*):34–36, 1977.

Loran, D. F. C.: Surface corrosion of hydrogel contact lenses, *Contact Lens*, *4*(*4*):3–8, 1973.

Lowther, G. E.: Effectiveness of an enzyme in

removing deposits from hydrophilic lenses, *Am. J. Optom. Physiol. Optics*, *54*(*2*):76–84, 1977.

MacKeen, D. L.: The safety and efficacy of chemical disinfection with hydrophilic gel contact lenses, *Cont. Lens J.*, *8*(*3*):17–21, 1974.

MacKeen, G. D., and Bulle, K.: Buffers and preservatives in contact lens solutions, *Contacto*, *21*(*6*):33–36, 1977.

Milauskas, A. T.: *Pseudomonas aeruginosa* contamination of hydrophilic contact lenses and solutions, *Trans. Am. Acad. Ophthalmol. Otolaryngol.*, *76*(*2*):511–516, 1972.

Moore, R., Satterberg, L. B., and Weiss, S.: Novel temperature-dependent model for examining soilant deposition deterrent action. I. Preserved thermal disinfecting solutions, *Contacto*, *24*(*2*): 23–30, 1980.

Morgan, J. F.: Evaluation of a cleaning agent for hydrophilic contact lenses, *Can. J. Ophthalmol.*, *10*(*2*):214–217, 1975.

Morgan, J. F. et al.: Blood constituents and hydrophilic lens coating, *Cont. Lens Forum*, *2*(*8*):50–51, 1977.

Morrison, R. J. et al.: The effectivity of hygiene procedures upon soft contact lens material, *Contacto*, *17*(*1*):23–27, 1973.

Pearson, R. M.: Hygienic care of soft contact lenses, *Contact Lens*, *4*(*8*):8–11, 1974.

Pedersen, N. B.: Allergy to chemical solutions for soft contact lenses, *Lancet*, *2*(*7999*):1363, 1976.

Penner, J. L., Jackson, D., and Dixon, W. S.: Inhibition of pseudomonas strains in two soft contact lens soaking solutions, *Can. J. Ophthalmol.*, *11*(*4*):323–326, 1976.

Phares, R. E.: Microbiology and hygienic care of hydrophilic lenses, *Contacto*, *16*(*3*):10–12, 1972.

Tragakis, M. P., Brown, S. I., and Pearce, D. B.: Bacteriologic studies of contamination with soft contact lenses, *Am. J. Ophthalmol.*, *75*(*3*):496–499, 1973.

Trager, S. Y.: Solutions for soft lenses, *Manufacturing Optics International*, *25*(*10*):403–405, 1972.

Chapter 22

SYMPTOMATOLOGY AND AFTERCARE

ADAPTIVE AND FOLLOW-UP CARE

The soft contact lens wearer should receive the same care and attention given to the hard lens wearer, and with the same frequency. The ease with which this lens is fitted has caused some to neglect the follow-up aspect of lens care.

After the initial lenses have been dispensed, the patient should be allowed to build wearing time to achieve maximum daytime wear of fourteen to eighteen hours. Adaptation is usually successfully completed during the first two weeks after dispensing. Some patients appear to adapt in only a few days, but some subclinical changes may still continue, which indicates that adaptation is not complete.

The patient should return for examinations at approximately the following times after the beginning of lens wear: three days, one week, two weeks, and one month. Depending upon the patient's progress, additional examinations should then be conducted at least on a semiannual basis.

EXAMINATION PROCEDURE

The following tests should be performed at each examination:

1. Visual acuity
2. Refraction over contact lenses
3. External observation with white light
4. Biomicroscopy with lenses
5. Biomicroscopy without lenses
6. Biomicroscopy with fluorescein

The following tests need not be performed at every visit:

1. Keratometry
2. Refraction without contact lenses
3. Ophthalmoscopy
4. Inspect contact lenses

SLIT-LAMP BIOMICROSCOPE EXAMINATION

When the patient has not been wearing contact lenses prior to the examination, the slit-lamp examination should be done using the following procedure:

A drop of sodium fluorescein is instilled in each eye in the normal manner, and the external examination is completed as follows:

Bulbar Conjunctiva

Using a parallelepiped and direct and indirect focal illumination, the temporal, inferior, nasal, and superior bulbar conjunctiva are examined for any abnormalities, including injection, thickening, or discoloration of tissue, and staining with fluorescein.

The injection is graded according to the following criteria: Grade 0, no injection, conjunctiva nearly white; Grade 1, mild injection in localized area; Grade 2, moderate, more diffuse injection; and Grade 3, severe injection.

If no other abnormalities are present, 0 is recorded. If any abnormalities are noted in any area of the conjunctiva, it is graded: Grade 1, slight; Grade 2, moderate; Grade 3, severe. All abnormalities should be fully described.

Palpebral Conjunctiva

The inferior and superior palpebral conjunctiva should be scanned for any abnormality, including injection, as performed for the bulbar conjunctiva (*see* preceding section).

The superior and inferior palpebral conjunctivas are examined for the presence of follicles, which are basically lymphoid hyperplasias with secondary vascularization. The lower lid is pulled down, and the palpebral conjunctiva is examined with a 2 to 3 mm. parallelepiped white beam.

The patient is told to gaze downwards, and the upper lid is gently everted using a clean cotton swab. The superior palpebral conjunctiva is examined with a 2 to 3 mm. wide beam of white light. The presence or absence of follicles is noted and graded: Grade 0, no follicles; Grade 1, few, slightly raised; Grade 2, few, moderately raised; Grade 3, large, raised follicles involving the complete conjunctiva.

The superior and inferior palpebral conjunctivas are also examined for the presence of papillary hypertrophy (or in severe cases, giant papillary conjunctivitis), which consists of folds or projections covered by hyperplastic epithelium and containing an arc of vessels surrounded by edematous subepithelial tissue infiltrate with chronic inflammatory cells—basically a vascular response with sec-

ondary lymphocyte and plasma cell infiltration.

The upper and lower palpebral conjunctivas are inspected as in the previous procedures used for the detection of follicles. The papillae are graded as follows: Grade 0, devoid of papillae and a smooth surface; Grade 1, small, 0.2 to 0.4 mm., elevated papillae; Grade 2, 0.4 to 0.8 mm. papillae; Grade 3, 1 mm. or greater over complete surface. The Grade 3 condition is usually accompanied by stringy or sheetlike mucoid exudates and mild itching.

Cornea

Using a parallelepiped and direct, indirect, and retroillumination, the cornea is scanned for any staining with fluorescein, signs of abnormalities, or edema.

Edema

Using direct focal illumination and a parallelepiped with at least 16× magnification, observe the cornea for any sign of reduced transparency and edema in the stroma and epithelium.

Use indirect illumination to observe edema. Use a small thin parallelepiped and focus upon the central epithelium. Instead of observing the area in the beam itself, observe the area of cornea illuminated by the light reflected off the iris. If edema is present, the area will look unclear and rough—a showerglass appearance.

Grade the edema using the following scale: Grade 0, no edema; Grade 1, just detectable haziness; Grade 2, moderate haziness, diffuse; and Grade 3, severe haziness indicating gross edema. For edema of Grades 1 to 3, describe the location.

Staining

With the blue filter, scan the cornea in a clockwise fashion using a parallelepiped and direct focal illumination. Note any staining, and grade according to the following criteria: Grade 0, no staining; Grade 1, very light pinpoint staining, very superficial; Grade 2, diffuse pinpoint staining and moderate stipple staining; Grade 3, heavy stippling, coalescing into areas of dense, deeper staining. If Grades 1, 2, or 3 are present, note the location using a drawing.

Striae

Observe the cornea for striae (folds in Descemet's membrane or the posterior stroma) using focal illumination and indirect retroillumination with at least 16× magnification. The lines usually orient vertically, but may run obliquely. Use a parallelepiped and scan back and forth. Striae can be counted and recorded as follows: if the stria is less than 1 mm. in length, it is counted as 0.5; if it is longer than 1 mm. it is counted as 1.0. The total number of striae using this counting procedure is recorded.

Scarring

Observe the cornea for scarring using direct focal illumination, indirect, and retroillumination with at least 16× magnification. Using a parallelpiped and optic section as necessary, scan back and forth looking for any corneal scars. Grade as follows: Grade 0, no scarring; Grade 1, light scarring (nebular—most light is transmitted); Grade 2, moderate scarring (macular—some light passed through); Grade 3, severe scarring (leucoma—no light transmitted through affected area).

Neovascularization

Observe the cornea for neovascularization using direct focal, indirect, and retroillumin-ation with at least ×16 magnification. Using a parallelepiped and optic section as necessary, scan back and forth, looking for any ingrowth of vessels into the cornea. The amount of neovascularization, the location, and depth of new vessels should be recorded. The amount is recorded in millimeters, always using the figure that corresponds to the greatest advance of infiltration. The location is recorded by clock meridian. If more than one location exists with interrupted normal areas, describe it fully. The depth is recorded as follows: Depth 1, epithelial and anterior stromal layers; Depth 2, midstromal; Depth 3, posterior stroma and endothelium.

Endothelium

Observe the endothelium with the same illumination techniques as described above, checking for any abnormalities. Record and grade: Grade 0, no abnormalities; Grade 1, minor; Grade 2, moderate; Grade 3, severe. Describe any abnormalities fully.

When the patient is wearing contact lenses upon arrival for the examination, the following examination should be performed.

1. The lens is examined using direct and indirect illumination for the presence of coating or defects.

2. As soon as possible after lens removal, the corneas are examined with retroillumin-ation to observe edema of the corneas as has been previously described.

3. The remainder of the procedure for examination of the cornea and conjunctiva as already described is performed on both the right and left eyes.

ADVERSE RESPONSES

If adverse responses occur, corrective procedures should be taken to alleviate the problem. These procedures may involve any of the following:

1. Exchanging the lens for another
2. Discontinuing lens wear for a short period of time
3. Permanently discontinuing lens wear

TABLE 22.1
LEVEL ONE ADVERSE RESPONSE

1. Corneal edema of less than grade 2. This may be observed as diffuse corneal clouding on slit-lamp biomicroscopy using indirect illumination.
2. Epithelial staining (central or limbal), grade 2.
3. Spectacle blur. Visual acuity with maximum subjective refraction of no more than 10 percent (Snell-Sterling visual efficiency scale) poorer than baseline corrected visual acuity.
4. Papillary and bulbar hypertrophy or follicles of less than grade 2.
5. Corneal striae: one to four striae.

Patients who exhibit adverse responses can be categorized at three levels. Depending upon the level of the adverse response, the patient will either be monitored by extra examination visits, given a lens change, or referred for medical care.

LEVEL ONE ADVERSE RESPONSES

Level one adverse responses are of minimum consequence, as they are commonly seen as part of the adaptive response to contact lens wear. They are listed in Table 22.1. When any of these responses are observed, the fitter should determine whether such responses are within the expected adaptation range or whether a change in the contact lens is needed. If an adverse response at level 1 is seen after the adaptation period, it should be managed in the same way.

LEVEL TWO ADVERSE RESPONSES

The second level of adverse response indicates a more severe reaction to lens wear and requires that the lens be changed. The grading system for these adverse responses is shown in Table 22.2. When the adverse response is diagnosed as level 2, contact lens wear is first discontinued, if necessary, until the eye has returned to normal. Additional examinations should be scheduled for the patient during the recovery process. When the adverse response has subsided, the patient can be refitted with a new lens and begin the adaptive phase again.

TABLE 22.2
LEVEL TWO ADVERSE RESPONSE

1. Corneal edema greater than or equal to grade 2, but less than grade 3.
2. Epithelial staining (central or limbal) of greater than or equal to grade 2, but less than grade 3.
3. Spectacle blur: visual acuity with maximum subjective refraction of 10 to 30 percent (Snell-Sterling visual efficiency scale) poorer than baseline corrected visual acuity.
4. Papillary and bulbar hypertrophy or follicles of greater than or equal to grade 3.
5. Corneal striae: four or more.
6. Corneal neovascularization: up to 1 mm. of vessel growth.
7. Endothelial changes of less than or equal to grade 1.
8. Minor ocular infection (conjunctivitis, keratitis, etc.).

LEVEL THREE ADVERSE RESPONSES

This constitutes extreme responses from lens wear, such as corneal abrasion, corneal infection, or other ocular involvement. Patients should be referred for immediate ophthalmological consultation and care.

SYMPTOMS AND SIGNS

A diagnosis of the patient's problem is based upon a careful evaluation of the patient's symptoms and the interpretation of various abnormal signs. Just as with hard contact lens wearers, patient symptoms generally may be categorized as visual problems or discomfort. In addition, there are various signs of adverse ocular effects.

Symptoms of Adverse Effects

Visual Symptoms

Visual acuity must remain at normal levels both during contact lens wear and when lenses are removed (spectacle acuity). Reductions in visual acuity with contact lenses may result from changes in the physical properties of the lens and/or alterations in the cornea. Loss of visual acuity with spectacles would suggest an ocular complication. It is therefore important to evaluate visual acuity both during contact lens wear and with best spectacle correction.

The patient may report that vision is reduced at all times or that there is intermittent blurring. Constant reduced vision during the adaptive phase is generally caused by an improper refractive correction or the presence of significant residual astigmatism. These may be differentiated by an overrefraction, and corrective measures may be taken. If the reduced vision cannot be explained on this basis, then the optical quality of the lens should be suspect. Gel lenses occasionally have reduced optical quality, which is very difficult to detect when the lens is off the eye. Trying a second lens on the patient may provide the most convenient diagnostic procedure. If the vision is improved immediately, then the original lens should be returned for replacement.

Reduced vision may also be caused by a lens that has changed its base curve, usually by steepening. This occasionally occurs in lathe-cut gel lenses as a consequence of strain remaining in the lens from poor manufacturing technique.

Another cause of reduced vision may be lenses that have been inverted. Remove the lens from the patient's eye and check its orientation using the "taco test" (*See* Figure 21.2).

Lenses that have been switched typically produce reduced vision in one eye. This is generally the eye with the least plus correction initially.

After the lenses have been worn for several months, reduced vision, which was not present previously, is generally caused either by a change in the base curve of the lens or by the accumulation of lens deposits. The latter problem may be detected most easily during slit-lamp examination while the lenses are being worn.

Occasionally, vision may become blurred under conditions of a dry environment. This may occur in areas of low humidity or as a consequence of exposure to hair dryers or other warm, dry air flow. Patients with dry eye conditions may also experience this problem.

Vision that blurs intermittently is usually caused by a lens that is too loose. This should be diagnosed from the external examination but may be aided by careful observation by the patient during the visual acuity testing. Increased blurring of the visual acuity target immediately after blinking is generally diagnostic of a lens that is fitted too loose.

Discomfort

Discomfort with gel lenses is generally related to lenses that are too loose. The problem is accentuated if the lens is of the smaller type. Occasionally, a lathe-cut lens may have an edge that is too thick, and this contributes to a mild discomfort. Small or

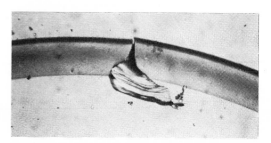

Figure 22.3. A lens that was caught in the carrying case cap while replacing the cap.

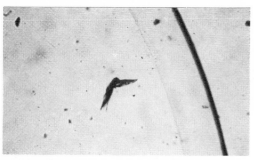

Figure 22.1. Sharp objects such as fingernails or poorly designed cases can puncture a lens.

large tears may occur in the lens edge or punctures may occur anywhere on the lens without the patient's knowledge, except for discomfort (Figures 22.1 to 22.3).

Burning and similar symptoms that occur immediately after lens insertion are generally related to one of the solutions used with lens care. Some patients show sensitivity or an allergic reaction to one of the various compounds in the solution. Burning may also occur as the result of poor hygiene, failure to remove all soap when washing the hands, or external noxious substances such as toxic fumes or poor air conditioners. A hypertonic saline solution or the accumulation of salt at the neck of the solution bottle may lead to temporary discomfort.

Photophobia

For the average patient, photophobia is not a significant problem, as it is with the hard contact lens wearer. When present, this symptom may indicate a low grade corneal infection or irritation from a lens that is loose or that has a bad edge.

Lens Ejection

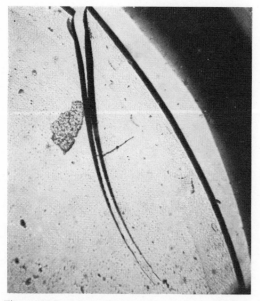

Figure 22.2. A lens that has been mishandled; it has been pried off the carrying case dome while in a dehydrated condition.

Under normal circumstances, it is rare to have gel lenses involuntarily ejected from the eyes, as occurs with hard corneal lenses. However, with a dry eye, sometimes the edges curl up sufficiently to allow ejection of the lens by the lid. Another cause of accidental ejection is an inside out lens.

Signs of Adverse Effects

The Red Eye

Five common causes of the red eye must be differentiated:

1. Infection
2. Corneal edema
3. Conjunctival compression
4. Chemical sensitivity
5. Allergy

CORNEAL INFECTION. Fortunately, true corneal infection is rare in soft contact lens wearers. However, cases of infection have been reported, which are usually associated with poor hygiene. If there is evidence of a viral infection, namely, corneal infiltrates and punctate staining, the lenses should be removed and appropriate treatment instigated. When the lenses are worn once again, the patient who is using a cold disinfection system should probably be switched to a heating system to avoid reinfection. There is some evidence that cold disinfecting systems are less effective against viruses than are hot systems.

CORNEAL EDEMA. In gel lens wearers a generalized epithelial edema occasionally occurs.[2] This edema cannot be detected by methods ordinarily used to find edema in a hard contact lens wearer.[3] This occurs because the edema is not confined to the central region of the cornea as occurs with a hard contact lens wearer, but instead the edema is spread uniformly throughout the corneal area (Figures 22.4 and 22.5).[4]

Many early investigators felt that no edema occurred in the cornea at all. However, several studies have shown that the edema is present to nearly the same degree as occurs for hard lenses and at about the same incidence. However, the edema is not detectable

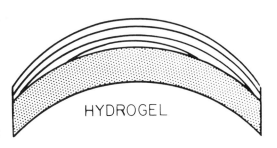

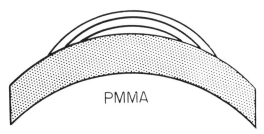

Figure 22.4. Edema in gel lens wearer is spread throughout the cornea, whereas P.M.M.A. lens edema is confined to the center.

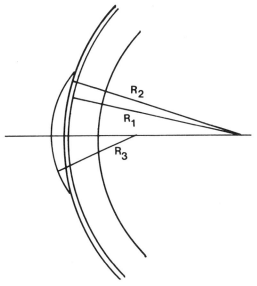

Figure 22.5. Gel lens edema does not produce a significant change in corneal radius: R_1 normal radius, R_2 radius from gel-induced edema, R_3 radius from hard lens-induced edema.

clinically by the usual techniques until swelling reaches about 6 percent. At this level, there are a number of clinical signs that allow the edema to be detected.

The earliest clinical clue to epithelial edema is direct observation with the biomicroscope. The edema can be detected by a technique in which the slit-lamp beam is directed at the limbal region to produce sclerotic scatter, while the microscope is directed at the epithelial layer (Figure 22.6). It is necessary to use magnification above $25 \times$ to achieve this. This edema may also be observed by indirect illumination or by retro-illumination.

When the epithelial edema reaches 8 to 10 percent, it is usually accompanied by circumcorneal injection.

The edema is not visible by the usual hard contact lens detection technique of sclerotic scatter and observation without magnification. This is because the border, which is ordinarily present to identify the edema of the hard lens wearer, is absent in the soft lens wearer. When the edema reaches a very advanced point, it may be detected by this method and has the appearance of a generalized haze. However, the absence of a border makes it very difficult to make a positive diagnosis.

When corneal edema reaches 6 to 8 percent, vertical striae begin to appear at the level of Descemet's membrane (Figure 22.7). These striae were first recognized by Sarver[5] as a separate entity in soft lens wear, but later their association with edema became apparent. As the edema increases, the number and size of the striae increase proportionately.

Vertical striae have been reproduced in subjects who did not wear contact lenses by exposing the cornea to 100 percent nitrogen (Figure 22.8).[6] The striae were again directly related to the amount of corneal edema, and it was assumed that their origin was a deficiency of the atmospheric oxygen supply. Further support for this hypothesis was derived from an experiment in which corneal striae were first produced by having subjects wear soft contact lenses and then making the striae

disappear by the application of hyperbaric oxygen while the lenses were worn. The striae could be made to appear, or to disappear, by simply controlling the oxygen concentration to the eye.

Vertical striae appear at the level of Descemet's membrane, although with the biomicroscope they may be localized in the deep stroma. They may be seen clinically at about the same time as the first detection of corneal edema. For some observers it is much easier to detect the vertical striae than to observe corneal edema, and hence, their appearance serves as a diagnostic sign of corneal edema. Furthermore, since vertical striae do not occur until corneal swelling reaches the 6 to 8 percent level, they indicate that significant edema has occurred, and corrective measures should be taken for its alleviation.

Vertical corneal striae are detected with the biomicroscope using a narrow parallelepiped.[7] The slit-lamp beam should be directed to the central area of the cornea, and a focusing adjustment made to observe the corneal surface (Figure 22.9). The biomicroscope is then moved forward until the portion of the beam intersecting the endothelium is in focus. The joystick is then moved from side to side so that the entire pupil area may be examined. Vertical corneal striae nearly always appear first in the central corneal area. In some cases, they must be differentiated from large nerve fibers. This is generally found to be a simple diagnosis. The nerve fibers can usually be followed all the way to the corneal periphery, whereas vertical striae extend 1 to 6 mm. and then terminate. Although vertical corneal striae may tend to bifurcate occasionally, the angle at division is very small compared to that found in most nerve fibers.

Tight Lens Relation to Edema. Actually, two distinct meanings are commonly applied to tight lens, and both are often used clinically without differentiation.[8] Usually when one says tight lens, it means a lens that does not

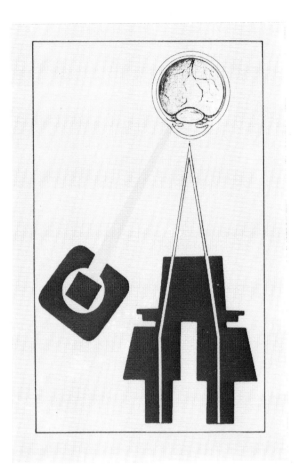

Figure 22.6a. Gel lens edema detection. The slit-lamp beam is directed at the limbus while the biomicroscope is directed at the epithelial layer.

move or, at the most, moves very little; in this sense, tight lens refers to the appearance of the lens fit. However, tight lens may also be used to describe a fitting relationship in which there is inadequate pumping of tears between the lens and cornea, detectable clinically only by its aftermath of corneal edema.

It is commonly assumed that a lens with inadequate movement also does not pump tears adequately. This association comes primarily from our hard lens experience, where it does indeed appear to be true (although it is not as closely related as some would have us believe). Some research shows that a hard lens that has a good fit can be made to move less by increasing the lens diameter or decreasing the radius of one of the posterior lens curves. Other evidence indicates that these same modifications which tend to reduce the hard lens movement also tend to reduce the lens tear pumping and increase the likelihood of corneal edema.

Soft contact lenses share many of the fitting relationships of hard contact lenses. A decrease in the base curve radius or an increase in the lens diameter will usually produce less lens movement. Modifications that reduce movement of a soft lens are also

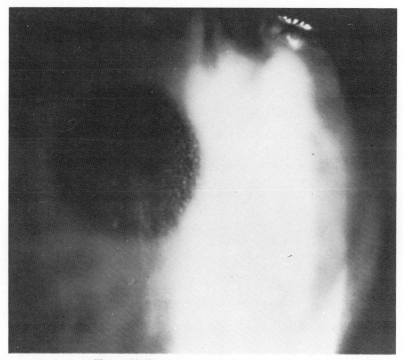

Figure 22.6b. Appearance of gel lens edema

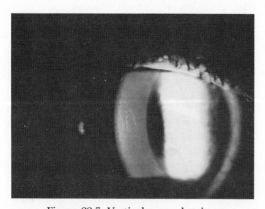

Figure 22.7. Vertical corneal striae.

assumed to reduce the lens tear pumping and increase the likelihood of corneal edema. Consequently, the usual recommendation is to change to a smaller or flatter lens to increase the lens tear pump. Measurements of the relationship between the base curve and edema in lathe-cut and spin-cast lenses have given the same results. Figure 22.10 shows a typical response for one subject, the corneal edema produced by wearing a series of AOSoft contact lenses on an alternating basis for a period of several months. Regardless of the base curve, the amount of edema produced remained essentially the same and was reduced only when the subject was switched to an ultrathin lens.

Mertz and his co-workers conducted a series of studies with the Bausch & Lomb Soflens.[9] They found that the only lens variable which had significant influence on the production of corneal edema was the lens thickness. The result was predictable on theoretical grounds, in that the amount of oxygen transmitted through a permeable material is always a function of its thickness.

The results obtained in these experiments

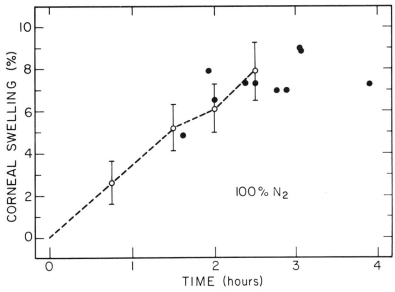

Figure 22.8. Change in corneal thickness for ten subjects. Vertical bars represent standard deviation. Individual points indicate time and corneal swelling when striae were first noted.

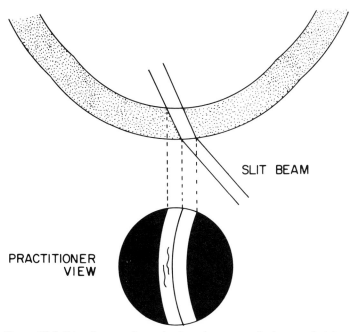

Figure 22.9. Biomicroscopic method to observe vertical corneal striae.

were in fact predicted by Hayashi and Fatt in 1976.[10] By a series of calculations, they showed that a soft contact lens should have only a fraction of the pumping efficiency of a hard lens and that it is probably an insignificant factor in bringing oxygen to the cornea. Because the tear pump is less efficient in a soft lens, oxygen must reach the cornea by passing directly through the lens material.

This prediction was proven by the work of Polse,[11] who measured the rate of pumping of tears under a soft contact lens experimentally. He found that a soft contact lens pumped only about 0.6 to 1.5 percent fresh tears with each blink, whereas a hard lens might pump up to 20 percent. All of this evidence supports the concept that the posterior curve of a soft contact lens has little effect on the amount of corneal edema produced.

The principal parameter of the soft contact lens that determines the amount of corneal edema is the lens thickness. Hence, true edema is an individual response dependent upon the oxygen permeability of the contact lens material, the thickness of the lens worn,

and the oxygen need of the individual cornea. If edema is present, it should be corrected by changing to a lens that provides more oxygen to the cornea either by greater permeability or reduced thickness.

CONJUNCTIVAL COMPRESSION. Conjunctival compression occurs when a lens grips tightly to the cornea in the manner of a suction cup. It is most often produced when a gel lens has either a base curve that is too steep or a diameter which is too large. When this effect is produced, there is minimal or no movement of the lens on the cornea. This effect rarely occurs, however, with ultrathin soft contact lenses. Even though the lens fits steeply and there is essentially no movement, there does not appear to be enough of a suction effect to interfere with blood circulation in the conjunctival vessels.

The conjunctival compression effect may be observed clinically with a slit-lamp bio-

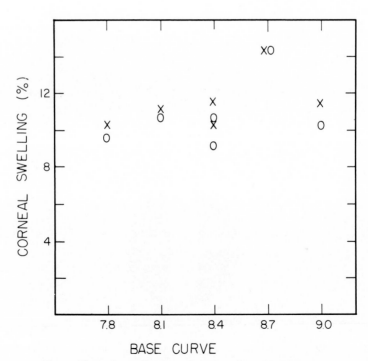

Figure 22.10. Corneal edema from a series of AO lenses.

microscope. Observation of the conjunctival vessels peripheral to the lens edge shows congestion, whereas there is blanching of the vessels immediately inside of the lens edge (Figure 22.11, Plate III). As the lens is moved during a blink, the conjunctival vessels may also be dragged with it. This effect is rarely seen with ultrathin soft contact lenses.

In the early stages, the only evidence of limbal compression by a soft contact lens is the observation of its direct effect upon the circumcorneal conjunctival vessels. At a later stage, there is a more generalized conjunctival injection, which is apparently a reaction to the limbal compression. The appearance of this generalized reaction is indistinguishable from the conjunctival injection that accompanies corneal edema.

It is necessary, then, to differentiate between conjunctival compression and corneal edema. A patient who has conjunctival compression associated with a lens that does not move should have the base curve of the lens flattened to relieve the condition. The alternative is to reduce the lens diameter if it appears to be excessive. This patient may or may not have an associated corneal edema, which must be considered separately. If corneal edema is observed and the lens appears to have adequate movement, it will not relieve the patient's problem simply to change to a flatter base curve. In this situation, the only solution is to switch to a thinner soft lens.

CHEMICAL SENSITIVITY. Almost any of the chemicals that are placed in the contact lens storage solution have the potential to cause ocular irritation, but the greatest problem occurs with the bactericidal agents thimerosal and chlorhexidine.[12] In order to kill the various microorganisms that may contaminate the storage solution, these agents must occur in concentrations which are just below the threshold for corneal irritation. If the concentration were raised slightly, a more effec-

tive germicidal solution would occur, but a much higher incidence of corneal irritation would accompany it. If the concentration of the germicidal agents were reduced, there will be less corneal irritation, but the solution will not be effective as a germicidal agent.

The eye's response to corneal irritation in mild form is conjunctival injection. This generally takes the form of a bulbar conjunctival injection, but the palpebral portion may also be affected. The injection is usually not as severe as that occurring in corneal infection, as only the larger vessels appear to be involved (Figure 22.12, Plate III). The diagnosis is usually made by switching the patient's storage solution to unpreserved saline, after which the signs generally disappear in a few days.

There has been much controversy over the incidence of eye irritation from contact lens storage solutions. Since the concentration of the germicidal agents is greatest in the cold storage solutions, they have generally been considered to produce the highest incidence of irritation. Estimates range from 10 to 50 percent. Probably about 30 percent of all patients experience mild ocular irritation from these solutions, and 10 percent show a moderate reaction.

In view of this, there would appear to be little justification for cold disinfection whenever a heating system can be effectively substituted.

ALLERGIC REACTIONS. True allergic reactions to contact lens storage solutions are rare but do occur. Most cases that are attributed to allergic reactions may in fact be due to chemical sensitivity. When allergic reactions do occur, they are very difficult to diagnose. Attempts to perform standard dermatological testing is time-consuming and inconvenient for the patient. If an allergic reaction is suspected, the patient should be switched to unpreserved saline, which generally will solve the problem.

Abnormal Tear Breakup Time

Occasionally the tear breakup time for a gel lens patient is reduced below ten seconds, indicating an abnormal condition.[13] This most often accompanies the wearing of lenses with coated surfaces and appears to be caused by an abrasive effect of the lens on the cornea. The condition may be alleviated by enzyme cleaning the gel contact lens.

Corneal Infiltrates

Occasionally infiltrates may occur at the peripheral cornea, which appear to have no relationship to any infection.[14] In some cases, the infiltrates have been thought to be due to chemical irritation (Figure 22.13, Plate III). They have also been reported in association with some of the older thicker lenses, which produce excessive compression in the limbal region. The lenses should be removed until the infiltrate is no longer present. An attempt should be made to locate the irritative stimulus and eliminate it.

Neovascularization

True neovascularization is not commonly seen in the cosmetic contact lens patient. The occurrence is more common in aphakic patients (*see* Chapter 27). Neovascularization may appear to have occurred, when in fact the circumcorneal vessels only show excessive engorgement as the result of either conjunctival compression or corneal edema (Figures 22.14 and 22.15, Plate III).[15]

Corneal Staining

The incidence of corneal staining has been reported to be very low. However, it is recognized that many practitioners do not routinely use fluorescein staining on their gel lens patients. Hence, there has been a tendency in some cases for practitioners to overlook the staining unless an additional problem occurs.

Fluorescein staining of the cornea should be made a routine part of the examination. The patient should be instructed at each visit that when he returns he will have a dye placed in the eyes and cannot wear his lenses until one hour after leaving the office. The fluorescein staining is usually done at the end of the examination. There are some types of staining that are pathognomonic of certain soft lens wearing problems.

PERIPHERAL STAIN. It is sometimes noted that an arcuate area of stippled stain occurs near the limbal region (Figure 22.16, Plate IV).[16] This is usually in an inferior or inferior-nasal position but may occur temporally or even superiorly in some cases. This stain almost always is associated with the lens that decenters on the eye and will be found in the corneal area exposed by the decentration. The staining occurs as a result of a drying effect, which may be accentuated by a mechanical trauma of the lens edge.

If a peripheral arcuate stain is allowed to remain on the cornea, it usually increases in severity with time, and over a period of months may lead to corneal breakdown and symptoms of an acute abrasion. At this point, the lens will no longer be tolerated by the patient, and he usually returns for care. The lens must be removed from the eye, and sufficient time allowed for healing to occur. The patient cannot be given the same lens again or else there will be a reoccurrence of the same problem. Another lens must be found that centers better on the eye.

It is advisable to first try another lens having the same specifications. There are sometimes variations in edge configuration or lens curvature that will make one gel lens center better than another. If this approach is not successful, then a lens of another type should be tried. It is not always predictable which lens will produce better centering, although lenses of larger diameter will usually tend to center better. A failure here will dictate that a hard lens must be used.

SCATTERED STIPPLING. Occasionally small

patches or areas of stippling occur over the cornea (Figure 22.17, Plate IV).[17] This is usually associated with a dirty contact lens or one that has been coated with foreign materials from the eye. This problem may be corrected by cleaning the lens thoroughly or by replacing the lens with a new one.

GENERALIZED STIPPLING. A cornea that shows a generalized stippling may indicate an infection or a chemical irritation (Figure 22.18, Plate IV).[17] If the patient is using a chemical disinfection system, this should be eliminated. The patient should be questioned to be sure that the eye has not been exposed to environmental chemicals which could cause this staining. A patient who mistakenly uses a soaking solution designed for hard contact lenses may have this staining.

FOREIGN BODY STAINS. Foreign body stains have much the same general appearance as for a hard contact lens. They may, however, be concentrated over a smaller corneal area because the gel lens moves less.

Corneal Curvature Changes

It is rare to find a significant change in the corneal curvature of a soft lens wearer as measured with a keratometer.[18-26] This is because, even though corneal edema may be present, its uniformity across the cornea causes a nearly insignificant change in corneal radius (*see* Figure 22.5). For the same reason spectacle blur is rarely found in a gel lens patient.

Sticking of Lenses

On very rare occasions a lens adheres to the cornea very tightly. The patient is not aware of any problem until an attempt is made to remove the lens. As the finger is placed on the lens, it is found that it cannot be moved at all.

This condition is only serious if an inept or naïve person attempts to remove the lens. If the lens is forcibly stripped from the cornea, it may do considerable damage to the epithelium (Figure 22.19, Plate IV). The lens should be removed by first irrigating the eye with normal saline solution or having the patient soak the eye with an eyecup filled with saline solution. After the lens has been saturated with saline for about five minutes, it will begin to loosen on the eye and can be removed easily.

This phenomenon is usually considered to be due to a drying of the lens on the eye. It is also thought to occur as a result of a hypotonic hydrating solution. However, the exact cause is not certain.

Giant Papillary Conjunctivitis*

Part of the normal (accepted) symptomatology associated with contact lens wearers has been increased amounts of ocular mucous secretions, itching with lens wear, and an increase in awareness of the lens with duration of lens wear. These symptoms have been universal in that no contact lens type, soft or hard, or variation in design has been spared of such responses.

Such symptomatology may, in a significant number of patients, be related to a syndrome first described by Spring and subsequently by Allansmith et al.[28] which, in the end stages, results in decreased contact lens wearing time and eventual intolerance of contact lenses. This condition has been termed giant papillary conjunctivitis, descriptive of the appearance of the upper palpebral conjunctiva in the acute stages.

SYMPTOMS. Four stages of symptoms in giant papillary conjunctivitis have been described. In stage I, a preclinical stage, a minimal increase in mucous secretion or ocular discharge present upon arising each morning is noted, along with mild itching upon lens removal. Such symptomatology can be elicited only by direct questioning and is not generally volunteered in the patient inter-

---

*The author has drawn extensively from the very complete discussion of this topic by Richmond.[27]

view as being significant.

Stage II, an early clinical stage, reflects increases in stage I symptomatology, as well as increased lens awareness, slight visual blurring, and mild itching while wearing the lens, all occurring toward the end of the wearing day.

In stage III, symptomatology again increases from that noted in stage II. Mucous secretions are common while the lens is being worn, with the secretions adhering to the lens surfaces, requiring frequent removal for cleaning; wearing time is decreased, and an increase in lens movement occurs.

In stage IV, the terminal stage, there is a total loss of lens tolerance and severe ocular discharge.

SIGNS. Allansmith et al. described the condition as giant papillary conjunctivitis when papillae were 1 mm. or greater in diameter, in order to distinguish this syndrome from other conditions.[28] It has become common practice, however, to use the term giant papillary conjunctivitis to describe the syndrome even when the papillae are less than 1 mm. in size.

Giant papillary conjunctivitis may be seen unilaterally or bilaterally. Clinically, the earliest signs are detectable only by biomicroscopic examination of the everted upper lid, often requiring fluorescein staining and cobalt blue light adjunctively to discern early changes. Only in the later stages of the syndrome are the clinical signs observable by gross examination of the everted lid.

The clinical signs can be correlated to the four stages of symptomatology presented previously. Stage I consists of symptomatology only, with the clinically observed conjunctiva appearing normal, with no papillae observable in the area of the tarsal plate.

Stage II involves the first appearance of papillae. In the earliest form, detection can only be made by biomicroscopic examination designed to reveal small, round light reflexes, which are reflected from the slightly and irregularly elevated conjunctiva covering the papillae (minute zones of irregular specular reflection). The conjunctiva is thickened, edematous, and moderately hyperemic (Figure 22.20, Plate IV). The conjunctiva, therefore, tends to obscure the finer vasculature, although the deeper vasculature is prominent. At the end of Stage II, the outlines of the early giant papillae become visible; however, observation of the form and outline of the giant papillae is only possible through the use of biomicroscopy and cobalt blue light after fluorescein staining.

Stage III signs show an increase in size, number, and elevation of abnormal papillae with cloverlike formations. The tops of the papillae will stain with fluorescein when the process is active, and there is heavy mucous secretion, often resulting in observable lens coatings (Figure 22.21, Plate V).

Stage IV is an exacerbation of the preceding symptoms, with a flattening of the tops of the papillae and elevations, often creating deep clefts between the papillae. The cornea is often involved via punctate fluorescein staining and occasionally shows white arcuate infiltrates superiorly. The lens is generally severely coated and, as a result, decenters frequently. Diagnosis can be made by gross examination with the naked eye.

The clinical appearance of giant papillary conjunctivitis is usually significantly different when it is associated with hard rather than soft contact lenses. The number of papillae are usually fewer with hard contact lenses, and the tops of the papillae tend to present a craterlike formation in contrast to a round or flattened appearance, which is present with soft contact lenses. The craterlike formation is particularly evident during the acute stages, when fluorescein staining at the top is severe. Fluorescein pooling also occurs in the depression (Figure 22.22, Plate V). Furthermore, papillae formation with hard lenses is usually confined to those areas of the palpebral conjunctiva covering the tarsal plate, with individual papillae frequently approaching the area of the lid margin. With soft contact lenses, the papillae usually are first observed in a confined area near the tarsal fold. The papillae associated with soft contact lens wear only approach the area of the lid margin in severe instances, usually stage IV. There are, however, many variations of appearance with both hard and soft lenses.

CAUSE. Giant papillary conjunctivitis appears to be closely related to vernal conjunctivitis. The cobblestone appearance, stringy mucus, and occasional corneal involvement in the acute stages are common to both. Evidence thus far indicates an immunologic basis for giant papillary conjunctivitis.

Lens-induced giant papillary conjunctivitis is also apparently not caused by a single factor. Protein buildup on the lens surface; mechanical irritation due to lens surface characteristics, lens edge, or fitting design; hypersensitivity to the lens polymer; and hypersensitivity to substances adhering to, or absorbed within, the lens have all been indicated as single or partial factors resulting in lens-induced giant papillary conjunctivities. As indicated previously, this syndrome is not isolated to any one contact lens design, polymer, or manufacturing technique.

THERAPY. Generally, lens removal results in resolution of giant papillary conjunctivitis. If this does not occur, a cause other than the contact lens is also present, although the contact lens may act to exacerbate the condition.

Resolution can be obtained in a high percentage of cases merely by having the patient clean the contact lenses more thoroughly. The use of papain with soft contact lenses has proven particularly effective and frequently has been directly responsible for allowing contact lens wearing to be maintained. Particular attention should also be directed to all aspects of the patient's general contact lens hygiene, since improvement in this area may

offer some resolution of the condition.

If removal of lens deposits is not possible, new lenses of the same design may be required. Failure of all attempts at resolution of the giant papillary conjunctivitis with the same lens design necessitates a change in lens design and/or polymer. Generally, if such a change is to be effective, it should be a dramatic change. This may then alter the causative factor, along with many other variables and/or factors. Certain patients may be unable to tolerate rigid lenses but may tolerate hydrogel lenses. The converse is also true. Resolution must, at present, be the subject of clinical trial procedures.

There is apparently a small percentage of patients who, once sensitized, are intolerant of any ocular foreign body, no matter how inoffensive. These patients then, for the present, are unable to wear contact lenses of any design.

Meibomian Gland Dysfunction

Korb and Henriquez describe a syndrome characterized by deficient or inadequate meibomian gland secretions, minimal or transient symptoms suggestive of ocular dryness, fluorescein staining of the cornea (often detected only after delayed observation or sequential instillation of stain), and contact lens intolerance.[29]

They investigated the meibomian glands of thirty-eight consecutive patients referred for evaluation of contact lens intolerance for which all conventional diagnostic techniques had failed to reveal a definitive cause.

While observation was made with 16× biomicroscopy, the meibomian glands in the area marked for study were gently expressed with the thumb against the lid surface to obtain secretions (Figure 22.23, Plate V). The results of expression were classified into three categories according to whether all, some, or none of the expressed glands released oil or thickened secretions. After instillation of topical 2% proparacaine into the inferior cul-de-sac, expression of the same meibomian glands was performed by compressing the lower lid with moderate force between a sterile cotton swab on the palpebral conjunctival surface and the thumb on the surface of the skin (Figure 22.24, Plate V). Expression of the same meibomian gland was then repeated with increased (forceful) pressure. The material recovered was classified in the same way as with gentle expression.

Expression with moderate and then with forceful pressure following topical anesthesia was effective in obtaining secretion from many orifices that did not yield with gentle expression. Clear oil was rarely obtained. With the application of forceful pressure, most orifices were observed to distend and to show elevation of the matrix from the lid surface. As forceful pressure was maintained, either of two phenomena would occur: the orifice would not yield, and no secretion would be obtained, or the orifice would release thickened secretions. Most, but not all, of the normal-appearing and elevated orifices would yield secretions if forceful pressure was maintained and combined with massaging of the meibomian glands by the thumb. Orifices that were receded into the lid margin, however, only rarely yielded secretion despite repeated forceful expression.

The thickened secretions released upon expression with increased pressure had different forms. A very fine filamentary secretion was apparently indicative of a stenotic orifice. Secretion in columnar form, resembling toothpaste squeezed from a tube, was apparently indicative of a less constricted orifice. Occasionally, the thickened secretion obtained only by forceful expression spread immediately over the lid surface. Creamy secretions appearing like pus (Figure 22.25, Plate V) were obtained from four of the thirty-eight symptomatic subjects after forceful expression. This finding was never observed in the twenty-nine patients of an asymptomatic control group after the same procedure.

Several mechanisms of contact lens intolerance associated with meibomian gland dysfunction are suggested. One appears to be due to the mechanical obstruction of the meibomian glands by keratotic plugs, which probably results in an alteration of their oily secretions. The second mechanism may be related to the release of bacteria or their toxic products, or both, from the meibomian glands into the precorneal tear film. The bacteriologic studies indicated that the most frequent organisms identified were *Staphylococcus epidermidis* and *Staphylococcus aureus*. The role of these bacteria in causing inflammation in the anterior segment has been demonstrated.[30]

The possibility of meibomian gland dysfunction is usually not investigated unless significant symptoms or gross signs are present. Symptoms are usually not present unless the integrity of the tear film is stressed, possibly by either a contact lens or by a dramatic change in the humidity or temperature of the environment. Thus, an apparently normal eye may unexpectedly manifest contact lens intolerance. The problem may be attributed to poor blinking, inadequate tear circulation, or other undesirable precorneal tear film characteristics. Yet, evaluation of all of these parameters may reveal no significant abnormality. The status of the meibomian glands as determined by the methods of expression appears to offer a method of evaluating both minimal and severe forms of meibomian gland dysfunction and possible related contact lens intolerance. Meibomian glands, to be considered normal, should yield oily secretions upon gentle expression.

Korb and Henriquez recommend that the treatment of meibomian gland dysfunction should be directed toward relieving the obstruction of the ducts and orifices, thus allowing normal flow of meibomian gland secretions onto the precorneal tear film. Treatment is best accomplished by multiple professional expressions of the meibomian glands at appropriate intervals. Home therapy consisting of hot compresses and scrubs of the lid margins should be instituted on a daily basis, particularly in the initial stages.

LENS PROPERTIES

When a lens is fitted successfully it should not change in its physical parameters. An alteration in the lens may affect vision and/or ocular health. It is therefore important to monitor lens parameters to determine if lens changes occur.

Hydrogel lenses sometimes alter their physical dimensions with time. The lens parameter that is most sensitive to change, in terms of its effect on lens fit, is the posterior curvature. Other lens parameters may also change, but none is significant without a concomitant change in posterior curvature. Hence, the stability of this parameter becomes of primary importance in assuring that a significant alteration in the fit of the lens has not been induced.

BASE CURVE

Changes of the posterior lens curvature are manifested clinically by a change in the apparent fit of the lens, either tightening or loosening. Visual acuity may also be affected due to a distortion effect, which is produced when the lens does not fit properly. Consequently, whenever vision is reduced as determined by examination or patient complaint, an additional measurement of lens curvature should be made.

Criteria for Lens Rejection

A change in posterior central curve radius greater than 0.1 mm. will require that the lens be changed.

LENS DISCOLORATION

Hydrogel contact lenses may become discolored with time because of the aging process of plastics, exposure to external dyes, or the introduction of drugs. There are variations in the quality of the plastics used for contact lenses from the various laboratories. Some lenses are more subject to aging processes, which result in the greying or brownish discoloration.

Many patients inadvertently transfer one of various common dyes to the lens from the fingers. An example of this would be a patient who has stamp pad ink on the fingers and handles the lens. Lenses may be discolored by various drugs, the most common of which is epinephrine, which imparts a brownish tint. Epinephrine is found in several over-the-counter decongestants, which are commonly used by patients.

LENS COATING

Several types of lens coatings have been reported to accompany soft lens wear.[31-49] These coatings may cause papillary conjunctivitis, discomfort, reduced visual acuity, and/or lowered oxygen transmissibility. The easiest method for analyzing lens coatings is by direct observation of the lens on the eye using the slit lamp.

The quality or grade of the coating can be identified by the following designation proposed by Koetting.[50] Grade 1 coating will not be recognized outside of the laboratory, so the designations 2, 3, and 4 are used in routine practice.

Grade 1. Films and deposits detectable by phase contrast microscopy.

Grade 2. Films and deposits that are visible only under certain conditions:

1. When the lens is removed from the eye and observed through an eyepiece of at least 7× magnifying power or under a powerful beam of light, preferably against a dark background.
2. Under biomicroscope examination with the lens in place on the eye, using direct illumination and viewing the lens against the dark background of the pupil or dark iris. A technique similar to that used in detecting central corneal clouding may also be employed.

Grade 3. Films or deposits that are visible under normal room lighting conditions, without any special equipment, on a dry lens (free of any water on the lens surface), but which are not visible as long as the lens is wet. This coating may also be observed using the biomicroscope when the lens is on the cornea. The patient is instructed not to blink, or the upper lid is held so that the surface is allowed to dry.

Grade 4. Films or deposits that are visible under normal room lighting conditions, with or without any special equipment, when the lens is wet or dry. These are easily seen with the biomicroscope, of course, but can also be detected without it.

The type of deposit can be classified by a letter, which generally corresponds to an abbreviation of the condition involved:

A. Abrasions—scrape marks.

C. Crystalline—crystal groups, which may be clustered together, scattered, or layered.

F. Films and hazes—coatings that are not granular or crystalline. The haze often has a bluish tint.

G. Granular—fine granulation, usually in mass form.

S. Speckles—Widely scattered small white specks.

The third step in the classification of films and deposits deals with determining the amount of area covered:

a. 0 to 25 percent
b. 25 to 50 percent
c. 50 to 75 percent
d. 75 to 100 percent

Criteria for Lens Rejection

A lens should be replaced if there is a grade 4 coating. If any of the following signs or symptoms appear to be associated with the coating, the lens should be replaced if there is a grade 3 coating:

1. Corneal staining
2. Discomfort
3. Allergic reaction
4. Visual acuity loss

Soft lens coating results in frequent replacement of lenses. Deposits on gel lenses can also reduce visual acuity and cause irritation that patients find very uncomfortable.

Extent of the Problem

A number of studies have been done to find out just how extensive is the surface coating problem on soft lenses.

In a study of 466 patients fitted between November, 1973, and July, 1974, Koetting found lens coating was the most important single reason for lens replacement.[50] About one-third of the patients he examined in the study needed a replacement pair of lenses as a result of the surface deposits.

In a retrospective study of three years' experience by patients fitted with the Bausch and Lomb Soflens contact lenses, Robbins found that some 70 percent of lenses worn more than three years had been replaced, 54 percent of two-year old lenses had been replaced, and 26 percent of lenses up to a year old had had to be replaced.[51]

In another study—as part of the development, testing, and evaluation of the enzyme cleaner by Allergan—Randeri and Cummings reported that some 51.3 percent of randomly selected used lenses had moderate to heavy deposits.[52] In a follow-up study, Randeri and Glicks found that some 65 percent of lenses worn more than one year had moderate to heavy deposits, which occurred in a majority of the lenses by the end of six months' wear.[53]

Lens coating is a major cause of lens replacement, and it occurs, to some degree, on all contact lenses. The degree of deposit and frequency of lens replacement appear to depend on the tear chemistry and amount of tear flow of the individual wearer. But, on the average, 20 to 30 percent of all lenses more than a year old will need to be replaced because of coating buildup.

Appearance

Gasset and Ruben found calcium spots on lenses, especially on lenses worn by aphakes and by people with pathological corneas (Figures 22.26 and 22.27, Plate VI).[54]

On lenses used on normal eyes for vision correction, Lowther found white crystalline deposits ascribed to the high calcium salt concentration in the artesian waters used by some wearers to prepare their saline solution for disinfection.[55] In addition, he found some diffuse deposits that develop slowly over several months' wear. He attributed this layer to some component of the tear film.

In another paper, Lowther reported that staining experiments identified the diffuse surface deposits as proteinaceous (Figures 22.28 to 22.30, Plate VI).[56]

Karageozian used amino acid analysis and UV spectroscopy to identify chemically the opaque deposits on lenses.[57] He found that they are proteinaceous, composed mostly of the tear protein lysozyme. Furthermore, he made up solutions of lysozyme with which he

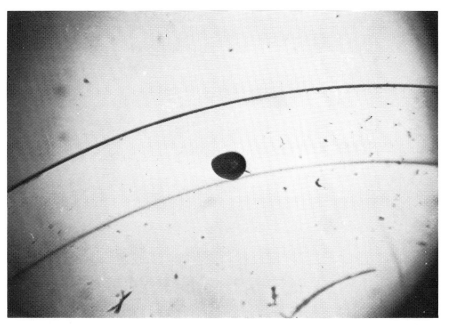

Figure 22.31. Moderate rust spot in the peripheral zone. Courtesy of Bausch & Lomb, Inc.

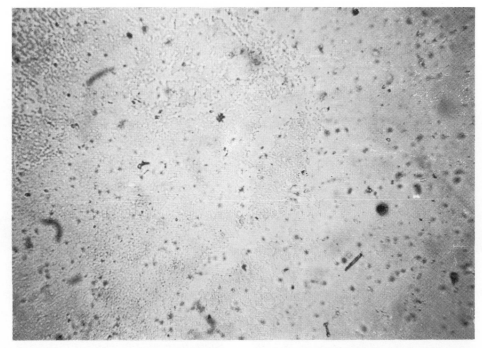

Figure 22.32. Light layer of surface film and small rust spot. The lens has not been properly cleaned, and a protein film has resulted. Courtesy of Bausch & Lomb, Inc.

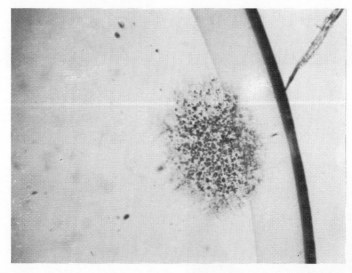

Figure 22.33. Large fungal growth in secondary and peripheral zone. Courtesy of Bausch & Lomb, Inc.

was able to simulate deposits on new lenses. Hathaway described how the precorneal tear film affects hydrophilic lens deposits.[58] He concluded that there was a relationship

PLATE III

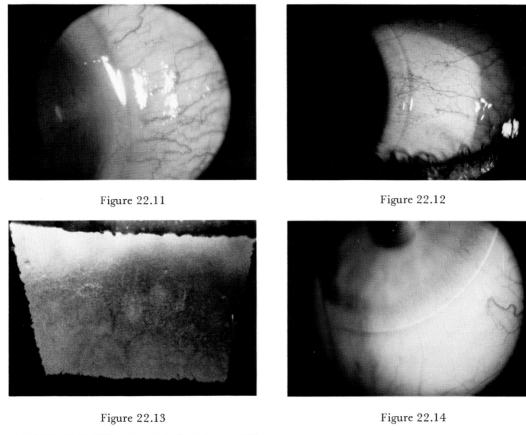

Figure 22.11

Figure 22.12

Figure 22.13

Figure 22.14

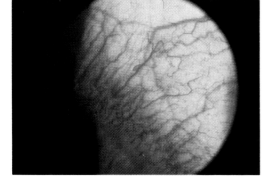

Figure 22.11. Blanching of the perilimbal vessels by the edge of the lens.

Figure 22.12. Conjunctival hyperemia.

Figure 22.13. Corneal infiltrates and exudates near the superior limbal region.

Figure 22.14. Neovascularization.

Figure 22.15. Engorgement of the perilimbal vessels.

Figure 22.15

Figures 22.11 through 22.15 courtesy of Doctor Joshua E. Josephson.

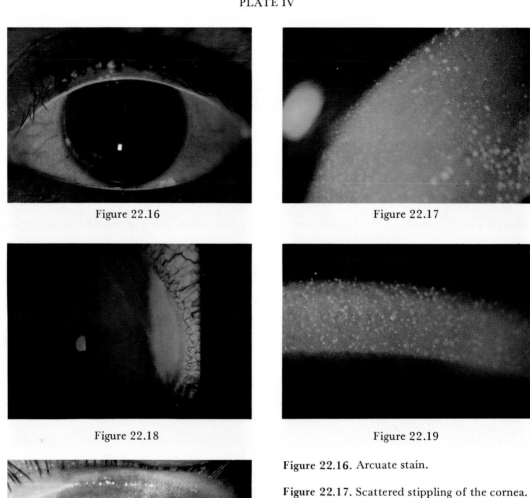

PLATE IV

Figure 22.16

Figure 22.17

Figure 22.18

Figure 22.19

Figure 22.20

Figure 22.16. Arcuate stain.

Figure 22.17. Scattered stippling of the cornea.

Figure 22.18. A lens that adheres to the cornea and if forcibly removed may do considerable damage to the corneal epithelium.

Figure 22.19. Stipple staining resulting from reaction to cold storage solution.

Figure 22.20. Stage II giant papillary conjunctivitis.

Figures 22.16 through 22.19 courtesy of Doctor Joshua E. Josephson.
Figure 22.20 from P.P. Richmond, Giant Papillary Conjunctivitis in Contact Lens Wearers, *American Journal of Ophthalmology*, *83(5):*697, 1977.

PLATE V

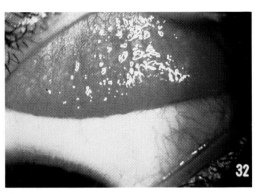

Figure 22.21

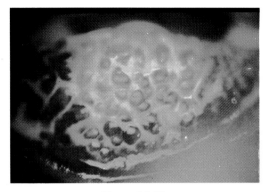

Figure 22.22

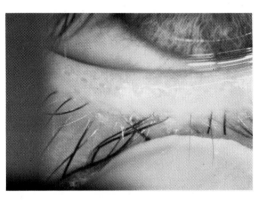

Figure 22.23

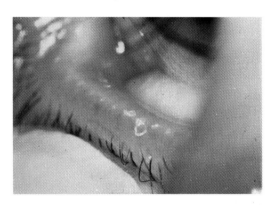

Figure 22.24

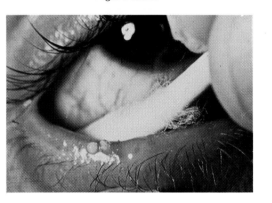

Figure 22.25

Figure 22.21. Biomicroscopic appearance of stage III giant papillary conjunctivitis. Papillae are present and vary in size from 0.3 to 0.8 mm.

Figure 22.22. Biomicroscopic appearance, as seen with black light, of a severe stage IV giant papillary conjunctivitis. In this instance, the giant papillae are numerous and cover almost the entire surface of the palpebral conjunctiva.

Figure 22.23. A number of meibomian gland orifices yield clear oil upon application of gentle pressure to the external surface of the lower lid with the thumb. Note the increase size of the meniscus as the result of the ex-pressed secretions.

Figure 22.24. Secretion is released upon force-ful expression between the sterile moistened swab and thumb. Secretions in the form of the columnar toothpaste phenomenon is obtained from one meibomian gland orifice.

Figure 22.25. Copious amounts of meibomian gland secretion are released upon forceful expression. Several glands release creamy thickened secretion appearing like pus.

Figures 22.21 and 22.22 from P.P. Richmond, Giant Papillary Conjunctivitis in Contact Lens Wearers, *American Journal of Ophthalmology, 83(5):*697, 1977.

Figures 22.23 through 22.25 from D.R. Korb and D.R. Henriquez, Meibomian Gland Dysfunction and Contact Lens Intolerance.*Journal of the American Optometric Association, 51(3):*243-251, 1980.

PLATE VI

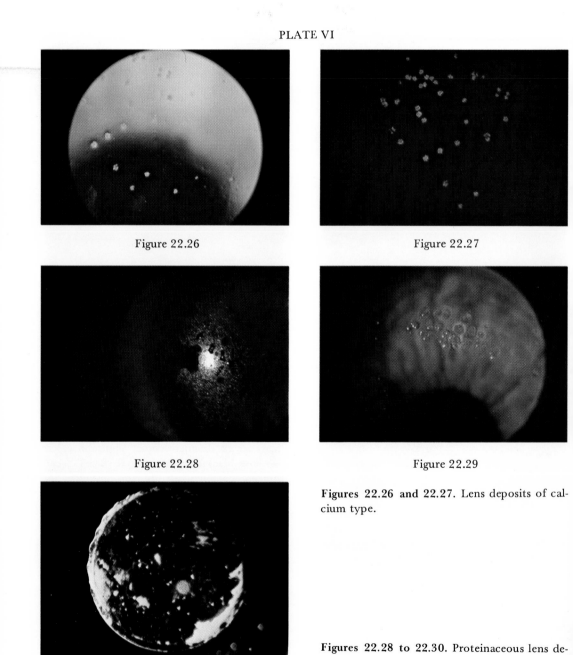

Figure 22.26

Figure 22.27

Figure 22.28

Figure 22.29

Figures 22.26 and 22.27. Lens deposits of calcium type.

Figure 22.30

Figures 22.28 to 22.30. Proteinaceous lens deposits.

Figures 22.26 through 22.30 courtesy of Doctor Joshua E. Josephson.

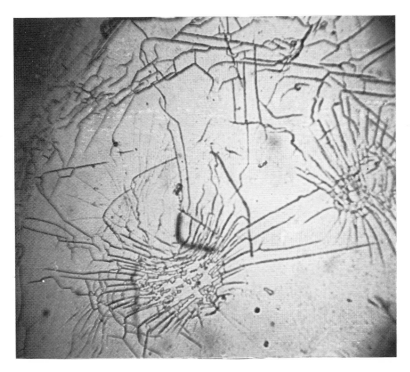

Figure 22.34. Heavy cracking surface film. Recommended cleaning procedures have not been followed, and protein and mucus have formed a film on the lens. Courtesy of Bausch & Lomb, Inc.

between the quantity of tears produced and the rate that deposits form. However, he could not establish a correlation between concentration of protein in the tears and the rate that deposits form.

Clinicians have found that protein coating is a problem with all soft lenses, although some lens materials seem to have a greater affinity for the protein than others. The proteins in the precorneal tear film are apparently the primary source of the diffuse coating buildup on lenses.

Red spots are visible with the biomicroscope using white light and direct illumination (Figure 22.31). They vary in size from 0.1 to 0.5 mm. and appear to have an irregular round shape. There is evidence that their usual origin is from iron-containing particles found in the normal daily environment. The small particles of iron find their way to the surface of the lens either through the air during wear or from the hands during lens handling. After attachment to the lens surface, the particles corrode to rust-colored spots following exposure to saline and heat. Red spots on lenses have been produced experimentally by rubbing lenses with iron powder or filings, followed immediately by a heat disinfection cycle.[59] Red spots could not be produced by soaking lenses in solutions of iron ions, indicating that their source is probably not improperly purified water. Red spots may in rare instances be formed of organic material. If rust spots are numerous or large in size, it may be necessary to replace the lens.

Attempts to remove red spots by rubbing the lens with saline solution or surfactant cleaners are usually unsuccessful. An occasional rust spot may be allowed to remain on

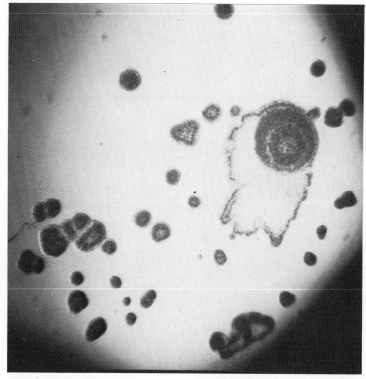

Figure 22.35. Dense round surface deposits. Lipid or mucopolysaccharide deposit buildup resulting from eye secretions. Courtesy of Bausch & Lomb, Inc.

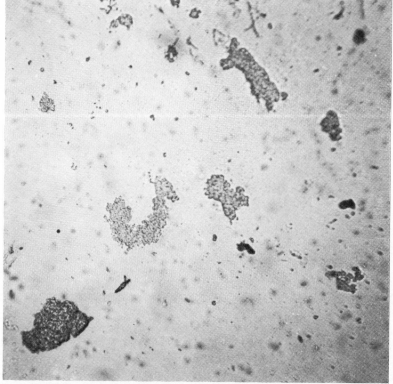

Figure 22.36. Small patches of surface deposits. Courtesy of Bausch & Lomb, Inc.

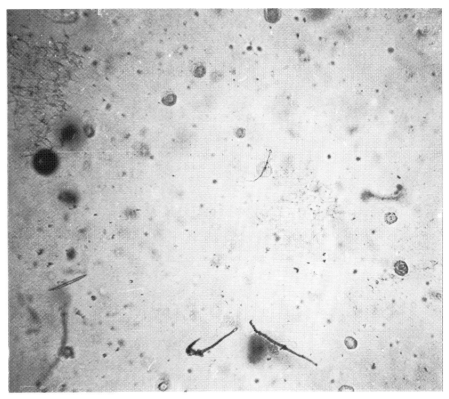

Figure 22.37. Several round deposits with light branching fungal growth. Courtesy of Bausch & Lomb, Inc.

the lens without causing any problems for the wearer but must be differentiated from fungal growths. This may be accomplished with a biomicroscope, using high magnification. A fungal growth will show outpouchings, whereas a rust spot has more regular edges and a rounder shape.

Some lens coatings can only be identified under light or phase contrast microscopy (Figures 22.32 to 22.37).

REFERENCES

1. Krachmer, J. H., and Purcell, J. J.: Bacterial corneal ulcers in cosmetic soft contact lens wearers, *Arch. Ophthalmol.*, *96*(*1*):57, 1978.
2. Mandell, R. B.: Corneal edema from hydrogel lenses, *Int. Cont. Lens Clin.*, *2*(*1*):88–98, 1975.
3. Mandell, R. B.: Corneal edema from hard and hydrogel contact lenses, *J. Am. Optom. Assoc.*, *47*(*3*):287, 1976.
4. Kame, R. T.: Clinical management of hydrogel-induced edema, *Am. J. Optom.*, *53*(*9*): 468–473, 1976.
5. Sarver, M. D.: Striate corneal lines among patients wearing hydrophilic contact lenses, *Am. J. Optom.*, *48*(*9*):762–763, 1971.
6. Polse, K. A., and Mandell, R. B.: Etiology of corneal striae accompanying hydrogel lens wear, *Invest. Ophthalmol.*, *15*(*7*):553–556, 1976.
7. Harris, M. G., Sarver, M. D., and Polse, K. A.: Vertical corneal striae among hydrogel lens wearers, *Int. Cont. Lens Clin.*, *2*(*4*): 50–55, 1975.

8. Mandell, R. B.: The "tight" soft contact lens, *Cont. Lens Forum*, 4(12):21–32, 1979.

9. Mertz, G.: When and why to use ultra-thin lenses, *Cont. Lens Forum*, 3(7):65, 1978.

10. Hayashi, T., and Fatt, I.: Lubrication theory model of tear exchange under a soft contact lens, *Am. J. Optom. Physiol. Opt.*, 53(4):101–103, 1976.

11. Polse, K. A.: Tear flow under hydrogel contact lenses, *Invest. Ophthalmol. Vis. Sci.*, 18(4):409–413, 1979.

12. Fichman, S., Baker, V. V., and Horton, H. R.: Iatrogenic red eyes in soft contact lens wearers, *Int. Cont. Lens Clin.*, 5(5):20–24, 1978.

13. Doughman, D. J.: Basic and clinical considerations of tear film stability, *Cont. Lens J.*, 10(4):25–31, 1977.

14. Josephson, J.: Infiltrative keratitis in hydrogel lens wearers, *Int. Cont. Lens Clin.*, 6(5): 47–67, 1979.

15. Bron, A. J., and Dixon, W. S.: Fluorescein angiographic demonstration of corneal vascularization in contact lens wearers, *Am. J. Ophthalmol.*, 75(6):1010–1015, 1973.

16. Kline, L. N., and DeLuca, T. J.: Arcuate staining, *J. Am. Optom. Assoc.*, 47(3):360, 1976.

17. Kline, L. N., and DeLuca, T. J.: Pitting stain with soft contact lenses—hydrocurve thin series, *J. Am. Optom. Assoc.*, 48(3):372, 1979.

18. Bailey, I. L., and Carney, L. G.: Corneal changes from hydrophilic contact lenses, *Am. J. Optom. Arch. Am. Acad. Optom.*, 50(4):299–304, 1973.

19. Barnett, W. A., and Rengstorff, R. A.: Adaptation to hydrogel contact lenses: variations in myopia and corneal curvature measurements, *J. Am. Optom. Assoc.*, 48(3): 363, 1977.

20. Baron, H.: Temporary changes in the ocular refractive system caused by contact lens wear, *Contacto*, 21(6):10, 1977.

21. Hill, J. F.: A comparison of refractive and keratometric changes during adaptation to flexible and non-flexible contact lenses, *J. Am. Optom. Assoc.*, 46(3):290–294, 1975.

22. Hill, J. F.: Effects of thin HEMA lenses on refractive error and corneal curvature, *Cont. Lens Forum*, 2(1):31–33, 1977.

23. Hill, J. F.: Changes in corneal curvature and refractive error upon refitting with flatter hydrophilic contact lenses, *J. Am. Optom. Assoc.*, 47(9):1214–1216, 1976.

24. Hill, J. F.: Variation in refractive error and corneal curvature after wearing hydrophilic contact lenses, *J. Am. Optom. Assoc.*, 46(11): 1136–1138, 1975.

25. Lebow, K. A.: Corneal changes associated with Gelflex hydrophilic contact lenses, *Int. Cont. Lens Clin.*, 3(4):48–53, 1976.

26. Baldone, J. A.: Corneal curvature changes secondary to the wearing of hydrophilic gel contact lenses, *Cont. Intraoc. Lens Med. J.*, 1(1–2):175–176, 1975.

27. Richmond, P. P.: Giant papillary conjunctivitis: an overview, *J. Am. Optom. Assoc.*, 50(3):343–347, 1979.

28. Allansmith, M. R. et al.: Giant papillary conjunctivitis in contact lens wearers, *Am. J. Ophthalmol.*, 83(5):697, 1977.

29. Korb, D. R., and Henriquez, D. R.: Meibomian gland dysfunction and contact lens intolerance, *J. Am. Optom. Assoc.*, 51(3):243–251, 1980.

30. Thygeson, P.: Bacterial factors in chronic catarrhal conjunctivities, *Arch. Ophthalmol.*, 18:373, 1937.

31. Allen, J. et al.: Deposits on contact lenses, *The Optician*, 175(4517):8, 1978.

32. Arons, I. J.: Soft lens coating—and what can be done about it, *Rev. Optom.*, 115(4):35, 1978.

33. Benjamin, W. J., and Hill, R. M.: Surface coating: the fatal facade, *Cont. Lens Forum*, 4(8):107–109, 1979.

34. Blaine, J. E. et al.: Blood constituents and hydrophilic lens coating, *Cont. Lens Forum*, 2(8):50, 1977.

35. Doughman, D. J. et al.: The nature of "spots" on soft lenses, *Ann. Ophthalmol.*, 7(3): 345–353, 1975.

36. Gyorffy, I.: Deposits on contact lenses as a cause of intolerance, *Contact Lens*, , 3(7): 19–20, 1972.

37. Hathaway, R.: Appearance of hydrophilic lens deposits as related to chemical etiology, *Int. Cont. Lens Clin.*, 3(3):27–35, 1976.

38. Hathaway, R. A., and Lowther, G. E.: Factors influencing the rate of deposit formation on hydrophilic lenses, *Austr. J. Optom.*, 61(3):92, 1978.

39. Hilbert, J., Lowther, G., and King, J.: Deposition of substances within hydrophilic lenses, *Am. J. Optom. Physiol. Opt.*, *53*(2): 51–54, 1976.

40. Hill, R. M.: Can you overcome the oily lens?, *Int. Cont. Lens Clin.*, *5*(4):32, 1978.

41. Josephson, J. E.: Hydrogel contact lens problem solving, *The Ophthalmic Optician*, *18*(22): 819, 1978.

42. Kanai, A.: Electron microscopic studies of deposits on the soft contact lens, *J. Jap. Cont. Lens Soc.*, *4*(3):19, 1977.

43. Kennedy, J. R.: Aftercare of soft contact lenses, *J. Am. Optom. Assoc.*, *47*(3):369, 1976.

44. Kleist, F.: Appearance and nature of hydrophilic contact lens deposits—Part 2: inorganic deposits, *Int. Cont. Lens Clin.*, *6*(4):44, 1979.

45. Kleist, F. D.: Appearance and nature of hydrophilic contact lens deposits—Part 1: protein and other organic deposits, *Int. Cont. Lens Clin.*, *6*(39):49–59, 1979.

46. Klintworth, G. K. et al.: Calcification of soft contact lenses in patient with dry eye and elevated calcium concentration in tears, *Invest. Ophthalmol. Vis. Sci.*, *16*(2):158–161, 1977.

47. Kreji, L., and Harrison, R.: Corneal pigment deposits from topically administered epinephrine, *Arch. Ophthalmol.*, *82*(6):836–839, 1969.

48. Loran, D. F. C.: Red (rust) spots in hydrogel contact lenses, *Am. J. Optom. Physiol. Opt.*, *54*(12):837–844, 1977.

49. McClure, D. A. et al.: The effect on measured visual acuity of protein deposition and removal in soft contact lenses, *Contacto*, *21*(2):8–12, 1977.

50. Koetting, R. A.: Predicting soft lens surface problems, *Cont. Lens Forum*, *1*(6):18–21, 1976.

51. Robbins, J. C.: A three year retrospective Soflens study, unpublished, August, 1975.

52. Randeri, K.: Development and efficacy aspects of a new soft lens cleaner, *Austr. J. Optom.*, *57*(12):392–398, 1974.

53. Randeri, K., and Glicksir, B.: A survey of the incidence of visible deposits on soft lenses, Allergan Report No. 121, 1975.

54. Ruben, M., Tripathi, R. C., and Winders, A. F.: Calcium deposition as a cause of spoilation of hydrophilic soft contact lenses, *Br. J. Ophthalmol.*, *59*(3):141–148, 1975.

55. Lowther, G. E., Hilbert, J. A., and King, J. E.: Appearance and location of hydrophilic lens deposits, *Int. Cont. Lens Clin.*, *2*(4): 30–34, 1975.

56. Lowther, G. E., and Hilbert, J. A.: Deposits on hydrophilic lenses: differential appearance and clinical causes, *Am. J. Optom. Physiol. Opt.*, *52*(10):687–692, 1975.

57. Karageozian, H. L.: Chemical identity of opaque deposits on human worn lenses, Allergan Report No. 92, 1974.

58. Hathaway, R. A., and Lowther, G. E.: Appearance of hydrophilic lens deposits as related to chemical etiology, *Int. Cont. Lens Clin.*, *3*(3):27–35, 1976.

59. Riedhammer, T. M.: Rust deposits on soft contact lenses, *Int. Cont. Lens Clin.*, *7*(1): 30–36, 1980.

ADDITIONAL READINGS

Allansmith, M. R., and Fowler, S.: Evolution of soft contact lens coatings, *Arch. Ophthalmol.*, *98*:95, 1980.

Allansmith, M. R., Greiner, J. V., and Covington, H. I.: Surface morphology of giant papillary conjunctivitis in contact lens wearers, *Am. J. Ophthalmol.*, *85*(2):242, 1978.

Bailey, I. L., and Carney, L. G.: Hydrophilic contact lenses—their effect on the cornea, *Austr. J. Optom.*, *55*(5):161–163, 1972.

Balik, J., and Kubat, Z.: Changes in tear proteins concentration in patients wearing gel contact lenses, *The Optician*, *155*(4013):205, 1968.

Black, C. J., and Dyer, J. A.: The effects of hydrophilic contact lenses on the human cornea, *Cont. Lens Med. Bull.*, *3*(1):8–11, 1970.

Brown, N. A., and Lobascher, D.: Complication of soft contact lens use in correction of simple refractive errors, *Proc. Soc. Med.*, 68–53, 1975.

Chappell, G. H.: General after-care procedures and the contact lens patient—Part 19, *The Optician*, *168*(4355):14–16, 1974.

Chin, G. N., and Carp, G.: Corneal "immunies" ring in a contact lens wearer, *Cont. Intraoc. Lens Med. J.*, *4(4)*:34, 1978.

Cooper, R. L., and Constable, I. J.: Infective keratitis in soft contact lens wearers, *Br. J. Ophthalmol.*, *61*:250, 1977.

Covington, H. I., Greiner, J. V., and Allansmith, M. R.: Surface morphology of giant papillary conjunctivitis in contact lens wearers, *Am. J. Ophthalmol.*, *85(2)*:242, 1978.

Cumming, J. S., and Karageozian, H.: "Protein" conjunctivitis in hydrophilic lens wearers, *Contacto*, *19(4)*:8–9, 1975.

Dada, V. K., and Zisman, F.: Contact lens induced filamentary keratitis, *Am. J. Optom. Physiol. Optics*, *52(8)*:545–546, 1975.

Fontana, F. D.: Follow-up routine for the soft lens et rationale, *Optom. Weekly*, *63(26)*:11–12, 1972.

Hill, J. F.: Variation in refractive error and corneal curvature after wearing ultra-thin hydrophilic contact lens, *Int. Cont. Lens Clin.*, *3(4)*:23–29, 1976.

Johnson, D. G.: Keratoconjunctivitis associated with wearing hydrophilic contact lenses, *Can. J. Ophthalmol.*, *8*:92–96, 1973.

Kame, R. T.: Striate keratopathy and hydrogel lenses: a case report, *Optom. Weekly*, *65(39)*:1074–1076, 1974.

Katz, H. H.: A hypothesis for the formation of vertical corneal striae as observed in the wearing of softlens contact lenses and in keratoconus, *Am. J. Optom.*, *53(8)*:420–421, 1976.

Kline, L. N., and DeLuca, T. J.: An analysis of arcurate staining with the B&L soflens—Part I, *J. Am. Optom. Assoc.*, *46(11)*:1126–1129, 1975.

Kline, L. N., DeLuca, T. J., and Fishberg, G.: Corneal staining relating to contact lens wear, *J. Am. Optom. Assoc.*, *50(3)*:353, 1979.

Koetting, R. A.: Tear film break-up time on hydrophilic lens surfaces, *Int. Cont. Lens Clin.*, *4(6)*:30, 1977.

Koetting, R. A., and Boyd, N. S.: Unexplained "red eye" in adapted soft lens wearers, *Int. Cont. Lens Clin.*, *5(3)*:66, 1978.

Krachmer, J. H., and Purcell, J. J.: Bacterial corneal ulcers in cosmetic soft contact lens wearers, *Arch. Ophthalmol.*, *96(1)*:57, 1978.

Krejci, L., and Krejcova, H.: Effect of conventional hard and hydrophilic soft contact lenses on the corneal epithelium, *Br. J. Ophthalmol.*, *57(9)*:675–680, 1973.

Krezanoski, J.: What are the implications of dirty soft contact lenses?, *Int. Cont. Lens Clin.*, *4(2)*:57–60, 1977.

Kroll, T., and Kroll, J.: Clinical evaluation and follow-up programs on soft contact lens patients, *Contacto*, *22(3)*:23–24, 1978.

Lowther, G. E.: Effectiveness of an enzyme in removing deposits from hydrophilic lenses, *Am. J. Optom. Physiol. Opt.*, *54(2)*:76–84, 1977.

Lowther, G. E., and Hilbert, J. A.: Deposits on hydrophilic lenses: differential appearance and clinical causes, *Am. J. Optom. Physiol. Opt.*, *52(10)*:687–692, 1975.

Mackie, I. A.: Giant papillary conjunctivitis (secondary vernal) in assocition with contact lens wear, *Trans. Ophthalmol. Soc. U.K.*, *98*:3, 1978.

Polse, K. A., Sarver, M. D., and Harris, M. G.: Corneal edema and vertical striae accompanying the wearing of hydrogel lenses, *Am. J. Optom. Physiol. Opt.*, *52(3)*:185–191, 1975.

Chapter 23

THERAPEUTIC APPLICATIONS

THE USE OF HYDROGEL contact lenses has proven to be a valuable therapy for a number of serious corneal diseases.[1-9] They can also be used for the optical correction of scarred irregular corneas, providing vision for cases where hard lenses would produce epithelial ulcers and damage. The drying syndromes, when severe and accompanied by conjunctival cicatrization, are usually difficult to manage, and gel contact lenses provide one of the few effective therapies for cases in which artificial tears alone are not satisfactory. Severe ulcers can be permitted to heal when a gel lens protects the epithelium from the action of the lids and permits it to grow across the denuded area. Epithelial breakdowns after herpes, bacterial ulcers, and other corneal insults can be made to heal. Pain can be prevented in patients with granular, macular, or lattice dystrophy, and the irregular astigmatism is optically corrected so that surgery is often unnecessary.

BULLOUS KERATOPATHY

Bullous keratopathy was the first pathological condition to receive F.D.A. approval for treatment with therapeutic gel lenses. There have been numerous reports on this technique[1-3,10-12] since its introduction by Kaufman and Gasset.[13]

PATHOLOGY

Bullous keratopathy is the most severe form of corneal edema. It always involves all three layers of the cornea and results from diseased corneal endothelium, caused by one or more of the following conditions:

1. Fuchs' endothelial dystrophy
2. Aphakic bullous keratopathy caused by trauma during surgery, vitreous touch, etc.
3. Postkeratoplasty bullous keratopathy caused by iris adhesion, retrocorneal membrane, and separation of Descemet's membrane
4. Long-standing uveitis
5. Glaucoma

The natural course of the disease can be divided into the following stages:

Degeneration of the Corneal Endothelium

The corneal endothelium progressively degenerates until it is not able to carry out its function as a mechanical barrier and pump.

The endothelium decompensates, and aqueous humor leaks into the corneal stroma.

Stromal Edema

The stromal edema usually mirrors the endothelial disease. In some cases it is a small, well-localized area; in other cases it involves a diffuse area from limbus to limbus. In some cases stromal edema is present for months or even years without scarring or epithelial edema.

Epithelial Edema

The edema begins in the basal cell layers spreading through the epithelium and occasionally forming subepithelial bullae. Often before epithelial bullae are noted, a fibrous overgrowth begins between Bowman's membrane and the epithelium. At first this may be visible as irregular moon-shaped reflections seen by specular reflection. Later this subepithelial overgrowth may be quite hazy and grayish, and occasionally it makes significant contribution to the reduction of vision. Later epithelial bullae and the irregular astigmatism caused by the bullae appear. Irregular astigmatism is often the major cause of vision loss in bullous keratopathy.

Stromal Scarring

Scarring results only after long-standing epithelial edema. Corneal scarring usually begins anterior to Descemet's membrane as a slightly yellowish density or as grayish strands forming a hazy star-shaped area.

Folds in Descemet's Membrane

Folds in Descemet's membrane are due to swelling and hydration of the corneal stroma. The stroma as it swells cannot proceed anteriorly and is thrown into folds. When these folds are present for a long time, they scar and become fixed folds in Descemet's membrane. These folds also seem clinically important in reducing vision.

Gel contact lenses have revolutionized the management of bullous keratopathy. They can be used for two purposes: relief of pain and improvement of vision. Relief of pain is nearly certain with the gel lenses, but cycloplegia is necessary to relieve the iritis frequently present in these patients. If the lens is properly fitted and the iris is well controlled, it is very rare for patients to have significant residual discomfort, provided that they wear the lens constantly (twenty-four hours a day for months at a time). It is important that the lens not be removed frequently.

The improvement in vision in bullous keratopathy can be just as important as the relief of pain but is a bit more unpredictable. In early cases where there are not many folds in Descemet's membrane, the soft contact lens will eliminate the irregular surface of the cornea and the resulting irregular astigmatism and will improve the vision. Stromal haze contributes little to the decrease in vision; the primary visual loss is caused by anterior or posterior irregular astigmatism.

Gel lenses can be equally beneficial in patients with edema covering a part of the pupil. When edema creeps down from a faulty cataract incision or from a localized area of vitreous contact, the resulting irregular astigmatism may distort the image, even though much of the cornea is normal. In these patients where part of the cornea is normal and part is irregular, gel contact lenses can generally be counted upon to bring a marked improvement in vision. For further improvement of vision, 5 percent NaCl drops can be used as needed.

In patients with advanced bullous keratopathy and with many folds in Descemet's membrane, the improvement in vision is erratic and unpredictable. Still, a small proportion of these severe cases may obtain improved vision with gel lenses and hypertonic saline. Gel lenses should be tried even though bullous keratopathy is relatively advanced, especially in patients who are monocular, or whose visual demands are limited.

The following conclusions are based on a

study of eighty-six eyes in eighty-one patients treated with Softcon® lenses (made by Warner-Lambert) by Gasset[14] and 388 eyes treated in 366 patients by fourteen other investigators (Table 23.1). A detailed description of these lenses has been presented in Chapter 19.

The beneficial effects of a bandage gel lens stems from the following:

1. It acts as a pressure bandage reducing the epithelial edema. It is the most comfortable pressure bandage that can be worn constantly.

2. It replaces the irregular corneal toricity with a smooth optically perfect surface.

3. It acts synergistically with osmotherapy. Hypertonic saline used in conjunction with the lenses is absorbed and released over long periods of time, therefore increasing the effectiveness of this form of therapy.

4. It protects bullae from the lids, preventing rupture, and provides already ruptured bullae with protection and relieves pain.

FITTING PROCEDURE

Fitting patients with bullous keratopathy is significantly more difficult than fitting patients for refractive errors, especially if good visual results are required. However, experienced gained from fitting patients for refractive errors is a valuable asset in the fitting of pathological corneas. It usually simplifies the fitting procedure and improves the therapeutic results in this type of patient.

Trial lens fitting of gel lenses is the easiest and often the only method by which these lenses can be fitted in patients with pathological corneas. Trial lens testing is done to find the proper base curve and diameter that will give the best vision and most stable performance. The proper fit is achieved with a lens that has both central and peripheral contact so that it does not flex in the center with each blink and yet is large enough in diameter not to move with each blink. However, this fitting relationship is not easily verified.

The first question that must be answered is how to select a gel lens of the proper curve and diameter for a given patient that will provide sufficient adherence to prevent movement without inducing too much apical clearance and consequent reduced vision.

The selection of any gel lens can result in only three possibilities:

1. The lens is too flat.
2. The lens is too steep.
3. The lens is of the proper curve and diameter.

The evaluation of this relationship is the same as for nonpathological eyes. If the lens

TABLE 23.1

COMPOSITION OF BULLOUS KERATOPATHY CASES STUDIED

I. *Incidence*				
A.		*Sex*		
		Male	*Female*	*No. of Eyes*
Gasset *et al.*		50.6%	49.4%	86
All		41.0%	59.0%	388
B. *Race*		(366 Patients)		
White		84%		
Negro		7%		
C.		*Eye*		
		Right	*Left*	*No. of Eyes*
Gasset *et al.*		60.6%	40.0%	86
All		54.0%	46.0%	388
D. *Age*			*Number of Patients*	
			All	
(Years)	*Gasset et al.*		*Male*	*Female*
Less than 51	7		27	18
51-55	1		9	12
56-60	8		16	26
61-65	11		23	25
66-70	14		27	35
71-75	23		25	45
76-80	8		10	29
Over 80	5		9	20
II. *Etiology*		*All*		
Aphakia		239		
Glaucoma		90		
Fuch's Dystrophy		102		
III. *Symptoms*				
Pain—Gasset *et al.*		81%		

is too flat (or too small), it will move up and down with each blink or will be displaced laterally on lateral gaze.

If the lens is too steep, there is alternate blurring and clearing of vision with each blink. This may be somewhat difficult to evaluate initially in a patient with bullous keratopathy. However, if there is any doubt that the lens might be steep, one should try the next flatter lens (or the next smaller diameter).

Never evaluate the results of a given trial lens until the lens has been on the eye for at least fifteen minutes. This rule is most important in patients with bullous keratophathy.

Once the fitter is satisfied that the proper curve and diameter have been determined, the refractive power of the lens should be determined. The use of plano trial lenses will simplify the procedure. The power can be determined by one of the following techniques:

1. Use the spectacle refraction, allow for the vertex distance, and then refine the refraction through a trial lens procedure.

2. Use plano trial contact lenses and refract over them.

A lens that is well fitted initially may appear faulty after a few days of wear. The base curve of the lens will need to be changed to correct for changes in the corneal curvature, and the refractive power may also be altered.

Patients with bullous keratopathy must have an overrefraction at each follow-up visit.

Large single bullae usually disappear within a few days of lens wear and result in a diffuse epithelial edema. The constant wear of these lenses also produces dehydration of the cornea, which causes a significant change in corneal shape. This change usually results in a reduction in visual acuity. It is not unusual to find a patient who was fitted initially with these lenses and achieved an improvement in vision from 20/200 to 20/40 to change after a few days to a visual acuity of 20/100 to 20/200. Biomicroscopy of the eye usually reveals a significant change in the cornea with a disappearance of the big bullae and diffuse epithelial edema. If, in these cases, the lens is changed properly, the visual acuity usually improves again to 20/40. This may require the addition of hypertonic saline. In some cases several changes in the lens are required.

BIOMICROSCOPY

Biomicroscopy must be done routinely after the patient is first fitted and then in each follow-up visit. The following points should be checked:

1. Relationship between the lens edge and the sclera; the lens should neither be lifted off the sclera nor pressed on it tightly.

2. Appearance of the lens surface.

3. Evaluation of the cornea; corneal architecture should be intact.

4. Evaluation of the conjunctiva; no ciliary flush, no enlarged vessels.

5. Lens centering.

6. Lid pressure.

USE OF MEDICATIONS

1. It is extremely useful in cases of chronic bullous keratopathy to institute lid hygiene techniques. Hexachlorophene (pHisoHex®) scrubs for five minutes daily, twice a day, have decreased the incidence of minor infections to an almost insignificant level.

2. Pupils are dilated in cases of chronic bullous keratopathy, especially with epithelial defects because of the concomitant iritis present in almost every case.

3. Antibiotics are used if secondary infections or chronic blepharitis is present at the time of the fitting.

4. A 5% hypertonic saline solution without preservative or methylcellulose is the most important medication used in combination with the lenses. Its use produces a significant improvement in vision of from two to three lines. In most cases it is used three to five times a day as necessary. However, it should be avoided in the beginning for patients who have a significant amount of discomfort. In these cases the application of gel lenses and pupillary dilatation should result in significant relief of pain within a few days. At that time the patient should be refitted, and hypertonic saline used for the improvement of visual acuity.

The advantages of gel lenses in the treatment of bullous keratopathy can be divided into two main categories:

1. *General.* The use of gel bandage lenses in the treatment of bullous keratopathy is a simple, safe, and efficacious technique for relieving pain and restoring visual acuity in this group of patients (Table 23.2).

2. *Selected cases.* In a selected group of patients the gel bandage lenses have been most useful because of the fact that they are the only therapeutic technique for pain relief as well as for improvement in visual acuity. For example, in cases of glaucoma and bullous keratopathy, and particularly in cases of congenital glaucoma where penetrating kerato-

TABLE 23.2

THERAPEUTIC RESULTS

	Gasset	All
	%	%
A. *Pain Relief*		
Complete	82.6	73.3
Control	11.6	20.0
None	3.5	3.0
Not Stated	2.3	3.0
B. *Biomicroscopy*		
Improved	67.4	66.4
Unchanged	15.1	25.3
Worsened	1.2	2.3
Not stated	16.3	5.9
C. *Wearing Experience*	(*number of eyes*)	
Worn continuously		
(24 hours)	79	353
Discontinued due to		
untoward experience	5	97

plasty is extremely difficult, bandage lenses have achieved relief of pain in almost all cases, and improvement in visual acuity in the great majority (Table 23.3). In aphakic bullous keratopathy, bandage lenses have eliminated the serious complication of penetrating keratoplasty such as glaucoma, macular edema, and graft reaction. Moreover, it does not preclude a later penetrating keratoplasty in cases where improvement of visual acuity is unsatisfactory. In addition, in this same group of patients whose visual acuity does not improve to a satisfactory level, gel bandage lenses have played a significant and important role in improving the cornea to such a point that fluorescein angiography can be performed. A significant number of these patients were found to have macular edema as the main cause for the decrease in visual acuity. In this manner, the bandage lenses eliminate the necessity of surgery for the patient.

RELIEF OF PAIN

In almost every case, total comfort is obtained within a week. In the few cases where the pain was not relieved by application of the bandage lenses, one or several of the following conditions were determined:

1. Improper fitting of the lens
2. Failure to dilate the pupil
3. Conjunctivitis, blepharitis
4. Elevation in intraocular pressure

VISUAL ACUITY

Visual acuity often improved after the insertion of the gel lenses and the application of hypertonic solution. However, in many cases, several weeks or even months are necessary before the best visual acuity can be obtained, and several fittings may be necessary for optimum acuity.

Visual acuity improved after the application of 5% hypertonic saline without preservative. An effective schedule for the application of hypertonic saline is one or two drops every two hours. Hypertonic saline is most needed during the morning hours. In the afternoon, visual acuity often clears somewhat even without the application of hypertonic saline.

An unexplained decrease in visual acuity is always a signal that an overrefraction or refitting of the lens is needed. In several cases the refraction and corneal curvature have changed after wearing the bandage lens for several days or weeks. In all cases, refitting with the proper dimension and power of the lens has resulted in improvement of the visual acuity.

The high rate of patients fitted years ago who are still wearing the lenses with complete comfort and visual acuity improvement makes this mode of therapy clinically useful. Although in advanced bullous cases the improvement of visual acuity is unpredictable, it is simple to try such a lens to determine the degree of visual improvement that can be obtained over refraction. If unsuccessful, it can be easily removed without any permanent damage or expense to the patient.

TABLE 23.3

LINE CHANGE IN VISUAL ACUITY CHART FOR
BULLOUS KERATOPATHY CASES

No. of Lines Changed	No. of Patients	
	Gasset	Others
+10 (20/20)	1	1
+ 9	2	2
+ 8	4	6
+ 7	7	4
+ 6	3	7
+ 5	13	23
+ 4	7	15
+ 3	7	13
+ 2	9	32
+ 1	3	20
–0– (no change)	17	141
– 1	0	16
– 2	0	5
– 3	0	2
– 4	0	0
– 5	1	1

DRYING SYNDROMES

Gel lenses have been used for drying syndromes since early 1969. For this type of gel contact lens therapy, it is helpful to separate the drying syndromes into two categories, simple keratitis sicca and conjunctival cicatrization.[15] The latter can be divided into progressive conjunctival cicatrization, such as ocular pemphigus, and nonprogressive conjunctival cicatrization, such as Stevens-Johnson disease.

Simple keratitis sicca without lid abnormalities is easy to fit and treat. As a rule, the lens is fitted as if for a refractive error. The main problem is to keep the lens moist. Frequent administration of either regular or hypotonic (0.45%) saline or one of the artificial tear preparations (for example, Adaptettes®, made by Burton Parsons and Co., Inc.) is necessary to keep the lens in place. Saline administration must be frequent in the beginning, but after a few weeks it can be diminished.

It is important to remember that there are other medical problems generally accompanying keratitis sicca. Simply inserting a soft lens will not cure all of these problems. For instance, almost all keratitis sicca patients have blepharitis of some degree, and lid hygiene is important for the patient's comfort as well as to prevent secondary infections. These patients must be instructed to scrub their lids with baby shampoo and cotton swabs once or twice a day. If meibomianitis is severe enough, antibiotics should be prescribed. Similarly, any other problem present, such as iritis, should be treated as indicated.

Conjunctival cicatrization is characterized by adhesions from palpebral conjunctiva to bulbar conjunctiva and sometimes results in immobile lids, severe trichiasis, and extremely dry corneas. If the symblepharon is small and present only in the periphery of the cul-de-sac, gel lens insertion is easy. If the symblepharon is extensive, a space must be made for the soft lens by surgery. This consists of cutting the adhesion and peeling off the fleshy conjunctiva that covers the cornea.

After the surgery a gel lens can be inserted. It is important to instill atropine in the eye to minimize the postoperative discomfort from iritis.

If trichiasis is minimal, a soft lens alone will prevent corneal damage. Sometimes it is necessary to remove the lashes by epilation or electrolysis if trichiasis is significant, and in severe cases, plastic surgery is generally indicated. In most cases severe blepharitis is present, and must be treated with lid scrubs and antibiotics.

Once the lens is inserted, it is worn twenty-four hours a day. However, because the eye is so dry, the lens tends to dry, stick to the lids, and pop out. To minimize this, very frequent application of saline or artificial tear preparations is necessary, sometimes as often as every five to ten minues. After a few days on this regimen, the frequency can be diminished.

EPITHELIAL EROSIONS AND RECURRENT ULCERS

In recurrent ulcers and epithelial erosions, gel contact lenses have provided the necessary protection required for healing. The normal corneal epithelium does not interdigitate with its basement membrane but rather attaches to it with structures called hemidesmosomes (*see* Chapter 2). If this basement membrane is damaged, the epithelium cannot spread over the defective area and attach. It is this failure which causes most recurrent erosions.

A gel lens placed over the ulcer and worn continuously to prevent the lid from rubbing will facilitate healing. It is important, however, to treat the accompanying iritis with cycloplegics; otherwise, the patient will have pain.

Gel lenses have been used in recurrent erosions. They have relieved pain from erosions and have strikingly improved vision in granular, macular, and lattice dystrophy. They have permitted healing of ulcers after herpes,[16] bacterial infections, or alkali burns, and in burns have been effectively used along with collagenase inhibitors. One of the great additional benefits of these lenses has been their ability to promote the healing of epithelial defects after keratoplasty. In both burned and nonburned corneas, this has significantly improved keratoplasty results.

DRUG DELIVERY

When a piece of hydrated hydrogel material is placed into a solution containing a drug, the drug is taken up by the gel. The concentration of the drug within the gel increases with time to a maximum and then remains fairly constant. The final concentration is usually considerably higher in the gel material than in the solution. The exact concentration depends upon the particular hydrogel that is used and on the drug and its original concentration in the solution.

In some cases the drug concentration within the gel is several times higher than existed in the original solution. If the piece of gel is now removed and placed in pure water, the drug begins to effuse. Again, the rate at which the drug is released from the polymer depends on which hydrogel material is used and the drug concentration. However, the drug release time is typically extended over a period of hours.

The initial drug loss from the gel is high and gradually drops with time. This ability of hydrogel material to release drugs over extended time periods has prompted the experimental use of this polymer as a drug delivery system. For the eye, this system has been formed from a hydrogel contact lens or by a small button of hydrogel material that is placed in the cul-de-sac. This mode of application has two potential advantages over the conventional application of topical drugs to the eye by drops every three or four hours during the day. First, the number of applications may be reduced, and second, the penetration to the internal eye may be kept at a more uniform level throughout the diurnal period.

There is considerable interest in the use of a gel lens as a drug delivery system for pilocarpine.[17-19] Podos et al. have studied the dynamics of pilocarpine release from the Softcon lens.[17] They found that the amount of pilocarpine taken up by five lenses varied with the concentration of the drug and duration of soaking (Table 23.4). There is some variation from lens to lens. About 90 percent of the pilocarpine concentration had effused from the lenses after four hours.

Podos et al. also studied the diurnal variation of pressure in ten selected patients with high ocular tension.[17] Their studies showed that pilocarpine 0.5% had little or no effect when given three times a day without a gel contact lens in place. However, with the gel lens soaked in pilocarpine 0.5% for two minutes and inserted for twenty-three hours, there was a significant reduction of intraocular pressure in the treated eye as compared to a saline treated contralateral eye.

In normal subjects, one drop of 1% pilocarpine over the Softcon lens produced miosis greater than that elicited by 8% pilocarpine and lasted approximately twenty-four hours. In another experiment, two drops of 5% phenylephrine over the Softcon lens produced significantly greater and more prolonged mydriasis than with the Bausch and Lomb Soflens gel lens, hard contact lens, or no lens at all.

Preliminary studies at the University of Florida have indicated that in a mild case of open angle glaucoma, intraocular pressure was reduced further with 1% pilocarpine and the Softcon lens than with pilocarpine alone. Twenty hours later the drug was still active as measured by pupillary reaction and intraocular pressure. In another case, 2% pilocarpine with a Softcon lens was more effective than 0.25% phospholine iodide.

Other drugs have been used experimentally with the Softcon lens. In rabbits infected with herpes virus, IDU and Softcon lens treatment healed the ulcer faster than in eyes treated with IDU alone. On the other hand, *Pseudomonas* ulcers treated with polymyxin B and Softcon lenses did not heal any faster than when treated with the drug alone, suggesting that once an effective antibiotic level is obtained, further concentration has no beneficial effect on the infection.

There is considerable difference between the amount of various drugs taken up by different gel lenses. For example, *in vitro* pilocarpine uptake was five times greater for the Softcon lens than for the Bausch and Lomb Soflens. Some of this may be attributed to size differences, but a large amount is due

TABLE 23.4

In Vitro Study of Pilocarpine and Five Soft Contact Lenses

Pilocarpine Concentration (%)	Soak Time* (minutes)	Mean and Range of Uptake (mg)	Mean Loss† (%)				
			Half Hour	One Hour	Two Hours	Three Hours	Four Hours
0.5	2	.40 (.37– .43)	—	76	95	100	—
0.5	4	.44 (.37– .51)	59	80	92	97	100
0.5	6	.82 (.72– .97)	56	73	86	93	96
0.5	10	.94 (.75–1.43)	49	75	86	93	98
0.5	30	1.18 (1.04–1.28)	38	57	77	87	93
0.5	60	1.08 (.98–1.16)	46	62	76	86	92
1.0	2	1.07 (.96–1.30)	58	75	86	92	96
1.0	10	1.51 (1.37–1.70)	52	67	80	87	93
4.0	2	2.66 (1.06–3.66)	61	74	83	89	94
4.0	10	3.11 (2.30–4.07)	65	76	84	90	94

* Soaked in 12 drops of pilocarpine by immersing the lens in contact lens case.
† Eluted into fresh 3 ml of distilled water, agitated and eluate read against fellow lens soaked in saline at designated times.

to basic structural differences of the the two hydrogels. The action of these and other gel lenses in the release of drugs to the eye is in the early stages of development and is considered an experimental procedure.

REFERENCES

1. Kaufman, H. E., and Gasset, A. R.: The new hydrophilic contact lenses (interview), *Highlights of Ophthalmology*, *12*(3):177–190, 1969.

2. Kaufman, H. E., and Gasset, A. R.: Therapeutic soft bandage lenses, *Int. Ophthalmol. Clin.*, *10*(2):379–385, 1970.

3. Kaufman, H. E. et al.: The medical uses of soft contact lenses, *Trans. Am. Acad. Ophthalmol. Otolaryngol.*, *75*(2):361–373, 1971.

4. Leibowitz, H. M., and Rosenthal, P.: Hydrophilic contact lenses in corneal diseases. I. Superficial, sterile indolent ulcers, *Arch. Ophthalmol.* , *85*(2):163–166, 1971.

5. Leibowitz, H. M.: Hydrophilic contact lenses in corneal disease. IV. Penetrating corneal wounds, *Arch. Ophthalmol.*, *88*(6):602–606, 1972.

6. Lerman, S., and Sapp, G.: The hydrophilic (hydron) corneoscleral lens in the treatment of corneal disease, *Can. J. Ophthalmol.*, *6*(1):1–8, 1971.

7. Buxton, J. N., and Locke, C. R.: A therapeutic evaluation of hydrophilic contact lenses, *Am. J. Ophthalmol.*, *72*(3):532–535, 1971.

8. Feldman, G. L. et al.: Clinical experiences with cosmetic and therapeutic soft lenses, *J. Contact Lens Soc. Am.*, *5*(3):11–16, 1971.

9. Gasson, A.: Clinical experience with the Bausch and Lomb Soflens, *The Ophthalmic Optician*, *13*(2):81–84, 1973.

10. Espy, J. W.: Management of corneal prob-

lems with hydrophilic contact lenses, a report of thirty cases, *Am. J. Ophthalmol.*, 72(3):521–526, 1971.

11. Lerman, S., and Sapp, G.: The hydrophilic (Hydron) corneoscleral lens in the treatment of bullous keratopathy, *Ann. Ophthalmol.*, 2(2):142–144, 1970.

12. Gasset, A. R., and Kaufman, H. E.: Bandage lenses in the treatment of bullous keratopathy, *Am. J. Ophthalmol.*, 72(3):376–380, 1971.

13. Gasset, A. R., and Kaufman, H. E.: Therapeutic uses of hydrophilic contact lenses, *Am. J. Ophthalmol.*, 69(2):252–259, 1970.

14. Gasset, A. R.: Treatment of bullous keratopathy with soft contact lenses, To be published.

15. Gasset, A. R., and Kaufman, H. E.: Hydro-

philic lens therapy of severe keratoconjunctivitis sicca and conjunctival scarring, *Am. J. Ophthalmol.*, 71(6):1185–1189, 1971.

16. Aquavella, J. V.: The treatment of herpetic stromal disease, *Eye, Ear, Nose and Throat Mon.*, 51(10):374–381, 1972.

17. Podos, S. M. et al.: Pilocarpine therapy with soft contact lenses, *Arch. Ophthalmol.*, 73(3):336–341, 1972.

18. Maddox, Y. T., and Bernstein, H. N.: An evaluation of the Bionite hydrophilic contact lens for use in a drug delivery system, *Ann. Ophthalmol.*, 4(9):789–802, 1972.

19. Waltman, S. R., and Kaufman, H. E.: Use of hydrophilic contact lenses to increase ocular penetration of topical drugs, *Invest. Ophthalmol.*, 9(4):250–255, 1970.

ADDITIONAL READINGS

Amos, D. M.: The use of soft bandage lenses in corneal disease, *Am. J. Optom. Physiol. Opt.*, 52(8):524–32, 1975.

Amos, D. M.: Soft lenses in anterior segment pathology, *J. Am. Optom. Assoc.*, 47(3):291, 1976.

Aquavella, J. V.: Bionite hydrophilic bandage lenses in treatment of corneal disease soft contact lens, in Symposium and Workshop of the University of Florida, Gainesville, Gasset, A. R., and Kaufman, H. E. (Eds.): *Soft Contact Lens: Proceedings*, St. Louis, C. V. Mosby, 1972, p. 190.

Aquavella, J. V.: Avoidance of complications in hydrophilic bandage lens therapy, *CILMJ*, 4(3): 66, 1978.

Becker, B., Podos, S. M., Asseff, C., and Hartstein, J.: Pilocarpine therapy with soft contact lenses, *Am. J. Ophthalmol.*, 73(3):336–341, 1972.

Berndt, K., Sundmacher, R., and Silbernagl, K.: A controlled comparison of two therapeutic soft lenses in a clinical model, *Invest. Ophthalmol.*, 16(6): 559–561, 1977.

Bernstein, H. N., and Maddox, Y.: An evaluation of the bionite hydrophilic contact lens for use in a drug delivery system, *Ann. Ophthalmol.*, 4(9):789–802, 1972.

Binder, P. S.: A continuous-wear hydrophilic lens. Prophylactic topical antibiotics, *Arch. Ophthalmol.*, 94(12):2109–2111, 1976.

Binder, P. S. et al.: The results of penetrating keratoplasty after chemical burns, *Trans. Am. Acad. Ophthalmol. Otolaryngol.*, 79(4):584–595, 1975.

Black, C. J., and Kearns, W. P.: Bullous keratopathy and the soft contact lens, *Contacto*, 18(1):7–8, 1974.

Bloomfield, S. E. et al.: Treatment of filamentary keratitis with soft contact lens, *Am. J. Ophthalmol.*, 76(6):978–980, 1973.

Boruchoff, S. A., Dohlman, C. H., and Mobilia, E. F.: Complications in use of soft contact lenses in corneal disease, *see* Dohlman, C. H. et al., *Arch. Ophthalmol.*, 90(5):367–371, 1973.

Breitfeller, J. M., and Krohn, D. L.: Quantitation of pilocarpine flux enhancement isolated rabbit cornea by Hydrogel polymer lenses, *Invest. Ophthalmol.*, 14(2):152–153, 1975.

Brettschneider, I., and Krejci, J.: Gel contact lenses and their use in the treatment of chemical burns of the eye, *Arbeitsmed. Fragen in der Ophthalmologa*, 4(4):195–204, Symposium Budapest, 1972 (Karger, Basel, 1974).

Brodrick, J. D.: The Bausch and Lomb "T" lens in the treatment of corneal disease, *Trans. Ophthalmol. Soc. U.K.*, 96:330, 1976.

Brown, S. I., Tragakis, M. D., and Pearce, D. B.: Treatment of the alkali-burned cornea with soft contact lenses, in Symposium and Workshop of the University of Florida, Gainesville, Gasset, A. R., and Kaufman, H. E. (Eds.): *Soft Contact Lens: Proceedings*, St. Louis, C. V. Mosby, 1972, p. 224.

Brown, S. I. et al.: Treatment of filamentary keratitis with the soft contact lens, *Am. J. Ophthalmol.*, 76(6):978–980, 1973.

Callender, M. G., and Woo, G.: Use of an ultra-thin soft contact lens for keratoconjunctivitis sicca, *Int. Cont. Lens Clin.*, 4(3):57, 1977.

Citron, J., and Dyer, J. A.: The use of therapeutic contact lenses in corneal disease, *Contacto*, 20(6): 13–23, 1976.

Dabezies, O. H.: Lost eye in association with a soft contact lens used in treatment of bullous keratopathy, *Cont. Lens Med. Bull.*, 5(34):3–6, Dec. 1972.

Devoe, A. G.: Keratoprosthesis: history, techniques, and indications, *Am. Acad. Ophthalmol. Oto Ophtha Trans.*, 83(2):249, 1977.

Dohlman, C. H.: Symposium: soft contact lenses complications in therapeutic soft lens wear, *Trans. Am. Acad. Ophthalmol. Otolaryngol.*, 78(3): 399–405, 1974.

Dohlman, C. H., Boruchoff, S. A., and Mobilia, E.: Complications in use of soft contact lenses in corneal disease, *Arch. Ophthalmol.*, 90(5): 367–371, 1973.

Dohlman, C. H., Mobilia, E. F., and Holly, F. J.: A comparison of various soft contact lenses for therapeutic purposes, *Cont. Lens Med. J.*, 3(1): 9–15, 1977.

Eiferman, R. A., Lindmark, R., and Hyndiuk, R. A.: Cosmetic use of epinephrine tinted soft contact lenses to conceal abnormalities of the anterior segment, *Cont. Intraoc. Lens Med. J.*, 2(4):53–54, 1976.

Emery, J. M., Schecter, D. R., and Soper, J. W.: Corneal vascularization in therapeutic soft-lens wear, *see* Schecter, D. R.: *Cont. Intraoc. Lens Med. J.*, 1(1–2):141–145, 1975.

Fontana, F.: Soft lenses to protect the cornea after fasanella ptosis surgery, *J. Am. Optom. Assoc.*, 49(3):316–318, 1978.

Francois, J., and Cambie, E.: New prospects in the treatment of corneal ulcer (A), *Excerpta Medica*, 27(3):158, 1973.

Ganju, S. N., and Cordrey, P.: Effect of some drugs on contact lens wearers, *Ophthalmol. Optom.*, 17(10):390, 1977.

Gasset, A., and Lobo, L.: Simplified soft contact lens treatment in corneal diseases, *Ann. Ophthalmol.*, 9(7):843, 1977.

Gasset, A. R.: Correction of bullous keratopathy with soft contact lenses, *Int. Cont. Lens Clin.*, 1(1):89–99, 1974.

Gasset, A. R., and Bellows, R. T.: Hydrophilic contact lenses in the treatment of shallow or flat chambers, *Ann. Ophthalmol.*, 6(10):996–998, 1974.

Gasset, A.R., and Katzin, D.: Antiviral drugs and corneal wound healing, *Invest. Ophthalmol.*, 14(8):628–630, 1975.

Girolamo, L. C.: Treatment of some corneal affections by means of soft contact lenses, *Cont. Lens J.*, 5(6):19–20, 1976.

Gould, H. L.: Symposium: Soft contact lenses. Therapeutic experience with soft contact lenses, *Trans. Am. Acad. Ophthalmol. Otolaryngol.*, 78(3): 391–398, 1974.

Gutierrez-Avello, F., and Cordero-Moreno, R.: Treatment of corneal lacerations with soft contact lenses, *Cont. Intraoc. Lens Med. J.*, 3(2):21–23, 1977.

Hillman, J. S.: Management of acute glaucoma with pilocarpine-soaked hydrophilic lens, *Br. J. Ophthalmol.*, 58(7):674–679, 1974.

Hull, D. S. et al.: Ocular penetration of prednisolone and the hydrophilic contact lens, *Arch. Ophthalmol.*, 92(5):413–416, 1974.

Hull, D. S. et al.: Clinical experience with the therapeutic hydrophilic contact lens, *Cont. Lens J.*, 9(1):9–16, 1975.

Hurwitz, J. J., Dixon, W. S., and Sloan, A.: Therapeutic soft contact lenses: a survey, *Can. J. Ophthalmol.*, 9(1):72–78, 1974.

Junge, J.: Therapeutic use of contact lenses. Some non-cosmetic uses of contact lenses, *Contact Lens*, 4(7):3, 1974.

Kaufman, H. E.: Past development and future needs for therapeutic corneal contact lenses, *Cont. Intraoc. Lens Med. J.*, 1(1–2):31–37, 1975.

Laibson, P. R.: Therapeutic soft contact lenses (annual review: cornea and sclera), *Arch. Ophthalmol.*, 88(5):553–574, 1972.

Langston, R. H., Machamer, J., and Norman, C. W.: Soft lens therapy for recurrent erosion syndrome, *Cont. Lens J.*, 12(2):9, 1978.

Leibowitz, H. M., and Rosenthal, P.: Hydrophilic contact lenses in corneal disease. II. Bullous keratopathy, *Arch. Ophthalmol.*, 85(3):283–285, 1971.

Leigh, E.: Therapeutic uses of the soft contact lens, *Contact Lens*, 4(7):4, 1974.

Lemp, M. A.: The role of bandage lenses in the management of recurrent erosions of the cornea, *Cont. Intraoc. Lens Med. J.*, 3(2):28–32, 1977.

Marmion, V. J.: Role of soft contact lenses and delivery of drugs, *Trans. Ophthalmol. Soc. U.K.*, 96:319, 1976.

Mizutani, Y., and Miwa, Y.: On the uptake and release of drugs by soft contact lenses, *Cont. Intraoc. Lens Med. J.*, 1(1–2):177–183, 1975.

Mobilia, E. F., Dohlman, C. H., and Holly, F. J.: A comparison of various soft contact lenses for therapeutic purposes, *Cont. Intraoc. Lens Med. J.*, 3(1):9–15, 1977.

Mobilia, E. F., and Foster, C. S.: The management of recurrent corneal erosions with ultra-thin lenses, *Cont. Intraoc. Lens Med. J.*, 4(1):25–29, 1978.

Philpotts, J.: Silver nitrate treatment for intolerance to contact lenses, *Cont. Lens J.*, 5(6):12, 1976.

Polito, E., and Frezzoti, R., and Troiano-Billi, M. J.: Use of hydrophilic contact lenses in the treatment of bullous/edematous keratopathy, *Contacto*, 22(4):15–23, 1978.

Chapter 24

EXTENDED WEAR

EXTENDED WEAR REFERS to the procedure whereby contact lenses are worn twenty-four hours per day for a finite number of days. It should be differentiated from permanent wear or continuous wear, which refers to placing a contact lens on the eye for an indefinite period.

It was not long after the introduction of hydrogel contact lenses that it was discovered they could be worn by patients during sleep without clinically obvious adverse effects. This discovery came about in the treatment of patients with anterior segment diseases, particularly bullous keratopathy.[1-6] For these patients, the benefits of wearing gel contact lenses overnight clearly outweighed the risks, and hence, the practice became accepted. Its success lead clinicians to try overnight wear with other pathologic conditions, and soon there was experimentation with cosmetic cases. It was not long, however, before it was noted that adverse effects occurred in some patients, whereas others appeared to be trouble free.[7-9] Because of this, extended wear lenses have usually been reserved for those patients who have the greatest need for them. They have been used extensively for the correction of aphakia and somewhat less for cosmetic cases.[10-25]

Patients who benefit greatly from extended wear are those who desire one or more of these advantages: (1) no need to remove lenses at night, (2) elimination of inconvenient, and sometimes difficult, cleaning and disinfecting procedures, (3) less chance of loss or damage to the lenses because of reduced handling, (4) long-range reduced cost because daily cleaning and disinfecting solutions need not be purchased, (5) normal vision all the time, (6) reduced lens handling for individuals who keep irregular hours and would be troubled by lens removal and insertion, (7) more convenient travel because special solutions and electrical and water requirements can be ignored, and (8) elimination of lens removal and insertion procedures for those patients who have difficulty handling lenses.

Many hydrogel contact lenses that have been manufactured for daily wear may also be used successfully for extended wear. However, other lenses do not fulfill the requirements for extended wear and are likely to produce adverse effects. Hence, a clear understanding of the basic requirements for an extended-wear lens should be recognized by the fitter.

The design requirements of an extended-wear lens are dictated by at least five major changes in the lens environment when the eyes are closed.

1. The action of the lids is eliminated.
2. There is a change in pH of the tears.
3. There is a temperature increase at the cornea.
4. There is a change in the tear osmolarity.
5. The oxygen supply to the cornea is reduced.

LID ACTION

The action of the lids provides several functions that are eliminated during eye closure. There is some pumping of tears beneath the contact lens, but as was shown in Chapter 17, this is minimal in terms of providing the oxygen supply needed by the cornea. However, a second function of this tear exchange has become more apparent with the use of extended-wear contact lenses. During eye clo-

sure, various forms of debris become trapped between the contact lens and the cornea, which ordinarily would be removed by a flushing effect of the tears during blinking. The stagnation of this debris may cause a mechanical irritation of the cornea and may also lead to other effects that are not well understood (Figure 24.1).[26]

PH CHANGES

There is a change in the pH of tears when the eyes are closed.[27] The average change is from 7.3 to 7.1, but there is considerable

individual variability, and the importance of this effect in terms of contact lens wear is not known.

TEMPERATURE INCREASES

There is a temperature increase of approximately 4°F whenever the eyes are closed.[28] Theoretically, this temperature change

should increase the metabolic activity of the cornea, but the effect of this change is difficult to evaluate.

TEAR OSMOLARITY CHANGES

The tear osmolarity is reduced during sleep.[29] This occurs because the normal tear secretion from the lacrimal gland has a lower salt content than the normal precorneal film in the open eye. The higher salt content of the open-eye film is due primarily to evaporation from the precorneal surface. In Chapter 6 it was shown that tear osmolarity changes during adaptation to hard contact lenses were

sufficient to produce measurable corneal edema. Also, subjects have been shown to experience a 3 to 5 percent edema during sleep even when contact lenses are not being worn. It is undetermined whether this effect is accentuated during lens wear. In any case, it is likely that osmolarity changes during sleep may cause significant amounts of corneal edema.

REDUCED OXYGEN SUPPLY TO THE CORNEA

Chapter 17 demonstrated that hydrogel contact lenses reduce the available oxygen supply to the cornea to nearly its minimum requirement when the eyes are open. Clos-

ing the eyes reduces the oxygen tension available at the anterior surface of the lens to approximately one-third of the normal atmospheric condition. Hence, only about

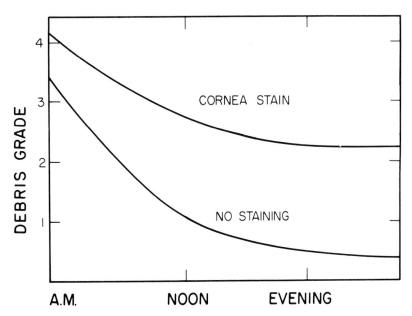

Figure 24.1. Hypothetical curves showing relationship between amount of debris and corneal staining. Patients with high levels of debris show less lens tolerance. Adapted from G. Mertz and B. Holden, Bausch & Lomb Research Conference, August 1980.

one-third of the oxygen reaches the cornea that would normally be supplied when the eyes are open. For many hydrogel contact lenses this reduces the oxygen level below the minimum corneal need and produces corneal edema. Hence, only those soft contact lenses which pass higher amounts of oxygen will suffice as extended-wear lenses.[30-33]

Contact lenses that pass high amounts of oxygen are generally those with higher water contents or minimum thicknesses. Unfortunately, the higher water content lenses tend to have lower mechanical strength, and hence, the lenses are generally made thicker to offset this disadvantage. The added thickness causes a further reduction in the oxygen transmission, but this is usually not enough to offset the advantages of higher water content on oxygen permeability. These lenses are particularly advantageous for high refractive correction where the lenses must have considerable thickness in any case.

Medium water content lenses can pass sufficient oxygen to supply the corneal needs if they are made thin enough. For lenses of 38 percent water content, the thickness must be 0.03 mm. Such lenses are prone to breakage and present difficult handling problems so that their use has been limited.

There are some practitioners who feel that lenses of higher water content are more compatible with the eye than lenses of lower water content, even when the two are equated for oxygen transmission. There is some clinical evidence to support this position, but it is not conclusive.

Another unresolved question for extended wear is to determine the oxygen requirement of the cornea during sleep.[34-36] Some experiments with extended-wear lenses have been conducted with eye closure during the awake state. It is possible that the oxygen use under these conditions is somewhat different from that required during sleep, when the metabolic activity level of the body has been reduced. Figure 24.2a shows the relationship between lens thickness and the oxygen level at the cornea for both the open– and closed-eye conditions. It is obvious that only the thinnest of lenses can allow oxygen levels above the minimum corneal need.[37,38] This suggests that most hydrogel contact lenses that are being used for extended wear do not provide the minimum corneal oxygen requirement. This is supported by studies that indicate that nearly all extended-wear lens patients show significant corneal edema during sleep.[39-40]

Leibowitz and Laing fitted one eye of ten normal subjects with a lens that was worn for ten days, while the other eye served as a control.[41] The average corneal swelling for the eyes wearing lenses was 21 percent in the morning and 15 percent in the afternoon. Most of the subjects had variable vision, deposits in the lens, and slight roughening of the epithelial surface. Polse et al. studied changes in corneal swelling of five subjects who wore ultrathin Bausch and Lomb soft lenses on one eye for 102 continuous hours.[42] An average 9 percent corneal swelling occurred overnight, which was accompanied by corneal striae. Each time after awakening (eyes open), the swelling decreased to about 3 percent over the next eight hours (Figure 24.2b). Mobilia, Dohlman, and Holly have measured corneal thickening upon the wearers' awakening in a study of thirty subjects who wore different hydrogel lenses.[43] Only sixteen subjects were able to complete the twenty-four hour wearing cycle, while the remaining fourteen dropped out of the study for reasons such as discomfort, punctate staining, and lens dislodging. For the sixteen successful subjects, it was found that ultrathin lenses caused little or no swelling, whereas thicker lenses caused significant increases in swelling (0.05 to 0.15 mm.). Sarver and his coworkers measured the corneal swelling resulting from three hours of lid closure.[44,45] They found that in all subjects the cornea

swelled, although there was considerable variability among subjects. These results suggest that the partial pressure of oxygen under the lens during sleep is insufficient to maintain normal corneal hydration, and that swelling under closed-eye conditions appears to be related to the oxygen transmissibility of the material.

Zantos and Holden have reported in a study on thirty-five patients that few patients on their first attempt were able to achieve successful continuous wear beyond one month and that every patient experienced some difficulty resulting in an interruption of lens wear.[46] Interruptions were due to (1) unsatisfactory lens fitting, (2) inadequate vision with lenses, and (3) disturbance to corneal integrity. The disturbances to corneal integrity were due to corneal edema (most patients), pannus (one patient), epithelial microvessicles (several patients), corneal ulceration (four patients), and red eye or nonulcerative keratitis (twelve patients). Zantos and Holden concluded that extended wear may be hazardous and open to abuse because the corneal epithelium beneath a continously worn lens is probably hypoxic and therefore less resistant to trauma and infection. They also suggested that corneal sensitivity is reduced, and patient response to early corneal damage is retarded. Holden and his coworkers have reported on short-term effects of extended wear.[47] They fitted ten subjects with Bausch & Lomb thin lenses (38% water, 0.03 mm.), Permalens® (75% water, 0.10 mm.), and Hydrocurve II® (55% water, 0.06 mm.). Patients wore these lenses for two weeks while corneal thickness and corneal response were monitored upon awakening and at three-hour and nine-hour intervals. Following this trial period, the patients were given a three-week period without lens wear, and the study was again repeated with another type of lens. With each type of lens, the cornea showed an average corneal swelling of 10 to 16 percent in the morning that did not decrease during the course of the study. This

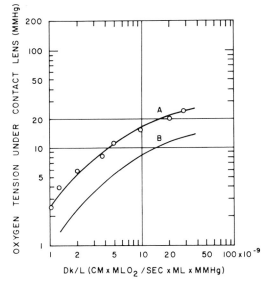

Figure 24.2a. Relationship between lens Dk thickness and oxygen level at the cornea for the open-eye (A) and closed-eye (B) conditions. Courtesy of K. Polse.

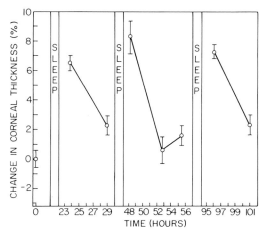

Figure 24.2b. Corneal swelling of a subject who wore soft lenses for 101 hours. From K. A. Polse, M. D. Sarver, and M. G. Harris, Effects of Soflens Parameters on Corneal Edema, *International Contact Lens Clinic*, Summer, 1976, pp. 35–41.

edema represented significant stress to the ocular system and probably could not have

been tolerated on a constant basis. However, when the eye was opened in the morning, the oxygen level was raised once again, and the edema was reduced. Hence, every extended-wear contact lens patient showed considerable diurnal fluctuation in the corneal thickness (Figure 24.3). For some subjects, this edema was responsible for a rejection of the lenses. In other patients, the edema caused significant symptoms, but the lenses continued to be tolerated for extended periods of time. Among those subjects who were asymptomatic, several showed epithelial staining, redness, specatacle blur, and infections requiring ophthalmological treatment. Holden's studies were limited by the small number of subjects, length of follow-up, and absence of concurrent controls; nevertheless, such information might suggest that some patients may develop more serious and perhaps permanent long-range effects from extended wear.

There is some evidence that subjects with higher amounts of corneal swelling during eye closure show a greater frequency of lens intolerance (Figure 24.4). This swelling is not detectable if patients are seen later in the day (Figure 24.5).

These results are in agreement with the experimental evidence that indicates extended-wear lenses will not supply sufficient oxygen to maintain normal corneal metabolism. Decker, Polse, and Fatt reported on the oxygen tension and oxygen flux at the corneal surface in both open and closed eyes covered by a hydrogel lens.[48] These values of oxygen tension (open eye 2 to 20 mm. Hg; closed eye 1 to 10 mm. Hg) indicate that, even with materials that have a high oxygen transmissibility, the partial pressure of oxygen under the lens during sleep is less than 11 mm. Hg, which would be insufficient to maintain normal corneal hydration.

The delivery of oxygen to the cornea covered by a contact lens may be further diminished by the buildup of materials on the front surface of the lens. Benjamin and Hill have

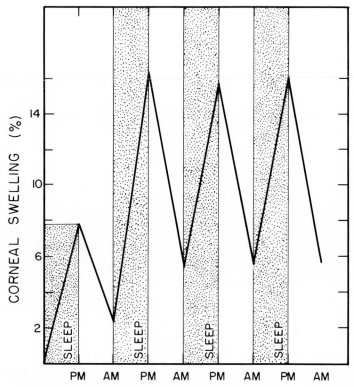

Figure 24.3. Diurnal fluctuation in corneal thickness with extended wear.

suggested that the coating of proteins and other material on the hydrogel lens may reduce the amount of oxygen transmissibility.[49] Fowler and Allansmith have shown that extended-wear lenses steadily build up coatings.[50] If oxygen transmissibility decreases with extended wear, late onset of problems related to reduced oxygen delivery to the cornea may result.

The laboratory studies seem to suggest that when a contact lens is worn during lid closure, corneal swelling that is most likely due to corneal hypoxia occurs. Presently available hydrogel materials will not supply enough oxygen during closed-eye conditions to prevent corneal swelling. Tear pumping under a lens is usually minimal; therefore, the contribution of additional oxygen by tear pumping is probably insignificant. The effect of reduced tear exchange on corneal function is not known. The effects of corneal hypoxia and low tear interchange over several months and/or years has not been studied.

SELECTION OF PATIENTS

The use of extended-wear contact lenses demands additional requirements on the part of the patient. He must understand the responsibilities and potential for complications if he does not follow good wearing habits. Some patients do not make good candidates for extended wear as outlined by Binder.[51] The guidelines include the following:

1. Good personal hygiene is a prerequisite for successful extended wear. Patients who have an anterior segment infection, blepharitis, abnormal eyelids, poor blinking responses, lagophthalmos,

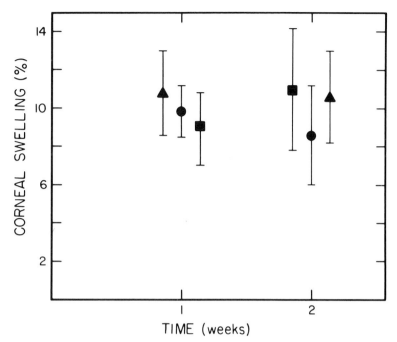

Figure 24.4. Corneal swelling of subjects who rejected extended wear lenses. Courtesy of Doctor D. Rorabaugh.

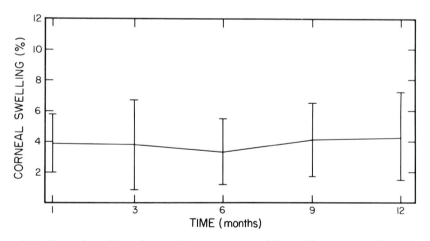

Figure 24.5. Corneal swelling of extended wear patients followed for one year. Measurements were made during the day and do not reflect overnight changes. Courtesy of Doctor D. Rorabaugh.

or dry eyes should not be considered as candidates because of an increased risk of infection.

2. Uncooperative and retarded patients, or those who might go unsupervised, should not be selected, because it will be difficult to obtain adequate examinations and followup evaluations.

3. Patients who cannot afford the expense or the time for multiple scheduled return office visits

must be excluded.

4. A successful daily wearer of a hard or soft contact lens should not be selected.

5. Patients in whom corneal edema develops with daily wear soft lenses are excluded.

6. Astigmatism greater than 2 diopters also eliminates many patients.

For these patients, some other choice should be made, e.g., no lens, glasses, tarsorrhaphy, conjunctival flap, intraocular lens implantation or a hard contact lens.

Inclusion Criteria — The following are suitable candidates:

1. A patient who fears damaging the eye during insertion and removal of a lens

2. A patient with a physical handicap (e.g., arthritis, Parkinson's disease, or following a stroke) preventing insertion and removal of a lens

3. An aphake who has poor vision in the other eye, e.g., cataract, macular disease, optic atrophy from any cause, etc.

4. Monocular aphakes who cannot tolerate a lens on a daily basis for physical or psychological reasons

5. A child with monocular aphakia whose parents are unable to insert and remove a daily wear lens

6. An intraocular lens candidate who did not have a lens implanted because of a contraindication at surgery

7. A monocular pseudophake who is now aphakic in the other eye (an extended wear lens in the aphakic eye will decrease the necessity for bilateral intraocular lens implantation)

8. Any candidate for a secondary intraocular lens implant. This patient should undergo a trial of extended wear before attempting surgery. (A patient who cannot afford the expense of a second surgical procedure is included in this group.)*

LENS DESIGN

Lenses for extended wear are usually designed to maximize the oxygen transmission. Other characteristics are typical of hydrogel lenses that are used for daytime wear. Some representative lenses are as follows:

Medium Water Content Lenses

1. The Hydrocurve II (Bufilcon A), a lathe-cut 45 percent hydrated lens, is available in diameters from 13.0 to 16.0 mm., base curves from 8.6 to 10.1 mm., and all powers. Its optical zone varies from 8.0 to 8.5 mm. and its center thickness from 0.06 to 0.7 mm. The Hydrocurve II–55 is a 55% hydrated lens which comes in diameters of 14.0 and 14.5 mm., base curves of 8.5 and 8.8 mm., and has a center thickness between 0.05 and 0.07 mm.

2. The CSI (Crofilcon A) is a thin lens, is 39 to 41 percent hydrated and its thickness varies between 0.03 and 0.08 mm.

3. Softcon (Vifilcon A) is a 55 percent hydrated lathe-cut lens which comes in powers from −6.00 to +18.00, base curves from 7.8 to 8.4, and diameters from 13.5 to 15.0. The optical zone is fixed at 8.0 mm. and the center thicknesses are found to vary between 0.28 and 0.70.

High Water Content Lenses — The following are included:

1. Sauflon 70 (Lidofilcon-A) and Sauflon PW (Lidofilcon-B) are lathe-cut lenses which are 70 to 85 percent hydrated. They come in diameters from 13.7 to 14.4 mm., all powers; base curves from 8.1 to 9.0 mm., and center thicknesses of 0.46 mm. to 0.67 mm.

2. The Permalens (Perfilcon-A) is a lathe-cut lens hydrated between 69 and 72 percent. It comes in diameters from 11.5 to 13.5 mm., base curves from 6.5 to 8.0 mm., center thicknesses from 0.24 to 0.43 mm., and all powers.*

FITTING PHILOSOPHY

In general, the approach to fitting an extended-wear lens is to provide lens movement and eliminate limbal pressure. It was originally thought that lens movement was

necessary in order to provide an additional

*From P.S. Binder, The Extended Wear of Soft Contact Lenses, *Journal of Continuing Education in Ophthalmology*, 4(6):15–32, 1979.

oxygen supply to the cornea. Evidence now shows, however, that the principal function of lens movement is to remove debris from beneath the lens surface. Retention of this debris will almost invariably lead to corneal problems.

A lens that applies pressure to the limbal region of the eye will also produce the effects which are typical of tight lens symptoms. The exact mechanism is unknown, but it is suspected to involve an interference with the limbal circulation. The effects that are produced are described under complications.

The evaluation of the lens fit should be made in the same way as for a daytime wear patient.

ADAPTATION

There are two modes that are practiced in adapting patients to extended-wear lenses. In the first, a lens is worn for a period of time as a day-wear lens and after a successful fitting is completed, the patient is shifted to extended wear. In the second, the patient begins immediately with extended wear and is treated accordingly. The first method has the advantage that the lenses may be evaluated independently of the extended-wear condition. Any necessary modifications can then be made before the patient is placed in a more stressful wearing condition. This approach has a disadvantage that lenses which are more fragile may not withstand the daily-wear routine.

The advantage of immediate twenty-four hour wear is that the patient does not necessarily need to learn lens insertion methods, although removal techniques should be taught for an emergency. The patient must be seen in the office at more frequent intervals to insure that complications are not occurring.

PATIENT CARE

Binder recommends that the patient be instructed to examine his eyes in a mirror while in the office to note the amount of conjunctival injection. The patient is informed that the eyes should not look more injected than at that time. The patient is instructed to return immediately if he has any combination of pain, redness, decreased vision, or increased tearing. The lenses for all patients will require cleaning at regular intervals. The exact time may vary with the patient and may be as frequent as once a week. Aphakic patients tend to have greater amounts of secretion and will require more frequent cleanings. In general, the same cleaners are used that are provided for daily-wear lenses.

Lenses may be disinfected by either chemical or standard heat systems. There is some evidence that the heat system is more effective against various pathogenic organisms and, hence, may be more efficacious for extended-wear lenses. However, many patients are successful with either heat or chemical disinfection, and both methods are used.

Some high water content lenses have handling characteristics that are significantly different from other lenses. High plus lenses (aphakia range) show a sagging effect, which is helpful in determining whether a lens is inside out (Figure 24.6).

The number of follow-up examinations should be increased over that which is used for daily wear. The patient should always be seen the day after the lenses are dispensed. Some practitioners prefer to follow the patient two or three days later, whereas others may wait as long as a week. The patient must then be seen on a weekly basis for two or three

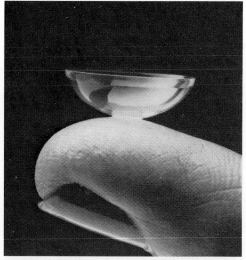

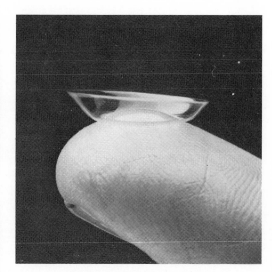

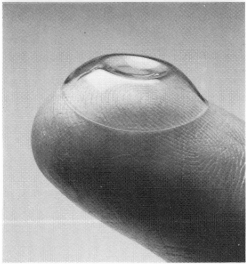

Figure 24.6. High water content lens in correct position for insertion (*a*). A lens that is inside out will sag in the center (*b* and *c*). Courtesy of Cooper Vision.

weeks and monthly thereafter. It is never possible to release an extended-wear patient for long periods of time without an examination.

For some patients, a physical disability makes it impossible for them to learn insertion and removal procedures. These patients may return to the practitioner's office periodically for lens removal and cleaning (Figure 24.7). It is always best if someone is available to the patient who can remove the lenses in the event of an emergency.

COMPLICATIONS

Several complications from using extended-wear lenses have been reported. Many of these reports were on aphakic patients because they were among the first patients to wear

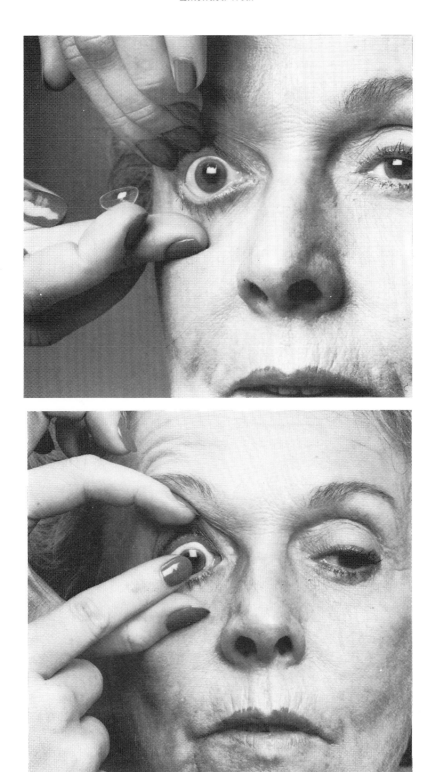

Figure 24.7. Insertion (*a*) and removal (*b*) for patients with a physical handicap may be carried out as a routine office procedure.

lenses on an extended basis. Nevertheless, the experience gained from the examination of extended wear on the aphakic eye probably provides a conservative model for extended wear on the phakic eye, because recent evidence suggests that the aphakic eye may tolerate extended wear better than the phakic eye.[52] Complications include corneal edema, neovascularization, infection, inflammation, increased superior tarsal papillary hypertrophy, epithelial necrosis, endothelial changes, mucus formation, lens deposits, and decreases in corneal sensitivity. Reports of the incidence of complications associated with extended wear are variable. Binder reported in a study of fifty-seven patients that there were four lens applications associated with significant corneal swelling, six with infections, five with corneal neovascularization, and fifteen with cases of injected eyes resulting in moderate to severe pain.[53] Gasset and his coworkers reported increased corneal swelling in aphakic patients wearing extended-wear contact lenses as compared to those wearing lenses on a daily basis.[54] In the same study, there was a high incidence of neovascularization (24.4%), conjunctivitis

(12.3%), and epithelial edema (12.2%). Highman studied forty-seven eyes fitted with Sauflon-85 lenses for three months.[55] He reported three eyes (two patients) with 2 mm. of neovascularization, one eye with a central corneal ulcer, four eyes with conjunctivitis, and numerous lenses with mucoprotein coating. Recently, McMonnies and Zantos have reported that some patients wearing hydrogel lenses develop a cluster of edematous droplets on the endothelium.[56] They describe these droplets as endothelium bedewing and suggest that they may be caused by a low grade anterior uveal response. Clinicians who fit extended-wear lenses have described a tight lens syndrome, which includes edema, keratitis, inflamed eye, and anterior uveitis.[57] This syndrome is apparently associated with a tight lens (no movement); however, its etiology is not known.

Most of the complications from extended-wear lenses may be attributed to partial corneal anoxia or inadequate tear pumping to remove debris trapped between the lens and cornea during sleep. These provide sources of corneal irritation, and the eye responds as follows.

LENS DEPOSITS

Excessive secretions and their entrapment beneath the contact lens lead to the accumulation of lens deposits to a greater degree than exists in daily-wear patients.[58] These deposits often present the major obstacle to the success of extended-wear lenses.[59,60] They may be composed of various substances including lipids, calcium, and protein.[61-63] They exist to some degree in nearly every patient and become a severe clinical problem in about

20 percent of the wearers. Only the most severe cases show an interference with vision, but many patients show corneal staining, conjunctival injection, and allergic reactions.

The tendency for ocular secretions to coat the lens appears to be an individual characteristic but has not been correlated with blood chemistry or tear composition. Its occurrence defies prediction before the fitting is accomplished.

LENS PROBLEMS

It has been argued that extended wear does not result in the theoretical expectation of longer lens life. These lenses are often

subject to loss, breakage, and splits, cracks, and tears. The lenses may become discolored and show degenerative changes.

ANOXIC SYNDROME

Patients who have a high oxygen minimum requirement are subject to a more severe reaction when extended wear is attempted. They show lens intolerance, which usually occurs after the first night of lens wear, but some delay may exist before the reaction is manifested. The syndrome may consist of all or any of the following: pain, photophobia, severe conjunctival injection, obvious edema and striae, and epithelial punctate staining. There may also be ciliary flush, anterior chamber flare, and/or visual loss. The possibility of this syndrome makes mandatory the examination of every patient on the day following the beginning of lens wear.

CONJUNCTIVAL COMPLICATIONS

Binder has described conjunctival complications during daily cosmetic soft lens wear including conjunctival injection, conjunctivitis, follicular conjunctivitis, perilimbal conjunctival edema, and giant papillary conjunctivitis.[64] These conjunctival complications have been reported during therapeutic lens wear,[65-70] and as expected, they have also been documented during extended wear.

A continuously worn soft lens does not affect the conjunctival flora in cosmetic[71] or therapeutic patients.[69] The infections or injection may be caused by contamination of the lens solutions, allergy to tear proteins on the lenses, undiagnosed dry eyes and blepharitis, abnormalities in the contact lenses, poor-fitting contact lenses, or toxic/allergic reactions to solutions associated with lens cleaning and sterilization.[72]

When an extended-wear patient presents with a red eye, one must assume he has an infection until proven otherwise. The lens should be inspected while on the eye to detect deformities. Questioning the patient about his methods of lens cleaning and disinfection may expose a break in accepted procedure. The eyelids should be everted to look for giant papillary changes. If a toxic reaction is suspected, the disinfection technique should be changed to a thermal type using saline *after a three-day wash in saline* to eliminate the chlorhexidine.[73] Routine bacteriologic cultures may be performed for a suspected infection.

CORNEAL INVOLVEMENT

Corneal punctate staining may indicate a dirty lens, severe edema, allergic reaction, or corneal infection. When due to a dirty lens, the punctate areas tend to coalesce into patches, but this is not always pathognomonic. Corneal edema must usually exceed 10 percent before staining occurs, but this is a function of whether the edema is more epithelial than stromal.

Infectious keratitis may be obvious if it is severe and other ocular signs are present such as conjunctivitis.[74,75] A viral keratitis may be more elusive and not accompanied by other signs. Stromal infiltrates may be present, but these are also known to occur as a result of mechanical lens irritation at the limbal region. Any patient who evidences signs of viral conjunctivitis is suggested to maintain his lenses on a heat disinfection regimen, which is thought to provide better efficiency than many cold-solution methods. Allergic reactions may occur from many of the cold storage solutions, but they are often particularly severe with lenses of high water content, which tend to absorb and concentrate many chemicals such as chlorhexidine.

REFERENCES

1. Rycroft, B. W.: Anterior segment lenses, *Highlights Ophthalmol.*, 7:253–256, 1964.

2. Kaufman, H. E., Gasset, A. R.: The new hydrophilic contact lenses, *Highlights Ophthalmol.*, 12:177–184, 1969.

3. Gasset, A. R., Kaufman, H. E.: Therapeutic uses of hydrophilic contact lenses, *Am. J. Ophthalmol.*, 69:252–263, 1970.

4. Leibowitz, H. M., and Rosenthal, P.: Hydrophilic contact lenses in corneal disease. I. Superficial, sterile, indolent ulcers, *Arch. Ophthalmol.*, 85:163–169, 1971.

5. Leibowitz, H. M., and Rosenthal, P.: Hydrophilic contact lenses in corneal disease. II. Bullous keratopathy, *Arch. Ophthalmol.*, 85:283–291, 1971.

6. Gould, H. L.: Therapeutic experience with soft contact lenses, *Trans. Am. Acad. Ophthalmol. Otolaryngol.*, 78:391–396, 1974.

7. Dohlman, D. H., Boruchoff, S. A., and Mobilia, E. F.: Complications in the use of soft contact lenses in corneal disease, *Arch. Ophthalmol.*, 90:367–378, 1973.

8. Sugar, J.: Adrenochrome pigmentation of hydrophilic lenses, *Arch. Ophthalmol.*, 91:11, 1974.

9. Palmer, E., Ferry, A. P., and Safir, A.: Fungal invasion of a soft (Griffin bionite) contact lens, *Arch. Ophthalmol.*, 93:278–282, 1974.

10. Binder, P. S.: Extended wear of three soft contact lenses, *Cont. Intraoc. Lens Med. J.*, 5:45–47, 1979.

11. Aquavella, J. V., Jackson, G. K., and Guy, L. F.: Therapeutic effects of bionite lenses: mechanisms of action, *Ann. Ophthalmol.*, 3:1341–1347, 1971.

12. Benson, C.: Continuous use of contact lenses, *Austr. J. Ophthalmol.*, 4:99–101, 1976.

13. Pierse, D., and Kersley, H. J.: Fitting "continuous wear" soft contact lenses at the time of cataract extraction, *Trans. Ophthalmol. Soc. U.K.*, 96:11–17, 1976.

14. Freeman, M. I.: Continuous wear of contact lens after cataract surgery, *Bull. Mason Clin.*, 30:145–152, Winter, 1976–77.

15. Kersley, H. J., Kerr, C., and Pierse, D.: Hydrophilic lenses for "continuous" wear in aphakia: definitive fitting and problems that occur, *Br. J. Ophthalmol.*, 61:38–43, 1977.

16. Gasset, A. R., Lobo, L., Houde, W.: Permanent wear of soft contact lenses in aphakic eyes, *Am. J. Ophthalmol.*, 83:115–122, 1977.

17. Leibowitz, H. M., Laing, R. A., and Sandstrom, M.: Continuous wear of hydrophilic contact lenses, *Arch. Ophthalmol.*, 89:206–209, 1973.

18. Hodd, N. F.: Some observations on 62 permanent wear soft lens cases, *The Ophthalmic Optician*, 15:1019, 1975.

19. de Carle, J.: Continuous wear contact lenses, *The Ophthalmic Optician*, 16:606–612, 1976.

20. Highman, V. N.: High water-content soft contact lenses for continuous wear, *Contact Lens J.*, 5:21–28, 1976.

21. Binder, P. S., and Worthen, D. M.: Clinical evaluation of continuous-wear hydrophilic lenses, *Am. J. Ophthalmol.*, 83:549–546, 1977.

22. Mobilia, E. F., Dohlman, C. H., and Holly, F. J.: A comparison of various contact lenses for therapeutic purposes, *Cont. Intraoc. Lens Med. J.*, 3:9–17, 1977.

23. Ganju, S. N., and Dreifus, D.: Prolonged-wear soft contact lenses, *The Optician*, 17:832–841, 1977.

24. Nesburn, A. B.: Prolonged-wear contact lenses in aphakia, *Trans. Am. Acad. Ophthalmol. Otolaryngol.*, 85:73–84, 1978.

25. Binder, P. S.: Extended wear of soft contact lenses, *Cont. Intraoc. Lens Med. J.*, 5:60, 1979.

26. Holden, B.: Extended Wear Contact Lenses, Paper read before the Bausch and Lomb Research Conference, Chicago, Aug. 1980.

27. Hill, R. M.: Escaping the sting, *Int. Cont. Lens Clin.*, 16:43, Jan/Feb, 1979.

28. Hill, R. M.: How the cornea "takes the heat", *Int. Cont. Lens Clin.*, 15:65–68, 1978.

29. Mandell, R. B., and Fatt, I.: Thinning of the human cornea upon awakening, *Nature*, 208(5007):292–293, 1965.

30. Phillips, A. J.: Extended-wear hydrogel lenses in the United Kingdom, *Int. Cont. Lens Clin.*, 6:54, 1979.

31. Refojo, M. F.: Materials in bandage lenses, *Cont. Intraoc. Lens Med. J.*, 5:34–49, 1979.

32. Holly, F. J., and Refojo, M. F.: Oxygen permeability of hydrogel contact lenses, *J. Am. Optom. Assoc.*, *43*:1173, 1972.

33. Morrison, D. R., and Edelhauser, H. F.: Permeability of hydrophilic contact lenses, *Invest. Ophthalmol.*, *11*:58, 1972.

34. Hill, R. M., and Carney, L. G.: Extended wear systems, *Cont. Lens Forum*, Jan. 1976, pp. 24–31.

35. Uniacke, C. A., Hill, R. M., and Greenberg, M. et al.: Physiological tests for new contact lens materials. I. Quantitative effects of selected oxygen atmosphere on glycogen storage, LDH concentration and thickness of the corneal epithelium, *Am. J. Optom.*, *49*:329–336, 1972.

36. Polse, K. A., and Mandell, R. B.: Critical oxygen tension at the corneal surface, *Arch. Ophthalmol.*, *84*:505–511, 1970.

37. Decker, M., Polse, K. A., and Fatt, I.: Oxygen flux into the human cornea when covered by a soft contact lens, *Am. J. Optom. Physiol. Opt.*, *55*:285–293, 1978.

38. Polse, K. A. and Decker, M.: Oxygen tension under contact lens, *Invest. Ophthalmol.*, *18*:188–206, 1979.

39. Binder, P. S.: Extended wear of soft contact lenses, *Cont. Intraoc. Lens Med. J.*, *5(1)*:60–75, 1979.

40. Hirjit, N. K., and Larke, J. R.: Corneal thickness in extended wear of soft contact lenses, *Br. J. Ophthalmol.*, *63*:272–276, 1979.

41. Leibowitz, H. M., and Laing, R. A.: Continuous wear of hydrophilic contact lenses, *Arch. Ophthalmol.*, *89*:306–310, 1973.

42. Polse, K. A., Sarver, M. D., and Harris, M. G.: Effects of Soflens parameters on corneal edema, *Int. Cont. Lens Clin.*, Summer, 1976, pp. 35–41.

43. Mobilia, E. F., Dohlman, C. H., and Holly, F. J.: A comparison of various soft contact lenses for therapeutic purposes, *Cont. Intraoc. Lens Med. J.*, *3(1)*:9–15, 1977.

44. Sarver, M. D., Baggett, D. A., Harris, M. D., and Louie, K.: Corneal edema with hydrogel lenses and eye closure: effects of lens thickness, *Am. J. Optom. Physiol. Opt.*, in press.

45. Sarver, M. D., Baggett, D. A., Harris, M. G., and Louie, K.: Corneal edema with hydrogel lenses and eye closure: effect of

oxygen transmissibility, *Am. J. Optom. Physiol. Opt.*, (in press).

46. Zantos, S. G., and Holden, B. A.: Ocular changes associated with continuous wear of contact lenses, *Austr. J. Optom.*, *61*: 418–426, 1978.

47. Holden, B. et al.: Paper presented at the International Contact Lens Society, Aug. 1980.

48. Decker, M., Polse, K. A., and Fatt, I.: Oxygen flux into the human cornea when covered by a soft contact lens, *Am. J. Optom. Physiol. Opt.*, *55(5)*:285–293, 1978.

49. Benjamin, R., and Hill, R. M.: Ultra-thins: the case for continuous care, *J. Am. Optom. Assoc.*, 277–278, 1980.

50. Fowler, S., and Allansmith, M.: Evolution of soft contact lens coatings, *Arch. Ophthalmol.*, *98*:95, 1980.

51. Binder, P. S.: The extended wear of soft contact lenses, *J. Cont. Ed. Ophthalmol.*, *4(6)*: 15–32, 1979.

52. Korb, D., Richmond, P. P., and Herman, J.: Physiological response of the cornea to hydrogel lenses before and after cataract extraction, *J. Am. Optom. Assoc.*, *51(3)*: 267–270, 1980.

53. Binder, P. S., and Worthin, D. M.: Clinical evaluation of continuous wear hydrophilic lenses, *Am. J. Ophthalmol.*, *83*:549–553, 1977.

55. Highman, V.: High water content soft contact lenses for continuous wear, *Cont. Lens J.*, *5(5)*:21–22, 1975.

56. McMonnies, C. W., and Zantos, S. W.: Endothelial bedewing of the cornea in association with contact lens wear, *Br. J. Ophthalmol.*, *63(7)*:478–481, 1979.

57. Binder, P. S.: Complications associated with extended wear of contact lenses, *Arch. Ophthalmol.*

58. Kline, L. N., and DeLuca, T. I.: Pitting stain with soft contact lenses-hydrocurve thin series, *J. Am. Optom. Assoc.*, *48*:372–379, 1977.

59. Klintworth, G. K., Reed, J. W., Hawkins, H. K. et al.: Calcification of soft contact lenses in patient with dry eye and elevated calcium concentration in tears, *Invest. Ophthalmol.*, *16*:158, 1977.

60. Rubin, M., Tripathi, R. C., and Winder, A. R.: Calcium deposition as a cause of

spoiliation of hydrophilic soft contact lenses, *Br. J. Ophthalmol.*, *59*:141–150, 1975.

61. Eriksen, S.: Cleaning hydrophilic contact lenses: an overview, *Ann. Ophthalmol.*, *7*:1223–1235, 1975.

62. Karageozian, H. L.: Use of the amino acid analyzer to illustrate the efficacy of an enzyme preparation for cleaning hydrophilic lenses, *Contacto*, *20*:5–13, 1976.

63. Refojo, M. F., and Holly, F. J.: Tear protein absorption on hydrogels: a possible cause of contact lens allergy, *Cont. Intraoc. Lens Med. J.*, *3*:23–33, 1977.

64. Allansmith, M. R., Korb, D. R., Greiner, J. V. et al.: Giant papillary conjunctivitis in contact lens wearers, *Am. J. Optom.*, *83*: 697–708, 1977.

65. Tripathi, R. C., and Ruben, M.: Degenerative changes in a soft hydrophilic contact lens, *Ophthalmol. Res.*, *4*:185–193, 1973.

66. Ruben, M.: Acute eye disease secondary to contact lens wear, *Lancet*, *1*:138–148, 1976.

67. Lemp, M. A.: An unusual keratoconjunctivitis occurring after long-time wearing of AO Softcon hydrophilic contact lens, *Ann. Ophthalmol.*, *7*:97–103, 1975.

68. Johnson, D. G.: Keratoconjunctivitis associated with wearing hydrophilic contact lenses, *Can. J. Ophthalmol.*, *8*:92–99, 1973.

69. Brown, S. I., Bloomfield, S., Pearce, et al: Infections with the therapeutic soft lens, *Arch. Ophthalmol.*, *91*:275–281, 1974.

70. Pederson, N. B.: Allergic contact conjunctivitis from merthiolate in soft contact lenses, *Cont. Dermatitis*, *4*:165–169, 1978.

71. Binder, P. S., and Worthen, D. M.: A continuous-wear hydrophilic lens, prophylactic topical antibiotics, *Arch. Ophthalmol.*, *94*: 2109–2117, 1976.

72. Fichman, S., Baker, V. V., and Horton, H. R.: Iatrogenic red eyes in soft contact lens wearers, *Int. Cont. Lens Clin.*, *15*:202–209, 1978.

73. Josephson, J. E.: The "multi-purge" procedure and its application for hydrophilic lens wearers utilizing preserved solutions, *J. Am. Optom. Assoc.*, *49*:280–292, 1978.

74. Cooper, R., and Constable, I. J.: Infective keratitis in soft contact lens wearers, *Br. J. Ophthalmol.*, *61*:250–258, 1977.

75. Freeman, H., and Sugar, J.: Pseudomonas keratitis following cosmetic soft contact lens wear, *Cont. Lens J.*, *10*:21–27, 1976.

Chapter 25

HYDROGEL LENSES FOR ASTIGMATISM

Spherical hydrogel contact lenses conform more or less to the corneal contour. If the conformation is perfect, the back surface of the contact lens is shaped into the toric form of the cornea. This can only be accomplished if the entire lens is bent, which results in nearly all of the corneal toricity being transferred to the front surface of the hydrogel lens.[1,2] The eye-lens system will now have nearly the same astigmatism as would be present before placing the contact lens on the eye. Hence, it would be predicted that the population of patients who wear hydrogel contact lenses will manifest nearly the same incidence of astigmatism as the uncorrected population.

In practice, the hydrogel contact lens does not conform precisely to the corneal contour; hence, a small difference exists between the predicted residual astigmatism and that which is actually found to occur. In most cases, the residual astigmatism that is measured is found to be less than predicted.[3] This indicates that the front surface of the hydrogel lens does not exhibit as much toricity as that which exists on the corneal surface. This conclusion is consistent with the lens-cornea bearing relationship seen with fluorexon. The pattern shows that the lens does not conform precisely to the cornea.

Sarver measured the astigmatism present with Bausch and Lomb Soflens contact lenses on 210 eyes.[4] He found that the mean residual astigmatism was about 84 percent of the refractive astigmatism. These results are in dramatic contrast to the relatively low residual astigmatism that is present with hard contact lenses (Figures 25.1 and 25.2).

The optical characteristics of spherical hydrogel contact lenses limit their use to that portion of the population which exhibits low refractive astigmatism. The limits of astigmatism that may be successfully accepted by the patient are somewhat arbitrary but are generally between 0.75 D. and 1.00 D. Above this, the patient often exhibits the signs and symptoms of an uncorrected residual refractive error. The tolerance for this residual astigmatism, however, varies greatly and is often related to the motivation of the patient. It is not unusual for a patient exhibiting 1.50 D. of residual astigmatism to accept hydrogel lenses if the need for them is compelling.[5,6] This was frequently experienced when only spherical hydrogel lenses were available so that no alternate choice existed.

The exact incidence of astigmatism in the population is somewhat difficult to determine. The data that are reported are generally taken from population samples which present themselves for eye examinations and do not represent the general population. Nevertheless, these data are important in establishing the general incidence of astigmatism (*see* Chapter 3). Approximately one-third of the population manifests astigmatism of 1.00 D. or more.[7] Thus, a significant portion of patients would not appear to be suitable for correction with spherical hydrogel lenses. For this reason toric hydrogel lenses were developed.

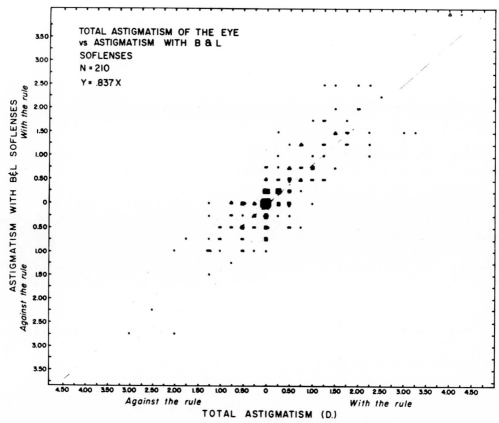

Figure 25.1. Soflens residual astigmatism. Courtesy of M. D. Sarver.

PRINCIPLES OF TORIC HYDROGEL LENSES

A toric hydrogel lens is designed basically like its toric hard lens counterpart.[8-15] The toric curve may be placed on either the front or back surface, and both designs are in common use. The principal difference from toric hard lenses is that a bitoric design is not needed. This occurs because the posterior surface of the hydrogel toric lens will tend to conform to the corneal toricity. Theoretically, if the corneal toricity is transferred to the front surface of the lens, the hydrogel cylinder power will remain the same whether the lens is in air or on the eye. This theoretical concept generally holds true in practice, providing that the refractive astigmatic axis coincides with the corneal axis of astigmatism. Hence, in many respects the optics of hydrogel toric lenses are simpler than the optics of toric hard contact lenses.

METHODS OF STABILIZING ROTATION

Just as with toric hard lenses, a major challenge with toric hydrogel lenses has been to develop a method for stabilizing rotational movements of the lens on the eye.[16-18] There

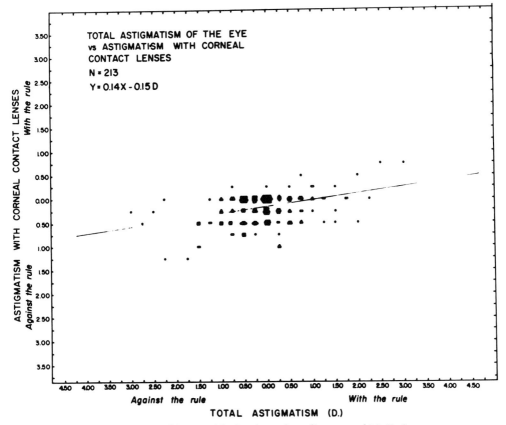

Figure 25.2. Hard lens residual astigmatism. Courtesy of M. D. Sarver.

are five basic designs that have received some acceptance as a stabilizing method. The major design features that have been tried follow.

Single and Double Truncation

A single truncation that is applied to the inferior portion of a hydrogel lens provides only minimal efficiency in stabilizing lens rotation.[19-20] A double truncation is more effective but has had limited success in practical use.[21] The lenses sometimes rotate 90 degrees from the desired position.

Prism Ballast

Just as with hard toric contact lenses, it is possible to use prism ballast to stabilize the rotation of a hydrogel lens.[22,23] The thicker portion (base) of the prism will move to a downward position as the result of gravity. Because of its effectiveness, this is the principal method in which most toric hydrogel contact lenses are designed. The prism ballast may or may not be combined with an inferior truncation. The truncation conforms to the lower lid margin and further stabilizes lens rotation (Figure 25.3).

Thinning of the Superior and Inferior Margins

The superior and inferior margin portions of the lens may be thinned by tapering or a slab-off technique to reduce the edge thickness.[24,25] This aligns the central area of the lens, consisting of a horizontal band, within the palpebral aperture (Figure 25.4). This lens design has variable results and is, at times, extremely successful. Unfortunately,

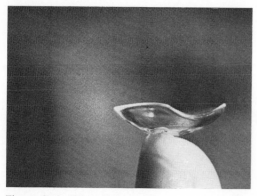

Figure 25.3. Prism ballast toric lens with truncation.

in some cases considerable rotation occurs with each blink, and in addition, the lens may stabilize off axis.

The Superior Slab-Off Lenticular

A design in which the superior half of only the lenticular carrier portion of the lens is slabbed off produces the same effect as that achieved with prism ballast. The superior half of the lens is thinned greatly, and a demarcation exists at the horizontal midpoint of the lens.

LENS FITTING CHARACTERISTICS

The performance of a toric hydrogel contact lens depends upon several factors including the following:[26-28]

1. Corneal topography
2. Limbal topography
3. Conjunctival characteristics
4. Lid shape, position, and tightness
5. Blinking characteristics

The following lens characteristics also contribute to the fit:

1. Lens design
2. Material from which the lens is made
3. Tightness of the lens fit

Corneal Topography

The influence of the corneal topography on the lens fit is not well understood. The corneal toricity that is measured in the central region with a keratometer does not necessarily indicate that the same characteristics exist in the corneal periphery. Since a hydrogel contact lens covers the entire corneal area, the peripheral cornea greatly influences its riding characteristics.

The most favorable patients for toric hydrogel lens success are those in which corneal astigmatism is near the 90 or 180 meridian. When corneal toricity is at an oblique axis,

the fitting of the contact lens becomes much more complex, and the success rate is reduced.

Attempts to measure corneal topography by photokeratoscopy and other methods has not proved to have an advantage in fitting. There is an inability to interpret the knowledge of the corneal contour in terms of what effect it has on lens positioning and rotation.

Limbal Topography

The shape of the limbus undoubtedly exerts considerable influence upon the positioning and rotation of the hydrogel lens. Unfortunately, little is known about the influence of this ocular structure. It may be seen that there is considerable variation from subject to subject in the curvature and depth of the limbal contour.

Conjunctival Characteristics

There is significant variation from patient to patient in the conjunctival characteristics, which seems to have some influence on the lens rotation and meridional stability. When the lens is tightly fitted to the eye, the conjunctiva beneath the lens edge may be moved during the blink. The resistance of the conjunctiva to lens movement appears to vary somewhat between different patients.

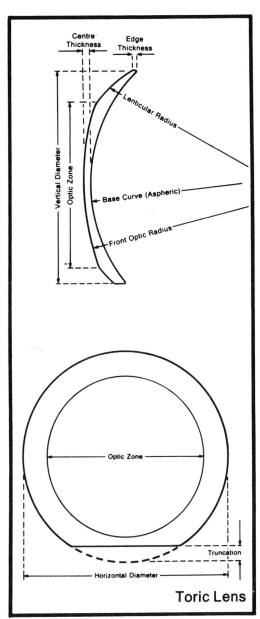

Toric Lens

Figure 25.4. Slab-off thinning of superior and inferior margins for lens stabilization.

major role in soft lens rotation, as is the case in hard toric lenses. Nevertheless, it does have some influence in relation to the truncation angle. The major influence of the lids appears to be attributable to the superior lid. As the superior lid moves down across the lens, it imparts a rotational movement. This seems to be influenced most by the edge thickness of the lens. If the edge thickness is the same on both sides of the lens at points of lid contact, then little or no rotational movement is imparted. This would occur when the axis of the lens toricity is perpendicular to the direction of lid movement. If the axis of the lens toricity is oblique, then the corresponding horizontal positions of the lens edge of the left and right sides are different in thickness. As the lid moves downward over the lens, it exerts a greater force on the side with the greatest thickness and imparts a rotational movement downward on that side. The edge thickness is also influenced by the angle of the lens prism.

Blinking Characteristics

There is obviously considerable variation in the blinking characteristics from subject to subject; however, these characteristics are very difficult to quantify. It may be noted whether the patient tends towards full or partial blinks. Some differences in the forcefulness of the blink may also be detectable. It is only after the toric lens is on the eye, however, that the full effects of the blinking action on lens positioning and movement can be detected. These effects are generally minimal as long as the prism and cylinder axis are near the vertical meridian. When the axis is oblique, the edge thickness differences on the two sides of the lens are more greatly affected by the lid action during blinking.

Lid Characteristics

The lid shape, position, and tightness have considerable influence on the riding characteristics of the hydrogel toric lens. It has been claimed that the lower lid does not play the

Lens Design

Various dimensions of the lens design have considerable influence on the fitting characteristics.[29] These include lens diameter, peripheral curve design, other lens curvatures, and amount of prism ballast. The basic fitting requisites of a hydrogel contact lens must be fulfilled (*see* Chapter 17).

Lens Material

The material from which the contact lens is made has some influence on the final fit. This is primarily a function of the lens flexibility and water content. Lenses with less flexibility must be fitted flatter to avoid limbal compression.

Tightness of the Lens Fit

Occasionally a lens rides off axis because the fit is too tight, and this hampers lens movement. The most frequent modification that must be made in fitting toric hydrogel lenses is to flatten the base curve of the lens so that the tightness of the fit is reduced.

FITTING METHODS

There is considerable variation in the fitting methods that have been used for various toric hydrogel lenses. These methods are based primarily upon the type of trial lens that is used for the fitting. Most of the methods that have been used fall under one of the following categories.[30]

SPHERICAL TRIAL LENSES

If the fitting method uses spherical trial lenses, a diagnostic fitting is achieved in the same way as when prescribing the spherical lenses. Under ideal conditions, the trial lens should have a power close to the spherical equivalent of the patient's refractive error. A complete overrefraction with spherocylindrical correction is then carried out. The result obtained is added to the trial lens power to arrive at the final prescription. A small compensation of 10° to 15° in lens prism axis from the vertical is made to allow for the usual rotational characteristics of the lens. The advantage of this method is that regular trial lenses, which are readily available, may be used. The disadvantages are that there is no opportunity for the fitter to evaluate the rotational characteristics of the lens on the eye. Since misalignment between the contact lens axis and the principal meridians of the astigmatism is the most common problem in toric hydrogel lens fitting, this constitutes a serious problem. In many cases, the final lens will not ride as predicted.

A common problem for many types of toric contact lenses is that only a few base curves are available, and these do not correspond to the base curves of the spherical series. Even when the base curves are matched, it is often found that the riding characteristics of the toric lens differs significantly from those of the spherical lens.

TRIAL LENS OF PLANO POWER, PRISM BALLAST, AND TRUNCATION

A set of trial lenses having the prism and truncation characteristics of the final lens is helpful in assessing the rotational stability and positioning of the lens upon the eye. This trial lens is particularly useful when there is low refractive error and low amounts of lens cylinder. If the lens assumes an acceptable riding position on the eye, then the final prescription may be obtained by overrefraction.

When a lens is ordered by this method, a compensation must be made for any rotation of the trial lens on the eye when calculating the axis of the final correction (Figure 25.5). Since the axis of the cylinder is located with respect to the base of the prism, it follows that when the lens is rotated the cylinder axis will also rotate the same amount and direction as the base. A compensation of the cylinder axis must then be made in the opposite direction so that the final lens will have the correct axis when it is on the eye. If the base of the prism rotates to the patient's right, the number of degrees of rotation must be added to the cylinder axis found in the overrefraction (Figure 25.6). This rule follows for both the right and left eye, since the axis designation is the same in each case. When rotation of the base of the prism is to the left, then the number of degrees of rotation are subtracted from the patient's cylinder axis found in the overrefraction (Figure 25.7).

If significant rotation of the trial lens occurs upon each blink, an attempt should first be made to find a trial lens that reduces or eliminates this rotation. If this is not successful, the patient should be considered an unlikely candidate for successful toric lens wear. Rotation of spherical prism ballast trial lenses is generally less than that of the final prescription which incorporates the cylindrical power.

TRIAL LENSES WITH PRISM BALLAST, TRUNCATION, AND TORIC SURFACES

The use of trial lenses that incorporate cylinder in addition to the prism ballast and truncation will often give further information as to how the final lens will ride on

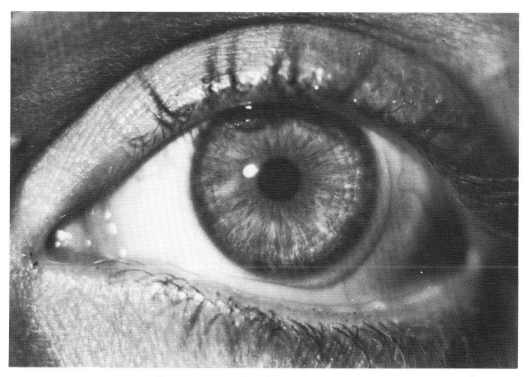

Figure 25.5. Rotation of toric lens on the eye.

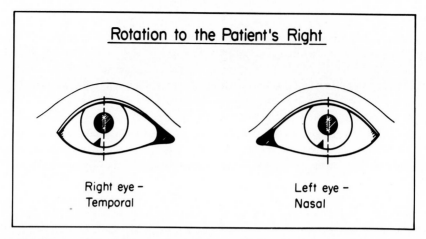

Figure 25.6. The number of degrees of rotation are added to the patient's cylinder axis when a lens rotates to the patient's right on either eye.

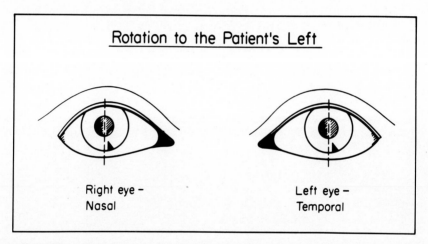

Figure 25.7. When rotation is to the patient's left, the number of degrees of rotation are subtracted.

the cornea. Such trial lenses generally have axes placed at or near the 90° or 180° meridians. A trial lens is selected with an axis as close as possible to that in the final correction. An assessment of the lens stabilization and movement then makes predictions for the final lens reasonably good.

When the fitting characteristics of the trial lens have been obtained and considered satisfactory, an overrefraction may be performed to find the spherocylindrical correction. Since the axis of the cylinder in the overrefraction does not usually coincide with that of the

trial lens cylinder axis, a computation of the resultant cylinder must be made for incorporation into the final prescription lens. In addition, the rotation of the lens upon the eye must be compensated for in the same manner as for a spherical prism ballast lens.

The use of a prism ballast trial lens that incorporates cylinder will sometimes improve the prediction of the final lens characteristics. This is particularly true when the cylinder axis and power are similar to that of the final correction. When significant differences exist, particularly when the final axis is more oblique, sometimes the corrective lens does not rotate to the same axis as did the trial lens.

TRIAL LENS THAT HAS PRISM BALLAST, TRUNCATION, AND OPTICAL POWER

A slight variation of the plano trial lens is one in which power is incorporated. Usually, an average power, for example −3.00 D., is chosen for this purpose. It has not been proven to provide a significant advantage over the plano trial lens.

ORDERING DIRECTLY

It is theoretically possible to order the final lens power on the basis of a simple refraction and keratometer reading. However, this procedure often results in a significant error, not only in the cylindrical correction or axis but also in the spherical power. With some lenses, there is a tendency for the prism ballast design to produce a minus tear lens up to 0.50 D. Such a tear lens is most accurately evaluated by the use of trial lenses.

The following rules should always be considered regardless of the fitting method that is used:

1. The higher the refractive correction that is necessary, the greater the amount of uncorrected cylinder which will be tolerated by the patient.

2. The cylinder of primary concern in dealing with the optics of toric hydrogel lenses is the refractive cylinder. The corneal cylinder is important only as it influences the fit of the lens.

3. The more cylinder that is present in the correction, the more critical will be the axis alignment and the greater the need for stability of the lens.

4. A tight lens fit may be used to aid in stabilizing a prism ballast lens. Unfortunately, this often results in the same physiological problems that are common to any tight lens fit.

CUSTOM OR STANDARD LENSES

Toric hydrogel contact lenses are available in both standard and custom designs. Most manufacturers prefer to use a standard lens design and may limit their availability to a narrow range of powers and axes (Table 25.1). This usually consists of cylinder axes near the horizontal or vertical meridian.

Whenever the patient requires a lens that falls in this category, it is probably simpler and less expensive than the custom design approach. However, custom-designed lenses must be used in more uncommon cases of astigmatism.

FITTING PROCEDURE

The fitting procedure usually consists of several parts.

Contact Lens Examination

A complete contact lens examination

TABLE 25.1
FEATURES OF SAMPLE TORIC SOFT LENSES

Lens	% Water	Power Range	Diameter	Base Curves.	Prism	Truncation
Durasoft	30	+20.00 to −20.00 DS +0.75 to 4.00 cyl	12.8, 13.5	7.6 to 8.8	0.75 to 1.50	1.0 at base of prism
Hydrocurve II Toric	46	−1.50 to −6.00 DS only −1.25 cyl axis 90 & 180 ± 25°	13.5	8.6 only	1.0	No
B & L	38	−1.25 and −1.75 cyl only in limited range	14.0	8.3 & 8.6	1.0	No
Hydron	38	+20.00 to −20.00 DS −0.50 to −6.00 cyl	13.5, 14.0, 14.5	7.7 to 8.7 aspheric	1.0	Yes

should be performed.

Measurements for Toric Correction

Note any unusual variation in the patient's lid configuration or position.

Select Trial Lens

Depending upon the trial set that is available, the lens which is nearest to the patient's refractive needs will be selected and placed on the eye. Follow the manufacturer's guide for the initial lens specifications.

Evaluate the Trial Lens

The initial evaluation of the lens can usually be made after twenty minutes of lens wear or whenever the patient stops tearing excessively. The usual criteria for hydrogel lens evaluation should be fulfilled. There should be definite movement of the lens following each blink. The prism angle should remain at a constant position and not rotate excessively following the blink. Measure the rotation of the lens.

Several methods may be used to determine accurately the amount of lens rotation on the eye. Trial lenses are usually marked to aid the fitter in locating the base position. This mark may consist of either a dot near the edge of the base position, or a vertical line. In some cases, horizontal lines are also indicated, dividing the lens into upper and lower halves. These lines are generally not carried

across the central portion of the lens. The amount of rotation of the base mark may be evaluated in one of the following ways:

1. Spectacle trial lens. A spectacle trial lens with axis lines and a trial frame may be used to determine the contact lens rotation. With the trial frame in place, rotate the lens until the axis lines are in alignment with the prism base marked on the contact lens. The amount of rotation may then be read from the scale on the trial frame.

2. Special protractor scales are available for some biomicroscopes, which allow the easy visualization of the lens rotation (Figure 25.8). The marks are usually in 5° intervals.

3. With some experience, an estimate of

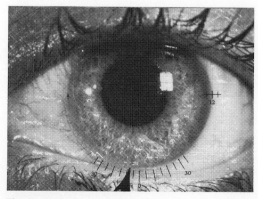

Figure 25.8. Protractor in biomicroscope allows direct viewing and measurement of lens rotation.

the lens rotation may be made without any guide. The fitter should imagine a clock superimposed upon the cornea with each hour indicating 30° of rotation. Hence, a base that is rotated about two-thirds of the way to the 5 o'clock position will be rotated 15°.

A further aid to the axis determination may be obtained by projecting a narrow slit, which is placed vertically and centered with respect to the slit lamp. This provides a vertical reference line on the cornea from which the rotation may be more easily located.

REFERENCES

1. Fink, M. J.: Residual astigmatism: a case study of hydrophilic lenses, *Rev. Optom.*, *114(6)*: 78–79, 1977.

2. Gerritson, F. F., and Colenbrander, M. C.: Residual astigmatism in wearers of contact lenses, *Ophthalmologica*, *173*:180–183, 1976.

3. Lee, A. N., and Sarver, D. S.: The gel lens—transferred corneal toricity as a function of lens thickness, *J. Opt. Arch. Am. Acad. Optom.*, *49(1)*:35–40, 1972.

4. Sarver, M. D.: Vision with hydrophilic contact lenses, *J. Am. Optom. Assoc.*, *43(3)*: 316–320, 1972.

5. Baron, H.: Observations concerning the fitting of astigmatic eyes with hydrophilic lenses, *Contacto*, *18(2)*:24–30, 1974.

6. Grosvenor, T.: Visual acuity, astigmatism and soft contact lenses, *Am. J. Optom.*, *49(5)*: 407–412, 1972.

7. Holden, B. A.: Correcting astigmatism with toric soft contact lenses, *Int. Cont. Lens Clin.*, *3(1)*:59–61, 1976.

8. Levin, B. J.: Toric soft lenses, *Contacto*, *21(4)*: 8–12, 1977.

9. Pennington, R. N.: Toric optic soft lenses, *The Optician*, Sept. 7, 1979, pp. 34–38.

10. Baronet, P.: Soft toric contact lenses fitting of the toric Gel 38 lenses, *Cont. Lens J.*, *5(5)*:12–13, 1976.

11. Bayshore, C. A.: Astigmatic soft contact lenses: a report of 88 patients, *Int. Cont. Lens Clin.*, *2(1)*:69–73, 1975.

12. Brown, S. I., and Tragakis, M. P.: Hydrophilic contact lenses for correcting irregular and high astigmatism, *Arch. Ophthalmol.*, *88(6)*: 596–601, 1972.

13. De Smedt-Houttequiet, and Missotten, L.: Mini semi-flexible lenses type Boyd and irregular corneal astigmatism, *Contact Lens*, *4(7)*:9–10, 1974.

14. Hodd, N. F. B.: Clinical experience with toric and tinted and cosmetic Weicons, *Cont. Lens J.*, *6(3)*:8, 1977.

15. Jurgensen, G.: Fitting the small, soft toric contact lens Hydroflex/ M–T, *The Ophthalmic Optician*, *17(14)*:539–540, 1977.

16. McMonnies, C. W., and Parker, D. P.: Predicting the rotational performance of toric soft lenses, *Austr. J. Optom.*, *60(4)*:130–138, 1977.

17. Bibby, M., Tomlinson, A., and Jurkus, J.: Evaluation and control of Durasoft lens rotation, *Am. J. Optom. Physiol. Opt.*, *55(6)*: 365–370, 1978.

18. Fanti, P.: The fitting of a soft toroidal contact lens, *The Optician*, *169(4376)*:8–16, 1975.

19. Harris, M. G., Laconic, M., and Ward, J.: Stability of back-toric prism-ballast hydrogel contact lenses, *Am. J. Optom. Physiol. Opt.*, *55(1)*:15, 1978.

20. Jurkus, J., and Tomlinson, A.: Prism-ballasted and truncated spherical trial lenses as indicators of toric soft lens rotation, *Am. J. Optom. Physiol. Opt.*, *56(1)*:16–17, 1979.

21. Bailey, N. J.: Two truncations can be better than none, *Cont. Lens Forum*, *1(4)*:50–51, 1976.

22. Hodd, N. B.: A comparison of toric soft lens success, *The Optician*, *173(4487)*:29, 1977.

23. Holden, B. A.: The principles and practice of correcting astigmatism with soft contact lenses, *Austr. J. Optom.*, *58(8)*:279–299, 1975.

24. Attridge, J. G.: Double slab off toric soft contact lens, *Can. J. Optom.*, *41(2)*:88–92, 1979.

25. Attridge, J. G.: Dominion double slab-off front surface toric soft contact lens, *Austr. J. Optom.*, *62(4)*:147–151, 1979.

26. Gasson, A.: The correction of astigmatism

and Hydroflex toric soft lenses, *The Cont. Lens J.*, 8(2):3, 1979.

27. Hodd, N. F. B.: How to fit soft lenses—10 toric soft lenses (Part 2), *The Optician*, 173(4483):8, 1977.

28. Lieblein, J.: A study of the Durasoft toric contact lens for astigmatism, and a fitting rationale, *Int. Cont. Lens Clin.*, 7(1):21–25, 1980.

29. Gasson, A.: Back surface toric soft lenses, *The Optician*, 174(4491):6–11, 1977.

30. Remba, M. J.: Clinical evaluation of F.D.A. approved toric hydrophilic soft contact lenses, Part 1, *J. Am. Optom. Assoc.*, 50(3):289–293, 1979.

SECTION IV

SPECIAL TOPICS

Chapter 26

CONTEMPORARY LENSES

NEW POLYMERS

VARIOUS POLYMER MATERIALS have been evaluated for possible use in the manufacture of contact lenses. Most lenses that are made from new polymers are an attempt to correct one or more of the deficiencies of the hydrogel contact lens. A few of the new polymers are designed as a replacement for the hard contact lens.

New polymers that have been investigated include numerous variations of hydrogel materials, vinyls, combinations of silicone and other polymers, and other materials (Figure 26.1). Many problems have been encountered when these lenses were tested on the eye. However, it may be anticipated that many of these materials will be found in future lenses.

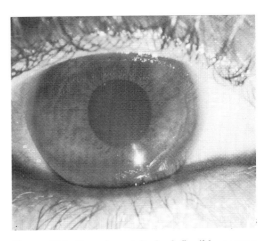

Figure 26.1 Experimental vinyl flexible contact lens.

HARD–SOFT COMBINATION LENSES

There have been several reports of combination hard and soft lenses used together in an attempt to correct the deficiencies of each lens type. When properly constructed, this combination lens has been reported to have the comfort of a gel contact lens and the good vision of a hard contact lens.[1] Baldone[1] has recommended that this technique be used in the following cases:

1. When visual acuity of an eye cannot be effectively improved with spectacles alone

2. When a hard contact lens cannot be fitted or cannot be tolerated

3. When the best fit with a soft gel lens is attained, and the resultant visual acuity is not adequate or optimum after the addition of a spectacle correction

Additional myopic or hyperopic correction can be used to augment the power of a soft gel lens, but usually the hard lens is fitted to eliminate irregular astigmia that is residual.[1]

Clinically these cases are usually patients with keratoconus; corneal irregularities from injury or ulcerations; postoperative cataract patients with a large amount of corneal astigmia; or warped corneas from the long-time wear of large, thick, hard contact lenses.

FITTING PROCEDURE

Keratometer readings are made from the anterior surface of the soft gel lens while it is on the eye.* From these readings one determines from which base curve to begin the hard trial lens fitting. It is advocated that hard lenses of 8.3 mm. size be used.[1] The movement and position of the first hard trial lens on the soft lens indicates what direction to take in the subsequent selection of a trial lens with regard to base curve and size (Figure 26.2).

If a hard lens does not glide gently for 1.0 to 1.5 mm. over the anterior surface of the soft gel lens at each blink, it will probably prove to be too tight. Tightness will be evidenced by limited wearing time of the combination lenses associated with the production of central corneal edema. Then a slightly flatter base curve is selected, and the power of the hard lens is compensated. Increments of 0.25 D. (0.05 mm.) in base curve are advocated. A looser fit can also be attained by fitting a smaller lens of the same base curve, but this is rarely necessary.

If the hard lens moves excessively (more than 1.5 to 2.0 mm.) with each blink or lags inferiorly markedly, then a steeper base curve or a larger size is indicated as the next step. Most often the size can remain fixed while only the base curve is varied.

The fit of the hard lens cannot be studied with fluorescein, as the dye is absorbed by the present-day hydrophilic gel lenses. A slightly loose fit is critical; otherwise, the presence of a hard lens will lead to hypoxia of the central corneal epithelium.

After the proper base curve and size of the hard contact lenses are determined, the necessary power is measured by over-refraction.

Baldone reported that three-fourths of the 8.3 mm. hard lenses that he used were fitted 0.50 D. (±0.25 D.) steeper than the front curvature of the fitted gel lens.[1]

In thirteen cases of Baldone,[1] the relationship of the hard lens base curve to the curvature of the anterior surface of the soft gel lens is given in Table 26.1. In some cases the anterior surface readings of the soft lenses were not possible, and the above relationship could not be established.

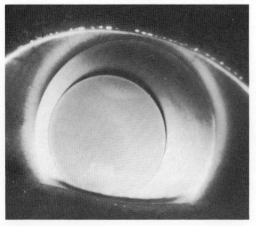

Figure 26.2 Hard-soft combination lens on the eye.

SILICONE CONTACT LENSES

From a theoretical standpoint, silicone presents the most promising new contact lens material. However, this material has been found to have more of a theoretical advantage than has been found to be true in practical application. The chief appeal of the silicone material is its high permeability for oxygen and other gases. This permeability is great enough that sufficient oxygen can pass from the atmosphere through the lens to the cornea to satisfy the needs of the corneal epithelium.[2-4] In fact, it has been shown that enough oxygen should pass through a silicone lens to satisfy the corneal needs even when the eyes are closed.

*Note: This report is based on studies using the Warner-Lambert Softcon.[1]

TABLE 26.1

No. of Cases	Flatter Than	Hard Lens Base Curve Parallel to *(The Anterior Surface of Soft Lens)*	Steeper Than
1	4 diopters		
1		on "K"	
1			0.12 diopter
1			0.25
5			0.50
1			0.37
2			0.75
1			0.87

From Baldone, J.: The fitting of hard contact lenses onto soft contact lenses in certain diseased conditions, paper read before Section on Ophthalmology, American Medical Association Convention, 1973.

The most serious problem encountered with silicone lenses has been a tendency for a lens to increase its adherence to the eye after a short wearing period. This problem generally occurs when lenses of large diameters are used and is attributed to the negative pressure effect created by the elastic properties of the lens material. In some cases the lens has adhered so tightly to the eye that epithelial damage occurred upon removal of the lens. This problem has been generally averted by adopting smaller lens designs.

SILSOFT® CONTACT LENS

The Silsoft contact lens is a silicone lens made by Dow-Corning. The lens is made from a special silicone rubber known as Silastic®, which is of medical grade and has been used in other medical applications.

The Silsoft contact lens is molded by conventional male and female dies, formed from highly polished stainless steel. The lens is molded under very high temperature and pressure, which is followed by a curing cycle. The quality of the lens is dependent upon the quality of the mold, and great care must be taken in its production.

Lens Design

The Silsoft lens can be made in any diameter but is usually formed in only two sizes, 11.3 and 12.5 mm. diameter (Figure 26.3). There are two peripheral curves so that the lens has the overall appearance of a hard corneal lens. The edges are formed mechanically and have presented many fabrication problems.

Coating

Since silicone is a very hydrophobic material, it has been necessary to treat the lens surfaces to make them hydrophilic. If this is not done, the lens is very resistant to rubbing across its surface and is uncomfortable in the eye.

Flexibility

The Silsoft lens is flexible, although some-

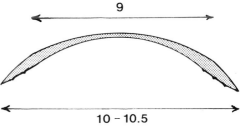

Figure 26.3 Dow-Corning Silsoft contact lens.

what less than a hydrogel contact lens. The lens can be folded in half and yet immediately springs back to its original shape when released. It is much stronger than the hydrogel material, and it takes considerable effort to split the lens.

Lens Verification

With the silicone lens it is possible to measure all of the dimensions except the base curve using the same techniques as can be used for hard lenses.

Fitting Procedure

The general procedure for fitting the Silsoft lens is identical to that for a hard contact lens. Usually the Silsoft lens is fitted on K or slightly flat. The lens may be fitted with or without the assistance of a trial set. The lens is available in base curves 7.3, 7.5, 7.7, 7.9, 8.1, and 8.3.

Astigmatism

The Silsoft lens appears to give somewhat better results than a hydrogel lens for cases of refractive astigmatism. Nevertheless, the Silsoft lens suffers from the same deficiencies as all flexible lenses in that it tends to conform to any corneal toricity, and the patient is often left with residual astigmatism.

Patient Complaints and Problems

The principal problem with the Silsoft lens has been lack of comfort. Many patients have found that these lenses are no more comfortable than a hard contact lens, and in a significant portion of patients, the discomfort is intolerable. Many of these problems have been associated with poor lens design in the past, and there is potential for their eventual solution.

Care and Storage

Special cold storage solutions have been prepared for Silsoft lenses. The patient should be advised to use only these solutions, as some chemicals found in common hard lens storage solutions will bind to the surface of a Silsoft lens and cause irritation.

REFERENCES

1. Baldone, J.: The Fitting of Hard Contact Lenses onto Soft Contact Lenses in Certain Diseased Conditions, paper read before Section on Ophthalmology, American Medical Association Convention, 1973.
2. Hill, R. M.: Effects of a silicone rubber lens on corneal respiration, *J. Am. Optom. Assoc.*, 37:1119–1121, 1966.
3. Hill, R. M., and Schoessler, J.: Optical membranes of silicone rubber; and their effects on respiration of human corneal epithelium, *J. Am. Optom. Assoc.*, 38:480–483, 1967.
4. Burns, R. P., Roberts, H., and Rich, L. F.: Effect of silicone contact lenses on corneal epithelial metabolism, *Am. J. Ophthalmol.*, 71:486–489, 1971.

ADDITIONAL READINGS

Arens, F. D.: One year of experience with silicon lenses, *Contacto*, 23(6):26, 1979.

Baszkin, A.: Silicone grafted with poly(vinyl pyrrolidone) for contact lenses. Surface properties and stability of thin tear film, *J. Bioeng.*, 2: 527–537, 1978.

Bernstein, H.: Extended wear silicone lenses in aphakia, *Cont. Intraoc. Lens Med. J.*, 5(3):31–36, 1979.

Bernstein, H. N.: Extended wear silicone lenses in aphakia, *Cont. Lens J.*, 12(4):19, 1979.

Black, C. J.: Silicone lens, in Gasset, A. R., and Kaufman, H. E. (Eds.): *Soft Contact Lens*, St. Louis, C. V. Mosby, 1972, p. 126.

Caudell, T. P.: Silicone rubber applied within the eye: a preliminary study, *Applied Optics, 18(9)*: 1305, 1979.

Cummings, D. G.: Facts about the hydrophilic and silicone contact lenses, *Mich. Optometrist, 48(11)*: 14–17, 1969.

Failla, J.: Silicone lenses for extended wear, *Cont. Lens Forum, 4(7)*:73, 1979.

Fanti, P., and Holly, F. J.: Silicone contact lens wear II. Clinical experience, *Cont. Intraoc. Lens Med. J., 6(1)*:25–32, 1980.

Forst, G.: Messverfahren fur silikon-contactlinsen (Engl. abstract), *Die Contactlinse, 11(2)*:9–13, 1977.

Gasson, A.: Preliminary observations in fitting Silflex silicone contact lenses, *The Optician, 174(4509)*:7, 1977.

Hamano, H.: Scanning electron microscope observation of corneal surface after wearing hard, soft, and silicon rubber lenses, *Contacto, 21(5)*:16, 1977.

Harwood, L. W.: Combination Soflens contact lens/hard lenses—use on high toric corneas, *Proc. Second Natl. Research Symp. on Soft Cont. Lenses*, Chicago, Ill., Aug. 1975.

Himi, T.: Clinical studies on silicone contact lenses (translation), *J. Jap. Cont. Lens Soc., 18(3)*:39–42, 1976.

Iwasaki, W.: Complication caused by silicon elastomer lenses in West Germany and Japan, *Folia Ophthalmol. Jap., 30(5)*:759, 1979.

Jacobs, H. A.: A new class of materials: silicone rubber contact lens, *Contacto, 19(5)*:21–23, 1975.

Kaye, A.: Aphakia: extended wear with silicone lenses, *The Optician, 177*:67–81, Oct. 5, 1979.

Lippman, J. I.: Silicone lenses in aphakia: fact vs. fancy, *Cont. Intraoc. Lens Med. J., 4(4)*:58–62, 1978.

Long, W. E.: An update of the silicone lens status, *Contacto, 18(3)*:35–37, 1974.

Majima, Y.: Continuous wear of a hydrophilic silicone rubber contact lens (HSRCL) in postoperative aphakic patients, *Folia Ophthalmol. Jap., 30(2)*:319, 1979.

Mizutani, Y.: Clinical investigations of hydrophilic silicone rubber contact lenses (Engl. abstract), *J. Jap. Cont. Lens Soc., 19(12)*:155, 1977.

Mizutani, Y., and Nobuhara, S.: Clinical investigations of hydrophilic silicone rubber contact lens "Hislic", *Austr. J. Optom., 62(4)*:143–146, 1979.

Mizutani, Y. et al.: Hydrophilic silicone rubber contact lens, *Contacto, 21(1)*:15–19, 1977.

Chapter 27

APHAKIA

KENNETH A. POLSE

ALTHOUGH COSMETIC considerations are of some importance to the aphakic patient, the main reason for prescribing contact lenses is the excellent visual performance.[1-5] A spectacle correction will not give the aphakic patient the visual function and comfort that is obtained with contact lenses.[6-8]

Fitting the aphakic patient with contact lenses represents one of the most interesting and challenging services that the contact lens practitioner can provide. The practitioner not only must have a high level of skill in fitting contact lenses but must have a solid foundation in binocular vision, ocular disease, and psychology of the geriatric patient.

To recognize fully what contact lenses mean to the aphakic patient, the visual difficulties encountered with spectacle lenses should be understood.

MAGNIFICATION

Most aphakic patients require approximately 10 to 14 D. at the spectacle plane to correct the ametropia that occurs following cataract surgery. A +10 D. lens placed 10 mm. in front of the eye will induce approximately 30 percent magnification.[9] In monocular aphakia, it is usually not possible for fusion to be maintained with such an induced size discrepancy between the two eyes.[10] Aniseikonic lenses cannot be designed to correct such a large image size difference between the two eyes. Although it has been reported that some patients with monocular aphakia have been able to adapt to a binocular spectacle correction,[7] the majority have difficulty in maintaining fusion.

A contact lens for aphakia typically causes a 5 to 9 percent magnification, and although this magnification may lead initially to some difficulty, it is usually well tolerated by the patient.[2,11,12] In cases of unilateral aphakia where the patient has difficulty accepting this amount of magnification, a size lens can be placed in front of the phakic eye to equalize the size differences.[13]

The bilateral aphakic patient who wears a spectacle correction encounters several perceptual problems caused by the increased magnification.[14] When a binocular aphakic puts on his spectacles for the first time, he is invariably astounded by the apparent increase in size of familiar objects around him.[15] Binocular vision and some degree of depth perception are present, but because objects are magnified, they appear closer than they actually are. Pouring water into a glass can become a difficult task; reaching for a cup of coffee often results in spillage. Each task performed for the first time after surgery becomes a new lesson in the aphakic patient's reorientation to his space perception. These conditions of image magnification and faulty spatial placement can be eliminated, or at least minimized, through the use of contact lenses.

VISUAL LIMITATIONS

The visual field of the spectacle-corrected aphakic patient is limited.[15-18] Due to the power of the lens, there is an increasing base-out prismatic effect from the optical center towards the periphery of the lens. This prismatic effect becomes great enough essentially to limit the overall field to approximately 30°.[17] Patients frequently complain about bumping into objects and feeling unsteady when walking around.

A contact lens of +14 D. gives almost normal visual fields.[17] There is still a slight reduction, but the patient is usually not bothered and is able to perform tasks such as driving with little or no difficulty.

A further problem caused by the increased prismatic effect towards the periphery of the aphakic spectacle lens is that light is deviated so that the patient actually has an uncorrected field of vision with a blind area in between (Figure 27.1).[9,15,18,19] This blind area, often referred to as a ring scotoma, moves when the patient moves his head. The movement of this scotoma with each head movement causes objects to jump in and out of the visual field of the patient. This is the so-called jack-in-the-box phenomenon and is a continual source of aggravation to the patient. The jack-in-the-box problem is eliminated with contact lenses.

FUSION

A spectacle correction for bilateral aphakia

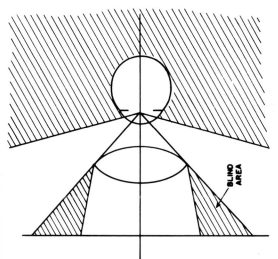

Figure 27.1. The prismatic effect at the periphery of high plus spectacle lenses causes a blind area in the visual field.

causes some fusion problems even though the image sizes are relatively equal between the two eyes. When the patient looks inward from the lens pole (as when converging during reading), there is an increasing amount of base-out prism (Figure 27.2). The base-out prism induces an exophoria that is significant in high plus lenses.[9,15,18] It is not uncommon for the binocular aphakic who is corrected with spectacle lenses to complain of difficulty in reading. Frequently, convergence insufficiency is found in the aging patient; this, added to the induced base-out prism, increases the magnitude of the problem.

Another difficulty that the bilateral aphakic encounters comes from the frequent difference in correction in each lens. This presents no difficulty when looking through the optical centers, but as the patient looks down through the bifocal or away from the optical centers, there is an induced anisophoria. When a contact lens is worn, this problem is essentially eliminated.

Several studies have shown that fair to excellent binocular vision can result when contact lenses are used for the correction of unilateral and bilateral aphakia.[1,2]

DISTORTION

There are variations in the magnification of the spectacle lens from center to edge. The degree of this aberration is directly proportional to the lens power; thus, a high plus cataract lens produces a distortion of disconcerting proportions.[9,15,18]

To the neophyte wearer, the world of straight lines no longer exists. In walking through a doorway, the sides of the doorway seem to bow in a pincushion manner until they almost touch each other. As he approaches the door, it appears to open. Not only do straight lines bow, but with eye movements they also appear to undulate. This undulating motion has been referred to as "withering snakes."[9,14,15] A contact lens eliminates most of these distortions.

OTHER SPECTACLE PROBLEMS

Even the most carefully fabricated aphakic spectacle lens will only give a fair cosmetic appearance. A high plus power causes the eyes to look large and alters the normal appearance of the patient.

The spectacle-corrected aphakic has a need for constant spectacle adjustments. To a greater extent than the average patient, the aphakic patient must have his glasses properly adjusted at all times if he is to function with any degree of efficiency. The weight of the spectacles causes them to slide down, and this movement will alter the effective power of the lens by as much as a diopter or more. If the temples are out of adjustment, even minimally, the patient may be seeing through a portion of the lens other than the optical center. The aforementioned aberrations will be compounded by each misalignment.

Because of his absolute dependence on a properly fitted pair of spectacles, the aphakic patient sometimes has four or five pairs of spectacles conveniently placed for easy and rapid location.

There is little doubt that if the aphakic patient, either monocular or binocular, can be fitted successfully with contact lenses, he will perform better visually and will have a more normal appearance. It is, therefore, worthwhile to try to encourage most aphakic patients to consider contact lenses, providing that the fitter feels the patient has sufficient dexterity and skills.

PRESURGICAL CONSIDERATIONS

PATIENT MANAGEMENT

There should be a complete discussion with the patient of the nature of a cataract and its management. There are many misconceptions regarding the causes and treatment of cataracts. It is a great help if the patient can comprehend his problem and the various methods of treatment. The use of illustrations, books, and audiovisual aids is helpful.[20]

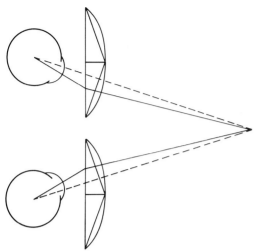

Figure 27.2. The induced base-out prism effect when looking inward from the optical center of a high plus lens.

Probably the most important part of the presurgical consultation is the discussion of the type of correction that the patient will need. The patient must understand why a contact lens is required. There is frequently a gross misunderstanding regarding this aspect of care. Some patients think that the eye will need no type of correction but that surgery or a simple conventional spectacle lens will correct their vision following surgery.

Frequently, the patient is confused about the time required following surgery before an optical correction can be prescribed. A detailed discussion of the expected postoperative course and the length of time required before a contact lens can be prescribed is helpful.

The practitioner should discuss and illustrate what the patient should expect as an end result (visual acuity, comfort, etc.).

During the initial presurgical consultation, the practitioner should attempt to determine whether the patient will tolerate a contact lens. If the cataract is monocular and visual acuity is good in the other eye, a contact lens will be required. Therefore, the practitioner must consider before surgery whether a contact lens will be tolerated. Considerations include the patient's psychological set, manual dexterity, corneal health, and certain ocular parameters such as corneal topography, refractive error, and lid characteristics. The patient must be willing to wear a contact lens. He must accept this as a necessary part of the visual rehabilitation. It is sometimes helpful to allow a patient who is extremely apprehensive about his ability to wear a contact lens to try on a lens at the time of this initial consultation. Many patients are surprised with the comfort of a lens and become more encouraged following this trial period. If the patient is absolutely opposed to the idea of a contact lens and the other eye has adequate vision, then only the intraocular lens (I.O.L.) can be used as an alternative. If there are contraindications to using an I.O.L. (Fuch's dystrophy, narrow angle glaucoma, etc.),[21] surgery should not be performed unless there are definite medical indications (hypermature cataract, phakolytic iritis, etc.).[22]

PREOPERATIVE PROCEDURES

Expected Visual Acuity

It is useful to have some clinical impression of what the vision will be after surgery. This will help when discussing visual rehabilitation with the patient and the results the patient should expect. There are a number of tests that can be done to estimate the prognosis for vision. Visual acuity measurements prior to the formation of cataracts is often of value. If acuity was relatively good one to two years prior to the formation of the cataract, probably the visual acuity will be normal following surgery. Generally, if no macular disease is present, the postoperative visual result is excellent. A survey of 2,875 eyes that had undergone phacoemulsification showed that approximately 87 percent had a corrected visual acuity of 20/40 or better following surgery.[23] Similar results have been found with intracapsular extraction.

The visual acuity with hard and soft contact lenses can also be expected to be quite good. Hard lens acuity in most aphakics is excellent without overcorrection; however, many patients wearing flexible lenses, i.e. hydrogels, require an additional spectacle correction for best acuity.[24] Figure 27.3 and 27.4 show the visual acuity of twenty-three aphakic patients wearing gel lenses with and without overcorrection. Shown in Figure 27.5 is the relationship between the best hard lens acuity (no overcorrection) and best soft lens acuity (with overcorrection). These data indicate that an overcorrection is required to achieve soft lens acuity equal to vision with hard lenses. Therefore, if a soft lens is likely to be prescribed, the patient should be informed of the need for an additional spectacle correction to achieve best acuity.

If the patient is new to the office and the previous visual acuity cannot be obtained or macular dysfunction is suspected, there are several tests that can be done to prognosticate useful vision after cataract extraction.

The first is the Petit macular function test.[25] This test is performed with a modified conventional flashlight (Figure 27.6). The flashlight has a black opaque front with five holes, each 1 mm. in diameter. The center hole is backed by a red filter, and all five apertures are backed by a frosted glass diffuser. The lights surrounding the central red point of fixation are at 1° each for the two lateral and 2° each for the two vertical lights. By using an attached shutter, the four peripheral white spots can be covered so that only the center red dot is exposed. The five points of light are uncovered and held 13 inches from the eye. If the patient can readily see the five points of light, the result is recorded as macular function is good at 1° and 2° for red and white.

If a cataract is so dense as to cause diffusion of light so that the five points of light are not individually resolved, the shutter may be closed, exposing only the red fixation point, and the accessory beam from a small penlight is also used. The approximate minimum

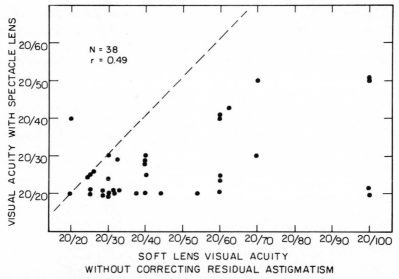

Figure 27.3. Scattergram of soft lens visual acuity without correcting residual astigmatism (*abscissa*) and visual acuity with aphakic spectacles (*ordinate*).

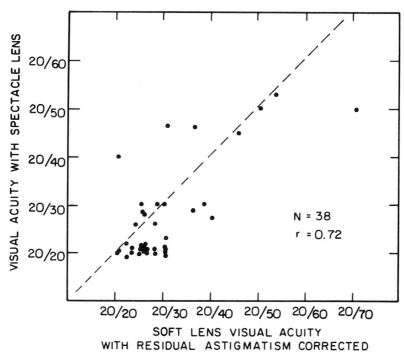

Figure 27.4. Scattergram of soft lens visual acuity with residual astigmatism corrected (*abscissa*) and visual acuity with aphakic spectacles (*ordinate*).

distance for which two lights are distinguished can be recorded. Each 6 mm. is equal to one degree.

Another test, which requires a good observer but which can be useful, is to allow the patient to view his own macular area entoptically. This is done by having the patient look down while a transilluminator light is rubbed gently back and forth over the eyelid (Figure 27.7). After this is done (for a moment or two), the patient will be able entoptically to view his own macula. If he is able to describe the retinal tree, with a macular area, the practitioner may presume that the macular region is intact. However, if he has difficulty describing it or notices many blotches or circles present, this may indicate the presence of macular degeneration, hemorrhages, etc.

The swinging flashlight test for Marcus Gunn pupil can also be used. If there is disturbance in the visual pathway anterior to the optic chiasma, the pupil on the affected side can be made to dilate while light is shined directly onto the eye. This test was described carefully by Levatin in 1959. He described the proper technique:

The lights are dimmed and the patient fixes his gaze on a spot on the opposite wall near the ceiling to eliminate the effect of accommodation on the pupils. A pocket flashlight with a bright light is passed back and forth from one eye to the other, the examiner noting the movement of the pupil in the eye that is illuminated. Normally, there is a slight, sometimes imperceptible, contraction of the illuminated pupil as the light strikes it. In an eye harboring diseases of the retina or optic nerve, the pupil dilates slowly while the light is still upon it. A striking contrast occurs as the light is swung back to the normal eye, which shows a marked pupillary contraction. Thus, instead of measuring the final size of the pupil, one observes the direction of movement of the illuminated pupil, which becomes larger in the abnormal eye and smaller in the normal eye. Several passes back and forth with the flashlight may be

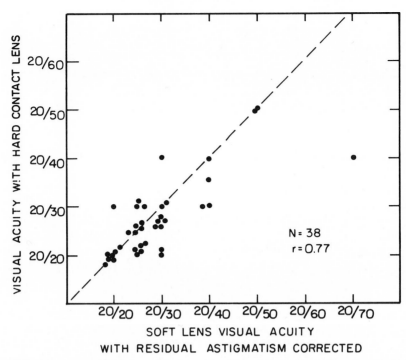

Figure 27.5. Scattergram of soft lens visual acuity with residual astigmatism corrected (*abscissa*) and visual acuity with a hard lens (*ordinate*).

required before the proper speed is found to bring out the dynamic anisocoria.[26]

There are many ocular abnormalities that may be identified by the swinging flashlight test.[27,28] A positive Marcus Gunn sign is found in such diseases as (1) optic neuritis, (2) retinal detachment, (3) optic atrophy, (4) direct pressure on the intraorbital or intracranial optic nerve, (5) occlusion of the central retinal artery or vein or their branches, (6) glaucoma, and (7) other widespread organic diseases

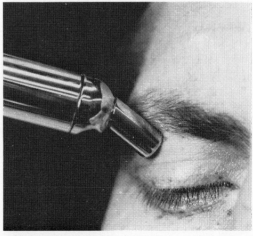

Figure 27.7. Procedure for eliciting entoptic imagery. Transilluminator light is rubbed gently back and forth over the eyelid.

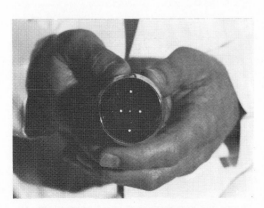

Figure 27.6. Petit macular function test.

of the retina. In all of these conditions, the more extensive the lesion, the greater the impairment of light sense and the more striking the Marcus Gunn sign. A negative response is obtained in amblyopia ex anopsia, cataract, and corneal disease. This important difference between positive and negative signs may help differentiate retinal and optic nerve diseases from other causes of reduced visual acuity.

Recently, the development of interferometry has made possible the prediction of visual acuity in some patients.[29] This technique projects a laser beam onto the retinal surface and creates interference fringes. Changes in the width of the interference bands (spatial frequency) have been shown to predict a visual acuity that correlates well with the acuity obtained postsurgically. Clinicians have reported that this technique does not work well with advanced cataract but is useful in patients with moderate changes and acuity lower than predicted by media changes.[29] A commercially available instrument for using this technique is made by Rodenstock.

Corneal Curvature

Presurgical keratometry readings provide the practitioner with information regarding any corneal distortions or irregularity. Some surgeons feels that postoperative astigmatism can be corrected by the position of the incision,[7] and therefore, it is useful to know the amount and type of preoperative corneal toricity. With the advancement of microsurgical techniques and the development of the surgical keratometer, it may become possible to control the magnitude and direction of corneal astigmatism accurately.

Original keratometry findings will also allow the clinician to evaluate surgically induced curvature changes.

Slit-Lamp Examination

A careful slit-lamp examination with fluorescein and rose bengal should be performed.[30] Listed in Table 27.1 are certain con-

TABLE 27.1
CONTRAINDICATIONS TO CONTACT LENS WEAR

1. Recurrent herpes keratitis
2. Uncontrolled glaucoma
3. Advanced keratitis sicca
4. Immunosuppressive therapy
5. Neuroparalytic keratitis
6. Active anterior segment disease

TABLE 27.2
RELATIVE CONTRAINDICATIONS TO
CONTACT LENS WEAR

1. Incomplete lid closure
2. Corneal guttata
3. Mild dry eye
4. Recurrent corneal erosion
5. Fuchs' dystrophy
6. Moderate ocular allergy
7. Epithelial dystrophy
8. Poorly controlled blepharitis
9. Nocturnal lagophthalmos

ditions that contraindicate contact lens wear. These conditions are considered so severe that the eye and/or vision might be compromised if a contact lens is worn. There are also conditions that are relative contraindications to contact lens wear, and although the patient may initially be fitted, the prognosis is guarded. These conditions are listed in Table 27.2.

Cornea guttata and Fuchs' dystrophy may reduce the physiological function of the endothelium so that the stress of a contact lens could not be tolerated. Patients with mild keratitis sicca may have inadequate tears to keep a hydrogel lens properly hydrated. If the lens dehydrates, the oxygen transmissability will decrease (*see* Chapter 17), and corneal edema may occur. Also, dry eye patients may have difficulty keeping the lens properly wetted. Methods of evaluating tear function are discussed later. Incomplete lid closure (nocturnal lagophthalmos[31]) may lead to chronic epithelial breakdown. Patients with chronic blepharitis are usually more susceptible to corneal infection[32] and may develop corneal ulcers. Recurrent corneal erosions may be aggravated during lens wear, although a continuously worn lens may also be therapeutically useful.

Refractive Error

The refractive error should be measured. In some cases it will give some indication of the postoperative correction required. For example, a highly myopic eye may only be slightly hyperopic following surgery, whereas a hyperopic eye may be extremely hyperopic after removal of the cataract. This information may prove helpful in evaluating possible complications that may be encountered with the postoperative prescription. For example, if high hyperopia is expected (20 D. or greater), it may be necessary to use a contact lens in combination with a spectacle lens, since contact lenses over 20 D. are sometimes difficult to fit. This type of information will prove useful in preoperative consultation with the patient.

Predictive Testing

Ideally, it would be advantageous to be able to predict which patients could physiologically tolerate contact lens wear, especially extended lens wear. Even the patient without the contraindications listed in Tables 27.1 and 27.2 may not tolerate lens wear. Presently there are no definitive tests that can be used to predict the ocular response to lens wear.

Some clinicians have suggested that it is possible to predict a patient's response to a contact lens by subjecting the eye to a short period of contact lens wear prior to surgery. The test requires wearing an aphakic hydrogel lens with the eyes closed for two hours. Slit-lamp inspection is done before and after wearing the lens. If there is only a minimal edematous response, it might be anticipated that the subject will not encounter marked edema during lens wear after surgery.

POSTSURGICAL CARE

CONSULTATION

Following surgery, the need for a contact lens should again be discussed. The aphakic patient usually needs a great deal of encouragement and understanding to acquire the motivation essential to successful contact lens wear. During this consultation, several specific points regarding time for fitting, expected visual acuity, complications, etc. should be reemphasized.

It may be necessary to explain again to the patient about the difficulties encountered with aphakic spectacles that can be eliminated by contact lenses. In extreme cases where the practitioner is having difficulty relating these points, it may be necessary first to prescribe spectacle lenses and allow the patient to experience some of the optical problems associated with cataract spectacle lenses.[7] Once the patient has encountered some of these problems, he will usually be more receptive to contact lens wear.

An appraisal of the time required to fit the contact lens is a necessary part of the consultation. Generally, patients take between two and four months to be completely comfortable with the lens. This will depend on a number of factors including the type of lens, postsurgical healing, and corneal adaptation. Since the contact lens must be accepted both psychologically and physiologically, and since many patients will adapt slowly at first, it is better to be conservative in estimating the time required to complete the fitting. The aphakic patient is anxious to regain normal vision. Without an understanding of the time involved, he may become discouraged.

The consultation should also include the patient's prognosis. This would include an appraisal of the expected visual acuity, hours of wear, and comfort. Finally, a discussion of the fees related to the fitting, lost lenses, and follow-up care will complete the consultation.

TIME OF FITTING

There are several factors that will determine when the contact lens can be fitted following surgery. Among the most important factors are the type of surgical procedure, the rate of healing, and postsurgical complications.

Two types of surgery are presently being used for senile cataract: intracapsular lens extraction (I.C.C.E.) and phacoemulsification. There are advantages and disadvantages to each procedure, and the decision of which procedure is preferred depends upon a number of factors such as corneal health and type of cataract.[33-34] Generally, eyes that have undergone phacoemulsification heal faster and are ready for contact lens fitting about four to six weeks following surgery, whereas patients who have had I.C.C.E. require about twelve weeks.[35]

There have been several reports of fitting patients within a few days following surgery.[36,37] The proponents of this approach suggest that the soft lens will not adversely affect healing, and the patient will be able to have usable vision shortly after surgery. Most surgeons and fitters, however, are more conservative in their fitting approach and prefer to wait until the eye has healed. This delay does not cause much difficulty as long as the patient has been properly counseled before surgery about the expected time delay between surgery and contact lens fitting.

In helping decide when the patient is ready for fitting, the clinician may find it useful to use keratometry readings and refraction as indicators of corneal stability.

Keratometry Readings

The practitioner should try to make several keratometry readings before proceeding with the fitting. Usually, the first reading can be taken one to three weeks after surgery. This can be followed by a reading at about two-week intervals until two readings are the same and the mires are not distorted. When this occurs, the corneal curvature has most likely stabilized.

It is sometimes difficult for the aphakic patient to fixate for the keratometry measurement. A device consisting of a small light can be set in the aperture of the keratometer, which assists the aphakic in holding fixation steady (Figure 27.8). This can be made by using a small flexible plastic rod (about 3 mm. in diameter), which is mounted on the inside edge of the keratometer housing. The keratometer light will illuminate the rod and thus provide a fixation for the patient.

Refraction

Refractive measurements are a very sensitive indicator of when the cornea has stabilized.[38] At the same visit when keratometry readings are made, a subjective refraction should be performed. Stabilization of the refractive measurement is an excellent indication of complete corneal healing.

Slit Lamp

Fluorescein and rose bengal dyes should be instilled in the eye, and the cornea should be examined for the presence of epithelial staining, edema, or dry spots. Any changes in the cornea that were not present presurgically indicate that the cornea is still healing. During the healing process, low tear film breakup time (*see* Chapter 2), conjunctival hyperemia, mild corneal staining, and edema are quite common. When these changes sub-side, the eye is usually healed sufficiently for the contact lens fitting to proceed.

When the cornea has stabilized, the prac-titioner is ready to begin fitting the contact lens. The fitting procedure can be divided into the examination and trial lens fitting.

EXAMINATION

Keratometric Readings

In aphakia, keratometric measurements taken in the conventional manner are often of little value in determining lens specifica-tions, due to distortion of the corneal sur-face. Nevertheless, it is important to obtain good readings to provide an approximate base curve for beginning the trial lens fitting pro-cedure. Three sets of measurements on each eye should be taken.

Refraction

A careful refraction should be done using a trial frame. The vertex distance and best visual acuity should be recorded. A refractive mea-surement is important even if glasses are not prescribed. This allows the practitioner the opportunity during the postfitting care to put on the trial frame and get an estimate of the induced spectacle blur. Also, if glas-ses are to be prescribed at a later date, the necessary information is already at hand.

Slit Lamp

The biomicroscope examination of the postsurgical patient provides essential infor-mation for the fitting procedure. All impor-tant findings should be carefully recorded. Listed below are some special areas of im-portance that must be checked in addition to the routine examination done on all con-tact lens patients (*see* Chapter 4).

Pupil

The shape, size, and position of the pupil should be recorded. Most cataract surgery done today leaves the patient with a normal-shaped round pupil. However, occasionally the surgeon must remove large amounts of iris, leaving a large pupil (full iridectomy) because of surgical complications or the need to make frequent fundus examinations in a patient who does not dilate well. Changes in the initial shape, size, or position of the pupil may indicate serious underlying pathology such as retinal detachment, iritis, or cystoid macular edema.[39]

Vitreous

The position of the vitreous should be examined. When an intracapsular extraction is done, the vitreous is free to move anteriorly. Since the vitreous is attached to the retina, it is desirable to have the vitreous not pull forward but remain essentially in the same location. However, the vitreous may pro-lapse and thereby cause a potential source of pathology (Figure 27.9).[40] If the vitreous face prolapses and adheres to the corneal endothelium, chronic corneal edema may

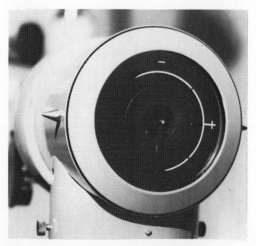

Figure 27.8. Auxiliary fixation device for kerato-meter.

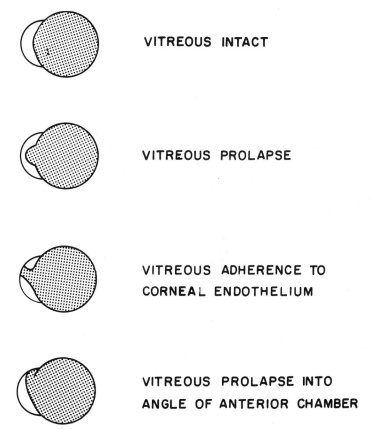

VITREOUS INTACT

VITREOUS PROLAPSE

VITREOUS ADHERENCE TO
CORNEAL ENDOTHELIUM

VITREOUS PROLAPSE INTO
ANGLE OF ANTERIOR CHAMBER

Figure 27.9. Schematic drawing of different vitreous positions following surgery.

result. The vitreous could also enter the angle of the anterior chamber, resulting in increased intraocular pressure. If the vitreous is drawn up into the wound, there is usually a change in pupil shape or position. In cases of vitreous loss, complications such as glaucoma, corneal edema, epithelial downgrowth, retinal detachment, or macular edema can develop.[41]

Iris

There is usually a small degree of iritis occurring after surgical trauma, which lasts from one to two weeks. However, persistent iritis can occur in cases with vitreous loss, residual lens material, foreign debris in the anterior chamber, iris prolapse, and glaucoma. A careful inspection for aqueous flare and ciliary injection should be made during the slit-lamp procedure.

Anterior Chamber

The depth and angle of the anterior chamber can be approximated with the slit lamp using direct illumination with an optic section.[42] Occasionally, the iris may prolapse, leading to a flat anterior chamber, which results in a serious medical emergency. The contact lens practitioner should note the angle and depth of the chamber. If changes occur, the patient should be referred for consultation. If the clinician suspects that vitreous may be in the angle, gonioscopy should be done.

Corneal Endothelium

Cataract surgery may induce morphological changes in the corneal endothelium.[43] In addition, a mild corneal dystrophy (corneal guttata) or more advanced Fuchs' dystrophy may be present. Many aphakic eyes show reduced cell density and pleomorphism.[44] The significance of these changes and their relationship to contact lens wear is not known; nevertheless, a careful inspection of the corneal endothelium is important. It is possible to observe directly the endothelial mosaic for these and other changes using specular reflection. High magnification and a good light source are required. This technique is described elsewhere.[45] Marked loss of cells, or corneal dystrophy may indicate when corneal complications from contact lens wear might be expected.

Corneal Staining and Edema

The cornea may be abnormal due to the surgical procedures or as a result of normal changes associated with aging.

Corneal edema can result from vitreous touching the corneal endothelium, endothelial dystrophy, excessive surgical trauma to the cornea, or glaucoma. Chronic corneal edema can lead to a number of fitting complications. Corneal dry spots (*see* Chapter 2) are sometimes observed following cataract surgery. The dry spots are usually related to insufficient mucin in the precorneal film. Following a blink, the film appears to break up quickly, and a small area that will not wet becomes observable. Minute stippling in this area may also be present. These dry spots may be the result of surgical trauma and frequently go away when healing is complete. The dry spots can also be caused by chronic loss of mucus-secreting goblet cells.[46] If dry spots were not noted presurgically, then they are probably due to the surgical trauma, and the practitioner should wait until the dry spots disappear before fitting the lens.

The cornea may also show chronic epithelial staining following surgery. This staining may be a result of partial loss of the protective reflex. Older patients usually have a loss of corneal sensitivity, which is further decreased following cataract surgery, for approximately one-half of the afferent sensory fibers are severed during the surgical procedure.[47] A loss in sensitivity may result in a loss of the protective mechanism. Staining may also indicate incomplete healing or active keratitis. If no staining was present presurgically, the cause should be determined, and appropriate treatment given.

KERATITIS SICCA. Insufficient tear production occurs frequently in the older age group and is more prevalent in females.[48] This condition may add difficulties to the fitting procedure. Keratitis sicca should be suspected if the patient complains of dryness or excessively red eyes or if the slit-lamp exam shows persistent corneal staining. The Schirmer test (*see* Chapter 2) is of diagnostic value; however, a negative result does not necessarily rule out this condition. The rose bengal stain is a more sensitive agent in detecting this condition. This stain is specific for devitalized cells and mucin. Thus, the dessicated epithelial cells will show up as extensive staining.

Other tests such as observations of the tear film meniscus, tear debris, and fluorescein dilution time may also be helpful in diagnosis.[49] The tear film meniscus should be at least 1 mm. wide and have a good convex surface. If it is scanty or if there are areas of discontinuity, keratitis sicca should be suspected. It is normal to have a few desquamated epithelial cells and a little mucin in the tear strip, but pronounced debris or mucin strands in the tear film indicate reduced flushing action of the tears suggestive of keratitis sicca.

The fluorescein dilution test measures tear production indirectly by measuring tear turnover. A known quantity of a known dilution of fluorescein is instilled in the eye, and its dilution by the tears is measured with a fluorophotometer. This gives an accurate measurement, but is not yet available for clinical use.

Conjunctiva

Following surgery there is usually marked

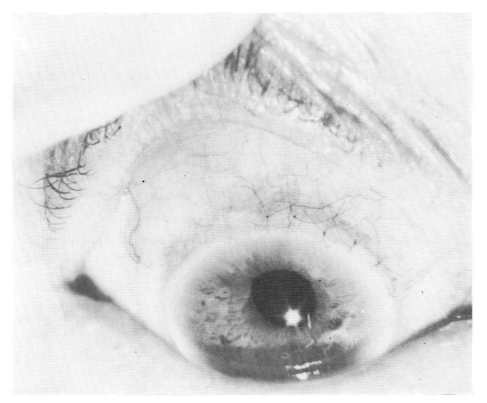

Figure 27.10. Examination of superior bulbar conjunctiva four to six weeks postsurgery. Note mild injection around the sutures.

conjunctival hyperemia. As the healing proceeds, the injection subsides. The upper lid should be retracted, and the superior bulbar conjunctiva investigated. Any marked redness may indicate that healing is not complete (Figure 27.10).

Most I.C.C.E. procedures leave the sutures in place, which are covered by the conjunctiva. Occasionally, one or more of these sutures may work its way up through the conjunctiva. These exposed sutures often catch mucus and can become local areas of infection or irritation. Usually the surgeon will want to remove these sutures if they are present. When a suture is exposed, extended wear should be discontinued, since the opportunity for infection increases.

Epithelial Downgrowth

Occasionally, following surgery, there is poor apposition of the wound margins. This allows the epithelium of the cornea to grow down into the wound and into the angle of the anterior chamber. This can result in a serious glaucoma and, even when treated promptly, may result in loss of the eye.

Filtering Bleb

Incomplete wound closure following surgery may cause aqueous to filter through the wound, creating a bleblike formation on the conjunctiva (Figure 27.11). These blebs provide a channel between the inner and outer eye and therefore can potentially provide a mechanism for intraocular inflammation, which may lead to an endophthalmitis. A rather minor bacterial conjunctivitis can be eye threatening in a patient who has a postoperative bleb. For this reason, most surgeons suggest that if the bleb does not spon-

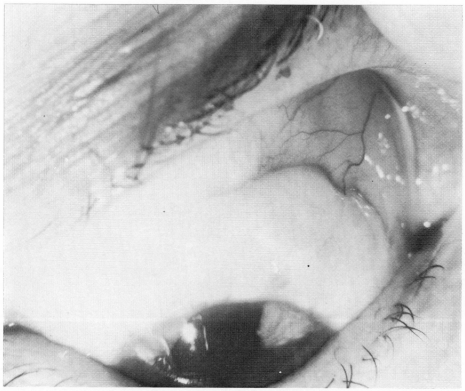

Figure 27.11. Large filtering bleb at superior limbal area.

taneously close within two to three months after surgery, a surgical procedure should be initiated to close the bleb. In any case, contact lens fitting should probably be delayed until the bleb is closed.

Visual Field

The aphakic patient is prone to develop certain pathologies that are detectable with field testing. It is therefore important to establish reliable baseline fields so that any early departures can be detected. The visual field should be done with a contact lens in place using a tangent screen, Goldmann perimetry, or other appropriate field-testing device.

Using an appropriate near point addition, an Amsler grid test should be done and recorded.[50] The use of these two tests may prove valuable in the early detection of retinal detachment or cystic macular edema, which are two relatively common pathologies occurring in surgical aphakia.

Tonometry

Occasionally, glaucoma may develop in the aphake. Persistent iritis, flat or narrow anterior chamber, and vitreous prolapse may be causes. It is therefore valuable to have baseline tonometric readings.

Ophthalmoscopy

Several months or years may have elapsed since an adequate view of the fundus was obtained. Since there are many retinal diseases that may have developed or may develop, a careful fundus evaluation should be done.

TRIAL LENS FITTING

In order to determine the correct power, lens construction, and base curve, it has long been recognized that a diagnostic contact lens fitting should be done prior to ordering.[51] The aphakic eye is usually 10 D. to 14 D. hyperopic in the spectacle plane. Even the most careful vertex measurements may yield incorrect power in the contact lens; a 1 mm. error could produce a 0.50 D. to 1.00 D. error in the required power. Incorrect power determination may also result from relying on keratometry readings, which are only an approximation of true corneal power.

A trial lens fitting must also be done to determine the type of lens (single cut, lenticular, hydrogel, etc.) that should be prescribed. This cannot easily be determined from keratometer readings or from other information, but only from observations using diagnostic lenses.

Finally, the base curve of the lens can best be determined using a trial lens. Keratometer readings do not give a true measurement, and diagnostic lenses provide the only method of determining the proper base curve required to achieve an optimum bearing relationship between the cornea and the contact lens.

Selection of Lens Type

There are several types of contact lens corrections available, and the choice of lens will depend on several factors, which include the postoperative refractive error, corneal health, and patient requirements. The current options available are hard lenses (P.M.M.A. and gas-permeable materials) and hydrogels (daily and extended wear). Each of these lens types has advantages and disadvantages. Listed below are the procedures to be followed for fitting each type.

Hard Lens Fitting Procedures (P.M.M.A. and Gas Permeable)

There are basically two designs of hard lenses used in fitting aphakic patients—the single cut and minus-carrier lenticular lenses. There are strong advocates of each type of lens. Both lenses are valuable, each having its own advantages and disadvantages, depending upon the particular patient.[52,53,54] The following factors should be evaluated when deciding whether a minus-carrier lenticular or single cut lens should be used.

Corneal Astigmatism

If the corneal curvature is flatter than 45.0 D. or if there is 1.50 D. or more against-the-rule toricity, a minus carrier lens usually gives better centration and movement.

If the corneal curvature is greater than 45.0 D. or if with-the-rule toricity is present, a single cut lens should be considered. A single cut lens can usually be fitted smaller than a lenticular lens and therefore may provide a better physiological result on steeper corneas where smaller lenses are often indicated. A single cut lens may ride centrally when with-the-rule toricity is present.

Palpebral Aperture

Large palpebral apertures or lower lid margins that touch below the inferior limbus are indications for using a minus carrier lens. The minus carrier lens will tend to ride up and not be as dependent on the lower lid for positioning as a single cut lens.

A minus carrier lens centers better when there is a loose upper lid, since there is some ability of the lid to grasp the minus carrier of the lens. However, a very tight upper lid may cause a minus carrier lens to ride too high, and a single cut lens should be tried.

Narrow palpebral apertures also are an indication for the single cut lens, which can more easily be fitted within the aperture.

Pupil Size and Shape

Lenticular lenses can be fitted to round, well-centered pupils. Large keyhole pupils,

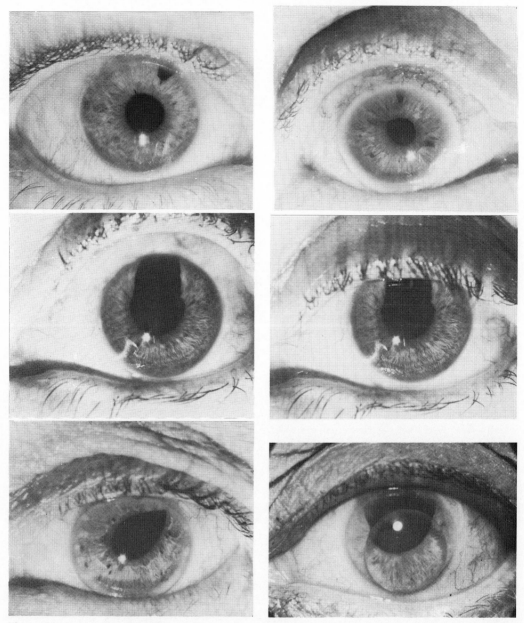

Figure 27.12. Examples of different pupil shapes following surgery: (*a*) round pupil with peripheral iridectomy at one o'clock position, (*b*) round pupil with slight asymmetry and peripheral iridectomy at twelve o'clock position, (*c*) keyhole pupil with upper lid retracted, (*d*) keyhole pupil on same patient as c with lid in normal position, (*e*) slightly peaked pupil following vitreous prolapse, and (*f*) full iridectomy with single cut contact lens in place.

wedge-shaped pupils, and irregular pupils (Figure 27.12) usually do better with single cut lenses because the junction zone of a minus carrier (*see* Chapter 15) may cross the pupil, causing some visual disturbances.

Lens Construction

MINUS CARRIER LENS. A basic problem of high plus contact lenses is that they are thick and heavy. This causes the lens to gravitate downward, frequently dropping unevenly over the cornea. If the lens tends to gravitate and stay downward, frequently there is poor tear circulation. The construction of the lenticular lens with a minus carrier (*see* Figure 27.13) greatly reduces the weight and center thickness.[55] The use of a minus carrier usually allows the lens to ride up and center on the eye (*see* Chapter 15). Using a minimum thickness junction zone and small optic cap, it is possible to construct a relatively thin, lightweight minus carrier lenticular lens that positions and moves very much like a well-fitted conventional contact lens. Shown in Figure 27.14 is a schematic drawing of the specifications for such a lens. Figure 15.7 showed a plot of power versus thickness for various size optic caps when the junction zone is kept at 0.13 mm. Tables 27.3 and 27.4 list the various parameters for a small and large trial set of minus carrier lenticular lenses based on a junction zone of 0.13 mm.

An approximate guide for choosing the initial trial lens specifications with minus

TYPES OF APHAKIC LENSES

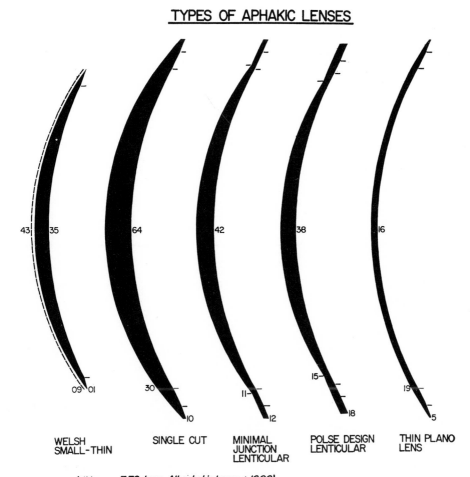

| WELSH SMALL-THIN | SINGLE CUT | MINIMAL JUNCTION LENTICULAR | POLSE DESIGN LENTICULAR | THIN PLANO LENS |

(all lenses 7.70 base. All aphakic lenses + 16.00)

Figure 27.13. Types of aphakic lenses compared to thin plano lens. Courtesy of D. Korb.

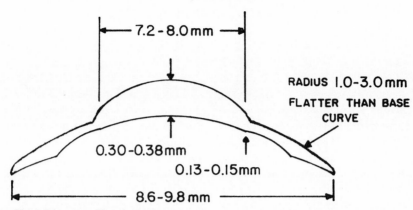

Figure 27.14. Diagram of lenticular lens showing range of specifications: (*a*) small diameter 8.6 mm. to 9.8 mm., (*b*) small optic cap 7.2 mm. to 8.0 mm., (*c*) minimum thickness of junction between outer flange and optic cap 0.13 mm. to 0.15 mm., (*d*) minimum center thickness varying between 0.30 mm. and 0.38 mm., depending upon optic cap size and power (12 D. to 15 D.), and (*e*) radius of second front curve should be 1.0 mm. to 3.0 mm. flatter than base curve.

TABLE 27.3
APHAKIA (MODIFIED CONTOUR, LENTICULAR, MINUS CARRIER)
DIAGNOSTIC LENS FITTING SET

Base Curve	O.Z.R.	Second Curve Radius	Second Curve Width	Blend Curve	Periph. Curve Radius	Periph. Curve Width	O.Z. Diam.	Lens Diam.	Thick.	Power (Front Vertex)	Optic Cap Diam.	Anter. Curve Radius
46.00	7.34	8.1	.5	9.0	10.0	.4	7.6	9.4	.37	+13.00	7.6	9.1
45.50	7.42	8.2	.5	9.0	10.0	.4	7.6	9.4	.37	+13.00	7.6	9.2
45.00	7.50	8.3	.5	9.0	10.0	.4	7.6	9.4	.37	+13.00	7.6	9.3
44.50	7.58	8.4	.5	9.5	10.5	.4	7.6	9.4	.37	+13.00	7.6	9.4
44.00	7.67	8.5	.5	9.5	10.5	.4	7.8	9.6	.38	+13.00	7.8	9.5
43.50	7.76	8.6	.5	9.5	10.5	.4	7.8	9.6	.38	+13.00	7.8	9.6
43.00	7.85	8.7	.5	9.5	10.5	.4	7.8	9.6	.38	+13.00	7.8	9.7
42.50	7.94	8.8	.5	9.5	10.5	.4	7.8	9.6	.38	+13.00	7.8	9.8
42.00	8.04	8.9	.5	10.0	11.0	.4	8.0	9.8	.39	+13.00	8.0	9.9
41.50	8.13	9.0	.5	10.0	11.0	.4	8.0	9.8	.39	+13.00	8.0	10.0
41.00	8.23	9.1	.5	10.0	11.0	.4	8.0	9.8	.39	+13.00	8.0	10.1
40.50	8.33	9.2	.5	10.0	11.0	.4	8.0	9.8	.39	+13.00	8.0	10.2
40.00	8.44	9.3	.5	10.0	11.0	.4	8.0	9.8	.39	+13.00	8.0	10.3

From Sarver, M. D.: *Contact Lens Syllabus,* University of California Alumni Association, 1973.

carrier lenses is given in following sections. It should be clearly understood that the final lens specifications cannot be determined by simple rules of thumb but rather by a careful diagnostic fitting.

Diameter. Overall diameter usually ranges from 8.3 mm. to 9.8 mm. In general, flatter corneal curvatures or larger corneal diameters require larger lenses. Also, if the lids are quite loose or the lower lid margins lie below the inferior limbus, a larger diameter lens

should be used. The diameter should be 1.5 mm. to 2 mm. larger than the optic cap. This gives an adequate lenticular flange so that the upper lid can grasp the flange portion of the lens to help with lens centering (*see* Chapter 15).

Base Curve. A base curve that is close to the flattest corneal reading provides a good starting point. For each diopter of corneal toricity, the base curve can be increased by 0.25 D. When high corneal toricity is pres-

TABLE 27.4
Aphakia (Small Lens, Lenticular, Minus Carrier)
Diagnostic Lens Fitting Set.

Base Curve	O.Z.R.	Second Curve Radius	Second Curve Width	Blend Curve	Periph. Curve Radius	Periph. Curve Width	O.Z. Diam.	Lens Diam.	Thick.	Power (Front Vertex)	Optic Cap Diam.	Anter. Curve Radius
46.00	7.34	8.1	.3	9.0	10.0	.4	7.2	8.6	.33	+13.00	7.2	9.1
45.50	7.42	8.2	.3	9.0	10.0	.4	7.2	8.6	.33	+13.00	7.2	9.2
45.00	7.50	8.3	.3	9.0	10.0	.4	7.2	8.6	.33	+13.00	7.2	9.3
44.50	7.58	8.4	.3	9.5	10.5	.4	7.2	8.6	.33	+13.00	7.2	9.4
44.00	7.67	8.5	.3	9.5	10.5	.4	7.2	8.6	.33	+13.00	7.2	9.5
43.50	7.76	8.6	.3	9.5	10.5	.4	7.4	8.8	.35	+13.00	7.4	9.6
43.00	7.85	8.7	.3	9.5	10.5	.4	7.4	8.8	.35	+13.00	7.4	9.7
42.50	7.94	8.8	.3	9.5	10.5	.4	7.4	8.8	.35	+13.00	7.4	9.8
42.00	8.04	8.9	.3	10.0	11.0	.4	7.4	8.8	.35	+13.00	7.4	9.9
41.50	8.13	9.0	.3	10.0	11.0	:4	7.4	8.8	.35	+13.00	7.4	10.0
41.00	8.23	9.1	.3	10.0	11.0	.4	7.4	8.8	.35	+13.00	7.4	10.1
40.50	8.33	9.2	.3	10.0	11.0	.4	7.4	8.8	.35	+13.00	7.4	10.2
40.00	8.44	9.3	.3	10.0	11.0	.4	7.4	8.8	.35	+13.00	7.4	10.3

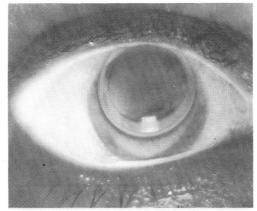

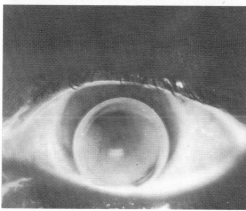

Figure 27.15. Effect of varying anterior flange radius on lens positioning: (*a*) lens rides too high, front radius should be reduced 1 to 2 mm., (*b*) lens positioning too low, front radius should be increased 1 to 2 mm.

ent, a toric base curve may be required. It should be reemphasized that the keratometer readings in aphakia are only an approximation, and the final base curve may differ significantly from the flattest keratometry reading.

Optic Zone Diameter. The optic zone should be slightly larger (2 mm. to 3 mm.) than the pupil size.

Front Optic Cap. The cap size should be very close to the O.Z.D., i.e. 7.0 mm. to 8.5 mm. The cap size limits the effective O.Z.D.; therefore, the cap is not usually made smaller than the O.Z.D. The larger the optic cap, the thicker will be the lens; therefore, a minimum cap size consistent with good vision should be selected.

Thickness. The center thickness is a function of lens power, cap size, and thickness of the junction. Minimum thickness should be used and can be chosen by referring to Figure 15.7, which gives a plot of center thickness with different powers and cap sizes.

Peripheral and Secondary Curves Based on fluorescein observation, the radii and width of the secondary and peripheral curves should be chosen. The peripheral curve must be flat enough to give a sufficient tear film reservoir to allow an adequate interchange of tears under the lens.

Anterior Curve Radii. The anterior curve of the lenticular flange should be 1 mm. to 3 mm. flatter than the base curve. This will provide an adequate edge thickness and outer flange radius to allow the upper lid to pick up and center the lens (*see* Figure 27.15) (*see* Chapter 15). It is important for the clinician to recognize that the positioning of the lens can be controlled by varying the flange width and/or radius. The longer the radius, the higher the lens tends to ride, and vice versa. Also, the width of the flange can influence positioning. Increasing the flange radius and/or width will position a lens higher, and a short radius or narrower flange will have the opposite effect.[56] (*See* Figures 15.8 and 15.9).

Power. Power is determined by doing a refraction over the trial contact lens. Residual astigmatism should be carefully noted. Frequently, the residual astigmatic error is incorporated into a spectacle correction. If the power needed over the trial lens is greater than ±4.00 D., a power conversion table (*see* Appendix 2) should be used; if added power is less than ±4.00 D., vertex distance can be disregarded.

Shown in Table 27.5 are approximate guides for selecting the diagnostic lens for a lenticular fitting.

SINGLE CUT LENS. When the fitter is presented with a large keyhole pupil, an irregular pupil, an excessively steep cornea, or a very tight upper lid, a single cut lens may be

TABLE 27.5

LENTICULAR LENS FITTING GUIDE

Flat K	Diam.	O.Z.D.	Cap	Periph. Curve/W	Secondary Curve/W
40-42	9.5	7.5	7.5	11.5/0.50	9.3/0.40
42-44	9.1	7.5	7.5	11.0/0.40	8.5/0.30
44-46	8.9	7.0	7.0	10.5/0.45	8.3/0.35
46-48	8.3	7.0	7.0	10.0/0.50	

1. Base curve
   a. Start with base curve = flat K
   b. For each 1 D. ΔK add +0.25 to base curve
2. Flange radius 1.5 mm. flatter than base curve
3. Thickness: refer to Figure 15.7

TABLE 27.6

SINGLE-CUT HIGH PLUS TRIAL SET

B.C.	D.	T.	O.Z.D.	P.C.W.	Power
42.00	8.5	.48	7.5	11.0/.45	+13.00
42.50	8.5	.48	7.5	11.0/.45	+13.00
43.00	8.5	.48	7.5	11.0/.45	+13.00
43.50	8.5	.48	7.5	11.0/.45	+13.00
44.00	8.0	.43	7.0	10.5/.45	+13.00
44.50	8.0	.43	7.0	10.5/.45	+13.00
45.00	8.0	.43	7.0	10.5/.45	+13.00
45.50	7.5	.39	6.5	10.0/.45	+13.00
46.00	7.5	.39	6.5	10.0/.45	+13.00
46.50	7.5	.39	6.5	10.0/.45	+13.00

best suited for the eye. Most advocates of single cut lens fitting tend to use a small single cut lens so that center thickness can be reduced.[57] Listed in Table 27.6 are parameters for a single cut high plus trial set. An approximate guide for choosing initial trial lens specifications are given in the following sections. Again, it should be noted that these serve only as guidelines, and a trial fitting should be done.

Diameter. The larger the diameter, the thicker will be the center of the lens; therefore, it is desirable to keep overall diameter at a minimum. Diameters usually range from 7.5 to 8.5 mm. The steeper the corneal curvature and the narrower the palpebral aperture, the smaller the overall diameter. Large and/or irregular pupils may necessitate a larger lens.

Base Curve. The proper base curve should give apical alignment or slight apical touch. This usually means fitting on or close to the flattest corneal curvature. For each diopter of corneal toricity, the base curve should be increased by +0.25 D. A toric base curve may be required if high corneal toricity is present. Care should be taken not to have a lens fitted too steep, since this will tend to cause the lens to gravitate down and also interfere with good tear interchange.

Optical Zone Diameter. The optical zone diameter should be selected on the basis of

pupil size. It is possible to use a large optic zone, which is helpful in large, irregular, keyhole or displaced pupils. The main limitation on the O.Z.D. is interference with corneal metabolism. Larger O.Z.D.s tend to produce tighter fitting lenses.

Thickness. Center thickness will be determined by the power and lens diameter. The smaller the diameter, the thinner the lens. The minimum center thickness that still produces a good edge should be used.

Peripheral and Secondary Curves. In most of the single cut lenses (< 8.5 mm.), only a single peripheral curve, i.e. bicurve lens, need be added. This must be flat enough to allow adequate tear film interchange. Larger diameter lenses will require an additional curve, i.e. tricurve lens.

Power. The same general rules, as with lenticular lenses, apply also for determining the power of a single cut lens.

Shown in Table 27.7 are approximate guides for selecting the first diagnostic lens for a single cut lens fitting.

Trial Lens Procedure

The criteria used in selecting the final lens specifications should be based on observations of the centration, movement, and fluorescein pattern. In general, the criteria should not differ significantly from nonaphakic contact lens patients (*see* Chapter 8). The lens should center well, ride slightly up

TABLE 27.7

SINGLE-CUT LENS FITTING GUIDE

Flat K	Diam.	O.Z.D.	Periph. Curve
42-43.50	8.5	7.5	10.5/0.45
44-45	8.0	7.0	10.0/0.45
45-50	7.5	6.5	9.5/0.45

1. Base curve
   a. Start with base curve = flat K
   b. For each 1 D. K add +0.25 to base curve
2. Center thickness (see Appendix 8)

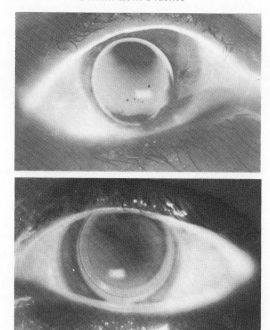

Figure 27.16. Different fluorescein patterns: (*a*) single cut lens riding inferiorly. Note nasal limbal stain from improper movement and positioning; (*b*) lenticular lens on same patient as in Figure 27.16a with proper positioning. Also note absence of limbal staining.

after the blink, and then slowly drop 1 mm. to 2 mm. The fluorescein pattern should show minimum apical clearance, good transition zone, and an adequate tear reservoir for optimum tear flow interchange. As with nonaphakics, several trial lenses may be required before an optimum fitting pattern is achieved.

Shown in Figure 27.16a and b are fluorescein patterns of two lenses fitted to an aphakic eye. Each picture was taken immediately after a blink.

Following the usual trial lens procedure, any additional tests should be done at the time of the diagnostic fitting. These tests should be done with the test lens on the eye. Also, trial lenses placed in a trial frame should be used to provide the maximum visual acuity.

Hydrogel Lens Fitting Procedures

Background

Hydrogel lenses for aphakia can be pre-scribed for daily or extended wear. Although ideally all aphakics would be suitable candidates for extended wear, there are at present problems that need to be solved before all aphakic patients can benefit. Such problems include lens spoilage, lens deposits, acute eye inflammations, corneal edema, neovascularization, increased superior tarsal papillary hypertophy, epithelial necrosis, mucus formation, decreased corneal sensitivity, and apparent increased susceptibility to infection.

Some of the physiological problems are related to the high plus powers that are necessary in the correction of aphakia. These lenses have relatively low oxygen transmissibility and might be insufficient to maintain normal corneal metabolism. The oxygen transmission through these lenses is lowered further during sleep because the partial pressure of oxygen at the lens surface is reduced by two-thirds during lid closure.[58] It is estimated that the oxygen tension at the corneal epithelium when covered by high plus lenses would be near zero during periods of prolonged lid closure.[59]

Laboratory studies suggest that when a contact lens is worn during prolonged lid closure, a significant amount of corneal swelling occurs, which most likely results from corneal hypoxia. The hypoxia results from two factors. First, the high plus lens must be relatively thick, and thus, the oxygen diffusing through the lens to the cornea during closed eye conditions will be very low. Second, the tear pumping is minimal or absent during sleep; therefore, no significant amount of oxygen will reach the cornea-lens interface by tear flow.[60]

These results are in agreement with experimental evidence that indicates most lenses used for extended wear do not supply sufficient oxygen to maintain normal metabolism during closed-eye conditions. Polse and Decker reported on the oxygen tension and oxygen flux at the corneal surface in both open and closed eyes covered by a hydrogel contact lens.[59] These values of oxygen tension (open eye, 2 to 20 mm. Hg; closed eye, 1 to 10 mm. Hg) indicated that even with materials that have high oxygen transmissibility, the partial pressure of oxygen under the lens during sleep is less than 11 mm. Hg, which would be insufficient to maintain normal corneal hydration.[61,62]

This evidence suggests that patients wearing a high plus lens during sleep should and do develop complications related to the reduced oxygen at the corneal surface. However, there are several clinical observations and some limited laboratory studies that suggest that the aphakic eye often tolerates a gel lens during extended wear without clinical evidence of edema or other complications. Although reports of the success vary, there seems to be sufficient clinical evidence to indicate that some patients tolerate extended wear.

There have also been some limited laboratory studies that indicate that the aphakic eye may respond differently from the phakic eye to high plus hydrogel lens wear. Polse, Sarver, and Harris measured the corneal swelling in five phakic and five aphakic patients wearing similar lenses.[63] They found that the aphakic eyes swelled 7.1 percent compared to 9.6 percent for phakic patients over a comparable wearing time. Holden and his coworkers have reported that, in monocular aphakics, the aphakic eye swelled 3 to 4 percent less over a five hour closed-eye wearing period than the phakic eye that was wearing an identical lens.[64] Recently, Korb and his coworkers measured the corneal swelling response of three patients wearing thick (0.35 mm.) hydrogel lenses overnight before and after surgery.[65] On one subject, prior to cataract surgery, the lens, when worn overnight, caused a 35 percent increase in corneal thickness. Following surgery, only a 10 percent swelling response was measured when the identical lens was worn overnight. Similar results were observed on the other two patients. This suggests that some process has occurred following surgery that allows the cornea to tolerate the lens better.

These laboratory results are limited, but they do suggest that there may be a different mechanism in aphakia that allows thicker lenses with reduced oxygen transmissibility to be tolerated by some individuals.

These reports suggest that the aphakic eye can tolerate wearing hydrogel lenses for extended periods without removal. Nevertheless, numerous complications have been reported, therefore, only some patients may be suitable candidates. The clinician should carefully monitor any patient who is fitted for extended wear.

Many of the procedures used in fitting hydrogel lenses to aphakic patients are similar to those used in fitting other gel lenses (*see* Chapters 18 and 19). There are some additional tests and procedures that should be done when fitting gel lenses to the aphakic eye.

Overrefraction

Most aphakic eyes have some corneal

astigmatism that must be incorporated into a spectacle prescription if best vision is to be obtained. Therefore, a careful overrefraction must be done over the hydrogel trial lens (which has parameters close to that which will be ordered) to correct the eye properly.

If the overcorrection is greater than ±4.00 D., a new trial contact lens should be used. Lens power will often affect the fitting characteristics; therefore, it is helpful to have a lens that is as close as possible to the final power. Following the refraction, the residual cylinder should be put into a trial frame, and the patient should be questioned about whether his vision is clear. Not infrequently, soft lens vision can be good when measured on the Snellen acuity chart, but the patient will still complain that his vision is not clear. This may be caused by aberrations or positioning of the lens. If satisfactory vision cannot be obtained with one lens type, a lens of different specifications, e.g. base curve, diameter, thickness, water content, should be tried.

Trial Lens Set

It is useful to have trial sets of two or three lens types with several base curves and diameters (Table 27.8). This gives the clinician the best chance of finding the lens that will provide best vision. The power of the lenses should be about +13.50, which will be within ±2.00 D. of most aphakic corrections.

Lens Fitting

It is important for the lens to center and to have about 0.5 mm. of movement following the blink. A lens that does not move may trap debris and cause anterior segment inflammation.[66] (*See* Chapter 24). The clinician should try to use a lens that is as thin as possible, since oxygen transmissibility will be increased as the lens is made thinner.[67]

Extended Wear

In addition to the procedures outlined previously, the patient using lenses under an extended-wear regime should undergo some additional procedures. These include twenty-four-hour, seventy-two-hour, and seven-day follow-up visits. After the lenses have been fitted, the patient should report the following day in the morning, as soon after awakening as possible. A slit-lamp inspection for edema, staining, striae, inflammation, trapped debris behind the lens, and lens deposits should be made. If findings show a clear lens and minimal corneal change, the patient may continue wearing the lenses and return at seventy-two hours and seven days for additional

TABLE 27.8
APHAKIC EXTENDED-WEAR LENSES

	Sauflon PW	Permalens	Hydrocurve
H₂O CONTENT	79%	71%	55%
O₂ PERMEABILITY (room temperature)	47	33	14
VISUAL ACUITY 20/40 or better:			
without overcorrection	76%	74%	60%
with overcorrection	88%	85%	N/A
MATERIAL	M.M.A. based copolymer	H.E.M.A. based copolymer	H.E.M.A. based copolymer
OPTICAL ZONE	8.0 mm.	6.6 to 7.4 mm.	7.0 mm.+
CENTER THICKNESS	.46 to .67	.43	.25 to .48 mm.
CHORD DIAMETERS	14.4 mm.	14.0, 14.5 mm.	13.5, 14.0, 15.5, 16.0 mm.
BASE CURVES	8.1, 8.4, 8.7	8.0, 8.3, 8.6	8.5, 8.6, 8.9, 9.2, 9.5, 9.8
POWERS	+10 to +17	+11 to +17	+10 to +20

examinations. If these are satisfactory, the patient may be dismissed for two weeks and seen again. Following these visits, the patient should be seen bimonthly. If possible, visits should be soon after awakening, since the morning effects of extended wear are likely to be more marked.

If the patient is not doing well with a particular lens type, a new lens can be tried; however, the prognosis is poor unless the fitter can order a new lens, which would substantially increase the oxygen transmissibility.

Additional Tests

Cover Test

Many monocular aphakic patients initially may have difficulty with fusion.[68,69] This may be due to the prolonged occlusion from the cataract or from the induced aniseikonia caused by the contact lens. If a large vertical or horizontal muscle imbalance is found, the patient should be told of the possibility of double vision. If no previous history of diplopia or strabismus exists, it is best to allow the patient to wear the new prescription one to two weeks before prescribing prism and/or orthoptics, since fusion may reestablish without additional treatment.

If a contact lens rides low, it may induce a significant vertical imbalance itself. This may interfere with fusion. If the lens cannot be made to center, it may be necessary to prescribe vertical prism for proper fusion to be maintained.

Reading Prescription

The patient is usually very anxious to be able to read. With the trial lens on, measurement for a reading addition can be made, and the reading lens ordered. In the case of unilateral aphakia, the phakic eye should also be checked and the prescription given for that eye so that a proper binocular balance is maintained.

Aniseikonia

An estimation of the induced aniseikonia is useful. It is probably best to wait before prescribing treatment, but any magnification over 7 to 8 percent may require treatment. This can usually be done by placing an overall *size* lens before the phakic eye.[13] The amount of aniseikonia can be determined with an eikonometer. It can also be estimated by having the patient compare the relative size of vertical bars using overall size lenses to equalize the difference.

Ordering and Verification

The same procedures that are employed in ordering and verification for regular contact lens patients should be used with the aphakic (*see* Chapter 13). Similar tolerances and ordering procedures should be followed.

Delivery of Lenses

Handling

One of the most difficult parts of the contact lens fitting for the aphakic patient is learning to insert, center, and remove his lenses properly. Many corneas have been traumatized through incorrect insertion and removal techniques. Even though the patient has appeared to master the technique, he may forget after several weeks or months and need additional instruction. The aphakic patient is difficult to teach proper technique because he is usually older and also has a great deal of apprehension during the first few weeks of wear. The ability to insert and remove the lens is one of the greatest fears the aphakic patient has. The mastering of the proper technique is greatly reassuring to the patient.

The training should begin by instructing the patient in a conventional technique (Figure 27.17). Lens removal is usually more difficult than insertion for the aphakic. Frequently the two-handed technique (*see* Chapter 11) is necessary for lens removal because

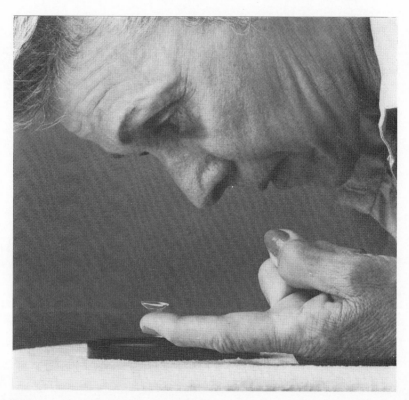

Figure 27.17. Insertion technique for the aphakic. A magnifying mirror provides a useful aid.

the lids have lost their muscle tone, and the one-handed technique will not properly remove the lens. There are a number of devices to assist the patient.[70] However, it is best if the patient can learn to insert and remove his lenses without the use of aids. The use of magnifying mirrors and good lighting will frequently help the patient. If all other techniques fail, it is possible for the patient to use a suction cup, although great caution must be exercised, since it is possible for the aphakic to apply the cup directly to the cornea if the lens has decentered off the cornea.

Insertion can be done in the conventional manner. If a hand tremor or poor manual dexterity is present, the patient can place the lens on the middle finger and the hand against the face for stabilization (*see* Chapter 11). It is

important to emphasize that the upper lid must be held firmly against the orbital rim and that the other eye must be kept wide open.

It is sometimes beneficial to train a member of the family to assist if the patient is having difficulty. Frequently the patient does not master the technique and then becomes extremely frustrated if the lens does not come out at the first attempt. This type of frustration can often be avoided if a member of the family can assist the patient during these minor crises.

It takes a great deal of patience to instruct the aphakic patient properly. The fitter should try to remain enthusiastic and give the patient a great deal of encouragement. Frequent reassurances are necessary for many of the patients to master the technique. Many problems can be avoided if the patient can initially learn the proper technique for insertion and removal.

Examination

Before allowing the patient to start wearing the lenses, visual acuity, fluorescein pattern, and slit-lamp examination should be evaluated. A wearing schedule similar to the nonaphakic patient's can be used (*see* Chapter 11).

Instructions to Patient

The aphakic patient should be carefully instructed about abnormal signs and symptoms (*see* Chapter 11). Because of the reduced corneal sensitivity and dependence on the lens, he is more likely to overwear his lenses

and tolerate a poor fit. The patient should be carefully instructed not to overwear the lenses.

Hygiene

Unfortunately, even after meticulous instruction, many contact lens wearers fail to follow good hygienic techniques in the handling and storage of their lenses. Since many of the aphakic patients are older and tend to forget earlier instruction, continued reminders may be necessary. Consultation in appropriate cleaners and disinfection procedures should frequently be reviewed. Corneal irritation often produces no symptoms because of reduced corneal sensitivity, and good hygienic procedures may reduce the chance of infection.

FOLLOW-UP CARE

Daily Wear

Similar postfitting visits and procedures to those which are used for nonaphakic contact lens wearers should be followed. However, because of the postsurgical problems aphakics are likely to encounter (*see* following section on postfitting complications), a three-month follow-up interval (rather than six months) is often used. Extra care should be used in going over proper cleaning and stor-

age techniques. Daily cleaning with a surfactant (*see* Chapter 21) is helpful in maintaining a clear lens. The patient should be cautioned to rinse the lens carefully after cleaning, since many cleaners are toxic to the cornea. Listed in Table 27.9 are ocular complications that occur in aphakics. The treatment of these complications is similar to that of nonaphakics (*see* Chapters 14 and 22).

Extended Wear

A detailed discussion of the complications resulting from extended wear appears elsewhere in the text (*see* Chapter 24); however, special care must be used in fitting the aphakic with extended-wear lenses. Most of the complications listed under daily wear may also result during extended wear; however, frequently they can be more marked and lead to serious corneal or ocular complications. The main complications seen in extended wear are gross edema, neovascularization,

TABLE 27.9
OCULAR COMPLICATIONS ACCOMPANYING HYDROGEL LENS WEAR

Corneal edema
Epithelial cell loss
Vertical striae
Change in corneal curvature
Increased breakup time
Neovascularization
Giant papillary conjunctivitis
Corneal infection

infection, and heavy lens deposits.[71]

Postfitting Complications

The aphakic patient may demonstrate signs and symptoms that are common to all contact lens wearers (*see* Chapter 14). The treatment of these problems is similar to that used for regular contact lens wearers. There are, however, some unique complications that tend to occur in aphakia.

Diplopia

During the first few weeks of contact lens wear, it is not uncommon for the monocular aphakic to experience diplopia. The patient should be made aware of this and instructed not to drive or engage in activities where diplopia could be dangerous. Every effort should be made to promote fusion. Often altered head positions or different viewing distance can give single binocular vision. If no previous history of strabismus or diplopia exists, the prognosis for return to good single binocular vision should be excellent.[10] Usually there is a steady improvement, and diplopia goes away completely in two to three weeks.

Nonaphakic Eye

If the patient is a unilateral aphakic, the other eye may be developing a cataract. Should the patient start to complain of blurred vision, one should suspect the possibility of blurring from the phakic eye. Often the decision to operate will depend on whether the cataract is interfering with efficient binocular vision.

Aniseikonia

There is usually between 5 to 9 percent image size difference between the phakic and aphakic eye.[11] Some patients can tolerate the aniseikonia quite well, while others cannot. Those patients who can tolerate the image size difference usually demonstrate reduced acuity in one eye, poor fusion, or suppression.[12] If the binocular vision is good, aniseikonia may be a significant problem. If treatment is indicated, a reverse Galilean telescopic system can be made by overplusing the contact lens and adding minus in a spectacle correction.[13,72] Also, it is possible to add an overall size lens to the phakic eye.[13] The latter choice is often the easiest to do and usually works quite well when aniseikonia is a problem.

Ocular Complications Not Related to Contact Lenses

There are several postoperative eye complications.[73,74] Some of the more common problems follow.

CYSTOID MACULAR EDEMA. In some cases following surgery, the macula becomes edematous and shows characteristic cystlike lesions, which are best demonstrated with fluorescein retinal angiography (Figure 27.18).[75,76] This condition results in lowered visual acuity. The patient will complain of slightly blurred vision, often stating that the contact lens has shifted position or that the lens seems dirty. At the early stages acuity may be as good as 20/20 or 20/25, and this condition can be easily overlooked unless further testing is performed. Even with good acuity, a central visual field performed with small isopters often demonstrates a relative scotoma. The Amsler grid will often show metamorphopsia. This condition can occur from a few weeks to several years following surgery. In any event, if one suspects visual changes that cannot be improved by refraction, the patient should be referred back to the surgeon.

RETINAL DETACHMENT. Retinal detachment occurs in approximately 2 percent of uncomplicated cataract surgical cases.[39,77] Where there has been a vitreous prolapse, vitreous loss, or other surgical complication, the incidence increases considerably. Often the patient will be asymptomatic as long as the macula remains attached, so the practitioner must be

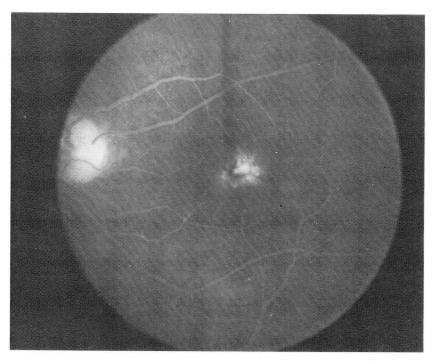

Figure 27.18. Retinal fluorescein angiogram showing fluorescence in macular area due to cystoid macular edema.

alert to other symptoms. These may include very slightly blurred vision, floaters, flashing lights, or a curtainlike cloud obliterating part of the visual field. A suspected visual change should be thoroughly investigated with visual fields and ophthalmoscopy. Since this condition warrants immediate attention, any suspicion of detachment should be referred back to the surgeon.

IRITIS. The small degree of iritis occurring after surgical trauma usually clears within several weeks after cataract surgery. However, persistent iritis is noted in cases with vitreous loss, residual lens material, foreign debris in the anterior chamber, iris prolapse, and glaucoma. Also, in cases of heterochromia with recurrent iritis that resulted in complicated cataract extraction, it is not uncommon for the iritis to continue intermittently after cataract extraction. The eye should be checked frequently for recurrence of the iritis and for increased intraocular pressure, which can result in glaucoma. Changes in intraocular pressure or in the quiescence of the eye should be referred for consultation.

GLAUCOMA. Glaucoma may result from a prolonged flat anterior chamber with resultant posterior and anterior synechia. Vitreous in the angle of the anterior chamber may also raise the intraocular pressure. Pupillary block may lead to an acute angle closure glaucoma. Persistent iritis may contribute to glaucoma in aphakia.

CORNEAL EDEMA. Persistent corneal edema can follow cataract surgery. It can result from vitreous touching the corneal endothelium, epithelial-endothelial dystrophy, excessive surgical trauma to the cornea, or glaucoma. This edema may be very difficult to control and may lead to numerous problems in the fitting of contact lenses. These eyes must be carefully watched because of the possibility of ulceration. Several cases of corneal vascularization have been noted, which might be related to gross corneal edema.[78,79]

VITREOUS PROLAPSE. Even after a successful intracapsular cataract extraction, the vitreous can prolapse and result in serious complications.[40] Vitreous prolapse can result in corneal edema, glaucoma, updrawn pupil, macular edema, and retinal detachment. The vitreous should be examined regularly, and any changes should be referred for consultation.

The postfitting care of the aphakic patient must continue at regular intervals. These patients always represent potential sources of pathology. Lens changes are usually infrequent, but if corneal changes are noted, new lenses should be prescribed.

ADDITIONAL TOPICS

PEDIATRIC CONTACT LENS FITTING

The child who has cataract surgery requires special considerations in contact lens fitting.[80,81] (*See* Chapter 31.)

SCLERAL CONTACT LENSES

For many years, scleral lenses were used in the correction of unilateral aphakia.[82,83] With the success of corneal lenses, and in particular soft lenses, scleral lenses lost their popularity among practitioners. The scleral lens frequently caused marked corneal edema and epithelial staining, and all-day wearing time was usually not achievable. Some cases, however, which also have conditions such as proptosis, ptosis, corneal grafts, anesthetic cornea, complete iridectomy, and updrawn pupil, may do better with a carefully fitted haptic lens.[84] In many cases, when a scleral type of fit is indicated, it is now possible to fit a large lenticular or hydrophilic lens.

INTRAOCULAR LENS

Ideally, the intraocular lens represents the best correction following surgery.[85,86] Over the past few years, thousands of I.O.L.s have been used in the correction of aphakia. Numerous complications have resulted; however, with improved lenses, manufacturing control, and better surgical techniques, some patients do very well. Which aphakic eyes should be fitted with intraocular lenses is presently a matter of considerable controversy among ophthalmic surgeons. Some ophthalmologists use this procedure for nearly all patients, while others are more conservative and only use I.O.L.s on a limited basis. The more conservative surgeon tends to prefer contact lenses for either daily or extended wear and only implant lenses when the contact lenses cannot be fitted.

REFRACTIVE KERATOPLASTY

The cornea represents about two-thirds of the total refractive power of the eye. Theoretically, small changes in corneal curvature could significantly change the refractive power. For about twenty years, work has been done on surgically changing the curvature of the cornea using a technique called *keratomileusis*, which was developed by Jose Barraquer.[87] This technique consists of removing part of the patient's cornea, freezing it, putting it on a precision lathe, and reshaping the curvature. The cornea is then sutured back in place. A modification of keratomileusis is called *keratophakia*, in which a thin disc of donor cornea is lathed to form a lens and then sandwiched into the recipient's cornea. This procedure is supposed to correct high hyperopia, as found in aphakia.

Recently, experiments with intralamellar corneal implants have been used to correct high plus refractive errors.[88,89] There presently is considerable research activity in refractive keratoplasty; however, it is too early to be able to evaluate either the safety or efficacy of these procedures.

REFERENCES

1. Hirtenstein, A.: Contact lens in unilateral aphakia, *Br. J. Ophthalmol.*, 668–674, 1950.
2. Constantine, E. F., and McLena, J. M.: Contact lenses in aphakia, *Arch. Ophthalmol.*, 51(2):212–215, 1954.
3. Little, M. F.: Treatment of unilateral cataract with contact glasses, *Arch. Ophthalmol.*, 11(4):646–650, 1934.
4. Town, A. E.: Contact glasses for correction of refractive errors in monocular aphakia, *Arch. Ophthalmol.*, 21(6):1021–1026, 1939.
5. Rosenbloom, A. A.: The correction of unilateral aphakia with corneal contact lenses, *Am. J. Optom.*, 30(10):536–542, 1953.
6. Berens, C., Girard, L. J., and Foree, K.: Corneal contact lenses: a clinical investigation, *Trans. Am. Ophthalmol. Soc.*, 50: 50–75, 1952.
7. Welsh, M. D., and Welsh, J.: *The Second Report on Cataract Surgery*, Miami, Ed. Press, 1971, pp. 23–37, 48–57.
8. Cassady, J. R.: Correction of aphakia with corneal contact lenses, *Am. J. Ophthalmol.*, 68(2):319–323, 1969.
9. Boeder, P.: Spectacle correction of aphakia, *Arch. Ophthalmol.*, 68(6):870–874, 1962.
10. Burian, H. M.: Optics: fusion in unilateral aphakia, *Trans. Am. Acad. Ophthalmol. Otolaryngol.*, 66:285–289, 1962.
11. Ogle, K. N., Burian, H. M., and Bannon, R. E.: On the correction of unilateral aphakia with contact lenses, *Arch. Ophthalmol.*, 59(5):639–652, 1958.
12. Dyer, J. A., and Ogle, K. N.: Correction of unilateral aphakia with contact lenses, *Am. J. Ophthalmol.*, 50(1):11–17, 1960.
13. Enoch, M. J.: An attempt to restore binocular stereoscopic vision in selected unilateral aphakia patients, in Becker, B., and Burde, M. D. (Eds.): *Current Concepts in Ophthalmology*, St. Louis, Mosby, vol. 2, 1969, pp. 236–247.
14. The adjustment to aphakia (editorial), *Am. J. Ophthalmol.*, 35(1):118–125, 1952.
15. Welsh, R. C.: *Post-operative Cataract Spectacle Lenses*, Miami, Ed. Press, 1961, pp. 1–34.
16. Massin, M., and Piot, J.: Recording of the visual field in aphakic eyes and in high myopia by the corneal lens, *Bull. Soc. Ophthalmol. Fr.*, 63:161–173, 1963.
17. Beasley, H.: The visual fields in aphakia, *Trans. Am. Ophthalmol. Soc.*, 63:363–416, 1965.
18. Benton, C. D., Jr., and Welsh, R. C.: *Spectacles for Aphakia*, Springfield, Thomas, 1971, pp. 5–35.
19. Isen, A. A.: Fitting contact lenses in aphakic patients, in *Encyclopedia of Contact Lens Practice*, South Bend, Indiana, International Optics, 1959–1963, Chap. 16, pp.

3–12.

20. Sloane, A. L. E.: *So You Have Cataracts: What You and Your Family Should Know.* Springfield, Thomas, 1970.

21. Roper-Hall, M. J.: Intraocular lenses, in Duane, T. (Ed.): *Clinical Ophthalmology,* Hagerstown, Harper & Row, 1979, p. 2.

22. Lerman, S.: *Cataracts: Chemistry Mechanisms and Therapy.* Springfield, Thomas, 1964, pp. 177–183.

23. Emery, J. M., and Paton, D.: Phacoemulsification: a survey of 2,875 cases, *Trans. Am. Acad. Ophthalmol. Otolaryngol.,* 78(1):31–34, 1974.

24. Polse, K. A.: Refitting aphakics with the Soflens, *Int. Cont. Lens Clin.,* 1(3):89–95, 1974.

25. *Petit Mascular Function — Directions of Use,* Parsons Optical Lab., San Francisco, Calif.

26. Levitan, P.: Pupillary escape in disease of the retina or optic nerve, *Arch. Ophthalmol.,* 62:768–779, 1959.

27. Levitan, P., Prasloski, P. F., and Collen, M. F.: The swinging flashlight test in multiphasic screening for eye disease, *Can. J. Ophthalmol.,* 8:356, 1973.

28. Levitan, P.: Unilateral papilledema and the swinging flashlight test, *Trans. Pacific Coast Oto-Ophthalmol. Soc.,* 1969, pp. 161–177.

29. Green, D. G., and Cohen, M. M.: Laser interferometry in the evaluation of potential macular function in the presence of opacities in the ocular media, *Trans. Am. Acad. Ophthalmol. Otolaryngol.,* 75(3):629–637, 1971.

30. Goldberg, J. B.: *Biomicroscopy for Contact Lens Practice,* Chicago, Professional Press, 1970.

31. Katz, J., and Kaufman, H. E.: Corneal exposure during sleep (nocturnal lagophthalmos), *Arch. Ophthalmol.,* 95(3):449–453, 1977.

32. Wilson, L. A.: Bacterial conjunctivities, in Duane, T. (Ed.): *Clinical Ophthalmology,* Hagerstown, Harper & Row, 1977, p. 12.

33. Kelman, C. D.: Phaco-emulsification and aspiration: the Kelman technique of cataract removal, in Duane, T. (Ed.): *Clinical Ophthalmology,* 5:8A, 2–4, Hagerstown, Harper & Row, 1979.

34. Kelman, C. D.: Phacoemulsification — indications, contraindications, and results, in

35. Floyd, G.: Changes in corneal curvature following cataract extraction, *Am. J. Ophthalmol.,* 34(11):1525–1533, 1951.

36. Englerth, F. L.: Immediate post-operative fitting in aphakia, *Contacto,* 11(4):13–15, 1967.

37. Koetting, R. A.: Advantages of contact lenses fitted early in aphakia, *J. Am. Optom. Assoc.,* 37(3):239–242, 1966.

38. Polse, K. A.: Changes in corneal hydration after discontinued contact lens wear, *Am. J. Optom.,* 49(6):511–516, 1972.

39. Corneal lenses in aphakia and molded scleral lenses in aphakia, complications after cataract surgery, *Int. Ophthalmol. Clin.,* 5:304–329, 1965.

40. Irvine, S. R.: A newly defined vitreous syndrome following cataract surgery, *Am. J. Ophthalmol.,* 36:599–619, 1953.

41. Vail, D.: After-results of vitreous lens, *Am. J. Ophthalmol.,* 59:573–586, 1965.

42. Herick, W. V., Schaffer, R. P., and Schwartz, A.: Estimation of the width of angle of anterior chamber, *Am. J. Ophthalmol.,* 69:626–633, 1969.

43. Bourne, W. M. et al.: Corneal endothelial cell damage from extracapsular versus intracapsular cataract extraction and lens implantation, ARVO Abstracts, 263–264, May 4–9, 1980.

44. Hoffer, K. J., and Phillippi, G.: A cell membrane theory of endothelial repair and vertical cell loss after cataract surgery, *J. Am. Intraoc. Implant Soc.,* 4(1):18–25, 1978.

45. Brandreth, R. H.: *Clinical Slit Lamp Biomicroscopy,* San Leandro, Ca., 1978, pp. 47–48.

46. Dohlman, C. H.: The function of the corneal epithelium in health and disease, *Invest. Ophthalmol.,* 10(6):383–407, 1971.

47. Shirmer, K. E., and Mellor, L. D.: Corneal sensitivity after cataract extraction, *Arch. Ophthalmol.,* 65:433–436, 1961.

48. Holly, F. J., and Lemp, M. A.: Tear physiology and dry eyes, *Survey Ophthalmol.,* 22(2):69–87, 1977.

49. Lemp, M. A.: Diagnosis and treatment of tear deficiencies, in Duane, T. (Ed.): *Clinical Ophthalmology,* Hagerstown, Harper & Row, 1979, pp. 5–6.

Symposium on Cataracts, *Trans. New Orleans Acad. Ophthalmol.,* St. Louis, C. V. Mosby, 1979.

50. Amsler, M.: Earliest symptoms of diseases of the macula, *Br. J. Ophthalmol.*, *37*:521–537, 1953.

51. Welsh, R. C.: Corneal contact lens trial sets for postoperative cataract patients, *Arch. Ophthalmol.*, *65(3)*:427–432, 1961.

52. Welsh, M. D., and Welsh, J.: *The Second Report on Cataract Surgery*, Miami, Ed. Press, 1971, pp. 23–37, 48–57.

53. Fraser, J. P., and Gordon, S. P.: The "apex" lens for binocular aphakia, *The Ophthalmic Optician*, *7(23)*:1190–1194, 1967.

54. Polse, K. A.: Contact lens fitting in aphakia, *Am. J. Optom.*, *46(3)*:213–219, 1969.

55. Mandell, R. B.: A method to determine the dimensions of a minus carrier contact lens, *J. Am. Optom. Assoc.*, *39(7)*:641–642, 1968.

56. Nelson, G., and Mandell, R. B.: The relationship between minus carrier design and performance, *Int. Cont. Lens Clin.*, *2(2)*: 75–81, 1975.

57. Girard, L. J.: Special designs and fitting techniques, in *Corneal Contact Lenses*, St. Louis, Mosby, 1970, pp. 305–311.

58. Hill, R. M., and Fatt, I.: Oxygen deprivation of the cornea by contact lens and lid closure, *Am. J. Optom. Arch. Am. Acad. Optom.*, *41(11)*:678–687, 1964.

59. Polse, K. A., and Decker, M.: Oxygen tension under a contact lens. *Invest. Ophthalmol. Vis. Sci.*, *18(2)*:188–193, 1979.

60. Polse, K. A.: Tear flow under hydrogel contact lenses, *Invest. Ophthalmol.*, *18(4)*:409–413, 1979.

61. Polse, K. A., and Mandell, R. B.: Critical oxygen tension at the corneal surface, *Arch. Ophthalmol.*, *84*:505–508, 1970.

62. Mandell, R. B., and Farrell, R.: Corneal swelling at low atmospheric oxygen pressure, *Invest. Ophthalmol.*, in press.

63. Polse, K. A., Sarver, M. D., and Harris, M. G.: Corneal effects of high plus hydrogel lenses, *Am. J. Optom. Physiol. Opt.*, *55(4)*: 234–237, 1978.

64. Holden, B. A., Mertz, G., and Guillon, M.: Corneal swelling response of the aphakic eye, *Invest. Ophthalmol.*, in press.

65. Korb, D. R., Richmond, P. P., and Herman, J. P.: Physiological response of the cornea to hydrogel lenses before and after cataract extraction, *J. Am. Optom. Assoc.*, *51(3)*:267–270, 1980.

66. Mertz, G. W., and Holden, B. A.: The overnight wear of very thin low water content hydrogel lenses, in press.

67. Fatt, I., and St. Helen, R.: Oxygen tension under an oxygen-permeable contact lens, *Am. J. Optom. Physiol. Opt.*, *48(7)*:545–555, 1971.

68. Gettes, B. C., and Ravdin, E. M.: Monocular aphakia and exotropia by contact lenses, *Am. J. Ophthalmol.*, *32(6)*:850–851, 1949.

69. Dixon, W. S. et al.: Unilateral aphakia and corneal contact lenses, *Can. J. Ophthalmol.*, *8*:97–105, 1973.

70. Breacher, L. L.: Insertion technique for aphakics, *Opt. J. Rev. Optom.*, *96(10)*:38–39, 1959.

71. Nesburn, A. B.: Prolonged-wear contact lenses in aphakia, *Trans. Am. Acad. Ophthalmol. Otolarygol.*, *85(1)*:1978.

72. Enoch, M. J.: A spectacle-contact lens combination used as a reverse Gallilean telescope in unilateral aphakia, *Am. J. Optom.*, *45*:231–240, 1968.

73. Chandler, P. A.: Symposium, Cataract extraction: complications after cataract extraction: clinical aspects, *Trans. Am. Acad. Ophthalmol. Otolaryngol.*, *58(3)*:382–396, 1954.

74. Goldsmith, A. J. B.: Late complications of aphakia, *Trans. Ophthalmol. Soc. U.K.*, *81*: 67–112, 1961.

75. Gass, J. D. M., and Morton, E. W. D.: Cystoid macular edema and papilledema following cataract extraction, *Arch. Ophthalmol.*, *76(5)*:646–661, 1966.

76. Zweng, H. C., Little, H. L., and Peabody, R. R.: Cystoid macular edema, in *Laser Photocoagulation and Retinal Angiography*, St. Louis, Mosby, 1969, pp. 102–112.

77. Shapland, D. C.: Retinal detachment in aphakia, *Trans. Ophthalmol. Soc. U.K.*, *54*: 176–196, 1934.

78. Mandelbaum, J.: Corneal vascularization in aphakic eyes following the use of contact lenses: a report of two cases, *Arch. Ophthalmol.*, *71(5)*:633–635, 1964.

79. Dixon, J. M., and Lawachek, E.: Corneal vascularization due to contact lenses, *Arch. Ophthalmol.*, *69(1)*:72–75, 1963.

80. Francois, J.: *Congenital Cataract Changes*, Springfield, Thomas, 1963, pp. 605–615.

81. Cowan, A.: Monocular aphakia, *Arch. Ophthal-mol.*, *49(4)*:473–474, 1953.

82. Ridley, F.: Contact lenses in unilateral aphakia, *Trans. Ophthalmol. Soc. U.K.*, *73*:373–386, 1953.

83. Ridley, F.: Scleral contact lenses: their clinical significance, *Arch. Ophthalmol.*, *70(5)*: 740–745, 1963.

84. Gould, H. L.: Molded scleral lenses in aphakia, *Int. Ophthalmol. Clin.*, *5(1)*:315–328, 1965.

85. Girard, L. J. et al.: Intraocular implants and contact lenses. A comparison of the visual functions of monocularly aphakic patients treated by pupillary intraocular lens implants and corneal contact lenses, *Arch. Ophthalmol.*, *68(6)*:762–775, 1962.

86. Guerry, D., III: Present status of the anterior chamber lens, *Am. J. Ophthalmol.*, *50(2)*: 250–258, 1960.

87. Barraquer, J. I.: Keratomileusis and keratophakia: indications, complications, and results, in Turtz, A. I. (Ed.): *Proceedings of the Centennial Symposium, Manhattan Eye, Ear and Throat Hospital*, vol. 1, *Ophthalmology*, St. Louis, C. V. Mosby Co., 1969.

88. McCarey, B. E., and Andrews, D.: Refractive keratoplasty with intralamellar hydrogel implants, ARVO Abstracts, p. 261, 1980.

89. Weston, J.H. et al.: Hydrogel intracorneal implants in rabbits, ARVO Abstracts, pp. 261–262, 1980.

Chapter 28

LOW VISION

Although the uses of contact lenses as aids for the low vision patient are limited, they are greater than is generally appreciated. Estimates of the number of low vision patients who could benefit from wearing contact lenses range from 0.6 percent[1] to 10 percent.[2] Bier feels that even the latter figure, which applies to children of school age, is too low.[3] Statistics on this topic are often misleading, as they compare groups that differ in age, visual acuity, and visual anomalies. Recent figures often exclude keratoconus, aphakia, and high myopia cases, which were formerly classed with the low vision group but which are now generally considered routine clinical cases when fitted with contact lenses.

In their application as corrective devices for low vision, contact lenses may be used independently or may be worn with spectacle lenses to form a telescopic optical system. Many low vision patients benefit from routine fitting of contact lenses. Often vision is restored to nearly normal, especially when the visual defect is due to an irregularity of the corneal curvature.[4]

When patients only partly benefit from wearing contact lenses or when telescopic systems are contemplated, it is important to give considerable attention to the special procedures of low vision examination and fitting.* Often, the psychological relationship between the practitioner and patient will be the most important factor in determining whether or not the aid will be accepted.[6]

The time and effort that must be expended in caring for a low vision person is usually two to three times that allotted the average patient. Patients who must wear telescopics or similar aids will require longer fitting periods. An estimate of the probability of success in fitting is made principally from the patient's case history (including age, motivation, cooperative attitude) and whether his vision can be corrected to a level that will fulfill his needs. To be successful, the patient must be well motivated, understand the limitations of his proposed visual aid, and have a definite purpose for which the aid is to be used.[7,8] Patients who just want to see better should be made to understand that any device that will be given to them is only applicable for certain tasks. Some people, because of long held beliefs that nothing further can be done for their vision, will need to be encouraged and reassured that improvement is possible, but extreme caution must be taken not to mislead the patient into expecting too much from his new correction.

If the patient's visual loss is recent, this may be a contraindication for fitting. These people are seldom satisfied with anything less than normal vision and do not adjust psychologically to the limited advantages of a low vision aid. Patients who have had their visual loss for at least a few years tend to be more successful. They have usually adjusted to their status emotionally, have become convinced that nothing can be done for their vision, and are satisfied with any improvement. Each case must be considered on its

---

*For this information the reader is referred to general discussions on low vision.[3,5]

689

own merits, however, and handled accordingly.

Care should be taken that the patient's motivation is genuine. Some individuals become so adapted to their "blind" status that they have no real wish to have their vision restored, especially if this would mean the loss of financial support or withdrawn attention of a relative or friend.[9]

In addition to his visual condition, the patient's mental and physical capabilities must be evaluated. Many older people do not have sufficient manual dexterity to handle small corneal lenses, and a scleral lens should then be considered. In a few cases, a relative can assist with the task of insertion and removal, but this arrangement often fails over a long term.

METHODS TO AID LOW VISION

As a correction for low vision, contact lenses have four important uses: (1) to eliminate or modify the effects of corneal irregularities as in keratoconus, irregular astigmatism, or corneal scarring; (2) to provide better visual function, including field of view, than that obtained with the ophthalmic lens counterpart, as in aphakia, high myopia, and high astigmatism; (3) to produce magnification as the ocular component of a telescopic lens system; and, finally, (4) to serve as a limiting aperture that will increase visual function and efficiency in patients with certain forms of ocular pathology.

TELESCOPIC SYSTEMS

Spectacle Telescopic Systems

Telescopic systems aid the partially sighted patient by producing a general magnification of the retinal image.* Usually, the principle used is that of the Galilean telescope, which has also found application in opera glasses and other familiar optical devices. The Galilean optical telescope has the advantages of producing an erect image, of being made in compact form, and of requiring a minimum number of components. Construction of the system is simple, as it requires only two lenses, one positive, the other negative and of higher power, positioned in such a way that their respective secondary and primary focal points coincide (Figure 28.1). For example, a Galilean telescope could consist of a +10.00 D. lens (focal length 10 cm.) and a −40.00 D. lens (focal length 2.5 cm.), separated by 7.5 cm. (This would be impractical for a spectacle device.) This separation can be found by subtracting the focal length of the negative power lens (eyepiece) from the focal length of the positive power lens (objective), which for the previous example would be 10 cm. − 2.5 cm. = 7.5 cm.

The magnification produced by a Galilean system is simply the ratio of the powers of the eyepiece (F_e) and objective (F_o).

$$\text{Mag} = \frac{\text{Power of eyepiece lens } (F_e)}{\text{Power of eyepiece lens } (F_o)}$$

Hence, a +10.00 D. objective and 30.00× D. eyepiece combination would give a magnification of 3×. A −40.00 D. eyepiece combined with the same +10.00 D. objective lens would increase the magnification to ±4, but the separation of the lenses would need to be changed from 6.67 cm. (10 cm. − 3.33 cm.) to 7.5 cm. (10 cm. − 2.5 cm.). This illustrates

---

*Magnification for a telescopic system is computed on an angular basis but is equally valid in terms of an apparent linear increase in object size. For example, a two times magnification (2×) literally means doubling the apparent size of an object.

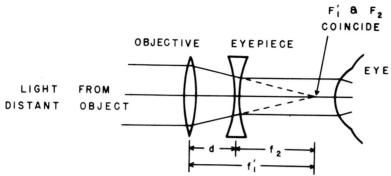

Figure 28.1. Construction of a Galilean telescope. The components are a plus lens objective and minus lens eyepiece positioned so their respective secondary and primary focal points coincide.

how one or the other of the components of the system may be varied to change the magnification and the separation of the lenses. To produce systems that are compact enough to be incorporated into spectacle devices, it is necessary to use lens powers of the order of 30.00 D. for the positive lens and 50.00 D. for the negative lens, which need be separated by only 1.33 cm. and give a ±1.67 magnification. This approaches the practical limit of a spectacle telescopic magnification, with an adequate field of view for general wear and with acceptable aberrations, although spectacle telescopics with magnifications up to 3.5× are available and often used for part-time wear.

Limited field of view presents one of the most serious handicaps of spectacle telescopics. In a 2.2× telescopic it is limited to about 20°, which is equivalent to seeing an area 3.48 feet in diameter at twenty feet. Obviously, walking, climbing stairs, and other mobile activities are made extremely difficult by the field limitations, and activities such as driving a vehicle become virtually impossible. In addition to the optical limitations, the poor cosmetic appearance of spectacle telescopics greatly reduce their more general acceptance.

Contact-Spectacle Telescopic

If a contact lens is used as a part of a Galilean telescopic, it is possible to reduce the objectionable cosmetic and optical features. Successful use of a spectacle-contact telescopic was reported by Bettman and McNair,[10] Ludlam,[11] and others.[12-16] The success ratio is probably very low, and the method should be used with reservation.

In the contact-spectacle lens Galilean telescopic, a high minus contact lens, which forms the eyepiece, is combined with a positive power spectacle lens, which forms the objective. A telescope of this type, which is composed of a −30.00 D. contact lens and a +20.00 D. spectacle lens separated 17 mm., will have a magnification of 1.50× and a theoretical field of about 43°17 if the spectacle lens has a 25 mm. diameter (in lenticular form), and it will have a 68° theoretical field if the spectacle lens has a 44 mm. diameter. In the latter case, the aberrations of the positive lens will reduce the usable field limits to about 50°. Table 28.1 (after Ludlam[11]) gives theoretical and practical characteristics of Galilean telescopes made from various combinations of lenses.

Aside from its larger field of view, the contact-spectacle lens telescopic offers a considerable cosmetic advantage over the spectacle telescopic. A lenticular spectacle lens can be used in combination with the contact lens to further reduce weight and improve the appearance of the system. A lenticular

TABLE 28.1
CONTACT-SPECTACLE TELESCOPE CONSTRUCTIONS

Dioptric Power of Contact Lens	Dioptric Power of Spectacles	Vertex Distance in mm.	Mag.	Monocular* Field of View in Degrees
−40	26.3	13	1.52	79
	23.8	17	1.69	61
	22.2	20	1.80	51
	21.1	23	1.91	43
−30	21.8	13	1.35	87
	20.0	17	1.50	68
	18.8	20	1.60	58
	17.7	23	1.68	50
−20	15.9	13	1.26	92
	14.9	17	1.33	76
	14.3	20	1.40	65
	13.7	23	1.46	58

* Assuming 44 mm. eye size.

lens actually gives little reduction in the usable field of view, since the area that is lost is highly aberrated. If a full diameter spectacle lens is used, it has been recommended that it be made from plastic to minimize the weight.

Limitations of the Contact-Spectacle Telescopic

It is regrettable that sometimes there has been a tendency to minimize the disadvantages of a contact lens telescopic system. Any movement of the contact lens on the cornea in a telescopic system will bring about an apparent movement of the visual field. This is caused by the high power of the contact lens, which produces large variations in prismatic effect when the lens is not centered on the line of sight. This movement is most noticeable during blinking, and its constant repetition can be very annoying to the patient. Normally a gel lens will move much less on the cornea, and for this reason, it is often the contact lens of choice when very high powers are needed to produce high magnification telescopics. As an alternative, a scleral lens presents the same advantages.

A certain proportion of patients are unable to tolerate the contact lens and are thereby eliminated as potential wearers. If the cornea is irregular or has been damaged severely, it may not be possible to fit the patient with a corneal type of contact lens, although he may be fitted successfully with a gel or haptic lens.

An additional problem that occurs when wearing any telescopic system, and for which the contact lens gives no relief, is that each time the patient turns his head there is a rapid movement of the visual field in the opposite direction. In addition, magnified objects appear to be much closer than they actually are, and the patient finds himself groping in space for door handles and other objects. An apparent increase (magnification) occurs in the speed of moving objects, which is psychologically disturbing.

A contact lens telescopic also presents various mechanical adjustment problems. It is sometimes difficult for a patient to keep his spectacle in the proper position on his face for the lenses of the telescopic system to have their correct separation. Any lateral movement of the spectacle lens will cause an apparent movement of the visual field. This movement is usually more pronounced when the spectacle lens is fitted far away from the face. A maximum vertex distance does allow the use of a weaker spectacle lens power, but this advantage may be offset by the unsteadiness of the spectacle lens. For this reason, various spectacles that have been designed to hold the spectacle lens at a large distance from the eye are often impractical.

A former difficulty in making a contact lens telescopic was to obtain a contact lens with sufficient power and with good optical characteristics. With modern manufacturing methods this is no longer a serious problem, and only first quality lenses should be accepted from the laboratory. High minus lenses must be of lenticular form. The size of the optical section will vary with the lens power. Table 28.2 gives the recommended front optical zone diameters for lenses of various powers.

TABLE 28.2

RECOMMENDED FRONT OPTICAL ZONE DIAMETERS FOR
HIGH MINUS LENTICULAR CONTACT LENSES. TOTAL
DIAMETER 9.5 MM.

Power	Front Optical Zone Diameter
–10 D.	8.0
–20 D.	7.4
–30 D.	7.0
–40 D.	6.6
(Pl front)	3.8

Patient Selection

It is difficult to state a definite range for the visual acuity of patients who respond best to correction with contact-spectacle lens telescopics. There must be sufficient vision after magnification for the patient to see well enough to perform a desired task. As a simple rule, the acuity that is expected after correction with the telescopic can be predicted by multiplying the magnification of the telescopic device by the Snellen acuity rating. For example, a patient with a 20/200 acuity who is to be given a 2× telescopic will be expected to achieve an acuity of 20/100. In practice the acuity will often improve a little more than was predicted, so the subject of this example might be expected to achieve 20/80.

There are occasional reports of patients who are given a contact-spectacle telescopic and who achieve unanticipated acuity improvements, e.g. from 20/200 to as high as 20/25. In such cases there is probably some corneal anomaly that is corrected principally by the contact lens, and the reader should not be misled into believing that the improvement was due totally to the telescopic system.

Patients with visual acuity below 20/400 will usually not derive enough benefit from a contact-spectacle telescopic system to warrant its use and will probably do better with other types of visual aids. Usually in such cases magnification of at least 4× is needed,

and this can only be achieved with hand held telescopes. If a pair of binoculars is disjoined, the monoculars can very often be of use to these patients. They can be carried in the pocket or purse and kept available for identifying bus numbers and other important features.

If the patient's acuity is between 20/50 and 20/100, it is often adequate for him, so he will not bother with the difficulties and inconveniences that accompany the wearing of a vision aid. A contact lens device is particularly poor for this patient because he will, on many occasions, prefer to have unmagnified vision, and his aid cannot be easily removed. People in this acuity group usually want to wear their low vision aid for special occasions. For example, college students need magnification for seeing the blackboard and can often get along with their low vision in other activities. The most useful type of correction for them may be a hand-held telescopic, which can be held to the eye only at those times needed, or a small segment telescopic mounted in the upper portion of a spectacle lens.

In any case, the primary criteria for the selection of the aid will be the task the patient wishes to accomplish and the magnification needed to perform this task. The absolute visual acuity of the patient plays a lesser role.

Monocular Correction

It is often best to correct only one eye with the telescopic system, even when both eyes have approximately the same acuity. Usually, the central vision of the uncorrected eye will be suppressed when the telescopic is used. Some patients can learn to alternate their vision between one eye and the other to see either with or without the telescopic.

Binocular Correction

Binocular correction with a contact-spectacle telescopic is possible in some cases where the visual acuity is nearly the same in both eyes and where only low magnification is required. Ludlam reported three patients who were able to wear low power binocular contact-spectacle telescopics for all daily activities.[11]

Correction for Near

Because of the effectivity of the very high powers of the lenses that make up a telescopic system, objects held at a near distance cannot be focused by the eye. Light from a near object that passes through the telescopic is made very divergent when it leaves the system (and strikes the eye), and since the patient cannot accommodate to overcome this vergence, the object will appear blurred. If an object is viewed at 20 cm. in front of the objective of a telescopic composed of a spectacle lens of +25.00 D. and a contact lens of −50.00 D. separated by 1.33 mm., the stimulus to accommodation is −12.40 D.*

If a plus lens is added to the front of the telescopic system, the system will be in focus for a position coinciding with the focal point of the plus lens. This becomes evident when it is realized that light from an object at the focal point of the plus lens will be made parallel by the lens (collimated) and will be refracted by the Galilean system in the same way as light received from distant objects (Figure 28.2). A distance telescopic may be converted into a near telescopic by simply adding a plus lens clip-on to the objective,

---

*The calculation of this problem can be most easily performed by finding the vergence of the light as it passes through each part of the telescopic system. Light from a point 20 cm. in front of the objective lens will have a vergence of −5.00 D. upon striking the plus lens. This vergence will be added to (+30.00 D.) the power of objective lens, so light leaving this lens will have a power of +25.00 D. The effective vergence of the light striking the eyepiece will be +37.6 D. (*see* Chapter 32) and, combined with the −50.00 D. of power of the eyepiece, will leave that lens with a vergence of −12.40 D. It is obvious that few people will be able to accommodate for this stimulus.

with the focal length corresponding to the distance at which the near task is to be placed. As the focal length is shortened, there is greater total magnification by the system. The approximate total magnification may be found by this simple formula. Magnification is one-fourth the dioptric power of the add times the magnification of the telescope.

$$\text{Mag} = \frac{F}{4} \times (M_t)$$

A +8.00 D. lens placed in front of a 2× contact-spectacle telescope will give a total reading magnification of four times, and the reading material must be held at about 5 inches from the spectacle lens.

Although a clip-on can be used for the reading aid, it is usually better to make up the objective lens for the reading system in another pair of spectacles. Sometimes it is preferable to order the spectacle lens in the form of a button, which can be cemented to a plano carrier in any position. Theoretically, a system could be devised in which the spectacle lens could have a superior button for distance and a separate button of higher power for near.

Because moving a plus lens away from the eye increases its effective power at the spectacle plane, it may be possible to focus a contact-spectacle telescopic for a near object by simply pushing the spectacles down the nose a little. This is only feasible for short reading periods.

Clinical Fitting Procedure

The general procedures used in low vision refraction will also apply to those cases in which a contact lens telescopic is contemplated. The patient should first be tested with a spectacle telescopic to insure that the improvement in acuity will be adequate for his needs.

OUTLINE OF CLINICAL FITTING PROCEDURE.

1. Determine magnification necessary for patient's needs using spectacle telescopic.

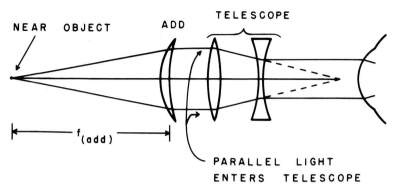

NEAR OBJECT   ADD   TELESCOPE

$f_{(add)}$

PARALLEL LIGHT
ENTERS TELESCOPE

Figure 28.2. The addition of a plus lens to a telescopic puts the system in focus for a near object.

2. Fit patient with conventional contact lenses.

3. From Table 28.1 determine approximate powers of spectacles and contact lenses and order final contact lenses from laboratory.

4. While the patient wears the final contact lens, determine, by trial and error, the plus spectacle lens that gives the best visual acuity, starting with the power of the lens in Table 28.1 and bracketing.

5. Correct for vertex differences between trial frame and spectacles, and order spectacle lens.

It is usually desirable to fit the patient with a conventional contact lens before attempting to fit the high minus lens for the telescopic.[18] There are three advantages to this procedure. It gives the wearer an opportunity to learn handling procedures for contact lenses and thereby reduces the difficulties he must surmount when adjusting to the telescopic system. All modifications of the contact lens can be completed so that it functions with maximum efficiency when incorporated into the telescopic system, recognizing the power change to be made. The examination for the telescopic system is simplified and is usually more accurate when the contact lens can be worn without any of the difficulties experienced by the new wearer.

If the patient is successful in wearing the trial contact lens, a high minus contact lens should be ordered. Its power is determined by estimating the magnification that the patient will need and selecting the power from the combination of lenses found in Table 28.1 which gives the desired magnification. After the contact lens is received, it should be worn by the patient during the remainder of the examination.

The objective lens is found by trial and error. Start with a lens having the recommended power found in Table 28.1, and place this in a trial frame. Then hold plus and minus 5.00 D. trial (spectacle) lenses in front of the tentative lens. If neither improves the acuity, try plus and minus 2.50 D. lenses, and proceed to bracket in smaller and smaller steps until the maximum acuity is obtained. Vertex distance should then be carefully measured. The frame that is to be used for the patient should be placed on his face, and the vertex distance again carefully measured. It is helpful if the trial frame can be adjusted on the patient's face until the vertex distance is the same as it will be in the spectacle frame so that no correction will be necessary for vertex depth differences. Otherwise, the power of the trial spectacle lens must be modified for any difference in vertex distance.

The trial and error fitting system described is rapid, requires no calculations for lens powers, and has the further advantage of being equally applicable to patients with ametropia; however, a slight modification in the system is helpful with ametropia for making a better estimate of the correct spectacle trial lens. The spherical correction for the ametropia is subtracted from the contact lens power; the remaining value represents the power of the eyepiece for the telescope. For example, a -10.00 D. myope who is to be given a -50.00 D. contact lens would have an effective eyepiece power of -40.00 D. A $+5.00$ D. hyperope would have an effective eyepiece power of -55.00 D. if the same contact lens were worn.

This relationship may be made clearer if the contact lens is considered as though it were two lenses, one having the power required to correct the ametropia and the other having the power necessary for the eyepiece of a Galilean telescope. The powers of the two lenses are then combined to form a single lens.

It should be noted, however, that the ametropic correction must be added to the eyepiece of the telescopic. If the power of the ametropia is added to the objective instead, its effective power value will not be correct, and the telescopic system will not be correct for the eye.

CYLINDRICAL CORRECTION. The contact lens' near elimination of the anterior surface of the cornea often corrects astigmatic ametropia for patients requiring contact-spectacle telescopics. Small, residual astigmatic errors (up to 1.00 D. and occasionally more) can usually be ignored, since their correction has no appreciable effect on the visual acuity. If it is found that a cylindrical correction is needed, it can be incorporated into the contact lens in one of the toric types of lenses (Chapter 9), or less satisfactorily, it can be placed in the spectacle correction. Due allowances must then be made for effective power differences.

SPECIAL OBJECTIVE HOLDERS. Some attempts have been made to attach special devices to the spectacles, which would support the objective lens in front of the frame and allow a greater separation between the two lenses of the contact-spectacle telescopic.[19] If the support is flimsy, however, it will allow the heavy plus lens to wobble and cause apparent motion.

Bivisual Telescopic Systems

It is possible to modify the contact-spectacle telescopic system so the contact lens can be worn alone for normal seeing when the telescopic system is not used.[20,21] This is accomplished by grinding a very small high-minus segment in the center of the contact lens, smaller in diameter than the patient's pupil.

Rays enter the eye through both the segment and the peripheral lens area, but they have different vergences. When the contact lens is worn alone, the peripheral rays focus at the retina and form a clear image. This is illustrated in Figure 28.3 by rays 1 and 2. Rays 3 and 4 pass through the high-minus button and are out of focus when they reach the retina, thus having little effect on the retinal image. If a plus power spectacle lens is now placed before the eye at the distance necessary to form a Galilean telescope with the contact lens button, rays passing through the telescopic (3 and 4, Figure 28.4) will be focused on the retina, and the highly convergent rays 1 and 2, which strike the peripheral area of the corneal lens, will be rendered out of focus. Hence, the wearer of this system can enjoy the advantages of contact-spectacle telescopics and of normal vision, the latter by simply removing his spectacles.

The disadvantages of the bivisual optical system is that neither the normal nor the telescopic optical systems will give optimum performance. If the contact lens is designed so the minus segment occupies one-half the area of the pupil, then 50 percent of the light that is available for vision will always be lost.* Furthermore, the veiling effect of the

---

*Under this condition a slightly greater loss will occur with unmagnified imagery, since rays entering the peripheral portion of the eye's optical system will be less effective in producing an image sensation due to the Stiles-Crawford effect.

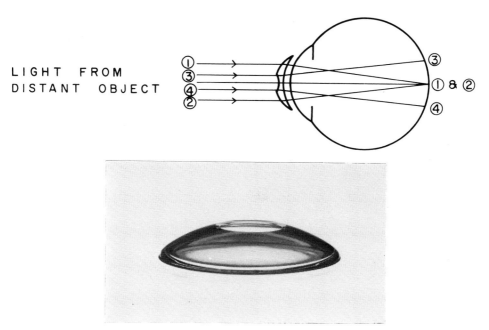

Figure 28.3. Contact lens designed for use in bivisual system.

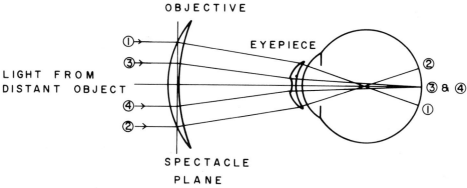

Figure 28.4. Bivisual contact-spectacle telescopic. System is in focus with or without objective. lens.

light that is out of focus will further reduce the effectiveness of the system, both as a telescopic and under normal viewing conditions.

A bivisual telescopic system by Filderman (called the Telecon® system) has proved very practical and makes it possible to have normal vision and telescopic vision with the same optical device.[21,22] The optical system is formed by a contact lens and a spectacle lens, each of which contains areas of two refractive powers.

The contact lens is first constructed so as to correct the patient's ametropia. It is then modified by cutting a small flat area in the center of the front curve. The recommended diameter of this area is 2.5 mm., but it can be enlarged if the lens rides eccentrically. The important factor is for this segment to be smaller than the entrance pupil of the eye so that only part of the ray bundle that ultimately enters the eye passes through this segment. The rest of the rays are refracted by the lens in a normal manner.

The second part of the system consists of a plano spectacle lens on which is cemented a high plus wafer 25 mm. in diameter in the central position (Figure 28.5). The wafer and the central portion of the contact lens have powers that produce a telescopic system. When the patient looks away from the wafer on the lens, he sees normally because the spectacle carrier has no power and the rays that have passed through the periphery of the contact lens form a focused image (Figure 28.6). Rays

that have passed through the plano part of the spectacle lens and through the central part of the contact lens are so greatly out of focus that they produce only a slight central blur on the image. This blur is distracting, however, and must be considered a definite disadvantage of this system.

In the original recommendation the spectacle wafer had a power of +25. D. and had to be worn 20 mm. from the contact lens. This is not usually practical, and it is best to fit this system by the same technique recommended for the contact lens telescopic and to determine the power of the spectacle lens by trial and error.

Usually Filderman's system is recommended

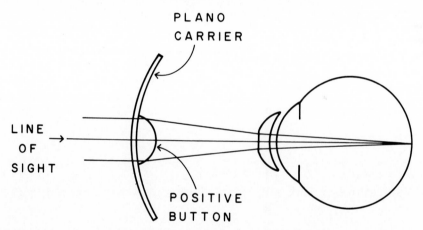

Figure 28.5. The Telecon system. Condition for viewing a distant, magnified object.

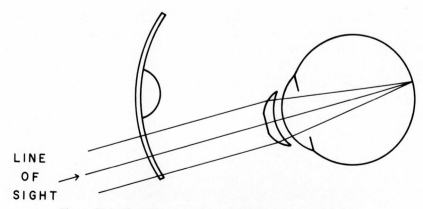

Figure 28.6. The Telecon system. Condition for normal vision.

to be fitted to only one eye so that the central blur would be filled in by the contralateral eye. Monocular correction is not always necessary, however, as this problem may be overcome by decreasing the size of the minus segment in the contact lens. A binocular correction by this system is definitely possible, although usually for only a young and adaptable patient.

It has been suggested that a lens system that would provide a telescopic system for both distance and near be constructed by putting a second wafer on the spectacle lens below the distance wafer, the near wafer having a power which would be greater by the amount of the near add.[23]

The approximate power of the contact lens with a flat front surface can be found very simply if the lens is considered (optically) as thin. In air, the lens will have all its power on the posterior surface; this can be calculated from the power formula for a single refracting surface.

$$F = \frac{n' - n}{r}$$

For a lens with base curve of 7.5 mm. and an index of 1.49, the power will be -65.3 D. A lens with base curve of 8.0 mm. will have a power of -61.3 D.

If the lens is to have a higher power, it follows that the front surface must be concave. Such a surface is undesirable because it is difficult to manufacture, and its optical quality is very poor when worn because the tears often do not make a smooth layer in the concavity.

Self-contained Contact Lens Telescopic

A contact lens telescopic was constructed by Feinbloom in which both lens elements of a Galilean system were placed in the same contact lens.[24] While it should have several advantages, this device actually is bulky (center thickness about 5 mm.) and is impractical for general use. A similar contact lens telescopic was made by Braff.[25]

Reverse Telescopic System

A reversed telescopic system, which minifies the retinal image, can be constructed simply by reversing a Galilean telescope. Since a larger area of the visual field is then condensed into a smaller image, this system has theoretical applications for those patients who have visual field constrictions, e.g. from retinitis pigmentosa. It is often unacceptable to the patient, however, because of the effective loss of acuity when viewing the minified image.

CONTACT LENS MICROSCOPIC

An attempt has been made to prescribe very high power plus lenses (or microscopics, as they are called) for low vision patients to aid reading or other near work. Part of this trend is due to an improvement in the optical qualities of high power lenses, but it also represents an increased acceptance by optometrists of this method of correction. A high plus power lens produces magnification of a near object because it allows the object to be held very near to the eye, namely, at the focal point of the lens.

A high plus power microscopic, up to +50.00 D., can be made in lenticular form in a contact lens and provides good optical characteristics. Such a lens cannot be easily removed, so it is only valuable for rare conditions where only near vision is necessary. If the acuity is nearly equal in the two eyes, one eye may be fitted with a high plus lens for near vision, and the other corrected for distance vision. This type of arrangement is best suited for a young adult.

Certain types of bifocal contact lenses can be ground with high adds and used as microscopics. However, fitting difficulties with this type of lens are great.

The magnification of a near object by a contact lens microscopic is found by the following formula:

$$\text{Mag} = \frac{\text{Power of lens in diopters}}{4}$$

This magnification expresses the relative size of an object as seen through the microscopic when compared with the same object held at a standard distance of 25 cm.

PINHOLE LENSES

Pinhole lenses are valuable corrective devices for low vision cases that are due to a variety of anomalies of the eye's optical system. Their uses have been discussed in Chapter 15. In many low vision patients, a larger than usual aperture may be considered, since the primary effect is not just to produce an optical pinhole but to restrict rays that may be dispersed by opacities of the media or an irregular pupil. Rosenbloom refers to these lenses as controlled-pupil contact lenses (Figure 28.7) and recommends their use for low vision patients with permanent mydriasis of the pupil, distorted pupil, scarred cornea resulting from ocular burns, diffuse corneal opacities, coloboma of the iris, aniridia, multiple disseminated opacities of the media, and certain kinds of cosmetic contact lens fittings.[26]

Several types of controlled-pupil contact lenses are manufactured. Probably the two most common designs involve a laminated lens with iris match and a solid color peripheral corneal lens with clear central zone.

The diagnostic procedure begins with the fitting of a single vision clear contact lens with the correct power. The lens is worn for about one month, during which time approx-

imate adjustments are made to achieve maximum comfortable wearing time. As an essential part of the determination of optimum pupil size, Rosenbloom uses a series of diagnostic control lenses of 11.0 mm. diameter with variable pupils ranging from 1.0 to 6.0 mm. in 1.0 mm. steps. The finished lenses are larger than conventional corneal lenses, by a difference of 0.5 to 2.0 mm. or more. After successful adaptation to the untinted lens has been demonstrated, the clear lens is returned to the laboratory with a detailed prescription of the precise design characteristics. The nature of the peripheral lens color and the size and position of the pupil are also reported. Although the finished controlled-pupil lens cannot be fully evaluated by fluorescein technique, the biomicroscope offers an adequate method of appraising the central lens-cornea relationship.

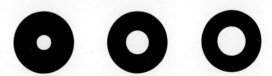

Figure 28.7. Controlled-pupil contact lenses.

SPECIAL PROCEDURES FOR PATIENT

Before the fitting of the contact lens has been completed, it is necessary to decide what procedure can best be used by the patient for lens insertion and removal. Every attempt should be made to teach the patient self-reliance when handling contact lenses. Many

patients who have extreme difficulty in the early wearing period (even to the point of spending hours inserting and removing the lenses) can, after a few weeks of practice, handle the lenses with a surprising degree of skill.

A low vision patient who must care for

his own lenses will be faced with a number of problems. If the lens is lost from the eye, he may be unable to find it. Patients who are also correctible by spectacles should probably be given a pair for just such emergencies. Patients not correctible with spectacles should carry spare contact lenses that may be worn to find any lost lenses. Tinting a lens may aid in locating it.

Elderly people, children, mentally retarded persons, and those with poor manual dexterity may find it necessary to depend upon a relative for all handling of the contact lens. If the assistant is suitable, this arrangement can be very satisfactory.

ASSISTANT

The ideal assistant is another person who wears contact lenses. Unfortunately this fortuitous arrangement seldom occurs.

If the assistant has no previous experience with contact lenses, he should be invited to accompany the patient throughout the various phases of fitting. He should be allowed to participate as soon as possible so that the practitioner can assess his proficiency and guide his training.

One difficulty that many laymen have is not being able to see the contact lens on another person's eye. For this reason it is best to tint the lenses so their location in the palpebral fissure is discernible.

INSERTION AND REMOVAL

Many patients can learn to insert and remove their lenses by feel. The clumsiness of the patient in his first attempts to do this

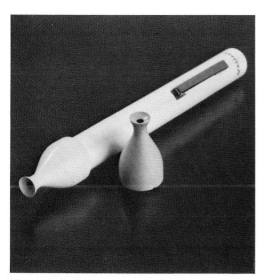

Figure 28.8. Suction cup mounted on a penlight for use in contact lens insertion and removal.

should not deter the practitioner from continuing to insist that the patient try. The patient must put on the lenses in a room where they can be easily retrieved if dropped.

A device that is often helpful for insertion and removal is a small penlight on which a suction cup is attached (Figure 28.8).

Light from the penlight passes through the hole in the suction cup. The contact lens is then attached to the cup and the patient fixates the bright light and moves the whole device toward the cornea until contact. The suction cup is then released. Some training is necessary before the patient learns when he has reached the eye, and caution is necessary in the early use of this device. Some patients prefer not to remove the lens from the eye but merely to push it off the cornea onto the sclera when sleeping. No deleterious effects appear to occur from this practice, but the lenses often become excessively coated with mucus and need to be cleaned often.

A magnifying mirror can also be of use

for certain patients when acuity is not too low.

It is occasionally recommended that spectacles be made which contain only one lens so that one eye can see, and the contact lens can be inserted in the other eye. These have the problem that the vision is often obscured, and the eyewire prevents free access to the eye. A section of the lower eyewire may be cut out to facilitate this.

REFERENCES

1. I. H. B., *Optical Aids Service Survey*, Brooklyn, The Industrial Home for the Blind, 1957, p. 23.
2. Chief Medical Officer of the Ministry of Education: *The Health of the School Child, Fifty Years of the School Medical Service*, London, Her Majesty's Stationery Office, 1958.
3. Bier, N.: *Correction of Subnormal Vision*, London, Butterworths, 1960, p. 83.
4. Neill, J. C.: Selection of the aid for the partially blind patient, *J. Am. Optom. Assoc.*, 29(11):719–723, 1958.
5. Rosenbloom, A. A.: The partially seeing child, in Hirsch, M. J., and Wick, R. E. (Eds.): *Vision of Children*, Philadelphia, Chilton, 1963, pp. 251–270.
6. Robbins, I., and Freudenberger, H. J.: Some clinical observations for optometrists working with low vision patients, *Am. J. Optom.*, 36(3):129–135, 1959.
7. Pascal, J. I.: Telescopic spectacles in ophthalmological practice, *Eye, Ear, Nose Throat Mon.*, 28:171–173, 1949.
8. Ellerbrock, V. J.: Selection of the partially blind patient, *J. Am. Optom. Assoc.*, 29(11):713–714, 1958.
9. Rosenbloom, A. A.: Principles and techniques for examining the partially blind patient, *J. Am. Optom. Assoc.*, 29(11):715–718, 1958.
10. Bettman, J. W., and McNair, G. S.: A contact-lens-telescopic system, *Am. J. Ophthalmol.*, 22(1):27–32, 1939.
11. Ludlam, W. M.: Clinical experience with the contact lens telescope, *Am. J. Optom.*, 37(7):363–372, 1960.
12. Sauter, H.: Modification of telescopic spectacles by the use of contact lenses, *Arch. Ophthalmol.*, 149:142–155, 1949.
13. Baglien, J. W., and Middleton, R. V.: A telescopic device with corneal contact lenses, *Optom. Weekly*, 43(2):39–41, 1952.
14. Abrams, B. S.: Contact lenses in sub-normal vision cases, *Optom. Weekly*, 45(20):827–830; 45(35):1383–1388, 1954.
15. Seitzman, I. D.: A special aid for subnormal vision, *Optom. Weekly*, 50(1):15, 1959.
16. Dupont, I.: A case in point; application of a contact lens-telescopic correction for subnormal vision, *Contacto*, 3(6):172–173, 1959.
17. Westheimer, G.: The field of view of visual aids, *Am. J. Optom.*, 34(8):430–438, 1957.
18. Williams, C. E.: The use of contact lenses in subnormal vision, in *Encyclopedia of Contact Lens Practice*, South Bend, Indiana, International Optics, 1959–1963, vol. 3, Chap. 16, pp. 63–76.
19. Bourquin, K. M., and Furie, A.: Contact lens telescope for reading, *Oregon Optometrist, July–October*, 1962.
20. Voss, E.: Demonstrated at the Research Study Group Meeting, Eye Research Foundation, Chicago, July, 1958.
21. Filderman, I. P.: The telecon lens for the partially sighted, *Am. J. Optom.*, 36(3):135–136, 1959.
22. Filderman, I. P.: The telecon lens system, a modified Galilean telescope, *Contacto*, 3(4):94–96, 1959.
23. Filderman, I. P.: Spectacle lens-contact lens system, *South. J. Optom.*, 4(6):5–7, 10, 30, 1962.
24. Isen, A.: Feinbloom miniscope contact lens, in *Encyclopedia of Contact Lens Practice*, South Bend, Indiana, International Optics, 1959–1963, vol. 3, Supp. 13, pp. 53–55.
25. Braff, S.: Calcon Contact Lens Co., personal communication.
26. Rosenbloom, A. A.: The controlled-pupil contact lens in low vision problems, *J. Am. Optom. Assoc.*, 40(8):836–840, 1970.

ADDITIONAL READINGS

Cohler, H. P.: Gel lens as an ocular, *Int. Cont. Lens Clin.*, *2(1)*:103, 1975.

Moore, L.: How to make the Moore contact lens-spectacle system work, *Contacto*, *21(5)*:32–37, 1977.

Chapter 29

PRESBYOPIA

THE PRESBYOPE REPRESENTS one of the greatest challenges to the contact lens practitioner.[1] His visual problem may be corrected by many approaches, but each involves special fitting techniques and requires considerable skill on the part of the practitioner. In addition, there is often a need for appreciable time and expense on the part of the patient.

Neither contact lenses nor spectacle lenses are totally satisfactory for the correction of all presbyopes.[2] Bifocal spectacles have the disadvantages of limited field of view and limited distances of clear vision. They require more critical placement and adjustment than single vision lenses. No single spectacle bifocal design can be said to be ideal for all wearers. A patient may need several types of lenses for the best performance of all his visual tasks. A large number of spectacle bifocals have been developed in an attempt to solve the problem of providing normal vision to the presbyope. That these are not entirely successful is evidenced by the common lay references to the difficulty of adjusting to bifocals and by the rejection of bifocals.[2]

Just as with spectacles, there is no single solution to the problem of correcting presbyopia with contact lenses. People vary in their working tasks, and the lenses must be designed accordingly. In addition, special attention must be given to the physical features of each patient's eyes and the fitting problems that they present.

The practitioner who cares for the presbyope must be prepared to use a number of approaches, only some of which will involve bifocal or other multifocal contact lenses. Four or five of the many techniques that have been tried in previous years have proven successful enough to be considered by the practitioner.

The care of presbyopia is often considered a specialized type of contact lens practice. If only a few patients in this category are contemplated, the practitioner might be wise to consider referring these cases. Otherwise, he may be tempted to seek the easiest method for the correction of the patient, rather than the method of most benefit to that patient.

Although the presbyope is not usually considered as the ideal contact lens patient, he does have several advantages over the younger patient:

1. Reduced sensitivity of the cornea and lid margins
2. Maturity to follow instructions
3. Greater dependence on visual correction
4. High motivation

With respect to the last advantage, it is important that the presbyope be more highly motivated than the average contact lens patient, since extra time and expense may be involved in his correction. Special care should be taken to insure that the patient understands the difficulties that are sometimes encountered with this type of lens so that he will not become disillusioned before the fitter has had a chance to reach an acceptable result.[3]

ACCOMMODATION AND PRESBYOPIA

An important consideration in fitting the presbyope is the effect that the substitution of contact lenses will have on the refractive correction for near vision.[4] In Chapter 4 it was shown that with spectacle lens correction, different amounts of accommodation were required of the ametrope than of the emmetrope. A myope must exert more accommodation, whereas a hyperope can exert less accommodation when wearing contact lenses rather than spectacles.

The difference in accommodation required by the hyperope and myope when wearing contact lenses rather than spectacles is of special importance for beginning presbyopes. Less of an add is necessary for a hyperope in the early stage of presbyopia if he wears contact lenses rather than spectacles (Figure 29.1). If he is an early presbyope, no add at all may be necessary when wearing contact lenses. It also may be possible to avoid the add temporarily by overplusing the distance correction, providing that the patient will tolerate the slight blur in his distance vision.

The myope, on the other hand, will always need to accommodate more through his contact lenses than through his spectacle lenses.[4,5] Consequently, a myopic patient who is approaching presbyopia and who does not yet need a spectacle bifocal may find himself with inadequate accommodation when wearing single vision contact lenses.

CONTACT LENSES FOR PRESBYOPIA

Various methods are available for correcting the presbyopic patient with contact lenses. They may be divided broadly into five approaches, only two of which involve bifocal

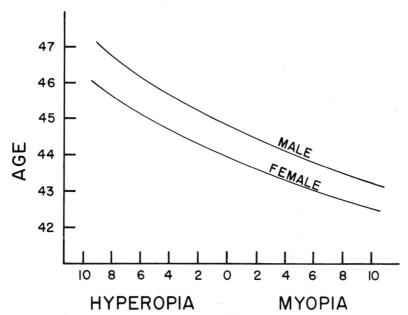

Figure 29.1. Hypothetical graph to show the change in onset of presbyopia when changing from spectacles to contact lenses. A myope manifests presbyopia one to two years earlier than normal, whereas a hyperope is delayed beyond normal.

contact lenses.

1. Single vision contact lenses for distance combined with a spectacle reading correction
2. Monovision contact lens correction
3. Pinhole lens

4. Concentric bifocal
5. Prism ballast bifocal

The difficult problem is to decide when each type of correction should be applied. An approach to aid in this decision will be discussed at the end of this chapter.

CONTACT LENSES AND AUXILIARY SPECTACLES

Very often the most satisfactory refractive correction for a presbyope is one in which contact lenses are worn to correct the distance refractive error and auxiliary spectacles are worn for near work.

This is the simplest form of presbyopic correction and produces the fewest fitting problems and fewest patient complaints. The near work spectacles may be single vision plus spheres, plano bifocals, or plano trifocals, with the necessary add. Of course, for the patient it is a compromise solution; he must be primarily concerned with his appearance when using distance vision or have little or no need for near vision. He must show little concern about using spectacles for reading. Unfortunately, for many presbyopes, the need to use a spectacle near correction may destroy the cosmetic advantage achieved by the contact lenses.

This may be the only satisfactory correction when the patient uses his eyes at near for prolonged periods. It is often the best form of correction under adverse viewing conditions, such as low illumination or glare sources.

MONOVISION WITH CONTACT LENSES

Single vision contact lenses may be prescribed for the presbyope by correcting one eye for distance vision and the other eye for near vision.[6,7,8] Refractionists are familiar with the occasional presbyope who is myopic in one eye and emmetropic or hyperopic in the other. He often learns to use one eye for his distance vision and the other eye for near vision. These patients are often surprisingly free of visual discomfort and seem to function reasonably well. Contact lenses may be used to create this situation artificially.

A monovision correction is produced by giving a contact lens that gives maximum near vision to only one eye. The chief advantage of this technique is that essentially the same fitting philosophies that are employed by the fitter for single vision contact lens patients may be used.

The principal decision that must be made in prescribing monovision lenses is which eye will be given the correction for distance vision. As a general rule, the dominant eye is selected; however, this is not an inviolable rule and may need to be reversed if comfort is not achieved following a trial period.

There is some disagreement as to how much the monovision correction interferes with stereopsis, visual fields, and other binocular functions. Many authors have reported that after their patients have gone through an adjustment period of three to fourteen days they do not feel disoriented, nor do they notice any loss of depth perception, peripheral vision, or other visual functions. This appears to be the common clinical impression, but subjects who were studied in depth reported some subjective decrease in depth perception and other problems.[9] For example, one patient studied by McLendon et al.

reported a slight feeling of loss of depth perception when driving her automobile and a greater loss of depth perception when landing the family's private airplane.[9]

A second patient had considerable inability to perform at near. His occupation required him to make minute wire connections, and he complained of inaccuracy and difficulty when doing so. Since so much of this patient's work was concentrated at the near point, the near point lens was switched to his dominant eye, and the far point lens to his nondominant eye. The response of the patient was poor, and the lenses were abandoned.

Another patient complained she developed severe headaches after wearing her monovision lenses. She had not experienced these headaches prior to wearing contact lenses, and they subsided only with rest or by putting distance contact lenses on both eyes.

McLendon et al. also found that the patients in their study frequently complained that their vision was hazy.[9] During the normal day-to-day routine, the conditions under which the haze was reportedly worse were (1) at a distance, (2) under decreased illumination, (3) indoors. The conditions in which the haze was less were (1) at near, (2) monocular occlusion, (3) good illumination.

When measurements of the patient's visual functions are taken after adaptation to the lenses, the following conditions are found:

1. Stereopsis is decreased in most patients.[9,10] The decrease is usually low but is occasionally annoying to the patient. Interestingly, the loss in stereopsis is greater when the same monocular add is given in spectacles.[11,12,13] The reports on the amount of loss are inconsistent, however, and may be related to the testing method. It is noteworthy that McLendon et al. did not find any correlation between the amount of add and the decrement in stereopsis.[9] However, a pilot study on two subjects by Christie and Sarver showed very little loss in stereopsis, if any, for low adds but a rapid loss in stereopsis for adds greater than 1.00 D.[12] They proposed that lower adds

are more easily accepted. Although their sample is too small to be conclusive, the evidence suggests that the power of the reading addition should be as low as possible for the patient's near requirements.

2. There is not a consistent effect on phorias or ductions, and any change is usually not significant.

3. Visual fields, as measured with a 3 mm. target, are decreased an insignificant amount for the eye with near correction (average 0.2°).[9] This is more than compensated by an average increase of 5° for the eye corrected with a contact lens for distance vision when compared to spectacles.[9]

In spite of the relatively good results demonstrated in several reports, the fitter should use the monovision technique with caution. There is always the possibility that this form of correction will interfere with many normal activities, such as driving a car, participating in sports, and any other tasks that require binocularity and stereopsis. Since the near vision correction is prescribed for the nondominant eye, there is occasionally a tendency to shift to the dominant eye even when it is not wanted. For example, when an individual reads and becomes engrossed in the subject matter, a shift may be made to the dominant eye. His vision becomes blurred, and confusion results.

In determining which presbyopic patients are to receive a monovision correction, the following should be considered:

1. Occupations that demand good acuity for long periods of time are contraindicated. Clerical and other types of desk work are acceptable as long as extended periods of time are not spent reading small print.

2. The visual task should be well illuminated.

3. The patient should not require maximum depth perception at near.

4. The patient should be willing to accept a blur or haze during the first two to four weeks of wearing. Also, during this time, he may have an occasional feeling of slight

imbalance.[9]

Occupations that seem most conducive to monovision correction are (1) stenographers and other indoor office workers who have good illumination, (2) housewives and others who do not have intense visual demands, (3) sales clerks.

There is also some indication that this might be an advantageous method of prescribing for tropias.[9]

Selection of Patients

Monovision contact lenses are recommended for the following:

1. Patients unable or unwilling to wear conventional bifocal contact lenses.

2. Previous single vision contact lens patients. Upon reaching presbyopia, they need change only one lens.

3. Patients who require a minimum fitting time or expense.

Fitting Procedure

The fitting procedure for monovision correction is as follows.[14] The patient is fitted with temporary distance contact lenses for both eyes. While the patient is adapting to these lenses, he is loaned a pair of reading glasses so that it is unnecessary to remove his contact lenses to read. After one to two weeks, a test is made to determine the minimum amount of plus that, when held in front of the nondominant eye, will permit clear vision of newspaper print or 20/40 equivalent. A trial frame may be used to determine whether this has any adverse effect on his distance vision.

The patient is allowed to keep the original pair of contact lenses and is advised that when any extensive amount of driving or far seeing is done, both distance lenses can be worn if desired.

There appears to be general agreement among clinicians that patients function better when the distance correction is placed before the dominant eye. There seems to be no evidence for the success of this procedure, and there are probably many exceptions.

Eye dominance may be defined in several ways, but in this application it usually refers to *sighting dominance*, that is, the eye a patient chooses when forced to view an object with only one eye. It is commonly tested by the following procedures.

A card with a small hole (about 1 cm. diameter) in the center is held at arm's length with both hands at a low position as the subject sights a fixation light. Upon command, the card is raised quickly to align the hole with the fixation target. The eyes are alternately covered, and the eye found to be viewing the target is the dominant eye (Figure 29.2).

There is considerable disagreement over the value of the dominance test.[15] In cases of anisometropia, the patient may be happier when a distance correction is given to the eye used previously for distance vision. If there is no preference, it should be considered that the eye with the most plus correction will need the lowest add and may do best with the near correction.[16]

The practitioners may prefer to fit the patient immediately with one distance and one near lens. In this instance, it may be necessary to supply a second contact lens for the eye that is given the near correction in order to provide an alternate correction for distance. Hence, when the patient needs good binocularity or maximum vision with both eyes, he can change lenses to achieve this.[17,18]

Instruct the patient first to remove the distance prescription and apply the near prescription in order to maintain clear near vision.

Patients should be informed that they may experience the following symptoms during adaptation, which are expected to subside within fourteen days.

1. Disorientation or feeling off balance
2. Intermittent haze or blur

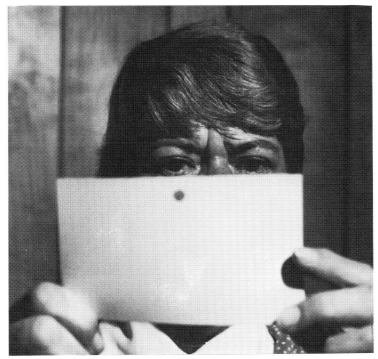

Figure 29.2. The dominant eye is viewing the target.

PINHOLE LENS

The principle of the pinhole lens for correcting refractive errors was presented in Chapter 15. This lens can be used equally well for correcting presbyopia.[19] If an emmetropic presbyope wears a pinhole contact lens with plano power, there is little or no effect on the clarity of distance objects.[20,21] There is, however, a great effect on the clarity of objects at near distances. With the pinhole, the blur circle formed by the light from an out-of-focus near object is reduced in size, and the object appears to be relatively clear.

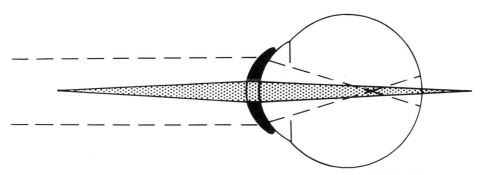

Figure 29.3. Pinhole contact lens used for the correction of presbyopia. The lens has an overcorrection of +1.00 D., which allows a minimum of image blurring for far and near viewing.

If the pinhole contact lens has, in addition, a plus refractive power, e.g. +1.00 D., the near object will be even clearer (Figure 29.3). The +1.00 D. would ordinarily make distant objects appear blurred to the emmetropic, but, because of the pinhole, distance blurring is not significant.

Ametropic presbyopes may be corrected with a pinhole contact lens by a principle similar to that used for the emmetrope. The power of the contact lenses in this case should be the algebraic sum of the ametropic correction and +1.00 D. For example, the −4.00 D. myope would have a correction in the pinhole lens of −3.00 D. of power. The +4.00 D. hyperope, on the other hand, should be corrected with +5.00 D. of power.

The optimum aperture diameter for a presbyopic pinhole lens is from 1 to 3 mm., with some preference toward the smaller. Larger pinholes are not effective in reducing the size of the blur circle, and smaller pinholes severely limit the illumination to the eye. A decrease in illumination is especially handicapping to the presbyopes; thus, pinhole lenses should not be worn at night.

The principal disadvantage of the pinhole lens is the undesirable cosmetic effect produced by the black annulus surrounding the pinhole. This disadvantage is eliminated if a cosmetic lens with a pinhole is used. Other disadvantages of a pinhole for presbyopia are the decrease of illumination and a vignetting effect on the subjective visual field.

A unique form of pinhole lens that has been recommended for presbyopes instead of a bifocal is the *Multi-Range® contact lens* (originally called the *Cosmetic Bifocal*).[22,23,24] The Multi-Range contact lens has a pinhole in the center that is surrounded by six radial slits placed in three meridians[25] (*see* Chapter 15). These slits serve to increase the field of view and act as stenopeic slits when the lens is decentered on the eye.[24] The principle of fitting the Multi-Range contact lens is similar to that for fitting a single vision lens, with a few additional measurements necessary for ordering the lens (*see* Chapter 15).

Diagnostic Lens Method

The fitting of a pinhole or Multi-Range contact lens may be facilitated by the use of a set of diagnostic contact lenses with pinholes of 1.0 and 1.5 mm. By varying the diameter of the pinhole, the best lens for achieving the greatest near point range can be determined.

The diagnostic pinhole lenses are usually manufactured in plano power. Spectacle trial lenses are then placed in front of the pinhole to achieve the best distance visual acuity. With the same spectacle trial lens in front of the pinhole, the gaze is directed towards the reading material, held at the normal reading distance. Normal illumination should be used when testing the near point acuity. If the patient is unable to read at near, a low plus power addition should be tried. If successful, the patient should be retested at distance to see if the pinhole will allow overplusing the distance correction.

BIFOCAL CONTACT LENSES

It is generally agreed that a successful bifocal contact lens presents the most desirable form of correction for the majority of presbyopic patients. However, the bifocal contact lens requires the most perfect fitting of any contact lens. A number of practitioners have adopted the attitude that a bifocal contact lens is too difficult to fit, and they will simply wait for a bifocal contact lens to be invented that is as simple to fit and as effective as a single vision lens. This attitude may have developed after they tried various bifocal contact lenses on a few patients and found a high percentage of failures. They usually became discouraged early and discarded the technique to wait for the development of the next panacea for correcting presbyopia.[17,18]

Unfortunately, several aspects of bifocal contact lenses make it unlikely they will ever be as simple to fit as single vision lenses. Bifocal contact lenses are usually divided into two power areas—an area for distance vision and an area for near vision. These areas must be crowded into the small optical zone of a contact lens; thus, each area is limited to a size that can barely cover the pupil of the eye. The sizes and positions of these power areas in relation to the pupil is most critical for the proper functioning of the lens, and the fit and movement of the lens must be carefully controlled.

Simultaneous versus Alternating Vision

A bifocal lens may be designed to function according to one of two different principles. The first principle is known as the *bivision* or *simultaneous vision* principle. When this principle of fitting is followed, the lens is designed so that light passes through both the near and distance power area simultaneously, and two bundles of light contribute to the retinal image at all times. If the patient views a distant object, the light passing through the distance power area forms a clear image on the retina, while the light passing through the near power area forms an image that is out of focus at the retina. If the patient views a near object, the light passing through the near power area is in focus, while the light passing through the distance power area is out of focus. Consequently, whenever the patient looks either distant or near, he has a clear image, but in addition, some blurring is formed by the light passing through the out-of-focus zone. For this reason, the patient never experiences vision without some blurring, which is the major drawback to this fitting principle.

The second principle that is used in fitting a bifocal contact lens is by *alternating vision*. Here the lens is designed to move to different positions on the cornea as the gaze is directed from distant to near so that either the distant or near power area completely or nearly covers the pupil.

Bifocal Lens Types

There have been many attempts to design bifocal contact lenses.[26,27] Only those which have achieved a fair degree of success will be discussed in detail.

Concentric (Annular) Bifocal

The concentric bifocal lens is produced in two general forms. In the first, a small distance power area in the center of the lens is surrounded by a concentric (annular) area, which contains the near prescription. The different power areas can be formed on either the front or back surface of the contact lens.[28,29]

In a second form of the lens, the zones are reversed so that the near power area is in the center.

FRONT SURFACE CONCENTRIC BIFOCAL. The front surface concentric bifocal contact lens consists of two distinct power areas, which are formed by two curves on the anterior surface.[30-33] The central portion of the optical zone contains the correction for the patient's distance ametropia; it is termed the *distance power area* (Figure 29.4a). Surrounding this area there is a concentric zone, which contains the near or reading correction. This concentric zone is also an optical zone and is called the *near power area*.

In fitting a front surface concentric bifocal lens by the principle of *simultaneous vision*, the usual techniques of fitting a single vision contact lens are used, with special attention given to the stability of the lens. The lens is designed to be as stable on the eye as possible. This can be achieved in a small lens by using an apical clearance fit or steep peripheral curves. A large lens can be fitted with corneal alignment and have sufficient stability. Usually this lens must be about 0.4 mm. larger than the single vision lens that would normally be used for a given eye. The distance power area is made smaller than the pupil of the eye so that light from the near power area also passes through the pupil simultaneously.

A second principle that may be used to fit the front surface concentric bifocal lens is by the principle of *alternating vision*. In this method the lens is usually increased in size so both the distant and near power areas may be made larger. The lens is also fitted so that it moves freely up and down on the eye. By varying the looseness of the fit and the sizes of the distance and near power areas, it is theoretically possible to make a lens center fairly well when a distant object is viewed and shift upward when the patient lowers his eyes to view a near object. The shifting of the contact lens is due principally to the lens's bumping against the lower lid on downward gaze. The failure of this lens to work well is usually due to inadequate movement.

The lens is normally fitted according to the following specifications:

1. Total diameter: 9.0 to 9.6 mm.
2. Optical zone radius: 0.05 to 0.15 mm. longer than the K radius
3. Optical zone diameter: 8.0 mm.
4. Distance power area diameter on front surface: average 4 mm. (range 3 to 6 mm.)

The lens thickness is slightly greater than for single vision lenses.[34] Several alternate forms have been tried.[35,36]

BACK SURFACE CONCENTRIC BIFOCAL. Another type of bifocal contact lens is very similar to the front surface concentric lens but differs in that the two power areas are formed by two different curves on the back surface of the lens (Figure 29.4b).[37-41] The back surface concentric bifocal lens may be fitted according to either the alternating or bivision principle, but the latter is usually the method of choice. In this lens the central distance power area is smaller than the pupil of the eye; thus, the patient looks through both the distance and near power areas at the

same time. The average distance power area is about 3 mm. in size but may be varied slightly according to the pupil diameter. Theoretically, the distance power area should be about one-half of the pupil area under conditions of average illumination.

General specifications for the bivision principle:

1. Total diameter: 8.5 to 10.5 mm.
2. Optical zone radius (distance portion) steeper than the base curve (near optical zone radius) by the amount necessary to provide add
3. Base curve (near optical zone radius): on K to steeper than K
4. Optical zone diameter: about 8 mm.
5. Distance power area: about 3 mm.

When the alternating principle is used, the central power area is larger, and the fit is modified so that lens movement is adequate for shifting the proper zone before the pupil.

General specifications for the alternating principle:

1. Total diameter: 8.5 to 10.5 mm.
2. Optical zone radius (distance portion) approximately equal to K
3. Secondary curve radius (near power area radius): flatter than the optical zone radius by the amount necessary to provide the add
4. Optical zone diameter: about 8 mm.
5. Distance power area diameter: about 5 mm.

In one unusual case a toric surface has been incorporated into this lens.[42]

REVERSE BIFOCALS. This lens is made either from a single piece of plastic or fused from plastic of two different indices of refraction to provide the optical properties.[43] The near power area of the lens is located in the center, with the distance power area immediately surrounding the near segment in concentric form (Figure 29.4c and d).

The lens is fitted in a low position so that when the patient looks at a distance, he views

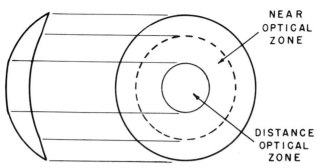

Figure 29.4a. Front-surface annular bifocal.

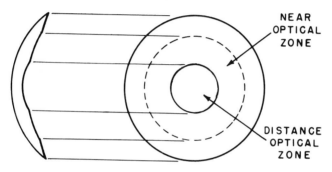

Figure 29.4b. Back-surface annular bifocal.

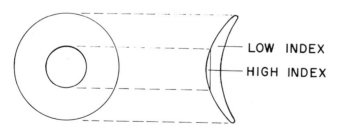

Figure 29.4c. Reverse centrad bifocal.

primarily through the concentric distance portion. When the gaze is directed from distance to near, the eye shifts down. Usually there is an accompanying small shift of the lens upwards, which more nearly places the pupil behind the center of the lens. At the same time, the pupil of the eye constricts and the lid aperture narrows so that vision is confined more to the central portion of the lens. The efficacy of this lens is enhanced if adequate lighting is provided for near viewing.

The lenses should be fitted the same in all specifications as a single vision lens, except that there must be reasonable centration and

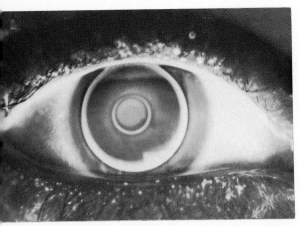

Figure 29.4d. One-piece central bifocal. Courtesy of ConCise Contact Lens Co.

stability of movement.

1. Distance power: the distance power is usually the same as that of the single vision lens.

2. Near power: the near power should be the same as in spectacles. The distance and near powers can be read accurately on the lensometer, as the mire image of each comes into focus sharply and clearly.

3. Near power area: the diameter of the near power segment, being located in the center of the lens, must be small enough so that there is little or no interference with distance vision. The near segment diameter is made equal to the pupil size under bright illumination, or 0.1 mm. to 0.2 mm. smaller. The diameter usually varies between 2.2 mm. and 3.0 mm., with the average about 2.6 mm. If the near segment is too large, a diplopia or overall blur develops for distance acuity. If the near segment is too small or gets decentered away from the pupil during near viewing, a diplopia results at near.

Use trial lenses and verify the centering of the lens using single vision lenses and modify accordingly to achieve good centering.

4. Optical zone diameter: the optical zone should be 1.4 mm. smaller than the overall size of the lens, but never smaller than 7.0 mm.

5. Lens diameter: the diameter of the lens must be small enough so that when the patient is looking straight ahead, the lens is within the palpebral aperture.

6. Thickness: the central thickness of the lens is based upon the power. The plano powered lens should be made 0.18 mm. central thickness. For every diopter of minus power, 0.01 mm. should be deducted from the plano powered central thickness down to a minimum of 0.10 mm. For every diopter of plus power on lenses up to 9.2 mm. size, add 0.025 mm. to the plano powered central thickness. For larger plus lenses, let the laboratory determine the thinnest lens practical for the particular size.

Prism Ballast Bifocal

Nonrotational bifocals are stabilized on the cornea by one of several possible methods. The majority fall in the class known as prism ballast bifocals.

Ballasted bifocal contact lenses, as the name implies, are those which are thicker and thus heavier at one edge than the other. This ballasting may be achieved in several ways.

One method is to produce a lens in a wedge or prism shape, with the thicker portion at the bottom.[44,45] A second method is to create a noncircular lens or to truncate the lens so that the lower portion is wider and heavier than the upper portion and thus able to maintain an erect position. Many other methods have been attempted with limited success.

Of the various forms of contact lenses for presbyopia, the prism ballast bifocal usually provides the best vision for both distance and near.

Prism ballast bifocal contact lenses have been made in several forms, and each has suffered various defects. The earliest problem that had to be solved was the quality of manufacture which for most bifocal lenses is now acceptable. The second problem was the presence of jump, the optical effect of a

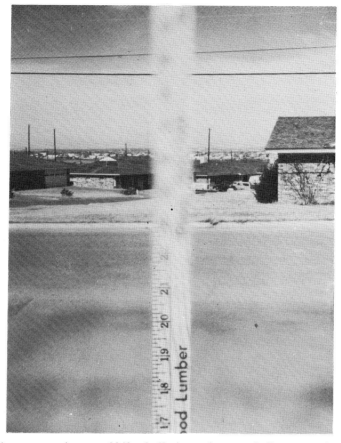

Figure 29.5. A monocentric type of bifocal eliminates jump and allows a continuous field of clear vision from distance to near.

displaced image as the eye shifts from distance to near and passes the segment line. It was found that any bifocal contact lens that had jump also had doubling of images for the patient. Although it was possible to have a few patients adapt to the presence of jump, it was never possible to get people to accept a bifocal contact lens that produced doubling. More recently, this problem was solved, and several new bifocals are now available that are made on a monocentric principle, which eliminates jump. It is recommended that only monocentric type of prism ballast bifocals be fitted (Figure 29.5).

Method of Performance

Prism ballast causes a contact lens to ride in an inferior position when the wearer is looking straight ahead. In this position the upper or distance portion of the lens is aligned in front of the pupil. As the eye moves to a downward position, the lens is pushed up by the lower lid, so the pupil becomes aligned with the lower portion of the lens, which contains the near power addition (Figure 29.6a). The eye excursion during this movement is limited to less than 4 mm. (Figure 29.6b).

Types of Prism Ballast Bifocals

The principal difference between the various prism ballast bifocals is in their construction. Some are fused, and others are one

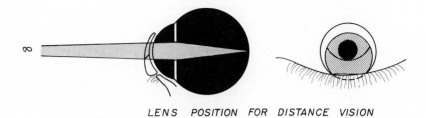

LENS POSITION FOR DISTANCE VISION

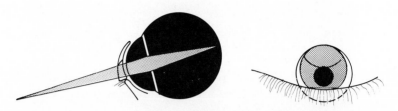

LENS POSITION FOR NEAR VISION

Figure 29.6a. Lens position for distance and near vision.

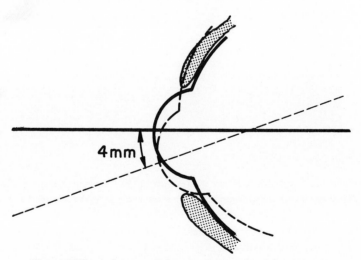

Figure 29.6b. A downward eye movement is less than 4 mm.

piece. Of the various one-piece bifocals, there are many different shapes for the segment line. However, they all have the common feature that the distance correction is always on the top and near correction is always on the bottom of the lens (Figure 29.7a). Many fitters consider the upsweep shape to have a distinct advantage (Figure 29.7b).

FUSED MONOCENTRIC BIFOCAL. Fused bifocal contact lenses are made with a single curve on both the front and back optical zone areas.[46-48] A segment that has a high index of refraction and that provides additional plus power to that portion of the lens is used. The lens is usually made with prism ballast (Figure 29.7c).

The advantages of the fused prism bifocal contact lens are the following:

1. There is a sharp transition between

the distance and near portions of the lens.

2. The lens can be made thinner than a one-piece bifocal.

3. Cylinder may be added to the lens.

The disadvantages of a fused bifocal are the following:

1. Lack of control of the segment upsweep.
2. Lens is subject to warpage.
3. An occasional segment separation.

The technique used for fitting the fused bifocal is similar to that used for fitting the one-piece prism ballast bifocal.

It is possible to dye the segment of a fused bifocal with a luminous dye that is colorless and transparent but which glows in ultraviolet light.[49] This has been an excellent aid with trial lenses in positioning the segment. However, fluorescent segments are often troublesome in regular lenses, as they glow and interfere with the vision of the patient.

ONE-PIECE MONOCENTRIC BIFOCAL. A one-piece monocentric bifocal contact lens has most of the advantages of a fused bifocal but in addition is less subject to warpage (Figure 29.7d). It became popular only after a monocentric design was introduced.[50] Its shape and average dimensions are shown in Figure 29.8.

It has the disadvantage that a front toric curve is not available for correcting residual astigmatism.

This lens can be made with any curvature for the segment line, and each lens is calculated so that no jump occurs anywhere along the segment line (Figure 29.9). Although usually a standard shape will be used, there are variations from this which are useful in some difficult cases. For example, a patient who must always look to the side when he observes a near object may benefit from a *concave* segment line. A patient with greater demands on his distance vision may benefit from a *flat* segment line.

Fitting Procedure

PATIENT SELECTION. The best patients for the prism ballast bifocal are those with a more or less average eye. The most important feature is the position of the lids. Watch out for patients with the following characteristics:

1. Low superior lids
2. Either a high or low inferior lid

In addition, check the following:

1. Be certain that the patient is motivated.

2. Do not start the patient with a single vision lens to build wearing time, but go right to the bifocal. Never put a single vision lens on the patient if you can avoid it. Fitting the single vision lens will not help you with the bifocal lens, and after the patient gets used to a single vision lens, he may not tolerate a bifocal lens with prism ballast. If you must start out with something besides a bifocal, use a single vision prism ballast contact lens.

3. Be leery of patients who do a great deal of close work or who work at odd angles.

4. Patients who are already wearing bifocal spectacle lenses make better patients.

The best results in fitting bifocal contact lenses have been found only to be achieved when bifocal trial lenses are used to obtain precise data for the final lens specifications. The following guide is used for the selection of the first trial lens ordered from the laboratory (Table 29.1):

1. Diameter and segment height: a trial lens having a diameter of 9.0 by 9.4 mm. is used. The diameter of the final lenses and the segment height are determined by observing the fitting characteristics of a trial lens.

2. Optic zone:

If vertical diameter is—	use O.Z. of—
8.8	7.6
9.0	7.8

3. Power: this needs to be only an approximation of final power. The power of the near segment should be the same as the add at near in spectacles. Do not make allow-

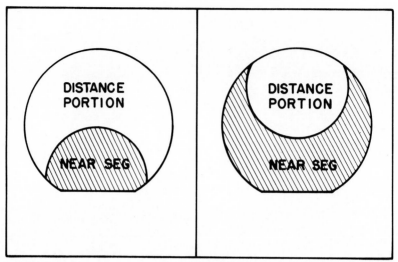

Figure 29.7a. The near segment assumes various shapes but is always placed at the lower portion of the lens.

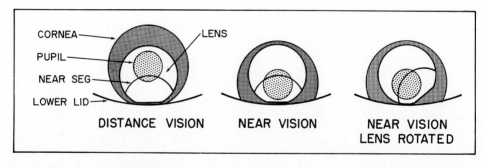

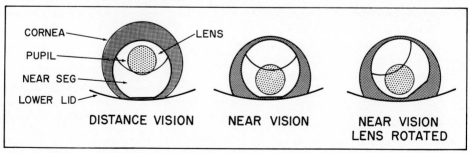

Figure 29.7b. Advantage of an upsweep segment occurs during near vision. The pupil is covered by near segment even during slight rotation of the lens.

ances for vertex distance at near.

4. Prism: normally 1.5 prism diopters is optimum, but powers from 1.0 to 3.0 prism diopters are found necessary to achieve sta-bility in some cases. Prism between 2.0 and 3.0 prism diopters is usually less comforta-ble, and prism over 3.0 prism diopters is usually not tolerated.

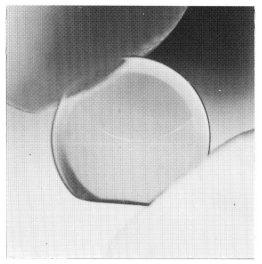
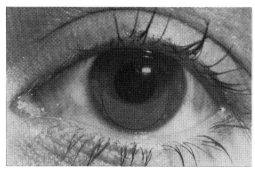

Figure 29.7c. Fused monocentric bifocal contact lenses. Courtesy of Neefe Optical Laboratory.

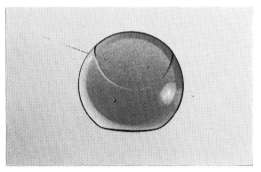

Figure 29.7d. One-piece monocentric bifocal. Courtesy of ConCise Contact Lens Co.

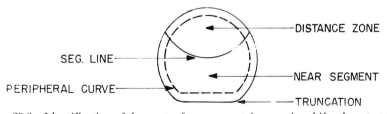

Figure 29.8a. Identification of the parts of a monocentric one-piece bifocal contact lens.

Lens Inspection for Trial Lenses and Final Lenses

LENS POWER. The distance power is determined in the same manner as for single vision contact lenses, that is, the powers of all prism ballast lenses are measured and recorded in terms of back vertex power. The lens is held in the lensometer with the concave surface against the lensometer stop (the convex surface of the lens faces the clinician). Other important considerations relative to accurate

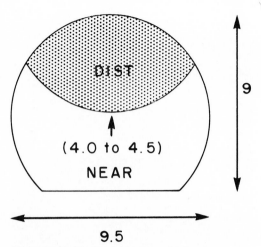

Figure 29.8b. Average dimension of a monocentric one-piece bifocal contact lens.

measurements follow.

1. To obtain a truer reading of lens power, a 3 to 4 mm. aperture may be used over the lensometer stop. This can easily be made by punching a hole in a piece of opaque tape and affixing this to the lensometer stop. This aperture is necessary due to the following:

a. The power in a prism lens is constantly changing due to the continuous variation in thickness going from top to bottom of the lens, becoming more plus powered towards the lens bottom.

b. Most lensometers have a stop of 6.5 to 7.0 mm. size, so too large an area is included to provide a clear focus on a lens of varying power.

c. The pupils of most presbyopes seldom measure more than 4 mm.; thus, a

TABLE 29.1

Base Curve Amount of Corneal Toricity	Base Curve Used
0.00 D.	0.50 D. flatter than "K"
0.25 D.	0.37 D. flatter than "K"
0.50 D.	0.25 D. flatter than "K"
0.75 D.	0.12 D. flatter than "K"
1.00 D.	On "K"
Over 1.00 D.	1/3 steeper than "K" difference

truer evaluation of what the patient is experiencing comes from using an aperture similar to his own pupil size.

2. A more accurate measurement of the power actually in front of the patient's eye with a bifocal lens is obtained by checking the portions of the lens that are really used by the patient for his distance and near seeing, as indicated in the following:

a. For distance seeing, the lens will be positioned low on the eye, so the patient will be looking through approximately the *center of the distance portion* of the lens. Therefore, when checking the distance power on the lensometer, one should put the same portion of the lens over the aperture-covered stop.

b. For near vision, the lower lid pushes the lens upward about 3 mm. Therefore, immediately after the distance power has been checked on the lensometer, the practitioner should move the lens up slowly, while he is still looking through the lensometer eyepiece, until the near focus *just comes into his field of view.* This procedure gives a close approxi-

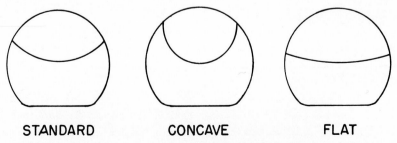

Figure 29.9. Variations in segment line curvature for a bifocal contact lens.

mation of the power with which the patient is corrected at near.

JUMP. Jump can be determined by either of two methods.

1. Measure the lens powers with a lensometer. Hold the lens so that the segment line is at the center of the lensometer stop and the base (truncation) is down (Figure 29.10).

Rotate the dial, starting from the minus direction, until the target comes into focus, indicating the distance-power. Note the amount of prism indicated by the target position on the scale.

Next, rotate the dial towards the plus power until the target comes into focus a second time, indicating the power of the near portion of the lens. The target should now be in the same position, indicating equal prism powers for the distant and near portions of the lens and insuring that no jump will be experienced by the wearer (Figure 29.11).

2. Hold the lens between the thumb and index finger with the base down. Viewing through the lens, observe a straight line on a piece of paper a few inches away. Move the lens up and down so that the segment line crosses the line on the paper. If the lens is not monocentric, the line will appear to jump each time the seg line is passed across it (Figure 29.12).

SEGMENT HEIGHT. This measurement is very critical. It can be most easily accomplished with a measuring magnifier. Measure from the truncation to the center of the segment line.

TRUNCATION. The truncation is usually 0.4 to 0.5 mm. and is responsible for the difference between the horizontal and vertical diameters, e.g. diameter 9.0 × 9.4 means the truncation is 0.4 mm. The truncation serves the following functions.

1. Thick edge for lens support
2. Reduce lens weight
3. Wider edge contacts lid

The truncation has the effect of adding ballast on a plus-power lens and reducing ballast on a minus-power lens (Figure 29.13). More or less prism is sometimes added to compensate for this (Table 29.2).

The shape of the truncation is important. The truncation should be nearly flat at the bottom with rounded corners (Figure 29.14). It should be rounded evenly on the front and back sides. If the truncation tapers toward the front surface, it will rub against the lower lid and cause severe discomfort. If the truncation tapers toward the rear surface, the lens will slip beneath the lower lid and not be supported in its proper position (Figure 29.15).

PERIPHERAL CURVE. The peripheral curve on the lens is made narrow (usually 0.5 mm.) and flat (12 mm.) so as to give a large optic zone. The most important area for checking the peripheral curve is at the truncation (Figure 29.16).

A lens is truncated after the peripheral curve is added, and the truncation removes the peripheral curve on the lower portion of the lens. If the lens is not rebeveled at this position, it causes tear stagnation in the lower lens position.

Procedure for Evaluating Trial Lenses to Obtain Exact Specifications for the Final Lenses

Do all tests monocularly, with the other eye under occlusion. A single cell trial frame is ideal for this. A recommended trial set is given in Table 29.3.

Place the trial lens on the eye; allow it to settle, and wait for any tearing to subside. Add fluorescein, and observe the lens under ultraviolet light. Be certain the patient is not tense or squinting.

RIDING POSITION. When the eye is in the primary position, the upper edge of the lens should be about 0.5 mm. or less above the top of the pupil. Any difference from this position should be corrected by ordering a different final lens diameter. Observe the position of the segment. The segment line will be outlined by fluorescein, which collects at the

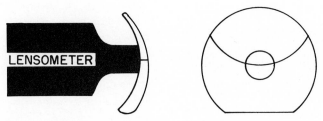

Figure 29.10. When checking for jump using the lensometer, the lens is held so that the segment line divides the lens stop of the lensometer.

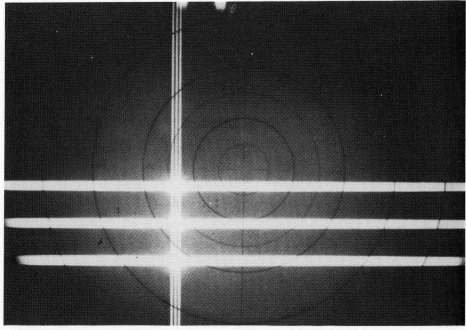

Figure 29.11. Prism power in a bifocal contact lens appears in the lensometer view in the same way as for a spectacle lens.

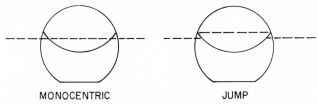

MONOCENTRIC   JUMP

Figure 29.12. If a bifocal lens is not monocentric, a line viewed through the lens will appear to jump each time the segment line passes across it.

TRUNCATION

ON PLUS AIDS BALLAST

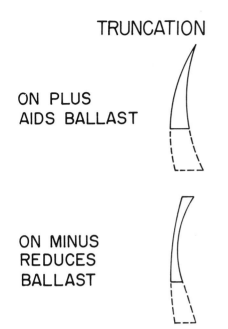

ON MINUS REDUCES BALLAST

Figure 29.13. A truncation is more or less effective, depending upon the refractive power of the lens.

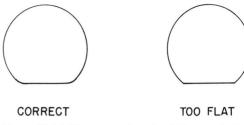

CORRECT   TOO FLAT

Figure 29.14. The truncation should be nearly flat at the bottom with rounded corners.

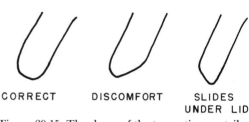

CORRECT   DISCOMFORT   SLIDES UNDER LID

Figure 29.15. The shape of the truncation contributes greatly to its comfort.

TABLE 29.2

Lens Power	Prism
+6.00	1 Δ
Pl	1.5 Δ
−6.00	2 Δ

junction of the distant and near sections. When the patient looks straight ahead and the lens is in its lowest riding position, the top of the segment should be tangent to or above the pupil margin in dim illumination. It may be necessary to make a small wax mark at top of the segment to make it more visible to the examiner. The lens should ride with its lower edge at or near the lower lid. If the lens does not position down, possible reasons are the following:

1. Lens is too tight, which can be corrected by—

    a. flattening the peripheral curves

    b. reducing the optical zone diameter

    c. Using a lens with a flatter base curve

    d. Reducing lens diameter, from top and sides (may damage lens)[51]

2. Lens has insufficient prism; in this case add ballast by—

    a. trying a lens with ½ D. more prism ballast

LENS MOVEMENT. With the patient fixating straight ahead, the lens should be picked up 1 mm. to 2 mm. on the blink and then drop back to a lower position. If lens is not picked up at all, tear stagnation under the lens may result. Possible reasons for this follow:

1. Lens is too heavy, which can be remedied by trying—

    a. a thinner lens, if present lens is not already as thin as possible

    b. a lens with ½ D. less prism

2. Lens is too flat; to correct or compensate, try—

    a. a lens with a steeper base curve

    b. a lens with a larger optical zone

LENS ROTATION. Lens should not rotate

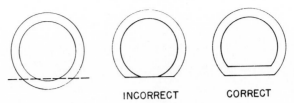

Figure 29.16. A lens is truncated after the peripheral curve is added, which removes the peripheral curve on the lower portion of the lens. This peripheral curve must be replaced to provide proper tear circulation under the lens.

TABLE 29.3

BIFOCAL TRIAL SET

Base Curve	Diameter	Power	Add	Seg. Height
40.00	9 × 9.5	+2.00	+2.00	4.5
40.50	8.8 × 9.2	−2.00	+2.00	4.3
41.00	9 × 9.5	+2.00	+2.00	4.5
41.50	8.8 × 9.2	−2.00	+2.00	4.3
42.00	9 × 9.5	+2.00	+2.00	4.5
42.50	8.8 × 9.2	−2.00	+2.00	4.3
43.00	9 × 9.5	+2.00	+2.00	4.5
43.50	8.8 × 9.2	−2.00	+2.00	4.3
44.00	9 × 9.5	+2.00	+2.00	4.5
44.50	8.8 × 9.2	−2.00	+2.00	4.3
45.00	9 × 9.5	+2.00	+2.00	4.5
45.50	8.8 × 9.2	−2.00	+2.00	4.3

between blinks. If there is rotation, it may be due to the following:

1. Lens's being too large, permitting maximum lid effect on it; therefore—

    a. reduce the lens diameter, from top and sides

2. Insufficient prism, in which case one can—

    a. try a lens with ½ D. more prism

    b. decenter the prism nasally

LENS SHIFT. Observe the patient from a low angle as he shifts his gaze from distance to a near point card. The lens should remain on the lower lid as the eyes shift down. Lift the upper lid and observe the lens shift as the patient lowers his gaze. (Be certain the patient's head remains erect—just as is necessary when using bifocal spectacle lenses.) There must be sufficient space between the top of lens and upper limbus to allow lens to slide up on the cornea when the eye moves down to read. If the lens strikes the upper limbus, it cannot slide up any farther. Hence, the lens is carried down with the eye, and the vision is not directed through the near portion of the lens (Figure 29.17).

REFRACTION. Unless the trial lens is a very poor fit (in which case another lens should be ordered), it should be possible to refract for distance vision through the lens. This correction should be placed in a trial frame (single cell), to be worn over the trial contact lens. The patient can now be shown a reading card and instructed to look from distance to near. Note whether the patient makes the transition quickly and smoothly or whether excessive head tilting is necessary.

Determine any power change needed in the add. This is most easily found by measuring the range of clear vision while adding plus or minus trial lenses. The form found in Figure 29.18 will help guide you in making lens modifications.

Subjective Visual Complaints and Their Correction

The patient's subjective reports are the best method of determining whether the reading segment is correctly positioned and has proper movement.

If the patient reports distance vision to be satisfactory but has difficulty in seeing near—

1. Patient may not be orienting his head properly for bifocal seeing at near, the same as with spectacles. If this is the cause, then

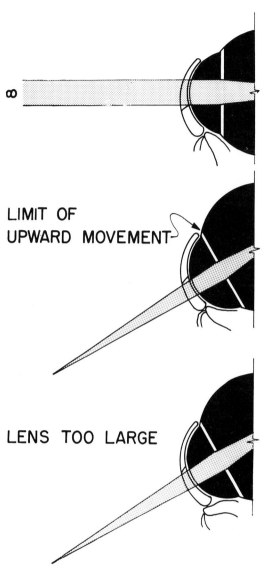

LIMIT OF
UPWARD MOVEMENT

LENS TOO LARGE

Figure 29.17. If a bifocal lens is too large, the top edge of the lens strikes the upper limbus as the eye begins to look downward. If the eye now continues its downward gaze, the lens will be forced beneath the lower lid, and the lid will cover the bifocal segment.

do the following:

    a. Instruct patient to hold head erect.

2. The vertical lens diameter may be too large, thus restricting the lens from moving

up sufficiently. This can be corrected by doing the following:

    a. Reducing lens diameter or more truncation.

3. The lens may be too tight, thus resisting the upward push of the lower lid. Adjust the lens in the following ways to obtain a looser fit:

    a. Flatten the peripheral curves.

    b. Reduce the optical zone diameter.

    c. Try a lens with a flatter base curve.

4. The lower edge of the lens may be sliding under the lower lid, instead of being pushed up by it.

    a. The lower lens edge may have been rounded too much, and if so, it should be flattened.

    b. The bottom truncation should be widened slightly, to present a broader bearing area to the lower lid.

    c. A lens with ½ D. more prism should be tried, since this will have a thicker bottom to contact the lid better.

5. The reading segment may not be high enough, in which case the following should be done:

    a. Order a lens with a greater seg height.

If the patient reports near vision to be satisfactory, but there is blurring at distance—

1. The lens may not be positioning low enough (if not touching the lid), and one can attempt to achieve proper low positioning by doing the following:

    a. Flattening the peripheral curves.

    b. Reducing the optical zone.

    c. Reducing the lens diameter, at top and sides.

    d. Trying a lens with a flatter base curve.

    e. Trying a lens with ½ D. more prism.

2. The seg height may be too high (be sure lens is riding at the lower lid). In order to reduce it one can do the following:

    a. Increase the truncation.

    b. Make diameter reduction to lens bottom and sides.

The following should be recorded:

		Lens Data		
Upper edge of lens R___mm (above, below) top of pupil			R	L
rests approx. L___mm (above, below) top of pupil				

Upper edge of   R___ mm (above, below) bottom of pupil

segment   L___ mm (above, below) bottom of pupil

Refraction (thru   R   Distance _____   Near _____

contacts)   L   Distant _____   Near _____

Rotation (Circle one)   Nil   Slight   Considerable

Lens Data	R	L
B.C.		
P.		
D.		
Seg.		
Add		
Psm.		

Draw lens in its riding position and carefully show the upper edge and segment position.

Figure 29.18. Example of follow-up form for bifocal contact lenses.

      c. Order a new lens with a lower seg height.

If the patient reports blurring following each blink—

1. Lens does not drop rapidly enough.
   a. Flatten peripheral curve.
   b. Flatten base curve.
   c. Increase prism ½ D.

Modification of Bifocal Contact Lenses

Bifocal contact lenses present special modification problems. With concentric simultaneous and alternating vision bifocals, it is possible to reduce the diameter of the distance optical zone, to increase the diameter of the distance optical zone, to decrease the total lens diameter, and/or to modify the

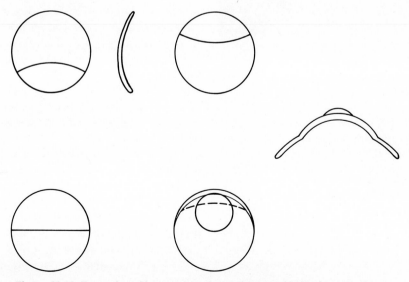

Figure 29.19. Examples of less commonly used types of bifocal contact lenses.

peripheral zones of the lens. With a noncon-centric bifocal, it is possible to alter the shape or truncation of the lens, to lower the height of the segment, and/or to change the periph-eral curve of the ocular surface.

The segment height of a nonrotational bifocal can be lowered by removing a sector from the lower border of the lens. Similar techniques to those of truncating a lens are used to remove the stock from one sector of the lens. If a prism ballast lens tends to rotate upward on the nasal side, the shape can often be modified to reduce the magnitude of the nasal torque (*see* Chapter 15).

It is almost impossible to change the power, the prism ballast, or the shape of the segment line on a nonrotational alternating vision bifocal. Generally all power changes, all segment size and height changes, and similar modifications should be made by the original fabricating laboratory.

Other Bifocals

A large number of other bifocal contact lenses have been invented, many of which present useful and novel forms of cor-rection for a limited number of patients. A few are listed here and are illustrated in Figure 29.19.

1. Variable power: An aspheric concen-tric lens with plus power increasing towards the periphery.[30]

2. Additive bifocal (Piggy Back): A sec-ond wafer, which provides the add, is placed on top of the distance lens.[52,53]

3. Paraseg K: An inside surface prism ballast one-piece bifocal.[54,55]

4. Multifocal or trifocal: Has two or more add areas.[56-60]

5. Pacific bifocal: A molded bifocal.[61]

6. Rectangular bifocal: Rectangular shape with or without a depression at top.[62-65]

7. Offset variable bifocal: Has parabola-like surfaces.[66]

8. Non-index bifocal: Formed from plas-tic of two colors.[67]

9. Biprofile: A concentric one-piece with zones on each surface.[68]

SELECTING THE PROPER PRESBYOPIC CORRECTION

From a practical standpoint, there are three factors of primary concern in selecting the proper contact lens correction for presbyopia.

1. Visual needs
2. Ocular structure
3. Cost and time of fitting

It is interesting to consider the three pri-mary factors in terms of the easiest and sim-plest form of correction. Consider again the five approaches to the correction of presbyopia.

1. Distance correction in contact lenses, near correction in spectacles
2. Monovision contact lens correction
3. Pinhole lens
4. Concentric bifocal
5. Prism ballast bifocal

The following gives the ranking of the preceding forms of correction when consid-ered from the standpoint of providing the simplest and least expensive solution to the problem of presbyopia.

1. Visual needs: 5, 4, 2, 1, 3
2. Ocular characteristics: 1, 2, 4, 5, 3
3. Cost and time of fitting: 1, 2, 3, 4, 5

It will be noted from these rankings that the correction that provides the optimum vis-ual performance ranks in reverse order to the correction which is suitable for the larg-est number of ocular characteristics and which is the cheapest and quickest to fit. In decid-ing on the form of correction for a new patient, the decision is based on the factors of greatest importance to the individual patient.

Although it is impossible to isolate the factors to be considered in selecting the mode of correction, it is often valuable to consider

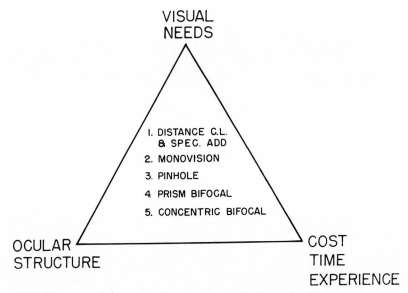

Figure 29.20. The type of correction for a presbyope is determined by the relative contributions of three factors.

first the needs of the patient.[16]

In general, if the patient has a need for considerable reading or other near work, the best solution may be reading glasses. If the patient is not content with wearing spectacles at any time, the best correction will be a prism ballast monocentric contact lens bifocal. If there is intermittent reading but a need for the best visual correction possible because of (1) poor lighting conditions, (2) small print or other requirement for good acuity, (3) frequent shifting of vision from distance to near, (4) residual astigmatism, then use a prism ballast bifocal contact lens. The decision for the type of correction to be used with a patient having heavy demands on his vision will also depend on the other two factors, which must be considered simultaneously.

If the ocular features are favorable for a prism ballast bifocal, it may tip the decision towards this type of correction. If the ocular structure does not favor the use of a prism ballast lens, then the decision must be made for one of the other forms of correction. If the cost or time of fitting is limited on the part of the patient, this will also be a factor

against the use of a prism ballast bifocal.

If a patient has only an occasional need to see near, then the problem of correction becomes easier. The choice of correction may depend somewhat on ocular structure, but probably one of the simpler types of correction, such as a concentric bifocal or pinhole lens, will work in this situation. The decision for the latter type of correction may be based on the lighting conditions for this particular patient. All the factors that contribute to the lens selection are summarized in Figure 29.20.

Other Factors

In addition to the factors already considered in the selection of a form of correction for presbyopia, one must also consider the following.

The personality of the patient is a primary consideration. Just how much of a nuisance the patient will be willing to accept is of prime importance. How the patient will respond if the fitting becomes more difficult than was anticipated is another consideration.

The amount of presbyopia should also be considered as a factor in the decision of the approach to the correction. A very early presbyope should not be considered a good candidate for bifocals or one of the more difficult fitting procedures. A simple temporary solution should be selected until the patient has progressed sufficiently so that he can fully appreciate the effect of a reading addition. If the advantage to the patient is minimal, he will certainly not be willing to accept more than a minimum of inconvenience during the fitting process.

Position of the patient's eyes during work is another factor to consider. If the patient is doing his near task in the reading position, any of the approaches to correction may be suitable. However, if he must read matter to the side or in the upward position, it may be possible to provide a better correction by use of a concentric bifocal or by the monovision technique. If the lighting is very good, this may also be a possible application for the pinhole, but a prism ballast contact lens will certainly not be adequate.

If the patient must work in low illumination but observe illuminated signs, it may present a very difficult problem for any bifocal contact lens correction. A pinhole lens cannot be considered because of the generally low illumination. A concentric bifocal will nearly always produce flare under these conditions. A prism ballast bifocal may be suitable if the lens has adequate shift so that the patient does not have the segment line across the pupil at any time.

If the patient is primarily concerned about the cost or time of fitting, then the correction of choice is probably a monovision. An alternate choice might be a concentric type of lens, but it is doubtful whether a prism ballast lens should be considered here. If the patient has worn regular contact lenses prior to the onset of presbyopia, it is often an intolerable adjustment if a change is made to a prism ballast bifocal lens.

REFERENCES

1. Mazow, B.: Visual problems of the aged, *Am. J. Optom.*, *35(7)*:360–368, 1958.
2. Allen, M. J.: Bifocal prescribing, *Optom. Weekly*, *49(49)*:2303–2306, 1958.
3. Schecter, L.: Some rules of thumb for bifocal contact lenses, *Optom. Weekly*, *50(20)*:1007–1008, 1959.
4. Hermann, J. S., and Johnson, R.: The accommodation requirement in myopia, *Arch. Ophthalmol.*, *76(1)*:47–51, 1966.
5. Neumueller, J.: The effect of the ametropic distance correction upon the accommodation and reading addition, *Am. J. Optom.*, *15(4)*:120–128, 1938.
6. Hersh, D.: A novel modality for management of presbyopia contact lens patients, *Opt. J. Rev. Optom.*, *106(6)*:35–40, 1969.
7. Fleischman, W. E.: The single vision reading contact lens, *Am. J. Optom.*, *45(6)*:408–409, 1968.
8. Ohlbaum, M. K.: Presbyopic contact lens patients, *Opt. J. Rev. Optom.*, *106(9)*:24–25, 1969.
9. McLendon, J. L., Burcham, J. L., and Pheiffer, C. H.: Presbyopic patterns and single-vision contact lenses — Part 2, *South. J. Optom.*, *10(4)*:7–10, 31, 36, 1968.
10. Koetting, R. A.: The importance of simplified procedure in fitting the geriatric contact lens patient, *Contacto*, *13(4)*:42–47, 1969.
11. Beddow, R. D., San Martin III, J., and Pheiffer, C. H.: Presbyopic patients and single vision contact lenses, *South. J. Optom.*, *8(11)*:9–11, 1966. Reprinted in *Mich. Optom.*, *46(3)*:6–9, 1967.
12. Christie, N., and Sarver, M. D.: The effect on stereopsis of a unilateral contact lens add for presbyopes, *O. D. Research Reports*, University of California, 1971.
13. Ong, J., and Burley, W. S., Jr.: Effect of induced anisometropia on depth perception, *Am. J. Optom.*, *49(4)*:333–335, 1972.
14. Cummings, D. G.: An unorthodox procedure which circumvents the necessity for bifocal contact lenses, *Mich. Optom.*, *45(10)*:3, 13, 1966.

15. Brungardt, T. F.: The monovision system for presbyopic contact lens fitting, *Optom. Weekly, 64(2)*:38, 1973.

16. Fonda, G.: Presbyopia corrected with single vision spectacles or corneal lenses in preference to bifocal corneal lenses, *Trans. Ophthalmol. Soc. Aust., 25*:78–80, 1966.

17. Bier, N.: Correction de la presbytie par verres de contact, *Cah. Verres Contact, 14*:6–18, 1967.

18. Bier, N.: Prescribing for presbyopia with contact lenses, *Am. J. Optom., 44(11)*:687–710, 1967.

19. Mazow, B.: The pupilens — a preliminary report, *Contacto, 2(5)*:128–131, 1958.

20. Bailey, N. J.: Special contact lenses and their applications. II. A brief résumé of pinhole contact lenses, *Opt. J. Rev. Optom., 97(1)*:32–33, 1960.

21. Freeman, E.: Pinhole contact lenses, *Am. J. Optom., 29(7)*:347–352, 1952.

22. Wesley, N. K.: A new concept in successful bifocal contact lens fitting, *Contacto, 11(1)*:71–73, 1967.

23. Sefcheck, M. R.: Latest cosmetic bifocal fitting technique, *Contacto, 12(4)*:52–53, 1968.

24. Sefcheck, M. R.: An interim report: field studies of cosmetic bifocal contact lens patients, *Contacto, 11(4)*:56–59, 1967.

25. Wesley, N. K.: *The Multi-Range Contact Lens*, The Contact Lens Publishing Company, 1969.

26. Bailey, N. J.: Special contact lenses and their applications. I. Bifocal lens design, *Opt. J. Rev. Optom., 96(24)*:41–50, 1959.

27. Danker, F. J.: Fitting bifocal contact lenses, *Guild Guide*, pp. 7–9, Dec., 1964.

28. Jessen, G. N.: Bifocal contact lenses — a survey, *Contacto, 6(2)*:53–56, 1962.

29. Goldberg, J. B.: A bifocal contact lens procedure, *Contacto, 5(6)*:218–225, 1961.

30. Jessen, G. J.: New bifocal lens technique results in more comfortable single vision lenses, *Contacto, 5(7)*:237–243, 1961.

31. Reynolds, A. E.: Fitting a bifocal contact lens, *Contacto, 2(2)*:64–66, 1958.

32. Wesley, N. K., and Jessen, G. N.: The sphercon bifocal contact lens, *Optom. Weekly, 49(13)*:583–585, 1958.

33. Davis, H. E.: Technique in the fitting of bifocal contact lenses, *Contacto, 3(3)*:70–71, 1959.

34. Jessen, G. N.: Recent developments in bifocal contact lenses, *Am. J. Optom., 37(8)*:379–387, 1960.

35. Arner, R. S.: A fitting procedure for the Moss-Arner bifocal contact lens, *Am. J. Optom., 42(8)*:464–472, 1964.

36. Arner, R. S.: A simplified design for the Moss Bifocal contact lens, *Am. J. Optom., 40(10)*:629–635, 1963.

37. Collins, I. W.: Preliminary report: A bifocal corneal contact lens, *J. Am. Optom. Assoc., 29(7)*:453–454, 1958.

38. Sellers, F. J. E.: Bifocal contact lenses for all? *Contacto, 7(6)*:27–29, 1963.

39. Morrison, R. J.: Some observations on bifocal contact lenses, *Opt. J. Rev. Optom., 98(7)*:32–35, 1961.

40. De Carle, J.: The De Carle bifocal contact lens, *Contacto, 3(1)*:5–9, 1959.

41. De Carle, J.: Further developments of bifocal contact lenses, *Contacto, 4(6)*:185–193, 1960.

42. Rubin, L.: Correcting residual astigmatism in the bifocal contact lens patient, *Aust. J. Optom., 51(5)*:136–137, 1968.

43. Bronstein, L.: Reverse centrad bifocal contact lenses, *Optom. Weekly, 59(25)*:45–48, 1968.

44. Baldwin, W.: The application of bifocal contact lenses to thirty presbyopes, *Optom. Weekly, 55(26)*:23–27, 1964.

45. Blackstone, M. R.: The fitting of bifocal corneal lenses, *The Optician, 157(4074)*:471–473, 1969.

46. Goldberg, J. B.: A comprehensive method for fitting monocentric crescent bifocal corneal lenses — Part 2, *Optom. Weekly, 60(24)*:23–31, 1969.

47. Goldberg, J. B.: A comprehensive method for fitting monocentric crescent bifocal corneal lenses — Part 3, *Optom. Weekly, 60(25)*:23–27, 1969.

48. Goldberg, J. B.: A comprehensive method for fitting monocentric crescent bifocal corneal lenses — Part 4, *Optom. Weekly, 60(26)*:29–32, 1969.

49. Ziff, S. L.: A new approach to the fitting of bifocal contact lenses, *Contacto, 9(2)*:15–17, 1965.

50. Mandell, R. B.: A no-jump bifocal contact lens, *Optom. Weekly, 58(22)*:19–21, 1967.

51. Gordon, S.: *Bifocal Fitting Manual*, Gordon Contact Lenses, Inc.

52. Taylor, C. McKay: The additive bifocal con-

tact lens, *The Ophthalmic Optician*, *2*(*13*): 637–646, 1962.

53. Breger, J. L.: A new concept in contact lenses for the presbyope, *Optom. Weekly*, *55*(*22*): 22–24, 1964.

54. Genevay, N. C.: Paraseg K inside segment bifocal contact lens, *Optom. Weekly*, *52*(*11*): 515–516, 1961.

55. Genevay, N. C.: A new inside segment bifocal contact lens, *Contacto*, *5*(*2*):59–60, 1961.

56. Jessen, G. N., and Wesley, N. K.: A new development in multifocal contact lenses, *Contacto*, *9*(*3*):11–14, 1965.

57. Soehnges, W. P.: Micro-pupil multifocal contact lenses, *Contacto*, *10*(*1*):4–8, 1966.

58. Soehnges, W. P.: Multifocal contact lenses, *Contacto*, *11*(*2*):7–8, 1967.

59. Soehnges, W. P.: Multifocal micro pupil lens, *Contacto*, *6*(*6*):156–159, 1962.

60. St. Palley, S. L.: The "polivision" multifocal lens—theory and design, *Opt. J. Rev. Optom.*,

96(*7*):40–42, 1959.

61. Green, M.: Preliminary report on a new bifocal lens, *Contacto*, *5*:83–89, 1961.

62. Akiyama, K.: Study of contact lenses for presbyopia, *Contacto*, *4*(*5*):149–152, 1960.

63. Akiyama, K.: Rectangular bifocal contact lens clinical application, *Contacto*, *5*(*11*):349–353, 1961.

64. Akiyama, K.: Clinical application of rectangular bifocal contact lenses (in Japanese), *J. Jap. Contact Lens Soc.*, *7*(*4*):49–53, 1965.

65. Akiyama, K.: The general study of rectangular bifocal contact lenses, *Contacto*, *4*(*10*): 461–467, 1960.

66. Taylor, C. McKay: The offset variable bifocal corneal lens, *The Optician*, *149*(*3860*):287–288, 1965.

67. Wesley, N. K.: Non-index bifocal, *Contacto*, *8*(*1*):22–23, 1964.

68. Moss, H. I.: The bi-profile corneal lens, *Optom. Weekly*, *54*(*18*):801–805, 1963.

ADDITIONAL READINGS

Bayshore, C. A.: You can fit that presbyope, *Cont. Lens Forum*, *2*(*12*):33, 1977.

Bayshore, C. A.: Presbyopia and contact lenses, *Cont. Lens J.*, *6*(*1*):24, 1977.

Beier, C. G.: A review of the literature pertaining to monovision contact lens fitting of presbyopic patients: clinical considerations, *Int. Cont. Lens Clin.*, *4*(*2*):49–56, 1977.

Bronstein, L.: Bifocal contact lenses—principles of fitting *J. Am. Optom. Assoc.*, *47*(*3*):319, 1976.

Brown, H. F.: Presbyopia and soft contact lenses, *Cont. Intraoc. Lens Med. J.*, *6*(*1*):18–21, 1980.

Bryant, P. G.: Construction and manufacture of a fused bifocal lens, *The Ophthalmic Optician*, *13*(*18*):1052–1056, 1973.

Dreyer, V.: The binocular as an indicator for the success and need for unilateral contact lenses, *The Optician*, *168*(*4345*):6–9, 1974.

El Hage, S. G.: Clinical evaluation of the presbycon aspheric contact lens, *Int. Cont. Lens Clin.*, *3*(*2*):65–74, 1976.

Evans, C. H.: Introducing a hydrogel for presbyopes, *Can. J. Optom.*, *41*(*2*):55–56, 1979.

Goldberg, J. B.: The asperic "biofocal" corneal lens—or is it? *Optom. Weekly*, *67*(*32*):885–887, 1976.

Goldberg, J. B.: Basic facts about multifocal corneal

lenses, *Optom. Weekly*, *68*(*27*):34, 1977.

Graves, O. M.: The soft lens for presbyopia, *Cont. Lens Forum*, *3*(*3*):38, 1978.

Hodd, F. A.: Bifocal contact lens practice part one, *The Ophthalmic Optician*, *14*(*7*):315–326, 1974.

Jaggs, M. R. M.: The use of bifocals in contact lens practice, *The Dis. Opt.*, *29*(*18*):67–69, 1977.

Kendall, C. A.: Ultrafocal bifocal contact lens, *Contacto*, *20*(*1*):31–35, 1976.

Koetting, R.: Contact lenses for the graying American, *J. Am. Optom. Assoc.*, *49*(*3*):287–289, 1978.

Kuhwald, E. P.: Bifocal contact lenses, *Cont. Lens J.*, *10*(*2*):18–20, 1976.

Lebow, K. A., and Goldberg, J. B.: Characteristic of binocular vision found for presbyopic patients wearing single vision contact lenses, *J. Am. Optom. Assoc.*, *46*(*11*):1116–1123, 1975.

Mandell, R. B.: A one-piece upsweep no-jump bifocal, *Int. Cont. Lens Clin.*, *1*(*4*):87–99, 1974.

Neefe, C. W.: Physiological optics multifocal aspheric contact lens, *Optom. World*, *64*(*2*):6–8, 1977.

Neefe, C. W.: Physiological optics of multifocal aspheric contact lenses, *The Optician*, *173*(*4485*): 19–20, 1977.

Neefe, C. W.: Prescribing bifocal lenses, *Cont. Lens Forum*, July, 1979, p. 19–21.

Chapter 30

KERATOCONUS

DESCRIPTION

KERATOCONUS IS A noninflammatory progressive conical deformity of the central portion of the cornea. It is characterized by corneal protrusion and thinning, with structural changes becoming apparent in the later stages. The conus varies in degree from a mild form, which may escape the attention of the less sophisticated practitioner, to a pronounced form, easily recognized by visual observation (Figure 30.1). The apex of the conus is usually displaced downward and temporally from the line of sight[1] and gives rise to an irregular astigmatism, which, in the more advanced condition, cannot be adequately corrected by spectacles but which responds favorably to correction by contact lenses. Some authors feel a different clinical form exists that is confined to the posterior cornea.[1-11]

The clinical manifestations of keratoconus most often begin in youth or adolescence, with the highest incidence found at about sixteen years of age.[12] Generally, following onset, there is progression for five or six years; the condition then often remains stationary. However, acute relapses are not uncommon, even in persons thirty-five to forty-five years of age.[13] However, the incidence of progressive cases reduces greatly with age of onset (Figure 30.2). Keratoconus is usually bilateral, with one eye advanced in relation to the other.[14] In unilateral cases, the condition often remains in a milder form.

PREVALENCE

Keratoconus is usually considered to be a very rare condition. Forrest found that at a large London eye hospital the average occurrence was one case in 7,000.[15] Since there is some self-selection by the patients who report to the hospital, it may be assumed that the incidence in the general population is less. However, in a keratoscopic survey of a selected population, the incidence found was 0.6 percent.[16] No follow-up was conducted to confirm the cases located in the survey, however, and it is questionable whether the figure found is at all representative, considering the difficulties encountered with this method of testing.[17]

It is often stated that women are more prone to keratoconus than men. Hall found that 56.7 percent of his cases were females,[18] and Thomas estimated that females comprised about 65 percent of the total cases.[19] However, most recent studies show no significant difference in the incidence between sexes.

ETIOLOGY

The cause of keratoconus is unknown. Several examples of familial incidence provide evidence in support of a hereditary factor;[20,21] but the mode of inheritance varies and is complicated by the possibility of mild forms, which remain undiagnosed. It may be due to a dystrophic condition[22] or to an endocrine or nutritional imbalance.[23-25] The view that an endocrine disturbance may sometimes be an etiological factor is supported by the development of the disease at about the time of puberty and the appearance of the condition in association with endocrine disturbances.[21] Keratoconus has often been associated with various diseases.[21-23,26-29] Many diseases were thought to be causes of keratoconus, but these were probably nothing more than chance relationships.[30] It might well be that keratoconus is a common result of any one of a number of different and separate etiological factors or perhaps a segment of a yet unidentified syndrome.* Ridley has advanced the theory that keratoconus is caused or at least triggered by eye rubbing.[32]

PATHOLOGY

From electron microscopy studies Teng has described the basic pathological processes that accompany the development of keratoconus.[33] In the early stages fragmentation of the basement membrane of the epithelium occurs along with fibrillation and breaks in Bowman's membrane. The death of the basal epithelial cells is very characteristic. The pathological picture is thought to be due to the liberation of proteolytic or autolytic enzymes upon the death of epithelial cells. These proteolytic enzymes affect the collagen fibers, keratocytes, monocytes, nerve fibers, and Descemet's membrane. The loss of collagen fibers may be the major cause of the weakening and protrusion of the cornea.[33]

As the pathological processes continue, the basement membrane and Bowman's membrane, as well as the anterior stroma, show actual destruction in places, with new-formed connective tissue filling these gaps (Figure 30.3).[34] There is marked thinning and bulging of the cornea. Teng states that the thinning is due to the stretching of the cornea and is not a fundamental process of the disease.[33]

CLINICAL APPEARANCE

The diagnosis of an advanced keratoconus is rather simple, but in the early stages it is very difficult.[35] More emphasis is now placed on the early recognition of the condition so that contact lenses may be fitted before significant progression has taken place.[36] Although the fundamental process of the disease is not changed by wearing contact lenses, there is some evidence that a lens will tend to prevent extreme bulging of the cornea and its resultant traumatic effects.[37,38]

Several clues may be discovered during a routine examination, which would lead the practitioner to suspect keratoconus. These are found by the following tests.

History and Symptoms

The main symptom of keratoconus is the decline of visual acuity. The patient may have had many changes in his spectacle lenses because he visited one practitioner after another in the hope of being helped, only to

---

*For a complete discussion, *see* reference 31.

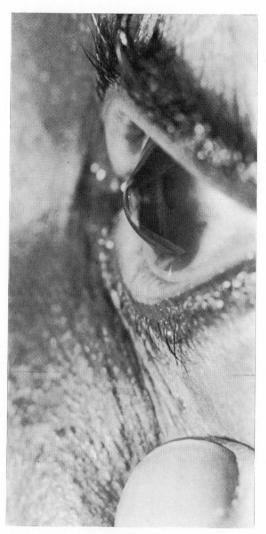

Figure 30.1. Advanced keratoconus. Courtesy of Obrig Laboratories, Inc.

be given another pair of glasses. Sometimes the new glasses do provide an improvement in acuity, but the acuity soon drops again. Changes in the cylindrical power and axis usually occur together with an increase in myopia. In the early stages of keratoconus, general symptoms of asthenopia have been reported; these are possibly due to the sub-

ject's attempts to improve visual acuity by squeezing his lids in order to make artificially a pinhole effect.[18] There may be photophobia or the appearance of halos around lights. In well-advanced keratoconus, monocular polyopia can occur when the irregular astigmatism is extreme; but this does not occur often.

External Examination

In its early stages the corneal apex will show a high brilliance. As the cone advances, its appearance becomes less brilliant and increasingly translucent.

Observing Corneal Profile

The outline of the corneal protrusion can be seen best by standing in front of the patient and raising his upper lid (Figure 30.4). The patient is asked to direct his fixation down until the lower lid margin bisects the cornea horizontally. The curve thus imparted to the lower lid by the cornea is an indication of the degree of conus. This cannot be seen in the early stages.

Ophthalmoscopy

Ophthalmoscopic examination will show a circular shadow separating the red reflex of the central and peripheral areas of the pupil. The fundus picture may be indistinct.

Biomicroscopy

In examination with a biomicroscope,[25,35] the following characteristics may be observed:

1. *Thinning of the cornea* occurs at the apex of the cone. When viewed in section, severe cases may show the anterior and posterior corneal surfaces nearly touching each other.

2. *The endothelial reflex.* The cupping of the endothelium at the cone sometimes induces a brilliant reflex.

3. *Striae.* Within the deep layers of the stroma may be seen a group of short, whitish,

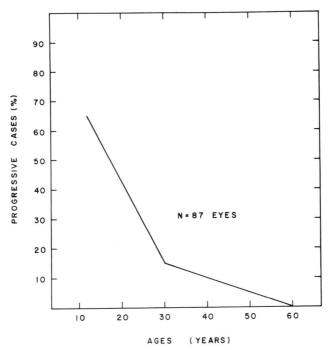

Figure 30.2. Percent of progressive cases of keratoconus. From F. Ridley, Contact Lenses in Treatment of Keratoconus, *British Journal of Ophthalmology, 40(5)*:295–304, 1956.

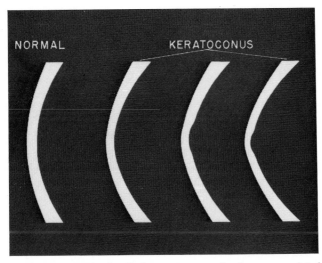

Figure 30.3. Types of corneal thinning in keratoconus varies from a restricted central area of thinning to a broad, general thinning.

vertical or oblique lines. These are probably tension lines caused by stretching the corneal lamellae.

4. *Fleischer's ring.* A yellow-brown or olive

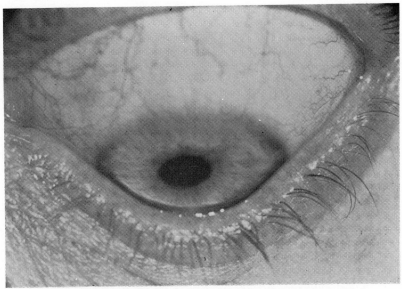

Figure 30.4. Observation of the corneal protrusion (Munson's sign).

green line forms an incomplete ring around the base of the cone in the zone of Bowman's membrane. It is not present in every case of keratoconus.

5. *Ruptures in Descemet's membrane.* When such ruptures occur, they are associated with ruptures of the endothelium and the imbibition of aqueous by the corneal tissues, producing edema and opacification. Upon regeneration of the endothelium, the edema and opacification subsides.

6. *Irregular superficial corneal opacities or scars.* In more advanced cases opacities may form at the apex of the cone. These opacities are found in Bowman's membrane and are due to ruptures in the membrane, which are later filled with connective tissue (Figure 30.5).

7. *Increased visibility of the nerve fibers.* With the beam of the slit lamp focused upon the corneal-scleral junction, many nerve fibers may be seen entering the cornea. It is not likely that the nerve fibers are actually more numerous but only that they are more easily seen due to changes in their density.[19] Since a similar picture is often seen in both the normal cornea and in keratitis, an increased visibility of the nerve fibers cannot be considered a singular distinction of keratoconus.

Retinoscopy

There is a bright central illumination moving against the direction of movement of the mirror. This movement of light is rapid at the periphery and slow at the center of the pupil. It appears to spin or swirl around a point corresponding to the apex of the cone.

Keratometry

In advanced keratoconus, the corneal curvature will usually be greater than 45.00 D., and the mire images usually appear irregular. With very advanced keratoconus, a reading may not be possible. In early keratoconus, the keratometer readings may fall within the normal range. At this stage, a diagnosis can be made by keratometry only on the basis of changes in the keratometry measurements over a period of months or years. Nevertheless, this usually provides

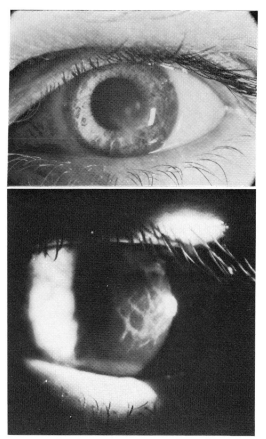

Figure 30.5. Corneal opacities that occur as a result of keratoconus. Courtesy of Obrig Laboratories, Inc.

the earliest diagnosis of beginning keratoconus.

The diagnosis of beginning keratoconus by keratometry may be delayed if the apex of the cone forms at some distance from the line of sight. In this case, the cone may develop considerably before the curvature of the corneal area near the line of sight is affected. Hence, there may be a delay before keratometry measurement changes are detected. In some cases, the earliest clue may come from the appearance of mire distortion rather than from any change in the actual corneal power.

The changes in keratometer readings over a seventeen-year period in a patient developing keratoconus are shown in Figure 30.6.*

Keratoscopy

Although it is not necessary, a verification of keratoconus can be made with a hand keratoscope, also known as a Placido's disc (Figure 30.7). This instrument consists of a target of concentric circle bull's-eye which is held in front of the patient's cornea so that an image of the target is formed by the cornea. The reflection of the target from the patient's cornea is viewed by the examiner through a hole in the center of the target. If the patient's cornea is spherical, or if the

---

*Data contributed by Doctor R. Newmaier.

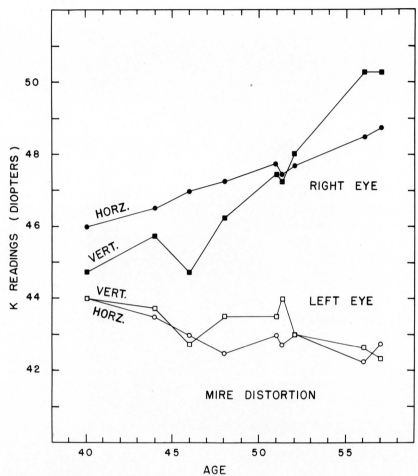

Figure 30.6. Keratometer readings over a seventeen-year period in a patient developing keratoconus.

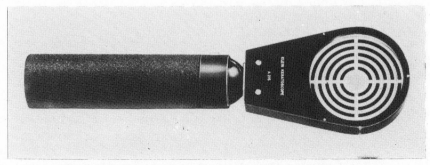

Figure 30.7. Hand keratoscope. Courtesy House of Vision, Inc.

keratoscope is used on a steel ball, the appearance of the reflected target will be that of

perfectly uniform concentric circles. If the cornea is toric, the appearance of the target reflection will be that of concentric ellipses with their long axes coincident to the meridian of flattest curvature. If the eye is keratoconic or irregular, the target reflection has an irregular appearance, which may take on many different shapes. In the early stages of keratoconus, the target reflection may have an egg-shaped appearance. In the later stages, the target has a wavy and very irregular appearance.

Keratoscopes are often recommended as an instrument in detection of keratoconus, but their value in early keratoconus is questionable. The principal problem is due to certain artifacts common to this technique. If the instrument is not held correctly but is tilted with respect to the optic axis of the cornea, an irregularity of the target reflection may be produced, even if the cornea is regular; it is difficult to differentiate this from a keratoconic cornea. It is impossible to make a positive diagnosis of keratoconus by this technique.

Subjective Refraction

The patient may appear to respond poorly to tests of astigmatism. This is due to the irregular astigmatism. Normal visual acuity cannot be obtained with spectacle lenses.

CLASSIFICATION

There is no generally accepted classification of keratoconus. Some authors have described variations in the appearance of keratoconic corneas, which they attributed to different etiology. An exact description of the corneal thickness may be of assistance in differentiating between various keratoconic conditions, if such do exist.

Attempts to classify keratoconus are usually based on a measure of corneal distortion. Amsler discovered the milder form of keratoconus and proposed a classification based on the corneal distortion observed with the keratoscope.[39] From a large series of photokeratographs, Amsler derived a classification of four degrees of keratoconus. First-degree keratoconus shows an angle of 1° to 3° between the two sides of the horizontal axis. Second-degree keratoconus shows an angle of 4° to 8° between the two sides of the horizontal axis. In third-degree keratoconus, skiascopy and ophthalmoscopy are abnormal. The biomicroscope reveals corneal thinning and opacities. In fourth-degree keratoconus, the condition can be diagnosed by simple inspection. Amsler's classification is seldom used. It is subject to some error because it is not only due to the advancement of the cone but to the position of the cone (Figure 30.8).

Haynes and others have pointed out some of the problems in interpreting the topography of the keratoconic cornea.[40] Haynes points out that in some cases, one can establish an approximate axis of symmetry of the cone, which is fairly symmetrical with the base of the cone.[40] He calls the angle between the line of sight and the axis of symmetry of the cone the angle of symmetry and says it is one reproducible characteristic of the cone (Figure 30.9). If one views the mire image reflected from a symmetrical cone, which has been aligned so that the axis of the cone coincides with the optical axis of the keratometer or photokeratoscope, one sees a more symmetrical image than can be obtained when the subject fixates the target directly. Haynes showed how one component of the mire image distortion is the result of the axis of symmetry of the cone not coinciding with the optical axis of the keratometer. This results from the fact that the primary line of sight, which does not coincide with the axis of symmetry, is aligned with the optical axis of the keratometer. If a fixation point is selected that is equal to the angle between the primary line of sight and the axis of symmetry, one can

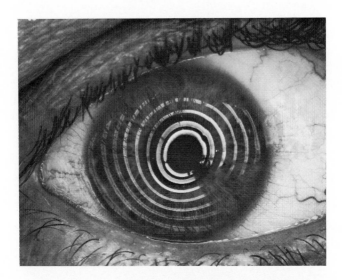

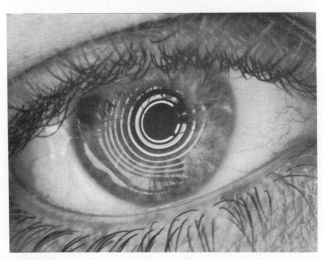

Figure 30.8. Photokeratograms of keratoconic eyes. (*a*) Early keratoconus. (*b*) Moderate keratoconus.

align the axis of symmetry of the cone with the optical axis of the keratometer. This can be accomplished with a small tangent screen wand or a small luminous source as a fixation point, which can be moved about by the examiner. This is more easily accomplished with a fixation device of commercial design.

Mandell and Polse feel that a classification system based on corneal distortion is invalid and that a more meaningful descrip-

tion of keratoconus can be given by the corneal curvature at the apex and the differential corneal thickness.[41] Measurement of changes of these variables provide quantitative evaluation of the conus progression. Corneal thickness measurements can be made with a pachymeter and slit lamp. Their conclusions, based on the use of this instrument are as follows. Their results of corneal thickness measurements on keratoconic corneas and

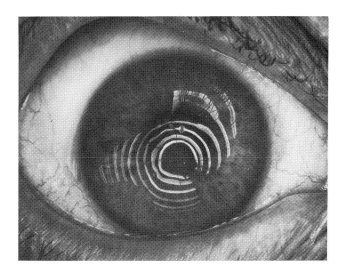

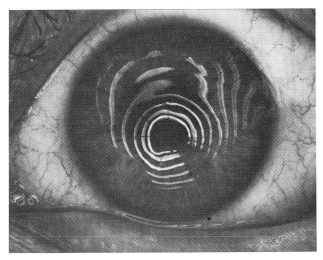

Figure 30.8. (*c*) Advanced keratoconus. (*d*) Approaching the need for keratoplasty.

normals are given in Figure 30.10.

The corneal thickness was measured at 5° intervals along the horizontal meridian of eighteen eyes of keratoconus patients. (From the total sample of twelve patients, six had only one eye included in the data. The other eye was not usable because of a keratoplasty, incomplete data, and two cases of monocular conus of long duration.)

The mean value for the central (minimum) thickness for the keratoconic patients was 0.377 mm. (range 0.13 to 0.505 and SD ±0.11), whereas the mean for the normals was 0.506 mm. (range 0.43 to 0.56 and SD ±0.04). The mean value for normal corneas is slightly lower than other figures that have been presented in the literature and probably occurs because they were using the minimum thickness measurement from each series on a cornea, whereas other studies have measured at a constant corneal position.

The corneal thicknesses for keratoconic

corneas varied considerably. Corneal thickness at its minimum was not pathognomonic, since many keratoconic corneas fell within the range of the normals. However, the differences between the central and peripheral corneal thicknesses were much greater for keratoconic corneas than for normals. This difference is particularly noticeable between the positions of minimum corneal thickness and 35° from this position, where a difference of greater than 0.085 mm. appears to be pathognomonic of keratoconus. The average difference at those positions was 0.165 mm. for keratoconic corneas and 0.062 mm. for normal corneas.

There is considerable variation in the area of corneal thinning. In many eyes the central 2 to 3 mm. of the cornea was very much thinner than the remaining cornea, but the exact point of departure from normal thickness is difficult to determine.

TREATMENT OF KERATOCONUS

MEDICAL TREATMENT

It is occasionally recommended that medical treatment should be given for the improvement of the patient's general health and for the correction of any disturbance of the endocrine system. Although various specific drugs have been reported as effective in the treatment of keratoconus, they are not generally advised, and their value is doubtful.[18]

Radiation has also been used.[42]

SURGICAL TREATMENT

With the success of current methods of fitting contact lenses to keratoconic corneas, surgery is seldom necessary. An operation is indicated, however, when satisfactory vision cannot be obtained by means of contact lenses. Leigh outlines the following indications for keratoplasty:

1. Failure of a contact lens to improve vision because of the development of opacities at the apex of the cone. The decision to operate will rest upon the degree of visual acuity that the patient requires for his work;

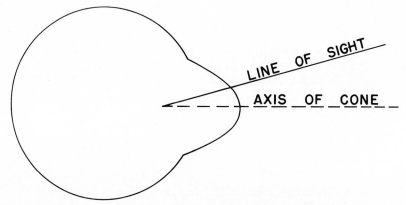

Figure 30.9. The axis of the cone usually does not correspond to the line of sight.

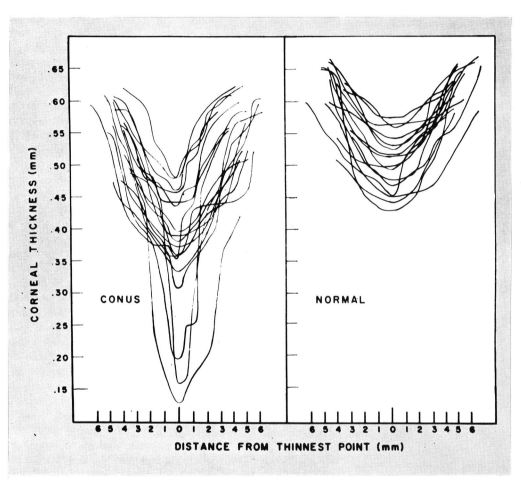

Figure 30.10. Corneal thicknesses along the horizontal meridian for normal and keratoconic eyes. From R. B. Mandell and K. A. Polse, Keratoconus: Spacial Variation of Corneal Thickness as a Diagnostic Test, *Archives of Ophthalmology*, 82:182–188, 1969.

each case must be assessed individually.

2. Thinning of the cornea with the rapid development of progressive ectasia. While perforation is extremely unlikely to occur, the ectasia may develop to such an extent as to involve the greater part of the cornea, producing a condition approximating keratoglobus.[21]

Many operations were formerly advocated for keratoconus, but usually keratoplasty is performed at present. Here the deformed central section of the cornea is replaced by clear corneal tissue that has been taken from another eye. Keratoplasty has proved to be a very successful treatment for keratoconus as evidenced by the high percentage of clear grafts that give excellent corrected vision and a minimum of myopia and astigmatism.[21] In fact, of all the conditions for which perforating keratoplasty is performed, results are most successful in cases of keratoconus.[43-45]

Occasionally, attempts have been made to scar the cornea thermally in a controlled manner to reduce the cone.

TREATMENT WITH CONTACT LENSES

Contact lenses are at present the preferred method of correction and treatment of keratoconus. A contact lens corrects keratoconus in the same way that it corrects other corneal irregularities, that is, by effectively replacing the conus with a regular optical surface. In addition, the pressure of the lens on the conus relieves the bulging of the cornea and also appears to improve the corneal clarity.

Scleral or Corneal Lens Selection

Before the introduction of corneal lenses, scleral lenses were commonly used for keratoconus.[46-52] While they provided good optical results, they often caused adverse physiological effects and were limited to a short wearing time. Zekman and Krimmer demonstrated the advantages of corneal lenses for keratoconus by making a comparison of patients fitted with both haptic and corneal lenses.[53] It was found that corneal lenses provided better visual acuity, reduced incidence of corneal hydrops, few subjective symptoms, and long wearing periods. Most later reports have confirmed their early conclusions, and it is the consensus that corneal lenses are preferable.[54-56]

Corneal Lens Fitting Technique

Early keratoconus can be fitted by standard procedures. The central aspherical area of the more advanced keratoconic cornea cannot be paralleled by a spherical base curve contact lens, so only three fitting relationships are possible. A flat lens may be used, which will rest heavily on the central cornea and have clearance in the periphery; a steep lens may be used, which will give apical clearance and rest entirely on the corneal periphery; or a lens may be used that will rest on both the central and peripheral cornea at the same time (Figure 30.11).[57] Each of these fitting relationships has been tried.

In the past, lenses were often fitted extremely flat in the hope that the pressure would flatten the conical portion of the cornea.[58] Usually good results were obtained when a flat lens was first worn, but ultimately the lens caused severe abrasions to the central cornea. Lenses fitted with apical clearance also produced ungratifying results. Very often the corneal curvature became steeper, and corneal hydrops occurred, which resulted in decreased visual acuity and shortened wearing time. The most successful technique has been one in which the lens is supported mainly by the peripheral cornea but touches the corneal apex lightly. Theoretically this bearing relationship is successful for two reasons. Most of the weight of the lens is supported by the peripheral cornea, where there has been little weakening and thinning. The central cornea is supported by

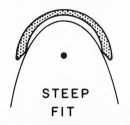 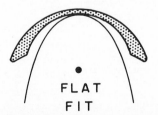 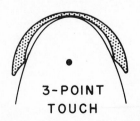

Figure 30.11. Possible bearing relationships of lens to keratoconic cornea.

the light touch of the lens, but the lens does not bear so heavily on the central cornea that it causes further abrasion. With minor variations, this fitting philosophy is represented by the techniques of Moss,[59] Chiquiar Arias,[60,61] and Isen and Filderman.[62] The lenses used are a type of tricurve and have the following average specifications.

Total Diameter

Lenses for keratoconus patients are usually slightly larger than average in order to provide lens support and stability. However, a smaller lens is preferred, providing it is stable. Excessive lens movement and its frictional effects on the central cornea are to be avoided. Average total diameter is approximately 9.0 mm. with most lenses being between 8.5 and 9.5 mm. A smaller lens may be used if it does not show excessive movement.

Optical Zone Radius

The optical zone radius does not have any established relationship to the central corneal curvature as determined by the keratometer. Attempts to measure the keratoconic cornea with a keratometer result in large errors, even when appropriate adjustments are made in the measurement technique for corneal curvatures beyond the range of the keratometer.[63] The separation of the mire reflection areas on the aspherical cornea of a keratoconic eye is too much to allow a valid reading. As mentioned previously, the central keratoconic cornea is aspherical and cannot be paralleled by the optical zone of a contact lens. In addition, the apex of the conus is soft and will easily conform to the shape of any contact lens having an optical zone radius that is approximately the same as the central corneal radius. The optical zone radius is determined by the area of corneal touch that the lens exerts and can be found accurately only by means of trial lenses and fluorescein.

Optical Zone Diameter

The diameter of the optical zone is usu-ally made smaller than average so that the zone can better conform to the aspherical central cornea. The normal range is from 6 to 7 mm., with a large proportion at 7 mm.

Intermediate Curve

The intermediate curve radius should be about 2 mm. flatter than the optical zone radius.

Peripheral Curve

The peripheral curve radius should be about 2 mm. flatter than the intermediate curve radius or 4 mm. flatter than the optical zone radius.

The peripheral curve width is found after the central and intermediate curves have been selected. It is usually approximately equal in width to the intermediate curve width. A fourth curve is sometimes found necessary from the examination of the fluorescein pattern.

Power

The lens power must be determined with the aid of trial lenses. The contact lens that best fits the cornea should first be selected, and then a refraction should be conducted while the lens is worn. Lens power will usually be between −5.00 D. and −15.00 D.

Color

Tinting the contact lens has not been shown to be of any advantage for the keratoconic patient. A light tint is sometimes used as an aid in locating the lens.

Trial Lens Fitting

Trial Lens Sets

Many practitioners attempt to fit keratoconus patients with a trial set having only three or four lenses, but this is not adequate. If only a few keratoconus cases are seen, it may be best not to buy any trial lenses, since a complete set can usually be borrowed from a laboratory.

TABLE 30.1a
KERATOCONUS TRIAL SET

Base Curve	O.Z.D.	I.C.R.	I.C.W.	P.C.R.	P.C.W.	Diam.	tc	Power
6.3	6.5	8.5	0.8	12.0	0.4	8.9	.09	−10.00
6.4	6.5	8.5	0.8	12.0	0.4	8.9	.09	−10.00
6.5	6.5	8.5	0.8	12.0	0.4	8.9	.09	−10.00
6.6	6.5	8.5	0.8	12.0	0.4	8.9	.09	−10.00
6.7	7.0	8.5	0.8	12.0	0.4	9.4	.09	−10.00
6.8	7.0	9.0	0.8	12.0	0.4	9.4	.09	−10.00
6.9	7.0	9.0	0.8	12.0	0.4	9.4	.09	−10.00
7.0	7.0	9.0	0.8	12.0	0.4	9.4	.09	−10.00
7.1	7.0	9.0	0.8	12.0	0.4	9.4	.09	−10.00
7.2	7.0	9.0	0.8	12.0	0.4	9.4	.09	−10.00
7.3	7.0	9.0	0.8	12.0	0.4	9.4	.09	−10.00
7.4	7.0	9.0	0.8	12.0	0.4	9.4	.09	−10.00
7.5	7.0	9.0	0.8	12.0	0.4	9.4	.09	−10.00

TABLE 30.1b
KERATOCONUS TRIAL SET

Base Curve	O.Z.D.	I.C.R.	I.C.W.	Blend	P.C.R.	P.C.W.	Diam.	tc	te	Power
60.00	5.63	6.6	7.5	0.3	8.5	9.5	0.4	8.0	.16	.06	−6.00
59.00	5.72	6.6	7.5	0.3	8.5	9.5	0.4	8.0	.15	.06	−6.00
58.00	5.82	6.6	7.5	0.3	8.5	9.5	0.4	8.0	.15	.07	−5.50
57.00	5.92	6.6	7.5	0.3	8.5	9.5	0.4	8.0	.14	.07	−5.50
56.00	6.03	6.6	8.0	0.3	9.0	10.0	0.4	8.0	.16	.07	−5.00
55.00	6.14	6.6	8.0	0.3	9.0	10.0	0.4	8.0	.15	.07	−5.00
54.00	6.24	6.6	8.0	0.3	9.0	10.0	0.4	8.0	.15	.07	−4.50
53.00	6.37	7.0	8.0	0.3	9.0	10.0	0.4	8.4	.14	.07	−4.50
52.00	6.49	7.0	8.0	0.3	9.0	10.0	0.4	8.4	.14	.07	−4.00
51.00	6.62	7.0	8.5	0.3	9.5	10.5	0.4	8.4	.15	.07	−4.00
50.00	6.75	7.0	8.5	0.3	9.5	10.5	0.4	8.4	.15	.07	−3.50
49.00	6.89	7.0	8.5	0.3	9.5	10.5	0.4	8.4	.14	.07	−3.50
48.00	7.03	7.0	8.5	0.3	9.5	10.5	0.4	8.4	.14	.07	−3.00
47.00	7.18	7.0	8.5	0.3	9.5	10.5	0.4	8.4	.14	.08	−3.00

Designed by Morton D. Sarver

Recommended trial sets are given in Table 30.1.

Trial Lens Fitting Procedure

1. An attempt should be made to make central keratometer measurements, which may serve as a guide in selecting the first trial lens to be used. If a reading is not possible, either because the cornea is too steep or too distorted, the conus is considered as advanced. In this case special corneal curvature measurement procedures need not be used, since the conus has progressed beyond the point where its curvature would provide any useful fitting information.

2. Begin with a trial lens having a base curve that is estimated to be too flat. Place the lens on the patient's eye and verify that

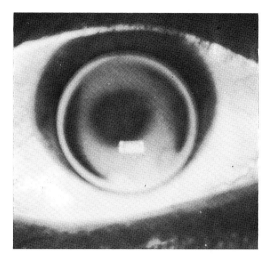

Figure 30.12. Correct fluorescein pattern for keratoconus — large lens.

the base curve is too flat by means of the fluorescein test. Then try a central corneal lens with a steeper base curve; repeat this until a lens is found that has a touch of 2 to 3 mm. as determined by the fluorescein test. With this lens in place observe the fluorescein pattern in the lens periphery. A narrow touch band should be evident at the position of the intermediate curve (Figure 30.12). If the fit is not correct for the intermediate curve, continue to change trial lenses until the proper fit is obtained. The lens that is ordered should have the optical zone radius of the trial lens which gave the correct central bearing and the intermediate curve of the trial lens which best fitted the cornea in the intermediate zone.*

3. The peripheral curve should be flat enough to provide a reservoir of tears around the outside portion of the lens. This curve is critical; if it is too flat, it will stand off the cornea resulting in lid irritation and excessive

---

*It may be noted that the relationship of the lens to the central cornea causes little effect on the fit of the intermediate curve. Even if the optical zone of the trial lens is much too flat for the central cornea, it is found that the thin central cornea is compressed sufficiently for the peripheral curve of the lens to be judged accurately.

lens movement. If it is too steep, it will not provide an adequate reservoir of tears.

4. If a proper fitting is achieved and the lens is nonetheless too loose and slips and slides over the corneal apex, it indicates that peripheral clearance is too great and should be corrected by a steepening of the secondary or tertiary radii. If excessive lens movement cannot be effectively controlled by steepening the trial lens peripheral curve, then the lens should be ordered approximately 0.4 mm. larger than the trial lens used.

Wearing Procedure

The wearing schedule for a keratoconic patient during his adaptation period should be at least as rapid as that of the usual patient. Some fitters feel that wearing time should be increased as rapidly as possible even though a few minor central abrasions are noted. Their purpose is to obtain settling of the lens so that it becomes stable and more easily worn.

Aftercare of Keratoconus Patients

Because of the molding effect of the contact lens on a keratoconic eye, the lens-cornea relationship is in perpetual change, and the fitting procedure is never really completed.

In the early wearing period following the completion of a satisfactory fit of the contact lens, the patient should be seen weekly. Observation should be made to determine if the apex of the cornea is flattening against the lens. This can be most easily determined by the fluorescein test. If the touch area has increased to 4 mm. or more, the lens should be changed to one with a steeper optical zone. Usually, a change of 0.50 to 1.00 D. in the optical zone will be necessary and is determined solely on the basis of the fluorescein pattern.

As the cornea becomes stabilized, the visits can be extended to a monthly basis.

Measurement of Corneal Curvature

Various methods have been used to obtain an accurate measurement of the corneal curvature in keratoconus, including modified ophthalmometry,[63,64] corneal molding, and photokeratoscopy.[65] As mentioned, these methods have little value for the fitting procedure but may be of help in charting the corneal changes that follow the wearing of contact lenses. These methods are discussed in detail in Chapters 3 and 33.

Other Lenses

Small Lenses

Small lenses have been used successfully in the fitting of keratoconus, especially for the milder form.[60] For the most part the general fitting philosophy parallels that used for larger lenses, that is, maintaining a light central corneal touch with a lens which bears mainly on a more peripheral area of the cornea. Since the small bicurve lens usually has a narrow peripheral curve, the principal bearing areas are at the center of the optical zone and near its limiting border. The peripheral curve should show definite clearance. Small lenses used for keratoconus have usually ranged in diameter from 7 to 8.5 mm.[60,64] with a peripheral curve 0.4 mm. wide and 10 mm. radius or flatter.

An advantage of using a small lens is that, because of its light weight, it may be fitted slightly flatter on the cornea without creating harmful pressure on the conus. Consequently, fewer lens changes may be necessary as the conus is reduced by the pressure of the lens. The disadvantage of a small lens for keratoconus is that often the lens is unstable, freely moved by the lids, and occasionally ejected. Such problems can usually be solved only by changing to a larger lens.

Multicurve Lenses

The multicurve contact lens was designed principally for use in cases of advanced keratoconus. Its posterior surface has four or five curves, which gradually flatten in an attempt to duplicate the general contour of a keratoconic cornea (Figure 30.13). They are usually fitted by a trial lens method. Originally the lenses were fitted very flat so that a 4 or 5 mm. central corneal touch was present. More recently, however, there has been a tendency to reduce the touch zone to 2 to 3 mm. by fitting the lenses relatively steeper.[66]

Conic Lenses

Conic lenses have been suggested for this condition.[67]

CONTACT LENSES AS A CAUSE OF KERATOCONUS

It has been suggested that contact lenses may actually be the cause of some cases of keratoconus.[58] There is actually no evidence to support this hypothesis other than that several contact lens wearers have been found to develop keratoconus while wearing contact lenses. Yet, by statistics alone one would expect that out of several million contact lens

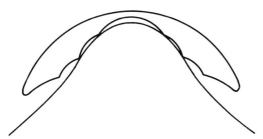

Figure 30.13. Bearing relationship of multicurve lens to keratoconic cornea.

wearers, a few hundred would be expected to develop keratoconus while wearing their lenses. In fact, the incidence of the onset of keratoconus would be expected to be higher in the contact lens population than in the general public for the following reasons:

1. The contact lens population is at the age where keratoconus usually begins.

2. Keratoconus patients usually become myopic before the keratoconus is manifested and may be corrected with contact lenses for the former condition.

REFERENCES

1. Butler, T. H.: Keratoconus posticus, *Trans. Ophthalmol. Soc. U.K.*, 50:551–556, 1930.

2. Tomlinson, A., and Schwartz, C. A.: Position of the corneal apex in keratoconus. *Am. J. Optom. Physiol. Opt.*, 57(1):29–32, 1980.

3. Goldsmith, A. J. B.: Bilateral circumscribed posterior conical cornea, *Trans. Ophthalmol. Soc. U.K.*, 63:180–181, 1943.

4. Butler, T. H.: Slit-lamp inspection, *Trans. Ophthalmol. Soc. U.K.*, 57:32–48, 1937.

5. Wolter, J. R., and Haney, W. P.: Histopathology of keratoconus posticus circumscriptus, *Arch. Ophthalmol.*, 69:357–362, 1963.

6. Leopold, I. H.: Keratoconus posticus circumscriptus, *Arch. Ophthalmol.*, 30(6):732–734, 1943.

7. Forsius, H., and Metsala, P.: Keratoconus posticus, *Survey Ophthalmol.*, 11(2):120–121, 1966.

8. Butler, T. H.: Two rare corneal conditions: I. Acute conical cornea, II. Keratoconus posticus circumscriptus, *Br. J. Ophthalmol.*, 16:30–35, 1932.

9. Jacobs, H. B.: Posterior conical cornea, *Br. J. Ophthalmol.*, 41(1):31–39, 1957.

10. Jacobs, H. B.: Traumatic keratoconus posticus, *Br. J. Ophthalmol.*, 41(1):40–41, 1957.

11. Karlin, D. B., and Wise, G. N.: Keratoconus posticus, *Am. J. Ophthalmol.*, 52(1):119–121, 1961.

12. Ridley, F.: Contact lenses in treatment of keratoconus, *Br. J. Ophthalmol.*, 40(5):295–304, 1956.

13. Hogan, M. J., and Zimmerman, L. E.: *Ophthalmic Pathology*, 2nd ed. Philadelphia, Saunders, 1962, pp. 330–332.

14. Jackson, J.: Conical cornea, or anterior myopia, *J.A.M.A.*, 69:793, 1917.

15. Forrest, J.: *The Recognition of Ocular Disease*, p. 77, cited by Hall, *see* reference 18.

16. Hofstetter, H. W.: A keratoscopic survey of 13,395 eyes, *Am. J. Optom.*, 36(1):3–11, 1959.

17. Levene, J. R.: An evaluation of the hand keratoscope as a diagnostic instrument for corneal astigmatism, *Br. J. Physiol. Opt.*, 19(3):123–138; 19(4):237–251, 1962.

18. Hall, K. C.: Keratoconus—with special reference to its treatment with contact lenses, *Transactions of the International Optometry Congress*, London, Hereford Times Ltd., 1951, pp. 369–389.

19. Thomas, C. I.: *The Cornea*. Springfield, Thomas, 1955, pp. 235–242.

20. Francois, J.: *Heredity in Ophthalmology*. St. Louis, Mosby, 1961, p. 297.

21. Leigh, A. G.: The problems of keratoconus, *Trans. Ophthalmol. Soc. U.K.*, 80:373–396, 1960.

22. Trevor-Roper, D.: *Ophthalmology: A Textbook for Diploma Students*. Chicago, Year Book,

1955, p. 440.

23. Perera, C. A.: *May's Manual of the Diseases of the Eye*, 22nd ed., Baltimore, Williams and Wilkins, 1957, pp. 167, 407.

24. Török, E., and Redway, L. D.: A preliminary report of 3 cases of keratoconus, *Arch. Ophthalmol.*, *57(1)*:19–37, 1928.

25. Appelbaum, A.: Keratoconus, *Arch. Ophthalmol.*, *15(5)*:900–921, 1936.

26. Knapp, A.: Etiology and the treatment of keratoconus, *Trans. Am. Ophthalmol. Soc.*, *27*:63–66, 1929.

27. King, E. F.: Keratoconus following thyroidectomy, *Trans. Ophthalmol. Soc. U.K.*, *73*:31–39, 1953.

28. Samuels, B., and Fuchs, A.: *Clinical Pathology of the Eye.* New York, Hoeber, 1952, p. 82.

29. Shank, W. R.: Monocular coexistence of anterior lenticonus, posterior keratoconus, and congenital nuclear cataracts, *Am. J. Optom.*, *31(12)*:646–651, 1954.

30. Hogan, M. J.: Atopic keratoconjunctivitis, *Trans. Am. Ophthalmol. Soc.*, *40*:265–281, 1952.

31. Duke-Elder, S.: *System of Ophthalmology*. Diseases of the outer eye; Part II: Cornea and sclera. St. Louis, Mosby, 1965, vol. III, pp. 964–976.

32. Ridley, F.: Keratoconus—etiology, pathology and treatment with contact lenses, in Girard, L. J. (Ed.): *Corneal and Scleral Contact Lenses—Proceedings of the International Congress*, St. Louis, Mosby, 1967, pp. 109–115.

33. Teng, C. C.: Electron microscope study of the pathology of keratoconus, *Am. J. Ophthalmol.*, *55(1)*:18–47, 1963.

34. Chi, H. H., Katzin, H. M., and Teng, C. C.: Histopathology of keratoconus, *Am. J. Ophthalmol.*, *42(6)*:847–860, 1956.

35. von der Heydt, R.: Slit-lamp observations on keratoconus, *Trans. Am. Ophthalmol. Soc.*, *28*:352–361, 1930.

36. Warren, E.: Detection of keratoconus, *Contacto*, *2(1)*:32–34, 1958.

37. Levey, E. M.: Contact lenses in 1967: Keratoconus, *The Optician*, *154(3990)*:292–294, 1967.

38. Morrison, R. J.: Keratoconus, aphakia and contact lenses, *J. Am. Optom. Assoc.*, *32(4)*:311–313, 1960.

39. Poster, M. G. et al.: An optical classification of keratoconus—a preliminary report, *Am. J. Optom.*, *45(4)*:216–230, 1968.

40. Haynes, P. R.: Fitting of contact lenses on patients manifesting keratoconus, in *Encyclopedia of Contact Lens Practice*, South Bend, Indiana, International Optics, 1959–1963, vol. 3, Chap. 16, pp. 13–30.

41. Mandell, R. B., and Polse, K. A.: Keratoconus: spacial variation of corneal thickness as a diagnostic test, *Arch. Ophthalmol.*, *82*:182–188, 1969.

42. Hilgartner, H. L., Hilgartner, H. L., Jr., and Gilbert, J. T.: A preliminary report of a case of keratoconus successfully treated with organotherapy, radium, and shortwave diathermy, *Am. J. Ophthalmol.*, *20(10)*:1032–1039, 1937.

43. Martin, W. R. J., and Smith, E. L.: Some points in the surgical technique of keratoplasty, *Am. J. Ophthalmol.*, *55(6)*:1199–1208, 1963.

44. Paton, R. T., and Swartz, G.: Keratoplasty for keratoconus, *Arch. Ophthalmol.*, *61(3)*:370–372, 1959.

45. Wachs, H.: Fitting a tri-curve lens to a conical cornea—case history, *Optom. Weekly*, *44(31)*:1288, 1953.

46. Fritz, A., and Fritz, R.: Fifteen years' experience in equipping keratoconuses with our thin and flexible contact lenses, *Survey of Ophthalmol.*, *9(3)*:357, 1964.

47. Cross, A. G.: Contact lenses: An analysis of the results of use, *Br. J. Ophthalmol.*, *33(7)*:421–445, 1949.

48. Kumar, D., Nath, K., and Nema, H.: Contact lenses in keratoconus, *Br. J. Physiol. Opt.*, *22(3)*:165–169, 1965.

49. Sitchevska, O.: Contact glasses in keratoconus and in ametropia, *Am. J. Ophthalmol.*, *15(11)*:1028–1038, 1932.

50. Golden, D. L.: Correction of keratoconus and high astigmatism with contact lenses, *Opt. J. Rev. Optom.*, *90(18)*:35–36, 1953.

51. Ridley, F.: Scleral contact lenses, *Arch. Ophthalmol.*, *70(6)*:740–745, 1963.

52. Hall, K. C., and Thompson, K.: Some aspects of keratoconus, *Contacto*, *6(7)*:207–211, 1962.

53. Zekman, N., and Krimmer, B. M.: The treatment of conical cornea, *Arch. Ophthalmol.*, *54(4)*:481–488, 1955.

54. Kemmetmuller: Corneal lenses and kerato-

conus, *Contacto,* 6(7):188–193, 1962.

55. Hersh, D.: Modern contact lenses for keratoconus, *Optom. Weekly,* 49(31):1397–1398, 1958.

56. Saliba, N. J.: A case of keratoconus fitted with micro lenses, *Opt. J. Rev Optom.,* 94(24):54, 1957.

57. Williams, C. E.: An interpretation of contact lens variables and a resultant keratoconus technique, *J. Am. Optom. Assoc.,* 31(8):613–616, 1960.

58. Hartstein, J.: Keratoconus that developed in patients wearing corneal contact lenses, *Arch. Ophthalmol.,* 80(3):345–346, 1968.

59. Moss, H.: The contour principle in corneal contact lens prescribing for keratoconus, *J. Am. Optom. Assoc.,* 30:570–572, 1959.

60. Chiquiar Arias, V. et al.: A new technique of fitting contact lenses on keratoconus, *Contacto,* 3(12):393–415, 1959.

61. Chiquiar Arias, V.: Reshaping the cornea in keratoconus, *Contacto,* 8(1):6–10, 1964.

62. Filderman, I., and Isen, A.: A suggested therapy for cases of keratoconus, *J. Am. Optom. Assoc.,* 31(8):623–626, 1960.

63. Haynes, R., and McEachern, C.: Keratometer readings for keratoconus, *Contacto,* 2(1): 35–38, 1958.

64. Williams, C. E.: An interpretation of contact lens variables and a resultant keratoconus technique, *J. Am. Optom. Assoc.,* 31(8):613–616, 1960.

65. Voss, E. H., and Liberatore, J. C.: Fitting the apex of keratoconus, *Contacto,* 6(7):212–214, 1962.

66. Wesley, N. K., and Jessen, G. N.: *Advanced Techniques in Contact Lens Fitting,* 2nd ed. Chicago, The Contact Lens Publishing Co., 1960, p. 45.

67. Thomas, P. F.: The keratoconus patient, *Austr. J. Optom.,* 49(12):364–366, 1966.

Chapter 31

SPECIAL FITTING PROBLEMS

CHILDREN

SELECTION OF PATIENT

AS A GENERAL RULE young children are not fitted with contact lenses simply as a cosmetic substitute for spectacles. If the need for contact lenses is not urgent, it is probably best to delay the fitting until the child is about eight years old.[1] This is a conservative approach and should be followed generally until further information is gathered. An exception might be made for a child actor or performer.

Contact lenses are indicated whenever they would be of advantage in assisting the development of normal binocular vision. They might be helpful for children with aphakia, certain types of strabismus, and the refractive type of anisometropia. Cosmetic contact lenses may have value in cases of ocular disfigurement, albinism, and aniridia.

Children may be divided into two groups: (1) infants and (2) elementary school children. By the time the child reaches high school, the examination and fitting procedures are essentially the same as for an adult, though the psychology of handling the patient may differ.

INFANTS

There are many reports of infants who have been fitted with contact lenses. Sato and Saito described cases of two babies less than a year old who were successfully fitted.[2] They point out that at this early age spectacles would be impractical. The measurements and fitting were done while the babies were under anesthesia. It was recommended that the lenses be worn continuously so that insertion and removal would not be necessary (see Chapter 24).

Fukai cites a number of reasons that would support the use of gas-permeable or conventional hard lenses.[3] First, there is often extreme mechanical difficulty in the insertion and removal of the larger soft lens through the newborn's small palpebral aperture. Since parental acceptance and compliance is the single most important factor in the successful wear of contact lenses by an infant, lens handling and care must be considered when selecting the lens design and material. Second, since the power of the contact lens is usually higher for aphakic infants than for the adult aphakic, hydrogel lenses can only be obtained in limited designs.

Fukai has also argued that metabolic and mechanical disturbance of the cornea are significantly less when employing hydrogel materials.[3] Insult to the cornea is a serious concern; however, it must not be assumed that the metabolic and mechanical disturbances are eliminated as a consequence of using hydrogel materials. The conventional hard material can be meticulously designed, manufactured, and fitted such that the doctor can monitor and manage any disturbance to the cornea. Finally, one must also consider the advantages of working with tinted, as opposed to clear, lenses; not having to contend with residual astigmatism; varying parameters in order to achieve an optimum fit; and providing a more durable and stable material.

It has been argued that, to insure the proper fitting of the complex parameters of contact lenses to a newborn's eye, the procedure must be carried out under general anesthesia. This has been found to be an unnecessary procedure by Fukai,[3] who claims that the clinician will find that, with a little patience (and a lot of careful manipulation), the fitting procedures can be carried out while the infant is asleep or feeding. In fact, the parents are instructed to insert and remove the contact lenses during these quiet times to avoid the possibility (probability) of resistance by the infant.

The optimum contact lens design has been a lenticular rather than a single-cut lens. The advantage of reducing the lens thickness is obvious, and there is the added advantage of having the latitude to maintain an effective diameter in order to achieve lens stability and a peripheral system. The power of the contact lens is prescribed approximately 3.00 D. over the compensating distance prescription so that vision will be at its optimum for near distance tasks.

The fitter must be aware that within the first year or two of life the infant's eye will undergo nearly its full growth to its adult size. Consequently, the relationship between the cornea and contact lens must be continually monitored and adjusted during this time of growth and change. Particular attention should be given to the increase in corneal diameter and the steepening of the corneal radius.

ELEMENTARY SCHOOL CHILDREN

By the time a child starts school, he has often matured sufficiently to participate in a fairly normal fitting routine. Here the problem lies in eliminating the child's fear. Care must be taken that the child has no painful experiences early in the fitting routine. Children's reactions differ, and great skill and psychology are needed by the fitter.

Even when the child is apparently able to take complete care of his contact lenses, the parent should be taught the procedures of contact lens care.

Handling procedure should be discussed in detail, and cleanliness should be stressed, since the child may not understand the necessity for this. It is best to schedule more frequent visits for children, since they are less likely to feel the urgency of any symptoms.

APHAKIA

If a child is to have cataract surgery, usually a contact lens will provide the best postoperative result. Several studies have shown that reasonable results can be achieved with contact lenses.[4] The decision to operate often is difficult to make. Recent studies indicate that the functional prognosis is poorer for total congenital cataracts than for incomplete cataracts.[4] Also, if evidence of good vision was present before the cataract, i.e. traumatic cataract, the prognosis for good vision postoperatively is favorable. Most of the modern operative techniques for juvenile cataracts allow the cornea to heal quite rapidly, and therefore, a contact lens can be fitted soon after surgery.

In fitting the child, it is important to start as soon as the healing is complete. This is so the child can use what vision he has and also to prevent the development of deep suppression or amblyopia.

Basically, the same measurements are required for the fitter (*see* Chapter 27) but may be much more difficult to determine. If the child is under three years of age, it may be necessary to make the initial measurements and tests under general anesthesia. If the child is older, it is usually possible to make measurements in the office. It may be necessary for the child to make one or two visits to the office before any tests are done. These trips are required to help familiarize the child with the office and fitter. Frequently, after the initial apprehensions subside, the child becomes fascinated by the lights and instruments and is most cooperative.

It is important to obtain the best distance correction possible. Any residual error should be incorporated into spectacle glasses. A large bifocal segment for near vision placed at about the inferior pupillary margin should be incorporated into the glasses.

Single cut, lenticular, or hydrogel lenses may be required. The same principles should be used as when fitting adults, except generally small diameter lenses will be required. This is because the child's palpebral aperture is frequently much narrower than the adult's and a larger lens may lead to metabolic interference.

After determining the initial specifications, the lens can be ordered. Usually, if the child is over six, he can be taught to handle the lens by himself. Children under six will usually require the assistance of one of the parents.

Follow-up care is important. A contact lens will probably be worn for the life of the patient; therefore, there can be no interference with the ocular physiology. Since the eye may be undergoing growth changes, it may be necessary to make periodic lens changes. Also, the practitioner must be alert for various postsurgical complications that can develop, such as glaucoma, retinal detachment, or uveitis.[5]

If the corrected visual acuity is relatively good (20/50 or better), an evaluation of binocular vision should be done. In the case of unilateral aphakia, i.e. trauma, the child may experience diplopia or have trouble maintaining fusion. Prisms, orthoptics, occlusion, aniseikonic aids, and/or surgery may be required to achieve the optimum functional result.

MYOPIA CONTROL

Occasionally, reports have been made in which the progression of myopia was said to be retarded when contact lenses were worn.[5-14] Bailey[15] lists various factors that may afford possible explanations for the apparent stability of prescriptions of myopic contact lens wearers: The effects on corneal curvature changes and axial length changes produced by the replacement of the flexible cornea by the rigid plastic material of either corneal or scleral contact lenses, ciliary spasm due to photophobia, settling effects, and common errors that occur in the fitting technique for contact lenses.

EFFECTS OF CORNEAL CURVATURE AND AXIAL LENGTH CHANGES

The factor that is immediately apparent when a contact lens is worn is that most of the power of the cornea as a refractive surface of the eye is eliminated. Hence, any change in the corneal curvature will not be manifested as a refractive change with the lens *in situ.* This in itself explains some reports of myopia control where the examiner merely checked the patient occasionally with the lenses in place, not bothering to do a refraction without the contact lenses. It does not explain, however, the few studies in which it has been claimed that refraction without the lenses was made and that this factor was still controlled.

After a contact lens is worn for an extended period, the cornea will sometimes be somewhat distorted. This distortion is not seen so much with present fitting techniques, but with earlier fitting methods there was a tendency for the lens to flatten the cornea, reducing its power

and effectively compensating for some or all of the myopia.[16] (In a study by Morrison,[5] it was reported that every patient was fitted with a lens of flatter inside-curve than the flattest meridian of the cornea by an amount that ranged from 1.62 D. for corneal type lenses and 2.50 D. for micro type lenses.) Whether the corneal change, which may be as high as 2.00 D., is permanent or not is open to question. It is likely that in most cases the cornea, if left for a sufficient time without lenses, would revert to its former curvature.[17] A corneal flattening would not in itself greatly affect the refractive status when the lens is worn, so it should not affect myopia control with the contact lenses in place.

PHOTOPHOBIA

It has been pointed out that photophobia may be accompanied by a spasm of accommodation, which, when present in the contact lens wearer at the early part of his fitting

period, could result in overcorrection of minus power. It is doubtful, however, that much overcorrection could be accounted for on this basis.

SETTLING EFFECTS

Occasionally, contact lenses appear to exert actual pressure effects on the cornea, which reduce the depth of the anterior chamber and, consequently, the axial length of the

eye. This would tend to produce an increase in the patient's hyperopia or decrease in his myopia. It cannot be said, however, whether these effects are permanent.

ERRORS IN TECHNIQUE

It is coincidental that most of the common clinical errors made during the fitting of contact lenses tend to make the initial correction for a myopic patient too strong. There is a tendency for such an error to go unnoticed by the patient, and it is often not corrected by the fitter. Hence, it may be found that at a later examination the patient does not require any further increase in his minus power. Such evidence is no proof that the contact lenses

have any influence on the rate of myopia progression, as has often been proposed. For example, in a report by Nupuf it was shown that there were few acuity changes in 100 of his contact lens cases over a period of years.[18] This does not prove his conclusion, however, that the contact lens tended to stabilize the myopia. Nupuf's data are plotted on the graph shown in Figure 31.1 along with data from a previous study by the author on the progres-

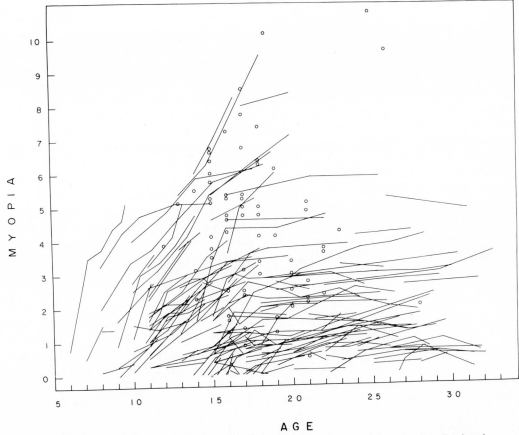

Figure 31.1. Progression of myopia for patients with spectacle correction (*lines*) and refractive errors of subjects of Nupuf (*circles*).

sion of myopia when full spectacle correction was worn. The majority of Nupuf's patients fall at positions on the graph where the rate of progression is also low for spectacle wearers.

A controlled study that will definitely establish the influence of contact lenses on refractive error has yet to be reported. Clinical experience reveals, however, that about 30 percent of patients will progress in myopia after the contact lenses are worn. Unfortunately, they are only occasionally reported in the literature.[19] Newer types of lenses do not exert as great a pressure on the central cornea, and the apparent myopia control will probably be noted less in the future. It is noteworthy that in those cases where myopia reduction was achieved with corneal distortion by the lens, the lenses could eventually not be worn.

Another factor that can be considered in the stability of refractive error is that even when a change in refraction is needed, it can often be made on the same lenses by a simple power modification, so new lenses are unnecessary.

ORTHOKERATOLOGY

Orthokeratology is a procedure for fitting contact lenses in which a deliberate attempt is made to flatten the corneal contour and reduce or eliminate the myopia. There are many variations in technique, but the approach usually consists of fitting a patient with a series of lenses over an extended period of time, each lens having a slightly flatter base curve. The criteria for when a lens change should be made varies considerably depending upon the individual technique of the fitter. Unfortunately, this procedure has suffered from the lack of a well-formulated and clearly defined approach.

The first orthokeratology technique that was introduced was by Jessen[20] and was called *orthofocus*. In this method, a plano lens was fitted flat enough to provide a correction for the refractive error by means of the fluid tear lens. The diameter of the lens was chosen as the minimum necessary to achieve adequate centration. Later techniques have been based on some definite lens-to-cornea relationship. Grant and May advocate fitting a lens initially that is on K to 0.37 D. flat.[21] The diameter is equal to the optic zone diameter plus 1.3 mm., and the center thickness about 0.18 mm. As the cornea flattens, a change in base curve is made, usually in 0.50 D. steps, until the need for a correction is eliminated or the patient requires a low plus power (+0.50 D.). At that point, the wearing time is reduced gradually until the lenses are eventually eliminated.

Several studies have shown that orthokeratology can be more or less successful.[22] There is a question, however, as to how well the procedure can be controlled and whether or not the results are predictable. Binder, May, and Grant found that the average uncorrected vision in a group of orthokeratology patients could be improved from an initial level of 20/120 to 20/40 in a period of twenty-four months.[23] Most of the improvement was actually obtained in the first months of the study. Unfortunately, a majority of the patients did not receive a full correction of their refractive error. Among the eyes whose average spherical equivalent was less than −3.78 D. of myopia, it was possible to reduce the minus power in their correction by 0.3 to 1.50 D. However, an average improvement in refraction by 1.52 D. produced an average improvement in visual acuity of five lines on the chart. This apparent inconsistency may be understood when it is realized that the cornea does not flatten in a regular fashion. Even when the patient is able to read 20/40 on the acuity chart, a loss in the quality of vision may occur.

There are often reports by orthokeratologists that the improvement in refractive error and visual acuity is far greater than that predicted by the change measured in the corneal curvature.[24] Various theories have been put forward to explain this on the basis of changes in other ocular structures, but these appear to be unnecessary. A remolding of the corneal curvature by orthokeratology will often produce an aspherical curve that cannot be easily measured by the usual clinical technique. Keratometry readings are invalid and may not be used as an index of the changing corneal contour. Measurements with small-mire keratometry or photokeratoscopy may be more informative for the important changes that occur in corneal contour. These measurements show that it is the central region of the cornea that is the major contributor to the refractive status of the patient. Measurements with the regular keratometer are sometimes too far in the corneal periphery to give a true indication of the refractive status.

In a study of twenty orthokeratology patients, nine patients were found to have a good response, six had a variable response, and five had no response to the treatment.[23] The variable response was characterized by an improvement in the unaided visual acuity initially but a later deterioration of vision. The patients never achieved an uncorrected visual acuity that would remain throughout the study. The patients who had the best responses tended to achieve their improved vision within the first nine months of the study. In a few cases, however, the best unaided acuity did not occur until eighteen months of lens wear. There were no characteristics among the three groups that would allow a practitioner to predict ahead of time who would respond best to the orthokeratology technique.

There have been few reports of complications with orthokeratology. There does not appear to be any severe physiological effects produced by a flat-fitting contact lens. It must be assumed that this occurs because the lens is fitted only slightly flatter than the cornea to begin with and that changes are made in the base curve at regular intervals. An attempt to fit a very flat lens initially might increase the chances of a central corneal abrasion. In some cases, it has been reported that high astigmatism was introduced as a side effect of orthokeratology. This is probably a function of a fitting relationship and shows the need for close monitoring of the orthokeratology patient. No significant differences have been found in the corneal sensitivity, corneal thickness, anterior chamber depth, or axial length during the orthokeratology process.

ANISOMETROPIA

Patients with anisometropia of moderate or high degree usually benefit greatly from wearing contact lenses. Spectacle lenses present many problems for the anisometrope. When the two eyes are not directed towards the optical centers of the lenses, unequal prismatic displacements of the images occur. To avoid this problem, often the anisometrope learns to turn his head rather than move his eyes. The anisometrope who wears spectacles must often tolerate differences in retinal image size. In addition, because varying degrees of aberration may be present for the two lenses, the general shape of the retinal images may differ.

Contact lenses, for the most part, eliminate the undesirable features of spectacle lenses for the anisometrope.

In fitting the anisometrope with contact lenses, some difficulty may be encountered in achieving a similar type of fit for the two eyes, due to differences in the lens powers.

ANISEIKONIA

Aniseikonia is defined as a difference in the perceptual or *ocular* images of the two eyes. It may be caused by a difference in the optical or retinal images formed by the refractive components of the two eyes[25] or by differences in the distribution of the retinal receptive elements and/or the physiological and cortical processes involved in vision.[26] Aniseikonia in any form will interfere with the ease of fusion of the images from the two eyes. If the aniseikonia is of high degree (over 5% difference in the two eyes), it may contribute to or be the etiological factor in strabismus. If it is of low degree, one eye may be suppressed or various symptoms of discomfort or spatial distortion may be caused. (The latter is more of a theoretical than practical problem.)

There is some disagreement on the incidence of aniseikonia and even more disagreement on when the need exists for its correction.[27] This has been discussed at length and requires no elaboration here. This chapter will be confined to the problem of finding the most suitable type of correction for aniseikonia when it exists to a degree that is clinically significant and requires correction.

Aniseikonia is of concern to the contact lens practitioner for two reasons:

1. Some cases of known aniseikonia (when spectacles are worn) will be relieved by contact lenses.

2. For some patients the fitting of contact lenses may induce aniseikonia where it was not present with spectacles.

SOURCES OF ANISEIKONIA

Very often aniseikonia is associated with anisometropia, but either can exist independently of the other.[28] Whether or not aniseikonia exists in a given case of optically corrected anisometropia depends upon which components of the two eyes cause the difference in refractive error and where the lenses are placed for the correction of the ametropias. If the anisometropia is due to a difference in the axial lengths of the two eyes, an ophthalmic lens correction in the spectacle plane will be very likely to produce retinal images of nearly the same size in both eyes.* If, however, the anisometropia is due to a difference in the refractive power of the two eyes, a correction in the spectacle plane will be likely to produce aniseikonia. Refractive aniseikonia can only be avoided by placing the corrective lenses at the secondary principal planes of the eyes. This can only be accomplished with intraocular lenses, although it can be partially accomplished with contact lenses because of their proximity to the secondary principal planes of the eyes. Consequently, it is of considerable interest to determine the amount of aniseikonia caused by axial differences or refractive differences in the two eyes.

The proportion of anisometropia attributable to either axial or refractive differences was studied by Sorsby, Leary and Richards.[29] They measured the optical components of eighty-seven patients who had anisometropias ranging from 2.00 to 15.00 D. From their measurements they determined what proportion of the anisometropia in each case would be attributed to differences in corneal power, lens power, or axial length. Their conclusions on the group as a whole (quoted verbatim) are of significant interest.

1. In sixty-five cases the axial length contributed to the anisometropia, being the predominant factor in sixty cases, in which it contributed over 50 percent of the anomaly. In no less than fifty-five cases the axial length accounted for at least 60 percent of the anisometropia.

2. In eleven cases the difference in axial length represented a greater difference in refraction than was actually observed. In these cases the cornea counteracted the tendency towards anisometropia; the lens also helped in one case.

3. The cornea by itself counteracted the tendency towards anisometropia in ten cases, but it added to it in another thirteen cases. In all but one of the fourteen cases in which it played a significant part, the lens increased the anisometropia.

There were no appreciable differences in the proportions of the various optical components of the eyes, which contributed to either hyperopic anisometropias or myopic anisometropias.

From the results of this experiment, it may be concluded that for anisometropia of more than 2.00 D., axial length difference is the major contributing factor. Whether these conclusions can be applied to lower anisometropia is not definitely known.

*This is assuming that the spectacle plane coincides with the anterior focal point of the eye. Errors from this source are not always negligible.

INSTRUMENTATION FOR DETECTION

A positive verification of aniseikonia can be made with various instruments that may be used to measure the aniseikonia directly. The instrument most commonly used clinically is the American Optical Eikonometer. It provides an accuracy of 0.25 to 0.75 percent. Unfortunately, few practitioners are sufficiently interested in the problem of aniseikonia to avail themselves of this or other instruments.

SYMPTOMS

The variety of symptoms associated with aniseikonia makes it difficult to attach diagnostic significance to any one of them. The symptoms cannot be distinguished from those arising from some types of ametropia or from accommodation or binocular coordination problems. Typical of the symptoms usually associated with aniseikonia are those reported by Bannon,[30] Table 31.1.

Many of these symptoms commonly occur because of contact lens wearing problems. Consequently, if a contact lens patient manifests aniseikonia, it may be very difficult to determine whether the symptoms should be attributed to the aniseikonia or to a contact lens problem.

METHOD OF CORRECTION

It has been shown that where anisometropia is due to axial differences in the two eyes, spectacle lenses are the method of choice to reduce aniseikonia to a minimum degree. However, where anisometropia is due to refractive differences, contact lenses are the

TABLE 31.1

CHARACTERISTIC SYMPTOMS REPORTED BY 500 PATIENTS REFERRED FOR ANISEIKONIC EXAMINATION

Asthenopia (local eye discomfort, such as fatigue, ache, pain, burning, pulling, tearing, etc.	67%
Headaches (all types)	67%
Photophobia	27%
Reading difficulty	23%
Nausea	15%
Motility difficulty (diplopia, etc.)	11%
Nervousness	11%
Vertigo and Dizziness	7%
General (physical) fatigue	7%
Subjective report of space perception difficulties	6%

From Bannon, R. E., and Triller, W.: Aniseikonia—a clinical report covering a ten-year period, *Am. J. Optom.*, 21(5):171-182, 1944.

method of choice. Since, in general, axial differences contribute most to anisometropia, the correction of choice on a chance basis would be spectacles.

In prescribing eikonic spectacle lenses for aniseikonia, it is usually found that greater success is achieved when the measured aniseikonia is consistent with the refractive error difference in the two eyes. (In other words, if the smaller image is associated with the more myopic or less hyperopic eye.) This information may provide some clue as to whether or not contact lenses will be beneficial in correcting the aniseikonia.

If the measured aniseikonia with spectacle lenses is consistent with the refractive error difference in the two eyes, one of two factors is responsible for the aniseikonia: (1) The difference in the two eyes is refractive (or, more likely, partially refractive), or (2) the anisometropia is axial, but the lenses are not worn at the anterior focal points of the eyes. The latter will be likely to cause less magnification; so large differences in magnification will probably indicate a refractive type of anisometropia, and contact lenses will be the correction of choice. Consequently, contact lenses are probably the best method of correction in cases where aniseikonia has been confirmed with spectacle lenses, but contact lenses are not the method of choice for the correction of anisometropia when no information is available about the aniseikonia.

If the patient manifests appreciable aniseikonia when wearing spectacles, he should be retested while wearing contact lenses. Trial contact lenses will usually suffice for this test, even if the patient has never worn lenses

before. Suitable trial lenses that closely meet the required specifications can be borrowed from the laboratory. The patient should wear the lenses approximately one hour before the eikonometer test is given.

Frequently, a reasonable prediction can be made about whether anisometropia is axial or refractive by comparing the keratometer readings with the refractive errors of the two eyes. If the corneal power is more in the more myopic or less hyperopic eye, it is assumed that the anisometropia is refractive, and the patient should be fitted with contact lenses.

MERIDIONAL ANISEIKONIA

When meridional aniseikonia occurs, it is often associated with differences in the powers or axes of the corneal astigmatism. If a refractive error exists that is consistent enough with high corneal astigmatism to be reasonably sure that the refractive astigmatism is caused by the corneal astigmatism, it may be assumed that any difference between the astigmatism of the two eyes is a refractive difference.

This usually occurs when one eye has astigmatism and the other does not, or when one eye has astigmatism of a greater magnitude than the other eye, or when both eyes have astigmatism with principal axes that do not coincide. If the astigmatism is oblique, with principal axes that do not coincide, a particularly annoying type of aniseikonia is produced which is best corrected with contact lenses.

APHAKIA

Since in aphakia the eye has lost a major refractive component, it may be assumed that the aniseikonia is refractive. Contact lenses

are therefore the most suitable correction (Chapter 27).

CONTACT LENSES VERSUS EIKONIC LENSES

When it has been determined that contact lenses provide the optimum optical correction for a patient, it must be decided whether the patient is a suitable candidate for contact lens wear. This is complicated because the patient is usually not seeking contact lenses and may not be motivated to wear them.

The decision to prescribe contact lenses

to an aniseikonic patient must be made with the same considerations as are made with any contact lens patient. The patient should be advised that contact lenses have these advantages over eikonic lenses.

1. Contact lenses have a better cosmetic appearance. Eikonic lenses are usually thick, heavy, and unsightly.

2. Contact lenses provide a much larger field of view and much less distortion than do eikonic lenses.

3. Contact lenses cost little more than do the eikonic lenses.

4. A large number of practitioners provide postfitting care for contact lenses, but only a few practitioners work with eikonic lenses; thus, postfitting care is more accessible for the patient with contact lenses.

STRABISMUS

Contact lenses have an important contribution to the total care of the strabismic patient, but the number of cases in which they provide a distinct advantage compared to spectacles is limited. It is important to differentiate clearly the types of strabismus that will or will not respond favorably to the use of contact lenses if the optometrist wishes to avoid a considerable number of failures. For example, if the strabismus is constant and combined with anomalous correspondence, there is little reason to anticipate that contact lenses will assist in a functional cure any more than do other methods of correction.

With a few exceptions, contact lenses are useful for the same types of strabismus that benefit from spectacle correction or occlusion. In some cases contact lenses may provide only the same correction as spectacles and are of value only if they also provide a cosmetic advantage over spectacles. In other cases contact lenses may provide a more efficient correction than spectacles. It is toward the latter instances that the major discussion will be directed.

The analysis of the various types of strabismus, their probability of correction, and their most favorable method of correction is too extensive to be covered here. The reader is referred to texts on this subject. A concise but comprehensive coverage has been presented by Flom.[31]

REFRACTIVE ERROR

Some cases of strabismus are corrected by simply making a proper spectacle lens correction. This often occurs (78% successful) when an esotropia is found in combination with hyperopia.[32] Because of the association between accommodation and convergence, the accommodation required to compensate the hyperopia is accompanied by unwanted convergence. If the fusional ability cannot overcome the excessive convergence, esotropia results. By correcting the hyperopia with spectacles or contact lenses, the convergence demand is lessened so that fusion may be possible.

An interesting variation of the preceding example occurs when there is a large amount of convergence, e.g. 8 Δ, associated with each diopter of accommodation (high AC/A). Here it may be found that spectacles or contact lenses correct the strabismus during distance fixation but an esotropia is present for fixation at near distances. The esotropia at near may be corrected by added correction of plus power above the distance correction. This reduces the accommodation necessary to view the near target, which results in less convergence. A correction of the type is commonly given in spectacle form by the use of bifocals. If contact lenses are desired for the distance correction, they may be given together with plus power reading glasses or bifocals with plano distance portion.

It is theoretically possible that an accommodative esotropia at near with hyperopia could be better corrected with single vision spectacle lenses than with contact lenses. This could occur because more convergence is required to fixate a near object with plus power spectacles than with contact lenses.

Since the patient is effectively overconverging, the greater convergence demand by spectacle lenses would require a lower divergence for fusion.

MINUS ADDS

For patients with extropia it is sometimes desired to provide an overcorrection of minus power to stimulate convergence. The minus lenses may be effective in reducing the exotropia in two ways. They may stimulate the accommodative convergence or may initiate reflex changes in the convergence. Usually, the range of added minus lenses prescribed for exotropia is between 1.00 and 3.00 D., with an average of about 2.00 D.[31]

Contact lenses have certain advantages over spectacle lenses when used as minus adds in that less minification of the retinal image is produced.* Contact lenses as minus adds have several disadvantages, however. Usually the minus add is a temporary type of correction, and a change in the contact lenses may entail considerable expense. A lesser problem, but one which might be considered, is that an exotropic myope will be required to converge more at near if contact lenses are worn rather than spectacles.

Regardless of the type of refractive error, proper correction will enhance the sharpness of the retinal images and may provide a greater stimulus to reflex fusional vergence.[31] If contact lenses provide better retinal imagery than spectacles, e.g. irregular astigmatism, it may be assumed they will be more effective in reducing the strabismus.

Monocular occlusion is commonly used as a form of treatment in strabismus. Perhaps its most common application is in treating suppression or amblyopia, but it may also be used to cover one eye in intractible diplopia. When it is anticipated that these treatments will be of short duration, it must be considered whether the problems associated with contact lens wear do not outweigh the advantages.

The contact lens occluder may be either a black lens or an opaque cosmetic lens.[33] The latter is much more expensive, and the fitting is more involved. It should be reserved for a permanent type of occluder. A contact lens occluder has several distinct advantages. It eliminates the cosmetic problem that is so important to children. With the cosmetic problem relieved, the child is more likely to wear the occluder, and better results can be anticipated from the occlusion. The child has no chance to look around his contact lens as he might with a spectacle occluder. In very small children their inability to remove the contact lenses will insure that they are worn.

ANISOMETROPIA

There is a large incidence of anisometropia

*As compared to the blurred image before correction. This effect is independent of whether the ametropia is axial or refractive.

that occurs in cases of strabismus. Flom found that 25 percent of all exotropias have anisometropia.[31] There are special considerations that apply to this group.

ANISEIKONIA

There is reasonable evidence that aniseikonia is an etiological factor in some cases of strabismus. If aniseikonia is present in the anisometropia, its correction might assist in helping the patient to retain fusion.

It is extremely difficult to identify aniseikonia in cases of strabismus. Special testing equipment is usually required, which is not readily available.

Only in anisometropia is it practical to make considerations as to the possibility of the existence of aniseikonia. Here the possible occurrence of aniseikonia is high. However, most anisometropia is of the axial type (*see* the previous section on aniseikonia). If the anisometropia is corrected with spectacle lenses, there is less chance of an aniseikonia being present than if a correction is made with contact lenses. Consequently, from the viewpoint of producing a minimum aniseikonia in an anisometropic-strabismus patient, he should be corrected with spectacle lenses.

On the other hand, other factors must be considered for the anisometropia, which have been discussed.

1. Differential magnification in spectacles may interfere with fusion.
2. Different prismatic effects to the two eyes.

It is not known how significant these factors are.

Often, simply making a proper optical correction with spectacles will assist materially in correcting the strabismus. Flom points out that this frequently occurs even though aniseikonia is present.[31] These patients, however, often show improved binocularity when contact lenses are worn. Flom suggests that because of the difficulty in measuring aniseikonia in children (where this is usually of value), it is best to prescribe spectacles and then observe their effects with time on the binocular anomaly.

One may draw these conclusions with respect to young anisometropes.

1. From the standpoint of aniseikonia, the best correction is probably spectacles.
2. From the standpoint of motor fusion demands and angular magnification, the best correction is probably contact lenses.

The evidence is incomplete on the relative contribution of these factors. On the whole, it cannot be said that there is any advantage to fitting contact lenses but in a few cases. This must be weighed against the problems of fitting contact lenses on children.

COSMESIS

If contact lenses should correct a strabismus, there is usually little need to worry about the motivation of the patient. A young child who has strabismus and must wear glasses, when relieved of both, will usually have such a psychological boost that no other stimulus is necessary. On the other hand, if the strabismic patient is fitted with contact lenses and they do not help to correct his strabismus, he may feel that his strabismus is even more apparent without the spectacles to cover his eyes partially.

CORNEAL TRANSPLANT

The usual indication for contact lenses following keratoplasty is to achieve better visual acuity than can be achieved with spectacle lenses.

The patient who has had a corneal graft presents two problems to the contact lens fitter: a visual problem and a physiological problem. Many transplants leave the patient with a high or irregular astigmatism in the graft. This may be surrounded by a host cornea with different shape characteristics.

Fortunately, in most cases a good optical result is possible with a spherical contact lens. It is rare that a toric design is needed, or even recommended, due to the difficulty in obtaining an acceptable fit.

A much more difficult problem with the graft patient is to obtain a fit that does not cause any physiological harm to the cornea. The difficulty of this task is closely dependent on the success of the graft in matching up with the surface of the cornea. If there is considerable scar tissue, or a significant difference in height between the graft and host tissue, the fitting problem becomes more complex.

It is not possible to describe one particular lens design that is optimum for all graft patients. Usually the lens should have a fairly small diameter, but this is not necessary. Some fitters have recommended that an attempt be made to fit a very small lens within the area of the graft. This is very difficult to achieve and serves no particular purpose, since the lens moves about on the cornea and must cross the scar area with this movement. It is probably wise, however, to have an interpalpebral fit, since the postoperative cornea seems particularly sensitive to pressure on the superior cornea, which is exerted by the lid via the upper portion of the lens. Undue pressure at this area would appear to contribute to neovascularization in some cases.

The primary consideration in the fitting of all graft cases is to find the lens that does not stagnate small pools of tears around the areas of scar tissue or irregular cornea. All other aspects of the fitting relationship are secondary to this consideration. This goal can only be achieved by the use of trial lenses. Keratometer readings serve only as a rough guide to the initial lens. In some cases it may be necessary to use an abnormally flat or abnormally steep lens to eliminate these areas of pooling. If small pockets of pooling are allowed to remain, over a period of time the cornea shows stippling and eventually breaks down with intolerable results.

The patient should be followed carefully during the adaptation period and observed for signs of abnormal staining and possible neovascularization. Other signs of graft rejection should also be looked for.

Since many grafts are performed on advanced keratoconus patients, these usually constitute the bulk of the fitted group. With the exception of the fitting principles described here, other considerations in the fitting routine are the same as for any keratoconic patient.

RED LENS FOR COLOR VISION

Occasionally a special red lens is prescribed for patients with color vision defects.[34,35] The basic concept of this lens is not particularly new. There have been numerous attempts for over one hundred years by various investigators to use spectacle red filters as an aid to the color deficient.[36]

In some cases it may be clearly demonstrated that the use of a red lens, as either spectacle or contact lens, in front of one eye will enhance the patient's ability to discriminate colors. However, this achievement only applies to patients with particular color defects and in a very limited set of circumstances. It by no means provides a correction for the color deficiency.

One situation in which a red lens before one eye is exceptionally helpful is in taking a color vision test using Ishihara plates.[37] The particular design of these plates lends themselves to a testing improvement when a red lens is worn before one eye. The apparent improvement is not nearly as great when the HRR testing plates are used. This occurs because the background of the HRR plates is composed of greyish toned circles that all appear darker when viewed through a red filter. The background of the Ishihara plates is composed of various colored circles, which appear relatively darkened or relatively lightened when viewed through a red lens.

A red filter before one eye appears to have a greater effect for those with green types of deficiencies (deutan) than for those with red deficiencies (protan).

A number of patients experience some benefits from the use of a red contact lens before one eye. This usually occurs under special conditions of color discrimination, and each situation must be evaluated on its individual merits. It should be understood that patients with severe red deficiency (protanopia) may suffer an extreme red loss and that the addition of the red lens may reduce the vision in that eye. If patients attempt to wear the lens under conditions such as operating trains and planes, there is a possible danger involved. Several authors have cautioned against the use of this lens under widespread conditions.[38] It remains a lens to be used for special situations only.

REFERENCES

1. Neill, J.: Contact lenses for young people, in Hirsch, M. J., and Wick, R. E. (Eds): *Vision of Children*, Philadelphia, Chilton, 1963, pp. 361–370.

2. Sato, T., and Saito, N.: Contact lenses for babies and children, *Contacto*, 3(12):419–424, 1959.

3. Fukai, M., and Pollack, S.: Contact lenses for the aphakic infant, *The Optometry Forum*, July/Aug. 1980, U. C. Berkeley School of Optometry.

4. Enoch, J. M.: The fitting of hydrophilic (soft) contact lenses to infants and young children, *Contact Lens Med. Bull.*, 5(3–4):36–47, 1972.

5. Morrison, R. J.: Contact lenses and the progress of myopia, *J. Am. Optom. Assoc.*, 28(12):711–713, 1957.

6. Dickinson, F.: The value of microlenses in progressive myopia, *The Optician*, 133(3443):263–264, 1957.

7. Morrison, R. J.: Observations on contact lenses and the progression of myopia, *Contacto*, 2(1):20–25, 1958.

8. Bier, N.: Myopia controlled by contact lenses, *The Optician*, 135:427, 1958.

9. Carlson, J. J.: Basic factors in checking the progression of myopia, *Optical J. Rev. Optom.*, 95(19):37–42, 1958.

10. Morrison, R. J.: The use of contact lenses in adolescent myopia, *Am. J. Optom.*, 37(3):165–168, 1960.

11. Barksdale, C. B.: The attrition and control of myopia in some selected cases, *Contacto*, 4(8):349–366. 1960.

12. Miller, B.: Can progressive myopia be prevented by corneal lenses?, *Contacto*, 6(7):196–199, 1962.

13. Neill, J.: Contact lenses and myopia, *Transactions of the International Ophthalmology and Optometry Congress*, London, Lockwood, 1962, pp. 191–197.

14. Nolan, J. A.: Progress of myopia and contact lenses, *Contacto*, 8(1):25–26, 1964.

15. Bailey, N. S.: Possible factors in the control of myopia with contact lenses, *Contacto*, 2(5):114–117, 1958.

16. Groppi, J. J., and Mandel, A. M.: Corneal curvature changes after fitting contact lenses, *Contacto*, 2(3):72–73, 1958.

17. Bier, N.: *Contact Lens Routine and Practice*, 2nd ed., London, Butterworths, 1957, pp. 138–140.

18. Nupuf, J. S.: Subjective responses to queries on changes in visual acuity while wearing contact lenses, *J. Am. Optom. Assoc.*, 34(4):297–306, 1962.

19. Stewart, C. R.: Corneal lens diameters and

vertical positioning, *J. Am. Optom. Assoc.*, *34(15)*:1223–1227, 1963.

20. Lilley, J.: Orthokeratology. Overview of eight techniques, *Calif. Optom.*, *6(8)*:7, 11, 1980.

21. Grant, S. C., and May, C. H.: Orthokeratology—a therapeutic approach to contact lens procedures, *Contacto*, 14:3, 1970.

22. Kerns, R. L.: Research in orthokeratology. Part VIII: results, conclusions, and discussion of techniques, *J. Am. Optom. Assoc.*, 49:308–314, 1978.

23. Binder, P. S., May, C. H., and Grant, S. C.: An evaluation of orthokeratology, *Am. Acad. Ophthalmol.*, *87(8)*:729–744, 1980.

24. Grant, S. C., and May, C. H.: Effects of corneal change on the visual system, *Contacto*, *16(2)*:65–69, 1972.

25. Lancaster, W. B.: Aniseikonia, *Arch. Ophthalmol.*, *20(6)*:907–912, 1938.

26. Bannon, R. E.: Space perception—some physiological and psychological aspects, *Am. J. Optom.*, 29:499, 1952.

27. Linksz, A.: Aniseikonia—with notes on the Jackson-Lancaster controversy, *Trans. Am. Acad. Ophthalmol. Otolaryngol.*, *63(2)*:117–140, 1959.

28. Bannon, R. E.: Developments in the field of aniseikonia, *Transactions of the International Optometry Congress*, London, Hereford Times Ltd., 1951, pp. 151–164.

29. Sorsby, A., Leary, G. A., and Richards, M. S.: The optical components in anisometropia,

Vision Res., 2:43–51, 1962.

30. Bannon, R. E., and Triller, W.: Aniseikonia—a clinical report covering a ten year period, *Am. J. Optom.*, *21(5)*:171–182, 1944.

31. Flom, M. C.: Treatment of binocular anomalies of vision, in Hirsch, M. J., and Wick, R. E. (Eds.): *Vision of Children*, Philadelphia, Chilton, 1963, pp. 197–228.

32. Lyle, T. K., and Foley, J.: Prognosis in cases of strabismus with special reference to orthoptic treatment, *Br. J. Ophthalmol.*, *41(3)*:129–152, 1957.

33. Bannon, R. E.: Diagnostic and therapeutic use of monocular occlusion, *Am. J. Optom.*, *20(10)*:345–358, 1943.

34. Zeltzer, H. I.: United States Patent, Method of Improving Color Discrimination, June 22, 1971, No. 3, 586, 423.

35. Zeltzer, H. I.: The X-chrom Contact Lens and Color Vision, *Opt. J. Rev. Optom.*, 110:15–19, 1973.

36. Schmidt, I.: Comments on the X-chrom lens, *J. Am. Optom. Assoc.*, *43(2)*:199–200, 1972.

37. Welsh, K. W., Rasmussen, P. G., and Vaughn, J. A.: Aeromedical Implications of the X-Chrom Lens for Improving Color Vision Deficiencies. Doc F A A-AM-78-22, 1978, U.S. Dept. Transport. Fed. Aviation Admin. Off. Aviation Med., Wash. D.C.

38. LaBissoniere, P. E.: The X-Chrom lens, *Int. Cont. Lens Clin.*, *1(4)*:48–55, 1974.

ADDITIONAL READINGS

Abrams, B. S., and Schmakel, J. G.: Contact lens fitting of infants and children, *Cont. Lens J.*, *8(4)*:6, 1979.

Arnold, S.: Children and contact lenses, *Cont. Lens J.*, *8(4)*:1979.

Baldone, J. A.: The fitting of hard contact lenses onto soft contact lenses in certain diseased conditions, *Cont. Lens Med. Bull.*, *6(23)*:15–17, 1973.

Berk, R. L.: The psychological impact of contact lenses on children and youth, *J. Am. Optom. Assoc.*, *34(15)*:1217, 1963.

Berry, R.: Contact lenses for contact sports, *Optom. Mgmt.*, *11(3)*:16–19, 1975.

Bertulis, A., and Guld, C.: Contact lenses for animals used in vision research, *Vis. Res.*, 15:441–

442, 1975.

Bier, N.: Contact lenses in the case of the very young child, *J. Am. Optom. Assoc.*, *50(11)*:1273, 1979.

Binkhorst, C. D.: Where contactology and pseudophakology meet. With special reference to aniseikonia. *Cont. Intraoc. Lens Med. J.*, *3(2)*:40–51, 1977.

Braff, S. M.: The king (Kong) and I, *Cont. Lens Forum*, *3(1)*:15, 1978.

Brungardt, T. F.: Orthokeratology: an analysis, *Int. Cont. Lens Clin.*, *3(1)*:56–58, 1976.

Cardona, H., and Trokel, S. L.: A soft vacuum lens for foreign body localization, *Trans. Am. Acad. Ophthalmol. Otoloaryngol.*, *76(2)*:521, 1972.

Carney, L. G.: Reshaping the cornea with contacts, *Cont. Lens Forum,* 1(2):16–21, 1976.

Carter, R. T.: Gas permeable lenses—orthokeratology, *Contacto,* 21(4):30–33, 1977.

Catford, G. V., and Mackie, I. A.: Occlusion with high plus corneal lenses, *Br. J. Ophthalmol.,* 52(4):342–345, 1968.

Clements, D. B., and Kauschal, K.: Contact lenses and children: conoid contact lenses in children, *Cont. Lens J.,* 4(6):13–15, 1974.

Cooper, J. S., and Baron, S. J.: Treatment of a divergence excess and amblyopia with orthoptic training and contact lenses, *J. Am. Optom. Assoc.,* 45(6):743–745, 1974.

Daniel, R.: Fitting contact lenses after keratoplasty, *Br. J. Ophthalmol.,* 60(4):263–265, 1976.

Daniel, R.: Post-keratoplasty fitting of contact lenses, *Cont. Lens J.,* 5(8):6–8, 1977.

Davis, H. F.: Use of contact lenses in infants and children *Int. Cont. Lens Clin.,* 2(3):31–38, 1975.

Dickinson, F.: Contact lenses and colour vision, *The Ophthalmic Optician,* 15(22):1001–1012, 1975.

Ditmars, D. L., and Keener, R. J.: A contact lens for the treatment of color vision defects, *Military Med.,* 141(5):319, 1976.

Dreifus, M.: Clinical findings with hydrophilic contact lens in unilateral aphakic children, *Ophthalmologica,* 161(8):279–285, 1970 (in French).

Edwards, K. H.: The management of ametropic and anisometropic amblyopia with contact lenses, *The Ophthalmic Optician,* 19(24):925, 1979.

Enoch, J.: Early surgery and visual correction of an infant born with unilateral eye lens opacity, Dept. of Ophthalmol., Univ. Florida College of Med. Res.

Erickson, P., and Thorn, F.: Does refractive error change twice as fast as corneal power in orthokeratology? *Am. J. Optom. Physiol. Opt.,* 54(9):581, 1977.

Firestone, L. E.: Contact lens use for sports, *J. Am. Optom. Assoc.,* 42(3):279, 1971.

Fonda, G.: Evaluation of contact lenses for central vision in high myopia, *Br. J. Ophthalmol.,* 58(2):141–147, 1974.

Fontana, A. A.: Should age be a factor in selecting candidates for an orthokeratology program?, *Contacto,* 20(1):39–40, 1976.

Fontana, A. A.: Using reverse cycons to control or eliminate corneal astigmatism in orthokeratology, *Contacto,* 22(1):21, 1978.

Freeman, R. A.: Orthokeratology: telling it like it is, *Cont. Lens Forum,* 1(5):43–45, 1976.

Garber, J. M.: Monocular high myopia, *Cont. Lens Forum,* 2(8):38–41, 1977.

Geyer, O.: Contact lenses in the treatment of anisometropia in children, *Contact Lens,* 4(6):24, 1974.

Goldberg, J. B.: Current commentary about contact lenses: corneal lens with opaque periphery, *Optom. Weekly,* 65(29):772–773, 1974.

Grant, S. C.: Philosophy of orthokeratology, *Optom. Weekly,* 66(30):811–813, 1975.

Greenspoon, M. K.: Contacting the incredible hulk, *Cont. Lens Forum,* 3(9):19, 1978.

Gregg, J. R.: Contact lenses for sportsmen, *Field and Stream,* July 1976, p. 96.

Grimm, W., Hilz, R., and Zoller, A.: Tinted contact lenses and color discrimination, *Contacto,* 21(5):9, 1977.

Harris, D. H.: Why orthokeratology is here to stay, *Optom. Weekly,* 66(43):1175–1179, 1975.

Hermann, J.: Traumatic aphakia in children and fusion in the monocular aphake, *Cont. Lens Med. Bull.,* 6(23):18–22, 1973.

Hermann, J. S.: Contact lenses in motor anomalies: practical application of experimental data in the myope, *Cont. Intraoc. Lens Med. J.,* 1(1–2):146–149, 1975.

Hie, O. H.: Soft lens wear in young children, *Cont. Lens J.,* 7(4):2, 1978.

Hirsch, J.: Prescribing contacts for kids, *Optom. Mgmt.,* 11(3):20–26, 1975.

Iwasake, W., and Kozaki, M.: The application of tinted soft contact lenses for children, *Cont. Lens Med. Bull.,* 6(1):25–27, 1973.

Kerns, R.: Orthokeratology, *Int. Cont. Lens Clin.,* 3(2):28–34, 1976.

Kerns, R. L.: Research in orthokeratology. Part I: Introduction and background, *J. Am. Optom. Assoc.,* 47(8):1047–1050, 1976.

Kerns, R. L.: Research in orthokeratology. Part II: Experimental design, protocol and method, *J. Am. Optom. Assoc.,* 47(10):1275–1285, 1976.

Kerns, R. L.: Research in orthokeratology. Part IV: Results and observations, *J. Am. Optom. Assoc.,* 48(2):227–238, 1977.

Kerns, R. L.: Research in orthokeratology. Part V: Results and observations—recovery aspects, *J. Am. Optom. Assoc.,* 48(3):345, 1977.

Kerns, R. L.: Reserach in orthokeratology. Part VII: Examination of techniques, procedures and control, *J. Am. Optom. Assoc.,* 48(12):1541, 1977.

Koetting, R. A.: A beginner's guide to orthokeratology, *Cont. Lens Forum*, 3(6):49, 1978.

Koetting, R. A.: Cosmetic contact lenses in the care of the child, *J. Am. Optom. Assoc.*, 50(11): 1245, 1979.

Koetting, R. A.: A new look at contact lens for the young athlete, *Optom. J. Rev. Optom.*, 111(21):7–9, 1974.

Kolles, B.: Ultrathin contacts in orthokeratology, *Contacto*, March, 1980, p. 31.

Kroll, J. R.: Preliminary report on refractive changes in orthokeratology. Patients using automated refractors, *Contacto*, 21(5):38, 1977.

Levinson, A.: Comparative study of the fitting of hard and Soflens (polymacon) contact lenses on infants and children, *The Optician*, (spec. suppl.), Jan., 1976, pp. 10–14.

Levinson, A., and Ticho, U.: The use of contact lenses in children and infants, *Am. J. Optom. Arch. Am. Acad. Optom.*, 49(1):59–64, 1972.

Lowther, G. E.: A new look at orthokeratology, *Cont. Lens Forum*, 4(3):57, 1979.

Maruo, T.: Application of soft contact lens to strabismus and amblyopia, *J. Clin. Ophthalmol.*, March 1976.

Mavani, M. R., and Mody, K. K.: The concept of the correction of high astigmatism with a combination of hard and soft lenses, *Contacto*, 20(6):31–33, 1976.

May, C. H., and Grant, S.: A three-eyed view of orthokeratology, *Cont. Lens Forum*, 2(3):33–40, 1977.

May, C. H., and Grant, S.: Orthokeratology today: Part II *Contact Lens Forum*, 2(4):25–27, 1977.

May, C. H., and Grant, S.: Orthokeratology today: Part III *Contact Lens Forum*, 2(5):39–41, 1977.

Morris, J.: Contact lenses in infancy and childhood, *Cont. Lens J.*, 8(4):15, 1979.

Nolan, J. A.: Orthokeratology and myopia control, Part IV, *The Optician*, 169(4380):31–35, 1975.

Polse, K. A.: Orthokeratology as a clinical procedure, *Am. J. Optom. Physiol. Opt.*, 54(6):345–346, 1977.

Chapter 32

SCLERAL LENSES

ROBERT FLETCHER AND SOLON M. BRAFF

THE SCLERAL CONTACT LENS was the first contact lens to be invented. However, with the introduction of the corneal lens in 1948, the scleral lens has assumed a lesser role in the contact lens armamentarium. It still fills an important place today, however, in certain cases. The scleral lens should therefore be considered a specialized type of contact lens.

The most important applications of scleral lenses today are the following: (1) advanced keratoconus, (2) cases of irregular cornea, and (3) corneal transplant.

Other applications of scleral lenses today are for the following:

1. The athlete or anyone engaged in sporting activities where significant refractive astigmatism is present. The soft lens will not work in such instances, and it is also possible that a hard corneal lens may be lost.

2. Unilateral aphakia. A corneal lens often drops and induces a base down effect and a vertical imbalance. The scleral lens remains centered.

3. Patients with residual astigmatism who do not respond well to corneal lenses. The scleral lens provides better meridional stabilization so that the axis of the cylinder remains stationary.

4. Cases of corneal toricity where corneal lenses cannot be used. The scleral lens can sometimes be used in these cases. In a scleral lens the base curve can be made spherical, even though the cornea has high toricity, because the lens is supported primarily by the scleral portion (haptic).

5. Lateral prism correction is possible with a scleral lens and not with a corneal lens.

6. In cases of lid pathology, the flange, or haptic section of the scleral lens, keeps the lid from contact with the cornea.

7. Scleral lenses are often useful as a cosmetic lens. An injured eye tends to be slightly smaller than the uninjured eye, and when the scleral lens is used, often there is equilization of eye size. Very often if the eye is not smaller, one tends to get an eye that appears slightly larger than the nonaffected eye. This may be a slight disadvantage.

Scleral lenses also have the advantage that they are easier to insert and remove, and if dropped, they are more easily located. They are often the lens of choice for the occasional wearer because there is much less sensation and less adaptation problem than for corneal lenses. It is difficult for foreign bodies to get under a scleral lens as often occurs with corneal lenses.

Disadvantages of scleral lenses include the following: (1) some types of scleral lenses have limited wearing time (fluid lens), (2) longer fitting times and greater expense, (3) limited availability of lenses and difficulty in lens reproducibility.

The original chapter was written by Robert Fletcher. Various additions have been made to the third edition by Solon M. Braff.

SCLERAL LENS TYPES

Scleral contact lenses are of two general types, impression lenses and preformed lenses .[1-5] The impression lens requires that an impression of the eye be taken, a positive eye model made from the impression negative, and a lens blank be formed to the contour of the eye model. The preform lens requires that the practitioner use numerous trial lenses, which vary in several dimensions.

Scleral contact lenses also may be classi-fied in terms of their intended fitting relationship to the eye, as fluid or minimum clearance lenses. Fluid scleral lenses are fitted so that there is assurance of full corneal clearance by the posterior surface of the lens. The minimum clearance lens is fitted to follow closely the corneal contour. It does not use an auxiliary fluid but depends for its function on the circulation of natural tear fluid.

DESCRIPTION

A typical scleral contact lens consists of three sections: a corneal section, a scleral section, and a transition section. The corneal section is approximately equal to the corneal diameter and provides the optical portion of the lens. The scleral section covers much of the scleral area and provides lens support. The transition connects the corneal and scleral sections and provides clearance at the limbal region, which is necessary for lens function. The transition is determined by a curve or a section of a cone on the posterior surface of the lens. Scleral lens nomenclature is illustrated in Figure 32.1.

EXAMINATION FOR SCLERAL CONTACT LENSES

The examination for scleral contact lenses is essentially the same as for corneal lenses.

After the examination is completed, a choice must be made as to which lens type will

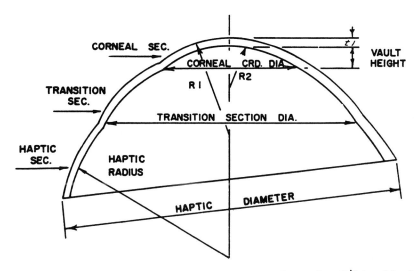

Figure 32.1. Scleral lens nomenclature. From M. D. Sarver, *Contact Lens Syllabus*, 5th ed., 1979. Courtesy of the University of California at Berkeley School of Optometry, Berkeley, California.

be used. This choice is usually based upon the following reasons:

A preformed lens is usually tried first because it is easier to fit. It is possible to judge immediately whether a good fit can be achieved. About the only time that the impression method would be used directly is if there is a highly toric globe. Even then it would probably be wise to try the preformed lens simply to determine whether or not it would fit properly.

Unfortunately, in the United States there is a very limited number of scleral lenses available. A number of lenses are available in England where this lens type remains more popular. Many different scleral contact lenses have been produced, but only a few are available today. A typical example of a modern scleral lens is the Lacrilens®.

FITTING SET

The fitting set consists of sixteen lenses with varying corneal and scleral curvatures. No optics have been ground into the lenses. The set consists of the corneal and scleral curves in Table 32.1.

Corneal Section

There are four curves within the corneal section. The primary curve (7.50, 7.70, 7.90, 8.10) has an 8.0 mm. optical zone or diameter. The second flatter curve has a 10.0 mm. diameter. The third flatter curve has a 12.0 mm. diameter, and the fourth flatter curve has a 14.50 mm. diameter, which is the overall diameter of the entire corneal section.

The preceding diameters are present in all lenses in the four series (Figure 32.2).

A 1 mm. fenestration is located between the primary and second curve at the temporal side of the corneal section.

The fitting lenses can be used for either the right or left eye.

Scleral Section

Each series has four scleral curves, which are progressively flatter ranging from A (steep) to D (flat) in steps of 0.25 mm. (Figure 32.3).

The overall diameter of the fitting lenses is 23.5 × 23.5 mm. The temporal scleral flange is wider than the nasal, superior, or inferior portion. This gives the appearance of an oval lens (Figure 32.4).

Identification

The lenses are identified by the series number (1, 2, 3, 4), which indicates the primary curve of the corneal section. The letters (A, B, C, D) indicate the scleral curvature.

For example, a lens marked 1-A will have a 7.50 primary curve and a 12.25 scleral curve.

TABLE 32.1

Series	Corneal section radius r_2	Haptic radius			
		A	B	C	D
1	7.50 mm	12.25 mm	12.50 mm	12.75 mm	13.00 mm
2	7.70	12.50	12.75	13.00	13.25
3	7.90	12.75	13.00	13.25	13.50
4	8.10	13.00	13.25	13.50	13.75

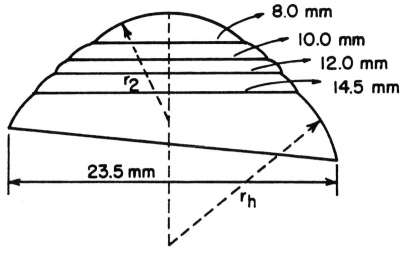

Figure 32.2. Construction of the Lacrilens. From M. D. Sarver, *Contact Lens Syllabus*, 5th ed., 1979. Courtesy of the University of California at Berkeley School of Optometry, Berkeley, California.

FITTING PROCEDURE

Salvatori has recommended the following fitting procedures:

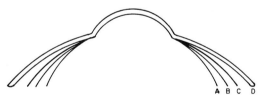

Figure 32.3. Four scleral curves of the Lacrilens.

1. Take keratometer measurements.

2. Select a lens from the fitting set corresponding to, or as near as possible to, the flattest corneal curve.

3. In spherical or nearly spherical corneas, select a lens having a primary curve approximately 0.20 mm. flatter than the corneal radius.

In astigmatic corneas of 3 D. or more, select a lens with a primary curve approxi-

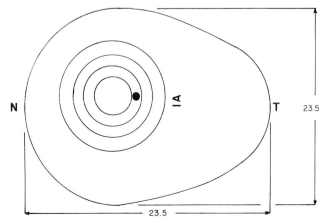

Figure 32.4. Overall dimensions of the Lacrilens.

mately 0.20 mm. steeper than the flattest corneal radius. In some instances the scleral fit from one series and the corneal fit from another series will achieve the desired criteria. It is possible to order a fitting lens with a combination of two series.

For example, if the 7.70 corneal radius (2-D) gives the proper apical and limbal clearance and if the 4-D scleral curve gives the best scleral fit, then the number 2 series with the 4-D scleral radius should be ordered.

4. In small, deep-set eyes, select a lens from the A group; in normal-size eyes, select a lens from the B group; and in large eyes, select a lens from either the C or D group.

5. Clean and thoroughly wet the lens before insertion.

6. Inserting the lens

a. Hold the lens between the thumb and second finger. The index finger rests under the corneal section. The fenestration points toward the temporal side.

b. Patient looks downward.

c. Retract the upper lid by placing the tip of the fingers under the eyelashes and hold firmly against the frontal bone.

d. Place the lens on the superior sclera and slide under the upper lid.

e. Hold the lens on the eye with the index finger only.

f. Gently push the upper lid over the lens and remove the index finger.

g. Hold the upper lid over the lens with the fingers.

h. Instruct the patient to look upward.

i. Retract the lower lid. Do not release the pressure on the upper lid until the lower lid has been retracted and the lens is in place.

7. Checking the lens for size

a. The lens should be kept as large as possible.

b. The lids should not catch the margin of the lens.

c. Upon excursions of the eyes, the lens should not strike the inner or outer canthus.

If a large bubble is present in the corneal

section and does not fill with tears, change to a lens in the same series but with a flatter scleral curve. If none of the flatter lenses eliminate the bubble, then change to a flatter primary curve and use the scleral radius that gave the best fit.

8. Observe the scleral fit under white light.

a. A blanched area at the periphery of the lens indicates that the scleral curve is too steep. A flatter radius should be tried.

b. A blanched area present between the transition zone and the periphery of the lens indicates that the scleral curve is too flat. A lens with a steeper radius should be tried.

9. The best scleral fit should be attained before attempting any adjustments or checking the corneal fit.

Bear in mind that any adjustments made on the scleral portion of the lens can change the corneal fit.

10. Checking the corneal fit

a. If the corneal section is filled with tears, allow the lens to settle for about ten minutes.

b. The tip of a fluorescein strip should be wetted with a solution and applied to the lower cul-de-sac.

Allow the patient to blink several times and to move the eyes up and down and horizontally.

c. Observe the fluorescein reflex with a cobalt light or slit lamp.

d. A greenish yellow reflex should be present between the cornea and the back surface of the lens and should extend to about 1.5 mm. beyond the limbus. The fluorescein reflex surrounding the limbus may be more pronounced than the apical clearance.

e. A dark area indicates a corneal touch or pressure.

f. Disregard any momentary corneal or limbal touches that may appear on excursions of the eyes.

g. If an apical corneal touch is present, change to a lens having a steeper corneal radius.

Changing to a steeper scleral curve will also raise the corneal portion. However, if the scleral fit is good, it is wise to leave it alone.

h. If the corneal clearance is too great and the scleral fit is good, use the lens in the next series having a steeper primary curve.

j. The lens should be completely filled with tears. On excursions of the eyes, bubbles of air will enter, and the lens will refill with tears when the eyes return to primary gaze.

k. Small bubbles are permissible so long as they move on excursions of the eyes.

l. If limbal touches are present, they can be eliminated by grinding with a carborundum stone then polishing with a felt disc and polishing compound.

m. The corneal section of the lens should center over the cornea. If it does not center, check the size. A wide flange can push the lens in the opposite direction thereby creating a corneal touch.

Note: If the fluorescein reflex shows a dumbbell pattern, the laboratory can supply fitting lenses with toric corneal curves.

In some instances the fitter can grind a toric corneal section with the carborundum stone and dental lathe. This is accomplished by grinding the areas of touch. For example, if touches are present nasally and temporally, the corneal section will appear oval in form when the areas of touch are ground and polished.

Scleral Adjustments

The scleral adjustment kit consists of a dental lathe with foot rheostat, several grinding tools, polishing pads, and polishing compound.

If tight areas are present, mark the exact areas of blanching (while the lens in on the patient's eye) with a red grease pencil (Dixon 71) using short straight strokes from the corneal section towards the periphery of the lens.

For pronounced tight areas, the carborun-dum stone is used, and for light tight areas, the rubber point impregnated with grit is used.

The grinding tool is inserted in the handpiece of the dental lathe.

A light rotary motion should be used when grinding. Do not exert pressure. Allow the tool to do the grinding.

To polish the ground areas, allow the felt disc to rotate on the polishing compound until the disc is completely covered with the polishing material.

When polishing the ground areas, do not exert undue pressure, as lens can be scorched.

Repeat this procedure until the tight areas have been eliminated.

Corneal Adjustments

Corneal touches around the limbal area can be eliminated by grinding and polishing. It is important that the exact areas be marked with the grease pencil. It is also important that no ridges be present after polishing the area.

If the diameter of the corneal section is too narrow, the transition zone can be extended by grinding and polishing.

Because the corneal portion has no optics, the fitter need not be concerned with the corneal surfaces.

Removal of Lens

The simplest method for the practitioner to remove the lens from the patient's eye is the hand method.

Removal of Right Lens

1. Instruct the patient to lower the gaze of the eyes.

2. Place the thumb of the left hand (starting at the inner canthus) under the lashes of the upper lid.

3. Raise the upper lid above the edge of the lens.

4. Slide the thumb along the margin of the upper lid toward the outer canthus.

5. While sliding the thumb along the margin of the upper lid, exert slight pressure towards the globe.

6. The upper portion of the lens will separate from the globe.

7. The lens should drop into the open right hand.

Removal of Left Lens

Use the right hand and follow the preceding instructions.

ORDERING LENSES

The fitting lenses are made without optics; therefore, it is impossible to refract the patient while he is wearing the fitting lenses.

The laboratory requires the following information:

Ordering Lenses:
Schedule No. 1

1. Ophthalmometer readings
2. The patient's spectacle prescription.
3. The vertex distance if the spectacle prescription is 5 D. or over
4. The series number of the fitting lens and the scleral curve

Ordering lenses: Schedule No. 2

1. In addition to the information required in Schedule No. 1, send the fitted lens to the laboratory.
2. If a cylinder is required, a horizontal line should be drawn (with a marking pencil) on the lens while it is on the patient's eye.

Note: The laboratory will, if possible, incorporate the prescription on the fitted lens. When the finished lens or lenses are returned, the laboratory will also include one or two fitting lenses to replace the ones used from the fitting set. In the event that it is impossible to incorporate the prescription on the fitted lens due to excessive adjustments, a copy will be made of the fitted lens, and the prescription will be ground on the new lens.

The laboratory will return the copied lens and a new fitting lens for the fitting set. Additional corrections can be added to the lenses if required.

Ordering lenses: Schedule No. 3

In the event an ophthalmometer is not available, the patient should be refracted while wearing a contact lens. Any contact lens, whether corneal or fluid type, will suffice.

The information required by the laboratory is as follows:

1. Radius of curvature of the contact lens
2. The power of the contact lens
3. The additional correction over the contact lens
4. The vertex distance if the power is 5 D. or over
5. The series number of the fitting lens

ENGLISH PREFORMED LENSES

The various dimensions of the back surface of a haptic lens are illustrated in Figure 32.5. The temporal part of the haptic portion is usually made larger than the nasal part in order to avoid contact with the caruncle and plica during convergence. The axis of symmetry joins the centres of curvature of the (spherical) optic and haptic portions. Along this axis the *primary sag* is measured. This sagitta of the back optic surface, which is erected upon the *basic optic diameter*, is a fundamental aspect of the lens geometry. The basic optic diameter is the diameter of the sharp junction between the haptic and optic. In practice, this sharp junction does not exist, as it is modified by the *transition* and by any

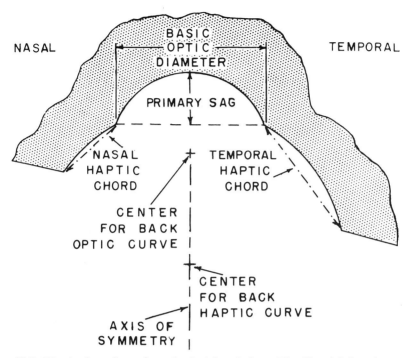

Figure 32.5. The back surface of a spherical haptic lens. The line joining the centers of curvature of the optic and haptic portions is the axis of symmetry.

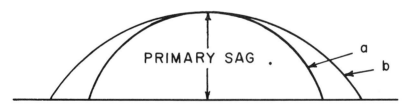

Figure 32.6. Two *optics* of equal primary sag. One (*a*) has a steep curve and a small B.O.D., the other (*b*) has a flat curve but large B.O.D.

peripheral optic flattening that may be employed. The primary sag must be related to the most central of the back optic curves and thus to any central corneal clearance.

The primary sag can be varied either (1) by changing the back central optic radius, (2) by changing the basic optic diameter, or (3) by making both types of changes (Figure 32.6). Figure 32.7 elucidates a simple rule by which different optics of the same primary sag can be identified. Equal additions to the radius and to the basic optic diameter will maintain

the primary sag at a specified value.

Two unequal haptic chords are shown in Figure 32.5. The displacement of the optic, abbreviated by D, is obtained by halving the difference between the two haptic chords. This was formerly called decentration, but it has been more properly called *displacement*, thus avoiding confusion with the usual connotation of decentration in ophthalmic work.

A standard method for the specification of a spherical haptic lens uses a sequence of dimensions that does not vary: (1) back haptic

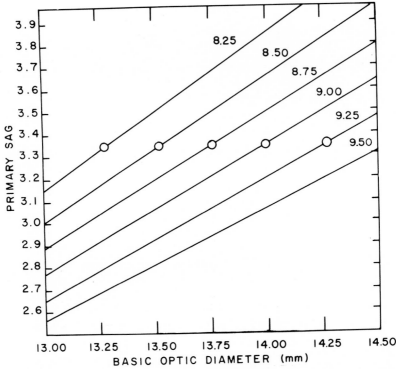

Figure 32.7. Primary sags (approximate) for back optic radii 8.25 to 9.50 in 0.25 mm. steps, each with basic optic diameters 13.00 to 14.50. Note that sags for 8.25/13.25, 8.50/13.5, 8.75/13.75, etc. are virtually identical.

radius, (2) back central optic radius, (3) basic optic diameter, (4) back haptic size, (5) displacement of optic.

A typical lens might be described as follows:

13.75 / 8.75 / 14.00 / 23.50 / D 2

The item *back haptic size* (B.H.S.) is suitably contrasted to overall size in Figure 32.8.

These two dimensions differ by twice the haptic thickness.

The lens in Figure 32.8 has the periphery of the back optic surface flattened; the original curvature remains (with the primary sag unaltered) within the *back central optic diameter.*

CONICAL LENS

A *conical lens* construction is shown in Figure 32.9. Such a lens may be varied in several ways; the *angle of the cone*, the radius of the spherical portion, the optic radius, and the primary sag may each be altered independently.

SPECIAL PREFORMED LENSES

Two preformed designs, in addition to the conventional spherical (or toroidal) design, warrant separate mention. Both can be used in fenestrated form. These are the *offset* and

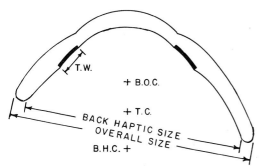

Figure 32.8. Lens with spherical curves. The basic optic diameter (but not the primary sag) has been obliterated by the peripheral flattening of the back optic surface and by adding a transition of width (T.W.) and center of curvature (T.C.) Back optic center (B.O.C.) and back haptic center (B.H.C.) remain as in Figure 32.5.

wide angle lenses. The former was developed by A. J. Forknall, who designed haptics with a series of well-blended curves.[6,7] Such spherical curves are successively flatter towards the periphery of the haptic. For each 1.50 mm.

further from the optic, the radius of the haptic increases 0.25 mm. Taken together they can be matched (in section) by a portion of a circle that has its center of curvature offset to a position distal to the axis of symmetry, hence the name. Haptics of this type are best made by molding to male forms. They are advantageous in several ways; they are relatively steep on the nasal side, and they are comparatively free from flattening of fit (if the back haptic size is reduced). McKellen described the offset lens as "the best preformed lens available."[7]

The wide angle lens combines the spherical or toroidal haptic with a conical transition that clears the globe and is 2 to 3 mm. in width. This departs from the more common *transcurve*, spherical transition favoured by Bier.[8] The wide angle lens differs from the conical lens by providing extensive spherical matching of the globe, even nasally. The cone of the conical lens lies in tangential contact with the bulbar conjunctiva.

SPECIAL APPLICATIONS

Practitioners dealing with a high proportion of pathological eyes almost invariably stress the great utility of haptics, as compared to corneal lenses.[9]

Several surveys of the special indications for these lenses have been made, such as the Doyne Memorial Lecture by F. Ridley,[10,11] which included contact lenses used in investigation and treatment. Corneal lesions caused by mustard gas keratitis, insensitive corneas in cases of facial nerve paralysis, and eyes with burns of all descriptions have benefited from the *protection* afforded by haptic lenses. Considerable assistance is rendered in the restoration of the conjunctival fornices when haptics of increasing diameter are employed. Frequently in pathological cases the physical aspects of the haptic contact lens dominate the optical, and in early stages at least, a shell without a front surface of precise curva-

ture is used.

A special cosmetic application of haptics enables ugly eyes to be covered or squints to be apparently corrected. Such devices strongly resemble artificial eyes. They are fitted over the eyeball, preferably with the aid of a preliminary transparent lens. From the latter, an opaque, painted model is prepared (Figure 32.10). Portions may be made transparent and even optically worked for vision. Albinos and people with aniridia benefit from masking devices in the form of contact lenses. Albinos are often provided with black-lined haptics, superficially resembling the sclera,[12] or with tinted optics. Aniridic cases may have pinhole constructions such as those described by Freeman.[13] Williamson-Noble utilized a haptic lens with a small steneopeic hole to avoid a corneal opacity.[14]

Tinting can be applied to the optic of a

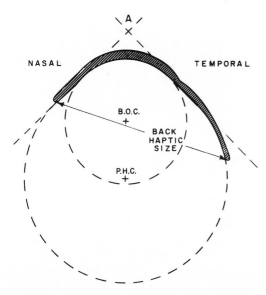

Figure 32.9. Cone lens. The back optic is spherical with its center at B.O.C. The central haptic is conical, of angle A, merging into a spherical peripheral haptic of center P.H.C. on the temporal side.

haptic lens. Dye may be used to color the surface layers, or a lamination of absorbing plastic material may be provided by cementing or by polymerization. In some techniques the appropriate portion of the optic is drilled away completely, a plug of dark material is cemented into place, and the optic is cut from this.

Ocular irradiation techniques employ haptics either by using lead shells with perforations in the required positions or by using an applicator for a radioactive source. The latter, a wire device, is imbedded in the contact lens, and suitable protection is given to other tissues by rings of tantalum wire.[15]

Electroretinography techniques employ haptic lenses fitted with electrodes.[16,17] The size of the lens, its fit, and the position of the electrode are factors that affect the recordings.

The x-ray localization of intraocular foreign bodies frequently demands the use of haptic lenses fitted with small lead inserts. Diagnostic contact lenses of this and other varieties are bulky and are sometimes difficult to keep in position. To overcome this problem, methods of producing a slight vacuum beneath the lens have been devised,[18,19] which gives greater stability and freedom from air bubbles.

Medicinal solutions are applied to the globe by being trapped beneath haptic lenses. J. M. Anderson used a simple design with a perforation,[5] and Klein fitted small tubes to the optic portion for the inlet and outlet of irrigation solutions.[20]

In the study of eye movements, special tight-fitting haptics have been used by Byford[21] and Riggs and Niehl.[22] Mirrors, optical systems, and even miniature lamps have been fitted to haptics for such studies, each moving in phase with the eyeball. Stabilization of the retinal image can be effected by similar means.[23,24]

PRINCIPLES OF HAPTIC FITTING

OPTICAL PRINCIPLES

Corneal and haptic lenses have almost identical optical principles and problems. Modern haptic lenses clear the cornea, leaving an insignificant thickness of tear liquid; consequently, variations in the tear lens thickness seldom arise. In the rare cases where deep liquid lenses are used, e.g. for refraction of eyes whose corneas come outside the trial set range of fittings, there is negligible error in assuming an increase of +0.12 D.S. in liquid lens power for every 0.10 mm. increase in liquid lens thickness. This approximation is suitable for average radii. A lens could have its clearance increased by grinding away the back surface, leaving the back radius the same. The decrease in the thickness of the plastic

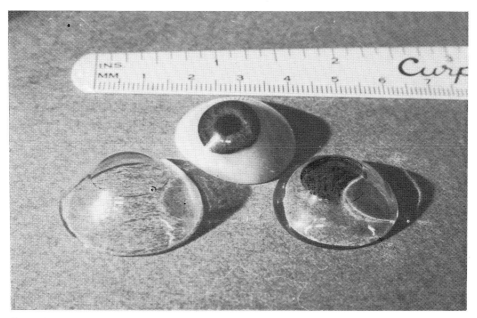

Figure 32.10. Three haptic contact lenses. A typical modern fenestrated preformed lens is on the left. In the center is a cosmetic lens with opaque white haptic complete with blood vessels; this has a painted pupil and iris lodged behind an anterior chamber of clear material, which is about 1.5 mm. thick.

material would account for about −0.25 D. per 0.1 mm.; therefore, if the liquid lens is thickened by the same amount, there would be a net gain of −0.12 D.

In general, considering the ease with which the final lens power can be made more minus, it is safe to add about +0.25 D. when writing the prescription.

Most haptic lenses have a liquid tear lens whose power lies between −2.00 D. and −4.50 D. In most corneal lenses fitted today, the tear lens is between −1.00 D. and +1.00 D.[25,26] The disposition of the liquid lens in the corneal lens thus scarcely alters as the lens moves across the cornea; the optic center of the plastic lens moves, but the optical center of the liquid lens remains stationary. When a haptic lens lags, both the contact lens and the liquid lens are decentered from the original axis; the haptic lens may slide down, resting on the part of the globe formed by the sclera. Figure 32.11 shows the difference that may be expected between the two lens types; a haptic

lens tends to produce more base down prism than the corresponding corneal lens, assuming that each drops by the same amount.

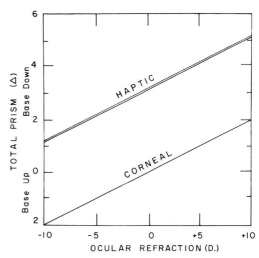

Figure 32.11. Prismatic effect due to drop of 2 mm. Haptic lens 8.50 back optic radius, liquid lens 3 D. Corneal lens liquid lens afocal.

FITTING THE HAPTIC PORTION

In fitting the haptic portion, an attempt is made to keep the pressure on the sclera uniformly distributed. Absence of tight areas when the eye is in the primary position is desirable. The insertions of the recti muscles exhibit variable areas that become slightly tight upon relaxation of the particular muscle. The lids should be separated in order to view the lens in position; gentle pressure from fingers or a small strip of transparent plastic material is applied to imitate lid pressure and to augment gravity. Arcs of pressure may be detected at a transition or at the edge; they must be eradicated. Upon removal of the lens, the bulbar conjunctiva should not exhibit a grossly marked and persistent pattern where the haptic has rested.

Looseness of the haptic is usually inadvisable, as bubbles, perhaps froth-forming, may occur. However, with nonfenestrated lenses, it is sometimes permissible to have a slight looseness; in some lenses channels are gouged in the back haptic surface to aid tear passage.

Edges of haptic lenses must not irritate the lids, nor must they persistently be caught by the lids.

FITTING THE OPTIC PORTION

Corneal clearance should exist, increasing slightly toward the periphery. Touch is normally objectionable due to the likelihood of corneal distortion and the possibility of corneal damage. The symptoms of corneal touch are similar to those of a foreign body in the conjunctival sac—pain, photophobia, and lacrimation, accompanied by injection of the bulbar conjunctiva and eventual swelling of the perilimbal tissues.

Excessive corneal clearance is unwarranted. It promotes annoying bubbles behind the lens. In a nonfenestrated lens, a tear lens that is too deep results, thus encouraging the formation of Sattler's veil.

FITTING THE TRANSITION

Clearance of the limbal tissues is of general importance. Clearance should be maintained during all but extreme eye movements. Care must be taken to avoid the superior (twelve o'clock) part of the limbus because such contact would transfer much of the total weight of the lens to the cornea. Caution must be taken to avoid slight edema or, alternatively, to avoid a mechanical bunching of the loose perilimbal conjunctiva. Lack of bridging in the limbus tends to cause inadequate diffusion and flow of fluids in and out of the optic. Excessive limbal clearance encourages bubbles to form in the optic and tends to cause lens lag.

ADDITIONAL FACTORS

Size

Too large a lens, even if it is presumed to fit, may restrict the field of fixation or of comfortable fixation. A very large lens will be awkward to insert into the conjunctival sac and exasperating to remove.

Too small a back haptic size tends to lack support, to promote undesirable cyclorotation of the lens, to catch the lower lid, and to create unpleasant visibility of the lens edges.

Displacement

The displacement of the optic is calculated by measuring half the difference between the two haptic cords. The optic concentric with a haptic (the two being projected into the same plane) is seldom used even in trial and diagnostic lenses. The nasal part of the haptic must be the smaller part except in atypical cases such as divergent squints. Testing with a reasonably fitting trial lens in place assists in the evaluation of the lag due to the lens inertia.

Bubbles

Monocular diplopia is a difficulty sometimes experienced when a bubble is large. It is related to the position, the mobility, and the size of the bubble and to the pupil size and position.

A bubble is produced behind a correctly fitting haptic lens. It is approximately the shape of a thin kidney bean, is restricted to the lower temporal transition (intruding slightly into the optic) in the primary position, and communicates with the atmosphere through the fenestration. During eye movements the bubble might shift away from the direction of gaze. Sometimes it rests higher than usual without any trouble. It should not cause a click sound when passing in and out of the fenestration.

Nonfenestrated lenses require much care in preventing excessive air bubbles from forming beneath the haptic in the space reserved for the liquid lens. Fenestrated lenses also require .care in controlling the formation of bubbles, especially in toroidal and irregular corneas. Not all bubbles are annoying, but the practitioner must introduce his patient to the bubble well before the patient takes the initiative and starts to comment, even to complain, about the appearance and subjective aspects of the bubble. Corneal respiration is certainly assisted by the bubble.

Fenestration

A lens fenestration must occupy a position that is exposed to the atmosphere. A position corresponding to the maximum limbal clearance within the palpebral aperture is preferred, which is usually temporal. Regard to cosmetic appearance locates the perforation almost at the lower rim of the upper lid, where it may be hidden by the cilia. If the lens rotates so that the lid seals the hole, this should be remedied by placing another hole in an exposed position. Nasal positioning of the hole may result in epithelial disturbance when the nasal optic touches heavily or frequently.

TOLERANCES

Suitable tolerances for dimensions are as follows (all in mm.):

Back haptic radius	±0.1
Back optic radius	+0.03 (flatter than ordered) to −0.05 (steeper than ordered)
Back optic diameter	+0.08 to −0.01
Back haptic size	+0.5 to −0.25

Displacement of optic	+0.3
Optic and haptic thickness	+0.25 to −0.1

Suitable tolerances for power (back vertex power) are the following:

+0.25 D. to −0.12 D.

THE ASSESSMENT OF FIT

The principles by which fit is judged apply to trial lenses and to lenses made to prescription.

White Light

1. Undue pressure on the bulbar conjunctiva produces *blanching*, a whitened area due to the emptying of small blood vessels. This frequently appears at the transition between haptic and optic or at the edge of the lens. In the latter position, some forms of edge combined with the adjacent tear liquid cause internal reflections that may imitate blanching.

2. Tendencies to lens tightness can be revealed by exerting force upon different parts of the haptic or the apex of the optic. A glass or plastic rod, well rounded at the end, serves as a suitable probe.

3. Areas of excessive lens clearance are revealed by bubbles forming beneath the haptic when the lens is displaced slightly or is lifted away from the globe very gently. As a lens (preferably dry) is lowered into position during insertion, a study of the order in which different parts wet as they contact the globe is most valuable.

Fluorescein

The haptic lens is placed upon the eye either dry or filled with a sodium bicarbonate solution. Fluorescein should be introduced into the lower fornix. Paper, wool, or rod applicators may be used, but a 2% sodium fluorescein solution is most popular for use with haptic lenses. Under ultraviolet irradiation, the stained tears can be seen intruding beneath the haptic through any channel that exists. If only slight traces intrude, for example, if the lens is truly sealed, movement of the globe frequently assists the fluorescein to reach the tear lens.

A lens fenestration readily admits the stained tears. Tears pooling beneath the haptic and optic show with characteristic green-yellow fluorescence.

Biomicroscope

An apical clearance between 0.05 and 0.15 mm. is satisfactory in fenestrated lenses. A considerable variation exists between patients as to the maximum extent of the clearance at which no air bubble forms. Probably 0.4 mm. is the extreme possibility for a fenestrated lens. The peripheral clearance of the optic may be up to three times the clearance at the corneal apex.[10,27-29]

Patient's Reaction

Care is needed in the evaluation of the immediate reaction to trial lenses and also of those lenses which are made to prescription. Conjunctival injection and swelling may be due to the wetting solutions, to clumsy or repeated insertion, or to a bad physical fit. Attention must be given to the possibility of accidentally using wrong lenses or solutions or of contamination of the tears by foreign bodies.

Lenses may become wrongly positioned on insertion; it is possible for a lens to lodge with the temporal part of the haptic pressing against the caruncle in a most uncomfortable manner. A careful check can be effected by asking the patient to look up and slightly retracting the lower lid.

FITTING PROCEDURE

The methods most applicable to present day practice have been fully described by Bier[27] and by Forknall and McKlellen.[29] These accounts tend to be complementary. They should be studied at length. Preformed lenses are fitted from sets of trial lenses. Haptic and optic fittings are best taken separately, using two sets of lenses (Table 32.2). If the haptic set contains 10 and the optic set 30 lenses, 300 combinations are possible. Alternately, but preferably in addition, a set of about fifty regular lenses may be employed. The latter must combine anticipated haptic and optic requirements and is best reserved for an approximate confirmation, on the eye, of the

TABLE 32.2
HAPTIC AND F.L.O.M. TRIAL SETS

A. Haptic

12.00/8.00/13.25/22 D. 1
12.50/8.00/13.25/22 D. 1
12.75/8.25/13.50/23.5 D. 1.5
13.00/8.25/13.50/22 D.1
13.50/8.25/13.50/22 D. 1
13.75/8.25/13.50/24 D. 2
14.00/8.25/13.75/23.5 D. 1.5
14.50/8.50/14.00/24 D. 2

with two toric haptics:

12.75 m 90, 13.25 m 180/8.25/13.50/23 D. 1 × 180
13.50 m 90, 14.00 m 180/8.25/13.50/23 D. 1 × 180

Other specifications:

1. Each to have a spherical transition with a radius which is midway between the haptic and optic radii and 2 mm. wide.
2. Non-fenestrated.
3. Thickness 0.6 mm.
4. Back vertex powers to be between −6.00 D. and +1.00 D.

B. Fenestrated Lenses for Optic Measurement (F.L.O.M.)

8.00/13.00	8.25/13.75	8.50/13.75	8.75/13.75
8.00/13.50	8.25/14.00	8.50/14.00	8.75/14.00
8.25/13.00	8.50/13.00	8.50/14.25	8.75/14.25
8.25/13.25	8.50/13.25	8.50/14.50	8.75/14.50
8.25/13.50	8.50/13.50	8.75/13.50	8.75/14.75
	9.00/13.50	9.00/15.00	
	9.00/13.75	9.25/14.00	
	9.00/14.00	9.25/14.50	
	9.00/14.25	9.50/14.50	
	9.00/14.50	9.50/14.75	
	9.00/14.75		

Other specifications:

1. Each to have a haptic radius of 13.00 mm. and back haptic size of 17 mm.
2. Fenestrated with 1 mm. hole just within optic.
3. Thickness 0.6 mm.
4. Transition barely polished.
5. Back vertex powers distributed between −10 D. and +2.00 D.

projected composite specification. The trial set consists of forty-six lenses with spherical haptics and four with toric haptics. The spherical lenses cover the eight haptic specifications of set A combined with the optics of set B (Table 32.2). The flatter optics are combined with the flatter haptics.

The toric lenses are as follows:

12.50 m 90, 13.00 m 180 / 8.50 / 13.50 / 23 D 1 × 180
12.75 m 90, 13.50 m 180 / 8.75 / 13.75 / 23 D 1 × 180
13.25 m 90, 13.75 m 180 / 8.50 / 13.50 / 23 D 1 × 180
13.50 m 90, 14.00 m 180 / 8.75 / 13.75 / 23 D 1 × 180

Each lens should be fenestrated with a 0.50 mm. hole in the transition, at its junction with the optic.

Stages in Fitting the Haptic

1. Assess palpebral aperture, exophthalmos, or enophthalmos.
2. Estimate initial conjunctival vascularity.
3. Note extent of fornices and restrictions due to check ligaments.
4. Start with small lens, 22 mm. B.H.S., estimated to fit.
5. Inspect lens to ensure it is the one required, before insertion.
6. Cleanse lens. Apply suction holder or arrange in fingers.
7. Retract patient's upper lid as he looks down.
8. Apply lens under upper lid first, retracting lower lid last. (Note that patient's head must be held horizontal if a complete liquid lens is desired, the lens being filled with sodium bicarbonate solution.)
9. Assess and record fit, initially judging whether globe is steeper or flatter than lens; if globe is toric, judge the flattest meridian and the difference between the principal meridians. Irregularity of the globe may be too great for fitting by modification of nearest preformed haptic available.
10. Apply fluorescein to conjunctival sac. Examine under ultraviolet light.
11. Sketch appearance, using green and blue pencils.

12. Remove lens, upper part first, with suction holder or upper lid.

13. Cleanse and replace lens in case.

14. Select and use alternate lenses until haptic fit is established. If necessary, increase B.H.S. to cover the anterior globe better.

The globe flattens, as does the cornea, with zones near the limbus tending to be steeper than zones nearer the equator. A spherical haptic of radius 13.00 mm. and B.H.S. 22 mm. may fit a certain eye, in which case a haptic 13.25 radius and 23.5 B.H.S. will likely also fit the same eye. As the B.H.S. is increased, the back haptic radius must be increased, and vice versa, when using spherical or toroidal haptics.

A globe having with-the-rule toricity may be matched in the horizontal meridian with a spherical haptic, but a pool of fluorescein will tend to extend from the optic portion upwards and downwards. Toric haptics, usually steeper in the vertical meridian by 0.50 mm. may be fitted to such toric eyes.

Stages in Fitting the Optic by F.L.O.M. Technique

The letters F.L.O.M. denote *fenestrated lens for optic measurement*, in the terminology used at Northampton College, London. Bier first described these fitting aids as *corneal ventilated trial contact lenses.*[8] The latter term is unsatisfactory due to confusion with a true *corneal* lens.

1. Select initial lens, judged from globe inspection; or by adding 0.75 mm. to flattest corneal radius and adding 1.00 mm. to the greatest diameter of the visible iris; or an average lens, e.g. 8.50/13.50.

2. Cleanse lens and apply to cornea with suction holder.

3. Ensure that the small haptic is not tight.

4. Inspect initial appearance of bubble, watch its diminution.

5. Assess bubble size, position, and mobility with slight eye rotations.

6. Apply fluorescein.

7. Inspect with ultraviolet lamp, prodding lens gently, right, left and up, in turn.

8. Assess bubble again.

9. Assess areas or arcs of corneal touch, pressing gently on lens apex.

10. Use alternate F.L.O.M. and repeat until best match for cornea is found.

11. Use F.L.O.M. 0.25 mm. flatter and 0.50 mm. steeper in B.O.D.

12. Use F.L.O.M. 0.50 mm. flatter and 0.75 mm. to 1.00 mm. steeper in B.O.D. Remember that two different F.L.O.M., although having the same primary sag, do not give equal clearance (Figure 32.12).

13. Decide upon the F.L.O.M. that gives optimum bubble, without apical touch.

14. Reassure patient, since F.L.O.M. is not comfortable.

Method of Combining Haptic and F.L.O.M. Requirements

Separate measurements have been obtained, e.g. —

Haptic radius 13.50
Back haptic size 24
Displacement 1.5
Optimum F.L.O.M. 8.75 / 13.75

These would be combined to give 13.50/8.75/13.75/24 D. 1.5, but it is best to add an extra 0.25 mm. to the B.O.D., since settling will probably take place. In a lens with a haptic radius over 14.00 mm., an extra 0.37 mm. is usually added. In the example given, the following should be ordered: 13.50/8.75/14.00/24 D. 1.5. This allowance is sufficient in most cases, provided that facilities are available for the subsequent grinding out of the back optic surface if corneal touch results from more than the usual amount of settling.

Double Curve Optics

About 10 percent of cases exhibit extreme peripheral flattening of the cornea. If a normal F.L.O.M. is used, the best attempt to match the cornea produces touch both at the apex and near the transition. In this event, a

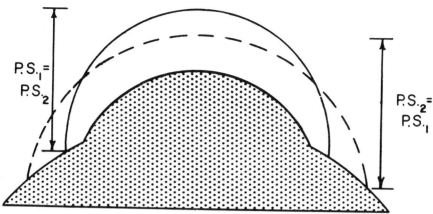

Figure 32.12. Two F.L.O.M. lenses as they fit onto a given eye, the latter shaded. The primary sag, P.S.$_1$ of the steeper lens equals that, P.S.$_2$, of the flatter lens. Due to the curvature of the globe, the flatter lens (with a greater B.O.D.) clears the cornea less than the steeper lens.

double curve construction is used, the back central optic radius being about 0.25 mm. steeper than the single curve, which gives the best approximation to a corneal match. The back central optic diameter is 6.00 mm., and the peripheral radius is 0.75 mm. flatter than the central radius. The two curves are blended slightly.

Toricity of the cornea calls for a steep optic that can be flattened during the final fitting in the flattest meridians of the cornea.

If the optic is fitted relatively steep, it simplifies subsequent modification: (1) the radii (central and peripheral) are readily flattened to meet individual requirements; (2) the back central optic diameter can be increased if necessary; (3) flattening the back central optic radius of a finished lens introduces plus power, which can be compensated by the simple process of flattening the front optic radius.

The Combined Method of Fitting

The required haptic is initially selected, taking account of any corneal touch. If the touch is heavy, as determined by the fluorescein test, it is probable that the haptic is not as close to the globe as is required.

Bubble characteristics and other factors must be judged in the same way as for the F.L.O.M. fitting, care being taken to note whether the fit of the haptic is interfering with the fit of the optic. Settling must be anticipated, and additions to the B.O.D. made in the same way as for F.L.O.M. fitting.

Refraction

As with corneal lenses, trial lenses are used to carry out the refraction. A trial contact lens of the same back optic radius as is to be prescribed may be used.

IMPRESSION TECHNIQUES

Every patient who is to receive haptic lenses may be fitted by the impression technique. Some practitioners insist that the use of this single method is best. Most, however, reserve impressions for unusual eyes and use

preformed lenses for the majority of cases. There is much to be said for a preliminary view of the fitting, as afforded by the preformed techniques.

Several authors have detailed the impression methods previously used. The contributions of Obrig and Salvatori,[30] Dickinson and Hall,[3] Freeman and Freeman,[31] Braff,[32,33] and Jenkin deserve study by all practitioners who intend to take eye impressions.

The term *impression* has been seldom used in earlier works, but in accordance with British Standard 3521:1962 it has been substituted for the word *moulding* in this context for good reasons.

MATERIALS

Dental impression materials have paved the way in this field, and some dental materials give rise to no ocular irritation. Irreversible hydrocolloidal gels are best, these commonly comprising calcium sulphate, a soluble alginate salt, a filler to give body and strength to the impression, and also a retarding salt. Cool storage, moisture-proof packing, and the careful trial of each batch of material are essential.

The impression is used for the preparation of a positive model in hard dental stone, called the *cast*. The dental stone power is added to a carefully estimated volume of water and mixed to a thin cream. Agitation of the rubber bowl removes bubbles of air. The creamy material is allowed to flow into the impression without trapping any air and is left to set for at least thirty minutes.

In addition to impression compounds, fluorescein and eye irrigation solutions should be provided. The latter are applied by means of an undine or irrigator syphon, at body temperature. Two percent centrimide or a similar agent is suitable for cleansing and sterilizing the small items of equipment. Mixing bowls, plastic spatulas, a well-rounded muscle hook, light mineral oil drops, and a mild bacteriostatic solution, e.g. 10% sodium sulphacetamide, complete the requirements.

Anaesthetic

It is sometimes convenient to use a surface anaesthetic and to reduce conjunctival injection with a vasoconstrictor. A solution of ½% amethocaine hydrochloride drops are

most common, but there are several suitable alternatives, which have a negligible effect upon the corneal epithelium, apart from anaesthesia. The vasoconstrictor most often chosen is adrenalin, 0.1%.

Impression Lens

Impression haptic lenses are produced from a cast of hard dental stone, itself derived from a soft impression of the eye. Figure 32.13 indicates the salient features of such a lens, as well as the wedge of stone added to level the cast for molding the plastic lens. In this instance the front central optic diameter is restricted to a relatively small lenticular portion. The back surfaces of impression lenses are often fairly irregular. Consequently, such lenses are often made about 1 mm. thick. Careful finishing and special molding of the final lens-blank can produce a haptic 0.4 mm. thick.

Impression Shells

A set is required of between six and ten pairs of *shells*, resembling haptic trial lenses with multiple perforations of about 1.25 mm. in diameter. It is necessary to anticipate a range of globe forms and palpebral aperture sizes in order to give an approximate fit and ready insertion and removal of the shells.

Some shells are provided with a tubular handle communicating with the optic portion, such shells being used with a syringe (Figure 32.14). Otherwise the shells have a nonperforated optic and are handled with a suction holder.

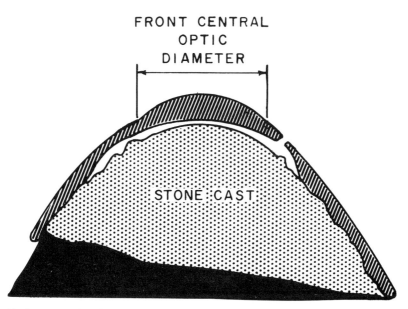

Figure 32.13. Impression lens resting on stone cast from which the back haptic surface was derived. The back optic is spherical, allowing a desired clearance from the cast. Note increasing clearance toward limbus. Note also ridge of conjunctival tissue reproduced at limbus of cast.

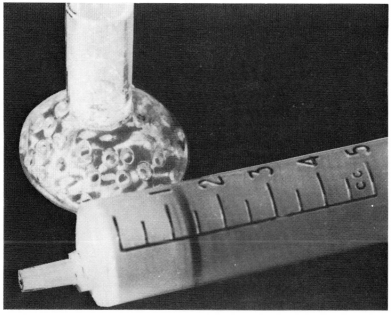

Figure 32.14. Injection impression shell with plastic syringe. The handle of the shell is a tube into which the nozzle of the syringe fits very loosely. A hole, slightly smaller than the bore of the handle, leads into the optic of the shell; from there the injected creamy material flows over the globe.

PREPARATION OF PATIENT

The patient usually sits erect with the head able to recline backwards on a rest. For injection fitting methods, a supine position is frequently used as an alternative.

Two drops of local anaesthetic are given to the eye that is to have the impression, one in each fornix, separated by an interval of about three minutes. The resulting corneal insensitivity can be confirmed with a wisp of cotton. It lasts about fifteen minutes.

The vasoconstrictor drops are applied after another three minutes, and a single drop of mineral oil is placed in the conjunctival sac before the impression material is mixed.

Special attention is paid to the cover test and to the visibility of the patient's fixation target. Where there is a deviation of the covered eye, the fixation position is suitably adjusted. It is necessary to ensure that the impression covers the temporal and superior aspects of the globe more than the inferior nasal area.

IMPRESSION PROCEDURE SUMMARY

1. Select shell and cleanse.
2. Add impression powder to water in bowl.
3. Spatulate material for thirty to forty seconds.
4. Fill shell or syringe for injection.
5. Insert shell.

Injection technique requires additional steps at this stage:

    a. Eliminate air from syringe filled with material.
    b. Lift shell 2 mm. from eye.
    c. Extrude material through shell handle.

6. Avoid pressure on shell or on eye.
7. Patient fixates steadily until impression solidifies.

8. Free lids from excess material.
9. Break suction at the caruncle.*
10. Remove shell as for a haptic lens.
11. Irrigate and inspect eye with ultraviolet light.
12. Pour the cast.

Figure 32.15 portrays a newly delivered impression lens with the original cast and a dental stone cast of the finished lens.

Optic Fitting

The eye must be fitted with an F.L.O.M. set as outlined previously to determine the correct back optic radius for the impression lens. It is hardly appropriate to include the basic optic diameter of the F.L.O.M. in the order.

CHECKING HAPTICS

BASIC APPARATUS REQUIRED

Dental stone
Millimeter scale
Magnifier, 4× to 10×
Spherometer based on Drysdale's method
Pinpoint dividers

Modeling clay

---

*Unless suction is broken, the shell and impression may separate. As the patient looks temporally, the plica is gently moved by stroking nasally with the muscle hook, stretching the conjunctiva and allowing tear liquid to flow beneath the impression.

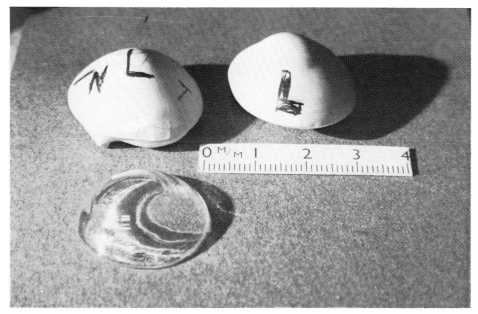

Figure 32.15. A new impression lens. Top left is the cast taken from the eye impression. The right dental stone cast is from the finished lens. The oblique illumination is an aid to understanding the contours, indicating how the transition between optic and haptic has been slightly blended, in anticipation of further blending as necessary.

METHODS

Initially the lens should be placed front side down on a small ball of modeling clay, avoiding distortion, then be filled to the brim with dental stone mixed to a thin cream. The resulting cast forms a permanent record and is used to measure several dimensions. It enables the transitions and the quality of polish to be examined.

SUBSEQUENT CHECKING PROCEDURES

Back Haptic Radius

The microscope movement of some (Drysdale method) optical spherometers permits the measurement of haptic radii and of transitions.

Alternatively, glass, steel, or plastic balls may be matched to the curve with sufficient accuracy.

Templates of plastic material can be used, edge on, scraping away a layer of polish, grease, or other marking material with which the haptic has been coated.

Some keratometers can be adapted for the measurement.

Back Optic Radius

An optical spherometer or keratometer may be used. Test plates are useful, since the optic of a haptic lens is thick enough to resist the slight pressure involved.

Basic Optic Diameter

If the transition is very sharp, the dividers may be applied to the cast for a direct measurement. This method is not accurate to more than 0.3 mm. A measuring microscope is best used if high accuracy is desired.

Back Haptic Size (B.H.S.)

The cast can be measured with the aid of dividers, or a scale can be applied to the back of the lens. In the latter case a slight allowance must be made for the rounding of the edge.

Displacement of Optic

The cast is measured with dividers along the maximum and minimum haptic chords. The difference is then halved to obtain the value of D.

Subsidiary Optic Dimensions

On a good cast both the back central optic diameter and the degree of blending are visible.

Transition

The cast shows the transition. Note the width, depth, and regularity of the transition area.

Thickness

A dial gauge is used.

Other characteristics such as power are checked in the same manner as for corneal lenses. It is helpful to make a checklist and sketch for each lens. On the sketch are recorded all identification marks, the position of holes, and thickness variations. Such sketches are valuable for reference when making lens modifications.

ADJUSTMENTS TO HAPTIC LENSES

Newly manufactured haptic lenses must be tried on the patient in the expectation that between one and two hours' work is needed before the initial period of wearing. Most patients are disappointed not to have their new lenses issued at once; hence, it is best to have adequate time and facilities available to deal with normal adjustments.

A motorized spindle capable of revolving at about 400 revolutions per minute, with interchangeable tools, is essential. An adjustable chuck to take the mandrels or spindles of the different tools may be convenient.

Tools should include mounted balls of stone 5 and 12 mm. in diameter, a small grinding disc, and a few abrasive-rubber dental points. Polishers of about the same sizes, in felt, should be supplied as well as a buffing compound of the wax base variety. A metal spatula resembling a teaspoon, bowl, fine-grade glass paper, a supply of modeling clay, and wax crayons in two colors must be available.

Optic grinding is best carried out with tools that are segments of spheres of different radii, coated with very fine diamond particles in a permanent bonding material. They should have a working face of about 12 mm. diameter. Optic polishing can be carried out with brass spherical tools covered with adhesive tape but is best done with hard wax.

Exact procedures for various modifications are too detailed for discussion here, and the reader is referred to more specialized coverage of this topic.[27,30]

CLINICAL PROCEDURES

INSTRUCTIONS FOR PATIENT

Insertion

Work over a table with a handkerchief or towel spread out to catch the lenses. Carry out the instructions very slowly. Identify the lenses by the R and L engraved on the part that rests beneath the lower lid.

Hold the lens with finger and thumb; a third finger may be used if this helps. Raise the upper lid with a finger of the other hand, looking downwards, at the chin. Gently place the lens close to the eye, near the lower lid. Still look down and slide the lens up underneath the upper lid. Support the lens with one hand while the other hand pulls the lower lid from beneath the lens. At this point look slowly and steadily upwards until the lens fully settles under the lids. Do not squeeze the eye shut; try to keep the eye open and relaxed. The hole in the lens should be on the side nearest your ear. Through this hole tears will flow beneath the lens to fill it almost completely. A bubble will remain, which should just avoid the pupil of the eye, to enable the surface of the eye to breathe naturally.

Removal

Look downwards at the chin, both eyes being kept open. Draw the upper lid up with the tip of one finger firmly placed on the edge of the lid, near the nose. Stretch the lid by pulling towards the top of the ear while sliding the finger slowly along the edge of the lid. The lid should be eased beneath the lens as the fingertip reaches the temporal part of the upper lid. Now slowly look up and catch the lens as it falls from the eye.

If the first attempt fails, repeat the procedure after a short interval, ensuring that the lids are dry.

The suction holder may be used for an alternative method of removal, placing the holder on the upper nasal area of the lens. Pull up the upper lid and look down. Place the holder on the lens with plenty of suction. Slightly twist the lens to move the nasal part upwards, at the same time tilting the whole lens away from the eye at the top. Immediately begin slowly to look up and take the lens away from the eye.

AFTERCARE

The patient should wear the lenses every day for three periods of two hours for about a week. He should then attend a session lasting some thirty minutes in order to enable the practitioner to reassess the situation. Notes must be made of the patient's reactions, commencing with the good and including the bad aspects. Refractive, phoria, and accommodative checks should be included. Residual errors of refraction should be attended to if at all possible, preferably by suitable recutting and polishing of the front optic surface. Minor adjustments should be completed.

During the second week, a patient should gradually build up to a wearing time of about twelve hours, broken into three periods by rests of about two hours each. The need for reporting after one, two, or three weeks will depend upon the individual circumstances, but within a month most patients will be in need of advice, if not attention.

The normal routine is to see the patient at least four times during the first three months and then to recall at intervals of six months until a pattern of yearly reexamination and attention is established, some two years after the first visit.

Settling, normally anticipated within six months, brings the back optic surface into contact with the corneal apex. Almost invariably in eyes with normal sensitivity, there follows the same type of reaction that accompanies a foreign body on the cornea. Pain, conjunctival redness and swelling, lacrima-tion, and some degree of photophobia are reported. Unless the patient is warned to expect the symptoms, he may be alarmed; alternately he may bravely try to ignore the symptoms and reduce his wearing time. Warnings must be used with care, since it is foolish to suggest trouble, yet unfair to pretend that settling is unlikely.

REFERENCES

1. *British Standard 3521: Glossary of Terms Relating to Ophthalmic Lenses and Spectacle Frames*, London, British Standards Institution, 1962.

2. Greenspoon, R.: A new trial set for fitting contact lenses, *Am. J. Optom.*, *20*(*9*):313–315, 1943.

3. Dickinson, F., and Hall, K.: *An Introduction to the Prescribing and Fitting of Contact Lenses*, London, Hammond, Hammond and Co., Ltd., 1946.

4. Bier, N., and Cole, P. J.: The transcurve contact lens fitting shell, *The Optician*, *115*:605 ff., 1948.

5. Anderson, J. M.: *Contact Lenses*, Hove, Courtenay Press Ltd., 1952.

6. Forknall, A. J.: Some notes on haptic lenses, *Br. J. Physiol. Opt.*, *16*(*2*):96–115, 1959.

7. McKellen, G. D.: The "offset" haptic lens, *The Optician*, *145*(*3749*):105–107, 1963.

8. Bier, N.: The practice of ventilated contact lenses, *The Optician*, *116*:497, 1948.

9. Hall, K. C.: A special contact lens for complete ptosis, *The Optician*, *135*(*3494*):245, 1958.

10. Ridley, F.: The contact lens in investigation and treatment, *Trans. Ophthalmol. Soc. U.K.*, *74*:377–410, 1954.

11. Ridley, F.: The contact lens in investigation and treatment, *Trans. Ophthalmol. Soc. U.K.*, *79*:533–549, 1959.

12. Dufour, R.: Indications particulières des verres de contact: keratite neuroparalytique, albinisime, *Acta Ophthalmol.*; *123*(*4–5*):290–294, 1952.

13. Freeman, E.: Pinhole contact lenses, *Am. J. Optom.*, *29*(*7*):347–352, 1952.

14. Williamson-Noble, F. A.: Experiences with early contact lenses and some of their later developments, *Br. J. Ophthalmol.*, *44*(*11*): 679–683, 1960.

15. Ridley, F.: Applicators for irradiation of the conjunctival sac, *Trans. Ophthalmol. Soc. U.K.*, *78*:171–178, 1958.

16. Sundmark, E.: Recording of the human electroretinogram with the contact glass, *Acta Ophthalmol.*, *36*(*2*):273–280, 1958.

17. Sundmark, E.: The contact glass in human electro-retinography, *Acta Ophthalmol.*, *37 Supp.*:52, 1959.

18. Worst, J. G. F.: A new method for fixing diagnostic contact lenses, *Am. J. Ophthalmol.*, *48*(*6*):849–850, 1959.

19. Worst, J. G. F., and Otter, K.: Low vacuum diagnostic contact lenses, *Am. J. Ophthalmol.*, *51*(*3*):410–424, 1961.

20. Klein, M.: Contact shell applicator for use as a corneal bath, *Br. J. Ophthalmol.*, *33*(*11*): 716–717, 1949.

21. Byford, G. H.: Eye movement recording, *Nature (Lond)*, *184, Supp. 19*:1493–1494, 1959.

22. Riggs, L. A., and Niehl, E. W.: Eye movements recorded during convergence and divergence, *J. Opt. Soc. Am.*, *50*(*9*):913–920, 1960.

23. Ratliff, F., and Riggs, L. A.: Involuntary motions of the eye during monocular fixation, *J. Exp. Psychol.*, *40*(*6*):687–701, 1950.

24. Ditchburn, R. W., and Pritchard, R. M.: Stabilized interference fringes on the retina, *Nature (Lond)*, *177*(*4505*):434, 1956.

25. Dickinson, F.: The value of microlenses in progressive myopia, *The Optician*, *133*(*3443*): 263–264, 1957.

26. Fletcher, R. J.: The ophthalmometer in contact lens fitting, *Br. J. Physiol. Opt.*, *12*(*1*):

37–41, 1955.

27. Bier, N.: *Contact Lens Routine and Practice*, 2nd ed., London, Butterworths, 1957.

28. Forknall, A. J.: Pre-formed lenses, corneal fit, with a note on the slit-lamp, *Br. J. Physiol. Opt.*, *10*(*1*):15–22, 1953.

29. Forknall, A. J., and McKellen, G. D.: Long tolerances with haptic lenses, *Br. J. Physiol. Opt.*, *19*(*2*):73–77, 1962.

30. Obrig, T. E., and Salvatori, P. L.: *Contact Lenses*, 3rd ed., New York, Obrig Laboratories, 1957.

31. Freeman, E., and Freeman, M.: The optometric impression technique in the fitting of contact lenses, *Am. J. Optom.*, *24*(*5*):203–238, 1947.

32. Braff, S. M.: Eye impressions without anaesthesia, *Optom. Weekly*, *36*(*6*):149, 1945.

33. Braff, S. M.: Eye impressions without anaesthesia, in *Encyclopedia of Contact Lens Practice*, South Bend, Indiana, International Optics, 1959–1963, vol. 4, Chap. 40, pp. 45–46.

34. Sarver, M. D.: *Contact Lens Syllabus*, 5th ed., UC Berkeley School of Optometry, Berkeley, Calif., 1979.

ADDITIONAL READINGS

Bier, N.: Treating monocular ptosis, *Cont. Lens Forum*, *3*(*9*):53, 1978.

Braff, S. M.: Scleral lenses, *J. Am. Optom. Assoc.*, *47*(*3*):321, 1976.

Braff, S. M.: Any future for scleral lenses? *Cont. Lens Forum*, *3*(*9*):39, 1978.

Gyorffy, I.: Past and future of plastic scleral lenses, *Contacto*, *21*(*6*):39, 1977.

Hirschhorn, H.: The art of making your own scleral lenses and shells, *Optom. Index*, *51*(*7*):36–44,1976.

Moss, H.: A minimum clearance molded scleral cosmetic-refractive contact lens, *J. Am. Optom. Assoc.*, *49*(*3*):277–279, 1978.

Nissel, G.: Re-discovering the scleral lens, *Optom. World*, *7*(*38*):16, 1978.

Chapter 33

CONTACT LENS INSTRUMENTS

BIOMICROSCOPE

DESCRIPTION

WITH THE SLIT–LAMP biomicroscope, it is possible to observe the transparent structures of the living eye under magnification of ten to fifty times. The instrument is composed of two parts: a stereomicroscope, which is mounted horizontally for direct viewing of the patient's eye, and a lamp, which is equipped with an optical system to project a slit of light upon the eye (Figure 33.1). The slit lamp may be adjusted to form a variety of light beams. By varying the light beam and viewing position, it is possible to enhance the visibility of various ocular structures. The small particles in the transparent structures of the eye reflect light in the direction of the biomicroscope (Tyndall phenomenon).

The biomicroscope is particularly useful for examining the cornea and, hence, has proved of invaluable assistance in contact lens work. Corneal manifestations of an improperly fitting contact lens can usually be detected first with a biomicroscope.

Biomicroscopes differ in the quality of the microscope, the illumination control, and the ease of handling the instrument. Specific manuals should be consulted for the directions for given instruments. The following outline is a guide to the use and application of all biomicroscopes. It is intended as a supplement to more extensive sources.[1-7]

OUTLINE OF PROCEDURE*

Diffuse Illumination (Figure 33.2a)

Description

A wide beam of light is directed obliquely at the cornea. No attempt is made to focus the light.

Procedure for Examination of the Cornea

1. Adjust the height of the instrument for patient comfort.

2. Position the microscope directly in front of the patient. Use low power.

3. Set the illuminating arm about 45° to the microscope.

4. Reduce the room illumination.

5. Turn on the illuminating system.

6. Open the slit.

7. Adjust the position of the illuminating arm so the whole cornea is illuminated.

8. Focus the microscope toward the cornea and away from the iris.

---

*Section on biomicroscopy was written by Doctor Roy Brandreth.

796

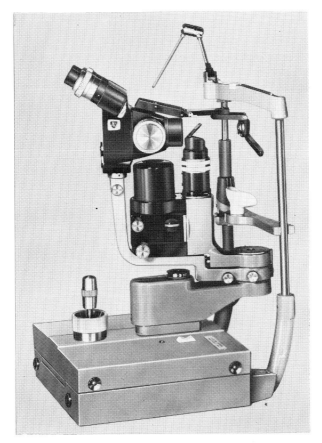

Figure 33.1a. Slit-lamp biomicroscope. Courtesy of American Optical Co.

Uses of Diffuse Illumination

1. Gives a good overall picture of the cornea, but no fine details. It is used primarily for a general survey of the eye.

    a. Can observe the entire extent of a corneal scar or infiltration.

    b. Folds in Descemet's membrane become visible.

    c. The presence of any invading blood vessels in the cornea is disclosed.

    d. Edema of the epithelium may be indicated by a hazy, grey, and somewhat granular appearance.

Direct Focal Illumination (Figure 33.2b)

Description

The beam of light and the microscope are sharply focused on the same area.

Three Types of Direct Focal Illumination

1. Optic section
2. Parallelepiped
3. Conical beam

Procedure for Obtaining Optic Section

1. Position the microscope directly in front of the eye to be examined.

2. Set the illuminating arm at an angle of about 45° to the microscope.

3. Adjust the microscope and the focusing lens to the click stop position. Use low power magnification first.

4. Narrow the slit to an almost closed position.

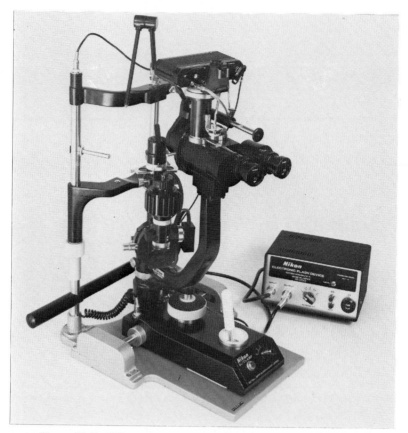

Figure 33.1b. Nikon photo slit lamp. Courtesy of Nikon, Inc.

5. Turn the illuminating system on.

6. Sighting from the side, position the beam on the cornea. Continue to move the unit forward (using the joystick when one is present) until the beam appears sharply defined.

7. Look into the microscope. An illuminated section of the cornea should be visible. Fine adjustments with the joystick, microscope, and/or focusing lens may be necessary to bring the illuminated section into very sharp focus.

8. The beam may be moved across the cornea by moving the joystick sideways or by moving the illuminating arm. The optic section should always be kept in sharp focus when sweeping across the cornea.

9. Increasing the angle between the microscope and the illuminating system will expose a greater area of stroma.

An Optic Section Allows One to See

1. The tear layer (the first bright zone).

2. The dark epithelial line (normal epithelium is usually considered as an optically empty space).

3. The brighter Bowman's zone.

4. The stroma—This appears as a grey, somewhat granular, area under low power, but shows nerve fibers, arachnoid corpuscles, and other anatomical components under higher power.

5. The endothelial zone, which appears brighter than the stroma.

DIFFUSE   DIRECT
FOCAL   INDIRECT

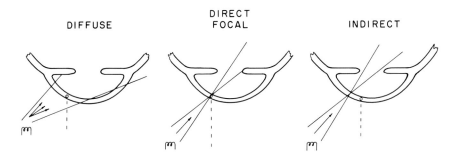

RETRO   SPECULAR   SCLEROTIC
SCATTER

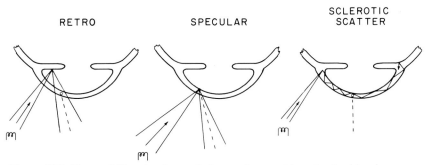

Figure 33.2. Types of illumination and observation positions for the biomicroscope.

Uses of Optic Section

1. To discover thickening, thinning, and distortions in the corneal contour.

2. To determine the depth of foreign bodies or opacities in the corneal substance. (The apparent depth is approximately two-thirds of its real depth.)

3. To see a wide section of stroma. (The angle between the microscope and illuminating arm can be increased.)

4. To perceive flare or relucency in the aqueous. The luminous beam is directed so that the upper portion of the beam enters the lower part of the pupil. This permits dark areas immediately above to serve as a dark contrasting background. The presence of appreciable flair is indicative of a pathological state. (*See also* Conical Beam.)

Procedure for Obtaining a Parallelepiped

1. Position the microscope directly in front of the eye to be examined.

2. Set the illuminating arm at an angle of about 45° to the microscope.

3. Use low power magnification.

4. Open the slit slightly.

5. Adjust the microscope and the focusing lens to the click stop position.

6. Turn the illuminating system on.

7. Align the beam of light on the cornea using the joystick. The beam should appear to be in sharp focus before looking into the microscope.

8. Look into the microscope. A wide block of the posterior surface, substantia propria, and anterior surface should be in view.

9. Fine adjustments with the joystick microscope and/or focusing lens may be necessary to sharpen the parallelepiped.

10. Using the joystick, move the parallelepiped across the cornea.

11. Increase or decrease the slit width as

desired. The angle between the microscope and illuminating arm may also be varied.

12. Change the power of the objectives and oculars if more magnification is desired for detail analysis.

Uses of Parallelepiped

1. Gives a broad view of the anterior and posterior corneal surfaces.

2. Gives a view of a wide block of substantia propria.

3. To determine anterior surface irregularities (*see* Specular Reflection for method of use).

4. Used to examine the endothelium (*see* Specular Reflection for method).

5. To make a general survey of cornea.

    a. Opaque features in the cornea such as scars, abrasions, nebulae, blood vessels, and folds in Descemet's membrane reflect the light and thus appear whiter than the surround. These should also be examined under retroillumination.

    b. Corneal nerves appear under higher magnification as fine white silk threads usually branching into a Y (seen mostly in middle third of stroma).

    c. Corneal epithelial edema is only seen poorly with a parallelepiped but gives an increased grey, whitish appearance in the affected area. The best method for seeing edema is by retroillumination.

6. Used to determine the fit of contact lens after fluorescein has been instilled in the eye.

7. With the aid of fluorescein, areas of epithelial embarrassment or erosion will stain and therefore appear much more green than the surround.

Conical Beam

The conical beam is obtained when the light is directed through a small circular aperture. This is the most sensitive method for observing aqueous flare (Tyndall phenomena) and requires bright illumination and greater magnification.

1. Align the microscope directly in front of the eye to be examined.

2. Position the illuminating arm about 45° to the microscope.

3. Use very reduced room illumination or a completely dark room. The observer should also become dark adapted.

4. Direct the light through the pupil.

5. Focus the microscope alternately on the posterior corneal surface and the anterior crystalline lens to determine the range of focusing.

6. Refocus the microscope into the anterior chamber.

7. Switch to higher magnification if necessary.

8. Rack the illuminating arm very gently from side to side.

9. If appreciable flare is seen, it is indicative of a pathologic state.

    a. Red blood cells appear as reddish-yellow dots.

    b. Larger clumps of white blood cells and fibrin appear greyish white.

    c. Pigment granules appear brown.

10. The beam and microscope should gradually be moved over as large an area as possible.

Indirect Illumination (Figure 33.2c)

Description

The observer focuses the microscope sharply on an area immediately adjacent to the illuminated position.

Procedure

1. Use a beam of moderate width.

2. The incident beam should be at a wide angle to the axis of observation.

3. The beam may be oscillated to give variable illumination. The other hand can be used to focus the microscope in short

back-and-forth movements if desired.

Uses of Indirect Illumination

1. Particularly valuable in studying the iris for pathology.

2. Any fine vesiculation of the corneal epithelium is easier to observe.

3. The only method by which the outer rim of the iris sphincter may be seen.

Retroillumination

Description (Figure 33.2d)

The light is focused on the deeper structures such as the iris, lens, or retina while the microscope is focused to study the more anterior structures in the reflected light. The most typical use is to study the cornea in light reflected from the iris.

Procedure

1. Use a parallelepiped focused on the iris.

2. If direct retroillumination is desired, the observed feature on the cornea is viewed in the direct pathway of the reflected light. The angle between the microscope and the illuminating arm is about 60°. Thus, the observed structure is directly in line with the illuminated background.

3. If indirect retroillumination is desired, the observed feature is not viewed in the direct pathway of the reflected light. Thus, the retroilluminated object is viewed against a dark nonilluminated background. The angle between the microscope and the illuminating system can be varied considerably.

Uses of Retroillumination

1. Especially useful in studying deposits on Descemet's membrane and blood vessels that have invaded the cornea.

2. The method of choice for the examination of epithelial edema, vacuoles, and delicate scars.

Optical Properties of Observed Features in Retroillumination

Features opaque to light that appear dark against a white background:

1. Scars
2. Pigment
3. Vessels containing blood

Features that scatter light which appear lighter than the dark background:

1. Edema of the epithelium
2. Corneal precipitates

Specular Reflection

Description (Figure 33.2e)

The illuminating arm and the microscope are positioned such that the beam of light, when reflected from the corneal surfaces, will pass through one of the oculars of the microscope. At this point the angle of incidence of the light will be equal to the angle of reflections.

Procedure

1. The angle between the illuminating arm and the microscope should be about 60°.

2. Use a magnification of about twenty or twenty-five times.

3. Use a fairly wide parallelepiped.

4. Locate the catoptric image of the illuminating lamp.

5. Move the illuminating arm until the catoptric image is just behind the posterior surface of the parallelepiped.

6. The dazzle from the precorneal fluid will be apparent. (Angle of incidence equals angle of reflection.)

7. Focus on the back of the parallelepiped. A mosaic of hexagonal cells will appear.

Uses of Specular Reflection

1. Elevations and depressions of the anterior surface appear as dark defects in the

brilliant zone of regularly reflected light.

2. Details of the precorneal fluid, mucus, meibomian secretion, and the corpuscular elements of the tears are seen.

3. The study of the posterior surface of the cornea, particularly the endothelium and deposits on the surface.

Sclerotic Scatter

Description (Figure 33.2f)

A broad beam of light is focused sharply at the limbus, and the microscope is focused sharply on the cornea.

Procedure

1. Align the microscope directly in front of the eye to be examined.

2. Use the lower power magnification.

3. The angle between the microscope and illuminating arm should be 45° or greater.

4. Focus the light sharply at the limbus.

5. A crescentic halo of light should be visible around the cornea, particularly noticeable at the opposite side.

Uses of Sclerotic Scatter

To observe whether a disturbance of the normal transparency is present. Nebulae, maculae, interstitial deposits, perforating scars, and pigmented areas will cause the light to scatter and therefore appear whiter.

Tangential Illumination

Description

A method of examination of the iris by using very oblique illumination when the microscope is aligned in front of the eye under observation.

Uses of Tangential Illumination

Shows up freckles, tumors, and integrity of the iris.

USE OF THE SLIT-LAMP BIOMICROSCOPE IN A CONTACT LENS PREFITTING EXAMINATION

Examination of the lids, lid margins, lashes, palpebral and bulbar conjunctiva, sclera, tears, and cornea should always precede a contact lens fitting.

The objective is to do the following:

1. Uncover any condition that may make the wearing of contact lenses inadvisable

2. Disclose conditions that may complicate the successful fitting of contact lenses

3. Insure that the tissue is healthy and free of any active pathology

4. Observe any anatomical variations that should be alleviated before fitting contact lens

5. Allow the clinician an easy means for noting preexisting conditions that should be accurately recorded, even though their presence may not alter the clinician's decision to fit the lenses

Examine the Lids

1. Use low magnification and diffuse illumination for an overall view of the external lid tissue and lid margins.

2. Note the palpebral aperture height.

3. Note the position of the upper and lower lid margins in relation to the limbus.

4. Observe the blink rate and length of time of lid closure.

5. Ask the patient to close his eyes. The upper and lower lid margins should meet uniformly over their entire length.

6. Note the general appearance of the lids for signs of edema, hyperemia, ectropion, entropion, ptosis, benign lumps or nodules, tumors, and verrucae.

Examine the Lashes, Lid Margins, and Tears Simultaneously

1. Use a moderately wide beam of light.
2. Increase the magnification.
3. Start at the outer canthus. Set the angle between the microscope and light source between 30° and 45°.
4. Move the stage laterally, using the joystick, toward the inner canthus keeping the margins, lashes, and tear layer in sharp focus.
5. Note the arrangement of the lashes. Look for any cilia growing in toward the eyeball.
6. Examine the lid margins, at the same time looking for signs of blepharitis, hordeola, cysts, and neoplasms.
7. Simultaneously concentrate on the appearance of the tear film covering the conjunctiva and cornea and the fluid meniscus formed between the lid margin and globe, with particular emphasis in the region of the lacrimal lake. Look for the presence of debris and sediment, mucous strands, excessive lacrimation, or dryness of the eyes. (Observation of the tear film can be enhanced by the use of fluorescein.) Examine the puncta and caruncle.

Examine the Palpebral and Bulbar Conjunctiva

1. Use a moderately wide beam of light.
2. Use about $16\times$ magnification.
3. Vary the angle between the light source and microscope.
4. Evert the lower lid. Look for follicles, cysts, concretions.
5. Evert the upper lid, looking for signs of follicles, papillae, concretions, scarring.
6. Examine the bulbar conjunctiva, looking for signs of conjunctival injection or ciliary injection. Note any pinguecula, pterygium, or pigmentation.

Examine the Sclera

1. Use the same type of illumination and magnification.

2. Look for signs of scleritis, necrotic conditions, sclerokeratitis, degenerative conditions, and neoplastic conditions.

Examine the Cornea

All the various types of illumination are used to examine the cornea. Low magnification is used for an overall view, high magnification for detailed study.

1. Start with diffuse illumination, and note any abnormalities to get an overall view of the cornea.
2. Narrow the vertical beam to a moderate width, and focus on the temporal limbus to illuminate the cornea by sclerotic scatter. This type of illumination is used to observe whether a disturbance of the normal transparency of the cornea is present. Nebulae, maculae, interstitial deposits, perforating scars, ghost vessels, and endothelial folds will cause the light to scatter and appear whiter.
3. Central corneal clouding is easily seen using a variation of this method of illumination and is discussed in detail in Chapter 14.
4. The detailed examination of the cornea is then begun to study any abnormalities noted in steps 1 and 2 and to look for other anomalies that may not be seen by the previous methods. This is accomplished by using direct focal illumination, at least $16\times$ magnification and a parallelepiped and focusing across the cornea, observing the cornea in direct illumination and retroillumination (both direct and indirect) simultaneously. A broad area of the anterior and posterior corneal surfaces and a wide block of stroma is visible.
5. Opaque areas in the cornea such as scars, infiltrates, nebulae, maculae, ghost vessels, and folds in Descemet's membrane reflect the light and therefore appear whiter than the surround. Corneal edema is easily seen in retroillumination. Foreign bodies in the cornea are easily seen.
6. Use an optic section to observe thickening, thinning, curvature variations, depths

of foreign bodies, and scars.

7. Use specular reflection to examine the anterior corneal surface for elevations and depressions and for minute debris in the precorneal fluid. Use the same illumination to examine the endothelium for signs of keratitic precipitates (K.P.).

8. Instill fluorescein in the eye. Interpose the blue filter. Ask the patient to blink sev-

eral times to spread the fluorescein uniformly over the cornea. Observe for dry spots. At times many small, round dots of fluorescein may be absorbed over a portion of all of the cornea. This stipple staining may indicate the presence of a keratitis. Contact lenses should not be fitted until appropriate therapy has been completed.

USE OF THE SLIT-LAMP BIOMICROSCOPE FOR THE CONTACT LENS FITTING EXAMINATION AND EVALUATION

The slit-lamp biomicroscope is used to evaluate the physical fit of a hard lens and the physiological response of the cornea, lids, and conjunctiva to the lens.

Physical Fit

The physical fit of the lens refers to the bearing relationship existing between the concave surface of the contact lens and the convex cornea.

Procedure

1. Instill fluorescein in both eyes.

2. Adjust the head rest position for patient comfort.

3. Reduce the room illumination.

4. Interpose the blue filter.

5. Place the microscope directly in front of the eye. Angle the light about 30° to the microscope.

6. Ask the patient to blink several times to insure adequate spreading the fluorescein. It may be necessary to wait briefly for any excess tearing to subside.

7. Use a broad beam of light to create diffuse illumination.

8. Use low magnification to obtain an overall view of the eye and the contact lens–cornea bearing relationship indicated by the fluorescein pattern.

9. Observe the lens centration.

a. The lens should center reasonably

well, relative to the pupil.

b. The lens should not rest on the lower lid with straight ahead fixation.

c. The lens should not rest beyond the corneal-scleral junction.

10. Observe the lens movement during and following each blink and on excursions of the eye.

a. A short downward movement of the lens should be observed as the lids begin to close during the first part of the blink. The lens should not be driven down so the edge strikes the lid margin.

b. A short upward movement of the lens should be observed as the upper lid rises ending the blink.

c. The lens should remain on the cornea and be reasonably well centered through all changes in the directions of eye gaze.

11. Observe the anterior and posterior lens surfaces for signs of dry areas, scratches, and mucus.

a. Lenses that are wetting poorly present a splotchy appearance (wetting in one area, and dry and hazy in another). Immediately after the blink the tear layer on the lens surface recedes from one or more areas as the hydrophobic characteristics of the plastic are exaggerated. Scratches, aerosol sprays, creams, oils, etc. can create this picture when present on the lens surface(s). If the patients complain that their vision is not clear or remains clear only a short time, then the lenses must be removed and cleaned repeatedly. The lenses need to be thoroughly cleaned and the surfaces reconditioned or polished.

b. It is usually possible to determine whether one or both surfaces are creating a wetting problem. Switch to a parallelepiped and increase the magnification, observing both the anterior and posterior lens surfaces as the stage is moved laterally. Sometimes switching to specular reflection and an optic section will also give additional information in determining the lens surface(s) involved.

c. Scratches on the lens surfaces are easily recognized, appearing as silvery, whitish, or greyish threadlike lines running haphazardly on the lens surface(s). Concentric scratches running around the periphery of the lens usually indicate areas of poor peripheral or secondary curve polishing or blending.

d. Debris on the lens surface is usually mucus, which stains readily with fluorescein and moves about with each blink. The presence of mucus may be an indication of decreased tear production, minor conjunctival infections, a minor palpebral conjunctival irritation, or a viscous tear film. The presence of sebaceous material is indicated by minute oil droplets glistening in the light beam. Occasionally associated with this will be minute foamy bubbles forming along the lid margins near the inner or outer canthus.

KERATOMETER

CALIBRATION PROCEDURE

Isen has described a procedure for measuring and improving the validity of a frequently used keratometer.[8] He illustrates that this instrument may be accurate for parts of the scale and inaccurate for the rest of the scale. This error can only be detected by test measurements made with a keratometer on a range of precision steel balls. These balls are usually available in the following radii with the corresponding dioptric values for the keratometer.

Radius (mm.)	Keratometer Reading
7.14	47.25 D.
7.54	44.75 D.
7.94	42.50 D.
8.38	40.25 D.
8.73	38.62 D.
9.13	37.00 D.

Each ball should be carefully measured three to five times, and an average taken of the values. The average values then can be graphed for easier reference. Place the values for the keratometer readings on one axis and the dioptric values for the steel ball (expected keratometer reading) on the other axis. An example of the preceding procedure is illustrated in Figure 33.3. For the illustrated keratometer, all of the readings are higher than they should be. Also, this error is greater for the higher powers than for the lower powers. From the graph it is possible to prepare a table of correction values for quick reference.

Method to Correct Keratometer

The simplest error to correct occurs when the keratometer consistently reads too high or too low by the same amount. This error can be corrected by changing the position of the keratometer power dial. The dial can be turned by loosening the two set screws and moving the dial an amount corresponding to the error.

Rapid Procedure for Calibration of a Keratometer

Making a precise setting of the power drum during the calibration of a keratometer

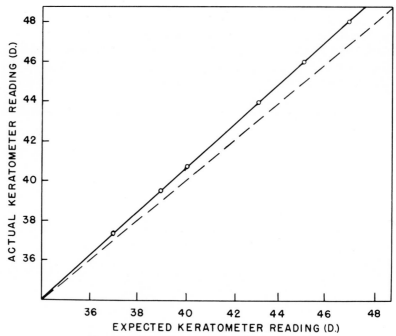

Figure 33.3. Plotting the keratometer curve.

is sometimes very tedious, and often the clinician does not have time to make such an adjustment. This is especially true when many individuals use the same instrument, as would perhaps occur in a clinic. Hence, the need arose for a rapid calibration of the keratometer. This can be accomplished in the following way.

Align and focus the keratometer for measuring a calibration ball of known radius. Then, without observing the keratometer mire image, set the power drum at the position that corresponds to the ball radius. For example, if the calibration ball has a radius of 7.94 mm., the power drum should be set for 42.50 D. Next, view the mire images in the instrument. If they are not aligned, make a few clockwise turns of the eyepiece, and refocus the instrument. The mires will now be either closer together or farther apart than they were for the previous adjustment. If they are farther apart, the eyepiece should be rotated in a counterclockwise direction, and the instrument should be refocused. By a system of

trial and error, it is possible to vary the position of the eyepiece and to focus the instrument until the mires coincide. The calibration is then completed.

The optical explanation of this technique may be of interest. In Figure 33.4a, light from the mires (not shown) forms the virtual corneal images m_1 and m_2. These images can be considered as objects in order to trace the rays through the telescope of the keratometer. Light from the virtual corneal images is refracted by the objective lens of the keratometer telescope to form the images m'_1 and m'_2. A doubling prism, P, intercepts a portion of the light passing through the objective and displaces the image, m'_2, so that it appears adjacent to the image m'_1. If the focal point of the eyepiece coincides with the images m'_1 and m'_2, light from the images will, after passing through the eyepiece, emerge parallel.

If the eyepiece is now turned counterclockwise (moved away from the objective) as in Figure 33.4b and if the keratometer is refocused, the distances are altered between the corneal image, the telescope objective, and the focal plane of the images formed by the objective. Using the ray tracing procedure followed previously and considering the virtual corneal image as an object to be focused by the objective, it is found that the object distance, s, is now shortened, and the image distance, s', is lengthened. Since magnification

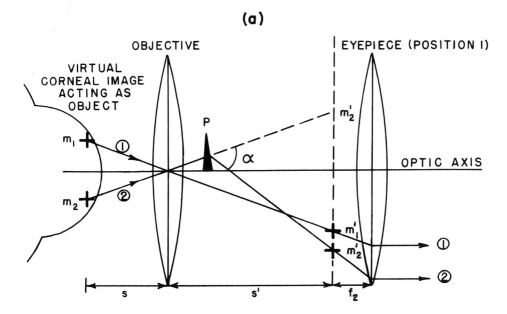

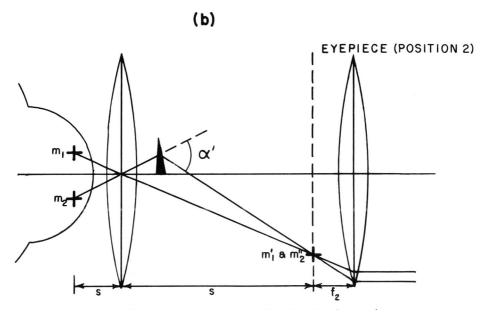

Figure 33.4. Calibration of the keratometer by adjusting the eyepiece.

by a lens is equal to the ratio of the image to object distance, the image m_1 will be formed at a greater distance from the optic axis. The chief ray from m_1 will leave the objective lens at a greater angle than under the conditions of Figure 33.4a because of the decreased object distance; also, the image m'_1 will have a larger angular subtense at the objective.

The question may now be asked whether the keratometer will still remain accurate for the measurement of powers other than that for which it has been calibrated. Moving the eyepiece position will vary the magnification of the keratometer telescope and change the relative size of the images that are measured by the keratometer doubling system. The scale on the power drum should no longer correspond to the amount of doubling and, hence, may be inaccurate. It is possible, however, that the error may be so small as to be negligible. This was tested by measuring the effect of this type of adjustment upon the accuracy of a keratometer in the following way.

A series of five precision steel balls were measured with a keratometer to determine its accuracy over the entire power range. Next the power drum was purposely offset 0.50 D. so that the keratometer would always read 0.50 D. higher than the true reading. The error in the keratometer was then corrected by changing the eyepiece by the method described previously. The series of steel balls

were then retested. Each ball was again measured five times, and the average value computed. No significant difference existed in the readings found for the steel balls after the instrument had been recalibrated. It is therefore concluded that the difference in readings, which theoretically should occur by adjusting the eyepiece, is not great enough to be of practical significance. Nevertheless, even though the method would appear to be reasonably accurate, there are two additional disadvantages to calibrating a keratometer by adjusting the eyepiece.

1. This method can only be used to correct for a calibration error in one of the two meridians in which a measurement is possible with the keratometer. If the dials for both meridians are out of adjustment, then only one can be corrected, and the other must be left in error.

2. The clinician using the keratometer will not be able to observe the cross hairs to insure that his accommodation is relaxed. Although such a check may not be necessary for an experienced operator, those who have not learned to keep their accommodation relaxed may find a significant error in their measurements due to this reason. It is therefore felt that the method of calibrating the keratometer by readjusting the position of the power drums is to be preferred over adjusting the eyepiece.

PROCEDURES TO INCREASE THE ACCURACY OF KERATOMETER MEASUREMENTS

Eyepiece Adjustment

If the keratometer is to be used by only one operator, then it is only necessary to adjust the eyepiece once, although an occasional check may be necessary to be certain no accidental change has been made. The adjustment should be made either by shining a light into the front of the instrument or by turning on the instrument and holding a card in front of the telescope to reflect the

light from the mires into the telescope. The instrument may have either cross hairs or a round circle to be focused. Begin by turning the eyepiece counterclockwise as far as it will go. Then slowly turn the eyepiece clockwise until the cross hairs come into best focus. Always approach from the counterclockwise to clockwise direction, as this will give greater accuracy than if the eyepiece is screwed back and forth until a focus is secured. This will help to keep accommodation relaxed at all times during the focusing. Always try to keep accommodation relaxed as much as possible by visualizing the target as being a great distance away.

A few of the older instruments have no focusing target. Such instruments should have their eyepieces converted if high accuracy is to be achieved. This conversion can be done either by the manufacturer or by any optical company that manufactures microscopes or telescopes.

Taking the Reading

1. Occlude the patient's eye that is not being measured. Many times this simple procedure is neglected because of lack of time. If the occluder is not used, the eye that is not being measured often becomes the fixating eye, so the eye being measured is not looking directly at the telescope of the instrument. The reading may actually be taken from a peripheral part of the cornea.

2. The instrument should constantly be refocused during the setting of the power dial. (It is recommended that this procedure be followed for both the American Optical Ophthalmometer and the Bausch and Lomb Keratometer.)

As a keratometer becomes worn some play will usually occur in the power wheel. This play can cause considerable error in the measurements. It can be effectively eliminated if the mire settings are always made by dialing from the same direction. If the final setting is made by turning the dial back and forth, the measurement will be less accurate.

Modifications to Instruments

The ability to achieve an accurate focus with the American Optical ophthalmometer can be improved by glueing a thin wire across one of the mires of the instrument. When the mire is viewed through the instrument, the wire appears as a thin, black line, which will fade from view when the instrument is out of focus. The focus should always be accomplished by moving the instrument towards the patient.

Shick has suggested a modification for the Bausch and Lomb keratometer that is designed to increase the accuracy and repeatability of the measurements.[9]

The mires are partially covered by black electrical tape. The top minus mire is shortened by covering the ends. The center of the bottom mire is also covered. A similar modification is made to the plus mires (Figure 33.5). This allows a vernier type alignment when the mires are viewed through the instrument.

INCREASING THE RANGE OF THE KERATOMETER*

Due to the individual calibration characteristics of each keratometer, a very small error occurs in the conversion chart to extend the range of this instrument. Rather, each owner can make his own calibration curve that will precisely extend the range of his individual instrument. The extended range as discussed here will be from approximately 31.00 D. to 61.00 D., which should be generally adequate.

Materials Needed

1. Four or five spherical surfaces of good quality fairly evenly spaced between 37.00 D. and 50.00 D. Steel ball bearings of the following diameters work well: 23/32 inch, 5/8 inch, 19/32 inch and 17/32 inch.

2. A +1.25 and a −1.00 D. sphere lens from a good test lens set. These lenses should be marked to be sure always to use the iden-

*Reprinted by permission of Mr. Keller from *Contacts*, vol. 1, No. 1, October 26, 1960.

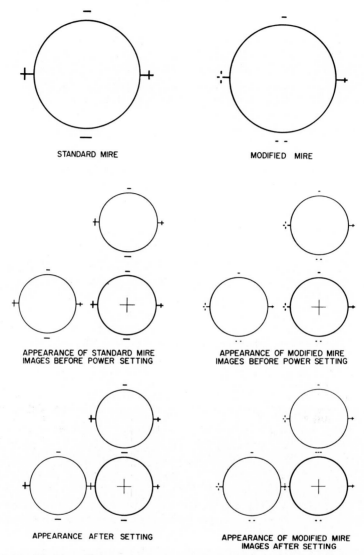

STANDARD MIRE   MODIFIED MIRE

APPEARANCE OF STANDARD MIRE   APPEARANCE OF MODIFIED MIRE
IMAGES BEFORE POWER SETTING   IMAGES BEFORE POWER SETTING

APPEARANCE AFTER SETTING   APPEARANCE OF MODIFIED MIRE
                                IMAGES AFTER SETTING

Figure 33.5. Modification of keratometer mires. From C. Shick, A Simple Mire Modification to Improve Keratometer Efficiency, *Journal of the American Optometric Association*, *34*(5):388–390, 1962.

tical lenses when reading the extended range of the individual keratometer.

3. Some suitable holder such as the Con-ta-Chek® for holding the balls in front of the keratometer.

4. Size 11 inches by 17 inches graph paper with ten divisions in one-eighth subdivisions on the ordinate and fifteen divisions in one-eighth subdivisions on the abscissa.

Procedure

1. Place the ⅝ inch steel ball on the Con-ta-Chek, and make five accurate readings of this ball. Take the average, and this is the true dioptral power of this ball (approximately 42.52 D.) (abscissa).

2. Now, without moving ball or keratometer adjustment, place the +1.25 D. sphere in front of the keratometer central aperture.

Hold lens handle between index finger and target plate, with finger at approximately 135° so as not to obliterate the plus or minus signs of the target. Center this lens over aperture by sliding with finger until reticle (cross hair) is again centered in the focusing circle.

Focus keratometer and take power readings with +1.25 sphere in place. Take five readings, and average as for true power previously. The resulting reading will be "keratometer reading" (ordinate). This indicated K reading for the ⅝ inch ball with the +1.25 sphere will be approximately 36.20 D.

The preceding will give one point for the graph extending range from 52.00 D. to 61.00 D., i.e. K reading (ordinate) 36.20 D./true power (abscissa) 42.52 D.

3. Using the same ⅝ inch ball and the −1.00 D. lens held in front of the keratometer, in place of the +1.25 D. lens, take five readings and average. This should give a K reading (ordinate) of approximately 49.70 D., for a true power (abscissa) of 42.52 D. This point is for your graph, extending the range from 36.00 D. to 31.00 D.

4. Repeat steps 1, 2, and 3 using the steel ball of 19/32 inch diameter. The true power (abscissa) should be approximately 44.76 D. and the K reading (ordinate) should be approximately 38.25 D. with the +1.25 D. lens and approximately 52.37 D. with the −1.00 D. lens.

5. Repeat the procedure using the 23/32 inch steel ball (true power approximately 37.00 D.) and the −1.00 D. lens only. (The +1.25 D. lens will give a reading off the range of the keratometer.) The K reading with the −1.00 D. lens will be approximately 43.25 D.

6. Repeat the procedure using the 17/32 inch ball (true power approximately 50.00 D.) and the +1.25 D. lens only. (The −1.00 D. lens will give a reading off the range of the keratometer.) The keratometer reading with the +1.25 D. lens will be approximately 42.60 D.

7. On the graph paper lay off the ordinate from 36.00 D. to 52.00 D. and label it "Keratometer Reading."

8. Lay off the abscissa from 30.00 D. to 62.00 D. and label it "True Dioptral Power."

9. You now have three points—Keratometer Reading/True Power—for the +1.25 D. lens as follows: 36.20/42.52, 38.25/44.76, and 42.60/50.00. Plot all three points, and if data have been accurately obtained, they will lie in a straight line. Extrapolate this curve to 61.00 D. true power.

10. Likewise for the −1.00 D. lens the three points are as follows: 43.25/37.00, 49.70/42.52, and 52.37/44.76. Plot, and extrapolate this curve to 31.00 D.

The foregoing is for convex surfaces.

To obtain a reading on a cornea too steep for the keratometer, simply place the +1.25 sphere in front of the keratometer, and take your reading through the +1.25 sphere. Look this value up on the chart under K reading (ordinate) and follow across to the plotted curve and follow down from the intersection to the true power (abscissa). For a flat cornea use the −1.00 D. lens and read true power from the calibration chart in a like manner.

A sample graph is presented in Figure 33.6. This graph may be used if only an approximate (± 0.50 D.) conversion is desired. A table gives better accuracy (*see* Appendix 7).

BASIC PRINCIPLES OF THE KERATOMETER

A Bausch and Lomb keratometer will be used to illustrate the general principles of a keratometer. Luminous mires at the front of the instrument are reflected by the cornea, which acts as a convex mirror and forms an image of the mires that is erect, virtual, and located about 4 mm. behind the corneal surface. The size of this image and the size of

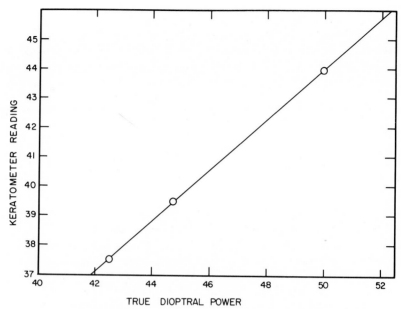

TRUE DIOPTRAL POWER

Figure 33.6. Extending the range of the keratometer.

the mires is sufficient information to calculate the radius of curvature of the cornea from optical mirror formulas. The size of the mires is fixed by the manufacturer, and the optical system of the keratometer is designed to give an accurate measurement of the image size, which is automatically converted into the radius of curvature for the cornea.

The size of the mire is too large to be considered as reflecting paraxial rays from the cornea, so this formula cannot be used in calculations where high precision is necessary. However, for the keratometer it is not necessary to know the exact image sizes but only the relative sizes of the images for various radii. Hence, the simple paraxial formula is used without fear of serious error. The derivation of this formula involves an approximation, which becomes very important for understanding the limitations of keratometry. Of the rays that can be constructed from the keratometer mire to the cornea in order to find the corneal image, the clinician should use the one that is directed at the focal point and which is reflected by the mirror so that it

is parallel to the optic axis (Figure 33.7). A second ray directed towards the center of curvature is reflected back along its own path. The extensions of these rays can be used to locate the position of the virtual corneal image.

h = size of the object (mire)

h′ = size of the image (corneal image)

r = radius of curvature of a mirror (cornea)

d = distance between the object and image

By similar triangles

$$\frac{h'}{h} = \frac{f'}{x} = \frac{r/2}{x}$$

To simplify the design of the keratometer, the following approximation is made.

The mire (object) is sufficiently far from the cornea that the virtual corneal image is formed very near to the focal plane of the cornea. The distance from the mire target to the focal plane is very little different from the actual distance, d, between the object (mire) and its corneal image.

Hence,

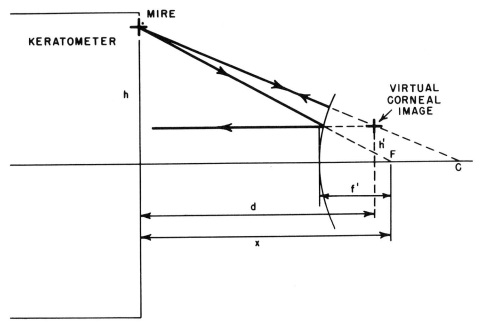

Figure 33.7. Basis of keratometer optics.

$$r \cong \frac{2dh'}{h}$$

The two mires, which are shaped as plus signs, represent the extreme points of an imaginary object in the horizontal meridian (Figure 33.8a). The distance between the two pluses represents the size of an object in the horizontal meridian. The size of the imaginary object is equal to the separation of the pluses, which in the keratometer is equal to 64 mm. The same distance separates the two minus sign mires, which represent an object in the vertical meridian. The distance from the mires to the corneal image is 75.0 mm.

Figure 33.8a shows the relation of the mires to the usual method of representing an object in an optical system by arrows. The image formed by the cornea is reduced in size and erect. Figure 33.8b shows the conventional optical construction of the image formation in the cornea.

The circle in the mire target does not contribute to the measuring operation of the keratometer but does provide a guide to irregularities in the curvature of the cornea. If the cornea is nearly spherical, the circle will be imaged in the cornea as a perfect circle. If the cornea has high astigmatism, the image of the circle will be an ellipse. Should corneal distortions occur, the circle is seen as irregular, blurred, doubled, or discontinuous.

The corneal image of the mire can be seen with the naked eye by looking from the side of the keratometer. In principle, the size of the image could be measured directly by holding a rule before the subject's cornea, except that the corneal image size is only about 3.0 mm.; and it would be difficult to measure with sufficient accuracy.

The keratometer provides an extremely accurate method to determine the size of the corneal image by combining a number of optical components into an elaborate measuring system. In order to understand this system, it may be conveniently divided into three parts, the illumination system, the telescopic system, and the doubling system.

Illumination System

Figure 33.9 shows a cutaway view of the

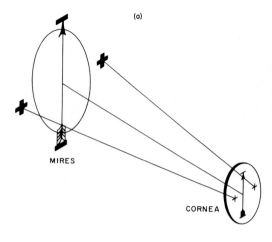

(a)

MIRES

CORNEA

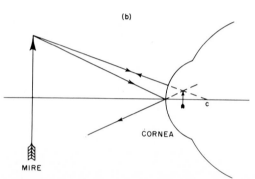

(b)

CORNEA

MIRE

Figure 33.8. Corneal image of the keratometer mires.

optical system of the keratometer. The illumination system begins at lamp I, from which rays are reflected by an elliptical reflector to pass through a filter and diffusing screen. They are then reflected by a silvered mirror, Z, to a condensing lens, R, through which they pass to illuminate the mires, M. Rays leaving the mires are reflected from the cornea and produce a virtual image whose size may then be measured to determine the radius of curvature of the cornea.

Telescopic System

The telescopic system of the keratometer consists of an ordinary astronomical refracting telescope, which is focused for a short viewing distance.

Light from the corneal image passes through an aperture between the mires to enter the telescope objective (L in Figure 33.9), composed of two doublet lenses. After traversing the objective, the light passes through a multiple aperture, which divides the light into four bundles that are focused at Y, the focal plane of the objective. The light from the image continues into the eyepiece, E.P., which has its anterior focal point at Y. Hence, the light that leaves the eyepiece is parallel. The eyepiece may be moved back and forth to compensate for the refractive error of the operator.

The function of the telescope is to magnify the corneal image. A simplified form of the telescopic system is illustrated in Figure 33.10. The virtual image of the mire that has been formed in the cornea is now treated as a new object, h_1, which will be imaged by the telescopic system. The mire image, h_1, is focused by the objective to form the image, h_1'. The size of this image is related to the object by the magnification of the objective. In the keratometer the magnification of the objective alone is 1.304, so $h_1' = 1.304h_1$.

The image, h_1', which is formed by the objective is further magnified by the eyepiece lens, which in the keratometer has a focal length of 16.7 mm. The total magnification of the keratometer is

$$\frac{103.4}{16.7} = 6.19 \times$$

If a scale were provided at the image plane, Y, both the scale and the image would be magnified by the eyepiece lens, and a fairly accurate measurement of the image could be read from the scale. However, the image would be constantly in motion due to small eye movements that are always present.

Doubling System

The problem of measuring a moving image is greatly reduced by incorporating a doubling system into the keratometer. The doubling principle was borrowed from astron-

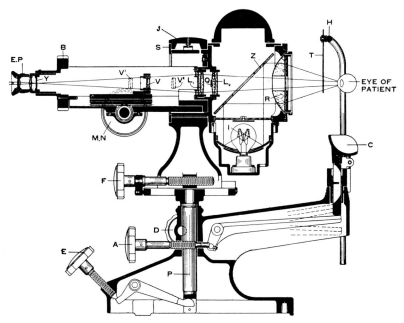

Figure 33.9. Optical system of the keratometer. Courtesy of Bausch and Lomb, Inc.

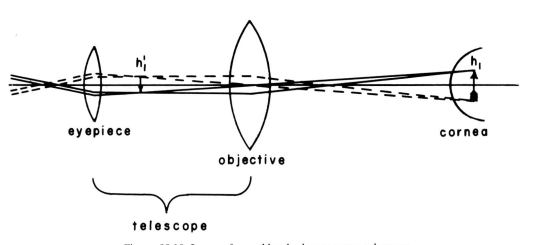

Figure 33.10. Images formed by the keratometer telescope.

omy, where it is used in the heliometer. It may be illustrated with a simple biconvex lens. In Figure 33.11a, a lens of 10 cm. focal length is used to focus an object at a distance of 20 cm. The image will be formed 20 cm. behind the lens. If a prism is placed 10 cm. behind the lens, the image will be displaced towards the direction of the prism base. A

prism of 10Δ will displace the image 1 cm. (Figure 33.11b). If the prism is moved towards the lens 1 cm. (and away from the image), the image will be displaced 1.1 cm. (Figure 33.11c).

If a smaller prism is placed behind the lens, which intercepts only part of the rays that pass through the lens, two images are formed, one at the usual position for the

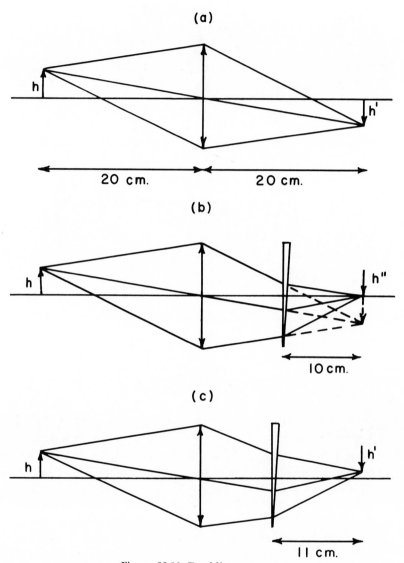

Figure 33.11. Doubling system.

image and another at a position which is determined by the power and position of the prism. Figure 33.12a shows the condition where a prism intercepts one-half of the light bundle that would form the image h' and produces a second image h''. If the object and image sizes are equal to 1 cm. and the prism is placed 11 cm. from the image plane, the ends of the two images will be separated by 0.1 cm. Changing the prism to a distance of 10 cm. from the image plane will move the images so the two ends touch, at which position the displacement of the image by the prism is equal to the image size. Consequently, if the size of the image were unknown, it would be determined by arranging the conditions of Figure 33.12a, moving the prism back and forth from the image plane until

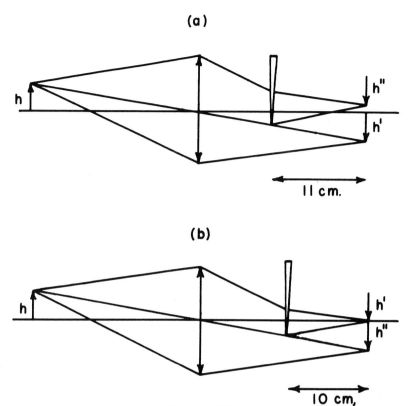

Figure 33.12. Doubling system.

the ends of the images touch (Figure 33.12b) and calculating the displacement of the image by the prism.

A doubling system may be incorporated into a telescope by interposing a prism into part of the light beam focused by the objective and forming two images in the image plane of the objective. If the prism is moved back and forth, a position may be found in which the ends of the images touch. In this position, the size of the image will be equal to the displacement by the prism. The additional magnification by the eyepiece lens will assist in the accuracy of aligning the images so that the ends of the images touch.

The most important attribute of the doubling system is that it is not materially affected by object movement. This is because the two images used to make the coincidence setting both move together as the object moves.

Formation of the View Seen by the Examiner

A front view of the multiple aperture used to break the rays into four bundles after passing through the objective is shown in Figure 33.13. The two smaller apertures, A and B, provide a very sensitive focusing mechanism based on Scheiner's principle, which doubles an image when it is not in focus. When the telescope is moved to its proper focus, the mire image is single. Apertures C and D are part of the doubling mechanism of the keratometer. The light bundle limited by aperture C passes through a base-in prism and forms a second mire image (G_2 in Figure 33.14) at Y. The light bundle that is limited by aperture D passes through a base-down prism and forms a third mire image (G_3) at Y. These prisms are shown in Figure 33.9 at positions V and V'.

The view to the examiner during a meas-

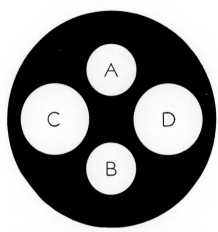

Figure 33.13. Keratometer aperture stop.

urement with the keratometer is illustrated in Figure 33.14. Figure 33.14a shows the appearance of a mire that is not in focus, shown by the double image G. The images that have been formed by the horizontal and vertical doubling prisms are found at G_2 and G_3 respectively.

In Figure 33.14b the instrument has been focused correctly, but the keratometer barrel must be rotated so that the pluses are in a direct line with each other, as in Figure 33.14c. This will occur only when the mires are aligned with the principle meridians of curvature of the cornea.

If the horizontal prism is moved back and forth from the focal plane, a position may be found in which the mire-crosses A and A' (Figure 33.14c) coincide as in Figure 33.14d. Since the mire-crosses represent the ends of an imaginary object in the horizontal meridian, the doubled images may be considered to be placed end to end when the opposite crosses are superimposed as in Figure 33.14d. The displacement of the image by the horizontal prism will now be equal to the size of the horizontal image. The size of the corneal image may be calculated from the magnification formula for the telescope objective. In the keratometer, the positions of the prisms are automatically converted into dioptric power values for the cornea, which appear on wheel M (*see* Figure 33.9) that moves the rack supporting the prism.

The size of the vertical image is measured in the same way.

OPTICAL SPHEROMETER

The optical spherometer, originally proposed by Drysdale as an instrument to measure surface curvatures of microscope objectives, has been successfully used in various surface radius measuring devices, e.g. radiuscope (Figure 33.15), for contact lenses. It is helpful first to review the principles of the optical spherometer and how it is used to measure a contact lens.

To produce an optical spherometer, an optical system is attached to an ordinary microscope, which projects an image of a target to a position about a centimeter below the microscope objective. This target is usually a pattern of lines arranged in a radial fashion. In most instruments the position at which the target is projected is coincident with the position at which an object must be held to be seen clearly by the observer when looking into the microscope. If the microscope is now focused upon the concave surface of a contact lens, the observer will see, in focus, both the surface of the lens and the target that is projected through the microscope (Figure 33.15).

If the microscope is now moved upward, a second position will be found at which the projected target is once again in focus. This occurs when the rays of the projected target strike the lens surface perpendicular to the surface and are reflected back along their own paths. A so-called aerial image is formed at the position for which the microscope is focused. Since the rays are now perpendicular to the surface of the contact lens, it means

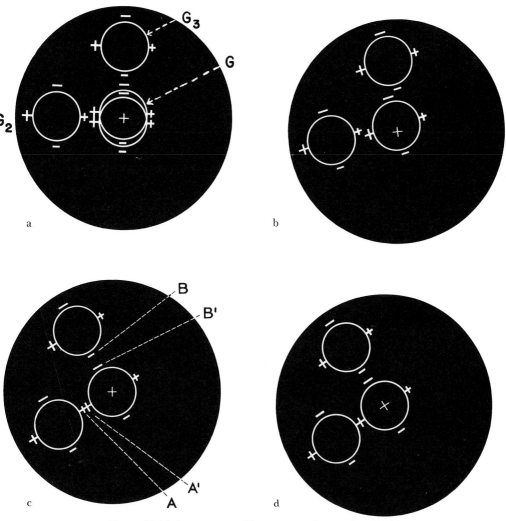

Figure 33.14. Appearance of keratometer images (*see* text).

that they pass through the center of curvature for the lens surface. The distance that the microscope must be moved to achieve first the focus on the lens surface and then the aerial focus will be equal to the radius of curvature of the lens surface. A measurement device is attached to the body of the microscope to measure the movement.

MEASUREMENT OF A CONTACT LENS CONCAVE RADIUS

The following procedure is used to measure the radius of the central curve concave side with an American Optical radiuscope (Figure 33.16).

1. Be certain that the contact lens is clean and dry.

2. Put a drop of water in the depression on the concave lens mount. Place the contact lens in the depression with the concave surface to be measured facing upward (Figure 33.17).

3. Position the lens mount in its support

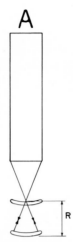

Figure 33.15. Optics of the optical spherometer.

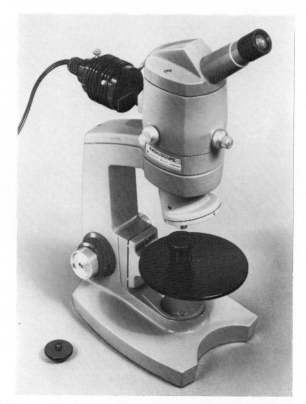

Figure 33.16. American Optical radiuscope. Courtesy of American Optical Co.

on the stage of the instrument. The mount should be reasonably level in its support, and the lens reasonably level in its mount in order that the center of the lens surface may be normal to the optical axis of the microscope.

4. Set the voltage selector at 5.0 V. (This is the most commonly used setting; however, others can be used depending on individual preference.)

5. Check the aperture selector of the illuminator to be certain that the *large* aperture is in working position. (When facing the instrument, push the selector to your left to position large aperture properly.)

6. Fully lower the objective of the microscope using a coarse adjustment knob.

7. Looking from the side, observe the beam of light coming from the objective, and move the stage until the beam appears to be centered on the contact lens. The stage can be rotated on its axis and moved in any horizontal direction by applying gentle pressure.

8. After visually centering the beam of light, *fully raise* the objective using a coarse adjustment knob. (Note: If using a binocular model, adjust the interpupillary distance of the eyepieces.)

9. Look into the eyepiece(s), and observe the scale on the right side of the field of view. Bring this scale into sharpest focus using scale focusing knob. (If the same practitioner always uses the instrument, it is not necessary to make this focusing adjustment each time the radiuscope is used. Merely check occasionally.)

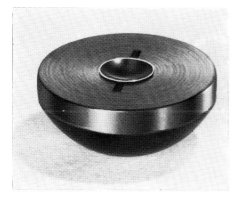

Figure 33.17. Concave lens mount with lens. Courtesy of American Optical Co.

10. While looking into the eyepiece(s), lower objective slowly, using a coarse adjustment knob, until you see light come into focus forming part or all of a spoke-patterned target.

11. Move the stage horizontally until the target is centered in the field of view. (Note: If using a binocular model, adjust the focus of the microscope for the right eye using a fine adjustment knob. Then with the right eye closed, adjust the left eyepiece tube. Refine interpupillary distance if necessary. Now both eyes should be properly focused for comfortable binocular vision.)

12. Now continue to lower objective. At one point the filament of the lamp will come into focus. Disregard and continue lowering objectives with a coarse adjustment knob.

13. The target will again come into view. (This is the real image of the target at the surface of the lens.) As focus begins to sharpen, change to a fine adjustment knob to bring target into critical focus.

14. When the target is in clear, sharp focus, use the index adjustment knob to move the index line to zero. On occasion, it may not be possible to move the index line to zero. In this case, set the index line to the nearest whole number.

15. Raise the objective until the upper (aerial) image of the target again comes into view. Raise the objective slightly beyond the point at which the image appears sharpest, then lower. (By focusing downward for final setting, more accurate readings are achieved.)

16. Bring the image of the target into sharp, clear focus using a fine adjustment knob.

17. If the original index line setting was at zero, read the radius of curvature directly from the scale at the position of the index line. If the original index line setting was at a plus whole number in the area on the scale below zero, add that whole number to the value shown by the index line at the aerial image.

Example

First setting (real image) index line at	+1
Second setting (aerial image) index line at	6.42
Radius of curvature	7.42

If the original index line setting was at a whole number in the main part of the scale above the zero setting, subtract this whole number from the value shown by the index line at the aerial image. The difference is the radius of curvature of the concave lens surface measured.

MEASUREMENT OF A CONTACT LENS CONVEX RADIUS

To measure the convex radius, the procedure is generally the same as for the concave radius, with one important exception: the position of the aerial and real images are reversed. When measuring a convex radius, the upper image is the real image and the lower, the aerial image.

1. Follow steps 1 through 5 used for concave measurement except that, in this case, the convex lens mount with the convex lens surface facing upward is used (Figure 33.18).

2. To center the beam of light on the convex lens surface (as described in step 7), the objective should be in the fully *raised* position. While in the raised position, bring the scale into sharpest focus using the scale focusing knob.

3. Fully lower objective, then raise until a spoke pattern target (the aerial image) comes into focus, and center target in the field of view.

4. Fully raise objective then lower until the other target (the real image) comes into focus. Move index line to zero (or the nearest whole number and note number).

5. Continue lowering objective to the lower target. Bring into sharp focus, using fine adjustment knob. Read scale at index line. Subtract this reading from previously noted whole number. The difference is the radius of curvature of the convex lens surface measured.

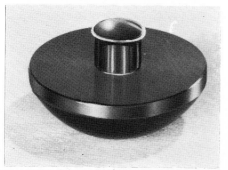

Figure 33.18. Convex lens mount with lens. Courtesy of American Optical Co.

MEASUREMENT OF TORIC BASE CONTACT LENSES

Follow steps 1 through 14 for a concave surface. Important: If the lens is not correctly positioned in its mount, the measurements cannot be taken, as target will appear fuzzy or distorted.

1. To orient the lens and mount properly, bring the target into the sharpest possible focus using a fine adjustment knob. Then slowly turn the mount in a horizontal circular direction until one of the spokes of the target becomes clearer than the remaining spokes. When turning, keep the whole target pattern centered in the field of view. It may be necessary to adjust focus with fine adjustment knob until this one spoke is in sharp focus. When this has been achieved, the lens is properly oriented for measurements.

2. Raise the objective until the upper (aerial) image of the target again comes into view. Bring the image of the same *spoke*, described in step 1, sharply into focus using a fine adjustment knob.

3. Read the radius of curvature from the scale, correcting for the original index line setting if necessary.

4. Next, using a fine adjustment knob, focus sharply on the spoke 90° away from the spoke previously in focus.

5. Repeat procedure in step 6 of previous section.

The *lowest reading* (smallest figure) is the meridian on the contact lens with the steepest curve. The *highest reading* is the meridian on the contact lens with the *shallowest* curve.

MEASUREMENT OF SECONDARY (PERIPHERAL) CURVE

The measurement of the secondary curve of a contact lens using the radiuscope is technically possible but only under *ideal* conditions. The secondary curve must be at least 1 mm. or wider and sufficiently well polished to reflect a measurable image. Otherwise, measurement is difficult or unattainable.

Use the same general procedure as previously outlined. However, in this case the stage is moved sufficiently to bring the peripheral curve portion of the test lens onto the optical axis of the microscope. Also, the lens and its mount are tilted in the lens mount support so that the secondary curve portion of the lens is normal (perpendicular) to the optical axis (Figure 33.19).

When measurement is possible, the secondary curve area can, generally, be more easily located and centered when the large aperture is used. It may be desirable to use the *small* aperture for the actual measurement, as its field of view is restricted to an area more nearly that of the secondary curve.

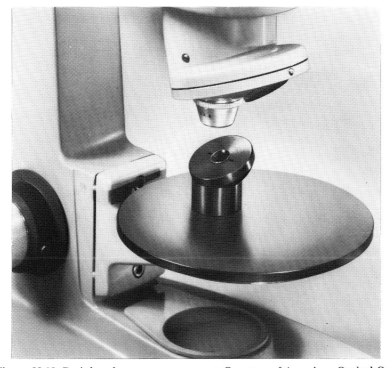

Figure 33.19. Peripheral curve measurement. Courtesy of American Optical Co.

CENTER THICKNESS MEASUREMENT OF CONTACT LENS

The radiuscope provides an optical method for measuring the thickness of a contact lens. This is particularly useful for flexible contact lenses where mechanical devices compress the lens.

Optical Principle

Assuming that the base curve (r_2) of the contact lens is spherical, optically it can be regarded as a concave reflecting surface and as a negative refracting surface. The radius of curvature of this surface determines the back reflecting and refracting powers. Since the American Optical radiuscope viewing system consists of a microscope, its front focal point can be positioned along the optical axis of the viewing system and the contact lens in such a way that point A_2, the back surface of the contact lens, can be viewed through the eyepiece. By advancing the radiuscope stage toward the microscope objective, a second focus (A_2), the image by the front surface, can be seen (Figure 33.20). This catadioptric image formed by the front surface of the lens is located within the lens. The distance of A_2 from A_3 provides the apparent depth or apparent thickness of the contact lens. The apparent thickness may be translated into the actual thickness by the following:

$$A^3A^2 = u' = \text{apparent thickness}$$
$$A^3A^1 = u = \text{actual thickness}$$

$$n = 1.49$$
$$n' = 1.00$$

From:

$$\frac{n'}{u'} = \frac{n}{u} + \frac{n' - n}{r}$$

Solve for u:

$$\frac{n}{u} = \frac{n'}{u'} - \frac{n' - n}{r} = \frac{n'}{u'} + \frac{n - n'}{r}$$

$$u = \frac{nu'r}{nr' + (n - n')u'} \text{ (exact)}$$

Substituting values:

$$u = \frac{1.49u'r}{r + 0.49u'}$$

Since $0.49u'$ in contact lenses is so small let it equal zero.

$$\therefore u = \frac{1.49u'r}{r}$$

And: $\underline{u = 1.49u'}$ (approximate)

Hence: actual thickness =
1.49 × apparent thickness

Procedure

Contact lens surfaces must be dry when measuring the center thickness. Place the lens with the concave surface up on the shoulder of the radiuscope lens holder. By elevating the radiuscope stage from its lowest position, the following will be seen successively through the eyepiece:

1. An aerial reflected image of the target formed by the back surface of contact lens.
2. Next, the lamp filament will appear in focus.
3. Finally, the target and back surface of

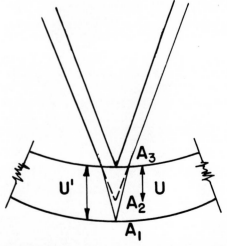

Figure 33.20. Measurement of contact lens thickness.

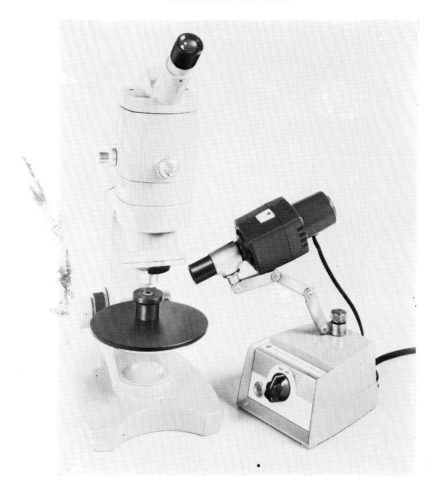

Figure 33.21. Use of radiuscope as a lens inspection instrument. Courtesy of American Optical Co.

the lens, when coincident, will appear in focus.

This last position (A_3) becomes the starting point in measuring the thickness of a contact lens. The stage is slowly elevated until the target is in focus as in step 3. Care must be exercised not to bypass point A_3 and focus on point A_2, the apparent point (Figure 33.20).

When point A_3 is in sharp focus, the indicator on the measuring gauge is adjusted to a zero reading. The stage is slowly and carefully elevated until the target is in focus at position A_2. (Note: A_3 will be only slightly out of focus; hence, a superficial image exists while viewing the lower image at A_2.)

The gauge reading is recorded in hundredths of a millimeter. This is the apparent thickness of the lens. The actual thickness is determined by multiplying the apparent thickness times the index of refraction:

Actual thickness = 1.49 × scale reading.

An alternate method, which requires no calculations, is borrowed from the industrial use of a measuring microscope. Place the lens on the platform and focus the target on the upper surface. Remove the lens and refocus on the platform. The distance traveled will equal the lens thickness.

TEST PLATE

A test plate is available and should be used periodically to verify the accuracy of the instrument.

CONTACT LENS INSPECTION

The radiuscope can also be used as an ordinary microscope for the examination of lens surfaces and edges. For this purpose it is recommended that the vertical illuminator be turned off and an inspection lamp be used. One method is to position the inspection lamp at a level just above that of the lens surface so as to provide grazing incidence of the light on the lens surface (Figure 33.21). Side illumination will cause the lens surface or edge characteristics to appear bright against a dark background when viewed through the instrument.

REFERENCES

1. Berliner, M. L.: *Biomicroscopy of the Eye*, New York, Hoeber, 1949.
2. Goar, E. L. et al.: *Slit Lamp Biomicroscopy—A Manual for Use of Graduates in Medicine*, Omaha, Douglas, 1954.
3. Mazow, B.: Slip-lamp microscopy in contact lens fitting, *J. Am. Optom. Assoc.*, 29(7):447–449, 1958.
4. Lester, R. W.: The use of the biomicroscope in contact lens fitting, *Optom. Weekly*, 50(46):2261–2270, 1959.
5. Neill, J. C.: Slit-lamp diagnosis and procedures in contact lens practice, *Am. J. Optom.*, 37(6):273–294, 1960.
6. Wachs, H.: Optometric slit-lamp procedures in contact lens practice, *Penn. Optometrist*, 21(3):16–20, 1961.
7. Goodlaw, E. I.: Use of slit lamp biomicroscopy in the fitting of contact lenses, in *Encyclopedia of Contact Lens Practice*, South Bend, Indiana, International Optics, vol. 3, Chap. 11, pp. 5–46, and vol. 4, Chap. 11, pp. 49–65.
8. Isen, A.: Methods that help achieve accurate ophthalmometry, *J. Am. Optom. Assoc.*, 30(10):723–724, 1959.
9. Shick, C.: A simple mire modification to improve keratometer efficiency, *J. Am. Optom. Assoc.*, 34(5):388–390, 1962.

ADDITIONAL READINGS

Brandreth, R. H.: Biomicroscopic techniques for hydrogel lenses, *Int. Cont. Lens Clin.*, 2(1):33–41, 1975.

Ciuffreda, K. J.: Understanding fluorescein contact lens photography: equipment and technique, *J. Am. Optom. Assoc.*, 46(7):706–713, 1975.

Crook, T. G.: Fluorescein as an aid in pachometry, *Am. J. Optom. Physiol. Opt.*, 56(2):124–127, 1979.

Estevez, J. M.: Poly (methyl methacrylate) for use in contact lenses, *Contact Lens*, 1(3):19, 1967.

Flower, F. C., and Hill, R. M.: Polymethylmethacrylate: measures of hydration, *Am. J. Optom. Arch. Am. Acad. Optom.*, 49(11):935, 1972.

Kaps, S. E.: Making the most of your slit lamp, *Cont. Lens Forum*, 2(10):15, 1977.

Ketelaars, H.: Measuring the power of wet contact lenses, *Ont. Optom.*, 8(5):12, 1976.

Chapter 34

OPTICS

S INCE THE INTRODUCTION of the corneal lens, there has been insufficient attention devoted to the purely optical aspects of contact lenses. Many of the optical principles that were developed previously for scleral lenses were applied to the corneal lenses without considering that in some respects the optics of the corneal lens are very different from a scleral lens and that varied approaches are necessary.

A complete knowledge of the theoretical optics of contact lenses is not absolutely necessary for a basic understanding of fitting procedures. However, much misinformation has permeated the contact lens field over the last decade that could have been avoided if more attention had been given to basic optics.

The sign convention used in this text is that of the Cartesian system,* in which light is considered as moving from left to right and in which all distances are measured from the lens, those to the left having a negative distance and those to the right being positive. Complex conditions with more than one lens will be explained as they occur.

OPTICAL CONSIDERATIONS FOR THE PRESCRIPTION

CONTACT LENS POWER

A contact lens is often treated as a thin lens so that thickness can be ignored and the simple formulas of thin lenses used. Although the contact lens is physically thin, it is not thin by the optical definition, and thick lens power formulas must be used. The error from making the thin lens assumption is very great for certain aspects of contact lens optics. For example, according to the thin lens formula for the optical power of a lens, one need only add the powers of the individual surfaces, F_1 and F_2, where

n' = index of refraction of the lens
n = index of refraction of the surrounding medium

The power of the front surface of the lens is

$$F_1 = \frac{n' - n}{r_1} \quad \text{(Formula 34.1)}$$

and the back surface

$$F_2 = \frac{n - n'}{r_2} \quad \text{(Formula 34.2)}$$

If F is the total lens power, then—

$$F = F_1 + F_2 \quad \text{(Formula 34.3)}$$

The following example will illustrate the error of the previous formula for contact lens calculations. A contact lens having surface powers of +70.00 D. and −65.00 D., by Formula 34.3, has a refractive power of +5.00 D.

---

*The Cartesian sign convention is well described in texts by Emsley[1] and Fincham.[2]

If, however, the thickness of the lens is 0.28 mm. and this factor is considered in the calculation, the power of the lens is found to be +5.86 D. The latter power is determined by the more accurate thick lens formula:

$$F_e = F_1 + F_2 - \frac{t}{n} F_1 F_2 \quad \text{(Formula 34.4)}$$

where

F_e = equivalent lens power in diopters
t = lens thickness in meters
n = index of refraction of lens material

For the previous example—

$$F_e = +70 + (-65) - \frac{.00028}{1.49} (70) (-65)$$

$$F_e = +5.855D.$$

From the equivalent power one may find the equivalent focal length of the lens, f_e, by the following formula:

$$f_e = -\frac{1}{F_e} \quad \text{(Formula 34.5)}$$

The equivalent focal length of a lens is measured from the principal planes (Figure 34.1). For most purposes it is correct to consider a thick lens as though it were replaced by a thin lens with a power equal to the equivalent power of the thick lens and placed in the position of the second principal plane.

The position of the principal planes of a contact lens will vary with the surface curvatures. It is therefore more useful, for practical purposes, to refer to the power of a contact lens as represented at one of the surfaces, a point that can be localized for various applications.

The power measured at the posterior surface, the back vertex power, is found by the following formula:*

$$F'_v = \frac{F_2}{1 - \frac{t}{n} F_1} + F_2 \quad \text{(Formula 34.6)}$$

This is the power obtained when a contact lens is measured with its posterior surface in the plane of the lensometer stop. (Anterior surface facing the telescope.) If the lens is reversed and held with the front surface facing the stop, one measures the front vertex power, given by the following formula:

$$F_v = F_1 + \frac{F_2}{1 - \frac{t}{n} F_2} \quad \text{(Formula 34.7)}$$

The variation in these powers is more pronounced when a plus lens of high power is considered. For example, given:

$$F_1 = 69.00 \text{ D.}$$
$$F_2 = 61.00 \text{ D.}$$
$$t = 0.30 \text{ mm.}$$

---

*Several alternate forms of this formula are commonly used.[1]

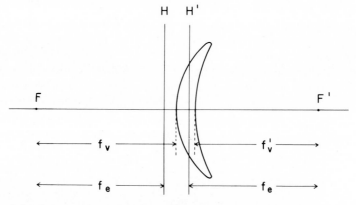

Figure 34.1. Comparison of the front vertex focal length (f_v), back vertex focal length (f_v'), and equivalent focal length of a contact lens.

$n = 1.49$

then

$$F_e = +8.842 \text{ D.}$$
$$F'_v = +8.966 \text{ D.}$$
$$F_v = +8.735 \text{ D.}$$

Hence, considerable error could occur if a lens were ordered on the basis of back vertex power and manufactured to give the power ordered in terms of front vertex power. This problem has indeed occurred in the contact lens field because there has not always been agreement as to which side of the lens should face the stop of the lensometer during its measurement.

The formulas previously discussed for lens powers apply when the lens is in air. When the lens is placed on the eye, the air is eliminated as an interface between the posterior surface of the lens and the cornea, but a thin layer of tears remains between the lens and cornea.

Consider two thin lenses, the first of which has a front surface power of $+10.00$ D. and a back surface power of -5.00 D. The second lens has a front surface power of $+6.00$ D. and a back surface power of $+10.00$ D. The entire combination appears in Figure 34.2.

The first lens has an index of 1.5, and the second lens an index of 1.6. If thicknesses are neglected, the power of the two lenses separated in air would be the sum of the powers of all the surfaces, or $F_{total} = +10 - 5 + 6 + 10 = +21$. If the lenses are joined together, their common surfaces are found to have the same radii of curvature so that the air surface

can be eliminated.

The radius of curvature for the back surface of the first lens is as follows:

$$F_2 = \frac{1 - n'_1}{r_2}$$

$$r_2 = \frac{0.50}{-5} = 0.1 \text{ M.}$$

The radius of curvature for the front surface of the second lens is as follows:

$$F_3 = \frac{n'_2 - 1}{r_3}$$

$$r_3 = \frac{0.6}{+6} = 0.1 \text{ M.}$$

Since the radii of the inside curves of the two lenses are the same, the two lenses may be joined together.

The total power of the lens is now the sum of the powers of the outside curves plus the power of the common interface, which is equal to the following:

$$F_{interface} = \frac{n'_2 - n'_1}{r_2}$$

$$= \frac{1.6 - 1.5}{0.1}$$

$$= \frac{0.1}{0.1} = 1.00 \text{ D.}$$

The total power of the outside surfaces is $+20.00$ D., making a total power for the lens of $+21.00$ D. This illustrates the very important principle that if two thin lenses each have a surface of the same curvature but opposite sign, it does not matter whether they are separated by a thin layer of air or placed together. The general expression for this relationship is easily derived. If F_1, F_2, F_3, and F_4 are the surfaces in order of the two lenses, the total power of the two lenses in air is

$$F_{total} = F_1 + F_2 + F_3 + F_4$$

If the inside surface radii of the lenses are represented by r_2 and r_3 and

$$r_2 = r_3$$

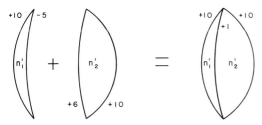

Figure 34.2. The power of two lenses joined together (*see* text).

then

$$F_2 = \frac{1 - n'_1}{r_2} \qquad\qquad F_3 = \frac{n'_2 - 1}{r_3}$$

When the lenses are joined together, the power of the common surface is

$$F_{3,2} = \frac{n'_2 - n'_1}{r_2}$$

Since the powers of the outside surfaces of the lenses will be the same regardless of whether the lenses are separated or not, the proposition will be proved if $F_{3,2} = F_2 + F_3$

$$F_2 + F_3 = \frac{1 - n'_1}{r_2} + \frac{n'_2 - 1}{r_3}$$

and since $r_2 = r_3$

$$F_2 + F_3 = \frac{1 - n'_1 + n'_2 - 1}{r_2}$$

$$= \frac{n'_2 - n'_1}{r_2} = F_{3,2}$$

If the refractive error of the eye is given with respect to the corneal plane, the following relationship holds. A contact lens that has an optical zone radius equal to the corneal curve will correct the eye's refractive error regardless of whether the lens is placed on the cornea or whether there was an infinitely thin air space between the lens and the cornea. Since this relationship is convenient only if the contact lens is expressed in terms of back vertex power, it is the method of choice to be used in most contact lens power calculations.

THE FLUID LENS

Even if the base curve of the contact lens has a radius of curvature equal to that of the cornea, a thin layer of tears is still found to lie between the two structures. The thickness of the tear layer is estimated to be less than 0.02 mm., which is too thin to have an appreciable effect on the power of the lens-eye optical system. If the optical zone radius of the lens is not equal to the corneal curve, however, as occurs in certain fitting techniques, the fluid lens must be considered in the contact lens power calculations.

If the parts of the contact lens-eye system are separated, there are three refractive elements—the contact lens, the tear layer, and the cornea—each of which may be considered as separated by an infinitely thin layer of air. The tear layer is often referred to as the *fluid lens* when considered in air. Its back curvature is fixed by the curvature of the cornea, and its front curvature is equal to the optical zone curvature of the contact lens.

The anterior and posterior powers of the contact lens surfaces are F_1 and F_2 respectively, and the powers of the fluid lens surfaces, F_3 and F_4. The back vertex power of the lens is F'_v and the power of the cornea-air surface is $F_{v_{cornea}}$ (Figure 34.3). In addition

r_1 = anterior surface radius of contact lens
r_2 = posterior surface radius of contact lens
r_3 = anterior radius of fluid lens
r_4 = posterior radius of fluid lens
$n_1 = 1.49$ = refractive index of lens
$n_2 = 1.3375$ = refractive index of tears

Consider the example where a trial lens with plano power is placed upon the cornea. The optical zone of the lens has a radius of 7.8 mm., and the curve of the cornea is 8.0 mm. The fluid lens now has a front curve of radius 7.8 mm. and a back curve with radius 8.0 mm. Its power, neglecting thickness (this will be justified later), is $F_1 + F_2$.

$$F_{f.l.} = \frac{1.3375 - 1}{0.0078} + \frac{1 - 1.3375}{0.008} =$$

$$43.27 - 42.19 = +1.08$$

When the optical zone of the contact lens differs in curvature from the cornea, the thickness of the tear layer becomes significant in contributing power to the contact lens–eye system.

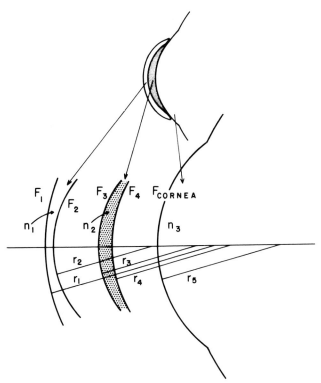

Figure 34.3. The contact lens–fluid lens–eye system.

Effect of Optical Zone Radius on Refraction

Occasionally it is necessary to change the optical zone radius of a lens in order to improve its fitting characteristics. If the optical zone radius of the contact lens is equal to the corneal radius and the contact lens corrects for the eye's ametropia, what effect will a change in the optical zone radius have on the total correction for the refractive error? This is most easily determined by reference to the fluid lens.

It should be recalled that when the cornea is measured with a keratometer only a radius measurement is obtained. This is converted (by the keratometer) into a dioptric value for the corneal power on the basis of an assumed index of 1.3375, which is very nearly the index of tears. When it is said that the optical zone radius of the lens is changed by some value, for example 0.50 D., this dioptric

value that is applied to the posterior lens surface is not correct. It too (by common faulty procedure) is based on a conversion of the radius for the posterior lens surface, which is incorrectly based on the index for tears of 1.3375, instead of the index of plastic, which is 1.49. However, this clinical error actually simplifies the calculation of effects on the refractive error caused by changing the optical zone radius.

The dioptric power that is incorrectly assigned to the optical zone radius of the lens is correct for the front surface of the fluid lens. Hence, any change in the power of the fluid lens will correspond to a change in the refractive status of the eye. For example, if the lens is fitted parallel to the cornea (so that the fluid lens has no power) and then steepened 0.50 D., the fluid lens now adds 0.50 D. too much plus power. The power of the lens must then be 0.50 D. more minus or less plus. Because it is the fluid lens that causes the changes in the refractive power and it does not depend on the refractive power of the contact lens, the simple rule still holds.

It is sometimes desired that a spectacle plane refraction be performed while a subject is wearing his contact lenses. This may be necessary in two situations: (1) when the fitting is accomplished by trial lenses and the refraction is taken through the lenses and (2) when the lenses have been fitted and it is necessary to modify the lens power. It is usually possible simply to determine the power of the spectacle lens needed to correct the ametropia, to make any allowance necessary for vertex distance from the spectacle plane to the cornea, and then to add the power of this correction algebraically to the refractive power of the contact lens that is being worn. If, however, the power of the contact lens is high, the simple relation previously described may not hold. Its failure is, once again, because the contact lens cannot be considered a thin lens and its back vertex power in combination with a spectacle lens will not be equivalent to the addition of the effective power of the spectacle lens with the back vertex power of the contact lens. For example, an aphakic is examined while wearing a +12.00 D. trial contact lens (0.4 mm. thickness) fitted on K, and it is found that an additional +3.00 D. is needed in the spectacle plane. If the vertex distance is 13 mm., the effective power of the +3.00 spectacle correction in the corneal plane is +3.12 D. The +3.12 D. diopters with +12.00 D. back vertex power of the contact lens gives a combined back vertex power for the spectacle and contact lens of +15.12 D.

If, instead of the method just described, light is passed through the same lenses using the vergence method, one finds the following:

Vergence of light striking spec. lens	0
Power of spec. lens	+3.00
Vergence leaving spec. lens	+3.00
Effective power vergence at C.L.	+3.12
Power of first surface C.L. (r = 7.849)	+72.97
Power at second surface C.L.	+77.62
Power leaving system F'_v	+15.24

Fortunately, for clinical purposes, the error is not significant.

The Fluid Lens Thickness

Measurements of the thickness of the tear layer range from 0.005 to 0.015 mm.[3] It is extremely difficult to make accurate measurements of the fluid lens thickness when the contact lens is *in situ*. However, it is possible to estimate the fluid lens thickness on a geometric basis if only a few assumptions are made. When a contact lens has an optical zone radius that is 0.1 mm. shorter than the corneal radius, the outer portion of the optical zone will rest on the cornea proper. If it is assumed that the lens does not compress the cornea, one may easily calculate the central clearance of the contact lens from the cornea.

It is possible to determine the heights of the cornea and base curve of the lens directly from the sagittal depth table. For example, a cornea of radius 8 mm. has a sagittal depth of 0.806 mm. for a 7 mm. cord width. The optical zone of the lens has a sagitta of 0.817 mm., so their separation is 0.11 mm.

Hence by geometry a fluid lens thickness of only 0.11 mm. is expected when the previous lens has been fitted 0.50 D. steeper than K. It may be argued that the lens is separated completely from the cornea by a layer of tears and that this value is too low. Clinical experience with fluorescein would indicate, however, that the lens does indeed rest on the cornea. Since the cornea is slightly compressible, the values calculated by geometry are high, if any appreciable error does exist.

If the contact lens optical zone radius deviates significantly from the corneal curve, it would be necessary to test whether the fluid lens must also be considered as a thick lens. The error due to neglecting the thickness of the fluid lens may be found by the vergence method shown previously.

For example, a contact lens with back vertex power of +4.00 D. and optical zone radius of 7.6 mm. is fitted 0.4 mm. steeper than the corneal curve. The optical zone is 7 mm. in diameter, the index of the lens 1.49, the fluid lens thickness equals 0.048 mm., and the index of the tears is 1.3375. Find the difference in the contact lens–fluid lens power when the fluid lens is considered as a thick and as a thin lens.

With the fluid lens considered thin, the procedure is as follows. Since the contact lens is given in terms of back vertex power, no calculation needs to be made for the power of the contact lens. The power of the fluid lens, considered to be thin, is simply the sum of its two surface powers.

The front surface of the fluid lens will have the same radius as the optical zone of the contact lens, or 7.6 mm. The power of this surface will be

$$F_3 = \frac{1.3375 - 1}{0.0076} = 44.408 \text{ D.}$$

The power of the posterior surface of the fluid lens is

$$F_4 = \frac{1 - 1.3375}{0.008} = -42.188 \text{ D.}$$

The power of the fluid lens is the algebraic sum of the surface powers, which equals

$$
\begin{array}{r}
+44.408 \\
-42.188 \\
\hline
+\ 2.220
\end{array}
$$

If the thickness of the fluid lens is now considered, the problem can be solved by the vergence method.

Light from a distant object leaves the contact lens with a vergence of +4.00 D. (the back vertex power). When the light strikes the front surface of the fluid lens, that surface imparts +44.408 D. of vergence, so the total vergence of light leaving the surface is

$$
\begin{array}{r}
+44.408 \\
+\ 4.000 \\
\hline
+48.408
\end{array}
$$

The effective vergence of this light at the position of the second surface of the fluid lens located 0.048 mm. away is

$$V = \frac{48.408}{1 - \dfrac{0.000048}{1.3375}(48.408)} = 48.492 \text{ D.}$$

If the vergence imparted by the second surface is now added, then

$$
\begin{array}{r}
48.492 \\
-42.188 \\
\hline
+\ 6.304 \text{ D.}
\end{array}
$$

The power of light leaving the fluid lens of +6.304 is the back vertex power of the contact lens–fluid lens system. Compared to the power of +6.220 D. obtained by considering the fluid lens as thin, there is a difference of +0.084 D. Such a difference is negligible for contact lens calculations.

It should be noted that the specifications of the contact lens were such as to create a rather thick fluid lens. Most of the time the lens will fit much closer to the curve of the cornea, and the power of the fluid lens becomes infinitesimal.

There has been concern over the effect of the fluid lens in corneal contact lens fitting. This appears to be a result of experience in fitting scleral lenses, where the fluid lens becomes significant in power. The tables for scleral contact lenses do not apply to corneal lenses.

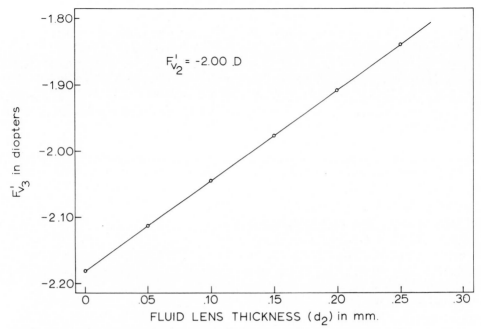

Figure 34.4. The contact lens–fluid lens back vertex power. From M. D. Sarver, Fluid Lens Power Effect with Contact Lenses, *American Journal of Optometry*, 39(8):434–437, 1962.

Calculation of the contact–fluid lens back vertex power can be made directly from the Gaussian formula for multiple surfaces, a technique used by Westheimer,[4] Sheard,[5] and Sarver.[6] Sarver determined (Figure 34.4) the relationship between fluid lens thickness and the back vertex power of the contact–fluid lens system (his F'_{v3}) for a contact lens of -2.00 D. back vertex power (F'_{v2}). He considered the base curve of the contact lens to be 0.03 mm. flatter than the corneal curve. In the range of fluid lens thicknessess to be expected for corneal lenses, that is, from 0 to 0.15 mm., the effect of the fluid lens is to add a small amount of minus power to the system. Actually, this amount of minus power is due principally to fitting the lens flatter than the corneal curvature, rather than to the thickness of the fluid lens system. It may be noted in passing that a contact lens fitted flatter than the cornea has a fluid lens that is of near zero center thickness and can always be neglected.

PRISMATIC EFFECTS

Corneal contact lenses remain centered with respect to the optical system of the eye for only a portion of the wearing time. With every blink or eye movement, there is an accompanying movement of the lens, then a compensatory movement while the lens comes to equilibrium with gravity. When the contact lens is not centered, there is an induced prismatic effect analogous to that which occurs when spectacle lenses are decentered from the line of sight.

If, as has previously been done, the contact lens is considered to be separated from the fluid lens by a thin layer of air, prismatic power may be computed in exactly the same way as for spectacles, using the well-known Prentice's rule, $\varDelta = Fd$, where

$\varDelta$ = prism induced in prism diopters
F = dioptric power of lens
d = decentration in centimeters

A lens of 9.0 mm. diameter, which moves to the limbus of a cornea 14 mm. in diameter, will be decentered approximately 0.25 cm. For each diopter of refractive power, the prism induced will be $\varDelta = 1(0.25) = 0.25\varDelta$.

It may therefore be concluded that prism effects are negligible for lower powers but may become significant in higher power contact lenses. Fortunately, the lens movement for the two lenses worn by a patient usually occurs together, so no relative prismatic difference occurs to interfere with binocular motor balance.

The effect of a vertical movement of a minus lens is to cause an apparent displacement of the visual field upward as the lens moves up on the eye and downward as the lens moves down. This apparent movement of the visual field during blinking can be somewhat disturbing when it is significantly high, as for a patient with high refractive correction.

As occasionally occurs after a blink in which the lenses are drawn high on the cornea, one lens may drop before the other, so significant vertical differences exist in the induced prism. If one lens is centered and the other touching the limbus, a lens of 6.00 D. will induce a difference of 1.5 $\varDelta$. There is sufficient vertical imbalance to cause fatigue.

It is sometimes desired that prism power be incorporated into the contact lens either for its optical effect or to act as a weight or prism ballast.

The prism power of a contact lens in air is not changed when the lens is placed on the eye. Bailey[7] and Mandell[8] have shown that the path of a ray through a prism incorporated into either a spectacle or a contact lens

can be found by the same formula. Consequently, prism power in a contact lens is not related to whether the lens is in air or on the eye, as has been claimed.[9,10]

Calculation of the contact lens prism can be most easily performed if the lens is considered to be composed of two elements, a prism and refractive part, separated by a thin layer of air.[8] The prism element will then be a thin meniscus, which can be considered as in air, and the usual formulas for spectacle prims can be used. This statement needs explanation.

The effectivity of a prism contact lens will vary according to its surrounding media. Four conditions must be considered.

1. A prism contact lens with plano power in air
2. A prism contact lens with plano power in water
3. A prism contact lens with plano power on the eye
4. A prism contact lens with significant refractive power on the eye

Each of these presents a unique optical problem.

Prism Contact Lens with Plano Power in Air

It has been standard practice to assume that the thin lens prism formula was applicable to contact lenses in air.[7-13] Strictly speaking, the use of this formula for contact lenses introduces an error due to the high surface curvatures (*see* the section Effect of Meniscus later in this chapter). Fortunately, the error does not affect the answer to the present problem, and the thin lens prism formulas can be used to simplify the discussion.

The well-known formula for the deviation produced by a prism of small apical angle is

$$d = \theta (n - 1)$$

where

d = angle of deviation of light
θ = apical angle of prism
n = index of refraction of prism

If the index of plastic is assumed to be 1.5, then

$$d = 0.5\,\theta$$

Prism Contact Lens with Plano Power in Water

The prism formula also applies, providing the relative index of water to plastic is used. Thus,

$$d = \theta \; \frac{1.5 - 1}{1.33} = 0.13\,\theta$$

Hence, the deviating capacity of a prism in water compared to the same prism in air is

$$\frac{0.13\,\theta}{0.5\;\theta} = 26\%$$

A Prism Contact Lens with Plano Power on the Eye

When a prism contact lens is placed on the eye, it forms a lens system consisting of a thin meniscus of tears, a prism contact lens, a second thin meniscus of tears, and the eye (Figure 34.5). If the posterior surface of the lens is equal in curvature to the cornea and the anterior surface is oriented at an angle θ to form a prism, both surfaces of the tear meniscus covering the front lens surface are also oriented at an angle θ with respect to the line of sight. A chief ray of light passes into the system at such an angle that it emerges along the line of sight. Assuming that the tear meniscus is thin, the normals n_1 and n_2 are parallel. Given:

n_1 = index of refraction of air
n_2 = index of refraction of tears
n_3 = index of refraction of lens
i_1 = angle of incidence of ray from air to tears
r_1 = angle of refraction of ray from air to tears
i_2 = angle of incidence of ray from tears to lens
r_2 = angle of refraction of ray from tears to lens
d_1 = deviation of ray from air to tears
d_2 = deviation of ray from tears to lens
d_3 = total deviation of ray from air passing into eye
θ = apical angle of prism

The total deviation of the ray is the sum of the deviations caused by refraction at the surfaces of the tears and contact lens. Hence,

$$d_3 = \theta\,(n_2 - 1) + \theta\,(n_3 - n_2) = (n_3 - 1)\,\theta$$

Since this is also the formula for the prism power in air, the deviating effect of a prism is

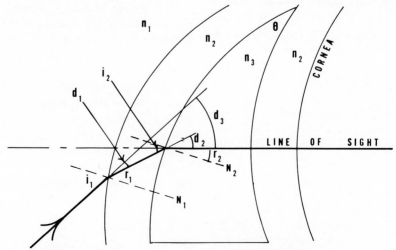

Figure 34.5. Deviation of a chief ray passing through tears, a prism contact lens, tears, and the eye.

not changed when it is placed on the eye. A proof can also be derived from the ray tracing of Figure 34.5 to prove

$$d_1 + d_2 = d_3$$

From the geometry it may be seen that the angles d_1 and d_2 form the acute angles of a triangle and that d_3 is the external angle of this triangle. Thus,

$$d_1 + d_2 = d_3$$

What is the effect of removing the tear layer covering the front lens?

From Snell's law

$$n_1 \sin i_1 = n_2 \sin r_1$$

which for small angles is

$$n_1 i_1 = n_2 r_1$$

and

$$n_2 i_2 = n_3 r_2$$

thus

$$\frac{n_1 i_1}{n_2 r_1} = \frac{n_3 r_2}{n_2 i_2}$$

Since n_2 factors from both sides, it is not effective. Consequently, the tear layer on the front of the lens has no effect on the total deviation of the ray.

A Prism Contact Lens with Significant Refractive Power on the Eye

Consider a prismatic contact lens as split into a refractive portion and a thin afocal prismatic portion so that their apposing surfaces, S_2 and S_3, have equal curvatures that are coaxial with surface S_4 but not surface S_1 (Figure 34.6). If two lenses each have an apposing surface of the same curvature but opposite sign, the optical power is not affected by separating the lenses by a thin layer of air or placing them together. Since every lens can be considered as an infinite number of prisms, the same reasoning should apply to a prism contact lens that is placed on the eye.

The effect of various refractive powers

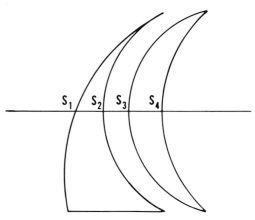

Figure 34.6. Prismatic contact lens considered as two parts, a prism and a lens.

combined with the prism power is illustrated in Figure 34.7.

In Figure 34.7a the lens has prism combined with plus power. If the lens is centered before the eye so that the line of sight is at LL', the prismatic effect would be equal to the prism component alone. If, however, as is usually the case, the lens rides down so that the line of sight passes through the top of the lens at PP', the prismatic effect is equal to the prism component plus the prism effect of a lens at a point away from the optical center. For the plus power lens (Figure 34.7a), this increases the effective prism power, base down, and for a minus lens (Figure 34.7b), it reduces the effective prism power. The total prism power may be calculated approximately by applying Prentice's rule to the refractive component and adding this to prism component of the lens. For example, a lens of $+5.00$ D. power combined with a 1.5Δ prism and riding 2 mm. below the line of sight would have an effective prism of 2.5Δ.

$$\text{induced } \Delta = d\,F$$
$$= 0.2\,(5) = 1$$
$$\text{total } \Delta = 1.5 + 1 = 2.5\ \Delta$$

A -5.00 D. lens with a 1.5Δ prism in the same position would have an effective prism power of 0.5Δ.

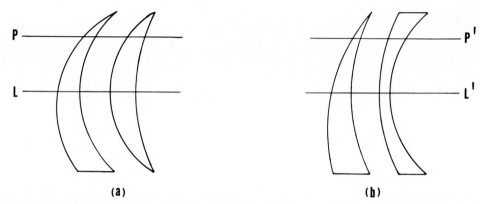

Figure 34.7. Effect of refractive power and lens position on prism power in a prism contact lens.

Effect of Meniscus

It cannot be assumed that the usual formula for the deviation of light by a flat prism of small apical angle θ always holds for a prism meniscus of small angle of inclination between two surfaces. Unlike a flat prism, a prism meniscus *in air* or *on the eye* has variable prism power, which is reduced at points away from the apex. The effective prism angle for any point on the prism meniscus is the angle of inclination of the two surfaces at the point of incidence of the ray of concern (Figure 34.8) and is found as follows:

Given:

γ = prism angle for incident ray
θ = apical angle
C_1 = center of curvature for front surface
C_2 = center of curvature for back surface
r = radius of curvature for prism surfaces

By dropping a perpendicular (ad) from a to the reference line and adding dC_1 parallel to bC_2, the following relationship holds:

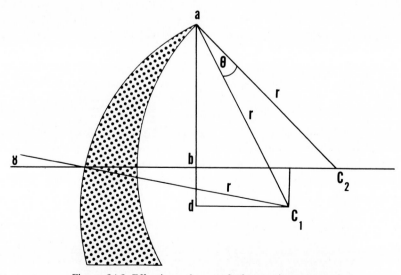

Figure 34.8. Effective prism angle for a prism contact lens.

$$\sin aC_2b = \frac{ab}{r}$$

$$\sin aC_1d = \frac{ad}{r}$$

$$\theta = aC_1d - aC_2b$$

$$\gamma = \arcsin \frac{bd}{r}$$

The standard prism formula

$$d = \theta (n - 1)$$

can be used for contact lenses if the apical angle is replaced by the angle of inclination of the two surfaces so that

$$d = \gamma (n - 1)$$

The effective prism power of a prism contact lens is always reduced at points away from the apex. If the prism power of a plano meniscus prism contact lens is measured at its geometric center on a lensometer and the lens rides down on the eye so that the line of sight passes above the geometric center, the effective prism power will be greater when the lens is on the eye than when it was measured in air.

Anisometropia

When an anisometrope has his contact lenses displaced from a centered position, there will be unequal prismatic effects induced. The prismatic imbalance will simply be the difference in prismatic power induced for the two lenses. In any case, the prismatic effect will always be less than would occur for the same subject wearing spectacles and making any significant excursion. Applying Prentice's rule for each lens

$$\Delta = dF$$

where

Δ = angle of deviation in prism diopters
d = distance (in cm.) contact lens is decentered
F = power of the lens

ACCOMMODATION

It was shown in Chapter 7 that the optical correction for the refractive error of the eye must have a slightly different power when it is in the corneal plane instead of the spectacle plane and that the difference is due to effective power. Refractive error is ordinarily referred to the spectacle plane as a matter of convenience and could be referred to the corneal plane or, if it were desired, to the second principal plane of the eye.

The stimulus to accommodation is usually specified with regard to the spectacle plane. If the stimulus to accommodation is referred to the corneal plane, it will have a slightly lower value. Obviously, the actual stimulus to accommodation has not changed because the object remained at the same position relative to the eye.

The actual accommodation that will be required by the eye can only be determined with reference to the first principal plane of the eye. Since the first principal plane is separated only about 1.35 mm. from the cornea, the accommodation required by the eye will be little different from that required at the corneal plane.

When an ametrope is corrected by spectacles, the stimulus to accommodation for an object at a given distance will be somewhat different from what it would be for an emmetrope looking at the same object.

It has already been discussed that a myope or hyperope of given refractive error in spectacle lenses would have different powers in their contact lenses. It is possible to determine the required refractive correction at the first principal plane by simply calculating the effectivity of the spectacle lenses using 15 mm. (distance from spectacle plane to principal plane) instead of the 13 mm. used for the distance from the spectacle plane to the cornea.

If one determines the corrective lens needed at the principal plane for two spectacle ametropes, one a −7.00 D. myope and the other a +7.00 D. hyperope, the effective corrections for the principal plane would be +8.47 D. for the hyperope and −6.33 D. for the myope. One can now calculate what stimulus to accommodation would occur for each of these subjects when they are viewing an object at 33.3 cm. away from the lens.

For the hyperope, the light striking the lens would have a vergence of −3.00 D. This combined with the +7.00 D. power of the lens would cause the light to leave the lens with a vergence of +4.00 D. The effectivity of this light in the principal plane would be +4.26 D. The subject would accommodate +4.26 − (+8.47) or −4.21 D. For the myope the light striking the lens would also have a vergence of −3.00 D. but in leaving the lens would have a vergence of −10.00 D. The effective power of this light at the first principal plane of the eye would be −8.70 D. The myope needs −6.33 D. of this to correct his

ametropia, which leaves an accommodative stimulus of −8.70 − (−6.33) or −2.37 D. It should be noted that an emmetrope looking at the same stimulus would be required to exert −2.87 D. of accommodation (1/34.83).

The previous calculations were performed with the assumption that thin lenses were used. If the form and thickness are considered, the results will differ little for minus lenses but may vary significantly for plus lenses.[14] This is because the first principal plane of a plus miniscus lens is always in front of the lens and gives the effect of moving the spectacle lens farther away from the eye. A slight shift of the principal planes may also occur during accommodation. Westheimer, using a vergence method, calculated the accommodation required for looking at a target for the distances of 33 and 50 cm. (Figure 34.9).[15] The spectacle plane was considered to be 14 mm. in front of the first principal plane.

Rather than calculate the preceding by the vergence method, it is possible, as Alpern has done,[16] to construct a formula for the same calculation.

CONVERGENCE

When converging to look at a near object, the angular rotation of the eyes depends upon the distance of the object fixated and the interpupillary distance of the subject. If the angle rotated by each eye is θ, then the total convergence is 2θ. Calling the distance of the object from the center of rotation of the eye u and one-half the interpupillary distance AC, then

$$\tan\theta = \frac{AC}{u}$$

If the subject is hyperopic and is corrected with spectacle lenses, he will need to converge more than an emmetrope to look at an object located at the same distance. This is so because as the eyes converge they look inwards

from the optic centers of the lenses and thus encounter what is effectively a base-out prism.

The calculation of the convergence required through positive spectacle lenses has been given by Alpern,[16] using methods suggested by Westheimer and Fry (Figure 34.10). The ray ADR is found, which, when refracted by the spectacle lens, passes through the center of rotation of the eye. The angle DRO then represents the rotation of the eye necessary to view the point A through the lens

$$\tan \dot{D}\dot{R}\dot{O} = \frac{DO}{OR}$$

DO is found first by locating the image of R as formed by the spectacle lens. Then by similar triangles

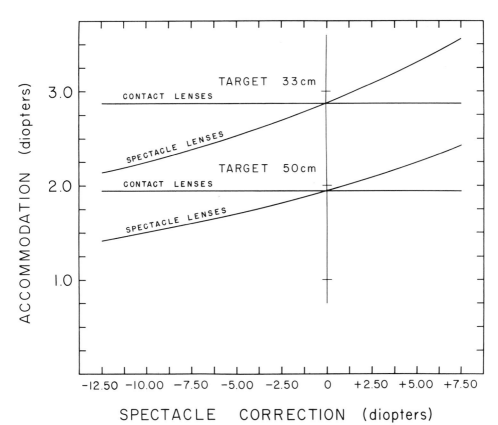

Figure 34.9. Ocular accommodation required when patient with the spectacle ametropia shown on the abscissa of the graph views a target 33.3 cm. and 50 cm., respectively, in front of the spectacle plane (14 mm. in front of the corneal vertex) when wearing spectacle lenses and contact lenses. From G. Westheimer, The Visual World of the Contact Lens Wearer, *Journal of the American Optometric Association, 34(2):*135–138, 1962.

$$\frac{DO}{AC} = \frac{s'}{CO + s'}$$

$$DO = \frac{s'AC}{CO + s'}$$

Since by the thin lens formula

$$\frac{1}{s'} - \frac{1}{s} = \frac{1}{f}$$

substituting

$$\frac{1}{s'} - \frac{1}{OR} = F$$

$$OR = \frac{s'}{1 - s'F}$$

If the same subject were wearing contact lenses instead of spectacles and they remained centered on his lines of sight, then each eye would only need to rotate through the angle ÁRĊ. The difference in rotation required when changing from spectacles to contact lenses would be

$$\text{ḊRȮ} - \text{ÁRĊ}$$

If the subject were myopic and wore minus lenses, it would be found that more convergence would be required when contact lenses were worn instead of spectacles.

Westheimer has calculated the convergence needed to bifixate targets at 33 and 50 cm. for various degrees of ametropia (Figure 34.11).[15]

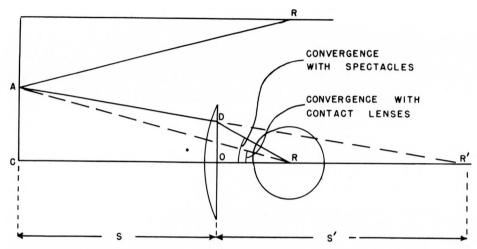

Figure 34.10. Calculations of the convergence required through a positive power spectacle lens. Adapted from M. Alpern, Accommodation and Convergence with Contact Lenses, *American Journal of Optometry, 26(9)*:379–387, 1949.

MANUFACTURER'S SPECIFICATIONS

FRONT SURFACE RADIUS

In the design and manufacture of a contact lens, the optical zone radius and power are specified in the prescription, while the refractive index and lens thickness are confined to narrow limits by the physical attributes of the lens material. The only lens dimension that can be varied to produce a large range of powers is the front surface radius.

To achieve the accuracy required in ophthalmic optics, the calculation of front surface radii for contact lenses must be accomplished by the use of the thick lens power formula. Since calculations by this formula are time-consuming, contact lens manufacturers depend upon rules derived from experience in making large quantities of lenses or books of tables, which give front surface curves for contact lenses of various dimensions.

Braff has shown that the calculation of front surface radius for a contact lens of given base curve and back vertex power can be greatly simplified by using the thin lens power

formula and adding correction factors that make it equivalent to the usual thick formula for back vertex power.[17] The correction factors were found by solving equations for front surface radius of a number of lenses using both thin and thick lens formulas and noting that for any given lens thickness the difference between the values found by the thin and thick lens formulas was constant. A table of such results was included in the paper.

It is possible to use a more general approach than that taken by Braff and show, by formal derivation, that the relationship between the thin and thick optics formulas holds for all lenses, regardless of their dimensions, and can be computed to any desired accuracy.[18]

Given:

r_1 = radius of front surface of thick lens
r'_1 = radius of front surface of thin lens
$k = r_1 - r'_1$ = correction factor

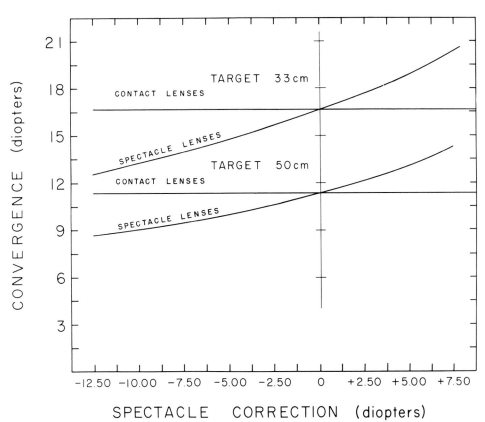

Figure 34.11. Convergence in prism diopters that has to be exerted by patient (P.D. 65 mm.) with the spectacle ametropia shown on the abscissa of the graph when viewing a target 33.3 cm. and 50 cm., respectively, in front of the spectacle plane when wearing spectacle lenses and contact lenses. From G. Westheimer, The Visual World of the Contact Lens Wearer, *Journal of the American Optometric Association, 34(2):*135–138, 1962.

From the thick lens formula for back vertex power it may be shown that

$$F'_v = \frac{F_1}{1 - \frac{t}{n}F_1} + F_2 = \frac{1}{\frac{1}{F_1} - \frac{t}{n}} + F_2$$

$$F_v - F_2 = \frac{1}{\frac{r_1}{n-1} - \frac{t}{n}}$$

$$= \frac{1}{\frac{nr_1 - t(n-1)}{n(n-1)}}$$

$$= \frac{n(n-1)}{nr_1 - t(n-1)} = \frac{n-1}{r_1 - \frac{t}{n}(n-1)}$$

Beginning again and using the thin lens formula for approximate power:

$$F = F_1 + F_2 \qquad \text{(Formula 34.3)}$$

If back vertex power can be found by adding a constant k to the front surface radius for the thin lens, then the same constant must be subtracted from the front surface radius of the thick lens:

$$F'_v = \frac{n-1}{r_1 - k} + F_2$$

$$F'_v - F_2 = \frac{n-1}{r_1 - k}$$

Taking both expressions equal to $F'_v - F_2$ as equal

$$\frac{n-1}{r_1 - k} = \frac{n-1}{r_1 - \dfrac{t}{n}(n-1)}$$

Thus:

$$k = \frac{t}{n}(n-1)$$

Therefore, the correction factor is a linear function of the refractive index of the lens and its thickness and, if these are fixed, will hold for any base curve or back vertex power.

Values for the thin lens front radius correction factor for various lens thicknesses (n = 1.49) appear in Table 34.1. Their application may be illustrated by the following problem.

Given these contact lens values:

$$n = 1.49$$
$$F_2 = -60$$
$$t = 0.18 \text{ mm.}$$

A lens is to be fabricated which will have a back vertex power of −4.00 D. What must be the radius of the front surface? If the thick lens formula for back vertex power is used

$$F_1 = \frac{F'_v - F_2}{1 + \dfrac{n}{t}(F'_v - F_2)}$$

$$= \frac{-4.00 - (-60)}{1 + \dfrac{0.00018}{1.49}(-56)}$$

$$= 55.624$$

$$r_1 = \frac{n-1}{F_1} = \frac{0.49}{55.624} = 0.008809$$

$$= 8.809 \text{ mm.}$$

in order to solve the same problem using the thin lens formula

$$F_1 = F - F_2$$

$$= -4.00 - (-60) = 56$$

$$r = \frac{1.49 - 1}{56} = \frac{0.49}{56} = 0.008750$$

$$= 8.750 \text{ mm.}$$

$$r_1 = r + k$$
$$r_1 = 8.750 + 0.059 = 8.809$$

If, in addition to Table 34.1, tables are used for power-radius conversions, it is possible to perform this calculation mentally. Such a table is given in Appendix 1.

EDGE THICKNESS

From a practical standpoint, the calculation of edge thickness for a contact lens is most often needed in determining whether it is possible to manufacture a lens of given specifications. It is not uncommon for contact lens manufacturers to receive orders for lenses that are impossible to make because they will not have sufficient edge thickness. A knowledge of edge thickness calculations is also valuable for determining the minimum center thickness of a positive power lens that will allow sufficient edge thickness.[19]

In all positive power lenses and in some negative power lenses with peripheral curves, the anterior and posterior surfaces approach each other in the periphery so that their intersection represents a theoretical limit to the total diameter (Figure 34.12a). At this limit, the lens has an edge thickness of zero. If the size of the lens is to be larger than its theoretical limit and the surface curvatures cannot be changed, the center thickness must be increased; otherwise, the lens cannot be made (Figure 34.12b). If the center thickness is reduced, the lens cannot be made unless it is also reduced in diameter. For practical purposes the possibility that a lens cannot be manufactured is controlled by choosing a center thickness that is more than the anticipated minimum. Unfortunately, this means that superfluous weight will be added to the positive power lenses, which in most cases are already heavier than that desired. Thus, it is important to choose the minimum cen-

TABLE 34.1

CENTER THICKNESS	ADD TO R
0.08	0.0263
0.10	0.0329
0.12	0.0395
0.14	0.0461
0.16	0.0526
0.18	0.0592
0.20	0.0658
0.22	0.0724
0.24	0.0789
0.26	0.0855
0.28	0.0921
0.30	0.0987
0.32	0.1052
0.34	0.1118
0.36	0.1184
0.38	0.1250
0.40	0.1316
0.50	0.1645
0.60	0.1973
0.70	0.2302
0.80	0.2631

be comfortable (knife edge). An edge thickness before finishing of approximately 0.12 mm. is optimal (Figure 34.12c).

In most cases, lenses of negative power will have sufficient edge thickness for any needed center thickness. An exception is found when a lens of low negative power has a very large diameter and a very flat peripheral curve. Here, again, it is possible to choose lens variables that make an impossible lens design.

The thickness of a contact lens edge varies as a function of every geometric variable of the lens, and its computation by usual methods is too lengthy to be of direct value to the practitioner or manufacturer. With the aid of sagittal depth tables, however, the calculation may be reduced to the simple addition and subtraction of the various sagitta of the lens curves. A number of sagittal depths for the curves in the range used for contact lenses have been compiled and are presented in Appendix 6.

The simplest illustration of the calculation for edge thickness of a contact lens occurs in the case of a monocurve lens, as shown in Figure 34.13. The sagittal depth of the front

ter thickness for a lens of positive power that will result in the minimum acceptable edge thickness.

Although an edge thickness of zero would be the theoretical minimum, practically speaking, a lens cannot be made with zero edge thickness, for the edge would be too sharp to

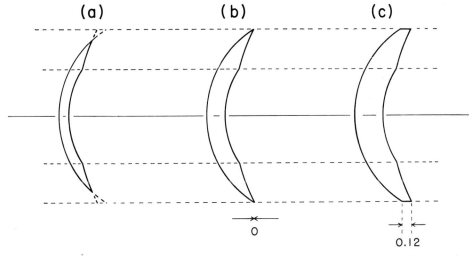

Figure 34.12. A contact lens is limited in diameter by the intersection of its surfaces (*a*). An increase in diameter can be achieved by increasing the center thickness (*b*). An increase in edge thickness can be obtained by increasing the center thickness (*c*).

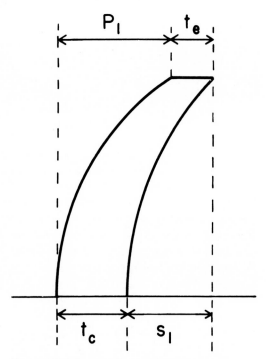

Figure 34.13. Sectional view of one-half of a mono-curve lens. Thickness of the edge varies as a function of every geometric variable of the lens.

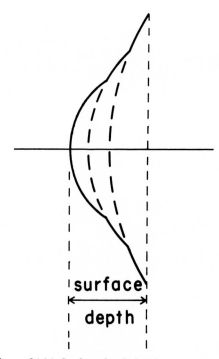

Figure 34.14. Surface depth for the posterior surface of a tricurve lens.

surface is P_1 and of the posterior surface is s_1. The edge thickness, t_e, is simply the sum of the center thickness, t_c, and the sagittal depth of the posterior surface, minus the sagittal depth of the anterior surface. This relationship may be expressed by the formula:

$$t_e = t_c + s_1 - P_1 \quad \text{(Formula 34.8)}$$

In multicurve lenses, where more than one curve is present on either the front or back surfaces of the lens, the total depths of the two surfaces (referred to hereafter as surface depth) may be substituted for the sagitta of Formula 34.8. Surface depth is measured from the apex of the most central curve to the plane passing through the periphery of the surface (Figure 34.14). The edge thickness for any lens will be equal to the sum of the center thickness and the posterior surface depth minus the anterior surface depth.

For a bicurve lens with a single curve front surface, the anterior surface depth will be equal to the sagittal depth of the anterior surface (Figure 34.15). The posterior surface depth must be calculated from the base and peripheral curves as follows: The sagittal depth of the optical zone, s_1, is found from Appendix 6 by using the diameter of the optical zone and the radius of the optical zone. The sagittal depth of the peripheral curve, s_2, is found by using the radius of the peripheral curve and the outside diameter of the peripheral curve, that is, the diameter of the optical zone plus twice the width of peripheral curve, which in this case is the total diameter of the lens. It may be noted from Figure 34.15 that the sagitta of the two posterior surface curves overlap by a distance m_1. The total surface depth will, therefore, be equal to the sum of the sagitta of the

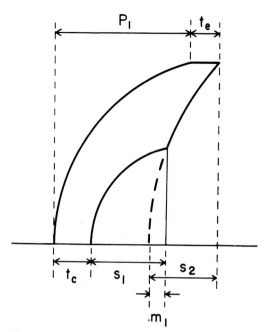

Figure 34.15. Sectional view of one-half of a bicurve lens.

central and peripheral curves minus the depth of their overlap. The overlap may also be determined from Appendix 6 since it is equivalent to the sagittal depth of the peripheral curve having a diameter equal to that of the optical zone. The edge thickness may now be found by adding the center thickness to the posterior surface depth and subtracting the anterior surface depth. This relationship may be expressed in terms of the following formula for the edge thickness of a bicurve lens:

$$t_e = t_c + s_1 + s_2 - m_1 - P_1 \quad \text{(Formula 34.9)}$$

For the tricurve lens the procedure for calculating edge thickness follows the same principle as described for the bicurve lens except that the sagittal depth of the third curve, s_3, is added, and the overlap between the second and third curves, m_2, is subtracted. The formula for a tricurve lens would be

$$t_e = t_c + s_1 + s_2 + \quad \text{(Formula 34.10)}$$

$$s_3 - m_1 - m_2 - P_1$$

The same method can be used for a lens with any number of posterior curves by adding to the right hand side of Formula 34.10 the sagittal depth of each additional curve and subtracting the length of its overlap with the previous curve.

Lenticular Lenses

If the front surface of a contact lens has more than one curve, as would occur in a lenticular lens, the sagitta of the curve(s) are subtracted, and the overlap(s) are added to the right side of any of the edge thickness equations. For example, Formula 34.8 would be modified for a two curve front surface to become

$$t_e = t_c + s_1 - P_1 - P_2 + n_2$$

where

P_2 = saggital depth of the peripheral anterior curve
n_2 = overlap between anterior curves.

For a lenticular bicurve lens, the formula would be

$$t_e = t_c + s_1 + s_2 - m_1 - P_1 - P_2 + n_2$$

Application of Formulas

The application of the edge thickness formulas may be illustrated by the following examples:

Example 1
Given a lens of the following specifications:

O.Z.R.	O.Z.D.	P.C.R.	P.C.W.	Dia.	Front Radius
7.00	7.00	7.50	1.0	9.00	7.60

Find the center thickness for the lens that will have an edge thickness of 0.12 mm.
From formula

$$t_e = t_c + s_1 + s_2 - m_1 - P_1$$

$$0.12 = t_c + 0.938 + 1.500 - 0.867 - 1.475$$

$$t_c = 0.216$$

Example 2
Given a lens of the following specifications:

O.Z.R.	O.Z.D.	P.C.R.	P.C.W.	Dia.	Front Radius	t_c
7.4	6.5	8.00	1.5	9.5	6.8	0.25

What is the edge thickness?

$$t_e = t_c + s_1 - s_2 + m_1 - P_1$$

$$t_e = 0.25 + 0.752 - 0.690 + 1.563 - 1.934$$
$$t_e = -0.059$$

Since the edge thickness has a negative value, it indicates that the lens cannot be made unless the center thickness is increased at least 0.059 mm. In order for the edge thickness to be 0.12 mm., the center thickness would have to be 0.429 mm.

MAGNIFICATION

In optics, magnification refers to the ratio of image to object size. For the eye, however, magnification may also refer to either the ratio of the sizes for the same ocular image under two different conditions or to the ratio of the image size for two eyes.

The corrected retinal image, which is in focus, is compared to one of two possible images:

1. *The blurred retinal image that was present before the correcting lens was placed before the eye.* The ratio of the size of the focused retinal image when an ametropic eye is corrected to the size of the blurred retinal image in the uncorrected eye will be called *magnification of correction.**

2. *The image size of a hypothetical emmetropic eye.* Calculations for relative comparisons of the image size between one eye and another may be simplified if each eye is compared to an emmetropic eye. The dimensions of the emmetropic eye may vary but are usually assumed to be equal to either the axial length or the refractive power of the ametropic eye, which is then considered to have either refractive or axial ametropia, respectively. The ratio of the size of the focused image in the corrected ametropic eye to the size of the focused image in the hypothetical emmetropic eye will be called *relative magnification.*

MAGNIFICATION OF CORRECTION

When the refractive error of an ametropic eye is corrected either by a contact lens or a spectacle lens, a change occurs in the size of the retinal image that corresponds to the power of the correcting lens, the lens position relative to the eye, and the shape of the lens. If the lens is thin, the shape can be ignored, and only the power and position need be considered.

With the standard method of Gaussian optics, it may be considered that light entering the eye is refracted at the first principal plane

and that light leaving the eye is refracted at the second principal plane. However, the principal planes are only of value when determining the size of a focused image. When the image is out of focus, it is necessary to calculate the retinal image size by measurements from the entrance and exit pupil of the eye.

The entrance pupil represents a hypothetical aperture, about 3 mm. behind the cornea, which limits the extent of the light bundle entering the optical system of the eye. This light bundle contains those rays which, after refraction, pass through the real pupil of the eye. The entrance pupil is defined as the image of the real pupil formed by the optics in front of it. The exit pupil limits the

---

*When spectacles are used to correct ametropia, magnification of correction is identical with what is commonly called "spectacle magnification."[1,14]

bundle of rays that leaves the optical system of the eye. The ray that passes from the object to the center of the entrance pupil (chief ray) represents the center of the light bundle which passes into the eye, and the ray from the center of the exit pupil to the image represents the center of the light bundle that passes from the optical system of the eye to the retina.

Geometric construction shows that when a blurred image is formed in the eye, the usual Gaussian ray trace does not give the true location of the retinal image. With the Gaussian system, when a blurred image is formed, the ray through the anterior focal point of the eye, which runs parallel to the axis from the principal plane to the retina, intersects the retina at a totally different position from the ray through the exit pupil, the chief ray (Figure 34.16). Therefore, the entrance and exit pupils can be used to determine the size of either a focused or out-of-focus image. The principal planes can only be used to determine an in-focus image size, but they may provide a more simplified calculation for this condition.

In Figure 34.17a a bundle of light limited by rays 1 and 3 enters a myopic eye. Ray 2 is the central or chief ray of the bundle and determines the center of the blur circle on the retina. The chief ray forms angle ω with the optic axis at the entrance pupil (E) and forms angle ω' with the optic axis at the exit pupil (E'). The ratio of angle ω' to angle ω is constant for any eye and has a value of approximately 0.8. The magnification of correction for this eye will equal the ratio of ω' after correction to ω' before correction. Since ω' is a constant function of ω, the magnification of correction will also equal the ratio of angle ω after correction to before correction. When the ametropia of the eye is corrected by the spectacle lens (Figure 34.17b), rays 1, 2, and 3 are refracted by the lens and enter the eye as though they had come from their virtual image at F'_s. Ray 4 represents a parallel ray from infinity, which passes through the optic center of the lens and thus enters the eye undeviated, forming angle μ with the optic axis. Angle μ is equal to angle ω before the lens was in place, as shown in Figure 34.17a by ray 2. With the lens in place (Figure 34.17b), ray 2 becomes the chief ray of the bundle entering E. Angle ω_1 subtended by ray 2 is the angle of the chief ray after the correcting lens is in place.

The magnification of correction can now be calculated.

If the height of the virtual image formed by the spectacle lens is I and the distance from the lens to E is called Z then

$$\text{M of C} = \frac{\omega_1}{u}$$

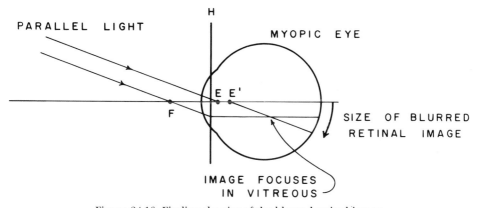

Figure 34.16. Finding the size of the blurred retinal image.

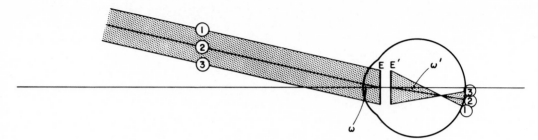

Figure 34.17a. Calculation of magnification of correction (*see* text).

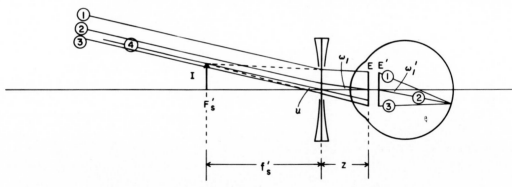

Figure 34.17b. Calculation of magnification of correction (*see* text).

$$\tan u = \frac{I}{-f'_s}$$

$$\tan \omega_1 = \frac{I}{-f'_s + Z}$$

The tangents of angles for paraxial optics are considered proportional to the angles themselves, thus

$$M \text{ of } C = \frac{\dfrac{I}{-f'_s + Z}}{\dfrac{I}{-f'_s}}$$

$$= \frac{-f'_s}{-f'_s + Z}$$

$$= \frac{1}{1 - \dfrac{Z}{f'_s}}$$

$$= \frac{1}{1 - ZF'_s}$$

This formula may be used to calculate the magnification of correction when either a contact lens or a spectacle lens is used to correct the eye's ametropia. The distance Z will be assumed to be 3 mm. for the contact lens and 16 mm. for the spectacle lens. Figure 34.18 shows curves for the ratio between the size of the retinal image with the contact lens and the image in the unaided eye and the

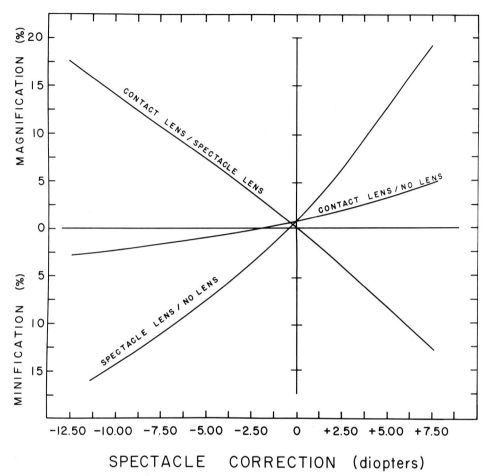

Figure 34.18. Magnifications of spectacle lens correction compared to unaided vision, contact lens correction compared to unaided vision, and contact lens correction compared to vision with the spectacle lens correction. Spectacle lenses have the powers and thicknesses of the orthogon series (Bausch and Lomb, Inc.). The contact lenses are fitted on *K* for 43.50 D. and have thickness of average values. Abscissa: spectacle ametropia in diopters. Effectivity has been allowed for so that all points on a vertical line refer to the same ametropia. From G. Westheimer, The Visual World of the Contact Lens Wearer, *Journal of the American Optometric Association, 34(2):*135–138, 1962.

corresponding curve for the spectacle lens. Due to differences in effectivity, the back vertex power differs for the two methods of correction. All figures in a vertical line refer to the same degree of ametropia.

To determine what relative difference there would be for an eye corrected with either a spectacle lens or a contact lens, one simply takes the ratio of the magnifications of correction. For a +10.00 D. spectacle lens and a +11.49 D. contact lens (the effective power of +10 at the cornea), the magnifications of correction are 1.19 (19%) and 1.04 (4%) respectively.

There is another, more direct method to find this result. To correct an ametropic eye, the secondary focal point of the correcting lens must coincide with the far point of the eye. The retinal image size is directly proportional to the image size formed at the far point of the eye.

This relationship is illustrated in Figure 34.19, where a hyperopic eye is shown with two possible correcting lenses, one at the spectacle plane and the other at the cornea. The focal point of either lens must coincide with the far point plane of the eye. By similar triangles, the image sizes formed by the lenses will be proportional to the images (I_s, I_c) formed in the eye when the same lenses are worn. If the size of the image formed by a lens of a distant object is inversely proportional to the power of the lens, then

$$\frac{\text{retinal image size with contact lens}}{\text{retinal image size with spectacle lens}} =$$

$$\frac{\dfrac{1}{F_c}}{\dfrac{1}{F_s}}$$

It may be shown that

$$F_c = \frac{F_s}{1 - d_1 F_s}$$

and

$$\frac{\dfrac{1}{F_c}}{\dfrac{1}{F_s}} = \frac{F_s}{F_c} = \frac{F_s}{\dfrac{F_s}{1 - d_1 F_s}} = 1 - d_1 F_s$$

This formula $(1 - d_1 F_s)$ may be applied in directly comparing the retinal image size of a contact lens to that of a spectacle lens. It may also be used in comparing the magnification properties of spectacles and contact lenses. For example, let the spectacle lens (F_s) be -15.00 D. and d_1 be 13 mm., then by substituting in $1 - d_1 F_s$, $1 - [(0.013)(-15.00)] = 1.195$, indicating that the contact lens produces a retinal image that is 19.5 percent larger than the spectacle lens. From this it may be concluded that for myopia the image magnification will be greater with contact lenses than with spectacles.

RELATIVE MAGNIFICATION

Relative magnification is the ratio of the corrected (thus focused) image size of an ametropic eye to the retinal image size of an emmetropic eye. If the ametropic eye is compared with an emmetropic eye of the same axial length, it is said to have a refractive type ametropia. If the two eyes differ in axial length and have the same equivalent power,

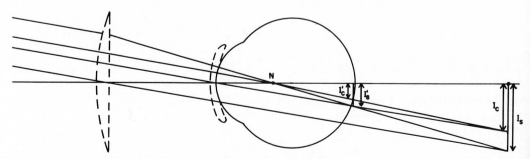

Figure 34.19. The image sizes formed by a spectacle lens (I_s) and a contact lens (I_c) off the eye are proportional to their respective image sizes (I'_s and I'_c) formed in the eye when the lenses are worn.

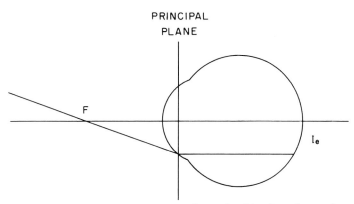

Figure 34.20. Retinal image size as determined by Gaussian optics.

the ametropia is axial.

Because all images involved in relative magnification are in focus, it is possible to use the more common method of Gaussian optics to find the image sizes. With this system the ray that passes from the object through the anterior focal point of an emmetropic eye will, upon reaching the first principal plane, be bent parallel to the optic axis. The size of the retinal image (I_e) is therefore equal to the distance between the axis and the point at which the ray strikes the first principal plane (Figure 34.20).

The size of the image for an ametropic eye viewing the same object can be found as follows. Locate the first principal plane and the anterior focal length of the system (f_h), which is composed of the ametropic correction lens and the eye. The ray through the anterior focal point of the system will strike the principal plane and be bent parallel to the optic axis. The distance from the optic axis at the position where the ray strikes the principal plane is equal to the image size. Thus, the image size is equal to the reciprocal of the anterior focal length.

$$I_a = \tan\alpha \, f_h = \frac{\tan\alpha}{F_h}$$

$$I_e = \frac{\tan\alpha}{F_e}$$

$$R.M. = \frac{I_a}{I_e} = \frac{F_e}{F_h}$$

$$F_h = F_s + F_a - dF_s F_a$$

$$R.M. = \frac{F_e}{F_s + F_a - dF_s F_a}$$

The relative magnification will vary depending upon whether the ametropic eye has an axial or refractive error.

AXIAL AND REFRACTIVE AMETROPIA

According to early theories, all emmetropic eyes had a single, ideal set of specifications. It was later shown that emmetropic eyes could have a large variation in the absolute values of their components as long as the components were properly coordinated. Hence, no single dimension can be considered as normal apart from the other ocular components. For example, an eye with an equivalent focal power of 60.00 D. would focus 20.58 mm. from the second principal plane. Another eye with an equivalent power of 65.00 D. and with the retina the same distance from the second principal plane would be myopic. When only this eye is considered, there is no possible way of saying whether it is refractive or axial myopia. If it is felt that the error should be considered refractive because it differed from the power of an emmetropic eye that had a corresponding axial length, then some difficulty will arise in comparing it with a third eye which has the same refractive power but a shorter axial length, thus making it emmetropic.

Consequently, when a given ametropic eye is said to have an axial error, it is implied that the error is axial if the eye is compared to an emmetropic eye with the same refractive power but different axial length. The same eye can be considered as having a refractive error if it is compared to an emmetropic eye with the same axial length.

Axial Ametropia

If the difference between an emmetropic and ametropic eye is purely axial, then their effective powers can be considered equal, so

$$R.M. = \frac{F_e}{F_s + F_e - dF_sF_e}$$

Dividing by F_e

$$R.M. = \frac{1}{\dfrac{F_s}{F_e} + 1 - dF_s}$$

and since $f_e = -1/F_e$ then

$$R.M. = \frac{1}{1 - dF_s - f_eF_s}$$

$$= \frac{1}{1 - (f_e + d)F_s}$$

If the sum of $f_e + d$ is made equal to p, then

$$R.M. = \frac{1}{1 + pF_s}$$

Since f_e is measured from the eye's first principal plane and is always negative and since d is considered positive, then p will equal the difference between f_e and d.

If the spectacle lens is placed at the anterior focal point of the eye, then p will be zero, and the R.M. will be 1; so no magnifica-

tion occurs. If the spectacle lens is placed within the anterior focal point of the eye, then p will be positive. If the lens is beyond the focal point, p will be negative. Hence, a positive power lens would magnify the retinal image of the ametropic eye if it were placed within the eye's anterior focal point, and it would reduce the retinal image if placed beyond the focal point.

Refractive Ametropia

If the difference between emmetropic and ametropic eyes is purely refractive, then

$$R.M. = \frac{F_e}{F_h}$$

If the difference in powers of the eye is A, then

$$R.M. = \frac{F_a + A}{F_h}$$

$$= \frac{F_a + A}{F_s + F_a - dF_sF_a}$$

And since A is simply the effective power of the spectacle lens at the principal plane,

$$A = \frac{F_s}{1 - dF_s}$$

Substituting

$$R.M. = \frac{F_a + \dfrac{F_s}{1 - dF_s}}{F_s + F_a - dF_sF_a}$$

$$= \frac{F_a - dF_aF_s + F_s}{(1 - dF_s)F_a - dF_aF_s + F_s}$$

$$= \frac{1}{a - dF_s}$$

Ametropia is rarely purely axial or purely refractive, but for purposes of comparison, the magnification produced by assuming either of these conditions is given in Figures 34.21 and 34.22.

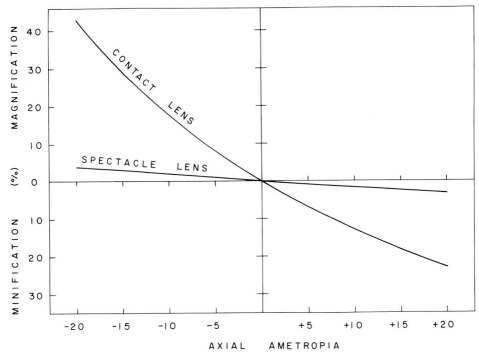

Figure 34.21. Relative magnification for an axial ametropia.

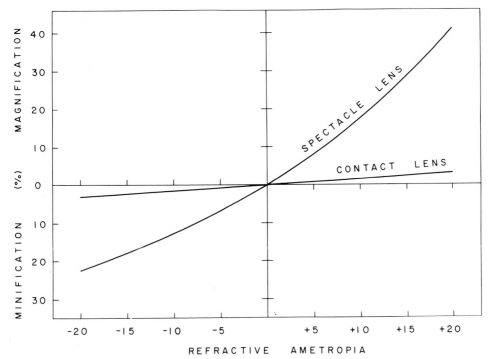

Figure 34.22. Relative magnification for a refractive ametropia.

REFERENCES

1. Emsley, H. H.: *Visual Optics*, 5th ed., London, Hatton, 1955.
2. Fincham, W. H. A.: *Optics*, 6th ed., London, Hatton, 1954.
3. Maurice, D. M.: Personal communication.
4. Westheimer, G.: *Studies in the Optical Theory of Contact Lenses*, Master's thesis, Sydney Technical College, 1949.
5. Sheard, C.: Optics: ophthalmic with applications to physiologic optics, in Glasser, O. (Ed.): *Medical Physics*, Chicago, Year Book Publisher, 1950, pp. 645–649.
6. Sarver, M. D.: Fluid lens power effect with contact lenses, *Am. J. Optom.*, 39(8):434–437, 1962.
7. Bailey, N. J.: Prism in a contact lens, *J. Am. Optom. Assoc.*, 37(1):44–45, 1966.
8. Mandell, R. B.: Prism power in contact lenses, *Am. J. Optom.*, 44(9):573–580, 1967.
9. Soper, J. W., Girard, L. J., and Sampson, W. G.: in Girard, L. J. (Ed.): *Corneal Contact Lenses*, St. Louis, Mosby, 1964, pp. 290–291.
10. Filderman, I. P.: The effect of surrounding media on prismatic contact lenses, *Optom. Weekly*, 56(26):19–24, 1965.
11. Mandell, R. B.: The prism controversy—or what's your angle? *J. Am. Optom. Assoc.*, 38(3):190, 1967.
12. Bennett, A. G.: *Optics of Contact Lenses*, 2nd ed., London, Association of Dispensing Opticians, 1956.
13. Westheimer, G.: *Studies in the Optical Theory of Contact Lenses, Master's thesis, Sydney Technical College, 1949, p. 71.*
14. Bennett, A. G.: *Optics of Contact Lenses*, 2nd ed., Kent, Walter E. English, 1956.
15. Westheimer, G.: The visual world of the contact lens wearer, *J. Am. Optom. Assoc.*, 34(2):135–138, 1962.
16. Alpern, M.: Accommodation and convergence with contact lenses, *Am. J. Optom.*, 26(9):379–387, 1949.
17. Braff, S.: Power determinations for contact lenses, in *Encyclopedia of Contact Lens Practice*, South Bend, Indiana, International Optics, 1959–1963, vol. 2, Chap. 32, pp. 27–29.
18. Mandell, R. B.: A simplified method to calculate front surface radius of contact lenses, *Am. J. Optom.*, 41(2):102–105, 1964.
19. Mandell, R. B.: The calculation of contact lens edge thickness, *Optom. Weekly*, 55(3):19–21, 1964.

ADDITIONAL READINGS

Allen, D. R., and Hoffer, K. J.: A simple lens power calculation program for the HP-67 and HP-97 calculators, *Am. Intraoc. Imp. Soc. J.*, 4(4):197, 1978.

Bauer, G. T.: Longitudinal spherical aberration of soft contact lenses, *Int. Cont. Lens Clin.*, 6(3):72–79, 1979.

Bennett, A. G.: Power changes in soft contact lenses due to bending, *The Ophthalmic Optician*, 16(22):939–945, 1976.

Brungardt, T. F., Carlson, N. J., and Kellogg, R.: Accommodative demand and vertex power compensation, *Cont. Lens Forum*, 3(2):23, 1978.

Creighton, C. P.: A computational form for contact lens thicknesses, *Optom. Weekly*, 55(45):34–36, 1964.

Dreifus, M.: Correction of axis myopic anisometropia with contact lenses, *Cont. Lens J.*, 5(5):27, 1976.

Dunn, M. J.: Factors influencing the specification of intraocular lens dioptric power, *Am. Intraoc. Imp. Soc. J.*, 3(2):130, 1977.

Dunn, M. J.: The resolving power of intraocular lens implants *Am. Intraoc. Imp. Soc. J.*, 4(3):126, 1978.

Fyodorov, S. N., Galin, M. A., and Linksz, A.: Calculation of the optical power of intraocular lenses, *Invest. Ophthalmol.*, 14(8):625–628, 1975.

Grosvenor, T. P.: Accommodative and fusional convergence with contact lenses, *J. Optom. (NZ)*, March/April, 1977, pp. 35–37.

Kaplan, M. M.: Optical considerations of hydrogel contact lenses, Part I., *Optom. Weekly*, p. 29, 1966.

Kline, S. L., and Holden, E. K.: *A Computer Program for the Design of Optimal Corneal Contact Lenses*, O.D. thesis, U.C. Berkeley School of Optometry, 1980.

Kollarits, C. R.: Calculation of intraocular lens power using the Texas Instruments. T. I. programmable 59 calculator, *Am. Intraoc. Imp. Soc. J.*, *4*(*3*):90, 1978.

Kollarits, F.: A FORTRAN IV program for intra-ocular lens power calculation, *Am. Intraoc. Imp. Soc. J.*, October, 1979, p. 330.

Neumueller, J. F.: The optics of contact lenses, *Am. J. Optom.*, *Arch. Am. Acad. Optom.*, *45*(*12*): 786–796, 1968.

APPENDICES

Appendix 1

SURFACE POWER—RADIUS CONVERSION

K	r A.O. (1.336)	r B&L (1.3375)	K	r A.O. (1.336)	r B&L (1.3375)	K	r A.O. (1.336)	r B&L (1.3375)
30.00	11.200	11.250	35.87	9.367	9.409	41.75	8.048	8.084
30.12	11.155	11.205	36.00	9.333	9.375	41.87	8.025	8.061
30.25	11.107	11.157	36.12	9.302	9.344	42.00	8.000	8.036
30.37	11.064	11.113	36.25	9.269	9.310	42.12	7.977	8.013
30.50	11.016	11.066	36.37	9.238	9.280	42.25	7.953	7.988
30.62	10.973	11.022	36.50	9.205	9.247	42.37	7.930	7.966
30.75	10.927	10.976	36.62	9.175	9.216	42.50	7.906	7.941
30.87	10.884	10.933	36.75	9.143	9.184	42.62	7.884	7.919
31.00	10.839	10.887	36.87	9.113	9.154	42.75	7.860	7.895
31.12	10.797	10.845	37.00	9.081	9.122	42.87	7.838	7.873
31.25	10.752	10.800	37.12	9.052	9.092	43.00	7.814	7.849
31.37	10.711	10.759	37.25	9.020	9.060	43.12	7.792	7.827
31.50	10.667	10.714	37.37	8.991	9.031	43.25	7.769	7.803
31.62	10.626	10.674	37.50	8.960	9.000	43.37	7.747	7.782
31.75	10.583	10.630	37.62	8.931	8.971	43.50	7.724	7.759
31.87	10.543	10.590	37.75	8.900	8.940	43.62	7.703	7.737
32.00	10.500	10.547	37.87	8.872	8.912	43.75	7.680	7.714
32.12	10.461	10.507	38.00	8.842	8.882	43.87	7.659	7.693
32.25	10.419	10.465	38.12	8.814	8.854	44.00	7.636	7.670
32.37	10.380	10.426	38.25	8.784	8.824	44.12	7.616	7.650
32.50	10.338	10.385	38.37	8.757	8.796	44.25	7.593	7.627
32.62	10.300	10.346	38.50	8.727	8.766	44.37	7.573	7.606
32.75	10.260	10.305	38.62	8.700	8.739	44.50	7.551	7.584
32.87	10.222	10.268	38.75	8.671	8.710	44.62	7.530	7.564
33.00	10.182	10.227	38.87	8.644	8.683	44.75	7.508	7.542
33.12	10.145	10.190	39.00	8.615	8.654	44.87	7.488	7.522
33.25	10.105	10.150	39.12	8.589	8.627	45.00	7.467	7.500
33.37	10.069	10.114	39.25	8.561	8.599	45.12	7.447	7.480
33.50	10.030	10.075	39.37	8.534	8.573	45.25	7.425	7.459
33.62	9.994	10.039	39.50	8.506	8.544	45.37	7.406	7.439
33.75	9.956	10.000	39.62	8.481	8.518	45.50	7.385	7.418
33.87	9.920	9.965	39.75	8.453	8.491	45.62	7.365	7.398
34.00	9.882	9.926	39.87	8.427	8.465	45.75	7.344	7.377
34.12	9.848	9.892	40.00	8.400	8.438	45.87	7.325	7.358
34.25	9.810	9.854	40.12	8.375	8.412	46.00	7.304	7.337
34.37	9.776	9.820	40.25	8.348	8.385	46.12	7.285	7.318
34.50	9.739	9.783	40.37	8.323	8.360	46.25	7.265	7.297
34.62	9.705	9.749	40.50	8.296	8.333	46.37	7.246	7.278
34.75	9.669	9.712	40.62	8.272	8.309	46.50	7.226	7.258
34.87	9.636	9.679	40.75	8.245	8.282	46.62	7.207	7.239
35.00	9.600	9.643	40.87	8.221	8.258	46.75	7.187	7.219
35.12	9.567	9.610	41.00	8.195	8.232	46.87	7.169	7.201
35.25	9.532	9.574	41.12	8.171	8.208	47.00	7.149	7.181
35.37	9.400	9.542	41.25	8.145	8.182	47.12	7.131	7.163
35.50	9.468	9.507	41.37	8.122	8.158	47.25	7.111	7.143
35.62	9.432	9.475	41.50	8.096	8.133	47.37	7.093	7.125
35.75	9.399	9.441	41.62	8.073	8.109	47.50	7.084	7.105

861

K	r A.O. (1.336)	r B&L (1.3375)	K	r A.O. (1.336)	r B&L (1.3375)	K	r A.O. (1.336)	r B&L (1.3375)
47.62	7.056	7.087	51.75	6.493	6.522	55.87	6.014	6.041
47.75	7.037	7.068	51.87	6.478	6.507	56.00	6.000	6.027
47.87	7.019	7.050	52.00	6.462	6.490	56.12	5.987	6.014
48.00	7.000	7.031	52.12	6.447	6.475	56.25	5.973	6.000
48.12	6.983	7.014	52.25	6.431	6.459	56.37	5.961	5.987
48.25	6.964	6.995	52.37	6.416	6.445	56.50	5.947	5.973
48.37	6.946	6.977	52.50	6.400	6.429	56.62	5.934	5.961
48.50	6.928	6.959	52.62	6.385	6.414	56.75	5.921	5.947
48.62	6.911	6.942	52.75	6.370	6.398	56.87	5.908	5.935
48.75	6.892	6.923	52.87	6.355	6.384	57.00	5.895	5.921
48.87	6.875	6.906	53.00	6.340	6.368	57.12	5.882	5.909
49.00	6.857	6.888	53.12	6.325	6.354	57.25	5.869	5.895
49.12	6.840	6.871	53.25	6.310	6.338	57.37	5.857	5.883
49.25	6.822	6.853	53.37	6.296	6.324	57.50	5.843	5.870
49.37	6.806	6.836	53.50	6.280	6.308	57.62	5.831	5.857
49.50	6.789	6.818	53.62	6.266	6.294	57.75	5.818	5.844
49.62	6.771	6.802	53.75	6.261	6.279	57.87	5.806	5.832
49.75	6.754	6.784	53.87	6.237	6.265	58.00	5.793	5.819
49.87	6.738	6.768	54.00	6.222	6.250	58.12	5.781	5.807
50.00	6.720	6.750	54.12	6.208	6.236	58.25	5.768	5.794
50.12	6.704	6.734	54.25	6.194	6.221	58.37	5.756	5.782
50.25	6.687	6.716	54.37	6.180	6.207	58.50	5.744	5.769
50.37	6.671	6.700	54.50	6.165	6.193	58.62	5.732	5.757
50.50	6.653	6.683	54.62	6.152	6.179	58.75	5.719	5.745
50.62	6.638	6.667	54.75	6.137	6.164	58.87	5.707	5.733
50.75	6.621	6.650	54.87	6.124	6.151	59.00	5.695	5.720
50.87	6.605	6.635	55.00	6.109	6.136	59.12	5.683	5.709
51.00	6.588	6.618	55.12	6.096	6.123	59.25	5.671	5.696
51.12	6.573	6.602	55.25	6.081	6.109	59.37	5.659	5.685
51.25	6.556	6.585	55.37	6.068	6.095	59.50	5.647	5.672
51.37	6.541	6.570	55.50	6.054	6.081	59.62	5.636	5.661
51.50	6.524	6.553	55.62	6.041	6.068	59.75	5.623	5.649
51.62	6.509	6.538	55.75	6.027	6.054	59.87	5.612	5.637
						60.00	5.600	5.625

Appendix 2

EFFECTIVE POWER OF SPECTACLE LENSES

EFFECTIVE POWER OF SPECTACLE LENSES AT THE CORNEAL PLANE FOR VERTEX DISTANCES
OF 11, 13, AND 15 MILLIMETERS. PLUS LENSES

Spectacle Lens Power	Vertex Distance 11 mm.	Vertex Distance 13 mm.	Vertex Distance 15 mm.	Spectacle Lens Power	Vertex Distance 11 mm.	Vertex Distance 13 mm.	Vertex Distance 15 mm.
0.25	0.25	0.25	0.25	10.25	11.55	11.83	12.11
0.50	0.50	0.50	0.50	10.50	11.87	12.16	12.46
0.75	0.76	0.76	0.76	10.75	12.19	12.50	12.82
1.00	1.01	1.01	1.02	11.00	12.51	12.84	13.17
1.25	1.27	1.27	1.27	11.25	12.84	13.18	13.53
1.50	1.53	1.53	1.53	11.50	13.17	13.52	13.90
1.75	1.78	1.79	1.80	11.75	13.49	13.87	14.26
2.00	2.04	2.05	2.06	12.00	13.82	14.22	14.63
2.25	2.31	2.32	2.33	12.25	14.16	14.57	15.01
2.50	2.57	2.58	2.60	12.50	14.49	14.93	15.38
2.75	2.84	2.85	2.87	12.75	14.83	15.28	15.77
3.00	3.10	3.12	3.14	13.00	15.17	15.64	16.15
3.25	3.37	3.39	3.42	13.25	15.51	16.01	16.54
3.50	3.64	3.67	3.69	13.50	15.85	16.37	16.93
3.75	3.91	3.94	3.97	13.75	16.20	16.74	17.32
4.00	4.18	4.22	4.26	14.00	16.55	17.11	17.72
4.25	4.46	4.50	4.54	14.25	16.90	17.49	18.12
4.50	4.73	4.78	4.83	14.50	17.25	17.87	18.83
4.75	5.01	5.06	5.11	14.75	17.61	18.25	18.94
5.00	5.29	5.35	5.41	15.00	17.96	18.63	19.35
5.25	5.57	5.63	5.70	15.25	18.32	19.02	19.77
5.50	5.85	5.92	5.99	15.50	18.69	19.41	20.20
5.75	6.14	6.21	6.29	15.75	19.05	19.81	20.62
6.00	6.42	6.51	6.59	16.00	19.42	20.20	21.05
6.25	6.71	6.80	6.90	16.25	19.79	20.60	21.49
6.50	7.00	7.10	7.20	16.50	20.16	21.01	21.93
6.75	7.29	7.40	7.51	16.75	20.53	21.41	22.37
7.00	7.58	7.70	7.82	17.00	20.91	21.82	22.82
7.25	7.88	8.00	8.13	17.25	21.29	22.24	23.27
7.50	8.17	8.31	8.45	17.50	21.67	22.65	23.73
7.75	8.47	8.62	8.77	17.75	22.06	23.07	24.19
8.00	8.77	8.93	9.09	18.00	22.44	23.50	24.66
8.25	9.07	9.24	9.42	18.25	22.83	23.93	25.13
8.50	9.38	9.56	9.74	18.50	23.23	24.36	25.61
8.75	9.68	9.87	10.07	18.75	23.62	24.79	26.09
9.00	9.99	10.19	10.40	19.00	24.02	25.23	26.57
9.25	10.30	10.51	10.74	19.25	24.42	25.68	27.07
9.50	10.61	10.84	11.08	19.50	24.82	26.12	27.56
9.75	10.92	11.17	11.42	19.75	25.23	26.57	28.06
10.00	11.24	11.49	11.76	20.00	25.64	27.03	28.57

863

EFFECTIVE POWER OF SPECTACLE LENSES AT THE CORNEAL PLANE FOR
VERTEX DISTANCES OF 11, 13 AND 15 MILLIMETERS. MINUS LENSES

Spectacle Lens Power	Vertex Distance			Spectacle Lens Power	Vertex Distance		
	11 mm.	*13 mm.*	*15 mm.*		*11 mm.*	*13 mm.*	*15 mm.*
− 0.25	− 0.25	− 0.25	− 0.25	−10.25	− 9.21	− 9.04	− 8.88
− 0.50	− 0.50	− 0.50	− 0.50	−10.50	− 9.41	− 9.24	− 9.07
− 0.75	− 0.74	− 0.74	− 0.74	−10.75	− 9.61	− 9.43	− 9.26
− 1.00	− 0.99	− 0.99	− 0.99	−11.00	− 9.81	− 9.62	− 9.44
− 1.25	− 1.23	− 1.23	− 1.23	−11.25	−10.01	− 9.81	− 9.63
− 1.50	− 1.48	− 1.47	− 1.47	−11.50	−10.21	−10.00	− 9.81
− 1.75	− 1.72	− 1.71	− 1.71	−11.75	−10.41	−10.19	− 9.99
− 2.00	− 1.96	− 1.95	− 1.94	−12.00	−10.60	−10.38	−10.17
− 2.25	− 2.20	− 2.19	− 2.18	−12.25	−10.80	−10.57	−10.35
− 2.50	− 2.43	− 2.42	− 2.41	−12.50	−10.99	−10.75	−10.53
− 2.75	− 2.67	− 2.66	− 2.64	−12.75	−11.18	−10.94	−10.70
− 3.00	− 2.90	− 2.89	− 2.87	−13.00	−11.37	−11.12	−10.88
− 3.25	− 3.14	− 3.12	− 3.10	−13.25	−11.56	−11.30	−11.05
− 3.50	− 3.37	− 3.35	− 3.33	−13.50	−11.75	−11.48	−11.23
− 3.75	− 3.60	− 3.58	− 3.55	−13.75	−11.94	−11.66	−11.40
− 4.00	− 3.83	− 3.80	− 3.77	−14.00	−12.13	−11.84	−11.57
− 4.25	− 4.06	− 4.03	− 4.00	−14.25	−12.32	−12.02	−11.74
− 4.50	− 4.29	− 4.25	− 4.22	−14.50	−12.51	−12.20	−11.91
− 4.75	− 4.51	− 4.47	− 4.43	−14.75	−12.69	−12.38	−12.08
− 5.00	− 4.74	− 4.69	− 4.65	−15.00	−12.88	−12.55	−12.24
− 5.25	− 4.96	− 4.91	− 4.87	−15.25	−13.06	−12.73	−12.41
− 5.50	− 5.19	− 5.13	− 5.08	−15.50	−13.24	−12.90	−12.59
− 5.75	− 5.41	− 5.35	− 5.29	−15.75	−13.42	−13.07	−12.74
− 6.00	− 5.63	− 5.57	− 5.50	−16.00	−13.61	−13.25	−12.90
− 6.25	− 5.85	− 5.78	− 5.71	−16.25	−13.79	−13.42	−13.07
− 6.50	− 6.07	− 5.99	− 5.92	−16.50	−13.97	−13.59	−13.23
− 6.75	− 6.28	− 6.21	− 6.13	−16.75	−14.14	−13.75	−13.39
− 7.00	− 6.50	− 6.42	− 6.33	−17.00	−14.32	−13.92	−13.55
− 7.25	− 6.71	− 6.63	− 6.54	−17.25	−14.50	−14.09	−13.70
− 7.50	− 6.93	− 6.83	− 6.74	−17.50	−14.68	−14.26	−13.86
− 7.75	− 7.14	− 7.04	− 6.94	−17.75	−14.85	−14.42	−14.02
− 8.00	− 7.35	− 7.25	− 7.14	−18.00	−15.03	−14.59	−14.17
− 8.25	− 7.56	− 7.45	− 7.34	−18.25	−15.20	−14.75	−14.33
− 8.50	− 7.77	− 7.65	− 7.54	−18.50	−15.37	−14.91	−14.48
− 8.75	− 7.98	− 7.86	− 7.73	−18.75	−15.54	−15.08	−14.63
− 9.00	− 8.19	− 8.06	− 7.93	−19.00	−15.72	−15.24	−14.79
− 9.25	− 8.40	− 8.26	− 8.12	−19.25	−15.89	−15.40	−14.94
− 9.50	− 8.60	− 8.46	− 8.32	−19.50	−16.06	−15.56	−15.09
− 9.75	− 8.81	− 8.65	− 8.51	−19.75	−16.23	−15.72	−15.24
−10.00	− 9.01	− 8.85	− 8.70	−20.00	−16.39	−15.97	−15.38

Appendix 3

THICKNESS CONVERSION

Inch	mm.	Inch	mm.	Inch	mm.	Inch	mm.	Inch	mm.
0.0010 = 0.0254		0.0056 = 0.1422		0.0101 = 0.2565		0.0147 = 0.3734		0.0193 = 0.4902	
0.0011 = 0.0279		0.0057 = 0.1448		0.0102 = .02591		0.0148 = 0.3759		0.0194 = 0.4928	
0.0012 = 0.0305		0.0058 = 0.1473		0.0103 = 0.2616		0.0149 = 0.3785		0.0195 = 0.4953	
0.0013 = 0.0330		0.0059 = 0.1499		0.0104 = 0.2642				0.0196 = 0.4978	
0.0014 = 0.0356				0.0105 = 0.2667		0.0150 = 0.3810		0.0197 = 0.5004	
0.0015 = 0.0381		0.0060 = 0.1524		0.0106 = 0.2692		0.0151 = 0.3835		0.0198 = 0.5029	
0.0016 = 0.0406		0.0061 = 0.1549		0.0107 = 0.2718		0.0152 = 0.3861		0.0199 = 0.5055	
0.0017 = 0.0432		0.0062 = 0.1575		0.0108 = 0.2743		0.0153 = 0.3886			
0.0018 = 0.0457		0.0063 = 0.1600		0.0109 = 0.2769		0.0154 = .0.3912		0.0200 = 0.5080	
0.0019 = 0.0483		0.0064 = 0.1626				0.0155 = 0.3937		0.0201 = 0.5105	
		0.0065 = 0.1651		0.0110 = 0.2794		0.0156 = 0.3962		0.0202 = 0.5131	
0.0020 = 0.0508		0.0066 = 0.1676		0.0111 = 0.2819		0.0157 = 0.3988		0.0203 = 0.5156	
0.0021 = 0.0533		0.0067 = 0.1702		0.0112 = 0.2845		0.0158 = 0.4013		0.0204 = 0.5182	
0.0022 = 0.0559		0.0068 = 0.1727		0.0113 = 0.2870		0.0159 = 0.4039		0.0205 = 0.5207	
0.0023 = 0.0584		0.0069 = 0.1753		0.0114 = 0.2896				0.0206 = 0.5232	
0.0024 = 0.0610				0.0115 = 0.2921		0.0160 = 0.4064		0.0207 = 0.5258	
0.0025 = 0.0635		0.0070 = 0.1778		0.0116 = 0.2946		0.0161 = 0.4089		0.0208 = 0.5283	
0.0026 = 0.0660		0.0071 = 0.1803		0.0117 = 0.2972		0.0162 = 0.4115		0.0209 = 0.5309	
0.0027 = 0.0686		0.0072 = 0.1829		0.0118 = 0.2997		0.0163 = 0.4140			
0.0028 = 0.0711		0.0073 = 0.1854		0.0119 = 0.3023		0.0164 = 0.4166		0.0210 = 0.5334	
0.0029 = 0.0737		0.0074 = 0.1880				0.0165 = 0.4191		0.0211 = 0.5359	
		0.0075 = 0.1905		0.0120 = 0.3048		0.0166 = 0.4216		0.0212 = 0.5385	
0.0030 = 0.0762		0.0076 = 0.1930		0.0121 = 0.3073		0.0167 = 0.4242		0.0213 = 0.5410	
0.0031 = 0.0787		0.0077 = 0.1956		0.0122 = 0.3099		0.0168 = 0.4267		0.0214 = 0.5436	
0.0032 = 0.0813		0.0078 = 0.1981		0.0123 = 0.3124		0.0169 = 0.4293		0.0215 = 0.5461	
0.0033 = 0.0838		0.0079 = 0.2007		0.0124 = 0.3150				0.0216 = 0.5486	
0.0034 = 0.0864				0.0125 = 0.3175		0.0170 = 0.4318		0.0217 = 0.5512	
0.0035 = 0.0889		0.0080 = 0.2032		0.0126 = 0.3200		0.0171 = 0.4343		0.0218 = 0.5537	
0.0036 = 0.0914		0.0081 = 0.2057		0.0127 = 0.3226		0.0172 = 0.4369		0.0219 = 0.5563	
0.0037 = 0.0940		0.0082 = 0.2083		0.0128 = 0.3251		0.0173 = 0.4394			
0.0038 = 0.0965		0.0083 = 0.2108		0.0129 = 0.3277		0.0174 = 0.4420		0.0220 = 0.5588	
0.0039 = 0.0991		0.0084 = 0.2134				0.0175 = 0.4445		0.0221 = 0.5613	
		0.0085 = 0.2159		0.0130 = 0.3302		0.0176 = 0.4470		0.0222 = 0.5639	
0.0040 = 0.1016		0.0086 = 0.2184		0.0131 = 0.3327		0.0177 = 0.4496		0.0223 = 0.5664	
0.0041 = 0.1041		0.0087 = 0.2210		0.0132 = 0.3353		0.0178 = 0.4521		0.0224 = 0.5690	
0.0042 = 0.1067		0.0088 = 0.2235		0.0133 = 0.3378		0.0179 = 0.4547		0.0225 = 0.5715	
0.0043 = 0.1092		0.0089 = 0.2261		0.0134 = 0.3404				0.0226 = 0.5740	
0.0044 = 0.1118				0.0135 = 0.3429		0.0180 = 0.4572		0.0227 = 0.5766	
0.0045 = 0.1143		0.0090 = 0.2286		0.0136 = 0.3454		0.0181 = 0.4597		0.0228 = 0.5791	
0.0046 = 0.1168		0.0091 = 0.2311		0.0137 = 0.3480		0.0182 = 0.4623		0.0229 = 0.5817	
0.0047 = 0.1194		0.0092 = 0.2337		0.0138 = 0.3505		0.0183 = 0.4648			
0.0048 = 0.1219		0.0093 = 0.2362		0.0139 = 0.3531		0.0184 = 0.4674		0.0230 = 0.5842	
0.0049 = 0.1245		0.0094 = 0.2388				0.0185 = 0.4699		0.0231 = 0.5867	
		0.0095 = 0.2413		0.0140 = 0.3556		0.0186 = 0.4724		0.0232 = 0.5893	
0.0050 = 0.1270		0.0096 = 0.2438		0.0141 = 0.3581		0.0187 = 0.4750		0.0233 = 0.5918	
0.0051 = 0.1295		0.0097 = 0.2464		0.0142 = 0.3607		0.0188 = 0.4775		0.0234 = 0.5944	
0.0052 = 0.1321		0.0098 = 0.2489		0.0143 = 0.3632		0.0189 = 0.4801		0.0235 = 0.5969	
0.0053 = 0.1346		0.0099 = 0.2515		0.0144 = 0.3658				0.0236 = 0.5994	
0.0054 = 0.1372				0.0145 = 0.3683		0.0190 = 0.4826		0.0237 = 0.6020	
0.0055 = 0.1397		0.0100 = 0.2540		0.0146 = 0.3708		0.0191 = 0.4851			
						0.0192 = 0.4877			

Inch	mm.	Inch	mm.	Inch	mm.	Inch	mm.	Inch	mm.
0.0238 =	0.6045	0.0251 =	0.6375	0.0264 =	0.6706	0.0277 =	0.7036	0.0290 =	0.7366
0.0239 =	0.6071	0.0252 =	0.6401	0.0265 =	0.6731	0.0278 =	0.7061	0.0291 =	0.7391
		0.0253 =	0.6426	0.0266 =	0.6756	0.0279 =	0.7087	0.0292 =	0.7417
0.0240 =	0.6096	0.0254 =	0.6452	0.0267 =	0.6782			0.0293 =	0.7442
0.0241 =	0.6121	0.0255 =	0.6477	0.0268 =	0.6807	0.0280 =	0.7112	0.0294 =	0.7468
0.0242 =	0.6147	0.0256 =	0.6502	0.0269 =	0.6833	0.0281 =	0.7137	0.0295 =	0.7493
0.0243 =	0.6172	0.0257 =	0.6529			0.0282 =	0.7163	0.0296 =	0.7518
0.0244 =	0.6198	0.0258 =	0.6553	0.0270 =	0.6858	0.0283 =	0.7188	0.0297 =	0.7544
0.0245 =	0.6223	0.0259 =	0.6579	0.0271 =	0.6883	0.0284 =	0.7214	0.0298 =	0.7569
0.0246 =	0.6248			0.0272 =	0.6909	0.0285 =	0.7239	0.0299 =	0.7595
0.0247 =	0.6274	0.0260 =	0.6604	0.0273 =	0.6934	0.0286 =	0.7264		
0.0248 =	0.6299	0.0261 =	0.6629	0.0274 =	0.6960	0.0287 =	0.7290		
0.0249 =	0.6325	0.0262 =	0.6655	0.0275 =	0.6985	0.0288 =	0.7315		
0.0250 =	0.6350	0.0263 =	0.6680	0.0276 =	0.7010	0.0289 =	0.7341		

Appendix 4

PHYSICAL PROPERTIES OF ELECTROGLAS '2'

Property	Average Values
Specific gravity	1.18
Abrasion resistance, Falling emery test (Times Methacrylate)	3
Water absorption, 24 hrs., 25°C.	
Water absorbed, percent	0.35
Soluble matter lost, percent	0.00
Ultra-violet transmittance, percent at 320 millimicrons	0

Odor	None
Taste	None
Solvent resistance, immersion at 77°F	
Acetone	Soft, Swollen
Ethyl Acetate	Soft, Swollen
Ethylene Dichloride	Soft, Swollen
Refractive index	1.49

Electroglas '2' is manufactured by Glasflex Inc., Stirling, N.J.

CONVERSION OF KERATOMETER DIOPTERS
TO MILLIMETERS

Dioptral Curvature	Radius in mm. Cx	CC	Dioptral Curvature	Radius in mm. Cx	CC
61.00	5.53	5.55	55.50	6.08	6.10
60.87	5.54	5.57	55.37	6.10	6.12
60.75	5.56	5.58	55.25	6.11	6.13
60.62	5.57	5.59	55.12	6.12	6.15
60.50	5.58	5.60	55.00	6.14	6.16
60.37	5.59	5.61	54.87	6.15	6.17
60.25	5.60	5.62	54.75	6.16	6.19
60.12	5.61	5.63	54.62	6.18	6.20
60.00	5.63	5.65	54.50	6.19	6.22
59.87	5.64	5.66	54.37	6.21	6.23
59.75	5.65	5.67	54.25	6.22	6.24
59.62	5.66	5.68	54.12	6.24	6.26
59.50	5.67	5.69	54.00	6.25	6.27
59.37	5.68	5.71	53.87	6.26	6.29
59.25	5.70	5.72	53.75	6.28	6.30
59.12	5.71	5.73	53.62	6.29	6.32
59.00	5.72	5.74	53.50	6.31	6.33
58.87	5.73	5.75	53.37	6.32	6.35
58.87	5.75	5.77	53.25	6.34	6.36
58.62	5.76	5.78	53.12	6.35	6.38
58.50	5.77	5.79	53.00	6.37	6.39
58.37	5.78	5.80	52.87	6.38	6.41
58.25	5.79	5.82	52.75	6.40	6.42
58.12	5.81	5.83	52.62	6.41	6.44
58.00	5.82	5.84	52.50	6.43	6.45
57.87	5.83	5.85	52.37	6.44	6.47
57.75	5.84	5.87	52.25	6.46	6.48
57.62	5.86	5.88	52.12	6.48	6.50
57.50	5.87	5.89	52.00	6.49	6.51
57.37	5.88	5.90	51.87	6.51	6.53
57.25	5.90	5.92	51.75	6.52	6.54
57.12	5.91	5.93	51.62	6.54	6.56
57.00	5.92	5.94	51.50	6.55	6.57
56.87	5.94	5.96	51.37	6.57	6.59
56.75	5.95	5.97	51.25	6.59	6.61
56.62	5.96	5.98	51.12	6.60	6.62
56.50	5.97	6.00	51.00	6.62	6.64
56.37	5.99	6.01	50.87	6.63	6.65
56.25	6.00	6.02	50.75	6.65	6.67
56.12	6.01	6.04	50.62	6.67	6.69
56.00	6.03	6.05	50.50	6.68	6.70
55.87	6.04	6.06	50.37	6.70	6.72
55.75	6.05	6.08	50.25	6.72	6.74
55.62	6.07	6.09	50.12	6.73	6.75
			50.00	6.75	6.77
			49.87	6.77	6.79
			49.75	6.78	6.80

Courtesy Bausch and Lomb Inc.

Dioptral Curvature	Radius in mm. Cx	CC	Dioptral Curvature	Radius in mm. Cx	CC
49.62	6.80	6.82	42.50	7.94	7.97
49.50	6.82	6.84	42.37	7.97	8.00
49.37	6.84	6.86	42.25	7.99	8.02
49.25	6.85	6.87	42.12	8.01	8.04
49.12	6.87	6.89	42.00	8.04	8.07
49.00	6.89	6.91	41.87	8.06	8.09
48.87	6.91	6.93	41.75	8.08	8.11
48.75	6.92	6.94	41.62	8.11	8.14
48.62	6.95	6.96	41.50	8.13	8.16
48.50	6.96	6.98	41.37	8.16	8.19
48.37	6.98	7.00	41.25	8.18	8.21
48.25	7.00	7.02	41.12	8.21	8.24
48.12	7.01	7.03	41.00	8.23	8.27
48.00	7.03	7.05	40.87	8.26	8.29
47.87	7.05	7.07	40.75	8.28	8.32
47.75	7.07	7.09	40.62	8.31	8.34
47.62	7.09	7.11	40.50	8.33	8.37
47.50	7.11	7.13	40.37	8.36	8.40
47.37	7.12	7.15	40.25	8.39	8.42
47.25	7.14	7.17	40.12	8.41	8.45
47.12	7.16	7.19	40.00	8.44	8.47
47.00	7.18	7.21	39.87	8.46	8.50
46.87	7.20	7.23	39.75	8.49	8.53
46.75	7.22	7.25	39.62	8.52	8.55
46.62	7.24	7.27	39.50	8.55	8.58
46.50	7.26	7.29	39.37	8.57	8.61
46.37	7.28	7.31	39.25	8.60	8.64
46.25	7.30	7.33	39.12	8.63	8.66
46.12	7.32	7.35	39.00	8.65	8.69
46.00	7.34	7.37	38.87	8.68	8.72
45.87	7.36	7.39	38.75	8.71	8.75
45.75	7.38	7.40	38.62	8.74	8.77
45.62	7.40	7.42	38.50	8.77	8.80
45.50	7.42	7.44	38.37	8.80	8.84
45.37	7.44	7.46	38.25	8.82	8.86
45.25	7.46	7.49	38.12	8.85	8.89
45.12	7.48	7.51	38.00	8.88	8.92
45.00	7.50	7.53	37.87	8.91	8.95
44.87	7.52	7.55	37.75	8.94	8.98
44.75	7.54	7.57	37.62	8.97	9.01
44.62	7.56	7.59	37.50	9.00	9.04
44.50	7.58	7.61	37.37	9.03	9.07
44.37	7.61	7.64	37.25	9.06	9.10
44.25	7.63	7.66	37.12	9.09	9.13
44.12	7.65	7.68	37.00	9.12	9.16
44.00	7.67	7.70	36.87	9.15	9.19
43.87	7.69	7.72	36.75	9.18	9.22
43.75	7.72	7.75	36.62	9.22	9.26
43.62	7.74	7.77	36.50	9.25	9.29
43.50	7.76	7.79	36.37	9.28	9.32
43.37	7.78	7.81	36.25	9.31	9.35
43.25	7.80	7.83	36.12	9.34	9.38
43.12	7.83	7.86	36.00	9.38	9.41
43.00	7.85	7.88	35.87	9.41	9.44
42.87	7.87	7.90	35.75	9.44	9.48
42.75	7.90	7.93	35.62	9.47	9.51
42.62	7.92	7.95	35.50	9.51	9.54

Dioptral Curvature	Radius in mm. Cx	CC	Dioptral Curvature	Radius in mm. Cx	CC
35.37	9.54	9.58	32.62	10.35	10.38
35.25	9.57	9.61	32.50	10.39	10.42
35.12	9.61	9.64	32.37	10.43	10.46
35.00	9.64	9.68	32.25	10.47	10.50
34.87	9.68	9.71	32.12	10.51	10.55
34.75	9.71	9.75	32.00	10.55	10.59
34.62	9.75	9.78	31.87	10.59	10.63
34.50	9.78	9.82	31.75	10.63	10.67
34.37	9.82	9.86	31.62	10.67	10.71
34.25	9.85	9.89	31.50	10.72	10.75
34.12	9.89	9.93	31.37	10.76	10.80
34.00	9.93	9.96	31.25	10.80	10.84
33.87	9.96	10.00	31.12	10.84	10.88
33.75	10.00	10.04	31.00	10.89	10.93
33.62	10.04	10.08	30.87	10.93	10.97
33.50	10.08	10.11	30.75	10.98	11.02
33.37	10.11	10.15	30.62	11.02	11.06
33.25	10.15	10.19	30.50	11.07	11.11
33.12	10.19	10.23	30.37	11.11	11.15
33.00	10.23	10.27	30.25	11.16	11.20
32.87	10.27	10.30	30.12	11.20	11.25
32.75	10.31	10.34	30.00	11.25	11.29

Appendix 6

SAGITTA TABLE

SAGITTA MEASUREMENTS IN MILLIMETERS
DIAMETER IN MILLIMETERS

RAD. MM.	R²	5.00	5.50	5.60	5.80	6.00	6.20	6.40	6.50	6.60	6.80	7.00	7.20	7.40	7.50	7.60	7.80	8.00	8.20
6.00	36.00	.546	.667	.693	.747	.804	.863	.925	.956	.989	1.056	1.127	1.200	1.277	1.316	1.357	1.440	1.528	1.619
6.05	36.60	.541	.661	.687	.741	.796	.855	.916	.947	.980	1.046	1.115	1.188	1.264	1.302	1.343	1.425	1.511	1.601
6.10	37.21	.536	.655	.681	.733	.789	.846	.907	.938	.970	1.035	1.104	1.176	1.250	1.289	1.328	1.410	1.495	1.583
6.15	37.82	.531	.649	.675	.727	.782	.839	.898	.929	.961	1.026	1.093	1.164	1.238	1.276	1.315	1.395	1.479	1.566
6.20	38.44	.526	.643	.668	.720	.774	.831	.890	.920	.951	1.015	1.082	1.152	1.225	1.262	1.301	1.380	1.463	1.549
6.25	39.06	.522	.638	.662	.714	.767	.823	.882	.911	.942	1.006	1.072	1.141	1.213	1.250	1.288	1.366	1.448	1.533
6.30	39.69	.517	.632	.656	.707	.760	.815	.873	.903	.933	.996	1.062	1.130	1.201	1.237	1.275	1.352	1.433	1.517
6.35	40.32	.513	.626	.651	.701	.754	.808	.865	.895	.925	.987	1.052	1.119	1.190	1.225	1.263	1.339	1.418	1.501
6.40	40.96	.508	.621	.645	.695	.747	.801	.857	.886	.916	.978	1.042	1.109	1.178	1.213	1.250	1.326	1.404	1.486
6.45	41.60	.504	.616	.640	.689	.740	.794	.850	.879	.908	.969	1.032	1.098	1.167	1.202	1.238	1.313	1.390	1.471
6.50	42.25	.500	.610	.634	.693	.734	.787	.842	.870	.900	.960	1.023	1.088	1.156	1.191	1.226	1.300	1.377	1.496
6.55	42.90	.496	.605	.629	.677	.728	.780	.835	.865	.892	.952	1.014	1.078	1.145	1.180	1.215	1.288	1.363	1.442
6.60	43.56	.492	.600	.623	.671	.721	.773	.827	.856	.884	.943	1.004	1.068	1.135	1.169	1.204	1.276	1.350	1.428
6.65	44.22	.488	.595	.619	.666	.715	.767	.821	.848	.877	.935	.996	1.059	1.125	1.158	1.193	1.264	1.338	1.415
6.70	44.89	.484	.590	.613	.660	.709	.760	.814	.842	.869	.927	.987	1.049	1.114	1.147	1.182	1.252	1.325	1.401
6.75	45.56	.480	.586	.608	.655	.703	.754	.807	.834	.862	.919	.978	1.040	1.105	1.137	1.171	1.241	1.313	1.389
6.80	46.24	.476	.58u	.603	.649	.698	.748	.800	.827	.854	.911	.970	1.031	1.095	1.127	1.161	1.230	1.301	1.375
6.85	46.92	.473	.576	.599	.644	.692	.742	.794	.820	.847	.904	.962	1.022	1.085	1.118	1.151	1.219	1.289	1.363
6.90	47.61	.469	.571	.594	.639	.686	.736	.787	.813	.840	.896	.954	1.014	1.076	1.108	1.141	1.208	1.278	1.350
6.95	48.30	.465	.567	.589	.633	.681	.730	.781	.807	.834	.889	.946	1.005	1.067	1.098	1.131	1.198	1.267	1.338
7.00	49.00	.462	.563	.584	.629	.675	.724	.774	.800	.827	.881	.938	.997	1.058	1.089	1.121	1.187	1.256	1.326
7.05	49.70	.458	.558	.580	.624	.670	.718	.768	.794	.820	.874	.930	.989	1.049	1.080	1.112	1.177	1.245	1.315
7.10	50.41	.455	.554	.575	.619	.665	.713	.762	.787	.813	.867	.923	.980	1.040	1.071	1.103	1.167	1.234	1.303
7.15	51.12	.451	.550	.571	.615	.660	.707	.756	.781	.807	.860	.915	.972	1.032	1.062	1.094	1.157	1.224	1.293
7.20	51.84	.448	.546	.567	.610	.655	.702	.750	.775	.801	.853	.908	.965	1.023	1.053	1.085	1.148	1.213	1.281
7.25	52.56	.445	.542	.563	.605	.650	.696	.745	.769	.795	.847	.901	.957	1.015	1.045	1.076	1.139	1.203	1.271
7.30	53.29	.441	.538	.558	.601	.645	.691	.739	.763	.788	.840	.894	.949	1.007	1.037	1.067	1.129	1.193	1.260
7.35	54.02	.438	.534	.554	.596	.640	.686	.733	.757	.783	.834	.887	.942	.999	1.029	1.059	1.120	1.184	1.250
7.40	54.76	.435	.530	.550	.592	.635	.681	.728	.752	.777	.827	.880	.935	.991	1.020	1.050	1.111	1.174	1.240
7.45	55.50	.432	.526	.546	.588	.631	.676	.722	.746	.771	.821	.873	.928	.984	1.012	1.042	1.103	1.165	1.230
7.50	56.25	.429	.522	.542	.584	.626	.671	.717	.741	.765	.815	.867	.921	.976	1.005	1.034	1.094	1.156	1.220
7.55	57.00	.426	.519	.539	.579	.622	.666	.712	.735	.759	.809	.860	.914	.969	.997	1.026	1.085	1.147	1.210
7.60	57.76	.423	.515	.535	.575	.617	.661	.707	.730	.754	.803	.854	.907	.961	.989	1.018	1.077	1.138	1.201
7.65	58.52	.420	.511	.531	.571	.613	.656	.702	.725	.749	.797	.848	.900	.954	.982	1.011	1.069	1.129	1.192
7.70	59.29	.417	.508	.527	.567	.608	.652	.696	.719	.743	.791	.841	.893	.947	.975	1.003	1.061	1.120	1.182
7.75	60.06	.414	.504	.524	.563	.604	.647	.692	.714	.738	.786	.835	.887	.940	.968	.996	1.053	1.112	1.174
7.80	60.84	.411	.501	.520	.559	.600	.642	.687	.709	.732	.780	.829	.880	.933	.961	.988	1.045	1.104	1.164
7.85	61.62	.409	.497	.517	.555	.596	.638	.682	.704	.727	.775	.824	.874	.927	.954	.981	1.037	1.096	1.156
7.90	62.41	.406	.494	.513	.552	.592	.634	.677	.699	.722	.769	.818	.868	.920	.947	.974	1.030	1.088	1.147
7.95	63.20	.403	.491	.510	.548	.588	.629	.673	.695	.717	.764	.812	.862	.914	.940	.967	1.023	1.080	1.139
8.00	64.00	.401	.487	.506	.544	.584	.625	.668	.690	.712	.758	.806	.856	.907	.933	.960	1.015	1.072	1.130
8.05	64.80	.398	.484	.503	.541	.580	.621	.664	.685	.708	.753	.801	.850	.901	.927	.954	1.008	1.064	1.123
8.10	65.61	.395	.481	.499	.537	.576	.617	.659	.680	.703	.748	.795	.844	.894	.920	.947	1.001	1.056	1.114
8.15	66.42	.393	.478	.496	.534	.572	.613	.655	.676	.698	.743	.790	.838	.888	.914	.940	.994	1.049	1.107
8.20	67.24	.390	.475	.493	.530	.568	.609	.650	.671	.693	.738	.784	.832	.882	.907	.934	.987	1.042	1.099
8.25	68.06	.388	.472	.490	.527	.565	.605	.646	.666	.689	.733	.779	.827	.876	.901	.927	.980	1.035	1.091
8.30	68.89	.385	.469	.487	.523	.561	.601	.642	.662	.684	.728	.774	.821	.870	.895	.921	.973	1.027	1.083
8.35	69.72	.383	.466	.484	.520	.558	.597	.638	.658	.680	.724	.769	.816	.865	.889	.915	.967	1.020	1.076
8.40	70.56	.381	.463	.480	.516	.554	.593	.634	.654	.675	.719	.764	.810	.859	.883	.909	.761	1.013	1.069
8.45	71.40	.378	.460	.477	.513	.551	.589	.630	.650	.671	.714	.759	.805	.853	.878	.903	.954	1.007	1.061
8.50	72.25	.376	.457	.474	.510	.547	.585	.625	.646	.667	.710	.754	.800	.848	.872	.897	.947	1.000	1.054
8.55	73.10	.374	.454	.472	.507	.544	.582	.622	.642	.663	.705	.749	.795	.842	.866	.891	.941	.994	1.047
8.60	73.96	.371	.451	.469	.504	.540	.578	.618	.638	.658	.701	.744	.790	.837	.860	.885	.935	.987	1.040

Table courtesy of Doctor F. U. Baublitz.

SAGITTA MEASUREMENTS IN MILLIMETERS
DIAMETER IN MILLIMETERS

RAD. MM.	8.40	8.50	8.60	8.80	9.00	9.20	9.40	9.50	9.60	9.80	10.00	10.20	10.40	10.60	10.80	11.00	11.20	11.40
6.00	1.715	1.764	1.816	1.921	2.031	2.148	2.270	2.334	2.400	2.537	2.683	2.842						
6.05	1.696	1.744	1.794	1.898	2.006	2.121	2.241	2.303	2.368	2.502	2.644	2.796						
6.10	1.676	1.724	1.773	1.875	1.982	2.094	2.212	2.272	2.336	2.467	2.606	2.753						
6.15	1.658	1.705	1.753	1.853	1.958	2.068	2.184	2.244	2.306	2.434	2.570	2.713						
6.20	1.639	1.686	1.733	1.832	1.935	2.043	2.158	2.215	2.276	2.401	2.534	2.674						
6.25	1.622	1.667	1.715	1.812	1.913	2.019	2.131	2.188	2.248	2.371	2.500	2.638						
6.30	1.604	1.649	1.696	1.791	1.891	1.995	2.105	2.161	2.220	2.340	2.467	2.601						
6.35	1.588	1.632	1.678	1.772	1.870	1.973	2.080	2.136	2.193	2.311	2.436	2.567						
6.40	1.571	1.615	1.660	1.752	1.849	1.950	2.056	2.110	2.167	2.283	2.405	2.533						
6.45	1.555	1.598	1.643	1.734	1.829	1.928	2.033	2.087	2.142	2.256	2.376	2.502						
6.50	1.540	1.582	1.626	1.716	1.810	1.908	2.010	2.063	2.117	2.229	2.347	2.470	2.600					
6.55	1.524	1.566	1.609	1.698	1.791	1.887	1.988	2.040	2.094	2.204	2.319	2.440	2.568					
6.60	1.509	1.550	1.593	1.681	1.772	1.867	1.967	2.018	2.070	2.179	2.292	2.411	2.536					
6.65	1.494	1.535	1.578	1.664	1.754	1.848	1.946	1.996	2.048	2.155	2.264	2.383	2.505					
6.70	1.480	1.520	1.562	1.647	1.736	1.829	1.925	1.975	2.026	2.131	2.230	2.355	2.475					
6.75	1.466	1.506	1.547	1.632	1.719	1.810	1.906	1.954	2.005	2.108	2.216	2.333	2.452					
6.80	1.452	1.492	1.532	1.616	1.702	1.792	1.886	1.934	1.983	2.085	2.191	2.302	2.418					
6.85	1.439	1.478	1.518	1.600	1.686	1.775	1.867	1.915	1.963	2.064	2.168	2.277	2.391					
6.90	1.426	1.464	1.504	1.585	1.669	1.757	1.848	1.895	1.943	2.042	2.145	2.252	2.365					
6.95	1.413	1.451	1.490	1.570	1.654	1.740	1.831	1.877	1.924	2.022	2.123	2.229	2.339					
7.00	1.400	1.438	1.476	1.556	1.638	1.724	1.813	1.858	1.905	2.001	2.101	2.205	2.314	2.427	2.546	2.670	2.800	2.937
7.05	1.388	1.425	1.463	1.542	1.632	1.708	1.796	1.840	1.887	1.982	2.080	2.183	2.290	2.401	2.518	2.640	2.767	2.902
7.10	1.375	1.412	1.450	1.528	1.608	1.692	1.778	1.823	1.868	1.962	2.059	2.160	2.266	2.376	2.490	2.610	2.735	2.867
7.15	1.364	1.400	1.438	1.514	1.594	1.677	1.762	1.806	1.851	1.943	2.039	2.139	2.243	2.351	2.464	2.582	2.705	2.834
7.20	1.352	1.388	1.425	1.501	1.580	1.661	1.746	1.789	1.834	1.925	2.019	2.118	2.220	2.327	2.438	2.554	2.675	2.801
7.25	1.341	1.376	1.413	1.488	1.566	1.647	1.730	1.773	1.817	1.907	2.000	2.097	2.198	2.303	2.413	2.527	2.646	2.770
7.30	1.330	1.365	1.401	1.475	1.552	1.632	1.714	1.753	1.800	1.889	1.981	2.077	2.177	2.280	2.388	2.500	2.617	2.739
7.35	1.318	1.353	1.389	1.463	1.539	1.618	1.699	1.741	1.784	1.872	1.963	2.058	2.156	2.258	2.364	2.475	2.590	2.710
7.40	1.308	1.342	1.378	1.450	1.526	1.604	1.684	1.726	1.768	1.855	1.945	2.038	2.135	2.236	2.340	2.449	2.563	2.681
7.45	1.297	1.331	1.367	1.438	1.513	1.590	1.670	1.711	1.753	1.838	1.927	2.020	2.115	2.215	2.318	2.425	2.537	2.653
7.50	1.286	1.320	1.355	1.426	1.500	1.576	1.655	1.696	1.737	1.822	1.910	2.001	2.095	2.193	2.295	2.401	2.511	2.626
7.55	1.276	1.310	1.344	1.416	1.488	1.563	1.642	1.682	1.723	1.806	1.893	1.983	2.076	2.173	2.274	2.378	2.486	2.599
7.60	1.266	1.300	1.334	1.403	1.476	1.550	1.628	1.667	1.708	1.791	1.876	1.965	2.057	2.153	2.252	2.355	2.462	2.573
7.65	1.256	1.289	1.323	1.392	1.464	1.538	1.615	1.653	1.695	1.776	1.860	1.948	2.039	2.134	2.232	2.333	2.438	2.548
7.70	1.246	1.279	1.313	1.381	1.452	1.525	1.601	1.640	1.679	1.760	1.844	1.931	2.021	2.114	2.211	2.311	2.415	2.523
7.75	1.237	1.269	1.303	1.370	1.441	1.513	1.588	1.629	1.666	1.746	1.829	1.915	2.004	2.096	2.191	2.290	2.393	2.499
7.80	1.227	1.259	1.292	1.360	1.429	1.501	1.575	1.613	1.652	1.731	1.813	1.898	1.986	2.077	2.172	2.269	2.370	2.476
7.85	1.218	1.250	1.283	1.349	1.418	1.489	1.563	1.600	1.640	1.717	1.799	1.883	1.970	2.059	2.153	2.249	2.349	2.453
7.90	1.209	1.240	1.273	1.339	1.407	1.477	1.550	1.587	1.626	1.703	1.784	1.867	1.953	2.042	2.134	2.229	2.328	2.430
7.95	1.200	1.231	1.264	1.329	1.396	1.466	1.538	1.575	1.613	1.690	1.769	1.852	1.937	2.025	2.116	2.210	2.307	2.408
8.00	1.191	1.222	1.254	1.319	1.386	1.455	1.526	1.563	1.600	1.676	1.755	1.836	1.921	2.008	2.097	2.191	2.387	2.387
8.05	1.183	1.213	1.245	1.309	1.376	1.444	1.515	1.551	1.588	1.663	1.741	1.822	1.905	1.991	2.080	2.172	2.267	2.366
8.10	1.174	1.204	1.236	1.300	1.365	1.433	1.503	1.539	1.576	1.650	1.727	1.807	1.890	1.975	2.063	2.154	2.248	2.345
8.15	1.166	1.196	1.227	1.290	1.355	1.423	1.492	1.527	1.564	1.638	1.714	1.793	1.875	1.964	2.046	2.136	2.229	2.325
8.20	1.157	1.189	1.218	1.281	1.345	1.412	1.481	1.516	1.552	1.625	1.701	1.779	1.860	1.943	2.029	2.118	2.210	2.305
8.25	1.150	1.179	1.209	1.272	1.336	1.402	1.470	1.505	1.540	1.613	1.688	1.765	1.845	1.928	2.013	2.101	2.192	2.286
8.30	1.141	1.170	1.201	1.262	1.326	1.391	1.459	1.493	1.529	1.601	1.675	1.752	1.831	1.913	1.997	2.084	2.174	2.267
8.35	1.133	1.163	1.193	1.254	1.317	1.382	1.449	1.483	1.518	1.589	1.663	1.739	1.817	1.898	1.981	2.067	2.156	2.248
8.40	1.125	1.154	1.184	1.245	1.307	1.372	1.438	1.472	1.507	1.577	1.650	1.725	1.803	1.883	1.966	2.051	2.139	2.230
8.45	1.118	1.147	1.176	1.236	1.298	1.362	1.428	1.462	1.496	1.566	1.638	1.713	1.790	1.869	1.951	2.035	2.122	2.212
8.50	1.110	1.139	1.168	1.228	1.289	1.353	1.418	1.451	1.485	1.555	1.626	1.700	1.776	1.855	1.936	2.019	2.105	2.194
8.55	1.103	1.131	1.160	1.219	1.280	1.343	1.408	1.441	1.475	1.544	1.615	1.688	1.763	1.841	1.921	2.004	2.089	2.177
8.60	1.095	1.123	1.152	1.211	1.271	1.334	1.398	1.431	1.464	1.533	1.603	1.675	1.750	1.827	1.907	1.989	2.073	2.160

SAGITTA MEASUREMENTS IN MILLIMETERS
DIAMETER IN MILLIMETERS

RAD. MM.	R²	5.00	5.50	5.60	5.80	6.00	6.20	6.40	6.50	6.60	6.80	7.00	7.20	7.40	7.50	7.60	7.80	8.00	8.20
8.65	74.82	.369	.449	.466	.501	.537	.575	.614	.634	.654	.696	.740	.785	.831	.855	.880	.929	.981	1.034
8.70	75.69	.367	.446	.463	.498	.534	.571	.609	.630	.650	.692	.735	.780	.826	.849	.874	.923	.974	1.027
8.75	76.56	.365	.443	.460	.495	.531	.568	.606	.626	.646	.688	.731	.775	.821	.844	.868	.917	.968	1.020
8.80	77.44	.363	.441	.457	.492	.527	.564	.602	.622	.642	.683	.726	.770	.816	.839	.863	.911	.962	1.013
8.85	78.32	.361	.438	.455	.489	.524	.561	.599	.618	.638	.679	.722	.765	.811	.834	.857	.906	.956	1.007
8.90	79.21	.358	.436	.452	.486	.521	.557	.595	.614	.634	.675	.717	.761	.806	.828	.852	.900	.950	1.001
8.95	80.10	.356	.433	.449	.483	.518	.554	.592	.610	.631	.671	.713	.756	.801	.823	.847	.895	.944	.994
9.00	81.00	.354	.430	.447	.480	.515	.551	.588	.607	.627	.667	.708	.751	.796	.818	.842	.889	.938	.989
9.05	81.90	.352	.428	.444	.477	.512	.548	.585	.604	.623	.663	.704	.747	.791	.813	.837	.884	.932	.982
9.10	82.81	.350	.425	.441	.474	.509	.544	.581	.600	.619	.659	.700	.742	.786	.808	.831	.878	.926	.976
9.15	83.72	.348	.423	.439	.472	.506	.541	.578	.597	.616	.655	.696	.738	.782	.804	.826	.873	.921	.970
9.20	84.64	.346	.420	.436	.469	.503	.538	.574	.593	.612	.655	.692	.734	.777	.799	.821	.868	.915	.964
9.25	85.56	.344	.418	.434	.466	.500	.535	.571	.590	.609	.648	.688	.729	.772	.794	.817	.862	.910	.958
9.30	86.49	.342	.416	.432	.464	.497	.532	.568	.586	.605	.644	.684	.725	.768	.789	.812	.857	.904	.953
9.35	87.42	.341	.414	.429	.461	.494	.529	.565	.583	.602	.640	.680	.721	.763	.785	.807	.852	.899	.947
9.40	88.36	.339	.411	.427	.459	.492	.526	.561	.580	.598	.636	.676	.717	.759	.780	.802	.847	.894	.941
9.45	89.30	.337	.409	.424	.456	.489	.523	.558	.576	.595	.633	.672	.713	.755	.776	.798	.842	.888	.936
9.50	90.25			.422	.453	.486	.520	.556	.573	.592	.629	.668	.709	.750	.771	.793	.837	.883	.930
9.55	91.20			.420	.451	.484	.517	.552	.570	.588	.626	.665	.705	.746	.767	.789	.833	.878	.925
9.60	92.16			.417	.448	.481	.514	.549	.567	.585	.622	.661	.701	.742	.763	.784	.828	.873	.920
9.65	93.12			.415	.446	.478	.512	.546	.564	.582	.619	.657	.697	.738	.758	.780	.823	.868	.914
9.70	94.09			.412	.444	.476	.509	.543	.561	.579	.615	.653	.693	.733	.754	.775	.819	.863	.909
9.75	95.06			.411	.441	.473	.506	.540	.558	.576	.612	.650	.689	.729	.750	.771	.814	.858	.904
9.80	96.04			.409	.439	.470	.503	.537	.554	.572	.609	.646	.685	.725	.746	.767	.809	.853	.899
9.85	97.02			.406	.437	.468	.501	.534	.552	.569	.606	.643	.682	.721	.742	.763	.805	.849	.894
9.90	98.01			.404	.434	.465	.498	.531	.549	.566	.602	.639	.678	.717	.738	.758	.801	.844	.889
9.95	99.00			.402	.432	.463	.495	.529	.546	.563	.599	.636	.674	.714	.734	.754	.796	.840	.884
10.00	100.00			.400	.430	.461	.493	.526	.543	.560	.596	.632	.670	.710	.730	.750	.792	.835	.879
10.05	101.00			.398	.428	.458	.490	.523	.540	.557	.593	.629	.667	.706	.726	.746	.788	.830	.874
10.10	102.01			.396	.426	.456	.488	.520	.537	.554	.590	.626	.663	.702	.722	.742	.783	.826	.870
10.15	103.02			.394	.423	.453	.485	.518	.534	.552	.587	.623	.660	.699	.718	.738	.779	.822	.865
10.20	104.04			.392	.421	.451	.482	.515	.531	.549	.583	.619	.656	.695	.714	.734	.775	.817	.860
10.25	105.06			.390	.419	.449	.480	.512	.529	.546	.580	.616	.653	.691	.711	.731	.771	.813	.856
10.30	106.09			.388	.417	.447	.478	.510	.526	.543	.577	.613	.650	.687	.707	.727	.767	.808	.851
10.35	107.12			.386	.415	.444	.475	.507	.523	.540	.574	.610	.646	.684	.703	.723	.763	.804	.847
10.40	108.16			.384	.413	.442	.473	.505	.521	.537	.571	.607	.643	.680	.699	.719	.759	.800	.842
10.45	109.20			.382	.411	.440	.471	.502	.518	.535	.569	.604	.640	.677	.696	.715	.755	.796	.838
10.50	110.25			.380	.408	.438	.469	.500	.515	.532	.566	.601	.636	.673	.692	.712	.751	.792	.834
10.55	111.30			.378	.407	.436	.467	.498	.513	.530	.563	.598	.633	.670	.689	.708	.747	.788	.829
10.60	112.36			.376	.405	.434	.464	.495	.511	.527	.560	.595	.630	.667	.685	.705	.743	.784	.825
10.65	113.42			.375	.403	.432	.462	.493	.508	.524	.557	.592	.627	.663	.682	.701	.740	.780	.821
10.70	114.49			.373	.401	.430	.460	.490	.505	.522	.554	.589	.624	.660	.679	.698	.736	.776	.817
10.75	115.56			.371	.399	.428	.458	.487	.503	.519	.552	.586	.621	.657	.675	.694	.732	.772	.813
10.80	116.64			.369	.397	.425	.456	.485	.500	.517	.549	.583	.618	.654	.672	.691	.729	.768	.808
10.85	117.72			.367	.395	.423	.453	.483	.498	.514	.547	.580	.615	.650	.669	.687	.725	.764	.805
10.90	118.81			.366	.393	.421	.450	.481	.496	.512	.544	.577	.612	.647	.665	.684	.722	.760	.801
10.95	119.90			.364	.391	.419	.448	.479	.493	.509	.541	.575	.609	.644	.662	.681	.718	.757	.798
11.00	121.00			.362	.389	.417	.446	.476	.491	.507	.539	.572	.606	.641	.659	.677	.715	.753	.793
11.05	122.10			.361	.387	.415	.444	.474	.489	.504	.536	.569	.603	.638	.656	.674	.711	.750	.789
11.10	123.21			.359	.385	.413	.442	.472	.486	.502	.534	.566	.600	.635	.653	.671	.708	.746	.785
11.20	125.44			.356	.382	.409	.438	.467	.482	.497	.529	.561	.594	.629	.646	.664	.701	.739	.778
11.30	127.69			.353	.378	.406	.433	.463	.477	.493	.524	.556	.589	.623	.640	.658	.694	.732	.770
11.40	129.96			.349	.375	.402	.430	.459	.473	.488	.519	.551	.583	.617	.634	.652	.688	.725	.763
11.50	132.25			.347	.371	.398	.425	.455	.469	.484	.514	.546	.578	.611	.628	.646	.681	.718	.756
11.60	134.56			.343	.369	.394	.422	.451	.464	.479	.509	.541	.573	.606	.623	.640	.675	.711	.750
11.70	136.89			.340	.365	.391	.419	.446	.460	.475	.505	.536	.568	.600	.617	.634	.669	.705	.742
11.80	139.24			.337	.362	.387	.415	.442	.456	.471	.500	.531	.563	.595	.612	.629	.663	.699	.734
11.90	141.61			.334	.359	.384	.411	.438	.452	.467	.496	.526	.558	.590	.606	.623	.657	.692	.727
12.00	144.00			.331	.356	.381	.408	.435	.448	.463	.492	.522	.553	.585	.601	.618	.651	.686	.721
12.10	146.41			.329	.353	.378	.404	.431	.445	.459	.487	.517	.548	.580	.596	.612	.646	.680	.716
12.20	148.84			.326	.350	.375	.401	.427	.441	.455	.483	.513	.543	.575	.591	.607	.640	.674	.710
12.25	150.06			.325	.348	.374	.399	.425	.439	.453	.481	.511	.541	.572	.588	.604	.637	.671	.707
12.50	156.25			.318	.341	.365	.390	.417	.430	.443	.471	.500	.530	.560	.576	.592	.624	.657	.693
14.00	196.00											.445	.471	.498	.512	.526	.555	.584	.614
17.00	289.00											.364	.386	.408	.419	.433	.453	.477	.502
		5.00	5.50	5.60	5.80	6.00	6.20	6.40	6.50	6.60	6.80	7.00	7.20	7.40	7.50	7.60	7.80	8.00	8.20
$\left(\dfrac{D}{2}\right)^2$		6.25	7.56	7.84	8.41	9.00	9.61	10.24	10.56	10.89	11.56	12.25	12.96	13.69	14.06	14.44	15.21	16.00	16.81

SAGITTA MEASUREMENTS IN MILLIMETERS
DIAMETER IN MILLIMETERS

RAD. MM.	8.40	8.50	8.60	8.80	9.00	9.20	9.40	9.50	9.60	9.80	10.00	10.20	10.40	10.60	10.80	11.00	11.20	11.40
8.65	1.088	1.116	1.145	1.203	1.263	1.325	1.389	1.421	1.454	1.522	1.592	1.664	1.738	1.814	1.893	1.974	2.058	2.144
8.70	1.081	1.109	1.137	1.195	1.254	1.316	1.379	1.411	1.444	1.511	1.580	1.652	1.725	1.801	1.871	1.959	2.042	2.127
8.75	1.074	1.101	1.130	1.187	1.246	1.307	1.370	1.402	1.434	1.501	1.570	1.640	1.713	1.788	1.865	1.945	2.027	2.111
8.80	1.067	1.094	1.122	1.179	1.238	1.298	1.362	1.392	1.424	1.491	1.559	1.629	1.701	1.775	1.852	1.931	2.012	2.096
8.85	1.060	1.087	1.115	1.172	1.230	1.290	1.351	1.383	1.415	1.481	1.548	1.617	1.689	1.763	1.839	1.917	1.997	2.080
8.90	1.053	1.080	1.108	1.164	1.222	1.281	1.342	1.373	1.405	1.470	1.537	1.606	1.677	1.750	1.825	1.903	1.983	2.065
8.95	1.047	1.073	1.101	1.157	1.214	1.273	1.334	1.365	1.396	1.461	1.527	1.595	1.666	1.738	1.813	1.890	1.969	2.050
9.00	1.040	1.067	1.094	1.149	1.206	1.263	1.325	1.356	1.387	1.451	1.517	1.584	1.654	1.726	1.800	1.876	1.954	2.035
9.05	1.034	1.060	1.087	1.142	1.198	1.257	1.316	1.347	1.378	1.442	1.507	1.574	1.643	1.714	1.788	1.863	1.941	2.021
9.10	1.027	1.053	1.080	1.135	1.191	1.248	1.308	1.338	1.369	1.432	1.497	1.563	1.632	1.703	1.775	1.850	1.927	2.006
9.15	1.021	1.047	1.074	1.128	1.183	1.240	1.300	1.330	1.360	1.423	1.487	1.553	1.621	1.691	1.764	1.838	1.914	1.992
9.20	1.015	1.040	1.067	1.120	1.176	1.233	1.291	1.321	1.352	1.414	1.477	1.543	1.614	1.680	1.752	1.825	1.901	1.979
9.25	1.009	1.034	1.060	1.114	1.169	1.225	1.283	1.313	1.343	1.405	1.468	1.533	1.600	1.669	1.740	1.813	1.888	1.965
9.30	1.002	1.028	1.054	1.107	1.161	1.217	1.275	1.304	1.335	1.396	1.459	1.523	1.590	1.658	1.728	1.807	1.875	1.952
9.35	.997	1.022	1.048	1.100	1.154	1.210	1.267	1.296	1.326	1.387	1.449	1.514	1.580	1.647	1.717	1.789	1.863	1.939
9.40	.991	1.015	1.041	1.093	1.147	1.202	1.259	1.288	1.318	1.378	1.440	1.504	1.569	1.637	1.706	1.777	1.850	1.925
9.45	.985	1.010	1.035	1.087	1.140	1.195	1.252	1.281	1.310	1.370	1.431	1.495	1.560	1.626	1.696	1.766	1.838	1.913
9.50	.979	1.004	1.029	1.080	1.133	1.188	1.244	1.273	1.302	1.361	1.422	1.485	1.550	1.616	1.684	1.754	1.826	1.900
9.55	.973	.998	1.023	1.074	1.127	1.181	1.237	1.265	1.293	1.353	1.414	1.476	1.540	1.606	1.673	1.743	1.814	1.888
9.60	.967	.992	1.017	1.068	1.120	1.174	1.229	1.257	1.286	1.345	1.405	1.467	1.530	1.596	1.663	1.732	1.803	1.875
9.65	.962	.986	1.011	1.062	1.114	1.167	1.222	1.250	1.279	1.337	1.397	1.458	1.521	1.586	1.653	1.721	1.791	1.863
9.70	.956	.980	1.005	1.055	1.107	1.160	1.215	1.243	1.271	1.329	1.388	1.449	1.512	1.576	1.642	1.710	1.780	1.851
9.75	.951	.975	1.000	1.049	1.101	1.154	1.208	1.235	1.264	1.321	1.380	1.440	1.503	1.566	1.632	1.700	1.769	1.840
9.80	.946	.969	.994	1.043	1.094	1.147	1.201	1.228	1.256	1.313	1.372	1.432	1.493	1.557	1.622	1.689	1.758	1.828
9.85	.940	.964	.988	1.038	1.088	1.140	1.194	1.221	1.249	1.306	1.364	1.423	1.485	1.548	1.612	1.679	1.747	1.817
9.90	.935	.959	.983	1.032	1.082	1.134	1.187	1.214	1.242	1.298	1.355	1.415	1.476	1.538	1.602	1.668	1.736	1.806
9.95	.931	.953	.977	1.026	1.076	1.127	1.180	1.207	1.235	1.290	1.348	1.407	1.467	1.529	1.593	1.658	1.726	1.795
10.00	.925	.948	.972	1.020	1.070	1.121	1.173	1.200	1.227	1.283	1.340	1.398	1.458	1.520	1.583	1.648	1.715	1.784
10.05	.920	.943	.967	1.015	1.064	1.115	1.167	1.193	1.221	1.276	1.332	1.390	1.450	1.511	1.574	1.639	1.705	1.773
10.10	.915	.938	.961	1.009	1.058	1.108	1.160	1.187	1.213	1.268	1.324	1.382	1.441	1.502	1.565	1.629	1.695	1.762
10.15	.910	.933	.956	1.004	1.052	1.102	1.154	1.180	1.207	1.261	1.317	1.374	1.433	1.494	1.556	1.619	1.685	1.752
10.20	.905	.928	.951	.998	1.046	1.096	1.147	1.173	1.200	1.254	1.310	1.367	1.425	1.485	1.547	1.610	1.675	1.741
10.25	.900	.923	.946	.993	1.041	1.090	1.141	1.167	1.194	1.247	1.302	1.359	1.417	1.477	1.538	1.601	1.665	1.731
10.30	.895	.918	.941	.987	1.035	1.084	1.135	1.161	1.187	1.240	1.295	1.351	1.409	1.468	1.529	1.591	1.655	1.721
10.35	.891	.913	.936	.982	1.030	1.079	1.129	1.154	1.180	1.234	1.288	1.344	1.401	1.460	1.521	1.582	1.646	1.711
10.40	.886	.908	.931	.977	1.024	1.073	1.123	1.148	1.174	1.227	1.281	1.336	1.393	1.452	1.512	1.573	1.636	1.701
10.45	.881	.903	.926	.972	1.019	1.067	1.117	1.142	1.168	1.220	1.274	1.329	1.386	1.444	1.503	1.565	1.627	1.692
10.50	.877	.899	.921	.966	1.013	1.061	1.111	1.136	1.161	1.213	1.267	1.322	1.378	1.436	1.495	1.556	1.618	1.682
10.55	8.72	.894	.916	.961	1.008	1.056	1.105	1.130	1.155	1.207	1.260	1.315	1.371	1.427	1.487	1.547	1.609	1.673
10.60	.868	.889	.911	.956	1.003	1.050	1.099	1.124	1.149	1.201	1.253	1.308	1.363	1.420	1.479	1.539	1.600	1.663
10.65	.863	.885	.907	.952	.998	1.045	1.093	1.118	1.143	1.194	1.247	1.301	1.356	1.413	1.471	1.530	1.591	1.654
10.70	.859	.880	.902	.947	.992	1.039	1.088	1.112	1.137	1.188	1.240	1.294	1.349	1.405	1.463	1.522	1.582	1.645
10.75	.855	.876	.898	.942	.987	1.034	1.082	1.106	1.131	1.182	1.234	1.287	1.341	1.397	1.455	1.514	1.574	1.636
10.80	.850	.871	.893	.937	.982	1.029	1.076	1.101	1.125	1.176	1.227	1.280	1.334	1.390	1.447	1.505	1.565	1.627
10.85	.846	.868	.889	.932	.977	1.024	1.071	1.095	1.120	1.170	1.221	1.273	1.327	1.383	1.439	1.497	1.557	1.618
10.90	.842	.863	.884	.928	.972	1.018	1.065	1.089	1.114	1.163	1.214	1.267	1.320	1.375	1.432	1.489	1.549	1.609
10.95	.838	.859	.880	.923	.967	1.013	1.060	1.084	1.108	1.158	1.208	1.260	1.314	1.368	1.424	1.482	1.540	1.601
11.00	.833	.854	.876	.918	.963	1.008	1.055	1.078	1.103	1.152	1.202	1.254	1.307	1.361	1.417	1.474	1.532	1.592
11.05	.829	.850	.872	.914	.957	1.003	1.050	1.073	1.097	1.146	1.196	1.247	1.300	1.354	1.409	1.466	1.524	1.584
11.10	.825	.846	.867	.910	.952	.999	1.044	1.068	1.092	1.140	1.190	1.241	1.293	1.347	1.402	1.458	1.517	1.575
11.20	.818	.837	.859	.901	.944	.989	1.034	1.057	1.081	1.129	1.179	1.229	1.280	1.333	1.388	1.443	1.501	1.559
11.30	.810	.830	.850	.892	.935	.979	1.024	1.047	1.071	1.118	1.167	1.216	1.268	1.320	1.374	1.429	1.485	1.543
11.40	.802	.822	.842	.883	.926	.969	1.016	1.037	1.060	1.107	1.155	1.205	1.255	1.307	1.360	1.415	1.470	1.527
11.50	.794	.814	.835	.876	.917	.960	1.006	1.027	1.050	1.096	1.144	1.193	1.243	1.294	1.347	1.401	1.456	1.512
11.60	.787	.807	.827	.868	.909	.951	.996	1.017	1.040	1.086	1.133	1.182	1.231	1.282	1.334	1.387	1.441	1.497
11.70	.780	.800	.819	.859	.901	.942	.986	1.008	1.030	1.075	1.122	1.170	1.219	1.269	1.321	1.373	1.428	1.482
11.80	.773	.793	.812	.850	.892	.932	.976	.998	1.020	1.067	1.112	1.159	1.208	1.257	1.309	1.360	1.413	1.468
11.90	.766	.785	.804	.844	.886	.925	.966	.989	1.011	1.056	1.102	1.148	1.195	1.245	1.296	1.347	1.400	1.454
12.00	.759	.777	.797	.835	.875	.916	.958	.980	1.003	1.046	1.091	1.138	1.186	1.234	1.284	1.335	1.387	1.441
12.10	.752	.771	.790	.829	.868	.909	.950	.972	.993	1.037	1.082	1.127	1.175	1.222	1.272	1.322	1.374	1.427
12.20	.747	.764	.783	.821	.860	.901	.942	.963	.986	1.028	1.071	1.117	1.164	1.212	1.261	1.310	1.361	1.414
12.25	.744	.761	.781	.818	.857	.897	.938	.959	.981	1.023	1.067	1.112	1.159	1.206	1.255	1.305	1.355	1.407
12.50	.727	.744	.764	.801	.838	.877	.917	.938	.959	1.000	1.044	1.087	1.133	1.181	1.227	1.275	1.325	1.375
14.00	.646	.658	.677	.710	.743	.778	.809	.831	.849	.886	.923	.962	1.002					
17.00	.527	.538	.553	.579	.606	.634	.663	.677	.692	.721	.752	.783	.814					
	8.40	8.50	8.60	8.80	9.00	9.20	9.40	9.50	9.60	9.80	10.00	10.20	10.40	10.60	10.80	11.00	11.20	11.40
	17.64	18.00	18.49	19.36	20.25	21.16	22.09	22.56	23.04	24.01	25.00	26.01	27.04	28.09	29.16	30.25	31.36	32.49

Appendix 7

DIOPTRAL AND MM. CURVES
FOR EXTENDED KERATOMETER RANGE

LOW POWER (−1.00 LENS)

Drum Reading	Corneal Power in Diopters	Radius in mm Cx	CC	Drum Reading	Corneal Power in Diopters	Radius in mm Cx	CC
36.000	30.874	10.931	10.964	39.125	33.554	10.058	10.088
36.125	30.981	10.893	10.926	39.250	33.662	10.026	10.056
36.250	31.089	10.856	10.889	39.375	33.769	9.994	10.024
36.375	31.196	10.819	10.851	39.500	33.876	9.963	9.993
36.500	31.303	10.782	10.814	39.625	33.983	9.931	9.961
36.625	31.410	10.745	10.777	39.750	34.090	9.900	9.930
36.750	31.518	10.708	10.740	39.875	34.198	9.869	9.899
36.875	31.625	10.672	10.704	40.000	34.305	9.838	9.868
37.000	31.732	10.636	10.668	40.125	34.412	9.807	9.837
37.125	31.839	10.600	10.632	40.250	34.519	9.777	9.806
37.250	31.946	10.564	10.596	40.375	34.626	9.747	9.776
37.375	32.054	10.529	10.561	40.500	34.734	9.717	9.746
37.500	32.161	10.494	10.526	40.625	34.841	9.687	9.716
37.625	32.268	10.459	10.491	40.750	34.948	9.657	9.686
37.750	32.375	10.425	10.456	40.875	35.055	9.628	9.656
37.875	32.482	10.390	10.421	41.000	35.162	9.598	9.627
38.000	32.590	10.356	10.387	41.125	35.270	9.569	9.598
38.125	32.697	10.322	10.353	41.250	35.377	9.540	9.569
38.250	32.804	10.288	10.319	41.375	35.484	9.511	9.540
38.375	32.911	10.255	10.286	41.500	35.591	9.483	9.511
38.500	33.018	10.221	10.252	41.625	35.698	9.454	9.483
38.625	33.126	10.188	10.219	41.750	35.806	9.426	9.454
38.750	33.233	10.155	10.186	41.875	35.913	9.398	9.426
38.875	33.340	10.123	10.153	42.000	36.020	9.370	9.398
39.000	33.447	10.090	10.121				

HIGH POWER (+1.25 LENS)

Drum Reading	Corneal Power in Diopters	Radius in mm Cx	Radius in mm CC	Drum Reading	Corneal Power in Diopters	Radius in mm Cx	Radius in mm CC
43.000	50.134	6.732	6.759	47.500	55.380	6.094	6.119
43.125	50.279	6.712	6.739	47.625	55.526	6.078	6.103
43.250	50.425	6.693	6.720	47.750	55.672	6.062	6.087
43.375	50.571	6.674	6.701	47.875	55.817	6.046	6.071
43.500	50.717	6.655	6.681	48.000	55.963	6.031	6.055
43.625	50.862	6.636	6.662	48.125	56.109	6.015	6.039
43.750	51.008	6.617	6.643	48.250	56.255	5.999	6.024
43.875	51.154	6.598	6.624	48.375	56.400'	5.984	6.008
44.000	51.299	6.579	6.605	48.500	56.546	5.969	5.993
44.125	51.445	6.560	6.587	48.625	56.692	5.953	5.977
44.250	51.591	6.542	6.568	48.750	56.838	5.938	5.962
44.375	51.737	6.523	6.550	48.875	56.983	5.923	5.947
44.500	51.882	6.505	6.531	49.000	57.129	5.908	5.931
44.625	52.028	6.487	6.513	49.125	57.275	5.893	5.916
44.750	52.174	6.469	6.495	49.250	57.421	5.878	5.901
44.875	52.320	6.451	6.477	49.375	57.566	5.863.	5.886
45.000	52.465	6.433	6.459	49.500	57.712	5.848	5.871
45.125	52.611	6.415	6.441	49.625	57.858	5.833	5.857
45.250	52.757	6.397	6.423	49.750	58.003	5.819	5.842
45.375	52.903	6.380	6.405	49.875	58.149	5.804	5.827
45.500	53.048	6.362	6.388	50.000	58.295	5.789	5.813
45.625	53.194	6.345	6.370	50.125	58.441	5.775	5.798
45.750	53.340	6.327	6.353	50.250	58.586	5.761	5.784
45.875	53.486	6.310	6.335	50.375	58.732	5.746	5.769
46.000	53.631	6.293	6.318	50.500	58.878	5.732	5.755
46.125	53.777	6.276	6.301	50.625	59.024	5.718	5.741
46.250	53.923	6.259	6.284	50.750	59.169	5.704	5.727
46.375	54.069	6.242	6.267	50.875	59.315	5.690	5.713
46.500	54.214	6.225	6.250	51.000	59.461	5.676	5.699
46.625	54.360	6.209	6.233	51.125	59.607	5.662	5.685
46.750	54.506	6.192	6.217	51.250	59.752	5.648	5.671
46.875	54.651	6.175	6.200	51.375	59.898	5.635	5.657
47.000	54.797	6.159	6.184	51.500	60.044	5.621	5.643
47.125	54.943	6.143	6.167	51.625	60.190	5.607	5.630
47.250	55.089	6.126	6.151	51.750	60.335	5.594	5.616
47.375	55.234	6.110	6.135	51.875	60.481	5.580	5.603
				52.000	60.627	5.567	5.589

Appendix 8

SINGLE CUT PLUS LENS THICKNESS CHART—DIAMETER

PLUS POWER (BACK VERTEX)		6.5 mm.	7.0 mm.	7.5 mm.	8.0 mm.	8.5 mm.	9.0 mm.	9.5 mm.
+20.00 to +20.75		.40/.016	.45/.018	.51/.020	.58/.023	.65/.026	.72/.028	.84/.033
+19.00 to +19.75		.38/.015	.43/.017	.50/.020	.56/.022	.63/.025	.70/.028	.81/.032
+18.00 to +18.75		.37/.015	.42/.017	.48/.019	.54/.021	.60/.024	.68/.027	.78/.031
+17.00 to +17.75		.36/.014	.41/.016	.46/.018	.52/.020	.58/.023	.65/.026	.75/.029
+16.00 to +16.75		.35/.014	.40/.016	.45/.018	.50/.020	.56/.022	.63/.025	.72/.029
+15.00 to +15.75		.34/.013	.38/.015	.43/.017	.48/.019	.53/.021	.60/.024	.68/.027
+14.00 to +14.75		.32/.013	.36/.014	.41/.017	.46/.018	.51/.020	.57/.022	.64/.025
+13.00 to +13.75		.31/.012	.35/.014	.39/.015	.44/.017	.49/.019	.55/.022	.61/.024
+12.00 to +12.75		.30/.012	.34/.013	.38/.015	.42/.017	.47/.019	.52/.020	.58/.023
+11.00 to +11.75		.28/.011	.32/.013	.36/.014	.40/.016	.44/.017	.49/.019	.55/.022
+10.00 to +10.75		.27/.011	.31/.012	.35/.014	.38/.015	.42/.017	.46/.018	.52/.020
+ 9.00 to + 9.75		.26/.010	.29/.011	.33/.013	.36/.014	.39/.015	.44/.017	.49/.019
+ 8.00 to + 8.75		.25/.010	.28/.011	.31/.012	.34/.013	.37/.015	.41/.016	.46/.018
+ 7.00 to + 7.75		.24/.009	.27/.011	.30/.012	.32/.013	.35/.014	.39/.015	.43/.017
+ 6.00 to + 6.75		.23/.009	.25/.010	.28/.011	.30/.012	.33/.013	.36/.014	.39/.015
+ 5.00 to + 5.75		.21/.008	.24/.009	.26/.010	.28/.011	.30/.012	.33/.013	.37/.015
+ 4.00 to + 4.75		.20/.008	.22/.009	.24/.009	.26/.010	.28/.011	.31/.012	.34/.013
+ 3.00 to + 3.75		.18/.007	.20/.008	.22/.009	.24/.009	.26/.010	.28/.011	.31/.012
+ 2.00 to + 2.75		.17/.007	.19/.007	.21/.008	.22/.009	.24/.009	.26/.010	.28/.011
+ 1.00 to + 1.75		.16/.006	.17/.007	.19/.007	.20/.008	.22/.009	.23/.009	.25/.010
0 to + .75		.16/.006	.16/.006	.17/.007	.18/.007	.19/.007	.21/.008	.22/.009

Appendix 9

CALCULATION OF TRUE LENS THICKNESS

CALCULATION OF TRUE LENS THICKNESS FROM OPTICAL THICKNESS
MEASURED WITH A RADIUSCOPE (n = 1.40)

Measured Thickness t	True Thickness 1.4t	Measured Thickness t	True Thickness 1.4t
10	14	28	39.2
11	15.4	29	40.7
12	16.8	30	42
13	18.2	31	43.4
14	19.6	32	44.8
15	21	33	46.2
16	22.4	34	47.6
17	23.8	35	49
18	25.2	36	50.4
19	26.6	37	51.8
20	28	38	53.2
21	29.4	39	54.6
22	30.8	40	56
23	32.2	41	57.4
24	33.6	42	58.8
25	35	43	60.2
26	36.4	44	61.6
27	37.8	45	63

Appendix 10

FRONT SURFACE RADIUS

To find front radius of a contact lens when base curve, power, and thickness are given, the following should be done:

Procedure

1. Find radius value in table under base curve and power.
2. Add correction factor below to radius value to find front radius of lens.

Lens Thickness	Correction Factor
0.08	0.0263
0.10	0.0329
0.12	0.0395
0.14	0.0461
0.16	0.0526
0.18	0.0592
0.20	0.0658
0.22	0.0724

Lens Thickness	Correction Factor
0.24	0.0789
0.26	0.0855
0.28	0.0921
0.30	0.0987
0.32	0.1052
0.34	0.1118
0.36	0.1184
0.38	0.1250
0.40	0.1316
0.50	0.1645
0.60	0.1973
0.70	0.2302
0.80	0.2631

Example

Base Curve = 8.05
Power = −3.00
Thickness = 0.2
Front Radius = 8.467 + 0.0658 = 8.533

r_2	-350 r_1	-325 r_1	-300 r_1	-275 r_1	-250 r_1	-225 r_1	-200 r_1
7.63	8.070	8.037	8.004	7.971	7.939	7.907	7.875
7.64	8.081	8.048	8.015	7.982	7.950	7.918	7.886
7.65	8.092	8.059	8.026	7.993	7.961	7.929	7.897
7.66	8.103	8.070	8.037	8.004	7.972	7.939	7.907
7.67	8.115	8.081	8.048	8.015	7.982	7.950	7.918
7.68	8.126	8.092	8.059	8.026	7.993	7.961	7.929
7.69	8.137	8.103	8.070	8.037	8.004	7.971	7.939
7.70	8.148	8.114	8.081	8.048	8.015	7.982	7.950
7.71	8.159	8.126	8.092	8.059	8.026	7.993	7.961
7.72	8.171	8.137	8.103	8.070	8.037	8.004	7.971
7.73	8.182	8.148	8.114	8.081	8.047	8.014	7.982
7.74	8.193	8.159	8.125	8.091	8.058	8.025	7.992
7.75	8.204	8.170	8.136	8.102	8.069	8.036	8.003
7.76	8.215	8.181	8.147	8.113	8.080	8.047	8.014
7.77	8.227	8.192	8.158	8.124	8.091	8.057	8.024
7.78	8.238	8.203	8.169	8.135	8.102	8.068	8.035
7.79	8.249	8.214	8.180	8.146	8.112	8.079	8.046
7.80	8.260	8.226	8.191	8.157	8.123	8.090	8.056
7.81	8.271	8.237	8.202	8.168	8.134	8.101	8.067
7.82	8.283	8.248	8.213	8.179	8.145	8.111	8.078
7.83	8.294	8.259	8.224	8.190	8.156	8.122	8.089
7.84	8.305	8.270	8.235	8.201	8.167	8.133	8.099
7.85	8.316	8.281	8.246	8.212	8.178	8.144	8.110
7.86	8.328	8.292	8.257	8.223	8.188	8.154	8.121
7.87	8.339	8.303	8.268	8.234	8.199	8.165	8.131
7.88	8.350	8.315	8.279	8.245	8.210	8.176	8.142
7.89	8.361	8.326	8.290	8.256	8.221	8.187	8.153
7.90	8.372	8.337	8.302	8.267	8.232	8.197	8.163
7.91	8.384	8.348	8.313	8.277	8.243	8.208	8.174
7.92	8.395	8.359	8.324	8.288	8.254	8.219	8.185
7.93	8.406	8.370	8.335	8.299	8.264	8.230	8.195
7.94	8.417	8.381	8.346	8.310	8.275	8.240	8.206
7.95	8.429	8.393	8.357	8.321	8.286	8.251	8.217
7.96	8.440	8.404	8.368	8.332	8.297	8.262	8.227
7.97	8.451	8.415	8.379	8.343	8.308	8.273	8.238
7.98	8.462	8.426	8.390	8.354	8.319	8.284	8.249
7.99	8.474	8.437	8.401	8.365	8.330	8.294	8.259
8.00	8.485	8.448	8.412	8.376	8.340	8.305	8.270
8.01	8.496	8.459	8.423	8.387	8.351	8.316	8.281
8.02	8.507	8.471	8.434	8.398	8.362	8.327	8.291
8.03	8.519	8.482	8.445	8.409	8.373	8.337	8.302
8.04	8.530	8.493	8.456	8.420	8.384	8.348	8.313
8.05	8.541	8.504	8.467	8.431	8.395	8.359	8.323
8.06	8.552	8.515	8.478	8.442	8.406	8.370	8.334
8.07	8.564	8.526	8.489	8.453	8.417	8.381	8.345
8.08	8.575	8.538	8.501	8.464	8.427	8.391	8.356
8.09	8.586	8.549	8.512	8.475	8.438	8.402	8.366
8.10	8.597	8.560	8.523	8.486	8.449	8.413	8.377
8.11	8.609	8.571	8.534	8.497	8.460	8.424	8.388
8.12	8.620	8.582	8.545	8.508	8.471	8.434	8.398
8.13	8.631	8.593	8.556	8.519	8.482	8.445	8.409
8.14	8.642	8.605	8.567	8.530	8.493	8.456	8.420
8.15	8.654	8.616	8.578	8.541	8.504	8.467	8.430
8.16	8.665	8.627	8.589	8.552	8.514	8.478	8.441
8.17	8.676	8.638	8.600	8.563	8.525	8.488	8.452

−175	−150	−125	−100	−0.75	−0.50	−0.25	pl
r_1	r_1	r_1	r_1	r_1	r_1	r_1	r_1
7.844	7.812	7.781	7.751	7.720	7.690	7.660	7.630
7.854	7.823	7.792	7.761	7.730	7.700	7.670	7.640
7.865	7.833	7.802	7.771	7.741	7.710	7.680	7.650
7.875	7.844	7.813	7.782	7.751	7.720	7.690	7.660
7.886	7.854	7.823	7.792	7.761	7.731	7.700	7.670
7.897	7.865	7.833	7.802	7.771	7.741	7.710	7.680
7.907	7.875	7.844	7.813	7.782	7.751	7.720	7.690
7.918	7.886	7.854	7.823	7.792	7.761	7.730	7.700
7.928	7.896	7.865	7.833	7.802	7.771	7.740	7.710
7.939	7.907	7.875	7.844	7.812	7.781	7.751	7.720
7.949	7.917	7.885	7.854	7.823	7.791	7.761	7.730
7.960	7.928	7.896	7.864	7.833	7.802	7.771	7.740
7.971	7.938	7.906	7.875	7.843	7.812	7.781	7.750
7.981	7.949	7.917	7.885	7.853	7.822	7.791	7.760
7.992	7.959	7.927	7.895	7.864	7.832	7.801	7.770
8.002	7.907	7.938	7.906	7.874	7.842	7.811	7.780
8.013	7.980	7.948	7.916	7.884	7.852	7.821	7.790
8.024	7.991	7.958	7.926	7.894	7.863	7.831	7.800
8.034	8.001	7.969	7.936	7.904	7.873	7.841	7.810
8.045	8.012	7.979	7.947	7.915	7.883	7.851	7.820
8.055	8.022	7.990	7.957	7.925	7.893	7.861	7.830
8.066	9.033	8.000	7.967	7.935	7.903	7.871	7.840
8.076	8.043	8.010	7.978	7.945	7.913	7.882	7.850
8.087	8.054	8.021	7.988	7.956	7.924	7.892	7.860
8.098	8.064	8.031	7.998	7.966	7.934	7.902	7.870
8.108	8.075	8.042	8.009	7.976	7.944	7.912	7.880
8.119	8.085	8.052	8.019	7.986	7.954	7.922	7.890
8.129	8.096	8.062	8.029	7.997	7.964	7.932	7.900
8.140	8.106	8.073	8.040	8.007	7.974	7.942	7.910
8.151	8.117	8.083	8.050	8.017	7.985	7.952	7.920
8.161	8.127	8.094	8.060	8.027	7.995	7.962	7.930
8.172	8.138	8.104	8.071	8.038	8.005	7.972	7.940
8.182	8.148	8.115	8.081	8.048	8.015	7.982	7.950
8.193	8.159	8.125	8.091	8.058	8.025	7.992	7.960
8.204	8.169	8.135	8.102	8.068	8.035	8.003	7.970
8.124	8.180	8.146	8.112	8.079	8.046	8.013	7.980
8.225	8.190	8.156	8.122	8.089	8.056	8.023	7.990
8.235	8.201	8.167	8.133	8.099	8.066	8.033	8.000
8.246	8.211	8.177	8.143	8.109	8.076	8.043	8.010
8.256	8.222	8.188	8.153	8.120	8.086	8.053	8.020
8.267	8.232	8.198	8.164	8.130	8.096	8.063	8.030
8.278	8.243	8.208	8.174	8.140	8.107	8.073	8.040
8.288	8.253	8.219	8.184	8.150	8.117	8.083	8.050
8.299	8.264	8.229	8.195	8.161	8.127	8.093	8.060
8.309	8.274	2.240	8.205	8.171	8.137	8.103	8.070
8.320	8.285	8.250	8.215	8.181	8.147	8.113	8.080
8.331	8.295	8.260	8.226	8.191	8.157	8.124	8.090
8.341	8.306	8.271	8.236	8.202	8.168	8.134	8.100
8.352	8.316	8.281	8.246	8.212	8.178	8.144	8.110
8.363	8.327	8.292	8.257	8.222	8.188	8.154	8.120
8.373	8.337	8.302	8.267	8.232	8.198	8.164	8.130
8.384	8.348	8.313	8.278	8.243	8.208	8.174	8.140
8.394	8.359	8.323	8.288	8.253	8.218	8.184	8.150
8.405	8.369	8.333	8.298	8.263	8.229	8.194	8.160
8.416	8.380	8.344	8.309	8.273	8.239	8.204	8.170

r_2	+0.25 r_1	+0.50 r_1	+0.75 r_1	+100 r_1	+125 r_1	+150 r_1	+175 r_1
7.63	7.600	7.571	7.542	7.513	7.484	7.456	7.42
7.64	7.610	7.581	7.552	7.523	7.494	7.465	7.43
7.65	7.620	7.591	7.561	7.532	7.504	7.475	7.44
7.66	7.630	7.601	7.571	7.542	7.513	7.484	7.45
7.67	7.640	7.610	7.581	7.552	7.523	7.494	7.46
7.68	7.650	7.620	7.591	7.561	7.532	7.504	7.47
7.69	7.660	7.630	7.601	7.571	7.542	7.513	7.48
7.70	7.670	7.640	7.610	8.581	7.552	7.523	7.49
7.71	7.680	7.650	7.620	7.591	7.561	7.532	7.50
7.72	7.690	7.660	7.630	7.600	7.571	7.542	7.51
7.73	7.700	7.670	7.640	7.610	7.581	7.551	7.52
7.74	7.710	7.679	7.649	7.620	7.590	7.561	7.53
7.75	7.719	7.689	7.659	7.629	7.600	7.570	7.54
7.76	7.729	7.699	7.669	7.639	7.609	7.580	7.55
7.77	7.739	7.709	7.679	7.649	7.619	7.589	7.56
7.78	7.749	7.719	7.688	7.658	7.629	7.599	7.57
7.79	7.759	7.729	7.698	7.668	7.638	7.609	7.57
7.80	7.769	7.738	7.708	7.678	7.648	7.618	7.58
7.81	7.779	7.748	7.718	7.687	7.657	7.628	7.59
7.82	7.789	7.758	7.728	7.697	7.667	7.637	7.60
7.83	7.799	7.768	7.737	7.707	7.677	7.647	7.61
7.84	7.809	7.778	7.747	7.717	7.686	7.656	7.62
7.85	7.819	7.788	7.757	7.726	7.696	7.666	7.63
7.86	7.829	7.797	7.767	7.736	7.705	7.675	7.64
7.87	7.839	7.807	7.776	7.746	7.715	7.685	7.65
7.88	7.848	7.817	7.786	7.755	7.725	7.694	7.66
7.89	7.858	7.827	7.796	7.765	7.734	7.704	7.67
7.90	7.868	7.837	7.806	7.775	7.744	7.713	7.68
7.91	7.878	7.847	7.815	7.784	7.754	7.723	7.69
7.92	7.888	7.857	7.825	7.794	7.763	7.733	7.70
7.93	7.898	7.866	7.835	7.804	7.773	7.742	7.71
7.94	7.908	7.876	7.845	7.813	7.782	7.752	7.72
7.95	7.918	7.886	7.854	7.823	7.792	7.761	7.73
7.96	7.928	7.896	7.864	7.833	7.802	7.771	7.74
7.97	7.938	7.906	7.874	7.842	7.811	7.780	7.74
7.98	7.948	7.916	7.884	7.852	7.821	7.790	7.75
7.99	7.958	7.925	7.893	7.862	7.830	7.799	7.76
8.00	7.967	7.935	7.903	7.871	7.840	7.809	7.77
8.01	7.977	7.945	7.913	7.881	7.850	7.818	7.78
8.02	7.987	7.955	7.923	7.891	7.859	7.828	7.79
8.03	7.997	7.965	7.933	7.901	7.869	7.837	7.80
8.04	8.007	7.975	7.942	7.910	7.878	7.847	7.81
8.05	8.017	7.984	7.952	7.920	7.888	7.856	7.82
8.06	8.027	7.994	7.962	7.930	7.898	7.866	7.83
8.07	8.037	8.004	7.972	7.939	7.907	7.875	7.84
8.08	8.047	8.014	7.981	7.949	7.917	7.885	7.85
8.09	8.057	8.024	7.991	7.959	7.926	7.894	7.86
8.10	8.067	8.034	8.001	7.968	7.936	7.904	7.87
8.11	8.077	8.043	8.011	7.978	7.946	7.914	7.88
8.12	8.086	8.053	8.020	7.988	7.955	7.923	7.89
8.13	8.096	8.063	8.030	7.997	7.965	7.933	7.90
8.14	8.106	8.073	8.040	8.007	7.974	7.942	7.91
8.15	8.116	8.083	8.050	8.017	7.984	7.952	7.91
8.16	8.126	8.093	8.059	8.026	7.994	7.961	7.92
8.17	8.136	8.102	8.069	8.036	8.003	7.971	7.93

+200 r_1	+225 r_1	+250 r_1	+275 r_1	+300 r_1	+325 r_1	+350 r_1	+375 r_1
7.400	7.372	7.344	7.317	7.289	7.262	7.236	7.209
7.409	7.381	7.353	7.326	7.299	7.272	7.245	7.218
7.418	7.390	7.363	7.335	7.308	7.281	7.254	7.227
7.428	7.400	7.372	7.344	7.317	7.290	7.263	7.236
7.437	7.409	7.381	7.353	7.326	7.299	7.272	7.245
7.447	7.418	7.390	7.363	7.335	7.308	7.281	7.254
7.456	7.428	7.400	7.372	7.344	7.317	7.290	7.263
7.465	7.437	7.409	7.381	7.353	7.326	7.299	7.271
7.475	7.446	7.418	7.390	7.362	7.335	7.308	7.280
7.484	7.456	7.427	7.399	7.372	7.344	7.317	7.289
7.494	7.465	7.437	7.409	7.381	7.353	7.326	7.298
7.503	7.474	7.446	7.418	7.390	7.362	7.335	7.307
7.512	7.484	7.455	7.427	7.399	7.371	7.343	7.316
7.522	7.493	7.464	7.436	7.408	7.380	7.352	7.325
7.531	7.502	7.474	7.445	7.417	7.389	7.361	7.334
7.541	7.512	7.483	7.455	7.426	7.398	7.370	7.343
7.550	7.521	7.492	7.464	7.435	7.407	7.379	7.352
7.559	7.530	7.501	7.473	7.444	7.416	7.388	7.361
7.569	7.540	7.511	7.482	7.454	7.425	7.397	7.370
7.578	7.549	7.520	7.491	7.463	7.434	7.406	7.378
7.588	7.558	7.529	7.500	7.472	7.443	7.415	7.387
7.597	7.568	7.538	7.510	7.481	7.452	7.424	7.396
7.606	7.577	7.548	7.519	7.490	7.462	7.433	7.405
7.616	7.586	7.557	7.528	7.499	7.471	7.442	7.414
7.625	7.596	7.566	7.537	7.508	7.480	7.451	7.423
7.634	7.605	7.575	7.546	7.517	7.489	7.460	7.432
7.644	7.614	7.585	7.555	7.526	7.498	7.469	7.441
7.653	7.623	7.594	7.565	7.536	7.507	7.478	7.450
7.663	7.633	7.603	7.574	7.545	7.516	7.487	7.458
7.672	7.642	7.612	7.583	7.554	7.525	7.496	7.467
7.681	7.651	7.622	7.592	7.563	7.534	7.505	7.476
7.691	7.661	7.631	7.601	7.572	7.543	7.514	7.485
7.700	7.670	7.640	7.610	7.581	7.552	7.523	7.494
7.710	7.679	7.649	7.620	7.590	7.561	7.532	7.503
7.719	7.689	7.659	7.629	7.599	7.570	7.541	7.512
7.728	7.698	7.668	7.638	7.608	7.579	7.550	7.521
7.738	7.707	7.677	7.647	7.617	7.588	7.559	7.530
7.747	7.717	7.686	7.656	7.626	7.597	7.568	7.538
7.756	7.726	7.696	7.665	7.636	7.606	7.577	7.547
7.766	7.735	7.705	7.675	7.645	7.615	7.585	7.556
7.775	7.744	7.714	7.684	7.654	7.624	7.594	7.565
7.785	7.754	7.723	7.693	7.663	7.633	7.603	7.574
7.794	7.763	7.732	7.702	7.672	7.642	7.612	7.583
7.803	7.772	7.742	7.711	7.681	7.651	7.621	7.592
7.813	7.782	7.751	7.720	7.690	7.660	7.630	7.601
7.822	7.791	7.760	7.729	7.699	7.669	7.639	7.609
7.831	7.800	7.769	7.739	7.708	7.678	7.648	7.618
7.841	7.810	7.779	7.748	7.717	7.687	7.657	7.627
7.850	7.819	7.788	7.757	7.726	7.696	7.666	7.636
7.860	7.828	7.797	7.766	7.735	7.705	7.675	7.645
7.869	7.837	7.806	7.775	7.745	7.714	7.684	7.654
7.878	7.847	7.815	7.784	7.754	7.723	7.693	7.663
7.888	7.856	7.825	7.794	7.763	7.732	7.702	7.672
7.897	7.865	7.834	7.803	7.772	7.741	7.711	7.680
7.906	7.875	7.843	7.812	7.781	7.750	7.720	7.689

Appendix 11

RADII VALUES FOR THE LENTICULAR FLANGE

RADII VALUES FOR THE LENTICULAR FLANGE EXPRESSED IN MM. OF
CURVATURE FLATTER THAN THE BASE CURVE OF THE LENS

L-2 KORB TECHNIQUE (LENTICULAR DESIGNS) (PLANO TO –3.00)

	Plano (.11 CT.)			*–1.00 (.10 CT.)*			*–2.00 (.09 CT.)*			*–3.00 (.08 CT.)*		
	8.2D	*8.6D*	*9.0D*	*8.2D*	*8.6D*	*9.0D*	*8.2D*	*8.6D*	*9.0D*	*8.2D*	*8.6D*	*9.0D*
Base	*7.4L*	*7.8L*	*8.0L*	*7.4L*	*7.8L*	*8.0L*	*7.4L*	*7.8L*	*8.0L*	*7.4L*	*7.8L*	*8.0L*
7.40	3.2	2.6	2.7	2.6	2.2	2.6	2.4	1.7	2.0	2.1	1.5	1.7
7.50	3.1	2.6	2.7	2.6	2.2	2.5	2.4	1.7	2.0	2.0	1.4	1.6
7.60	3.0	2.5	2.6	2.5	2.1	2.4	2.3	1.6	1.9	2.0	1.4	1.6
7.70	2.9	2.4	2.5	2.5	2.0	2.3	2.2	1.5	1.8	1.9	1.3	1.5
7.80	2.8	2.4	2.4	2.4	1.9	2.2	2.2	1.5	1.8	1.8	1.2	1.4
7.90	2.7	2.3	2.3	2.4	1.9	2.0	2.1	1.4	1.7	1.7	1.2	1.3
8.00	2.6	2.2	2.2	2.3	1.8	1.9	2.0	1.4	1.6	1.7	1.2	1.3
8.10	2.6	2.1	2.2	2.3	1.8	1.8	2.0	1.4	1.6	1.7	1.2	1.3
8.20	2.5	2.0	2.1	2.2	1.7	1.7	1.9	1.3	1.5	1.6	1.2	1.2
8.30	2.4	1.9	2.0	2.1	1.6	1.5	1.8	1.2	1.4	1.5	1.2	1.2
8.40	2.4	1.8	1.9	2.0	1.5	1.4	1.8	1.2	1.3	1.5	1.2	1.2
8.50	2.3	1.7	1.8	1.9	1.4	1.3	1.7	1.2	1.2	1.4	1.2	1.2
8.60	2.2	1.6	1.7	1.8	1.3	1.2	1.6	1.2	1.2	1.3	1.2	1.2
8.70	2.1	1.5	1.6	1.8	1.2	1.0	1.5	1.2	1.2	1.2	1.2	1.2

The D refers to diameter, the L to lenticular diameter: i.e. 8.6D = 8.6 mm. diameter, 7.8L = 7.8 lenticular zone.

All lenses have been designed and calculated for an edge thickness of .075 with a maximum deviation of .005 mm. except the following lenses:

8.6 diameters, –2.00 power, 8.50, 8.60, 8.70 bases

8.6 diameters, –3.00 power, 8.20, 8.30, 8.40, 8.50, 8.60, 8.70 bases

9.0 diameters, –3.00 power, 8.40, 8.50, 8.60, 8.70 bases

The latter lenses have a maximum edge thickness of .09 mm. rather than the preferable .075 mm. This was necessitated by designing an adequate lenticular flange which would support the lens high on the cornea.

Prism tolerance—no prism tolerance is allowed to –2.00 diopters. Over –2.25 diopters to –4.00 diopters, 1/8th of a prism diopter tolerance is permitted. Above –4.00 diopters of power, some flexibility and tolerance is permitted up to an absolute maximum of 1/4th of a diopter of prism.

Over –3.00 in power, flatten the lenticular radius .15 mm. for each additional diopter of minus power.

Appendix 12

KORB TECHNIQUE LENTICULAR DESIGNS

	Diam.	O.Z.	R2	Blend	Edge	plano to −2.50		−2.75 to −6.00		+.25 to +4.00		+4.25 to +7.00		+7.25 up	
						D	C	D	C	D	C	D	C	D	C
	9.8	8.2	1.4	.7	4/12	8.2	1.5	8.6	1.5	8.2	2.0	8.2	2.0	8.2	2.2
	9.6	8.0	1.4	.7	4/12	8.2	1.5	8.4	1.5	8.2	2.0	8.2	2.0	8.2	2.2
	9.4	7.8	1.4	.7	3/12	8.0	1.6	8.2	1.5	8.0	2.0	7.8	2.0	7.8	2.2
	9.2	7.6	1.4	.7	3/12	8.0	1.6	8.2	1.5	8.0	2.0	7.8	2.0	7.8	2.2
I	9.0	7.5	1.4	.7	3/12	7.8	1.7	8.0	1.5	7.6	1.8	7.5	1.8	7.5	2.0
	8.8	7.4	1.4	.7	2/12	7.8	1.7	7.8	1.5	7.6	1.8	7.5	1.8	7.5	2.0
II	8.6	7.2	1.5	.8	2/12	7.6	1.7	7.6	1.5	7.4	1.8	7.3	2.0	7.2	2.2
	8.4	7.0	1.9	.9	2/12	7.4	1.9	7.4	1.5	7.2	2.0	7.1	2.0	7.0	2.2
III	8.2	6.8	2.3	1.0	1/12	7.2	2.0	7.2	1.7	7.0	2.0	6.9	2.0	6.9	2.5
	8.0	6.7	2.4	1.0	1/12	7.0	2.0	7.2	1.7	7.0	2.0	6.9	2.0	6.9	2.5
	7.8	6.5	2.4	1.0	1/12	6.8	2.0	6.8	1.7	6.8	2.2	6.6	2.5	6.5	2.5
	7.6	6.3	2.4	1.0	1/12	6.6	2.0	6.6	1.7	6.6	2.2	6.4	2.5	6.3	2.5

R2 = posterior peripheral curve.
C = anterior carrier radius above curves and blend expressed as mm. flatter than base curve.

Appendix 13

BLINKING INSTRUCTIONS

(The following is a copy of the instructions on correct blinking given by Korb in pamphlet form to every new contact lens patient.)

While the act of blinking is defined and thought of as an involuntary response, the type and frequency of blinking varies from one person to the next, and poor blinking habits are often acquired. Investigation reveals that almost all infants are excellent blinkers; investigation also reveals, however, that nearly everyone with visual problems develops an incorrect blink. Even as poor blinking habits may have been acquired, it is possible to achieve correct blinking habits again through the use of special exercises. It is imperative that all contact lens wearers develop good blinking habits, for correct blinking frequently makes the difference between success and failure with contact lens.

Although special and improved contact lens designs which facilitate correct blinking are used routinely, total success with contact lenses can only be achieved by a strong personal desire and an enlightened effort to practice blinking exercises.

Effects of Blinking on the Eye

The important function of blinking is the spreading of the tear film across the cornea and the maintenance of a natural moist condition which protects the eye from the irritating effects of dryness. During a blink the upper lid moves downward to contact the lower lid; the lower lid does not move up. If the upper lid does not move down sufficiently to contact the lower lid, a portion of the cornea will remain exposed and will not be moistened by the tears. As a result of this "partial" blinking, the exposed area of the cornea will dry and will cause itchiness, scratchiness, redness, burning and/or a tired, heavy feeling. Drying of the eyes often becomes a severe problem for contact lens wearers. Modern contact lenses position themselves on the upper portion of the cornea. That portion of the cornea covered by the contact lens is obviously protected from drying; but the area of the cornea surrounding the lens tends to dry very quickly, especially if blinking is not perfect. Although drying may sometimes make contact lenses difficult to wear from the beginning, the irritating effects of dryness do not usually develop until after months or even years of successful wearing. If the irritation becomes severe, it may require discontinuing contact lens wear.

The Blinking Exercise

The development of correct blinking for contact lens wearers has been pioneered by four contact lens specialists:

886

Dr. Ian Mackie of London, England; Dr. Donald R. Korb of Boston, Massachusetts; Dr. Charles R. Stewart of Waco, Texas; and Dr. C. Edward Williams of Denver, Colorado. The exercises prescribed are designed to eliminate faulty blinking by substituting a fully relaxed and normal appearing blink, as found with infants. These exercises have been developed over a six-year period and have been used successfully with thousands of patients.

There are two sets of muscles in the eyelids, which we will term the "heavy" and "light" muscles. The purpose of the heavy muscles is to close the eyelids quickly in the event of an emergency. These heavy muscles force the lids together with a crashing motion, and they should not be used for normal blinking. If through faulty habits the heavy muscles are utilized for "squinting" or for partial blinking, these undesirable habits must be eliminated in order for contact lenses to be worn with maximum success. The tension created by the heavy muscles can be appreciated by utilizing a method of placing your two index fingers at the extreme outer corners of your eyes, at the angle of the lids. When positioning your index fingers, gently move them so that they rest on the heavy muscles in order that the maximum tension created when a "forced" blink is made will be felt. While monitoring your blinking in this manner, you probably will at first feel muscle tension or pulling during blinking actions, since most people do not have the most desirable blinking habits for contact lens wear. However, a strong personal effort to improve blinking by practicing blinking

exercises can eliminate tension through relaxation of the heavy muscles, while learning to use the light muscles correctly. This usually requires a two- to eight-week period of intensive practice. After this time, a reduced maintenance program can be followed.

Steps for Correct Blinking Exercise

1. Relax. In order to relax the eye muscles you must totally relax and be at ease. It is very important not to force any eye movement throughout the entire exercise. A forced movement causes muscle tension and pull, which can be sensed through the fingertips. Instead, the eyes should close and open naturally with a smooth, fluid motion. The correct posture for the exercise is simple. The head should be straight and erect, and the eyes directed straight ahead. Do not concentrate on looking ahead when the eyes are closed, this tends to force unnatural eye movement.

2. Close. The eyes should be closed slowly and gently, in a fluid motion, as if you were closing them to fall off to sleep. If you are relaxed, as advised in step 1, this should not be a difficult task to perform. The fingertips will detect any deviation from this correct closing procedure as unwanted muscle tension. If tension is sensed, concentrate on "closing in slow motion" as if slowly falling asleep.

3. Pause. At the completion of the closure, pause for approximately a three count. This will allow the upper lid to complete a full closure. Thus, you will begin to learn the feeling of complete closure of the eyelids. A "hidden movement" of the eyes during the pause will

be appreciated, if the exercise is performed properly.

4. Open. Open slightly wider than normal. This should not be accented to the point of a wrinkled brow, open only *slightly* wider.

5. Pause. In the wide open position pause for a moment.

Quickly reviewing: head straight, look straight, fingertips at the corner of the lids, relax, close slowly, pause, open wide, pause. The timing of the complete exercise should be as follows: Blink . . . pause, pause, pause . . . open ¡ . . pause . . . blink . . . pause, pause, pause . . . open . . . pause . . . etc. . . .

This exercise should be performed regularly fifteen times a day, or as prescribed by your doctor, with each practice period consisting of ten correct blinks. This will require no more than ten to fifteen minutes of your time per day. Blinking exercises should be carried on in this manner until our office staff suggests alterations in either the amount of practice blinking, or the method which you employ. Within three to eight weeks your blinking habits should improve greatly, and you will then be placed on a maintenance program of five to six practice periods per day. You should make an effort to incorporate these exercise periods into your daily schedule, much the same as brushing your teeth. Progress evaluation of blinking are performed at office visits, when you will be advised if any changes are required to assist you in becoming a perfect blinker.

The exercises should be done with and without contact lenses on, but should *not* be done while engaged in situations requiring concentrated attention such as reading or driving.

The Ideal Blink

If this program is followed explicitly and you are faithful in your exercises, within a few weeks the partial, squinting blink will become a full, fluid, natural-appearing blink. This is the goal of our efforts. For assistance, watch other people blink; it is particularly valuable to observe trained actors in movies or on television. Notice *how* they blink and *when* they blink. In order to look attractive one normally does not blink while looking directly at a person or when conversing with the person, rather blinking is performed while looking from side to side or from one object to another. Practice concentrating on blinking while changing direction of gaze. Learn to look straight at people without blinking. Learning to blink when changing directions of gaze will help in the development of a natural-appearing and beneficial blink.

The frequency of blinking varies from one person to another; however, for most people a blink every five seconds is required. Learn to blink at approximately five-second intervals. Each blink will automatically become complete and smooth and attractive as a result of the training by the blinking exercises.

There is one caution for the new contact lens wearer. During the first four weeks of lens wearing, vision may blur temporarily as a full, correct blink moves excess tears over the contact lens. There may be a temptation to inhibit blinking or to partially blink in order to prevent this blurring of vision. If this occurs, it is essential to continue working for an ideal blink to prevent eventual eye drying symptoms. Within four weeks, your vision will become clear and constant.

The rewards gained through correct blinking are sharp vision, improved eye health, reduced eye redness, and maximum contact lens comfort. Remember, correct blinking frequently makes the difference between success and failure with contact lenses.

Appendix 14

ACCESSORY SOLUTIONS

Contact Lens Solutions

Product	Manufacturer	Vis¹	Chlorobutanol	Benzalkonium	EDTA	Thimerosal (Merthiolate)	Zinc	Naphazoline (Privine)	Phenylephrine (Neosynephrine)	Tetrahydrozoline (Tyzine)	Buffers²	Osmolarity	pH	Other Ingredients
(A) Wetting														
Contique	Alcon	A	—	.004	—	—	—	—	—	—	—	—	7.2	—
Liquifilm	Allergan	B, C	—	.013 phenylmercuric nitrate	—	—	—	—	—	—	—	—	—	—
Wetting Solution	Barnes-Hind	—	—	.004	*	—	—	—	—	—	—	—	6.5	NaCl, KCl
HyFlow	Flow	—	—	.01	.025	—	—	—	—	—	—	1.1	5.5-6.0	—
Rexall		—	—	.01	.01	—	—	—	—	—	—	—	7.7	—
(B) Soaking														
Contique	Alcon	—	—	.01	.01	—	—	—	—	—	—	—	—	—
Soakare	Allergan	—	0.3	.004	*	—	—	—	—	—	—	—	4.4	—
Soquette	Barnes-Hind	—	0.3	.004	—	—	—	—	—	—	—	—	4.3	—
(C) Soaking and Cleaning														
CleanNSoak	Allergan	—	—	.004	0.1	—	—	—	—	—	—	—	7.0	—
Cleaning and Soaking														
Duo-Flow	Barnes-Hind	—	—	.01	0.2	—	—	—	—	—	—	—	8 to 9	—
	Flow	—	—	.013	.25	—	—	—	—	—	—	—	—	Nonionic surfactant

(D) Lens Cleaning

Product	Company										pH	Remarks
LC-65	Allergan	—	—	—	—	.001	—	*	—	—	6.8	—
Titan	Barnes-Hind	.01	.02	—	—	—	.02	—	—	—	9.5	—
Clens	Burton, Parsons	.01	.02	—	—	—	.02	—	—	—	6.7	—
Contique	Alcon	—	—	—	—	—	—	—	—	—	—	—

Cleaning Gels

Product	Company										pH	Remarks
d-Film	Flow	.02	—	.25	—	—	—	—	.02	—	—	Nonionic detergent
Gel Clean	Barnes-Hind	—	—	—	—	.004	—	—	—	—	—	—

(E) Combination Wetting, Soaking and Cleaning

Product	Company										pH	Remarks
One Solution	Barnes-Hind	0.01	—	0.02	—	—	—	—	0.02	0.9	7.4	Nonionic surfactant
Lensine	Murine	0.01	0.01	0.1	—	.004	—	—	0.1	0.86	8.2	Sodium borate, Sodium bicarbonate
Soaclens	Burton, Parsons	0.01	0.01	0.1	—	.004	—	—	0.1	—	7.0	—
PCL	W-J	.01	.01	—	—	.004	—	—	—	1.04	7.6	—
Lens-Mate	Alcon	.004	.025	—	—	.004	—	—	—	0.9	6.2	PVA 2%
Total	Allergan	.004	0.1	—	—	—	—	—	0.1	1.4	7.1	PVA 2.4%

Decongestants (Ophthalmic)

Product	Company											Remarks
Allerest	WTS-Pharmcraft	.01	—	—	—	.0025	—	*	—	—	1	Camphor, KCl
Collyrium	Wyeth	.05	—	—	—	.002	—	—	.012 (Ephedrine 0.1)	—	4	Antipyrine 0.1%
Degest	Barnes-Hind	.01	—	—	—	.004	—	—	0.2	—	—	Sodium bisulfite 0.1%
Eye-Gene	Pearson Pharmaceutical	—	—	—	—	.004	—	*	*	—	4	$NaHSO_3$, camphor, peppermint, NaCl
Eyelo	Rexall	B	.004	—	—	.004	.001	*	—	—	4	Berberine
Eye-Mo	Winthrop	—	.013	—	—	.013	.001	*	**	—	5	Benzethonium
Isoptofrin	Alcon	A	—	—	—	.004	—	—	.12	—	7	
Murine	Murine Company	—	.004	—	—	.004	.001	*	—	—	2	Hydrastine, berberine, glycerin
Neosynephrine	Winthrop	.013	—	—	—	—	—	*	—	.125	3	
Neozin	Professional Pharmaceutical	.004	—	—	—	—	—	.21	—	.125	—	
Ocusol	Norwich	—	—	—	—	.001	—	—	.001 (Ephedrine)	—	4	Rose H_2O, camphor, witch hazel, glycerine, NaCl
Oph	Winthrop	0.13	—	—	—	.06	—	—	.08	—	5	

Product	Manufacturer	Vis[1]	Preservatives				Vasoconstrictors					Buffers[2]	Other Ingredients
			Chlorobutanol	Benzalkonium	(EDTA)	Thimerosal (Merthiolate)	Zinc	Naphazoline (Privine)	Phenylephrine (Neosynephrine)	Tetrahydrozoline (Tyzine)			
Op-isophrin	Broemmel	B	.10	—	—	—	—	—	.125	—	—	—
Op-isophrin M	Broemmel	—	.10	—	—	—	—	—	.125	—	—	—
Op-isophrin Z	Broemmel	—	.10	—	—	—	Sulfanilate	—	.125	—	—	—
Op-isophrin ZM	Broemmel	B	.10	—	'	—	Sulfanilate .25	—	.125	—	—	—
Prefrin	Allergan	C	—	.004	*	—	—	—	.12	—	8	Antipyrine 0.1%, NaS_2O_3, sodium acetate
Prefrin Z	Allergan	C	—	.004	*	—	*	—	—	—	1	$NaHSO_3$ 0.1%, KCl
Phenylzin	Crookes-Barnes	B	—	.01	.01	.002	.25	—	.12	—	—	Camphor .01%, KCl
Soothe	Burton, Parsons	—	—	—	—	—	—	—	.15	—	—	$NaHSO_3$ .05%, NaCl
Tearefrin	Crookes-Barnes	B-.45	—	.01	.01	—	.25	—	.12	—	5	$NaHSO_3$, KCl
Vas-i-zinc	Ayerst	B	.25	—	.01	—	.25	—	.125	—	6	—
Visine	Pfizer	A	—	.1	—	—	—	—	.12	.05	5	—
Zincfrin	Alcon	—	—	.01	.01	.0025	.25	—	.12	—	—	KCl
20-20	S.S.S.	—	—	—	—	—	*	.012	—	—	—	—
ARTIFICIAL TEARS												
Buf Opto Methulose	Professional Pharmaceutical	B	—	—	—	—	—	—	—	—	—	—
Isopto Alkaline	Alcon	A-1%	—	.15	.004	—	—	—	—	—	—	—
Isopto Plain	Alcon	A-½%	—	—	.002	—	—	—	—	—	—	—
Isopto Tears	Alcon	A-½%	—	—	.01	—	—	—	—	—	—	—
Lacril	Allergan	B,D	—	0.5	—	—	—	—	—	—	—	Acetic acid, polysorbate 80, Na acetate, borate, Cl, citrate; Ca, K, Mg;Cl; dextrose
Liquifilm Tears	Allergan	C	—	0.5	—	—	—	—	—	—	—	NaCl
Lytears	Barnes-Hind	*	—	—	.01	.05	—	—	—	—	—	NaCl, KCl
Methisol	Ayerst	B-½%	—	0.5	.01	.05	—	—	—	—	—	NaCl
Tearisol	Crookes-Barnes	B-.45%	—	—	.01	.01	—	—	—	—	—	NaCl, Kcl, $CaCl_2$

EYE WASHES

Product	Manufacturer	Vis[1]	Preservatives	Buffers[2]	Other Ingredients
Blinx	Barnes-Hind	—	Phenylmercuric acetate .004%	4	—
Collyrium	Wyeth	—	Thimerosal .002%	4	Antipyrine 0.4%
Dacriose	Crookes-Barnes	—	Benzalkonium .01% EDTA .01%	1	KCl
Eyelo	Rexall	—	Thimerosal .005%	4	Camphor
Lavoptik	Lavoptik	—	Benzalkonium .01%	5	Camphor, hydrastine, NaCl
Ocusol	Norwich	—	Benzalkonium .01%	4	Phenylephrine, berberine, rose water

* Present in product but quantity not stated
[1] Vis = viscosity agents
  A—hydroxypropylethylcellulose
  B—methylcellulose
  C—polyvinyl alcohol (1.4%)
  D—gelatin

[2] Buffers
  1 = boric acid + sodium carbonate
  2 = potassium borate + potassium bicarbonate
  3 = boric acid + sodium phosphate
  4 = boric acid + sodium borate
  5 = boric acid
  6 = barbital + sodium barbital
  7 = sodium citrate, sodium phosphate, sodium biphosphate
  8 = disodium phosphate + sodium acid phosphate

Appendix 15

CONTACT LENS MATERIALS (PARTIAL LIST)

Material[1]	Registered Name or Trademark	% H_2O[2]	USAN Council[3] and Other Names	Manufacturer
poly (hydroxyethyl methacrylate-co-ethylene dimethacrylate)	Hydron Soflens	39 39	 polymacon	National Patent Development Corp. Bausch & Lomb
poly(hydroxyethyl methacrylate-co-sodium methacrylate-co-2-ethyl-2-(hydroxymethyl)-1,3-propanediol trimethacrylate)	Hydro-Marc	52	etafilcon A	Frontier Contact Lens, Inc.
poly(hydroxyethyl methacrylate-co-ethoxyethyl methacrylate)	DuraSoft Phemecol	30	phemfilcon A	Wesley-Jessen, Inc.
poly(vinylpyrrolidone-g-hydroxyethyl methacrylate)	Softcon[5]	55	vifilcon A	American Optical Corp.
poly(hydroxyethyl methacrylate-co-vinylpyrrolidone-co-ethylene dimethacrylate)	HydroCurve I Naturvue PHP	45	hefilcon A	Soft Lenses, Inc. Milton Roy Soft Contact Lens, Inc. Automated Optics, Inc.
poly(hydroxyethyl methacrylate-co-methacrylic acid-co-vinylpyrrolidone)	PermaLens	68	prefilcon A; DeCarle	Global Vision (UK) Ltd.
poly(vinylpyrrolidone-co-methylmethacrylate-co-allylmethacrylate-co-ethylene dimethacrylate)	Sauflon-70 Sauflon-85	70 85	lidofilcon A lidofilcon B	Sauflon International
poly(hydroxyethyl methacrylate-co-methyl methacrylate-co-vinylpyrrolidone-co-divinylbenzene)	Aquaflex Aosoft	42	tetrafilcon A	UCO Optics, Inc. American Optical Corp.
poly(hydroxyethyl methacrylate-co-vinylpyrrolidone-co-ethylenebis(oxyethylene) dimethacrylate)	Hydralens	47	droxifilcon A	Ophthalmos, Inc.
poly(hydroxyethyl methacrylate-co-pentyl methacrylate-co-vinyl acetate-co-3-hydroxy-2-napthyl methacrylate)	N & N Lens	31	mafilcon A	N & N Menicon, Inc.

From N. F. Refójo, Materials in Bandage Lenses, *Contact Lens,* 5(1):34–44, 1979.

Material[1]	Registered Name or Trademark	% H_2O[2]	USAN Council[3] and Other Names	Manufacturer
poly(hydroxyethyl methacrylate-co-methyl methacrylate-co-ethylenebis(oxyethylene) dimethacrylate)	Gelflex	36	dimefilcon A	Calcon Labs.
poly(hydroxyethyl methacrylate-co-methacrylic acid-co-ethylene dimethacrylate)	Tresoft	48	ocufilcon A	Urocon Internat.
poly(hydroxyethyl methacrylate-co-N-(1,1-dimethyl-3-oxobutyl) acrylamide-co-1,3-propanediol trimethacrylate)	HydroCurve II	45	bufilcon A	Soft Lenses, Inc.
poly (2,3-dihydroxypropyl methacrylate-co-methyl methacrylate	CS-Membranes	39	crofilcon A, CSI, CS-151	Corneal Sciences, Inc.

[1]When the crosslinking agent is not given, it is ethylene dimethacrylate or a similar compound.
[2]The lens hydrations are only approximate values, and can vary several percentage points depending on conditions.
[3]United States Adopted Name Council.

Appendix 16

DIMENSIONS OF SOME HYDROGEL LENSES

TRADE NAME	INDEX	DIAMETER(s)	THICKNESS	BASE CURVES	POWERS
ACCUGEL (dexifilcon A)	1.45	13.1, 13.5, 13.9 14.0	.16 .07	8.1 to 9.4	−20 to +20
AMSOFT (deltafilcon A)	1.43	13.5	.10 − .20	7.8 to 9.0 7.8 to 8.8	−0.25 to −10.00
			.23 .06	7.8 to 8.8 8.3, 8.6, 8.9	plano to +5.00 −0.50 to −7.00
AOSOFT (tetrafilcon A)	1.43	13.0 13.8	.12 − .28 .07	7.8, 8.1, 8.4, 8.7, 9.0 8.3, 8.6, 9.0	−9.75 to +6.50 −0.25 to −7.75
AQUAFLEX (tetrafilcon A)	1.43	13.0 13.8 13.8	.10 − .22 .46 − .49 .05 − .07	7.8, 8.1, 8.4, 8.7, 9.0 8.28, 8.58, 8.88, 9.18, 9.48 8.5, 8.8	−20 to plano +10 to +20 −1.25 to −6.00
AQUASOFT (deltafilcon A)	1.43	14.00	.14	8.65, 8.33, 8.03 7.85, 7.67, 7.50	−8 to +6 +11 to +17
CIBASOFT	1.43	13.8	.10	8.6, 8.9, 9.2,	P1 to −20.
CIBATHIN (Tefilcon)	1.43	13.8	.035	8.9	P1 to −20
FLEXLENS (hefilcon A)	1.43	12.5 − 1.65	.10 − 1.0	6.0 to 11.0	−20 to +20
GELFEX (dimefilcon A)	1.43	13.4	.14 .06	7.6 to 8.6 8.0, 8.3, 8.6	−20 to +20 plano to −10
HYDROCURVE II (bufilcon A)	1.43	13.5 15.0, 15.5, 16.0	.05 .05	8.3, 8.6, 8.9 9.2, 9.5, 9.8, 10.1	−20 to +20 −20 to +20
	1.43	14.0	.05	8.5	−12 to +7

896

TRADE NAME	INDEX	DIAMETER(s)	THICKNESS	BASE CURVES	POWERS
	HYDROMARC				
(etafilcon A)	1.43	13.5 to 15.0	.07 to .65	8.15 to 9.05	−20 to +20
		14.0	.06	8.4, 8.8	−0.75 to 5.75
					+1.00 to +4.50
HYDRON					
(polymacon)	1.43	13.0	.12	8.1 to 8.9	−20 to +20
		15.0	.12	9.0, 9.3, 9.6	−30 to +30
		14.0	.06	8.4, 8.7, 9.0	plano to −6
METROSOFT					
(deltafilcon A)	1.43	13.5		8.3, 8.6, 8.9	−0.50 to 7.00
SOF–FORM					
(deltafilcon A)	1.43	14.0	.07	8.3, 8.5, 8.7, 8.9	−20 to +20
SOFLENS					
(polymacon)	1.43	12.5, 13.5, 14.5,	spherical .15 .07 (U) .04 (O)	−20 to +20 front (series) aspheric back power	
SOFTCON					
(vifilcon A)	1.40	13.5, 14.0, 14.5.	.17 to .27	7.8, 8.4, 8.7	−8 to +18
SOFTTINT	1.43	13.0	0.10	8.3, 8.6, 8.9	Pl to −20
		13.8	0.10	8.6, 8.9, 9.2	Pl to −20
SOFT FLOW					
(deltafilcon A)	1.43	13.5, 14.0, 14.5	8.0, 8.4, 8.8	−20 to +20	
SOFTICS					
(deltafilcon A)	1.43	13.5		8.0 to 9.1	−25 to +25
TRESOFT					
(ocufilcon A)	1.405	13.5 to 15.0	.10 to .50	8.6, 8.8, 9.0, 9.2	−20 to +20
TRI–POL 43					
(deltafilcon A)	1.44	13.5	.05 to .19	38, 39, 40, 41, 42D	−1.00 to −10

INDEX

A

A lens, 291
Abnormal symptoms, 309, 383, 388
Abrasions, corneal
    detection of, 48, 386
    fluorescein and, 321, 386
    foreign body, 412
    infection of, 321, 426
    insertion, 410
    overwear, 310, 410
    soft lenses and, 573
    types, 387
Abrasive stone
    conical, 474, 486
    spherical, 476
Absorption of light by tinted lenses, 431
Accessory contact lens devices, 334
    cleaning and storage devices, 334
    cleaning units, 334
    disposable soaking kits, 334
    lens holder, 303, 334
    mailing devices, 334
    soaking kits, 334
Accessory lacrimal glands, 41, 42
Accessory solutions, 337
Accommodation
    contact lens effect on, 107, 392, 839
    excessive, 241
    in hyperopia, 705, 840
    in myopia, 107, 705, 840
    presbyopia and, 705
    signs and symptoms and, 392
    and suitability for contact lens wear, 96, 107
Accommodative insufficiency, 392, 416
Acetone, 335
Adaptation, 160
    blinking and, 162, 165
    corneal changes with, 160, 161
    corneal sensitivity and, 39
    lids, neural adaptation of, 161
    mechanism, 160
    physiology of, 35
    symptoms and signs, 305
Adaptation period, 89
    driving in, 311
    length of, 90
    optimum, 310
    rapid, 166, 311

Adhesive tape, 479
    Adjustment period (*see* Adaptation period), 89
Adjustments
    to corneal lens, 464
    to haptic lens, 775, 795
    (*see also* Modification procedures)
Adolescents, 752
Advantages
    of corneal lenses, 89
    of gel lenses, 498
    of scleral contact lenses, 770
Aesthesiometer, 39
Aftercare
    gel lenses, 579
    hard lenses, 384
Against-the-rule astigmatism, 253
Agents for wetting and soaking contact lenses (*see also* Solutions), 313
Albinism, 110, 779
Alcohol, 335
Allergy
    to contact lenses, 111
    to contact lens solutions, 111, 591
    to plastics, 111, 595
Alignment, corneal, 169
Alternating vision bifocal (*see also* Bifocal contact lens), 711
Amblyopia, 110
American Optical Co. Radiuscope, 819
Ametropia
    axial, 854
    refractive, 854
    (*see also* Astigmatism and Myopia)
Amsler grid test, 668
Amsler's classification of keratoconus, 739
Anatomical considerations for fitting, 107
Anatomy of cornea, 16
Anesthesiometer, 98
Angle, contact or wetting, 315
Aniridia, 110, 779
Aniseikonia
    in aphakia, 679, 682, 761
    contact lenses for, 107, 759
    meridional, 761
    refractive, 759
    in strabismus, 764
Anisometropia
    contact lenses for, compared to spectacles, 758
    prismatic effects, 839